2024

3-2-1
CODE IT!

Michelle A. Green
MPS, RHIA, FAHIMA, CPC

 Cengage

Australia • Brazil • Canada • Mexico • Singapore • United Kingdom • United States

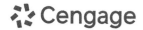

3-2-1 Code It!: 2024, 12th edition
Michelle A. Green

SVP, Product: Cheryl Costantini

VP, Product: Thais Alencar

Portfolio Product Director: Maureen McLaughlin

Senior Portfolio Product Manager:
Stephen G. Smith

Product Assistant: Madison Muschalek

Senior Learning Designer: Kaitlin Schlicht

Learning Designer: Jarmila Sawicka

Senior Content Manager: Kara A. DiCaterino

Digital Project Manager: Andy Baker

Senior Director, Product Marketing: Neena Bali

Product Marketing Manager:
Joann M. Gillingham

Content Acquisition Analyst: Erin McCullough

Production Service: MPS Limited

Designer: Gaby McCracken

Cover Image Source:
vs148/Shutterstock.com

Interior Image Source:
vs148/Shutterstock.com

For product information and technology assistance, contact us at
Cengage Customer & Sales Support, 1-800-354-9706
or support.cengage.com.

For permission to use material from this text or product, submit all requests online at **www.copyright.com.**

Library of Congress Control Number: 2023922798

ISBN: 978-0-357-93220-9

Cengage
5191 Natorp Boulevard
Mason, OH 45040
USA

Cengage is a leading provider of customized learning solutions. Our employees reside in nearly 40 different countries and serve digital learners in 165 countries around the world. Find your local representative at **www.cengage.com.**

To learn more about Cengage platforms and services, register or access your online learning solution, or purchase materials for your course, visit **www.cengage.com.**

Notice to the Reader
Publisher does not warrant or guarantee any of the products described herein or perform any independent analysis in connection with any of the product information contained herein. Publisher does not assume, and expressly disclaims, any obligation to obtain and include information other than that provided to it by the manufacturer. The reader is expressly warned to consider and adopt all safety precautions that might be indicated by the activities described herein and to avoid all potential hazards. By following the instructions contained herein, the reader willingly assumes all risks in connection with such instructions. The publisher makes no representations or warranties of any kind, including but not limited to, the warranties of fitness for particular purpose or merchantability, nor are any such representations implied with respect to the material set forth herein, and the publisher takes no responsibility with respect to such material. The publisher shall not be liable for any special, consequential, or exemplary damages resulting, in whole or part, from the readers' use of, or reliance upon, this material.

Printed in the United States of America
Print Number: 02   Print Year: 2024

Table of Contents

List of Tables

Preface

Introduction

Accurate coding is crucial to the successful operation of any health care facility or provider's office because reported codes determine the amount of reimbursement received. Semiannual revision of codes, coding guidelines, and payer requirements challenge coders because edits to encounter forms and chargemasters must be made and revised coding guidelines need to be interpreted. Those responsible for assigning and reporting codes in any health care setting require thorough instruction in the use of the ICD-10-CM, ICD-10-PCS, CPT, and HCPCS Level II coding systems. Students who are completing formal coursework as part of an academic program and experienced coders who are already employed in the health care field will find that *3-2-1 Code It!* provides the required information in a clear and comprehensive manner.

Due to the comprehensive nature of the *3-2-1 Code It!* textbook, including coding practice, instructors may choose to cover its content in more than one course to allow enough time for student mastery.

- Chapters 1 through 5 would be taught in a course that includes outpatient and physician office ICD-10-CM coding.

- Chapters 6 and 7 would be taught for an inpatient hospital coding course, which covers ICD-10-PCS coding and inpatient hospital ICD-10-CM/PCS coding guidelines (in addition to Chapters 1 through 5, ICD-10-CM coding).

- Chapters 8 through 19 could be taught in a CPT and HCPCS Level II coding course.

Instructors for medical assistant (MA) and medical office administration (MOA) programs may choose to cover the following chapters *only* in their coding course(s):

- Chapters 2 through 5, and 8 in an ICD-10-CM and HCPCS Level II coding course (because ICD-10-PCS and inpatient hospital ICD-10-CM/PCS coding guidelines are *not* used for outpatient and physician office coding, and ICD-10-CM/PCS inpatient hospital coding is covered in Chapters 6 and 7)
- Chapters 9 through 19 in a CPT coding course

Chapter 20 could be included as required reading in a coding course or for an insurance and reimbursement course, either as an introductory or summary chapter.

 NOTE:

Your academic program's community of interest (e.g., employers of graduates) will determine which sections of Chapters 12 through 16 (CPT Surgery) should be covered in your CPT coding course. If your graduates obtain employment assigning and submitting CPT Anesthesia codes, your course should include Chapter 11. If your graduates do not assign radiology or pathology/laboratory codes during their employment, Chapters 17 and 18 can be excluded from your CPT coding course.

The *3-2-1 Code It!* textbook requires users to have access to paper-based coding manuals (ICD-10-CM, ICD-10-PCS, HCPCS Level II, and CPT) because they are used as references when coding rules are explained and for completing exercises and reviews in each chapter. (Academic programs also make software, such as Optum *EncoderPro.com Expert* as an online coding and reference tool designed to enhance your coding capabilities, available to students.) Employers expect graduates to know how to use paper-based coding manuals and encoder software.

The intended use of *3-2-1 Code It!* is for:

- Academic programs in coding and reimbursement, health information management, medical assisting, medical office administration, and so on
- In-service education programs in health care facilities (e.g., physicians' offices, hospitals, nursing facilities, home health agencies, hospices), health insurance companies, quality improvement organizations, and so on
- Health care professionals who need a comprehensive coding reference to assist them in accurately assigning codes

It is recommended that students complete the following course work prior to and/or during the semester they are learning concepts presented in *3-2-1 Code It!*:

- Essentials of health information management
- Medical terminology
- Anatomy and physiology
- Essentials of pharmacology
- Human diseases/pathophysiology

The text was designed to support core learning objectives for the medical coder. Chapter objectives, content, and assessments are aligned to ensure that students learn and practice concepts and skills needed on the job. Student learning is supported by chapter outlines and measurable objectives located at the beginning of each chapter, as well as chapter headings and assessments that map to chapter outlines and objectives.

Special attention was focused on selecting appropriate Bloom's taxonomy levels for each chapter and when mapping assessment items (e.g., exercises, exam questions) to each objective.

Organization of This Textbook

This textbook is organized into 20 chapters.

- Chapter 1 includes an overview of coding systems used to report inpatient and outpatient diagnoses and procedures and services to health plans. It also focuses on coding career opportunities in health care, the importance of joining professional organizations and obtaining coding credentials, the impact of networking with other coding professionals, and the development of opportunities for career advancement. Coding manuals, encoders, and computer-assisted coding (CAC) are also covered.

- Chapter 2 covers ICD-10-CM coding concepts, an overview about coding guidelines, ICD-10-CM general coding guidelines, and ICD-10-CM coding conventions, and it provides coding practice. Chapters 3 and 4 cover ICD-10-CM chapter-specific coding guidelines and provide coding practice. Chapter 5 covers outpatient ICD-10-CM coding concepts and official outpatient guidelines, including assigning codes in the physician office and hospital emergency and outpatient department health care settings. (ICD-10-CM chapters are sequenced before HCPCS Level II and CPT chapters in this textbook because diagnosis codes are reported to justify the medical necessity of procedures and services.)

- Chapter 6 covers ICD-10-PCS coding concepts, general coding guidelines, coding conventions, and section coding guidelines, and it provides coding practice. Chapter 7 covers inpatient hospital coding concepts, which apply to acute care hospitals (and is not typically covered by academic programs that focus on outpatient and physician coding); this chapter requires students to assign ICD-10-CM and ICD-10-PCS codes to inpatient hospital diagnoses and procedures, respectively.

- Chapter 8 covers the HCPCS Level II coding system, which was developed by the Centers for Medicare & Medicaid Services.

- Chapters 9 through 19 cover CPT coding concepts, which were developed by the American Medical Association. Each CPT section has its own chapter, except for the Surgery section, which requires five separate chapters.

- Chapter 20 contains a detailed discussion of insurance and reimbursement concepts. (For comprehensive coverage of third-party payers and reimbursement methodologies, refer to Cengage's *Understanding Health Insurance: A Guide to Billing and Reimbursement*, by Michelle A. Green.)

Features of the Textbook

Each textbook chapter contains the following elements:

- List of chapter headings
- Chapter learning objectives
- Key terms
- Introduction
- Exercises
- Summary
- Internet links
- Review

Textbook features include

- Learning objectives and key terms located at the beginning of each chapter to help organize the material

- Boldfaced key terms throughout each chapter to assist students in learning the technical vocabulary associated with coding systems

- Coding tips and notes that highlight important concepts presented in each chapter

- Exercises after each chapter section that reinforce content presented

- Multiple choice and coding practice reviews that allow for mastery of coding concepts

New to This Edition

- The textbook and its ancillaries, including MindTap activities, have been updated to include the latest ICD-10-CM, ICD-10-PCS, CPT, and HCPCS Level II code sets, conventions, and guidelines.

- Textbook coding assignments, examples, exercises, and reviews have been updated to include the most recent ICD-10-CM, ICD-10-PCS, CPT, and HCPCS Level II codes.

- Answer keys have been updated in the *Solution and Answer Guide to Accompany 3-2-1 Code It!* The guide and other instructor resources for this product are available online. Sign up or sign in at www.cengage.com to search for this product and its online resources.

NOTE:

Chapter exercises and reviews were updated, and the *Solution and Answer Guide* contains detailed analysis about correct answers, including code paths.

- ICD-10-CM code answers include the code path from index to tabular list; coding conventions, general coding guidelines, and chapter-specific guidelines are included to clarify code answers.

- HCPCS Level II codes include the code path from index (when applicable), along with the section name where the code is located.

- CPT codes include the code path from index to the applicable section, subsection, category (or heading), and subcategory (or subheading), along with clarification about notes that apply to code answers.

Chapter-Specific Updates

- Chapter 1 includes new content about essential skills for a medical coding and reimbursement specialist as well as updated content about coding careers, professional associations, systems, and processes; risk adjustment/HCC coding and the AAPC's CRC credential; other classification systems, databases, and nomenclatures; documentation as the basis for coding; and health data collection. Examples, exercises, and the chapter review were also updated.

- Chapter 2 contains updated ICD-10-CM content and ICD-10-CM coding conventions. Examples, exercises, and the chapter review were also updated.

- Chapter 3 contains updated chapter-specific coding guidelines for ICD-10-CM Chapters 1 through 10, and Chapter 4 contains updated chapter-specific coding guidelines for ICD-10-CM Chapters 11 through 22. Examples, exercises, and chapter reviews were also updated in both chapters.

- Chapter 5 contains updated content about ICD-10-CM outpatient (and physician office) diagnosis coding guidelines. Examples, exercises, and the chapter review were also updated.

- Chapter 6 contains updated ICD-10-PCS coding concepts, conventions, and section coding guidelines. Examples, exercises, and chapter reviews were also updated.

- Chapter 7 contains updated content about inpatient hospital ICD-10-CM diagnosis coding guidelines and inpatient hospital ICD-10-PCS procedure coding guidelines. Examples, exercises, and chapter reviews were also updated.

- Chapter 8 contains updated content about HCPCS Level II coding. Examples, exercises, and the chapter review were also updated.

- Chapter 9 contains updated introductory content about CPT coding. Examples, exercises, and the chapter review have also been updated.

- Chapter 10 contains updated content about CPT's evaluation and management (E/M) section. Examples, exercises, and the chapter review were also updated.

- Chapter 11 contains updated content about CPT's Anesthesia section. Examples, exercises, and the chapter review were also updated.

- Chapters 12 through 16 contain updated content about CPT's Surgery section. Examples, exercises, and the chapter review were also updated.

- Chapter 17 contains updated content about CPT's Radiology section. Examples, exercises, and the chapter review were also updated.

- Chapter 18 contains updated content about CPT's Pathology and Laboratory section. Examples, exercises, and the chapter review were also updated.

- Chapter 19 contains updated content about CPT's Medicine section. Examples, exercises, and the chapter review were also updated.

- Chapter 20 contains new content about risk adjustment coding and updated content about insurance and reimbursement. The chapter review was also updated.

Instructor Resources

Additional instructor resources are available online. Instructor assets include an Instructor's Manual, Educator Guide, Solution and Answer Guide, PowerPoint® slides, a test bank powered by Cognero®, and curriculum/competency maps.

Sign up or sign in at www.cengage.com to search for and access this product and its online resources.

MindTap

ISBNs: 2-Semester Instant Access Code: 978-0-357-93225-4

2-Semester Printed Access Code: 978-0-357-93226-1

MindTap is a fully online, interactive learning experience built upon authoritative Cengage content. By combining readings, multimedia activities, and assessments into a singular learning path, MindTap elevates learning by providing real-world application to better engage students. Instructors customize the learning path by selecting Cengage resources and adding their own content via apps that integrate into the MindTap framework seamlessly with many learning management systems.

The MindTap includes

- Auto-graded Exercises, Chapter Reviews, and Coding Practices from the textbook

- Knowledge Checks that introduce each chapter through real-world examples and low stakes quizzing

- Video Quizzes that walk students step-by-step through coding patient cases

- Chapter Quizzes

- Additional Resources requiring both diagnostic and procedural coding: Coding Case Studies, Coding with Encoder Software practice, and Computer-Assisted Coding Case Studies

The 2024 edition has been updated to follow the most current ICD-10-CM, ICD-10-PCS, CPT, and HCPCS Level II code sets available at the time of publication. The Medical Coding Trainer app has been removed from this edition. Advanced coding activities similar to those found in Medical Coding Trainer are now available with additional resources in *MindTap for Advanced Medical Coding Practicum*.

To learn more, visit www.cengage.com/training/mindtap.

Optum EncoderPro.com

Enhance your course with Cengage materials and an online coding tool from Optum. *EncoderPro.com Expert* is an online coding and reference tool designed to enhance your coding capabilities.

- Using online coding tools can help by saving you time and money;
- Increasing accuracy, reducing denials, and ensuring you receive complete reimbursement; and
- Reducing required storage space and paper.

Features of *EncoderPro.com Expert* include

- ICD-10-CM, HCPCS Level II, and CPT code content search, and an ICD-10-PCS code builder tool
- ICD-10 mapping tools
- Coders' Desk Reference
- Complete code history
- Local Coverage Determinations (LCDs) and Medicare Pub. 100 access
- Medicare national correct coding initiative (NCCI) edits
- Enhanced compliance editor
- Enhanced LCD/NCD policy searching
- Cross-coder relationships from seven coding and billing specialty reference books

To make the switch and start saving on coding materials with Cengage and Optum®, contact your Cengage Consultant today at cengage.com/repfinder.

A Note About CPT Coding Manual Editions

Every attempt is made to make the material within this textbook and its ancillary products (e.g., Solution and Answer Guide, Educator Guide) as current as possible by updating to CPT 2024 just prior to publication.

About the Author

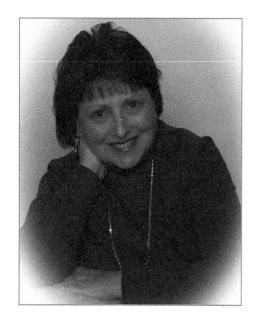

Michelle A. Green, MPS, RHIA, FAHIMA, CPC, is an educational consultant for health information management academic programs, which involves mentoring program directors as they pursue CAHIIM accreditation, building new online courses (e.g., Blackboard, Brightspace/D2L, Moodle, TopClass), and revising existing online course content. She taught traditional classroom-based courses at Alfred State College from 1984 through 2000, when she transitioned all of the health information management and coding courses to an Internet-based format and continued teaching full-time online until 2016. Upon relocating to Syracuse, New York, she began teaching for the health information technology program at Mohawk Valley Community College, Utica, New York in 2017. Prior to 1984, she worked as a director of health information management at two acute care hospitals in the Tampa Bay, Florida, area. Both positions required her to assign codes to inpatient cases. Upon becoming employed as a college professor, she routinely spent the semester breaks coding for a number of health care facilities so that she could further develop her inpatient and outpatient coding skills.

Content Reviewers

Dr. Laura Clifford-Podolsky, CPC, CPMA, CCS, CHDA, CPCO
Adjunct Faculty
Jackson College
Jackson, MI

Martha Davis
Lead Faculty
Ultimate Medical Academy
Tampa, FL

Lisa DeBroka, MPM, RHIT, CCS-P
Program Director
Sullivan University
Louisville, KY

Sonya Sample, MHRD
Professor
Greenville Technical College
Greenville, SC

Carlos Vargas
Program Director
Monroe College
Bronx, NY

Technical Reviewers

Terissia Bell, MHIIM, BBA, RHIA, CPC, COC, CIC
Health Information Management Program Director
Associate Professor of Health Information Management
University of Alaska Southeast Sitka Campus
Sitka, AK

Linda Coyne, CPC, CRC, RHIT
Risk-Adjustment Coding Professional
OS2 Healthcare Solutions
Killeen, TX

Digital Contributors

Traci Brochard, MBA, HCA, RHIA, CPC
Instructor
Health Sciences Department
College of Nursing & Health Sciences
University of Louisiana at Lafayette
Lafayette, LA

Lindsey Maass, CPC, CIMC
Instructor and Program Lead
Healthcare Administrative Programs
Alexandria Technical and Community College
Alexandria, MN

Lisa Riggs, CPC, CPC-I, AAS
Lead Curriculum and Instructional Design Specialist
Ultimate Medical Academy
Tampa, FL

Donna Sue M. Shellman, EdD, CPC
Instructor
Office Systems Technology Department
Career and Technical Education Division
Gaston College
Dallas, NC

Dr. Julie Storts, MSACN, CPC
Franklinville, NY

Acknowledgments

In memory of my son, Eric, who always kept me "on task" by asking, "How much did you get finished in the chapter today, Mom?" Thank you for truly understanding my need to pursue my passion for teaching and writing. You always proudly introduced me as your mom, the teacher and writer. You remain forever in my heart, Eric.

To my students, located throughout the world! You always ask me the toughest coding questions, and you also make me want to find the answers. You are truly critical thinkers!

To my technical reviewer, Linda Coyne, thank you for your incredible attention to detail!

To Kaitlin Schlicht, Senior Learning Instructional Designer, for her invaluable support, patience, and guidance!

To Stephen Smith, Senior Portfolio Product Manager, for patiently listening to all of my concerns about the revision process!

To the incomparable Kara DiCaterino, Senior Content Manager, what can I say? You are simply the best!

To my mom, Alice B. Bartholomew, for her support and assistance. Between writing real-life case studies for my textbooks and having originally helped me select a health care career, your guidance has been appreciated beyond words and I miss you.

Special appreciation is expressed to Optum® Publishing Group for granting permission to reprint selected images, tables, and pages from:

- *Coders' Desk Reference for Diagnoses*
- *Coders' Desk Reference for Procedures*
- *Coding & Payment Guide for Anesthesia Services*
- EncoderPro.com
- *HCPCS Level II Professional*
- *ICD-10-CM Professional*
- *ICD-10-PCS Professional*

Michelle A. Green, MPS, RHIA, FAHIMA, CPC

Feedback

Contact the author at michelle.ann.green@gmail.com with questions, suggestions, or comments about the text or its supplements. Please realize that the publisher (www.cengage.com) authorizes the release of the Solution and Answer Guide to educators only.

How to Use This Text

Chapter Outline and Key Terms

The Chapter Outline organizes the chapter material at a glance. The Key Terms list represents new vocabulary in each chapter. Each term is highlighted in color in the chapter, where it is also defined and used in context. A complete definition of each term appears in the Glossary at the end of the textbook.

Objectives

The Objectives list the outcomes expected of the learner after a careful study of the chapter. Read the objectives before reading the chapter content. When you complete the chapter, read the objectives again to see if you can say for each one, "Yes, I know that." If you cannot say this about an objective, go back to the appropriate content and reread. These outcomes are critical to a successful career as a coder.

Chapter Outline

Career as a Coder
Professional Associations
Coding Systems and Coding Processes
Other Classification Systems, Databases, and Nomenclatures
Documentation as the Basis for Coding
Health Data Collection

Chapter Objectives

At the conclusion of this chapter, the student should be able to:

1. Define key terms related to the overview of coding.
2. Summarize the training, job responsibilities, and career path for a coder.
3. Identify professional associations available to coders and medical assistants.
4. Summarize coding systems and processes.
5. Identify other classification systems and databases.
6. Explain how documentation serves as the basis for assigning codes.
7. Describe health data collection for the purpose of reporting hospital and physician office data.

Key Terms

assumption coding
Centers for Medicare & Medicaid Services (CMS)
classification system
clinical documentation improvement (CDI)
CMS-1500
code
coder
coding
coding system
computer-assisted
Diagnostic and Statistical Manual of Mental Disorders (DSM)
downcoding
encoder
encoding
HCPCS national codes
Healthcare Common Procedure Coding System (HCPCS)
Health Insurance Portability and Accountability Act

Introduction

The *International Classification of Diseases (ICD)* is published by the World Health Organization (WHO) and is used to classify *mortality* (death) data from death certificates. WHO published the tenth revision of ICD in 1994 with a new name, *International Statistical Classification of Diseases and Related Health Problems*, and reorganized its three-digit categories.

The *International Classification of Diseases, Tenth Revision, Clinical Modification* (ICD-10-CM) was developed in the United States and implemented in 2015. It is used to code and classify *morbidity* (disease) data from inpatient and outpatient records, including physician office records. ICD-10-CM is a closed classification system that is used in the United States to classify diagnoses, which means that ICD-10-CM provides just one place to classify each condition. All health care settings use ICD-10-CM to report diseases, injuries, and reasons for an encounter.

ICD-10-CM Official Guidelines for Coding and Reporting are used as a companion to ICD-10-CM to ensure accurate coding. This chapter includes an overview about *ICD-10-CM Official Guidelines for Coding and Reporting*, general diagnosis coding guidelines, and coding conventions. ICD-10-CM chapter-specific diagnosis coding guidelines are covered in Chapters 3 and 4.

 NOTE:

When reviewing examples and completing exercises and review questions in this chapter, use your ICD-10-CM coding manual to locate index entries and verify codes in the tabular list.

Introduction

The Introduction provides a brief overview about major topics covered in the chapter. The introduction (and the objectives) provides a framework for your study of the content.

Notes

Notes appear throughout the text and serve to bring important points to your attention. The notes clarify content, refer you to reference material, provide more background for selected topics, or emphasize exceptions to rules.

⚠ HIPAA Alert!

The HIPAA regulations for electronic transactions require providers and third-party payers, including Medicare administrative contractors (MACs), to adhere to the *Official Guidelines for Coding and Reporting*. Thus, a violation of the coding guidelines is technically a HIPAA violation. Because some third-party payers and MACs do not appear to be aware of (or understand) this HIPAA provision, to obtain appropriate reimbursement for submitted ICD-10-CM codes, bring specific provisions in the regulation that reference the coding guidelines to the attention of third-party payers. For example, the Z51 (Encounter for other aftercare and medical care) codes in ICD-10-CM can be reported as a first-listed code for outpatient care. If third-party payers and MACs deny claims that report Z51 codes, contact the regional CMS office or HIPAA enforcement office (located at CMS) for resolution.

HIPAA Alerts

The HIPAA Alert feature highlights issues related to the privacy and security of personal health information.

Coding Tips

The **Coding Tips** feature provides recommendations and hints for selecting codes and for the correct use of the coding manuals.

⚠ **Coding Tip**

Make sure you read CPT code descriptions carefully. When the code description states "with or without" another procedure, that other procedure is *not* reported separately.

Example: Patient underwent anterior colporrhaphy, repair of cystocele, and cystourethroscopy. Report code 57240. Do not report a separate code for the cystourethroscopy.

Examples

Examples appear throughout the text to promote understanding of presented concepts.

Example 1: For "metastatic carcinoma from left female breast to lung," assign two codes.

- Primary malignant neoplasm of left female breast (C50.912)
- Secondary neoplasm of lung (C78.00)

Exercises

Exercises reinforce chapter content.

Exercise 2.4 – ICD-10-CM Official Guidelines for Coding and Reporting

Instructions: Complete each statement.

1. The *ICD-10-CM Official Guidelines for Coding and Reporting* are approved by the _____ parties for ICD-10-CM to accompany and complement the official conventions and instructions provided within ICD-10-CM.
2. Official coding guidelines use the term _____ when referring to face-to-face contact between patients and health care providers in all health care settings, including inpatient hospital admissions.
3. Official coding guidelines use the term _____ when referring to a physician or any qualified health care practitioner who is legally accountable for establishing a patient's diagnosis.
4. HIPAA regulations for electronic _____ require providers and third-party payers, including Medicare administrative contractors (MACs), to adhere to the *ICD-10-CM Official Guidelines for Coding and Reporting.*
5. Section I of the *ICD-10-CM Official Guidelines for Coding and Reporting* includes ICD-10-CM's coding _____, general coding guidelines, and chapter-specific guidelines.
6. Section II of the *ICD-10-CM Official Guidelines for Coding and Reporting* covers selection of the _____ diagnosis (and secondary diagnoses) for inpatient hospital admissions.
7. Section III of the *ICD-10-CM Official Guidelines for Coding and Reporting* covers reporting of additional diagnoses for inpatient hospital settings, which are also called

Summary

The **Summary** at the end of each chapter recaps the key points of the chapter. The summary also serves as a review aid when preparing for tests.

Summary

The *International Classification of Diseases, 10th Revision, Clinical Modification* (ICD-10-CM) replaced ICD-9-CM effective October 2015 and includes many more codes because it is designed to collect data on every type of health care encounter (e.g., inpatient, outpatient, hospice, home health care, and long-term care). ICD-10-CM disease and injury codes contain at least three characters, but most have three characters followed by a decimal point and between one and four additional characters. There are two main parts of the ICD-10-CM manual: the alphabetic index and the tabular list. ICD-10-CM Index to Diseases and Injuries entries are organized according to main terms, subterms, second qualifiers, third qualifiers, and fourth qualifiers. The ICD-10-CM Tabular List of Diseases and Injuries contains 22 chapters. It is a sequential list of codes contained within chapters based on body system or condition, and codes are then organized within major topic headings, categories, subcategories, and codes.

Medical necessity is the measure of whether a health care procedure or service is appropriate for the diagnosis or treatment of a condition. This decision-making process is based on the payer's contractual language and the treating provider's documentation. Generally, the following criteria are used to determine medical necessity: purpose, scope, evidence, and value. The DHHS agencies CMS and NCHS prepare guidelines for coding and reporting using ICD-10-CM, which are approved by the four organizations that comprise the cooperating parties for the ICD-10-CM/PCS and include the AHA, AHIMA, CMS, and NCHS. The ICD-10-CM guidelines are used as a companion document when assigning ICD-10-CM codes. The ICD-10-CM guidelines are rules that were developed to accompany and complement the official conventions and instructions provided in ICD-10-CM. They are based on coding and sequencing instructions in ICD-10-CM, but provide additional instruction.

Internet Links

AHA Coding Clinic Advisor: www.codingclinicadvisor.com
ICD-10-CM: Go to **www.cms.gov**, click on Medicare, click on ICD-10 under Coding, and click on links in the first column to locate coding manual PDF files, general equivalence mappings (GEMs), and more.
ICD-10-CM search tool: https://icd10cmtool.cdc.gov
ICD-10-CM updates: Go to **www.cms.gov**, click on the Medicare link, click on the ICD-10 link under Coding, and scroll down to click on this year's ICD-10-CM link.
JustCoding News free e-newsletter: Go to **www.justcoding.com**, and click on the eNewsletter Signup link at the top of the page.

Internet Links

Internet Links are provided to encourage you to expand your knowledge at various state and federal government agency, commercial, and organization sites.

Review

2.1 – Multiple Choice: Format of the ICD-10-CM Index to Diseases and Injuries

Instructions: Select the most appropriate response to indicate the format used in the ICD-10-CM Index to Diseases and Injuries.

ICD-10-CM Index to Diseases and Injuries

Abnormal, abnormality, abnormalities
  —*see also* Anomaly
chromosome, chromosomal Q99.9
  sex Q99.8
    female phenotype Q97.9

Review

Each chapter **Review** includes multiple-choice questions and coding practice cases that will test your understanding of chapter content and critical thinking ability.

Notes

Part

I

Coding Overview

1 Overview of Coding

Chapter Outline

Career as a Coder

Professional Associations

Coding Systems and Coding Processes

Other Classification Systems, Databases, and Nomenclatures

Documentation as the Basis for Coding

Health Data Collection

Chapter Objectives

At the conclusion of this chapter, the student should be able to:

1. Define key terms related to the overview of coding.
2. Summarize the training, job responsibilities, and career path for a coder.
3. Identify professional associations available to coders and medical assistants.
4. Summarize coding systems and processes.
5. Identify other classification systems and databases.
6. Explain how documentation serves as the basis for assigning codes.
7. Describe health data collection for the purpose of reporting hospital and physician office data.

Key Terms

assumption coding

Centers for Medicare & Medicaid Services (CMS)

classification system

clinical documentation improvement (CDI)

clinical documentation integrity (CDI)

CMS-1450

CMS-1500

code

coder

coding

coding system

computer-assisted coding (CAC)

concurrent coding

Current Procedural Terminology (CPT)

Diagnostic and Statistical Manual of Mental Disorders (DSM)

downcoding

encoder

encoding

evidence-based coding

evidence-verification coding

HCPCS Level II

HCPCS national codes

Healthcare Common Procedure Coding System (HCPCS)

Health Insurance Portability and Accountability Act of 1996 (HIPAA)

institutional coding

International Classification of Diseases for Oncology, Third Edition (ICD-O-3)

International Classification of Diseases, 11th Revision (ICD-11)

International Classification of Diseases, Tenth Revision, Clinical Modification (ICD-10-CM)

International Classification of Diseases, Tenth Revision, Procedure Coding System (ICD-10-PCS)

International Classification of Functioning, Disability and Health (ICF)

jamming

Logical Observation Identifiers Names and Codes (LOINC®)

medical necessity

medical nomenclature

Medicare Prescription Drug, Improvement, and Modernization Act (MMA)

National Drug Codes (NDC)

overcoding

physician query process

professional coding

RxNorm

single-path coding

specialty coders

Systematized Nomenclature of Medicine Clinical Terms (SNOMED CT)

unbundling

Unified Medical Language System (UMLS)

upcoding

Introduction

This chapter focuses on coding career opportunities in health care, the importance of joining professional associations and obtaining coding credentials, the impact of networking with other coding professionals, and the development of opportunities for career advancement. It also provides a coding overview that explains clinical documentation improvement, the physician query process, and the use of computer-assisted coding (CAC) and encoder software. The documentation as a basis for coding section includes patient record formats and the importance of establishing medical necessity. The health data collection section covers the reporting of hospital and physician office data using abstracting software, medical practice management software, and CMS-1500 and UB-04 claims.

Essential skills needed to become a medical coding and reimbursement specialist include:

- *Attention to detail*, which means an individual uses a meticulous and precise approach when completing tasks, such as assigning medical codes, to ensure that results are perfect. Attention to detail is crucial to avoid making errors, such as reporting incomplete medical codes that result in denied claims.
- *Effective communication*, which relies on *active listening* to interact with patients, providers, third-party payers, and others when determining and resolving issues. Excellent writing skills are also needed to appeal denied claims or generate physician queries to assign accurate medical codes.
- *Knowledge about coding systems*, which requires medical coders to participate in continuing education programs to learn about the most up-to-date official coding guidelines, coding revisions, and software technology.
- *Problem solving*, which uses analytical, critical, and creative thinking to identify problems in the workplace and implement effective solutions. Medical coding and reimbursement specialists do more than just assign/report codes and submit claims. They work with others to address issues that need resolution, such as using available resources (e.g., medical records) as evidence to support the appeal of a denied claim.
- *Time management*, which requires individuals to establish goals, prioritize tasks, and meet deadlines. Making a to-do list of daily tasks to be completed along with a time estimate for each task can be helpful.

Additional professional skills are covered throughout this chapter.

NOTE:

This chapter does *not* require the use of ICD-10-CM, ICD-10-PCS, CPT, or HCPCS Level II coding manuals. However, later chapters in this textbook do require them because learning how to code is easier when you use paper-based coding manuals. (According to CAHIIM/AHIMA requirements, students should also learn how to use encoder software and interpret the results of computer-assisted coding [CAC] software.)

Career as a Coder

A **coder** acquires a working knowledge of coding systems (e.g., CPT, HCPCS Level II, ICD-10-CM, ICD-10-PCS), coding conventions and guidelines, government regulations, and third-party payer requirements to ensure that all diseases, injuries, reasons for an encounter, services (e.g., office visits), and procedures (e.g., surgery, x-rays) documented in patient records are coded accurately for reimbursement, research, and statistical purposes. Excellent interpersonal skills are required of coders because they communicate with providers about documentation and compliance issues related to the appropriate assignment of ICD-10-CM and ICD-10-PCS or CPT/HCPCS Level II codes.

Education and Training

Training methods for those interested in pursuing a coding career include college-based programs that contain coursework in medical terminology, anatomy and physiology, health information management, pathophysiology, pharmacology, ICD-10-CM, ICD-10-PCS, HCPCS Level II, and CPT coding, and reimbursement methodologies. Many college programs also require students to complete a nonpaid internship (e.g., 120 hours) at a health care facility. Professional associations (e.g., the American Health Information Management Association) offer noncredit-based coding training, usually as distance learning (e.g., Internet-based), and some health care facilities develop internal programs to retrain health professionals (e.g., nurses) who are interested in a career change.

 NOTE:

Pharmacology plays a significant role in accurate and complete coding. Coders review the medication administration record (MAR) to locate medications administered that impact ICD-10-CM coding. For example, upon review of the MAR the coder notices that the patient received a course of Librium (chlordiazepoxide) during inpatient hospitalization. Librium is classified as an antianxiety medication, but it can be also used to counteract alcohol withdrawal symptoms. If a physician documents that the Librium was administered to counteract alcohol withdrawal symptoms, the coder can assign an appropriate alcohol dependence ICD-10-CM code as well as alcohol detoxification ICD-10-PCS codes.

Coding Internship

The coding *internship* benefits the student and the facility that accepts the student for placement. Students receive on-the-job experience prior to graduation, and the internship assists them in obtaining permanent employment. Facilities benefit from the opportunity to participate in and improve the formal education process. Quite often, students who complete professional practice experiences (or internships) are later employed by the facility at which they completed the internship.

The *internship supervisor* is the person to whom the student reports at the site. Students are often required to submit a professional résumé to the internship supervisor and to schedule an interview prior to being accepted for placement. While this experience can be intimidating, it is excellent practice for the interview process that the student will undergo prior to obtaining permanent employment. Students should research the résumé writing and interview technique services available from their college's career services office. This office will review résumés and will provide interview tips. (Some even videotape mock interviews for students.)

 NOTE:

Breach of patient confidentiality can result in termination from the internship site, failure of the internship course, and even possible suspension and/or expulsion from your academic program. Make sure you check out your academic program's requirements regarding this issue.

The internship is on-the-job training even though it is nonpaid, and students should expect to provide proof of immunizations (available from a physician) and possibly undergo a preemployment physical examination and participate in facility-wide and department-specific orientations. In addition, because of the focus on privacy and security of patient information, the facility will likely require students to sign a nondisclosure agreement (to protect patient confidentiality), which is kept on file at the college and by the professional practice site.

During the internship, students are expected to report to work on time. Students who cannot attend the internship on a particular day (or who arrive late) should contact their internship supervisor and program faculty. Students are also required to make up any lost time. Because the internship is a simulated job experience, students are to be well groomed and should dress professionally. Students should show interest in all aspects of the experience, develop good working relationships with coworkers, and react appropriately to constructive criticism and direction. If any concerns arise during the internship, students should discuss them with their internship supervisor and/or program faculty.

Professional Credentials

The American Health Information Management Association (AHIMA) and the AAPC (previously called the American Academy of Professional Coders) offer certification in coding. Credentials available from AHIMA include the following:

- Certified Coding Associate (CCA)
- Certified Coding Specialist (CCS)
- Certified Coding Specialist—Physician-based (CCS-P)

The AAPC offers the following core coding certification exams:

- Certified Professional Coder (CPC)
- Certified Inpatient Coder (CIC)
- Certified Outpatient Coder (COC)
- Certified Risk Adjustment Coder (CRC)

The AAPC also offers specialty certification credentials in response to a demand for **specialty coders** who have obtained advanced training in medical specialties and who are skilled in compliance and reimbursement areas, such as the Certified Ambulatory Surgical Center Coder (CASCC) credential.

The type of setting in which you seek employment will indicate which credential(s) you should pursue. Inpatient and/or outpatient coders obtain CCS and CIC certification, and physician office coders choose the CCS-P and CPC credential. Outpatient coders also have the option of selecting the COC credential.

Risk adjustment/HCC coders would obtain the CRC credential. (HCC refers to hierarchical condition category.) *Risk adjustment coding* (or *HCC coding*) requires the assignment of ICD-10-CM codes based on patient record documentation. It is part of a risk adjustment program that calculates predictive risk scores based on HCCs so that providers are properly reimbursed according to the medical complexity and utilization of health care resources required for a managed care patient population.

Those who have not met requirements for field experience as a coder can seek apprentice-level certification by pursuing AHIMA's CCA credential; after obtaining necessary coding experience, candidates can pursue other coding credentials. Once certified, professional associations require maintenance of the credential through continuing education (CE) recertification per two-year cycle.

Employment Opportunities

Coders can obtain employment in a variety of settings, including clinics, consulting firms, government agencies, hospitals, insurance companies, nursing facilities, home health agencies, hospice organizations, and physicians' offices. Coders also have the opportunity to work at home for employers that partner with an Internet-based *application service provider (ASP)*, which is a third-party entity that manages and distributes software-based services and solutions to customers across a *wide area network (WAN)* (computers that are far apart and are connected via the Internet) from a central data center. Remote medical coders may be provided with necessary equipment to work from home (e.g., laptop computer), or they might be required to provide some of the necessary equipment. The Internet is used to access software (e.g., encoder) using an employer-based secure login process, and proper equipment must be in place to ensure a secure connection (e.g., cabled or wireless router). Typically, the remote medical coder signs a telecommuting agreement, which allows an employer to inspect the home-based workspace via videoconference (e.g., Zoom).

Other Professions Related to Coding

One profession that is closely related to a coder is that of a *health insurance specialist* (or *claims examiner*). When employed by third-party payers, these specialists review health-related claims to determine whether the costs are reasonable and medically necessary based on the patient's diagnosis reported for procedures performed and services provided. This process involves verification of the claim against third-party payer guidelines to authorize appropriate payment or to refer the claim to an investigator for a more thorough review.

Another profession that is closely related to a coder is the *medical assistant*. When employed by a provider, this person performs administrative and clinical tasks to keep the office and clinic running smoothly. Medical assistants who specialize in administrative aspects of the profession answer telephones, greet patients, update and file patient medical records, complete insurance claims, process correspondence, schedule appointments, arrange for hospital admission and laboratory services, and manage billing and bookkeeping.

When employed by a physician's office, health insurance specialists and medical assistants perform medical billing, coding, record keeping, and other medical office administrative duties. Health insurance specialists (or claims examiners) and medical assistants receive formal training in college-based programs or at vocational schools. They also receive on-the-job training.

- Health insurance specialists (or claims examiners) often become certified as a Certified Professional Biller (CPB) (through the AAPC).
- Medical assistants often become credentialed as a Certified Medical Assistant (CMA) through the American Association of Medical Assistants (AAMA) or as a Registered Medical Assistant (RMA) through the American Medical Technologists (AMT).

Health insurance specialists (or claims examiners) and medical assistants obtain employment in clinics, health care clearinghouses, health care facility billing departments, insurance companies, physicians' offices, and with third-party administrators (TPAs). When employed by clearinghouses, insurance companies, or TPAs, they often have the opportunity to work at home, where they process and verify health care claims using an Internet-based application service provider (ASP).

Exercise 1.1 – Career as a Coder

Instructions: Complete each statement.

1. A coder is required to have a working knowledge of the CPT, HCPCS Level II, ICD-10-CM, and _____ coding systems.

2. The complexity and intensity of procedures performed and services provided during an outpatient or physician office encounter are captured as part of _____ coding.

3. The intensity of services and severity of illness associated with inpatient care are captured as part of _____ (or facility) coding.

4. When a multi-hospital system provides physician office services along with traditional inpatient, outpatient, and emergency department hospital care, the concept of _____ coding is adopted to facilitate professional and institutional billing.

5. A profession that is closely related to that of a coder is health _____ specialist (or claims examiner) who review health-related claims to determine whether the costs are reasonable and medically necessary based on the patient's diagnosis reported for procedures performed and services provided.

Professional Associations

Students are often able to join a professional association (Table 1-1) for a reduced membership fee and receive most of the same benefits as active members (who pay much more!). Benefits of joining a professional association include the following:

- Eligibility for scholarships and grants
- Opportunity to network with members (for internship and job placement)
- Publications (e.g., professional journals)
- Reduced certification exam fees
- Website access for members only

Attending professional association conferences and meetings provides opportunities to network (or interact) with professionals, which can facilitate being placed for an internship or being considered for employment after graduation. Another way to network is to join an *online discussion board* (or *listserv*) (Table 1-2), which is an Internet-based discussion forum that covers a variety of professional topics and issues.

TABLE 1-1 Professional Associations

Career	Professional Association
Coder	AAPC (previously called American Academy of Professional Coders) American Health Information Management Association (AHIMA)
Medical Assistant	American Association of Medical Assistants (AAMA) American Medical Technologists (AMT)

TABLE 1-2 Internet-Based Discussion Boards (Listservs)

Discussion Board	Website
AHIMA Access	AHIMA members can log in at www.ahima.org.
AAPC	Go to www.aapc.com, click on Resources, click on the Forums link located below News/Networking, and scroll down to Medical Coding.

Exercise 1.2 – Professional Associations

Instructions: Complete each statement.

1. Students who become members of _____ association(s) usually pay a reduced membership fee and receive most of the same benefits as active members.

2. Attending professional association conferences and meetings provides opportunities to _____ (or interact) with other professionals, which can facilitate being placed for internship or job placement.

3. A medical assistant usually joins the American Medical Technologists (AMT) or the _____.

4. An Internet-based discussion forum that covers a variety of professional topics and issues is called an online discussion board or _____.

5. A coder usually joins either the American Health Information Management Association (AHIMA) or the _____.

Coding Systems and Coding Processes

Coding systems and medical nomenclatures are used by health care facilities, health care providers, and third-party payers to collect, store, and process data for a variety of purposes (e.g., health care reimbursement). A **coding system** (or **classification system**) organizes a medical nomenclature according to similar conditions, diseases, procedures, and services, and it contains codes for each (e.g., ICD-10-CM arranges these elements into appropriate chapters and sections). A **medical nomenclature** includes clinical terminologies and clinical vocabularies that are used by health care providers to document patient care. *Clinical terminologies* include designations, expressions, symbols, and terms used in the field of medicine, such as "pupils equal, round, and reactive to light," commonly abbreviated as PERRL in a patient's physical examination report. *Clinical vocabularies* include clinical phrases or words along with their meanings, such as "myocardial infarction," which is defined as the sudden deprivation of blood flow to the heart muscle due to coronary artery blockage resulting in tissue damage (necrosis) and commonly called a "heart attack." A **code** includes numeric (e.g., CPT) and alphanumeric (e.g., ICD-10-CM) characters that are reported to health plans for health care reimbursement, to external agencies (e.g., state departments of health) for data collection, and internally (acute care hospital) for education and research. **Coding** is the assignment of codes to diagnoses, services, and procedures based on patient record documentation.

 NOTE:

You are already familiar with a well-known coding system called the United States Postal Service ZIP Code system, which classifies addresses as numbers (e.g., 12345-9876).

Coding Systems

- The *International Classification of Diseases, Ninth Revision, Clinical Modification (ICD-9-CM)* was adopted in 1979 to classify diseases, injuries, reasons for an encounter (Volumes 1 and 2), and procedures (Volume 3). The ***International Classification of Diseases, Tenth Revision, Clinical Modification* (ICD-10-CM)** (and ICD-10-PCS) replaced ICD-9-CM on October 1, 2015, to classify all diseases, injuries, and reasons for an encounter whether patients are treated as inpatients or outpatients.

- The ***International Classification of Diseases, Tenth Revision, Procedure Coding System* (ICD-10-PCS)** was developed by the National Center for Health Statistics (NCHS) to classify inpatient hospital procedures and services, and it was implemented on October 1, 2015 (replacing Volume 3 of ICD-9-CM).

 NOTE:

ICD-10-CM/PCS is the abbreviation used by the Centers for Medicare & Medicaid Services to identify both classification systems.

- The ***Current Procedural Terminology* (CPT)** is published by the American Medical Association annually. CPT classifies procedures and services, and it is used by physicians and outpatient health care settings (e.g., the hospital ambulatory surgery department) to assign CPT codes for reporting procedures and services on health insurance claims. CPT is considered Level I of the Healthcare Common Procedure Coding System (HCPCS).

- The **Healthcare Common Procedure Coding System (HCPCS)** also includes Level II (national) codes, called **HCPCS Level II** (or **HCPCS national codes**), which are managed by the **Centers for Medicare & Medicaid Services (CMS)**, an administrative agency in the federal Department of Health & Human Services (DHHS). HCPCS Level II classifies medical equipment, injectable drugs, transportation services, and other services not classified in CPT. Physicians and ambulatory care settings use HCPCS Level II to report procedures and services.

NOTE:

HCPCS Level III local codes were discontinued in 2004. They had been managed by Medicare carriers and fiscal intermediaries (FIs). You might come across their legendary use in health care facility or insurance company databases. Some payers still use them.

The **Health Insurance Portability and Accountability Act of 1996 (HIPAA)** is federal legislation that amended the Internal Revenue Code of 1986 to

- improve portability and continuity of health insurance coverage in the group and individual markets;
- combat waste, fraud, and abuse in health insurance and health care delivery;
- promote the use of medical savings accounts;
- improve access to long-term care services and coverage;
- simplify the administration of health insurance by creating unique identifiers for providers, health plans, employers, and individuals;
- create standards for electronic health information transactions; and
- create privacy and security standards for health information.

To facilitate the creation of standards for electronic health information transactions, HIPAA requires two types of code sets to be adopted for the purpose of encoding data elements (e.g., procedure and service codes). This type of **encoding** is a process of standardizing data by assigning alphanumeric values (codes or numbers) to text and collecting other information (e.g., gender). (The concept of a medical *encoder* is covered later in this chapter.)

Large code sets encode:

- diseases, injuries, impairments, and other health-related problems and their manifestations;
- causes of injury, disease, impairment, or other health-related problems;
- actions taken to prevent, diagnose, treat, or manage diseases, injuries, and impairments; and
- substances, equipment, supplies, or other items used to perform these actions.

Example: The diagnosis of *essential hypertension* is assigned ICD-10-CM code I10.

Small code sets encode:

- race/ethnicity and sex;
- type of facility; and
- type of unit.

Example: A patient's sex is assigned 1 if male, 2 if female, 3 if nonbinary, and so on.

HIPAA also requires the following code sets to be adopted for use by clearinghouses, health plans, and providers:

- *International Classification of Diseases, Tenth Revision, Clinical Modification* and *Procedure Coding System* (ICD-10-CM/PCS)
- *Current Procedural Terminology* (CPT)
- *HCPCS Level II* (national codes)
- *Current Dental Terminology* (CDT)
- *National Drug Codes* (NDC)

A *clearinghouse* is a public or private entity (e.g., billing service) that processes or facilitates the processing of health information and claims from a nonstandard to a standard format. A *health plan* (or *third-party payer*) (e.g.,

Blue Cross/Blue Shield, a commercial insurance company) is an insurance company that establishes a contract to reimburse health care facilities and patients for procedures and services provided. A *provider* is a physician or another health care professional (e.g., a nurse practitioner or physician assistant) who performs procedures or provides services to patients. Adopting HIPAA's standard code sets has improved data quality and simplified claims submission for health care providers who routinely deal with multiple third-party payers. The code sets have also simplified claims processing for health plans. Health plans that do not accept standard code sets are required to modify their systems to accept all valid codes or to contract with a health care clearinghouse that does accept standard code sets.

 NOTE:

A health care clearinghouse is not a *third-party administrator (TPA)*, which is an entity that processes health care claims and performs related business functions for a health plan. The TPA might contract with a health care clearinghouse to standardize data for claims processing.

The **Medicare Prescription Drug, Improvement, and Modernization Act (MMA)** requires all code sets (e.g., ICD-10-CM, ICD-10-PCS) to be valid at the time services are provided. This means that midyear (April 1) and end-of-year (October 1) coding updates must be implemented immediately so accurate codes are reported on claims. However, coding updates do not require payment adjustments (e.g., diagnosis-related groups) until the next fiscal year.

The purchase of updated coding manuals and updating of billing systems with coding changes is crucial so that billing delays (e.g., due to waiting for new coding manuals to arrive) and claims rejections are avoided. If outdated codes are submitted on claims, providers and health care facilities will incur administrative costs associated with resubmitting corrected claims and delayed reimbursement for services provided.

- For manual coding, coders should consider using updateable coding manuals, which publishers offer as a subscription service. These *coding manuals* are usually stored in a three-ring binder so that coders can remove outdated pages and add newly printed pages provided by the publisher.

- Another option is to purchase *encoder* software, which publishers offer as a subscription service. Coders have access to the most up-to-date encoder software, which contains edits for new, revised, and discontinued codes. An *encoder* automates the coding process using computerized or web-based software; instead of manually looking up conditions (or procedures) in the coding manual index, the coder uses the software's search feature to locate and verify diagnosis and procedure codes.

- Automating the medical coding process is the goal of *computer-assisted coding (CAC)*, which uses a natural language processing engine to "read" electronic health records and generate ICD-10-CM, ICD-10-PCS, HCPCS Level II, and CPT codes. Because of this process, coders become coding auditors (or coding editors), responsible for ensuring the accuracy of codes reported to payers. (CAC can be compared to speech recognition technology that has impacted the role of medical transcriptionists.)

 NOTE:

Coding manuals, encoders, and computer-assisted coding (CAC) are discussed in more detail later in this chapter.

Coding References

Professional organizations that are recognized as national authorities on CPT, HCPCS Level II, ICD-10-CM, and ICD-10-PCS coding publish references and resources that are invaluable to coders. To ensure the development of excellent coding skills, make sure you become familiar with and use the following references and resources:

- *AHA Coding Clinic for ICD-10-CM and ICD-10-PCS,* and *AHA Coding Clinic for HCPCS*, quarterly newsletters published by the American Hospital Association and recognized by the CMS as official coding resources

- *Conditions of Participation* (CoP) and *Conditions for Coverage* (CfC), Medicare regulations published by CMS

> **NOTE:**
>
> - Official coding policy is published in the AHA *Coding Clinic for ICD-10-CM and ICD-10-PCS*, AHA *Coding Clinic for HCPCS*, and AMA *CPT Assistant*, and as National Correct Coding Initiative (NCCI) edits.
> - The AAPC and AHIMA publish coding newsletters, journals, and so on, but such publications do not contain official coding policy.

- *CPT Assistant Online*, a monthly newsletter published by the AMA and recognized by CMS as official coding resource
- *National Correct Coding Initiative* (NCCI), code edit pairs that cannot be used in the same claim (developed by CMS and published by the federal government's National Technical Information Service [NTIS])
- Compliance program guidance documents, guidelines published by the DHHS OIG
- *ICD-10-CM Official Guidelines for Coding and Reporting*, guidelines provided by CMS and NCHS to be used as a companion document to the official version of ICD-10-CM
- *ICD-10-PCS Official Guidelines for Coding and Reporting*, guidelines provided by CMS and NCHS to be used as a companion document to the official version of ICD-10-PCS
- *Outpatient Code Editor with Ambulatory Payment Classification* (OCE/APC), software developed by CMS, distributed by NTIS, and used by hospitals to edit outpatient claims to help identify possible CPT/HCPCS Level II coding errors and assign Ambulatory Payment Classifications (APCs) that are used to generate reimbursement

Avoiding Fraud and Abuse in Coding

Incorporating the use of coding references and resources assists coders in avoiding the following abusive and fraudulent (dishonest and illegal) coding practices, depending on intent. (Abuse involves mistakenly submitting incorrect codes, and fraud involves intentionally submitting incorrect codes to increase reimbursement.)

- **Unbundling**: Reporting multiple codes to increase reimbursement when a single combination code should be reported.
- **Upcoding**: Reporting codes that are not supported by documentation in the patient record for the purpose of increasing reimbursement.
- **Overcoding**: Reporting codes for signs and symptoms in addition to the established diagnosis code.
- **Jamming**: Routinely assigning an unspecified ICD-10-CM disease code instead of reviewing the coding manual to select the appropriate code.
- **Downcoding**: Routinely assigning lower-level CPT codes for convenience instead of reviewing patient record documentation and the coding manual to determine the proper code to be reported.

ICD-11 Classification System

The **International Classification of Diseases, 11th Revision (ICD-11)** was developed by the World Health Organization (WHO) and released in 2018 to facilitate the implementation process, such as translation into languages other than English. Implementation of ICD-11 for member states was on January 1, 2022. (A planned USA implementation date has not been announced.)

ICD-11 was revised for the purpose of recording, reporting, and analyzing health information. It contains improved usability, which means it contains more clinical detail and requires less training time. Other improvements include classifying all clinical detail, readying eHealth for the electronic health record, linking to other classifications and terminologies (e.g., SNOMED-CT), multilingual support, and updating scientific content.

The structure of ICD-11 is different from ICD-10, with the biggest changes focused on stem codes; extension codes; a supplementary section for the assessment of (patient) functioning; multiple parenting; and precoordination, postcoordination, and cluster coding. The number of chapters was expanded from 22 in ICD-10-CM to 26 in ICD-11, and while the ICD-11 *coding scheme* remains alphanumeric, codes range from 1A00.00 through ZZ9Z.ZZ. The second character of ICD-11 always contains a letter to differentiate the codes from ICD-10, and the third character is always a number (referred to as a *forced number*) so that the spelling of "undesirable words" is prevented. The first character of an ICD-11 code indicates the related chapter, and letters "I" and "O" are omitted to prevent confusion with numbers "1" and "0" (just like in ICD-10-PCS).

Multiple parenting allows a condition to be correctly classified in two different places (e.g., site or etiology). For example, esophageal cancer is classified in both the neoplasm chapter and the digestive system chapter. Thus, stem code 2B70.Z (malignant neoplasms of esophagus) appears in each chapter.

Stem codes are clinical conditions described by one single category to ensure the assignment of one code per case, resulting in the (data) collection of a *meaningful minimum of information*. *Precoordination coding* is the assignment of stem codes, which contain all pertinent information in a pre-combined manner. For example, pneumonia due to *Mycoplasma pneumoniae* includes the disease and its histopathology in ICD-11 stem (or standalone) code CA40.04.

Extension codes standardize the way additional information (e.g., anatomy, histopathology) is added to a stem code, begin with the letter "X," and can never be reported without a stem code. *Cluster coding* is used to indicate that more than one code is reported together using either a forward slash (/) or an ampersand (&) to separate multiple codes that describe a clinical case. *Postcoordination coding* is the process of combining or linking multiple (stem and extension) codes to completely describe a clinical case. For example, duodenal ulcer with acute hemorrhage is classified as stem codes DA63 (duodenal ulcer) and ME24.90 (acute gastrointestinal bleeding, NEC), and extension code XA9780 is added to indicate duodenum as the anatomic location. The codes are reported as DA63/ME24.90&XA9780.

Coding conventions such as code also, use additional code, includes, excludes, NEC, NOS, residual categories (e.g., certain, other, unspecified), and/or, due to, and with also appear in ICD-11 to provide additional information.

While ICD-11 was ready for distribution in 2018 and adopted by member states for implementation on January 1, 2022, there is no time line established for its adoption by the United States.

Medical Coding Process

The *medical coding process* requires the review of patient record documentation to identify diagnoses, procedures, and services for the purpose of assigning ICD-10-CM, ICD-10-PCS, HCPCS Level II, and/or CPT codes. Each health care covered entity (e.g., hospital, medical clinic, physician office) implements a unique medical coding process, which requires adherence to the following:

- Code of ethics
- Accurate coding
- Coding quality
- Avoiding assumption coding

- Professional, Institutional, and Single-Path Coding
- Physician query process
- Clinical documentation improvement
- Coding compliance programs

Code of Ethics

Professional associations establish a *code of ethics* to help members understand how to differentiate between "right" and "wrong" and apply that understanding to decision making. The AAPC publishes a code of ethics, and AHIMA publishes standards of ethical coding; both serve as guidelines for ethical coding conduct, and they demonstrate a commitment to coding integrity.

Accurate Coding

Regardless of health care setting, the *steps to accurate coding* begin with a review of the entire patient record (manual or electronic) before selecting diseases, injuries, reasons for an encounter, procedures, and services to which codes are assigned. Depending on the setting, coders perform retrospective coding, concurrent coding, or a combination of both.

Retrospective coding is the review of records to assign codes after the patient is discharged from the health care facility (e.g., hospital inpatient) or released from same-day outpatient care (e.g., hospital outpatient surgery unit). It is most commonly associated with inpatient hospital stays because accurate coding requires verification of diagnoses and procedures by reviewing completed face sheets, discharge summaries, operative reports, pathology reports, and progress notes in the patient records.

Concurrent coding is the review of records and use of encounter forms and chargemasters to assign codes during an inpatient stay (e.g., hospital) or an outpatient encounter (e.g., hospital outpatient visit for laboratory testing or x-rays, physician office visit). It is typically performed for outpatient encounters because encounter forms (e.g., physician office) and chargemasters (e.g., hospital emergency department visit, hospital outpatient visit for laboratory testing) are completed in "real time" by health care providers as part of the charge-capture process.

- *Encounter forms* are used to record data about procedures and services provided to patients.
- *Chargemasters* contain a computer-generated list of procedures, services, and supplies, and corresponding revenue codes along with charges for each.

 NOTE:

Information about encounter forms and chargemasters is located in Chapter 20 of this textbook, along with samples of each.

Professional, Institutional, and Single-Path Coding

Professional coding captures the complexity and intensity of procedures performed and services provided (CPT and HCPCS Level II) during an outpatient or physician office encounter. **Institutional coding** captures the severity of illness (ICD-10-CM) and the intensity of services (ICD-10-PCS), both of which are used to justify an inpatient facility admission, such as to an acute care hospital.

- *Severity of illness (SI)* is the extent of organ system loss of function or physiological decompensation, and it establishes an inpatient's physiologic status or "how sick the inpatient is." Severity of illness is an indicator that is used to estimate an inpatient facility length of stay and justify a patient's need for that level of care. For example, a patient diagnosed with end-stage renal disease (ESRD) and kidney failure would be classified as having a severe acuity of illness that justifies inpatient admission to an acute care hospital.
- *Intensity of services (IS)* includes the frequency, number, and type of procedures and services needed to diagnose and treat patients during an inpatient facility stay and is based on an established acuity of illness. For example, a patient diagnosed with a severe acuity of illness (e.g., ESRD and kidney failure) would require an increased level of services, such as inpatient dialysis and kidney transplant surgery.

SI/IS criteria is used by utilization management review specialists to review patient record documentation when assessing inpatient medical conditions. For example, Interqual® publishes SI/IS criteria as part of an "evidence-based clinical decision support solution to ensure clinically appropriate medical utilization decisions." SI/IS criteria is used to to determine patient evaluation and treatment plans, medical and surgical interventions, and anticipated outcomes.

An increase in multi-hospital systems that provide physician office services (along with traditional inpatient, outpatient, and emergency department hospital care) has resulted in the introduction of a concept called **single-path coding**, which combines professional and institutional coding to improve productivity and ensure the submission of clean claims, leading to improved reimbursement. Instead of employing separate professional and institutional coders (who are typically employed at different health care settings), a *single-path coder* manages both professional and institutional coding for the same patient using computer-assisted coding (CAC) software and accessing all documents required for inpatient institutional (ICD-10-CM and ICD-10-PCS) and outpatient professional (ICD-10-CM, CPT, and HCPCS Level II) coding. This process also facilitates professional and institutional billing by the organization, resulting in increased coding accuracy and reduced claims denials.

Example: Early in her career, as a health information manager in Florida, your author implemented a process to provide the hospital's medical staff with copies of discharged inpatient record face sheets, which contained diagnosis (and procedure) codes that were reported on the hospital's UB-04 institutional claim. Physician offices generated CMS-1500 claims to obtain reimbursement for professional services provided to hospital inpatients, and these professional claims

(continues)

(continued)

> reported the same diagnosis codes assigned by the health information management (HIM) department's coders. The hospital's HIM committee approved the process because it improved the accuracy of reporting diagnosis codes on CMS-1500 claims. (Physicians and outpatient settings report CPT and HCPCS Level II codes for procedures and services, while inpatient hospitals report ICD-10-PCS codes.)

Inpatient Hospital Coding Quality

According to the American Hospital Association, "The importance of understanding and following the basic ICD-10-CM, and ICD-10-PCS coding principles cannot be overemphasized in the training of coders and in quality control activities undertaken to improve the accuracy of data reported for internal and external hospital use. The measures for coding accuracy include (a) adherence to ICD-10-CM and ICD-10-PCS coding principles and instructions, (b) attention to specificity in code selection where indicated by physician documentation in the medical record [patient record], (c) grasp of medical terminology, and (d) absence of clerical-type errors, such as those due to carelessness in reading or in transposing [letters and] numbers. Auditing of coded diagnostic and procedural information for accuracy should not be confused with the review for relevancy in sequencing of the codes at hand. They are separate tasks linked together in the data reporting process."

The statement located in (b) of the aforementioned quote is significant because it means that coders are expected to review the *entire* record when assigning codes to diagnoses and procedures/services documented on the face sheet and in the discharge summary, which are located in the hospital inpatient record. Thus, coders should review the face sheet, discharge summary, and other documentation (e.g., progress notes, operative reports, pathology reports, laboratory data) to assign the most specific codes possible.

EHR Results in Greater Implementation of Concurrent Coding

Concurrent coding was introduced for inpatient coding just after the inpatient prospective payment system (using diagnosis-related groups) was implemented on October 1, 1983. Coders from the health information department worked part of the day on nursing units, accessing paper-based manual medical records to begin the process of assigning codes to diagnoses and procedures. On discharge of the patient from the hospital, the coders performed a final review of the patient record to ensure accuracy of reported codes. Because the paper-based manual patient record can be handled by just one individual at a time, coders "competed" with nurses, physicians, and other health care providers for access to the record. As a result, concurrent coding as a process was discontinued in some facilities because it was inefficient.

Today, implementation of the electronic health record (EHR) has resulted in a resurgence of concurrent coding practices because coders (still located in the health information department) access patient records in an electronic format. They no longer "compete" with other health care providers for access to the record and, as a result, efficiency associated with the concurrent coding concept has been realized. In practice, coders remain at their work stations in the health information department (and *remote coders* use their at-home work stations) to access patient EHRs to begin the discharge coding process. Rising health care costs created an impetus for concurrent coding processes because it is a much faster method for coders to review and verify the accuracy of codes on discharge of inpatients based on concurrent coding work performed (according to an established schedule) up until the date of discharge. For tertiary-care facilities that provide complex health care (e.g., transplant surgery) and quaternary-care facilities that provide highly specialized care (e.g., experimental medicine), both of which are also characterized as providing high-cost care (e.g., transplant surgery), having the ability to submit codes for reimbursement purposes within hours (instead of days) of inpatient discharge significantly and positively impacts their accounts receivables (and their "bottom line"). In addition, community-based hospitals also realize the benefits of concurrent coding.

Remember! Coders must avoid assumption coding, and when a problem with documentation quality is noted (e.g., conflicting diagnostic statements on the discharge summary, face sheet, and elsewhere in the record) the physician query process is initiated (discussed below).

Example 1: The provider documented *congestive heart failure* on the face sheet of the patient record. On review of progress notes that document the patient's response to treatment, the coder finds documentation of *acute and chronic diastolic and systolic congestive heart failure* in the discharge progress note. Instead of reporting a code for *congestive heart failure*, report the more specific code for *acute and chronic diastolic and systolic congestive heart failure*.

Example 2: The provider documented *malnutrition* on the discharge summary in the patient record. On review of progress notes, the coder finds documentation of *moderate malnutrition*. Instead of reporting the nonspecific code for *malnutrition*, report the more specific code for *moderate malnutrition*.

Assumption Coding

Coders are *prohibited* from performing **assumption coding**, which is the assignment of codes based on the presumption, from a review of clinical evidence in the patient's record, that the patient has certain diagnoses or received certain procedures/services even though the provider did not specifically document those diagnoses or procedures/services. According to the *Compliance Program Guidance for Third-Party Medical Billing Companies*, published by the Department of Health and Human Services' Office of the Inspector General, assumption coding creates risk for fraud and abuse because the coder assumes certain facts about a patient's condition or procedures/services, although the physician has not specifically documented the level of detail to which the coder assigns codes. *Coders can avoid fraudulent assumption coding by implementing the physician query process discussed in the following section.*

Example: An older adult patient is admitted to the hospital for treatment of a fractured femur. Upon examination, the physician documents that the skin around the fractured femur site has split open. X-ray of the left femur reveals a displaced fracture of the shaft. The patient underwent fracture reduction and full-leg casting. The physician documents *open Type I fracture of shaft, left femur* as the final diagnosis.

The coder assigns code S72.302B for the *open Type I fracture of shaft, left femur*, which is correct. The coder assigns code 0QS90ZZ for the *fracture reduction and full leg casting procedure*, which is incorrect because its code description is *reposition left femoral shaft, open approach (no device), femur (shaft)*. Although the patient has an open fracture, the physician did *not* perform an open reduction procedure. (An open reduction involves making a surgical incision to align displaced bones, and it may require external fixation to heal properly.) In this case, the coder incorrectly "assumed" that an open reduction was performed because the patient's open fracture was treated. The code that should be assigned for this procedure is 0QS9XZZ because its code description is *reposition left femoral shaft, external approach*. (A closed reduction involves casting the affected limb to stabilize the fracture for healing, and it might also require the physician to pull back two ends of bone that are touching each other and/or to correct any wide angles.)

Physician Query Process

When coders have questions about documented diagnoses and procedures or services, they use a **physician query process** to contact the responsible physician to request clarification about documentation and the code(s) to be assigned. The electronic health record (EHR) allows for development of an *automated* physician query process, which is used by utilization managers (or case managers), clinical documentation improvement specialists, and coders to obtain clarification about patient record documentation. Integrating the automated physician query process with the EHR allows physicians to more easily receive and reply to queries, which results in better and timely responses from physicians.

NOTE:

The query should not lead the physician to a desired outcome.

- A leading query would be phrased as, "Is the patient's anemia due to blood loss?" and leads the physician to add due to blood loss to the anemia diagnosis for more specific code assignment and possible increased reimbursement.
- A nonleading query would be phrased as, "Can the cause of the patient's anemia be specified? The history documents symptoms of fatigue, headaches, inflamed tongue, and lightheadedness. The CBC reveals low hemoglobin levels." This query allows the physician to determine whether the anemia can be qualified according to type.

The following guidelines should be followed when activating the physician query process:

- Establish a policy to indicate when a coder should generate a physician query, such as when documentation in the patient's record fails to meet one of the following five criteria (according to AHIMA's practice brief, entitled *Managing an Effective Query Process*):
  - *Legibility* (e.g., illegible handwritten patient record entries)
  - *Completeness* (e.g., abnormal test results but clinical significance of results is not documented)
  - *Clarity* (e.g., signs and symptoms are present in the patient record, but a definitive diagnosis is not documented)
  - *Consistency* (e.g., discrepancy among two or more treating providers regarding a diagnosis, such as a patient who presents with shortness of breath and the consulting physician documents pneumonia as the cause while the attending physician documents congestive heart failure as the cause)
  - *Precision* (e.g., clinical documentation indicates a more specific diagnosis than is documented, such as a sputum culture that indicates bacterial pneumonia and the diagnosis does not indicate the cause of the pneumonia)
- Query the physician when the following are noted by the coder and when provider documentation in the patient record is not present (according to AHIMA's practice brief, entitled *Managing an Effective Query Process*):
  - Clinical indicators of a diagnosis (e.g., lab, x-ray) but the diagnosis is not documented
  - Clinical evidence for a higher degree of specificity or severity (e.g., progress notes) but specificity or severity is not documented in the diagnosis
  - Cause-and-effect relationship between two conditions but the relationship is not documented in the diagnosis (e.g., due to, with)
  - An underlying cause when a patient is admitted with symptoms (e.g., shortness of breath is documented instead of diagnosed pneumonia)
  - Treatment is documented without a corresponding diagnosis for medical necessity (e.g., antibiotics for a secondary diagnosis of UTI, which is not documented as a diagnosis)
  - Lack of present on admission (POA) indicator status (e.g., history did not indicate diagnoses that were present on admission, such as chronic asthma) (The POA indicator status is discussed in Chapter 20 of this textbook.)

 NOTE:

Utilization managers (or case managers) are responsible for coordinating inpatient care to ensure the appropriate utilization of resources, delivery of health care services, and timely discharge or transfer. They usually have a bachelor's degree (e.g., nursing), professional licensure (e.g., RN), and clinical practice experience.

Utilization managers work closely with physicians on a daily basis, and they are a logical choice to facilitate the physician query process. In this role, they serve as the liaison for coders (and physicians) by helping coders write appropriate queries and clarifying queries for physicians so that responses are timely and complete.

- Determine whether the query will be generated concurrently (during inpatient hospitalization) or retrospectively (after patient discharge).
- Designate an individual who will serve as the physician's contact during the physician query process (e.g., coding supervisor, utilization manager). Remember that the coder's role is to assign codes based on documentation and that asking for clarification is appropriate, but making an assumption about codes to be assigned is considered fraud. That means that coders should ask physicians open-ended questions to avoid leading the physicians by indicating a preference for a particular response. Coders do not make clinical assumptions—that is the sole responsibility of the physician.

Use a physician query form (Figures 1-1A and 1-1B), not scrap paper, to document the coder's query and the physician's response. If the completed query form is filed in the patient's record, determine whether it is considered an official part of the record and subject to disclosure by those requesting copies of records or whether it is an administrative form that is not subject to disclosure. The query form could also be stored in an administrative file in the coding supervisor's office and the information resulting from the query documented kept in the patient record by the physician (e.g., as an addendum to the discharge summary). The length of time that the completed query form is retained is determined by each health care organization.

PHYSICIAN QUERY FORM

Patient Name: John Public
Admission Date: 03/30/YYYY
Patient Number: 123456

Date: April 14, YYYY
Coder: Lynn Smith
Email Address: lsmith@clinic.org
Office Number: (101) 555-1234

Dear Dr. Hughes ,

The diagnosis or procedure of pneumonia requires more specific information in order to assign the most accurate and complete code. The following information is documented in the discharge summary.
The patient had signs and symptoms of upper respiratory infection upon admission.

I have the following question(s) about this record:
RSV testing was positive for respiratory syncytial virus. Based on your clinical judgment, can you provide a diagnosis that represents the RSV positive finding? If so, please document the condition and causative organism (if known) in the patient record.

Please respond to this question in the space below, and also document an amendment in the patient record (if appropriate):
Patient has RSV. This is now documented in an addendum to the discharge summary in the patient record.

FIGURE 1-1A Sample open-ended physician query form

Example: A patient is admitted with severe dyspnea (shortness of breath), chest pain, and fever. Upon physical examination, the physician documents rhonchi (gurgling sound in the lungs), wheezing, and rales (clicking, bubbling, or rattling sounds in the lungs). Laboratory data during the hospitalization include a culture and sensitivity report of sputum that documents the presence of gram-negative bacteria. A review of the physician orders reveals documentation of appropriate medications to treat *pneumonia due to gram-negative bacteria*. The medication administration record (MAR) documents administration of the medications, and the physician progress notes document the patient's positive response to medications (and resolution of the pneumonia). The physician documents *viral pneumonia* as the final diagnosis. Generate a physician query to request clarification about the diagnosis of viral pneumonia, given patient record documentation that pneumonia due to gram-negative bacteria appears to have been treated.

Depending on the health care facility's coding policy and procedure, the coder has two options.

1. If the coding policy and procedure allow coders to use the entire patient record as the basis of assigning codes to final diagnoses and procedures, because documentation in the record supports a final diagnosis of *pneumonia due to gram-negative bacteria* (instead of viral pneumonia), the coder would assign the code for that condition.

PHYSICIAN QUERY: CHEST PAIN DIAGNOSIS CLARIFICATION

Hospital:	ANYWHERE CLINIC	Patient Number:	123456
Physician:	Dr. Hughes	Admission Date:	03/31/YYYY
Patient Name:	John Public	Discharge Date:	04/04/YYYY
Doctor:	Hughes	Date of Query:	April 5, YYYY

The patient record reflects the following clinical finding(s) (to be completed by coder):

Clinical Indicators:

Clinical Indicators	Location of Documentation in current record:
Chest pain (e.g., description, location, level of exertion)	History and Physical Examination
Signs/Symptoms (e.g., diaphoresis, palpitations, etc.)	Admission Progress Note
Shortness of breath (e.g., respiratory rate, activity)	History and Physical Examination
Abnormal test results (e.g., EKG, cardiac cath, chest x-ray)	EKG report and Chest x-ray report (negative)
Abnormal lab findings (e.g., troponin, CK and CK-MBs)	Laboratory report (cardiac enzymes negative)
Abnormal EGD (e.g., esophagitis, esophageal varices)	Not applicable
Treatment prescribed (e.g., nitroglycerine)	Not applicable

TO THE PHYSICIAN: The following may be a factor in determining and reporting the severity of illness of your patient (to be completed by physician, if applicable).

There is clinical documentation of **chest pain** in the patient record. Clarification of documentation is initiated to the provider when there is conflicting, incomplete, or ambiguous information in the patient record. Please use your clinical judgment in responding to this query. (**Note:** This physician query does not imply that any particular answer is desired or expected.)

Please respond to **ALL 4 sections below**. Per CMS guidelines or facility policy, please document your response in the patient record (e.g., progress note, dictated report).

Section 1: Specificity
- ☐ Cardiac
- ☐ Chest wall
- ☐ Musculoskeletal
- ☒ Psychogenic
- ☐ Atypical
- ☐ Traumatic
- ☐ Other:
- ☐ Unknown

Section 2: Etiology
- ☐ Unstable angina
- ☐ Acute MI
- ☐ Costochondritis
- ☐ Exacerbation of COPD
- ☐ Pneumonia
- ☒ Anxiety
- ☐ GERD
- ☐ Other:
- ☐ Unknown

Section 3: Acuity
- ☐ Acute
- ☐ Acute on chronic
- ☐ Chronic
- ☒ Other: *related to Anxiety*
- ☐ Unknown

Section 4: Present on Admission (POA)
- ☒ Yes
- ☐ No
- ☐ Clinically undetermined
- ☐ Unknown

Coder Name:	Sally Smith, CCS	Extension: 1234	Date: April 5, YYYY
Physician Signature:			Date: *April 6, YYYY*
	Mark Hughes, M.D.		

FIGURE 1-1B Sample multiple choice physician query form

2. If the coding policy and procedure require coders to generate a *physician query* when the final diagnosis (on the face sheet or in the discharge summary) differs from documentation found in the patient record, the coder would submit the following query to the physician, which allows the physician an opportunity to correct the documented final diagnosis if warranted. In this case, the physician changed *viral pneumonia* to *pneumonia due to gram-negative bacteria* (using the proper procedure for amending the patient record).

The assignment of a code to pneumonia due to *gram-negative bacteria* results in reimbursement of about $3,500, and the assignment of a code to *viral pneumonia* results in reimbursement of about $2,500. Not querying the physician would have resulted in a loss of $1,000 to the facility.

This case also includes documentation of signs and symptoms, which are due to the pneumonia. Thus, the coder would *not* assign codes to symptoms of dyspnea, chest pain, fever, or signs of rhonchi, wheezing, and rales.

Clinical Documentation Improvement

Clinical documentation improvement (or **clinical documentation integrity**) (**CDI**) helps ensure accurate and thorough patient record documentation and identifies discrepancies between provider documentation and codes to be assigned. Coders who have questions about documented diagnoses, procedures, and services use a *physician query process* to request clarification about documentation that impacts appropriate code assignment. For the physician query process, medical coders may coordinate with utilization management employees who routinely meet with providers about the medical necessity of continued patient stays. Thus, it is easier for utilization management employees to meet with providers for CDI purposes. (Medical coders are routinely located in a remote part of a facility, including off site buildings, or they work from home.) The result is a resolution of documentation and coding discrepancies. (Coders also review patient record documentation and use coding guidelines and other guidance, such as the NCCI program, to assign the most specific codes possible.)

The purpose of a *clinical documentation improvement (CDI) program* is to help health care facilities comply with government programs (e.g., RAC audits) and other initiatives (e.g., Joint Commission accreditation) with the goal of improving health care quality. As part of a CDI program, the CDI specialist initiates concurrent and retrospective reviews of inpatient and outpatient records to identify conflicting, incomplete, or nonspecific provider documentation. Concurrent reviews are performed on patient care units (to access paper-based patient records) or remotely (to access EHRs). The CDI program helps ensure that patient diagnoses and procedures are supported by ICD-10-CM and ICD-10-PCS codes, and CDI specialists use a physician query form to communicate with physicians (and other health care providers) with the intended result of improving documentation, coding, reimbursement, and severity of illness (SOI) and risk of mortality (ROM) classifications. CDI programs are usually associated with acute health care facilities; however, they are also implemented in alternate health care settings (e.g., acute rehabilitation facility, skilled nursing facility). A *clinical documentation improvement (CDI) specialist* is responsible for performing inpatient record reviews for the purpose of:

- implementing documentation clarification and specificity processes (as part of the physician query process);
- using and interpreting clinical documentation improvement statistics;
- conducting research and providing education to improve clinical documentation; and
- ensuring compliance with initiatives that serve to improve the quality of health care, which include:
  - complying with fraud and abuse regulations;
  - enforcing privacy and security of patient information; and
  - monitoring a *health information exchange (HIE)*.

Coding Compliance Programs

A *coding compliance program* ensures that the assignment of codes to diagnoses, procedures, and services follows established coding guidelines, such as those published by the Centers for Medicare & Medicaid Services (CMS). Health care organizations write *policies* (guiding principles that indicate "what to do") and *procedures* (processes that indicate "how to do it") to assist in implementing the coding compliance stages of detection, correction, prevention, verification, and comparison.

- *Detection* is the process of identifying potential coding compliance problems. For example, a coder notices that some patient records contain insufficient or incomplete documentation, which adversely impacts coding specificity. The coder brings these records to the attention of the coding compliance officer (e.g., coding supervisor), who implements the next stage of the coding compliance program.

- *Correction* is based on the review of patient records that contain potential coding compliance problems, during which specific compliance issues are identified and problem-solving methods are used to implement necessary improvements (corrections). For example, the coding compliance officer conducts a careful review of the patient records that contain insufficient or incomplete documentation. It is determined that all of the records are the responsibility of a physician new to the practice. Educational material specific to documentation issues noted during the review process is then prepared.

- *Prevention* involves educating coders and providers so as to avoid coding compliance problems from recurring. For example, the coding compliance officer schedules a meeting with the physician responsible for insufficient or incomplete documentation, and educates the physician about the specific areas of insufficient or incomplete documentation that adversely impact medical coding. This meeting is conducted in a nonconfrontational manner, with education and correction as its goals.

- *Verification* provides an "audit trail" that the detection, correction, and prevention functions of the coding compliance program are being actively performed. For example, the coding compliance officer maintains a file that contains the following:
  - Original codes assigned based on insufficient and incomplete documentation
  - Educational materials prepared specific to the documentation issues
  - Minutes of the educational meeting with the responsible physician
  - Final codes assigned based on sufficient and complete documentation
  - Remittance advice from third-party payer, which contains adjudication (decision about reimbursement, including possible claims denial)

- *Comparison* requires the analysis of internal coding patterns over specified periods of time (e.g., quarterly) as well as the analysis of external coding patterns by using external benchmarks (trends). For example, the coding compliance officer reviews reports of quarterly medical audits to determine whether the new physician's documentation has improved. Such reports contain the results of claims submission, which indicate the number of claims denials based on nonspecific codes submitted as a result of insufficient and incomplete documentation. In addition, the coding compliance officer obtains benchmark data (reports) from third-party payers and compares the coding practices in the facility with those of similar providers; if reimbursement to similar providers is significantly higher (or lower) than that paid to the provider, the *detection* process is initiated in an attempt to identify related coding compliance problems.

An effective coding compliance program monitors coding processes for completeness, reliability, validity, and timeliness.

- *Completeness* ensures that codes are assigned to all *reportable* diagnoses, procedures, and services documented in the patient record. For example, coders review the entire patient record to assign the most specific codes possible.

- *Reliability* allows for the same results to be consistently achieved. For example, when the same patient record is coded by different coding professionals, they assign identical diagnosis and procedure/service codes.

- *Validity* confirms that assigned codes accurately reflect the patient's diagnoses, procedures, and services. For example, coders do *not* assign codes to diagnoses that were not medically managed or treated during an encounter.

- *Timeliness* means that patient records are coded in accordance with established policies and procedures to ensure timely reimbursement.

Coding Manuals, Encoders, and Computer-Assisted Coding

Many publishers produce their own versions of the ICD-10-CM, ICD-10-PCS, and HCPCS Level II coding manuals. (The AMA publishes CPT.) Companies also publish **encoders**, which automate the coding process by using the search feature to locate and verify medical codes.

Computer-assisted coding (CAC) uses software to automatically generate medical codes by analyzing clinical documentation located in the electronic health record (EHR) or electronic medical record (EMR) (and provided by health care practitioners) (Figure 1-2). CAC uses "natural language processing" technology to generate codes that are reviewed and validated by coders for reporting on third-party payer claims. Similar to the medical editor's role in ensuring the accuracy of reports produced from speech recognition technology, the coder's role changes from that of data entry to validation or audit. The coder reviews and approves the CAC-assigned codes, improving efficiency and offering expanded career opportunities for enthusiastic coders.

Example: ICD-10-CM codes are assigned to justify the medical necessity of procedures and services provided by physicians, which are reported with CPT and HCPCS Level II codes. (ICD-10-PCS codes are reported for inpatient hospital procedures only.) If the reason for a patient encounter is the "flu," the patient's respiratory symptoms are also documented. Optum360's *EncoderPro.com Expert* software can be used to select ICD-10-CM as the Code Set Search, entering "flu" in the search box. A list of ICD-10-CM codes generated results in selection of "J11.1 Influenza due to unidentified influenza virus with other respiratory manifestations" based on review of its tabular list entry. The tabular entry includes the J11.1 code and its description and notes (e.g., Use additional code). J11.1 is then selected as the code to be reported on the claim. (Codes associated with the "Use additional code" notes were not documented in the patient record and, thus, not reported.)

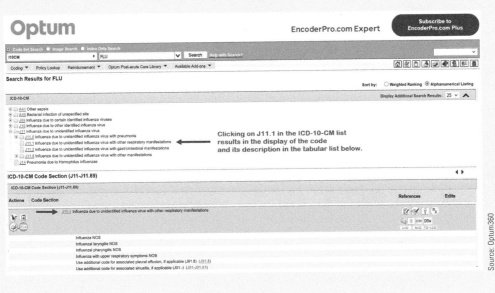

Coders use data analytic skills to review CAC-generated codes and determine which are to be reported. Data analytic skills allow coders to review codes generated by CAC software, compare codes to documentation in the electronic health record, and select appropriate codes to report for reimbursement purposes. Thus, coders use basic data analytic skills to turn data (e.g., CAC-assigned code) into action (coder-reviewed and approved code) using a logical and efficient method.

Coding auditors perform **evidence-based coding**, also referred to as **evidence-verification coding**, which involves clicking on codes that CAC software generates (Figure 1-3) to review electronic health record documentation (evidence) used to generate the code. When it is determined that documentation supports the CAC-generated code, the coding auditor clicks to accept the code. When documentation does not support the CAC-generated code, the coding auditor replaces it with an accurate code. For example, when the CAC-generated ICD-10-CM code does not indicate laterality or does not include a manifestation code, the coding auditor edits codes to ensure accurate reporting.

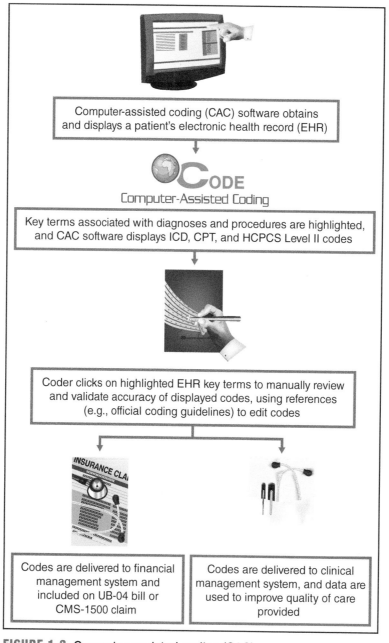

FIGURE 1-2 Computer-assisted coding (CAC)

Example of Computer-Assisted Coding: A physician office EMR note is pasted into the *Code-A-Note* CAC product (published by Find-A-Code, LLC), and the *Scan Notes* link in the software is clicked to generate a list of possible ICD-10-CM, CPT, and HCPCS Level II codes. The software's list of ICD-10-CM codes requires the coder to compare patient record documentation of diagnoses and conditions to select codes for reporting on the health insurance claim. Likewise, the software's list of CPT and HCPCS Level II codes requires the coder to compare patient record documentation of procedures and services to select codes for reporting on the health insurance claim. (In this case, the provider had already selected the appropriate CPT evaluation and management service code from the encounter form.)

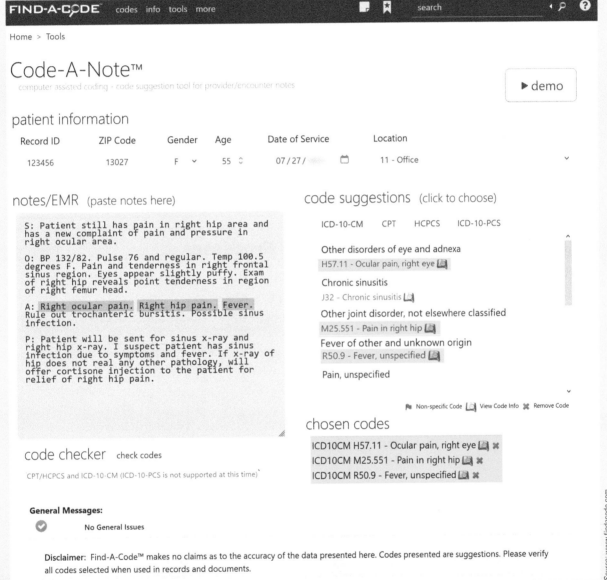

FIND-A-CODE   codes info tools more   search

Home > Tools

Code-A-Note™
computer assisted coding - code suggestion tool for provider/encounter notes

▶ demo

patient information

Record ID	ZIP Code	Gender	Age	Date of Service	Location
123456	13027	F ⌄	55 ⌃	07/27/	11 - Office

notes/EMR (paste notes here)

S: Patient still has pain in right hip area and has a new complaint of pain and pressure in right ocular area.

O: BP 132/82. Pulse 76 and regular. Temp 100.5 degrees F. Pain and tenderness in right frontal sinus region. Eyes appear slightly puffy. Exam of right hip reveals point tenderness in region of right femur head.

A: Right ocular pain. Right hip pain. Fever. Rule out trochanteric bursitis. Possible sinus infection.

P: Patient will be sent for sinus x-ray and right hip x-ray. I suspect patient has sinus infection due to symptoms and fever. If x-ray of hip does not real any other pathology, will offer cortisone injection to the patient for relief of right hip pain.

code suggestions (click to choose)

ICD-10-CM   CPT   HCPCS   ICD-10-PCS

Other disorders of eye and adnexa
H57.11 - Ocular pain, right eye

Chronic sinusitis
J32 - Chronic sinusitis

Other joint disorder, not elsewhere classified
M25.551 - Pain in right hip

Fever of other and unknown origin
R50.9 - Fever, unspecified

Pain, unspecified

🏳 Non-specific Code   View Code Info   ✖ Remove Code

chosen codes

ICD10CM H57.11 - Ocular pain, right eye ✖
ICD10CM M25.551 - Pain in right hip ✖
ICD10CM R50.9 - Fever, unspecified ✖

code checker   check codes

CPT/HCPCS and ICD-10-CM (ICD-10-PCS is not supported at this time)

General Messages:

✔   No General Issues

Disclaimer: Find-A-Code™ makes no claims as to the accuracy of the data presented here. Codes presented are suggestions. Please verify all codes selected when used in records and documents.

Source: www.findacode.com

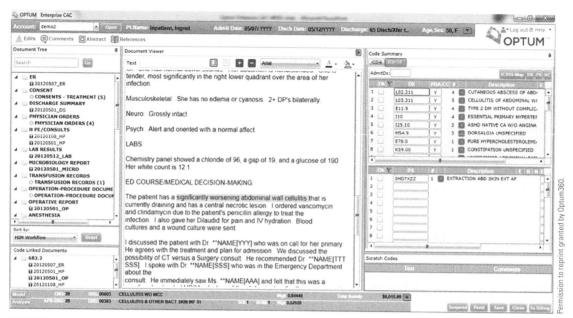

FIGURE 1-3 Sample screen from Optum360 Enterprise computer-assisted coding (CAC) software

Exercise 1.3 – Coding Systems and Processes

Instructions: Complete each statement.

1. A medical nomenclature that is organized according to similar conditions, diseases, procedures, and services, and contains codes for each is called a _____ (or classification) system.

2. All diseases, injuries, and reasons for an encounter, whether patients are treated as inpatients or outpatients, are coded using the _____ classification system.

3. Inpatient hospital procedures and services are coded using the _____ classification system.

4. A public or private entity that processes or facilitates the processing of health information and claims from a nonstandard to a standard format is called a health care _____.

5. Routinely assigning lower-level CPT codes for convenience instead of reviewing patient record documentation and the coding manual to determine the proper code to be reported is called _____.

6. Reporting codes that are not supported by documentation in the patient record for the purpose of increasing reimbursement is called _____.

7. Reporting codes for signs and symptoms in addition to the established diagnosis code is called _____.

8. Reporting multiple codes to increase reimbursement when a single combination code should be reported is called _____.

9. Coders should always avoid assumption coding, and can do so by generating a physician _____ when documentation needs clarification prior to the assignment of codes.

10. Software that automatically generates medical codes by analyzing clinical documentation in the electronic health record or electronic medical record is called _____.

Other Classification Systems, Databases, and Nomenclatures

In addition to the ICD-10-CM, ICD-10-PCS, HCPCS Level II national, and CPT coding systems, health care providers use the following classifications, clinical vocabularies, databases, and nomenclatures:

- *Alternative Billing Codes*
- *Clinical Care Classification System*
- *Current Dental Terminology*
- *Diagnostic and Statistical Manual of Mental Disorders*
- *Health Insurance Prospective Payment System* Rate Codes
- *International Classification of Diseases for Oncology, Third Edition*
- *International Classification of Functioning, Disability and Health*
- Logical Observation Identifiers Names and Codes
- *National Drug Codes*
- RxNorm
- *Systematized Nomenclature of Medicine Clinical Terms*
- Unified Medical Language System

 NOTE:

A *database* allows for the storage of comprehensive and accurate information that serves a critical function in health care, including

- Administration (e.g., financial data)
- Education and research (e.g., cures for disease)
- Patient care (e.g., improving treatment methods)

Alternative Billing Codes

The *Alternative Billing Codes (ABC codes)* classify services not included in the CPT manual to describe the service, supply, or therapy provided; they may also be assigned to report nursing services and alternative medicine procedures. Codes are five characters in length, consisting of letters, and are supplemented by two-digit code modifiers to identify the practitioner performing the service.

HIPAA authorized the Secretary of DHHS to permit exceptions from HIPAA transaction and code set standards to commercialize and evaluate proposed modifications to those standards. The ABC code set was granted that exception in 2003, and the codes were being commercialized and evaluated through 2005. The intent was for ABC codes to be adopted as part of the electronic code set (as HCPCS Level I and Level II were in 2000); however, in 2006, ABC codes could no longer be used in electronic claims processing.

Example: During an office visit, an acupuncture physician assessed the health status of a new client and developed a treatment plan, a process that took 45 minutes. ABC code ACAAC-1C is assigned.

Clinical Care Classification System

The *Clinical Care Classification (CCC) System* includes care components that classify each of three interrelated CCC terminologies:

- CCC of Nursing Diagnoses
- CCC of Nursing Interventions and Actions
- CCC of Nursing Outcomes

CCC care components represent behavioral, functional, physiological, and psychological patterns of clinical nursing care. CCC codes classify the standards of the American Nurses Association (ANA), which include assessment, diagnosis, evaluation, implementation, outcome identification, and planning.

> **Example:** 73-year-old female patient discharged from the hospital after treatment for acute myocardial infarction presents today for the scheduled outpatient cardiac rehabilitation sessions. Assign CCC code C08.1.4 (manage cardiac rehabilitation).

Current Dental Terminology

The *Current Dental Terminology* (CDT) is published by the American Dental Association (ADA) as an annual revision. It classifies dental procedures and services. Dental providers and ambulatory care settings use the CDT to report procedures and services. CDT codes are also included in HCPCS Level II, beginning with the first digit of D. The CDT also includes the Code on Dental Procedures and Nomenclature (Code), instructions for use of the Code, questions and answers, ADA dental claim form completion instructions, and tooth numbering systems.

> **Example:** Patient underwent incision and drainage of intraoral soft tissue abscess. CDT code D7510 is assigned.

Diagnostic and Statistical Manual of Mental Disorders

The **Diagnostic and Statistical Manual of Mental Disorders** (DSM) is published by the American Psychiatric Association as a standard classification of mental disorders used by mental health professionals in the United States. The first edition was published in 1952, and the most current edition (DSM-5) was published in 2014.

DSM-5 is designed for use in a variety of health care settings and consists of three major components:

- Diagnostic classification
- Diagnostic criteria sets
- Descriptive text

According to the Substance Abuse and Mental Health Services Administration (**www.samhsa.gov**), DSM-5 focuses on a "lifespan perspective [by] recognizing the importance of age and development on the onset, manifestation, and treatment of mental disorders." DSM-5 eliminates "the multi-axial system, removing the *Global Assessment of Functioning (GAF score)* and reorganizing the classification of disorders and changing how disorders that result from a general medical condition are conceptualized." DSM-5 categorizes "disorders into *classes* with the intent of grouping similar disorders (particularly those that are suspected to share etiological mechanisms or have similar symptoms) to help clinicians and researchers use the manual. [In] DSM-5, there has been a reclassification of many disorders that reflects a better understanding of the classifications of disorders from emerging research or clinical knowledge."

> **Example:** DSM-5 separately classifies *bipolar and related disorders, depressive disorders,* and *anxiety disorders* (instead of incorporating them as *mood disorders* in a previous edition of DSM).
>
> DSM-5 eliminated the class of *disorders usually first diagnosed in infancy, childhood, or adolescence* and placed such disorders within other classes. For example, *Tic Disorders* are classified as *Neurodevelopmental Disorders* in DSM-5 (instead of *Disorders usually first diagnosed in infancy,* as in a previous edition of DSM).

Health Insurance Prospective Payment System Rate Codes

The *Health Insurance Prospective Payment System (HIPPS) rate codes* are alphanumeric codes consisting of five digits. Each HIPPS rate code contains intelligence, with certain positions of the code indicating the case-mix group itself and other positions providing additional information (e.g., information about the clinical assessment used to arrive at the code). HIPPS was created as part of the prospective payment system for skilled nursing facilities in 1998. Additional HIPPS rate codes were created for other prospective payment systems, including a system for home health agencies in October 2000, and one for inpatient rehabilitation facilities in January 2002. HIPPS represents specific sets of patient characteristics (or case-mix groups) on which payment determinations are made under several prospective payment systems. HIPPS rate codes are not assigned from a coding manual; they are created when information for a data set is entered into software.

> **Example:** The home health prospective payment system (HHPPS) requires entry of the Outcome and Assessment Information Set (OASIS) data set into grouper software, which generates the five-digit alphanumeric HIPPS code that is entered on the UB-04 claim. For example, HIPPS rate code HAEJ1 is entered on the UB-04 claim.

International Classification of Diseases for Oncology, Third Edition

The *International Classification of Diseases for Oncology, Third Edition* **(ICD-O-3)** was implemented in 2001 as a classification of neoplasms used by cancer registries throughout the world to record incidence of malignancy and survival rates. The data produced are used to provide information for cancer control programs (e.g., National Comprehensive Cancer Control Program), research activity, treatment planning, and health economics. (The first edition of ICD-O was published in 1976, and a revision of topography codes was published in 1990.) ICD-O-3 codes classify a tumor in the following way:

- Primary site (four-character topography code)
- Morphology (six-character code)
  - Four-digit histology (cell type) code
  - One-digit behavior code (such as malignant, benign, and so on)
  - One-digit aggression code (differentiation or grade)

> **Example:** Fibrosarcoma of the left knee. ICD-O-3 codes C49.2 (Knee, NOS) and M8810/39 (Fibrosarcoma, NOS) are assigned.

The *International Classification of Diseases for Oncology, Fourth Edition (ICD-O-4)* will publish in 2023 and includes new codes, such as the addition of fifth-digit "0" where there is no need for a more specific code and other fifth-digit values to indicate a more specific code. The new fifth digits allow codes to collapse to ICD-O-3 edition categories and subcategories so as to ensure ease of conversion and consistency with ICD-O-3. *It is unknown when the United States will adopt ICD-O-4.*

ICD-O Morphology Codes

ICD-O morphology codes indicate the type of cell that has become neoplastic and its biologic activity; in other words, the kind of tumor that developed and how it behaves. There are three parts to a complete morphology code:

- M as the first character of each morphology code
- 4-digit cell type (histology) (e.g., 8010)
- 1-digit behavior (e.g., /o)
- 1-digit grade, differentiation, or phenotype (e.g., /x1)

A common root codes the cell type of a tumor, an additional digit codes the behavior, and yet another additional digit codes the grade, differentiation, or phenotype to provide supplementary information about the tumor.

Cancer and Carcinoma

The words *cancer* and *carcinoma* are often (incorrectly) used interchangeably. For example, squamous cell cancer is often used for squamous cell carcinoma. Both conditions happen to have the same ICD-10-CM code.

However, a condition such as "spindle cell cancer" could refer to "spindle cell sarcoma" or "spindle cell carcinoma." Each condition has an entirely different ICD-10-CM code assigned to it.

Behavior

The behavior of a tumor is the way it acts within the body. Pathologists use a variety of observations to characterize the behavior of a tumor. A tumor can grow in place without the potential for spread (/0, benign); it can be malignant but still growing in place (/2, noninvasive or in situ); it can invade surrounding tissues (/3, malignant, primary site); or it can disseminate from its point of origin and begin to grow at another site (/6, metastatic).

Fifth-Digit Behavior Codes for Neoplasms

Code	Behavior of Neoplasm
/0	Benign
/1	Uncertain whether benign or malignant Borderline malignancy Low malignant potential Uncertain malignant potential
/2	Carcinoma in situ Intraepithelial Noninfiltrating Noninvasive
/3	Malignant, primary site
/6	Malignant, metastatic site Malignant, secondary site
/9	Malignant, uncertain whether primary or metastatic site

 NOTE:

Cancer registries collect data on malignant and in situ neoplasms, or /2 and /3 behavior codes. They do not collect data about behavior codes /6, malignant, metastatic site, or /9, malignant, uncertain whether primary or metastatic site. For example, carcinoma that has spread to the lung and for which the site of origin is unknown is assigned ICD-10-CM code C80.1 (unknown primary site) and ICD-O code M-8010/3 (carcinoma). (The /3 signifies the existence of a malignant neoplasm of a primary site.)

Use of Behavior Code in Pathology Laboratories

Pathologists are usually interested in "specimen coding" (whereas a cancer registry identifies just the primary tumor). A pathologist receives the following tissue specimens on the same patient:

- Biopsy of supraclavicular lymph node
- Resection of fundus of stomach
- Resection of upper lobe bronchus

The pathologist has to track each of these specimens (while the cancer registry tracks only the primary cancer). Each pathological specimen is coded with the appropriate topography and morphology; for example, the term "metastatic" in the pathological diagnosis for tissue specimen, "supraclavicular lymph node (biopsy)," results in assignment of behavior character /6.

Tissue Specimen	Pathological Diagnosis	Codes
Supraclavicular lymph node (biopsy)	Metastatic signet ring cell adenocarcinoma, most likely from stomach (metastatic site)	C77.0 M8490/6
Fundus of stomach (resection)	Signet ring cell adenocarcinoma (primary site)	C16.1 M8490/3
Upper lobe bronchus (resection)	Metastatic signet ring cell adenocarcinoma (metastatic site)	C34.10 M8490/6

Code for Histologic Grading and Differentiation

The highest grade code is assigned according to the description documented in the diagnostic statement. The sixth digit of the morphology code is a single-digit code number that designates the grade of malignant neoplasms. Only malignant tumors are graded. The practice of assigning codes for histologic grading varies greatly among pathologists throughout the world, and many malignant tumors are not routinely graded.

Sixth Digit Code for Histologic Grading and Differentiation

Code	Grade	Differentiation
1	I	Well differentiated Differentiated, NOS
2	II	Moderately differentiated Moderately well differentiated Intermediate differentiation
3	III	Poorly differentiated
4	IV	Undifferentiated anaplastic
9		Grade or differentiation not determined, not stated or not applicable

Differentiation describes how much or how little a tumor resembles the normal tissue from which it arose. There is great variability in pathologists' use of differentiation descriptors. In general, adverbs such as *well, moderately,* and *poorly* indicate degrees of differentiation, which map to grades I, II, and III. Adjectives such as *undifferentiated* and *anaplastic* usually map to grade IV. Grading codes are assigned to all malignant neoplasms listed in ICD-O *if the diagnosis documents the grade and/or differentiation*.

> **Example:** The diagnosis *squamous cell carcinoma, grade* II, which is described as *moderately well differentiated squamous cell carcinoma*, is assigned morphology code M-8070/32.

When a diagnosis indicates two different degrees of grading or differentiation, the higher number is assigned as the grading code.

> **Example:** *Moderately differentiated squamous cell carcinoma with poorly differentiated areas* is assigned grading code 3, and the morphology code is M-8070/33.

This same sixth-digit column is also used to indicate cell lineage for leukemias and lymphomas, which provides useful ICD-O-3 comparison data (with ICD-O-2). Cell lineage is implicit in the four-digit histology code, and an additional grade of differentiation (sixth digit) code is not required. However, some registries assign the sixth digit to identify cases in which the diagnosis is supported by immunophenotypic data. In such instances, the immunophenotype code takes precedence over other diagnostic terms for grade or differentiation (e.g., well differentiated, grade III).

Sixth Digit for Immunophenotype Designation for Lymphomas and Leukemias

Code	Designation
5	T-cell
6	B-cell
	Pre-B
	B-precursor
7	Null cell
	non-T, non-B
8	NK cell
	Natural killer cell
9	Cell type not determined, not stated, or not applicable

International Classification of Functioning, Disability and Health

The *International Classification of Functioning, Disability and Health* (ICF) classifies health and health-related domains that describe body functions and structures, activities, and participation. (The ICF was originally published as the *International Classification of Injuries, Disabilities, and Handicaps [ICIDH]* in 1980.) The ICF complements ICD-10, looking beyond mortality and disease.

> **Example:** A trauma patient is evaluated two years after the initial injury, and the physician determines that the patient has a severe impairment in mental function as well as a severe impairment of the upper extremity. The patient experiences moderate difficulty in bathing without the use of assistive devices. Products for education are a moderate barrier for this patient. The following ICF codes are assigned:
>
> - b175.3 (severe impairment in mental function)
> - s730.3 (severe impairment of the upper extremity)
> - a5101.2 (moderate difficulty bathing without use of assistive devices)
> - e145.2 (products for education are a moderate barrier)

Logical Observation Identifiers Names and Codes

Logical Observation Identifiers Names and Codes (LOINC®) is an electronic database and universal standard that is used to identify medical laboratory observations and for the purpose of clinical care and management. Developed in 1994, it is currently maintained by the Regenstrief Institute, a U.S. nonprofit medical research organization. Health care providers use LOINC® codes when reportable disease results are sent to state and federal public health laboratories.

The Centers for Disease Control and Prevention (CDC) has developed a LOINC® panel specifically for public health case reporting called the Reportable Condition Mapping Tool (RCMT). This panel should be of considerable assistance to health care providers in identifying the correct LOINC® code for their reports. Laboratories are also required to archive LOINC® codes for test results they receive from other laboratories to which they have referred specimens and, similarly, referral laboratories should provide their clients with LOINC® codes when sending results.

> **Example:** The complete blood count (CBC) laboratory test of blood (without differential) is assigned LOINC® code 24317-0.

National Drug Codes

The *National Drug Codes* (NDC) is published by a variety of vendors, and the coding system is in the public domain. It is managed by the Food and Drug Administration (FDA) and was originally established as part of an out-of-hospital drug reimbursement program under Medicare Services as a universal product identifier for human drugs. The current edition is limited to prescription drugs and a few selected over-the-counter (OTC) products. Pharmacies use NDC to report transactions, and some health care professionals also report NDC on claims.

> **Example:** Aspirin tablets, 800 milligrams, is assigned NDC code 64125-*106-01. (There are many different NDC codes for aspirin, depending on dosage, manufacturer, and so on.)

RxNorm

RxNorm is a nomenclature that provides normalized names for clinical drugs and links drug names to many of the drug vocabularies commonly used in pharmacy management and drug interaction software, including those of First Databank, Micromedex, MediSpan, Gold Standard Drug Database, and Multum. By providing links among these vocabularies, RxNorm can mediate messages among systems that do not use the same software and vocabulary.

RxNorm is a normalized naming system for generic and branded drugs, and it is a tool for supporting semantic interoperation among drug terminologies and pharmacy knowledge base systems. The National Library of Medicine (NLM) produces RxNorm. The NLM receives drug names from many data sources, analyzes and processes the data, and outputs the data into RxNorm files in a standard format.

Purpose of RxNorm

RxNorm is a terminology built on and derived from other terminologies. RxNorm reflects and preserves the meanings, drug names, attributes, and relationships from its sources. Hospitals, pharmacies, and other organizations use computer systems to record and process drug information. Because these systems use many different sets of drug names, it can be difficult for one system to communicate with another. To address this challenge, RxNorm provides normalized names and unique identifiers for medicines and drugs. The goal of RxNorm is to allow computer systems to communicate drug-related information efficiently and unambiguously.

Scope of RxNorm

RxNorm contains the names of prescription and many OTC drugs available in the United States.

RxNorm includes generic and branded:

- Clinical drugs (pharmaceutical products given to or taken by a patient with therapeutic or diagnostic intent)
- Drug packs (packs that contain multiple drugs, or drugs designed to be administered in a specified sequence)
- Radiopharmaceuticals, bulk powders, contrast media, food, dietary supplements, and medical devices, such as bandages and crutches, which are out of scope for RxNorm

 NOTE:

RxNorm also includes the National Drug File—Reference Terminology (NDF-RT), created for the Veterans Health Administration. NDF-RT is a terminology used to code clinical drug properties, including mechanism of action, physiologic effect, and therapeutic category.

Example: When Synthroid is entered in the RxNorm database, results display levothyroxine as the ingredient and levothyroxine sodium as the precise ingredient. In addition, all possible dosages of the ingredient and brand name are listed under the clinical drug component, branded drug component, clinical drug or pack, and branded drug or pack. Oral product or pill is listed below the dose form group, with expanded information listed below the clinical dose form group and branded dose form group.

Systematized Nomenclature of Medicine Clinical Terms

The *Systematized Nomenclature of Medicine Clinical Terms* (SNOMED CT) is a comprehensive and multilingual clinical terminology of body structures, clinical findings, diagnoses, medications, outcomes, procedures, specimens, therapies, and treatments. It combines the content and structure of a previous revision of SNOMED with the following medical nomenclatures:

- United Kingdom's *National Health Service's Clinical Terms Version 3* (formerly called *Read Codes*, developed in the early 1980s by Dr. James Read to record and retrieve primary care data in a computer)
- *Logical Observation Identifier Names and Codes (LOINC®)* database, which provides a universal code system for reporting laboratory and other clinical observations

SNOMED CT supports the development of comprehensive high-quality clinical content in patient records; it provides a standardized way to represent clinical phrases documented by clinicians, facilitating automatic interpretation (e.g., computer-assisted coding).

Unified Medical Language System

The **Unified Medical Language System (UMLS)** is a set of files and software that allows many health and biomedical vocabularies and standards to enable interoperability among computer systems. UMLS can be used to enhance or develop applications, including electronic health records, classification tools, dictionaries, and language translators. The UMLS is used to link health information, medical terms, drug names, and billing codes across different computer systems.

> **Example 1:** UMLS is used to link billing codes, drug names, medical terms, and health information across different computer systems, such as among a patient's health care provider, pharmacy, and third-party payer or patient care coordination among several departments within a hospital.

> **Example 2:** UMLS uses include search engine retrieval, data mining, public health statistics reporting, and medical terminology research.

The UMLS contains three tools, called Knowledge Sources, which include the following:

- Metathesaurus (terms and codes from many vocabularies, including CPT, ICD-10-CM, LOINC®, MeSH®, RxNorm, and SNOMED CT) (MeSH is the National Library of Medicine's controlled vocabulary thesaurus.)
- Semantic network (broad categories, which are semantic types, and their relationships, which are semantic relations)
- SPECIALIST lexicon and lexical tools (natural language processing tools)

Exercise 1.4 – Other Classification Systems and Databases

Instructions: Complete each statement.

1. The classification of neoplasms used by cancer registries throughout the world to record incidence of malignancy and survival rates is called the _____.
2. Specific sets of patient characteristics (or case-mix groups) on which payment determinations are made under several prospective payment systems are represented by the _____.
3. The set of files and software that allows many health and biomedical vocabularies and standards to enable interoperability among computer systems is called the _____.
4. The coding system that is used to classify dental procedures and services is called the _____.
5. The system that classifies health and health-related domains to describe body functions and structures, activities, and participation is called the _____.
6. The system that classifies services not included in the CPT manual to describe the service, supply, or therapy provided and may also be assigned to report nursing services and alternative medicine procedures is called _____.
7. The nomenclature that provides normalized names for clinical drugs and links its names to many of the drug vocabularies commonly used in pharmacy management and drug interaction software is called _____.

Exercise 1.4 – continued

8. An electronic database and universal standard that is used to identify medical laboratory observations and for the purpose of clinical care and management is called the _____.

9. The American Psychiatric Association published a standard classification of mental disorders called the _____-5.

10. The system that provides a new standardized framework and a unique coding structure for assessing, documenting, and classifying home health and ambulatory care is called the _____ System.

Documentation as the Basis for Coding

Documentation includes dictated and transcribed, keyboarded or handwritten, and computer-generated notes and reports recorded in patient records by a health care professional. Documentation must be dated and authenticated (with a legible signature or electronic authentication). Health care providers are responsible for documenting and authenticating legible, complete, and timely patient records in accordance with federal regulations (e.g., Medicare CoP) and accrediting agency standards (e.g., The Joint Commission). The provider is also responsible for correcting or editing errors in patient record documentation.

A *patient record* (or *medical record*) is the business record for a patient encounter (inpatient or outpatient) that documents health care services provided to a patient. It stores patient demographic data and documentation that supports diagnoses and justifies treatment provided. It also contains the results of treatment provided. (*Demographic data* include patient identification information that is collected according to facility policy and includes information such as the patient's name, date of birth, and mother's maiden name.) The primary purpose of the record is to provide for *continuity of care*, which involves documenting patient care services so that others who treat the patient have a source of information on which to base additional care and treatment. The record also serves as a communication tool for physicians and other patient care professionals. It assists in planning individual patient care and documenting a patient's illness and treatment. Secondary purposes of the record do not relate directly to patient care and include:

- Evaluating the quality of patient care
- Providing data for use in clinical research, epidemiology studies, education, public policy making, facilities planning, and health care statistics
- Providing information to third-party payers for reimbursement
- Serving the medicolegal interests of the patient, facility, and providers of care

Documentation for Teaching Hospitals

In a teaching hospital, documentation must identify the service provided, how the teaching physician participated in providing the service, and whether the teaching physician was physically present when the service was provided. A *teaching hospital* is engaged in an approved graduate medical education (GME) residency program in medicine, osteopathy, dentistry, or podiatry. A *teaching physician* is a physician (other than another resident physician) who supervises residents during patient care. A *resident physician* is an individual who participates in an approved GME program. A *hospitalist* is a physician who provides care for hospital inpatients. They are often internists (e.g., internal medicine specialists) who handle a patient's entire admission process, including examining the patient, reviewing patient history and medications, writing admission orders, counseling the patient, and performing other tasks that would have required the primary care physician to travel to the hospital to coordinate the inpatient admission. Similar to the concept of emergency physicians practicing in the hospital's emergency department, hospitalists are based in the hospital and provide inpatient care. Thus, their practice is location-based instead of body system-centered (e.g., neurology) or age-centered (e.g., gerontology).

Medical Necessity

Documentation in the patient record serves as the basis for coding. The information in the record must support codes submitted on claims for third-party payer reimbursement processing. The patient's diagnosis must also justify diagnostic and therapeutic procedures or services provided. This is called **medical necessity** and requires providers to document services or supplies that are proper and needed for the diagnosis or treatment of a medical condition; provided for the diagnosis, direct care, and treatment of a medical condition; consistent with standards of good medical practice in the local area; and not mainly for the convenience of the physician or health care facility.

It is important to remember the familiar phrase, "If it wasn't documented, it wasn't done." The patient record serves as a medicolegal document and a business record. If a provider performs a service but does not document it, the patient (or third-party payer) can refuse to pay for that service, resulting in lost revenue for the provider. In addition, because the patient record serves as an excellent defense of the quality of care administered to a patient, missing documentation can result in problems if the record has to be admitted as evidence in a court of law.

> **Example of Missing Patient Record Documentation:** A representative from XYZ Insurance Company reviewed 100 outpatient claims submitted by the Medical Center to ensure that all services billed were documented in the patient records. Upon reconciliation of claims with patient record documentation, the representative denied payment for 13 services (totaling $14,000) because reports of the services billed were not found in the patient records. The facility must pay back the $14,000 it received from the payer as reimbursement for the claims submitted.

> **Example of Medical Necessity:** The patient underwent an x-ray of the right knee, and the provider documented "severe right shoulder pain" in the record. The coder assigned a CPT code to the "right knee x-ray" and an ICD-10-CM code to the "right shoulder pain." In this example, the third-party payer will deny reimbursement for the submitted claim because the *reason* for the x-ray (shoulder pain) does not match the *type* of x-ray performed. For medical necessity, the provider should have documented a diagnosis such as "right knee pain."

Patient Record Formats

Health care facilities and physicians' offices usually maintain either manual or automated records, and sometimes they maintain a hybrid record. A *manual record* is paper-based, while an *automated record* is computer-based. A *hybrid record* contains both paper-based and computer-based (electronic) documents. This means the facility or office creates and stores some reports as paper-based records (e.g., handwritten progress notes, physician orders, and graphic charts) and some documents using a computer (e.g., transcribed reports and automated laboratory results). A variety of formats are used to maintain manual records, including the source-oriented record (SOR), problem-oriented record (POR), and integrated record. Automated record formats include the electronic health record (EHR) (or computer-based patient record, CPR), electronic medical record (EMR), and document imaging (to scan paper-based reports, such as patient-signed consent forms). Hybrid records use a combination format, such as the POR for paper-based reports and EMR for computer-based reports.

 NOTE:

True EHRs are generated by multiple providers using specialized software, and results are stored electronically in a format that is easily retrievable and viewable by users.

Manual Record Formats

Manual record formats include the source-oriented record (SOR), problem-oriented record (POR), and integrated record.

Source-Oriented Record

Source-oriented record (SOR) (or *sectionalized record*) reports are organized according to documentation (or data) source (e.g., ancillary, medical, and nursing). Each documentation (or data) source is located in a labeled section.

Problem-Oriented Record

The *problem-oriented record (POR)* systematic method of documentation consists of four components:

- Database
- Problem list
- Initial plan
- Progress notes

The POR *database* contains the following patient information collected on each patient:

- Chief complaint
- Present conditions and diagnoses
- Social data
- Past, personal, medical, and social history
- Review of systems
- Physical examination
- Baseline laboratory data

The POR *problem list* serves as a table of contents for the patient record because it is filed at the beginning of the record and contains a numbered list of the patient's problems, which helps to index documentation throughout the record. The POR *initial plan* contains the strategy for managing patient care and any actions taken to investigate the patient's condition and to treat and educate the patient. The initial plan consists of three categories:

- *Diagnostic/management plans*: Plans to learn more about the patient's condition and the management of the conditions.
- *Therapeutic plans*: Specific medications, goals, procedures, therapies, and treatments used to treat the patient.
- *Patient education plans*: Plans to educate the patient about conditions for which the patient is being treated.

The POR *progress notes* are documented for each problem assigned to the patient, using the SOAP structure:

- *Subjective (S)*: Patient's statement describes how the patient feels, including symptomatic information (e.g., "I have a headache.").
- *Objective (O)*: Observations about the patient, such as physical findings, or lab or x-ray results (e.g., chest x-ray negative).
- *Assessment (A)*: Judgment, opinion, or evaluation made by the health care provider (e.g., acute headache).
- *Plan (P)*: Diagnostic, therapeutic, and education plans to resolve the problems (e.g., patient to take Tylenol as needed for pain).

A *discharge note* is documented in the progress notes section of the POR to summarize the patient's care, treatment, response to care, and condition on discharge—documentation of all problems is included. A *transfer note* is documented when a patient is being transferred to another facility. It summarizes the reason for admission, current diagnoses and medical information, and reason for transfer.

Integrated Record

Integrated record reports are arranged in strict chronological date order (or in reverse date order), which allows for observation of how the patient is progressing (e.g., responds to treatment) based on test results. Many facilities integrate only physician and ancillary services (e.g., physical therapy) progress notes, which require entries to be identified by appropriate authentication (e.g., complete signature of the professional documenting the note such as Mary Smith, RRT).

Automated Record Formats

The *electronic health record (EHR)* is a collection of patient information documented by a number of providers at different facilities regarding one patient. It is a multidisciplinary (many specialties) and multienterprise (many facilities) approach to record keeping. The EHR provides access to complete and accurate health problems, status, and treatment data; it contains alerts (e.g., of drug interaction) and reminders (e.g., prescription renewal notice) for health care providers. According to the *Journal of Contemporary Dental Practice*, February 15, 2002, some professionals prefer to "use *electronic* instead of the earlier term *computer-based* because *electronic* better describes the medium in which the patient record is managed."

The *electronic medical record (EMR)* is created on a computer, using a keyboard, a mouse, an optical pen device, a voice-recognition system, a scanner, or a touch screen. Records are created using vendor software, which also assists in provider decision making (e.g., alerts, reminders, clinical decision support systems, and links to medical knowledge). Numerous vendors offer EMR software, mostly to physician office practices that require practice management solutions (e.g., appointment scheduling, claims processing, clinical notes, patient registration).

Document imaging often supplements the EHR or EMR by converting paper records (e.g., consent to treatment signed by patients) to an electronic format using laser technology to create the image; a *scanner* is used to capture paper record images onto the storage media. The paper record must be prepared for scanning (e.g., removal of staples) so documents can pass through the scanner properly using a document feeder that is attached to the scanner; each report is pulled through the scanner so the image is saved. Each scanned page is *indexed*, which means it is identified according to a unique identification number (e.g., patient record number). A unique feature is that documents for the same patient do *not* have to be scanned at the same time. Because each scanned page is indexed, the complete patient record can be retrieved even when a patient's reports are scanned at a later time.

Documentation Cloning Is an EMR/EHR Concern

Electronic Health Records Provider Fact Sheet. (Permission to reuse in accordance with http://www .cms.gov content reuse and linking policy.)

Medicare administrative contractors noted the frequency of electronic medical records (EMRs) and electronic health records (EHRs) that contain identical documentation across services. This was likely the result of *documentation cloning*, which involves using the EMR or EHR to bring information from previous patient encounters forward to the current encounter without updating that information. Documentation must reflect patient conditions and treatment for each encounter. Bringing forward previous documentation and simply changing the date in the EHR or EMR is unacceptable. U.S. Department of Health and Human Services, Office of Inspector General (HHS-OIG) staff continue to closely monitor EMR and EHR documentation cloning.

Exercise 1.5 – Documentation as Basis for Coding

Instructions: Select the most appropriate response.

1. Continuity of patient care is considered a _____ purpose of the patient record.
   a. primary
   b. secondary

2. Evaluating quality of patient care is considered a _____ purpose of the patient record.
   a. primary
   b. secondary

3. Which is an example of patient demographic data?
   a. date of birth
   b. discharge diagnosis

4. Medical necessity requires providers to document procedures, services, and supplies that are proper and needed for the
   a. convenience of the physician or health care facility.
   b. diagnosis or treatment of a patient's medical condition.

5. Which is the business record for a patient encounter because it documents health care services provided?
   a. demographic data collected on admission
   b. patient record housed in the facility

Health Data Collection

Health data collection is performed by health care facilities and providers for the purpose of administrative planning, submitting data and statistics to state and federal government agencies (and other organizations), and reporting health claims data to third-party payers. *Administrative planning* requires health data analysis to determine employee staffing levels, services offered, and more. *Submitting data and statistics* to state and federal government agencies is mandated and includes cancer registry data, reportable events, reportable diseases, morbidity data, and more. *Reporting health claims data to third-party payers* uses data collected from patient records and assigned medical codes, which helps ensure the financial viability of the health care facility or medical practice.

Reporting Hospital Data

Hospitals and other health care facilities use *automated case abstracting software* to collect and report inpatient and outpatient data for statistical analysis and reimbursement purposes. Data are entered in an abstracting software program (Figure 1-4), and the facility's billing department imports it to the *UB-04* (or *CMS-1450*) claim (Figure 1-5) for submission to third-party payers. The facility's information technology department generates reports (Figure 1-6), which are used for statistical analysis. The UB-04 (or CMS-1450) is a standard claim (uniform bill) submitted by health care institutions to payers for inpatient and outpatient services.

> **Example:** Procedure data reports, profit and loss statements, and patient satisfaction surveys are used by health care planning and forecasting committees to determine the types of procedures performed at their facilities and the costs associated with providing such services. As a result of report analysis, procedures that contribute to a facility's profits and losses can be determined; in addition, some services may be expanded while others are eliminated.

Reporting Physician Office Data

Computerized physicians' offices use medical practice management software to enter claims data and either electronically submit CMS-1500 claims data to third-party payers or print paper-based CMS-1500 claims that are mailed or faxed to clearinghouses or payers for processing. The *CMS-1500* is a standard claim submitted by physicians' offices to third-party payers. *Medical practice management software* (e.g., e-Medsys, MediSoft) is a combination of medical practice management and medical billing software that automates the following daily workflow and procedures of a physician's office or clinic:

- Appointment scheduling (e.g., initial and follow-up appointments) (Figure 1-7)

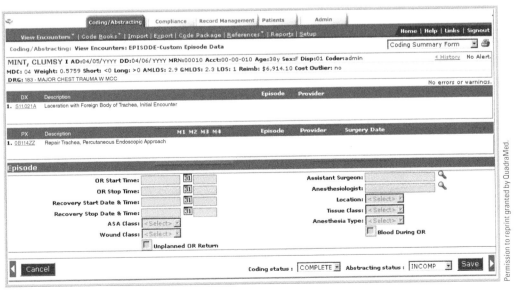

FIGURE 1-4 Sample data entry screen with ICD-10-CM and ICD-10-PCS codes and descriptions for automated case abstracting software

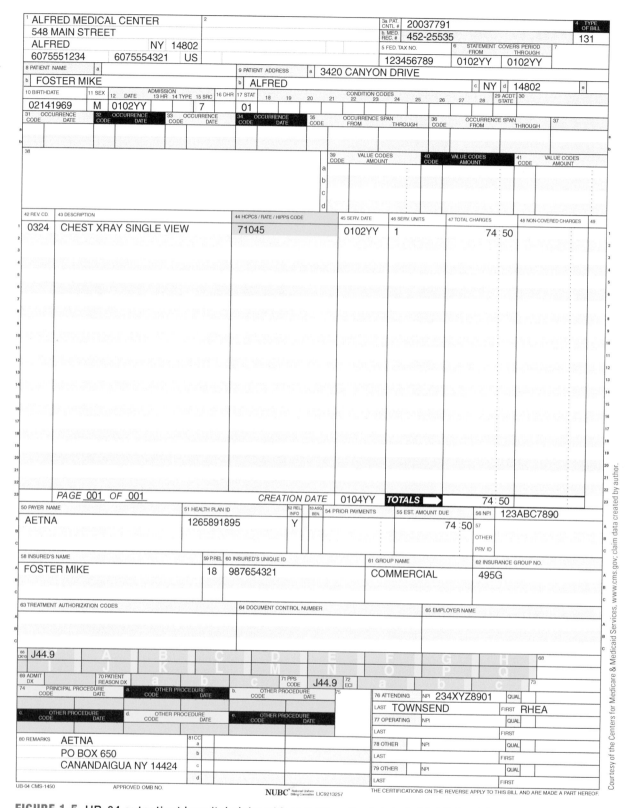

FIGURE 1-5 UB-04 outpatient hospital claim with sample patient data in highlighted form locators that also contain ICD-10-CM and CPT codes

Cengage Medical Center

Procedure Data Report

Reporting Period   0301YYYY–0301YYYY   Date Prepared 03-02-YYYY

                                                           Page 1 of 5

Principal Procedure	Secondary Procedures	Attending Physician	Age	Gender	Payer	Patient Number
CLOSED BIOPSY OF BRAIN 00B03ZX		248	42	F	01	562359
CRANIOTOMY 0N800ZZ		235	56	F	03	231587
0N800ZZ		326	27	M	02	239854
0N800ZZ		236	08	F	05	562198
0N800ZZ		236	88	M	05	615789
DEBRIDEMENT OF SKULL 0NB00ZZ		326	43	M	03	653218

FIGURE 1-6 Sample procedure data report containing ICD-10-PCS codes

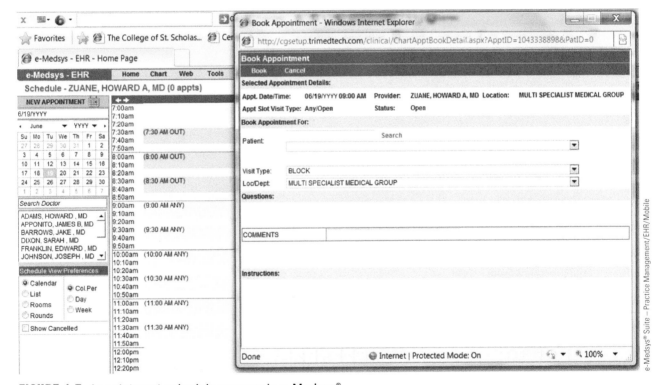

FIGURE 1-7 Appointment schedule screens in e-Medsys®

- Claims processing (e.g., CMS-1500 claims processing) (Figure 1-8)
- Patient invoicing (e.g., automated billing) (Figure 1-9)
- Patient management (e.g., patient registration) (Figure 1-10)
- Report generation (e.g., accounts receivable aging report) (Figure 1-11)

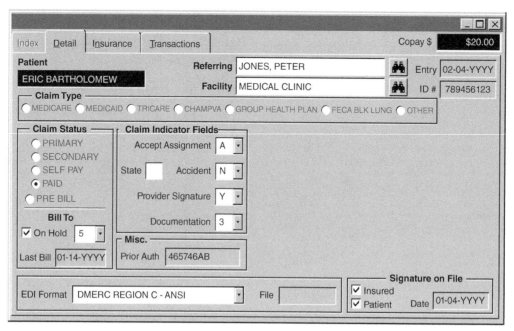

FIGURE 1-8 Claims processing screen

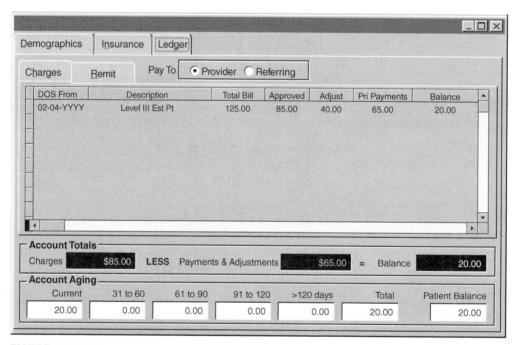

FIGURE 1-9 Billing screen

Medical assistants and insurance specialists use medical practice management software to collect physician office data for reimbursement purposes by locating patient information, inputting ICD-10-CM, CPT, and HCPCS Level II codes for diagnoses and procedures/services, and generating and processing CMS-1500 claims. Medical practice management software generates claims for a variety of medical specialties, and claims can be printed and mailed to clearinghouses, TPAs, or third-party payers for processing. The software also allows for submission of HIPAA-compliant electronic claims to clearinghouses, TPAs, or third-party payers.

When records are reviewed to select ICD-10-CM, CPT, and HCPCS Level II codes for reporting to third-party payers, documentation in the physician office patient record serves as the basis for coding. Coders are

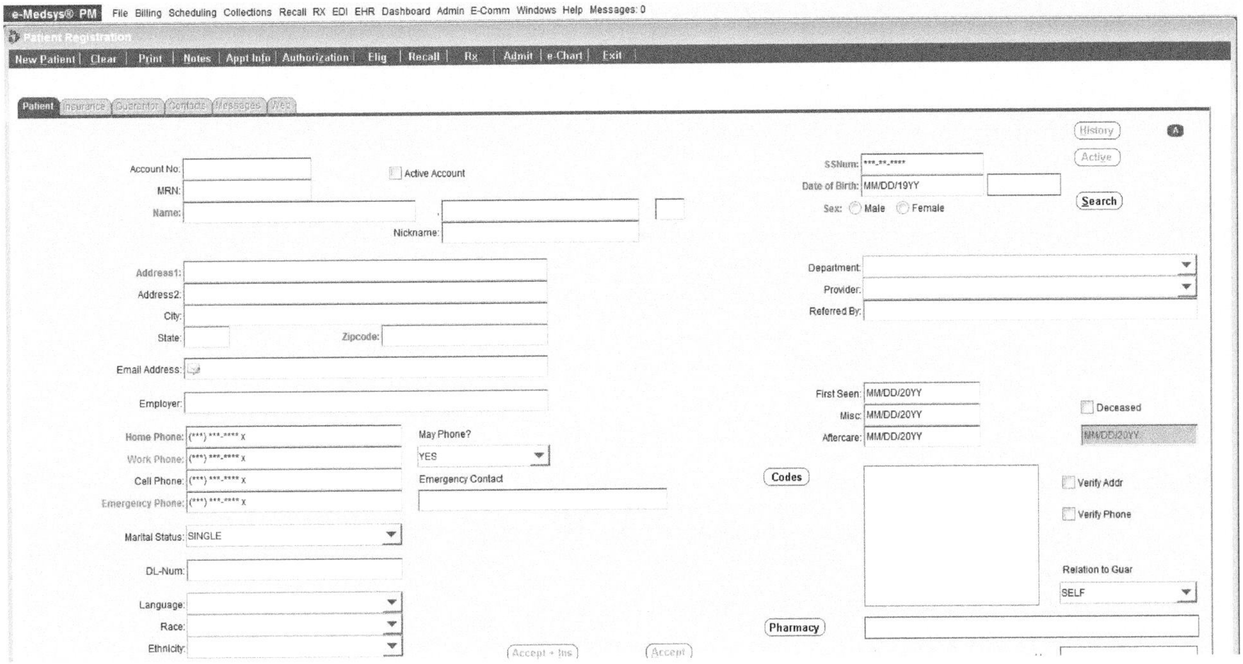

e-Medsys® Suite – Practice Management/EHR/Mobile

FIGURE 1-10 Patient registration screen in e-Medsys®

Payer
03/19/YYYY

Dates of Service: 03/01/YYYY to 03/10/YYYY

	Claim ID	Last Bill	Current	31 to 60	61 to 90	91 to 120	>120
AETNA							
Adams, Cynthia 800123456	243567	03/05/YYYY	160.00	0.00	0.00	0.00	0.00
AETNA			160.00	0.00	0.00	0.00	0.00
BLUE CROSS BLUE SHIELD							
Zhou, Jin 800234567	345678	03/01/YYYY	160.00	0.00	0.00	0.00	0.00
Zhou, Jin 800234567	345678	03/01/YYYY	240.00	0.00	0.00	0.00	0.00
Zhou, Jin 800234567	345678	03/10/YYYY	80.00	0.00	0.00	0.00	0.00
Zhou, Jin 800234567	345678	03/04/YYYY	113.00	0.00	0.00	0.00	0.00
BLUE CROSS BLUE SHIELD			593.00	0.00	0.00	0.00	0.00
MEDICAID							
Clark, Matthew 800345678	456789	03/03/YYYY	1,580.00	0.00	0.00	0.00	0.00
MEDICAID			1,580.00	0.00	0.00	0.00	0.00

Current	31 to 60	61 to 90	91 to 120	>120	Grand Total
2,393.000	0.00	0.00	0.00	0.00	2,393.00
100.00%	0.00%	0.00%	0.00%	0.00%	

FIGURE 1-11 Accounts receivable aging report

responsible for reviewing patient records to select the appropriate diagnoses and procedures/services to which codes are assigned. Information in the record must support the codes submitted on claims for third-party payer reimbursement processing. The patient's diagnosis must justify diagnostic or therapeutic procedures or services provided (medical necessity), and the provider must document services or supplies that:

- are proper and needed for the diagnosis or treatment of a medical condition;
- are provided for the diagnosis, direct care, and treatment of a medical condition;

- meet the standards of good medical practice in the local area; and
- are not mainly for the convenience of the physician or health care facility.

Claims can be denied if the medical necessity of procedures or services is not established. Each procedure or service reported on the CMS-1500 claim must be linked to a condition that justifies the necessity for performing that procedure or providing that service. If the procedures or services delivered are determined to be unreasonable and unnecessary, the claim is denied. On the UB-04 claim, procedures or services are not linked; however, payers often request copies of patient records to review documentation to verify diagnoses, procedures, and services reported on the claim.

Exercise 1.6 – Health Data Collection

Instructions: Complete each statement.

1. Appointment scheduling and claims processing are processes associated with medical _____ software.
2. Hospital coders and abstractors use automated case _____ software to collect and report inpatient and outpatient data for statistical analysis and reimbursement purposes.
3. Physicians' offices submit data to third-party payers on the _____ claim.
4. Hospitals submit data to third-party payers on the _____ (or CMS-1450) claim.
5. Claims are denied if _____ necessity of procedures or services is not established.

Summary

A coder is expected to master the use of coding systems, coding principles and rules, government regulations, and third-party payer requirements to ensure that all diagnoses, services, and procedures documented in patient records are accurately coded for reimbursement, research, and statistical purposes. To prepare for entry into the profession, students are encouraged to join a professional association. Students usually pay a reduced membership fee and receive most of the same benefits as active members. The benefits of joining a professional association include eligibility for scholarships and grants, opportunity to network with members, free publications, reduced certification exam fees, and website access for members only.

Coding systems and medical nomenclatures are used by health care facilities, health care providers, and third-party payers to collect, store, and process data for a variety of purposes. A coding system organizes a medical nomenclature according to similar conditions, diseases, procedures, and services; it contains codes for each. A medical nomenclature includes clinical terminologies and clinical vocabularies that are used by health care providers to document patient care; *clinical terminologies* include designations, expressions, symbols, and terms used in the field of medicine, and *clinical vocabularies* include clinical phrases or words along with their meanings. Codes include numeric and alphanumeric characters that are reported to health plans for health care reimbursement and to external agencies for data collection and internally for education and research. Coding is the assignment of codes to diseases, injuries, reasons for an encounter, services, and procedures based on patient record documentation. *Encoder* software automates the medical coding process, allowing coders to use a search function to locate and verify codes. *Computer-assisted coding (CAC)* software analyzes EHR or EMR documentation to generate codes for terms and phrases, and coders use data analytic skills to review and determine which CAC-generated codes are to be reported.

Health care providers are responsible for documenting and authenticating legible, complete, and timely patient records in accordance with federal regulations and accrediting agency standards. The provider is also responsible for correcting or editing errors in patient record documentation. Health data collection is performed by health care facilities to do administrative planning, to submit statistics to state and federal government agencies, and to report health claims data to third-party payers for reimbursement purposes.

Internet Links

Alternate Billing Codes (ABC codes): **www.abccodes.com**

AHA Coding Clinic Advisor: **codingclinicadvisor.com**

AAPC: **www.aapc.com**

American Association of Medical Assistants (AAMA): **www.aama-ntl.org**

American Health Information Management Association (AHIMA): **www.ahima.org**

American Medical Technologists (AMT): **www.americanmedtech.org**

Clinical Care Classification System: **careclassification.org**

Current Dental Terminology (CDT): Go to **www.ada.org**, scroll over Publications, and click on CDT coding.

Diagnostic and Statistical Manual of Mental Disorders (DSM): **https://dsm.psychiatryonline.org**.

ICD-10-CM and ICD-10-PCS encoder (subscription-based): **www.encoderpro.com** (free trial available)

Health Insurance Prospective Payment System (HIPPS) Rate Codes: Go to **www.cms.gov**, click on the Medicare link, scroll to the Medicare Fee-for-Service Payment heading, click on the Prospective Payment Systems - General Information link, and click on the HIPPS Codes link.

International Classification of Diseases for Oncology (ICD-O-3): Go to **https://training.seer.cancer.gov**, click on Resources, click on Links to Reference Materials, and scroll down and click on the ICD-O-3 Training module link. The international version of the ICD-O-3 coding manual is available by going to **www.iacr.com.fr**, scrolling over Support for Registries, and clicking on International Classification of Diseases for Oncology (ICD-O).

National Drug Codes (NDC): Go to **www.fda.gov**, and use the Search feature to enter National Drug Code Directory to navigate to the online NDC Directory.

National Cancer Institute's Surveillance, Epidemiology, and End Results (SEER) Training Modules: Go to **https://training.seer.cancer.gov**, click on the Cancer Registration & Surveillance Modules link, and click on the Coding Primary Site & Tumor Morphology link.

RxNorm: Go to **https://uts.nlm.nih.gov**, and click on the RxNorm link.

SNOMED CT: Go to **https://uts.nlm.nih.gov,** and click on the SNOMED CT link.

Unified Medical Language Systems (UMLS): Go to **https://uts.nlm.nih.gov**, and click on the Unified Medical Language System (UMLS) link.

Review

Multiple Choice

Instructions: Select the most appropriate response.

1. The Health Insurance Portability and Accountability Act of 1996 (HIPAA) requires two types of code sets, large code sets and small code sets, to be adopted for the purpose of _____ data elements.
    a. decrypting
    b. encoding
    c. interpreting
    d. translating

2. Which is considered to be a small code set according to HIPAA?
    a. Actions taken to prevent, diagnose, treat, and manage diseases and injuries
    b. Causes of injury, disease, impairment, or other health-related problems
    c. Diseases, injuries, impairments, and other health-related problems
    d. Race, ethnicity, type of facility, and type of unit

3. Which is a code set adopted by HIPAA for use by clearinghouses, health plans, and providers?
   a. CDT
   b. CMIT
   c. ICD-9
   d. SNOMED CT

4. The purpose of adopting standard code sets was to
   a. establish a medical nomenclature to standardize HIPAA data submissions.
   b. improve data quality and simplify claims submission for providers.
   c. increase costs associated with processing health insurance claims.
   d. regulate health care clearinghouses and third-party administrators.

5. According to HIPAA, health plans that do not accept standard code sets are required to modify their systems to accept all valid codes or to contract with a(n)
   a. electronic data interchange.
   b. health care clearinghouse.
   c. insurance company.
   d. third-party administrator.

6. Which type of clinical terminologies and clinical vocabularies are used by health care providers to document patient care?
   a. Classification system
   b. Demographic data
   c. Medical nomenclature
   d. Patient record

7. The requirement that patient diagnoses justify diagnostic and/or therapeutic procedures or services provided is called
   a. continuity of care.
   b. facilities planning.
   c. medical necessity.
   d. policy making.

8. Which is the business record for a patient encounter (inpatient or outpatient) that documents health care services provided to a patient?
   a. Demographic data
   b. Financial record
   c. Health care statistics
   d. Medical record

9. The primary purpose of the patient record is _____, which involves documenting patient care services so that others who treat the patient have a source of information on which to base additional care and treatment.
   a. continuity of care
   b. medical necessity
   c. medicolegal
   d. quality of care

10. Which is a secondary purpose of the medical record that does not relate directly to patient care?
    a. Clinical research
    b. Continuity of care
    c. Discharge note
    d. Hybrid record

11. Which type of medical record format stores documentation in labeled sections?
    a. Integrated record
    b. Problem-oriented record
    c. Source-oriented record
    d. SOAP notes

12. A progress note contains diagnoses of muscle strain and weakness. This statement would be located in the _____ portion of the POR progress note.
    a. Assessment
    b. Objective
    c. Plan
    d. Subjective

13. A progress note contains documentation that the patient is to be followed up with in the physician's office two weeks after discharge from the hospital. This statement would be located in the _____ portion of the POR progress note.
    a. Assessment
    b. Objective
    c. Plan
    d. Subjective

14. A progress note contains documentation that the EKG showed elevated T-wave changes. This statement would be located in the _____ portion of the POR progress note.
    a. Assessment
    b. Objective
    c. Plan
    d. Subjective

15. Which is documented in the progress notes section of the POR to summarize the patient's care, treatment, response to care, and condition on release from the facility?
    a. Demographic data
    b. Discharge note
    c. Medical necessity
    d. Transfer note

16. Which is used to capture paper record images onto storage media?
    a. EHR
    b. EMR
    c. Documentation cloning
    d. Scanner

17. To provide the maximum benefit to students, internships are typically _____ work experiences that are arranged by academic program faculty.
    a. elective
    b. nonpaid
    c. optional
    d. voluntary

18. To whom does the student report at the professional practice experience (or internship) site?
    a. Human resources
    b. PPE or internship supervisor
    c. Program faculty
    d. Volunteer department

19. Which is a benefit of joining a professional association?
    a. Free certification examination fees
    b. Opportunities to network with other members
    c. Reduced benefits as compared with nonmembers
    d. Website-only access to professional journals

20. Which processes health care claims and performs related business functions for a health plan?
    a. Health care clearinghouse
    b. Health care provider
    c. Third-party administrator
    d. Third-party payer

21. Which classifies outpatient hospital and physician office procedures and services?
    a. CDT
    b. CPT
    c. ICD-10-CM
    d. ICD-10-PCS

22. Which is a standard classification of mental disorders used by mental health professionals in the United States?
    a. ABC
    b. CCC
    c. DSM
    d. ICF

23. Which is an electronic database and universal standard used for clinical care and management?
    a. LOINC®
    b. SNOMED CT
    c. READ
    d. UMLS

24. Hospitals and other health care facilities use automated case abstracting software to
    a. collect and report data for statistical analysis and reimbursement purposes.
    b. generate claims data for electronic submission to health care providers.
    c. justify diagnostic or therapeutic procedures or services provided to patients.
    d. submit standard claims to providers for inpatient and outpatient services.

25. Which is the standard claim submitted by physicians' offices to third-party payers?
    a. CMS-1450
    b. CMS-1500
    c. UB-04
    d. UB-92

Part

II

ICD-10-CM Coding System

Part II of *3-2-1 Code It!* contains the following individual chapters that cover ICD-10-CM coding:

 NOTE:

ICD-10-CM coding is also included in the following textbook chapters:
- Chapter 5: ICD-10-CM Outpatient and Physician Office Coding
- Chapter 7: ICD-10-CM and ICD-10-PCS Inpatient Hospital Coding

2 Introduction to ICD-10-CM Coding and Conventions

Chapter Outline

Overview of ICD-10-CM

ICD-10-CM Index to Diseases and Injuries

ICD-10-CM Tabular List of Diseases and Injuries

ICD-10-CM Official Guidelines for Coding and Reporting

ICD-9-CM Legacy Coding System

ICD-10-CM Coding Conventions

General ICD-10-CM Diagnosis Coding Guidelines

Chapter Objectives

At the conclusion of this chapter, the student should be able to:

1. Define key terms related to the introduction of ICD-10-CM coding and coding conventions.
2. Explain the purpose of assigning ICD-10-CM codes.
3. Locate main terms for diagnostic statements using the ICD-10-CM Index to Diseases and Injuries.
4. Assign diagnosis codes using the ICD-10-CM Index to Diseases and Injuries and the ICD-10-CM Tabular List of Diseases and Injuries.
5. Explain the purpose of ICD-10-CM official guidelines for coding and reporting.
6. Use general equivalence mappings (GEMs) as part of the ICD-9-CM legacy coding system.
7. Assign diagnosis codes according to ICD-10-CM coding conventions.
8. Assign diagnosis codes according to general ICD-10-CM diagnosis coding guidelines.

Key Terms

category

coding conventions

  abbreviations

    NEC (not elsewhere classifiable)

    NOS (not otherwise specified)

  and

boxed note

code also

cross references

  see

  see also

  see category

  see condition

default code

due to

eponym

etiology and manifestation convention

  code first underlying disease

code, if applicable, any causal condition first

in diseases classified elsewhere

use additional code

excludes1 note

excludes2 note	parentheses	encounter	multiple codes
format	syndrome	essential modifier	nonessential modifier
in	tables	etiology	placeholder
includes note	trust the index	ICD-10 Coordination and Maintenance Committee	residual effect
inclusion term	typeface		sequela
manifestation	unspecified code	*ICD-10-CM Official Guidelines for Coding and Reporting*	subcategory
modifier	with		subterm
other code	combination code	Index to Diseases and Injuries	Tabular List of Diseases and Injuries
other specified code	Cooperating Parties for the ICD-10-CM/PCS	laterality	
punctuation		main term	
brackets			
colon			

Introduction

The *International Classification of Diseases (ICD)* is published by the World Health Organization (WHO) and is used to classify *mortality* (death) data from death certificates. WHO published the tenth revision of ICD in 1994 with a new name, *International Statistical Classification of Diseases and Related Health Problems*, and reorganized its three-digit categories.

The *International Classification of Diseases, Tenth Revision, Clinical Modification* (ICD-10-CM) was developed in the United States and implemented in 2015. It is used to code and classify *morbidity* (disease) data from inpatient and outpatient records, including physician office records. ICD-10-CM is a closed classification system that is used in the United States to classify diagnoses, which means that ICD-10-CM provides just one place to classify each condition. All health care settings use ICD-10-CM to report diseases, injuries, and reasons for an encounter.

ICD-10-CM Official Guidelines for Coding and Reporting are used as a companion to ICD-10-CM to ensure accurate coding. This chapter includes an overview about *ICD-10-CM Official Guidelines for Coding and Reporting*, general diagnosis coding guidelines, and coding conventions. ICD-10-CM chapter-specific diagnosis coding guidelines are covered in Chapters 3 and 4.

 NOTE:

When reviewing examples and completing exercises and review questions in this chapter, use your ICD-10-CM coding manual to locate index entries and verify codes in the tabular list.

Overview of ICD-10-CM

ICD-10-CM is a clinical modification of WHO's *International Classification of Diseases, Tenth Revision* (ICD-10). The term *clinical* is used to emphasize the modification's intent. This means that the coding system serves as a useful tool in the classification of morbidity data for indexing of patient records, reviewing quality of care, and compiling basic health statistics. Used to describe the clinical picture of the patient, ICD-10-CM codes are more precise than those needed for statistical groupings and trends analysis. ICD-10-CM enhances accurate payment by supporting the medical necessity of procedures and services provided and facilitating the evaluation of medical processes and outcomes.

 NOTE:

ICD-10-CM Official Guidelines for Coding and Reporting, which serve as a companion document to ICD-10-CM, are discussed later in this chapter.

Example 1: For a patient's annual physical without abnormal findings, report ICD-10-CM diagnosis code Z00.00, Encounter for general adult medical exam without abnormal findings.

Example 2: For a patient who presents with headache and cough, report ICD-10-CM symptom code R51.9, Headache, and sign code R05.9, Cough.

ICD-10-CM is the disease classification system developed by the Centers for Disease Control and Prevention (CDC) for use in *all* U.S. health care treatment settings. ICD-10-CM codes require up to seven characters, are entirely alphanumeric, and use coding conventions (e.g., Excludes1 and Excludes2 notes) to ensure coding specificity.

ICD-10-CM incorporates specificity and clinical information, resulting in

- Decreased need to include supporting documentation with claims
- Enhanced ability to conduct public health surveillance
- Improved ability to measure health care services
- Increased sensitivity when refining grouping and reimbursement methodologies

ICD-10-CM also provides codes to allow comparison of mortality and morbidity data, and provides data for

- Conducting research
- Designing payment systems
- Identifying fraud and abuse
- Making clinical decisions
- Measuring care furnished to patients
- Processing claims
- Tracking public health

ICD-10-CM classifies health-related conditions using three to seven characters, plus a decimal. Greater specificity is provided at the fourth, fifth, and sixth character levels, and a seventh character extension is added for some codes.

Example: The diagnosis is stage 3 pressure ulcer of the right lower back. In ICD-10-CM, assign combination code L89.133 to classify the condition (category L89 for pressure ulcer) along with its location (subcategory L89.1 for back), laterality (subcategory L89.13 for right lower back), and depth (code L89.133 for stage 3). Valid code L89.133 is reported for "Pressure ulcer of right lower back, stage 3."

ICD-10-CM Tabular List of Diseases and Injuries
L89.133 Pressure ulcer of right lower back, stage 3
Healing pressure ulcer of right lower back, stage 3
Pressure ulcer with full thickness skin loss involving damage or necrosis of subcutaneous tissue, right lower back

Sixth and seventh characters must be added to an ICD-10-CM code when applicable to fully report information documented in the patient record. Seventh characters that indicate the type of encounter (e.g., initial encounter) associated with a patient's injury are found in the tabular list; they are not included in the index.

Example: The diagnosis is mechanical breakdown of right femoral arterial graft, initial encounter. In ICD-10-CM, combination code T82.312A is reported. Notice that 7th character A (initial encounter) is selected from the tabular list entry for this category T82 code.

ICD-10-CM Tabular List of Diseases and Injuries

The appropriate 7th character is to be added to each code from category T82

   A   initial encounter

   D   subsequent encounter

   S   sequela

T82.3   **Mechanical complication of other vascular grafts**

    T82.31   **Breakdown (mechanical) of other vascular grafts**

        T82.310   Breakdown (mechanical) of aortic (bifurcation) graft (replacement)

        T82.311   Breakdown (mechanical) of carotid arterial graft (bypass)

        T82.312   Breakdown (mechanical) of femoral arterial graft (bypass)

        T82.318   Breakdown (mechanical) of other vascular grafts

        T82.319   Breakdown (mechanical) of unspecified vascular grafts

---

ICD-10-CM is divided into two main parts, both of which must be used to assign valid codes.

- Index to Diseases and Injuries, which is an alphabetical list of terms and their corresponding codes (and includes a Table of Neoplasms, Table of Drugs and Chemicals, and an Index of External Cause of Injuries)
- Tabular List of Diseases and Injuries, which is a sequential, alphanumeric list of codes organized according to chapters based on body system or condition

Updating ICD-10-CM

The National Center for Health Statistics (NCHS) and the Centers for Medicare & Medicaid Services (CMS) are the U.S. Department of Health & Human Services (DHHS) agencies that comprise the **ICD-10 Coordination and Maintenance Committee**, which is responsible for overseeing all changes and modifications to ICD-10-CM. The NCHS works with the WHO to coordinate official disease classification activities for ICD-10-CM. Activities include the use, interpretation, and periodic revision of the classification system. CMS is responsible for annually updating the ICD-10-PCS procedure classification. The Committee also updated the general equivalency mappings (GEMs) through 2018 for ICD-10-CM (and ICD-10-PCS).

The *Medicare Prescription Drug, Improvement, and Modernization Act (MMA)* of 2003 requires all code sets (e.g., ICD-10-CM, ICD-10-PCS) to be valid at the time services are provided. This means that April 1 and October 1 coding updates for ICD-10-CM/PCS must be implemented immediately so accurate codes are reported on claims. (HIPAA legislation also requires the reporting of codes on health insurance claims.) New diagnosis and procedure code releases in April each year are related to new technologies (and resultant new diseases) only. In 2021, CMS began exploring possible implementation of releasing updated codes, guidelines, and changes to Medicare Severity-Diagnosis Related Groups (MS-DRGs) in April (as well as October) of each year. At the time this textbook was published, CMS had not made a decision.

Mandatory Reporting of ICD-10-CM Codes

The Medicare Catastrophic Coverage Act of 1988 mandated the reporting of diseases, injuries, and reasons for an encounter codes on Medicare claims; in subsequent years, private third-party payers adopted similar requirements for claims submission.

Reporting ICD-10-CM codes on submitted claims (Figure 2-1) ensures the medical necessity of procedures and services provided to patients during an encounter. An **encounter** is a face-to-face contact between a patient and a health care provider (e.g., physician, nurse practitioner) who assesses and treats the patient's condition. Medicare defines *medical necessity* as "the determination that a service or procedure rendered is reasonable and necessary for the diagnosis or treatment of an illness or injury."

21. DIAGNOSIS OR NATURE OF ILLNESS OR INJURY Relate A-L to service line below (24E)				ICD Ind. **0**	22. RESUBMISSION CODE	ORIGINAL REF. NO.
A. **S63501A**	B. **E119**	C.	D.			
E.	F.	G.	H.		23. PRIOR AUTHORIZATION NUMBER	
I.	J.	K.	L.			

	24. A. DATE(S) OF SERVICE From / To (MM DD YY)	B. PLACE OF SERVICE	C. EMG	D. PROCEDURES, SERVICES, OR SUPPLIES (Explain Unusual Circumstances) CPT/HCPCS | MODIFIER	E. DIAGNOSIS POINTER	F. $ CHARGES	G. DAYS OR UNITS	H. EPSDT Family Plan	I. ID. QUAL.	J. RENDERING PROVIDER ID. #
1	05 01 YY	11		99214	AB	125 00	1		NPI	
2	05 01 YY	11		82947	B	95 00	1		NPI	
3	05 01 YY	11		S8451	A	105 00	1		NPI	
4									NPI	
5									NPI	
6									NPI	

FIGURE 2-1 CMS-1500 claim Blocks 21 (ICD-10-CM codes) and 24E (Diagnosis Pointer for CPT codes in 24D) illustrate medical necessity of procedures and services

NOTE:

The Administrative Simplification subtitle of the Health Insurance Portability and Accountability Act of 1996 (HIPAA) mandated the adoption of code set standards in the Transactions and Code Sets final rule published in the *Federal Register*. The final rule modifies the standard medical data code sets for coding diagnoses and inpatient hospital procedures by concurrently adopting the *International Classification of Diseases, 10th Revision, Clinical Modification* (ICD-10-CM) for diagnosis coding (including the *ICD-10-CM Official Guidelines for Coding and Reporting*, as maintained and distributed by the U.S. Department of Health and Human Services) and the *International Classification of Diseases, 10th Revision, Procedure Coding System* (ICD-10-PCS) for inpatient hospital procedure coding (including the *ICD-10-PCS Official Guidelines for Coding and Reporting*, as maintained and distributed by the HHS).

Medical Necessity

Today's concept of medical necessity determines the extent to which individuals with health conditions receive health care services. (The concept was introduced in the 1970s when health insurance contracts intended to exclude care, such as voluntary hospitalizations prescribed primarily for the convenience of the provider or patient.) *Medical necessity* is the measure of whether a health care procedure or service is appropriate for the diagnosis and treatment of a condition. This decision-making process is based on the payer's contractual language and the treating provider's documentation. Generally, the following criteria are used to determine medical necessity:

- *Purpose:* The procedure or service is performed to treat a medical condition.
- *Scope:* The most appropriate level of service is provided, taking into consideration potential benefit and harm to the patient.

- *Evidence:* The treatment is known to be effective in improving health outcomes.
- *Value:* The treatment is cost-effective for this condition when compared to alternative treatments, including no treatment.

NOTE:

Cost-effective does not necessarily mean least expensive.

Example: A 70-year-old patient with type 1 diabetes mellitus is treated at the physician's office for severe wrist pain resulting from a fall. When the physician asks whether the patient has been regularly taking insulin and checking blood glucose levels, the patient says "most of the time." The physician orders a blood glucose test to be done in the office, which reveals elevated blood glucose levels. The physician provides counseling and education to the patient about the importance of taking daily insulin and checking blood glucose levels. The physician also orders an x-ray of the wrist, which proves to be negative for a fracture. The physician provides the patient with a wrist brace and instructs the patient to follow up in the office within four weeks.

The insurance specialist reports ICD-10-CM codes for type 1 diabetes mellitus and sprained wrist along with CPT and/or HCPCS Level II codes for an office visit, blood glucose lab test, and the wrist brace. If the only diagnosis reported on the claim (Figure 2-1) was a sprained wrist, the blood glucose lab test would be rejected for payment by the insurance company as an unnecessary medical procedure.

Exercise 2.1 – Overview of ICD-10-CM

Instructions: Complete each statement.

1. The ICD-10 Coordination and _____ Committee is responsible for overseeing all changes to ICD-10-CM (and ICD-10-PCS).

2. The National Center for Health Statistics (NCHS) is responsible for overseeing all changes and modifications to the official _____ disease and injury classification, while CMS is responsible for annually updating the ICD-10-PCS procedure classification.

3. Reporting ICD-10-CM codes on submitted claims ensures the medical _____ of procedures and services provided to patients during an encounter, which is defined as "the determination that a service or procedure rendered is reasonable and necessary for the diagnosis or treatment of an illness or injury."

4. A patient is seen in the office for treatment of asthma and hypertension, and a chest x-ray and EKG are performed. For medical necessity purposes, the chest x-ray would be linked to the _____.

5. A patient is seen in the hospital emergency department for treatment of lacerations; the patient also complains of dizziness and a headache that is unrelieved by pain medications. The emergency department physician orders a brain scan and performs extensive suturing. For medical necessity, the suturing would be linked to the _____.

ICD-10-CM Index to Diseases and Injuries

The ICD-10-CM **Index to Diseases and Injuries** (Figure 2-2) is an alphabetical list of main terms, subterms, qualifiers, and their corresponding codes. Main terms are printed in boldfaced type, and subterms and qualifiers are indented below main terms. The ICD-10-CM index is subdivided into two parts (Table 2-1).

- Index to Diseases and Injuries, which includes a Table of Neoplasms and a Table of Drugs and Chemicals
- Index of External Cause of Injuries

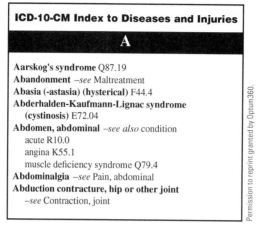

FIGURE 2-2 ICD-10-CM Index to Diseases and Injuries (partial)

TABLE 2-1 ICD-10-CM Index to Diseases and Injuries

Index to Diseases and Injuries (contains two tables)
Table of Neoplasms
Table of Drugs and Chemicals
Index of External Cause of Injuries

Courtesy of the Centers for Medicare & Medicaid Services, www.cms.gov.

Main terms in the Index to Diseases and Injuries are listed in alphabetical order, which means hyphens within main terms are ignored, but a single space within a main term is not ignored. When numerical characters and words appear below a main term, they are listed in alphabetical order. A code listed next to a main term in the index is referred to as a *default code*. The *default code* represents the code for the condition most commonly associated with the main term, or it may represent an unspecified code for the condition. (The Tabular List of Diseases and Injuries must always be referenced so that the most accurate and complete code is assigned.) If a condition is documented in a medical record (for example, appendicitis) without any additional information, such as acute or chronic, the default code should be assigned (after reviewing the Tabular List of Diseases and Injuries).

The Table of Neoplasms is organized alphabetically according to anatomical site. For each site, there are six possible code numbers according to whether the neoplasm in question is malignant, benign, in situ, of uncertain behavior, or of unspecified nature. The Table of Drugs and Chemicals is an alphabetic index of medicinal, chemical, and biological substances that result in poisonings (and associated external causes) and external causes of adverse effects. The Index of External Cause of Injuries is a separate index (from the Index to Diseases and Injuries) that contains main terms for external causes of morbidities (diseases) (e.g., burns) and injuries (e.g., motorcycle accident) in alphabetic order. (The Table of Neoplasms, Table of Drugs and Chemicals, and Index of External Cause of Injuries are described in more detail in Chapter 3 of this textbook.)

Example 1: ICD-10-CM Index to Disease and Injuries main terms are listed in alphabetical order, such as:

> `Catatonic`
>
> `Cat-scratch`

The hyphen in "Cat-scratch" is ignored, resulting in sequencing of that main term after "Catatonic".

> `Bee sting (with allergic or anaphylactic shock) —see` `Toxicity, venom,`
>   `arthropod, bee`
>
> `Beer-drinkers' heart (disease) I42.6`
>
> `Begbie's disease (exophthalmic goiter) —see` `Hyperthyroidism, with, goiter`

The space between "bee" and "sting" is considered, so main term "Bee sting" is sequenced above "Beer-drinkers' heart (disease)".

Example 2: ICD-10-CM Index to Diseases and Injuries numbered cranial nerves are listed in alphabetical order below the main term "Disorder", subterm "nerve", and second qualifier "cranial".

> `Disorder (of) —see also Disease`
>   `nerve G58.9`
>   `cranial G52.9`
>   `eighth —see subcategory H93.3`
>   `eleventh G52.8`
>   `fifth G50.9`
>   `first G52.0`
>   `fourth NEC —see Strabismus, paralytic, fourth nerve`
>   `multiple G52.7`
>   `ninth G52.1`
>   `second NEC —see Disorder, nerve, optic`
>   `seventh NEC G51.8`
>   `sixth NEC —see Strabismus, paralytic, sixth nerve`
>   `specified NEC G52.8`
>   `tenth G52.2`
>   `third NEC —see Strabismus, paralytic, third nerve`
>   `twelfth G52.3`

Main Terms, Subterms, and Qualifiers

ICD-10-CM index **main terms** (e.g., conditions) are printed in boldfaced type and are followed by the code. Main terms may or may not be followed by a listing of parenthetical terms, which serve as nonessential modifiers of the main term. **Nonessential modifiers** are qualifying words contained in parentheses after the main term that do not have to be included in the documented diagnostic or procedural statement for the code listed after the parentheses to be assigned.

Subterms (or **essential modifiers**) qualify the main term by listing alternative sites, etiology, or clinical status. A subterm is indented two spaces under the main term. Second qualifiers are indented two spaces under a subterm, and third qualifiers are indented two spaces under a second qualifier (Figure 2-3). Care must be taken when moving from the bottom of one column to the top of the next column or when turning to the next page of the index. The main term will be repeated and followed by —continued. When moving from one column to another, watch carefully to determine whether the subterm has changed or new second or third qualifiers appear.

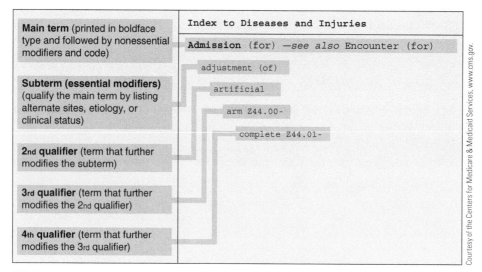

FIGURE 2-3 Display of main terms, subterms (nonessential modifiers), and qualifiers in the ICD-10-CM Index to Diseases and Injuries

Example: CONTINUATION OF TERMS IN ICD-10-CM INDEX TO DISEASES AND INJURIES: ICD-10-CM Index to Diseases and Injuries entries are organized according to main terms, subterms, second qualifiers, and third qualifiers. Refer to the index entry for "stricture, anus (sphincter) K62.4" and note the indented subterm and qualifiers. Notice that when the main term continues at the top of a column (or on the next page of the Index to Diseases and Injuries), the word —*continued* appears after the main term. The subterms and qualifiers are indented below the main term.

Start of Main Term in ICD-10-CM Index		Continuation of Main Term (Next Page)	
Main term:	Osteonecrosis M87.9	**Main Term:**	Osteonecrosis *–continued*
Subterm	secondary NEC M87.30	**Subterm:**	secondary NEC M87.30
Second qualifier:	due to	**Second qualifier:**	in
Third qualifier:	drugs M87.10	**Third qualifier:**	caisson disease T70.3 *[M90.50]*
Fourth qualifier:	carpus M87.13-	**Fourth qualifier:**	carpus T70.3 *[M90.54-]*

Basic Steps for Using the ICD-10-CM Index and Tabular List

It is important to remember that you should never code directly from the Index to Diseases and Injuries. After locating a code in the index, go to that code in the Tabular List of Diseases and Injuries to find important instructions (e.g., includes notes) and to verify the code selected. Instructions may require the assignment of additional codes or indicate conditions that are classified elsewhere.

Step 1   Review patient record documentation to locate the main term in the ICD-10-CM Index to Diseases and Injuries.

Begin the coding process in the Index to Diseases and Injuries by locating the condition's boldfaced main term and then reviewing subterms and qualifiers listed below the main term to locate the proper disease or injury. Refer to the patient record to locate documentation that supports the selection of subterms and qualifiers.

Example: The underlined terms in the following conditions are main terms:

```
Verbal agnosia
Intussusception, ileocolic
Status (post) angioplasty
```

Step 2   When the instructional phrase *–see* condition is found after the ICD-10-CM index main term, the coder has mistakenly referenced a descriptive term or an anatomical site instead of the condition or disease that was documented in the diagnostic statement.

Example: The provider's diagnostic statement is "upper respiratory infection." In the ICD-10-CM Index to Diseases and Injuries, look up the phrase *upper respiratory*. Notice that the term *–see* condition appears next to the phrase *upper respiratory*. This instruction directs you to the condition, which is main term *Infection* in the ICD-10-CM index.

Step 3   When the condition in the diagnostic statement is not easily found in the index, use the main terms below to locate the code.

Abnormal	Findings	Neoplasm
Anomaly	Foreign body	Obstruction
Complication	Infection	Pregnancy
Delivery	Injury	Sequelae
Disease	Late effect(s)	Syndrome
Disorder	Lesion	Wound

Step 4   Select and verify the code in the ICD-10-CM Tabular List of Diseases and Injuries, following coding instructions (e.g., code also, excludes1).

 NOTE:

- When the ICD-10-CM index entry includes a hyphen, such as Abruptio placentae O45.9-, review of the tabular list is required to assign the fifth character.
- To locate a code that describes an external cause of illness or injury, refer to the separate Index of External Cause of Injuries, such as "car sickness" as the cause of "vomiting."

Exercise 2.2 – ICD-10-CM Index to Diseases and Injuries

Instructions: Complete each statement.

1. The alphabetical listing of main terms or conditions printed in boldfaced type that may be expressed as nouns, adjectives, or eponyms is called the ICD-10-CM _____ to Diseases and Injuries.

2. Adverse effects and poisonings associated with medicinal, chemical, and biological substances are located in the ICD-10-CM Table of _____ and Chemicals.

3. Main terms in the ICD-10-CM Index to Diseases and Injuries are listed in _____ order, which means hyphens within main terms are ignored, but a single space within a main term is not ignored.

(continues)

Exercise 2.2 – continued

4. When numerical characters and words appear under a main term, subterm, or qualifier, they are listed in _____ order.

5. ICD-10-CM index main terms appear in _____ type.

6. Qualifying words that are contained in parentheses after the ICD-10-CM index main term, which do not have to be included in the diagnostic statement for the code listed after the parentheses to be assigned, are called _____ modifiers.

7. ICD-10-CM index subterms and qualifiers are considered _____ modifiers because they qualify the main term (or subterm and qualifier) by listing alternative sites, etiology, or clinical status.

8. When the provider documents "congenital asplenia," the ICD-10-CM index main term is _____.

9. When the provider documents "history of malignancy," the ICD-10-CM index main term is _____.

10. The patient is diagnosed with right lower quadrant abdominal pain, and the coder locates ICD-10-CM index main term Abdomen, abdominal –*see also* condition. This cross reference instructs the coder to go to ICD-10-CM index main term _____ instead.

ICD-10-CM Tabular List of Diseases and Injuries

The ICD-10-CM **Tabular List of Diseases and Injuries** (Table 2-2) contains 22 chapters. Chapters in ICD-10-CM classify diseases and injuries according to specific body systems as well as **etiology** (cause of disease). In addition, ICD-10-CM classifies external causes of morbidity, factors influencing health status, and contact with health services.

 NOTE:

ICD-10, created by the WHO, has 22 chapters. ICD-10-CM excludes the ICD-10 chapter, *Codes for Special Purposes, U00–U99*.

ICD-10-CM disease and injury codes consist of three characters, and most are followed by a decimal point and between one and four additional characters. The ICD-10-CM Tabular List of Diseases and Injuries is a sequential list of alphanumeric codes contained within chapters that are organized according to body system or condition. The ICD-10-CM Tabular List of Diseases and Injuries (Figure 2-4) uses an indented format for ease of reference and contains category codes, subcategory codes, and codes. Organization of the tabular list includes

- Major topic headings, which are printed in bold uppercase letters and followed by groups of ICD-10-CM three-character disease categories within a chapter (e.g., Intestinal Infectious Diseases, A00–A09). *The first character of an ICD-10-CM code is always a letter.*

- Categories, subcategories, and codes, which contain a combination of letters and numbers.
   - A **category** contains three characters.
   - A three-character category code that has no further subdivision is a valid code. For example, code I10 (hypertension) has no further subdivisions and is a valid code.
   - A **subcategory** contains four, five, or six characters. Subcategory codes that require additional characters are invalid if the fifth, sixth, and/or seventh character(s) are absent.

TABLE 2-2 ICD-10-CM Tabular List of Diseases and Injuries

Chapter Number	Range of Codes	Chapter Title
Chapter 1	A00–B99	Certain Infectious and Parasitic Diseases
Chapter 2	C00–D49	Neoplasms
Chapter 3	D50–D89	Diseases of the Blood and Blood-forming Organs and Certain Disorders Involving the Immune Mechanism
Chapter 4	E00–E89	Endocrine, Nutritional, and Metabolic Diseases
Chapter 5	F01–F99	Mental, Behavioral, and Neurodevelopmental Disorders
Chapter 6	G00–G99	Diseases of the Nervous System
Chapter 7	H00–H59	Diseases of the Eye and Adnexa
Chapter 8	H60–H95	Diseases of the Ear and Mastoid Process
Chapter 9	I00–I99	Diseases of the Circulatory System
Chapter 10	J00–J99	Diseases of the Respiratory System
Chapter 11	K00–K95	Diseases of the Digestive System
Chapter 12	L00–L99	Diseases of the Skin and Subcutaneous Tissue
Chapter 13	M00–M99	Diseases of the Musculoskeletal System and Connective Tissue
Chapter 14	N00–N99	Diseases of the Genitourinary System
Chapter 15	O00–O9A	Pregnancy, Childbirth, and the Puerperium
Chapter 16	P00–P96	Certain Conditions Originating in the Perinatal Period
Chapter 17	Q00–Q99	Congenital Malformations, Deformations, and Chromosomal Abnormalities
Chapter 18	R00–R99	Symptoms, Signs, and Abnormal Clinical and Laboratory Findings, Not Elsewhere Classified
Chapter 19	S00–T88	Injury, Poisoning, and Certain Other Consequences of External Causes
Chapter 20	V00–Y99	External Causes of Morbidity
Chapter 21	Z00–Z99	Factors Influencing Health Status and Contact with Health Services
Chapter 22	U00–U85	Codes for Special Purposes

Courtesy of the Centers for Medicare & Medicaid Services, www.cms.gov.

- Codes may contain three, four, five, six, or seven characters.
  - The final level of subdivision is a code.
  - All codes and descriptions in the ICD-10-CM tabular list are boldfaced.
- Codes that have an applicable seventh character are referred to as codes (not subcategories).
- Codes that have applicable seventh characters are invalid if the X placeholder(s) and/or the seventh character are missing. (A **placeholder** involves use of the letter X in certain ICD-10-CM codes to allow for future expansion, and it is used when a code contains fewer than six characters and a seventh character applies, such as T36.0X6A.)

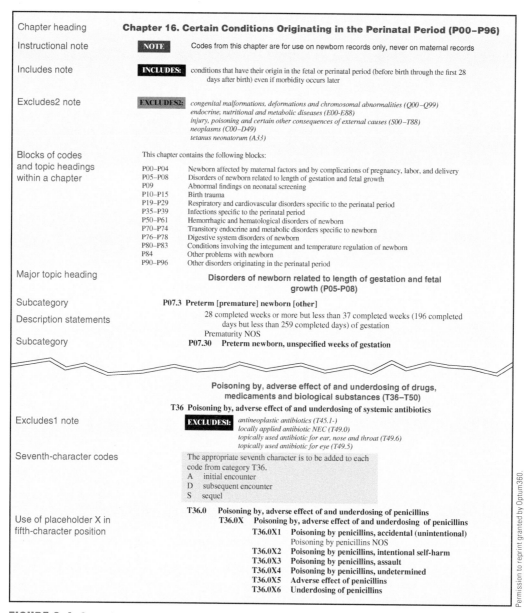

FIGURE 2-4 Sample page from ICD-10-CM Tabular List of Diseases and Injuries

Example 1: ICD-10-CM CATEGORY AND SUBCATEGORY CODES: Go to Figure 2-4, refer to the *Disorders of newborn related to length of gestation and fetal growth (P05–P08)* range of codes, and locate the 4-character subcategory code (P07.3) and the 5-character subcategory code (P07.30).

Example 2: ICD-10-CM 6-CHARACTER CODES: Go to Figure 2-4, refer to the *Poisoning by, adverse effects of and underdosing of drugs, medicaments and biological substances (T36–T50)* range of codes, and locate the 6-character subcategory codes (T36.0X1, T36.0X2, T36.0X3, T36.0X4, and T36.0X5), which also contain X as a placeholder to allow for future expansion. Then, locate the seventh characters (A, D, and S), one of which is to be added to each code from category T36 (depending on status of encounter or whether the condition is a sequela) (e.g., T36.0X1A).

Example 3: USE OF PLACEHOLDER X IN ICD-10-CM CODES: Go to Figure 2-4, and refer to code *T36.0X1 Poisoning by penicillins, accidental (unintentional)*. Code T36.0X1A requires X as a placeholder in the fifth-character position. Thus, reporting the code as T36.01A (without the X placeholder in the fifth-character position) makes it an invalid code, which is incorrect if reported and results in a denied claim for third-party payer reimbursement.

Exercise 2.3 – ICD-10-CM Tabular List of Diseases and Injuries

Instructions: Complete each statement.

1. The ICD-10-CM _____ List of Diseases and Injuries arranges codes and descriptions in alphanumerical order, and it contains 22 chapters.
2. The first character of an ICD-10-CM code is always a _____.
3. ICD-10-CM code I10 is an example of a three-character _____ code, which is defined as having no further subdivisions and is a valid code.
4. ICD-10-CM subcategory codes require additional characters and are considered _____ (or incomplete) when fourth, fifth, sixth, and/or seventh character(s) are absent from reported codes.
5. Letter X in the fifth and sixth character positions are entered as _____ in code O40.1XX0 to allow for future code expansion.

ICD-10-CM Official Guidelines for Coding and Reporting

The Centers for Medicare & Medicaid Services (CMS) and the National Center for Health Statistics (NCHS) are the agencies in the U.S. Department of Health & Human Services (DHHS) that develop official guidelines for coding and reporting using ICD-10-CM (and ICD-10-PCS). The **ICD-10-CM Official Guidelines for Coding and Reporting** (and the *ICD-10-PCS Official Guidelines for Coding and Reporting*) are approved by the four organizations that make up the **Cooperating Parties for the ICD-10-CM/PCS**. They include the American Hospital Association (AHA), American Health Information Management Association (AHIMA), CMS, and NCHS. The guidelines are a set of rules developed to accompany and complement the official conventions and instructions provided within ICD-10-CM. They clarify the coding and sequencing instructions in ICD-10-CM and provide additional coding guidance. The health care provider is responsible for complete and accurate patient record documentation, and the coder is responsible for assigning complete and accurate codes that are supported by documentation. Coders review the entire patient record to determine the reason for an encounter and the conditions treated. This means that if the provider documents a disease (or procedure) on the face sheet or in the discharge summary, the coder reviews other reports (e.g., progress notes, laboratory data, operative report, pathology report) to assign appropriate codes, including level of specificity. Quite often the provider will document additional information about a disease (or procedure) elsewhere in the patient record that contributes to the assignment of a specific code (e.g., laterality, acute or chronic nature).

The ICD-10-CM *Official Guidelines for Coding and Reporting* are organized into four sections and one appendix.

- Section I includes ICD-10-CM coding conventions, general coding guidelines, and chapter-specific guidelines.
- Section II includes guidelines for selection of the principal diagnosis in inpatient hospital settings. (The selection of principal diagnosis is discussed in Chapter 7.)
- Section III includes guidelines for reporting additional diagnoses (e.g., coexisting conditions, complications) in inpatient hospital settings. Additional diagnoses are also called *secondary diagnoses*, and they include *comorbidities* (co-existing conditions, such as chronic asthma) and *complications* (conditions that arise during inpatient hospitalization, such as a postoperative wound infection). (The coding of additional diagnoses is discussed in Chapter 7.)
- Section IV includes diagnostic coding and reporting guidelines for outpatient services. (Outpatient diagnosis coding is discussed in Chapter 5.)
- Appendix I includes present on admission (POA) reporting guidelines. (POA reporting is discussed in Chapter 20.)

A joint effort between the health care provider and the coder is essential to achieving complete and accurate documentation, code assignment, and reporting of diagnoses and procedures. The coding guidelines were developed to assist both the health care provider and the coder in identifying diagnoses and procedures that are to be reported. The importance of consistent, complete documentation in the patient record is crucial because without such documentation, accurate coding cannot be achieved. In addition, the entire record must be reviewed to determine the specific reason for the encounter and the conditions treated. (The term *encounter* is used in the coding guidelines for all health care settings, including inpatient hospital admissions. The term *provider* is used in the coding guidelines to mean physician or any qualified health care practitioner who is legally accountable for establishing the patient's diagnosis.)

 HIPAA Alert!

The HIPAA regulations for electronic transactions require providers and third-party payers, including Medicare administrative contractors (MACs), to adhere to the *Official Guidelines for Coding and Reporting*. Thus, a violation of the coding guidelines is technically a HIPAA violation. Because some third-party payers and MACs do not appear to be aware of (or understand) this HIPAA provision, to obtain appropriate reimbursement for submitted ICD-10-CM codes, bring specific provisions in the regulation that reference the coding guidelines to the attention of third-party payers. For example, the Z51 (Encounter for other aftercare and medical care) codes in ICD-10-CM can be reported as a first-listed code for outpatient care. If third-party payers and MACs deny claims that report Z51 codes, contact the regional CMS office or HIPAA enforcement office (located at CMS) for resolution.

Exercise 2.4 – ICD-10-CM Official Guidelines for Coding and Reporting

Instructions: Complete each statement.

1. The *ICD-10-CM Official Guidelines for Coding and Reporting* are approved by the _____ parties for ICD-10-CM to accompany and complement the official conventions and instructions provided within ICD-10-CM.

2. Official coding guidelines use the term _____ when referring to face-to-face contact between patients and health care providers in all health care settings, including inpatient hospital admissions.

3. Official coding guidelines use the term _____ when referring to a physician or any qualified health care practitioner who is legally accountable for establishing a patient's diagnosis.

4. HIPAA regulations for electronic _____ require providers and third-party payers, including Medicare administrative contractors (MACs), to adhere to the *ICD-10-CM Official Guidelines for Coding and Reporting*.

5. Section I of the *ICD-10-CM Official Guidelines for Coding and Reporting* includes ICD-10-CM's coding _____, general coding guidelines, and chapter-specific guidelines.

6. Section II of the *ICD-10-CM Official Guidelines for Coding and Reporting* covers selection of the _____ diagnosis (and secondary diagnoses) for inpatient hospital admissions.

7. Section III of the *ICD-10-CM Official Guidelines for Coding and Reporting* covers reporting of additional diagnoses for inpatient hospital settings, which are also called _____ diagnoses and include comorbidities and complications.

8. Inpatient hospital admissions require the reporting of secondary diagnoses that include comorbidities and _____.

Exercise 2.4 – continued

9. Section IV of the *ICD-10-CM Official Guidelines for Coding and Reporting* covers diagnostic coding and reporting for _____ services.

10. Appendix I of the *ICD-10-CM Official Guidelines for Coding and Reporting* covers present on _____ reporting guidelines.

ICD-9-CM Legacy Coding System

As a result of implementing the ICD-10-CM and ICD-10-PCS coding systems, the *International Classification of Diseases, Ninth Revision, Clinical Modification* (ICD-9-CM) became a *legacy coding system* (or *legacy classification system*), which means it is used to archive data but is no longer supported or updated by the ICD-9-CM Coordination and Maintenance Committee. However, because ICD-9-CM was used since 1979 in the United States to classify inpatient and outpatient/physician office diagnoses (Volumes 1 and 2) and inpatient procedures (Volume 3), *general equivalence mappings (GEMs)* (discussed below) were published. The GEMs facilitate the collection of data, including ICD-9-CM data, especially as its codes compare to ICD-10-CM and ICD-10-PCS.

ICD-9-CM was over 30 years old, had outdated and obsolete terminology, used outdated codes that produced inaccurate and limited data, and was inconsistent with current medical practice. It did not accurately describe diagnoses or inpatient procedures of care delivered in the 21st century. ICD-9-CM did not provide the necessary detail about patients' medical conditions or procedures performed on hospitalized inpatients; thus, effective October 1, 2015, provider offices and health care facilities (e.g., hospitals) adopted ICD-10-CM to code diagnoses. ICD-10-PCS is used to code inpatient hospital procedures. Provider offices and outpatient health care settings use CPT and HCPCS Level II to code procedures and services.

General Equivalence Mappings (GEMs)

General equivalence mappings (GEMs) are translation dictionaries or crosswalks of codes that can be used to roughly identify ICD-10-CM and ICD-10-PCS codes for their ICD-9-CM equivalent codes (and vice versa). (GEMs do not contain code descriptions.) GEMs facilitate the location of corresponding diagnosis codes between the code sets. In some areas of the classification, the correlation between codes is close, and since the two code sets share the conventions of organization and formatting in common, translating between them is straightforward. Although ICD-9-CM and ICD-10-PCS do not share the conventions of organization or formatting in common, the crosswalk between these two code sets is equally straightforward.

Example 1: There is straightforward correspondence between the code sets for *Salmonella meningitis*.

ICD-9-CM to ICD-10-CM General Equivalence Mapping

ICD-9-CM Diagnosis Code and Description	ICD-10-CM Diagnosis Code and Description
003.21 Salmonella meningitis	A02.21 Salmonella meningitis

Example 2: In other areas of the code sets, such as obstetrics, entire chapters are organized according to a different axis of classification, and translating between them offers a series of possible codes that must be verified in the appropriate tabular list to identify the correct code. (Think about translating the English language into Chinese or any other foreign language, and you will see the problems inherent in such translation.)

ICD-9-CM to ICD-10-CM General Equivalence Mapping

ICD-9-CM Disease Code and Description	ICD-10-CM Disease Code and Description
649.51 Spotting complicating pregnancy, delivered, with or without mention of antepartum complication	O26.851 Spotting complicating pregnancy, first trimester
	O26.852 Spotting complicating pregnancy, second trimester
	O26.853 Spotting complicating pregnancy, third trimester

Exercise 2.5 – ICD-9-CM Legacy Coding System

Instructions: Use the *ICD-9-CM to ICD-10-CM General Equivalency Mapping (GEM)* depicted in the table below to complete each statement. Enter the code from the table as your answer. Do *not* enter the description of the code in your answer.

ICD-9-CM to ICD-10-CM General Equivalence Mapping (GEM)

ICD-9-CM Diagnosis Code and Description	ICD-10-CM Diagnosis Code and Description
078.81 Epidemic vertigo	A88.1 Epidemic vertigo
078.82 Epidemic vomiting syndrome	R11.11 Vomiting without nausea
078.88 Other specified diseases due to *Chlamydiae*	A74.89 Other chlamydial diseases
078.89 Other specified diseases due to viruses	A98.3 Marburg virus disease A98.4 Ebola virus disease B33.8 Other specified viral diseases

1. ICD-9-CM code 078.82 maps to ICD-10-CM code _____.
2. ICD-9-CM code 078.81 maps to ICD-10-CM code _____.
3. ICD-9-CM code 078.88 maps to ICD-10-CM code _____.
4. ICD-10-CM code A74.89 maps to ICD-9-CM code _____.
5. ICD-10-CM code B33.8 maps to ICD-9-CM code _____.

ICD-10-CM Coding Conventions

The ICD-10-CM coding conventions (rules) can usually be found at the beginning of any ICD-10-CM coding manual. Coders are required to reference this material when reviewing case scenarios (and patient records) to assign ICD-10-CM codes. It is also helpful to coders when health care providers become familiar with coding conventions (and guidelines). When a coder initiates a physician query, an understanding of coding conventions and guidelines helps ensure the assignment of accurate codes for certain conditions and diagnoses.

Coding conventions for ICD-10-CM are general rules used in the classification, and they are independent of the coding guidelines (covered in Chapters 3–5 of this textbook). The conventions are incorporated into ICD-10-CM as instructional notes. For example, the ICD-10-CM index contains instructional notes that are *cross references* (e.g., *see, see also, see* category, *see* condition). The ICD-10-CM tabular list also contains instructional notes (e.g., includes, excludes, code also, code first underlying disease, code if applicable any causal condition first, and use additional code as).

Specific ICD-10-CM coding conventions include the following:

- The alphabetic index and tabular list
- Format and structure
- Use of codes for reporting purposes
- Placeholder character
- Seventh characters
- Abbreviations
- Punctuation
- Other and unspecified codes

- Includes note
- Inclusion terms
- Excludes notes
- Etiology and manifestation convention
- And
- With
- Cross references
- Code also note
- Default codes
- Code assignment and clinical criteria

The Alphabetic Index and Tabular List

ICD-10-CM is divided into the alphabetic index, which contains an alphabetical list of terms and corresponding code(s), and the tabular list, which is a structured list of codes divided into chapters based on body system or condition. The alphabetic index consists of the following parts: the Index of Diseases and Injuries, the Index of External Cause of Injuries, the Table of Neoplasms and the Table of Drugs and Chemicals. (Official coding conventions also provide direction to *See Section I.C.2. Neoplasms and Section I.C.19. Adverse effects, poisoning, underdosing and toxic effects*, covered in textbook Chapter 3 and Chapter 4, respectively.)

Eponyms

Eponyms are diseases or syndromes that are named for people. They are listed in alphabetical order as main terms in the ICD-10-CM Index to Diseases and Injuries. They are also listed as subterms below main terms *Disease* and *Syndrome* in the index. A description of the disease, syndrome, or procedure is usually included in parentheses following the eponym.

> **Example:** ICD-10-CM INDEX TO DISEASES AND INJURIES—EPONYM: The Index to Diseases and Injuries entry for *Christmas disease* can be located in alphabetical order. It can also be located under main term *Disease*. (Upon review of code D67 and its description in the Tabular List of Diseases and Injuries, Christmas disease is included as a synonym below the code description.)

Boxed Notes

Certain main terms in the ICD-10-CM index, including the Table of Neoplasms, are followed by **boxed notes**, which define terms and provide coding instruction.

> **Example:** The ICD-10-CM Index to Diseases and Injuries main term *Epilepsy* contains a boxed note that includes terms that are to be considered equivalent to intractable, such as *pharmacoresistant*. The ICD-10-CM Table of Neoplasms contains a boxed note that clarifies how to use the columns and rows in the table.

Tables

The ICD-10-CM index includes **tables**, which organize subterms, second qualifiers, and third qualifiers and their codes in columns and rows to make it easier to select the proper code. ICD-10-CM organizes the following main terms in tables, which are located at the end of the Index to Diseases and Injuries (before the Index of External Cause of Injuries):

- Table of Neoplasms
- Table of Drugs and Chemicals

The *Table of Neoplasms* (Figure 2-5) is an alphabetic index of anatomical sites for which there are six possible codes according to whether the neoplasm in question is malignant, benign, *in situ*, of uncertain behavior, or of

	Malignant Primary	Malignant Secondary	Ca *in situ*	Benign	Uncertain Behavior	Unspecified Nature
Notes—						

The list below gives the code numbers for neoplasms by anatomical site. For each site there are six possible code numbers according to whether the neoplasm in question is malignant, benign, *in situ,* of uncertain behavior, or of unspecified nature. The description of the neoplasm will often indicate which of the six columns is appropriate; e.g., malignant melanoma of skin, benign fibroadenoma of breast, carcinoma *in situ* of cervix uteri.

Where such descriptors are not present, the remainder of the Index should be consulted where guidance is given to the appropriate column for each morphologic (histological) variety listed; e.g., Mesonephroma *–see* Neoplasm, malignant; Embryoma *–see also* Neoplasm, uncertain behavior; Disease, Bowen's *–see* Neoplasm, skin, *in situ*. However, the guidance in the Index can be overridden if one of the descriptors mentioned above is present; e.g., malignant adenoma of colon is coded to C18.9 and not to D12.6 as the adjective "malignant" overrides the Index entry "Adenoma *–see also* Neoplasm, benign."

Codes listed with a dash -, following the code have a required additional character for laterality. The tabular must be reviewed for the complete code.

	Malignant Primary	Malignant Secondary	Ca *in situ*	Benign	Uncertain Behavior	Unspecified Nature
Neoplasm, neoplastic	C80.1	C79.9	D09.9	D36.9	D48.9	D49.9
abdomen, abdominal	C76.2	C79.8-	D09.8	D36.7	D48.7	D49.9
cavity	C76.2	C79.8-	D09.8	D36.7	D48.7	D49.89
organ	C76.2	C79.8-	D09.8	D36.7	D48.7	D49.89
viscera	C76.2	C79.8-	D09.8	D36.7	D48.7	D49.89
wall *-see also* Neoplasm, abdomen,						
wall, skin	C44.509	C79.2-	D04.5	D23.5	D48.5	D49.2
connective tissue	C49.4	C79.8-	—	D21.4	D48.1	D49.2
skin	C44.509	—	—	—	—	—
basal cell carcinoma	C44.519	—	—	—	—	—
specified type NEC	C44.599	—	—	—	—	—
squamous cell carcinoma	C44.529	—	—	—	—	—

FIGURE 2-5 ICD-10-CM Table of Neoplasms (partial)

unspecified nature. The description of the neoplasm will often indicate which of the six columns is appropriate (e.g., malignant melanoma of skin, benign fibroadenoma of breast, carcinoma *in situ* of cervix uteri).

The *Table of Drugs and Chemicals* (Figure 2-6) in ICD-10-CM is an alphabetical index of medicinal, chemical, and biological substances that result in poisonings and adverse effects as well as underdosings. The first column of the table lists generic names of drugs and chemicals (although some publishers have added brand names) with six columns for

- *Poisoning: Accidental (Unintentional)* (poisoning that results from an inadvertent overdose, wrong substance administered/taken, or intoxication that includes combining prescription drugs with nonprescription drugs or alcohol)

Substance	Poisoning, Accidental (unintentional)	Poisoning, Intentional Self-harm	Poisoning, Assault	Poisoning, Undetermined	Adverse Effect	Underdosing
1-Propanol	T51.3X1	T51.3X2	T51.3X3	T51.3X4	—	—
2-Propanol	T51.2X1	T51.2X2	T51.2X3	T51.2X4	—	—
2, 4-D (dichlorophen-oxyacetic acid)	T60.3X1	T60.3X2	T60.3X3	T60.3X4	—	—
2, 4-toluene diisocyanate	T65.0X1	T65.0X2	T65.0X3	T65.0X4	—	—
2, 4, 5-T (trichloro-phenoxyacetic acid)	T60.1X1	T60.1X2	T60.1X3	T60.1X4	—	—
3, 4-methylenedioxymethamphetamine	T43.641	T43.642	T43.643	T43.644	—	—
14-hydroxydihydro-morphinone	T40.2X1	T40.2X2	T40.2X3	T40.2X4	T40.2X5	T40.2X6
ABOB	T37.5X1	T37.5X2	T37.5X3	T37.5X4	T37.5X5	T37.5X6
Abrine	T62.2X1	T62.2X2	T62.2X3	T62.2X4	—	—
Abrus (seed)	T62.2X1	T62.2X2	T62.2X3	T62.2X4	—	—
Absinthe	T51.0X1	T51.0X2	T51.0X3	T51.0X4	—	—
beverage	T51.0X1	T51.0X2	T51.0X3	T51.0X4	—	—
Acaricide	T60.8X1	T60.8X2	T60.8X3	T60.8X4	—	—
Acebutolol	T44.7X1	T44.7X2	T44.7X3	T44.7X4	T44.7X5	T44.7X6
Acecarbromal	T42.6X1	T42.6X2	T42.6X3	T42.6X4	T42.6X5	T42.6X6
Aceclidine	T44.1X1	T44.1X2	T44.1X3	T44.1X4	T44.1X5	T44.1X6
Acedapsone	T37.0X1	T37.0X2	T37.0X3	T37.0X4	T37.0X5	T37.0X6
Acefylline piperazine	T48.6X1	T48.6X2	T48.6X3	T48.6X4	T48.6X5	T48.6X6

FIGURE 2-6 ICD-10-CM Table of Drugs and Chemicals (partial)

- *Poisoning: Intentional Self-harm* (poisoning that results from a deliberate overdose, such as a suicide attempt, of substance[s] administered/taken or intoxication that includes purposely combining prescription drugs with nonprescription drugs or alcohol); *Poisoning: Assault* (poisoning inflicted by another person who intended to kill or injure the patient)

- *Poisoning: Undetermined* (subcategory used if the patient record does not document whether the poisoning was intentional or accidental); *Adverse Effect* (development of a pathological condition that results from a drug or chemical substance that was properly administered or taken)

- *Underdosing* (taking less of a medication than is prescribed by a provider or a manufacturer's instruction).

Format and Structure

The ICD-10-CM Tabular List contains categories, subcategories, and codes. Characters for categories, subcategories, and codes may be either a letter or a number. All categories contain three characters. A three-character category that has no further subdivision is equivalent to a code. Subcategories contain either four or five characters. Codes may contain three, four, five, six, or seven characters. Thus, each level of subdivision below a category is a subcategory. The final level of subdivision is a code. Codes that have applicable seventh characters are referred to as codes, not subcategories. A code that has an applicable seventh character is considered invalid without the seventh character.

The ICD-10-CM index uses an indented **format** for ease in reference (Figure 2-7). All ICD-10-CM Index to Diseases and Injuries subterms associated with an index entry's main term are indented two spaces, with any second and third qualifiers associated with the main term further indented by two and four spaces, respectively. In addition, if an index entry requires more than one line, the additional text is printed on the next line and indented five spaces.

ICD-10-CM also makes use of the boldface and italic **typeface** for ease in reference. Boldface type is used for main term entries in the ICD-10-CM index and all codes and descriptions in the ICD-10-CM tabular list. Italicized type is used for all ICD-10-CM tabular list excludes1 and excludes2 notes and to identify manifestation codes, which are codes that should not be reported as the first-listed or principal diagnoses.

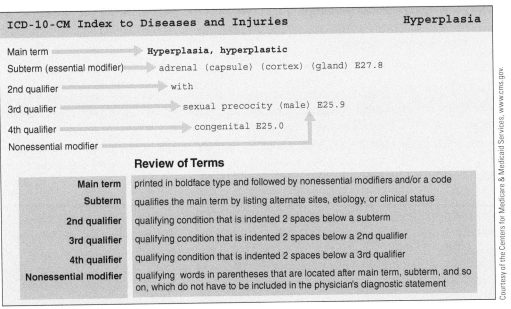

FIGURE 2-7 Display of main terms, subterms, qualifiers, nonessential modifiers in ICD-10-CM Index to Diseases and Injuries

Additional terms are indented below the term to which they are linked in the ICD-10-CM tabular list; if a definition or disease requires more than one line, that text is printed on the next line and indented five spaces.

Example 1: ICD-10-CM INDEX TO DISEASES AND INJURIES—INDENTED FORMAT AND BOLDFACE: Locate main term *Ulcer* in the ICD-10-CM Index to Diseases and Injuries, and notice that it is boldfaced. Also, notice that subterm *aphthous (oral) (recurrent) K12.0* is indented two spaces below the "U" of main term *Ulcer*. Then, notice that second qualifier *genital organ(s)* is further indented two spaces.

Example 2: ICD-10-CM TABULAR LIST OF DISEASES AND INJURIES—INDENTED FORMAT AND BOLDFACE: Locate *code K12.0 Recurrent Oral Aphthae* in the ICD-10-CM Tabular List of Diseases and Injuries, and notice that it is in boldface and its synonyms (e.g., Bednar's aphthae) are indented.

Use of Codes for Reporting Purposes

For reporting purposes, only (valid) codes are permissible. Categories or subcategories (that require additional characters) are not reportable. Any applicable seventh character is also required (to create a valid code).

Placeholder Character

The ICD-10-CM utilizes a *placeholder*, which requires entry of alphabetic character X for certain codes to allow for future expansion. For example, codes reported for poisonings, adverse effects and underdosings (categories T36-T50) often require entry of placeholder X to create a valid code.

Example: Code T36.0X1A, Poisoning by penicillins, accidental (unintentional), requires the entry of X as a placeholder in the fifth-character position. Thus, reporting T36.01A (without the X placeholder in the fifth-character position) is an invalid code, which will result in a denied claim for third-party payer reimbursement.

Seventh Characters

Certain ICD-10-CM categories have applicable seventh characters, which are required for all codes within a category *or* as instructed by notes in the tabular list. The seventh character must always be entered in the seventh character data field, and if a code that requires a seventh character does not contain six characters, placeholder X is entered to fill in the empty character(s).

Abbreviations

The ICD-10-CM index and tabular list contain **abbreviations** to save space. The ICD-10-CM index and tabular list contain the abbreviation **NEC (not elsewhere classifiable)**, which means "other specified" and identifies codes that are to be assigned when information needed to assign a more specific code cannot be located in the coding manual (or encoder). When a specific code is not available in the index for a condition, the coder is directed to the "other specified" code in the tabular list.

Example 1: ICD-10-CM INDEX TO DISEASES AND INJURIES—NEC ABBREVIATION: The Index to Diseases and Injuries entry for *aberrant, artery, basilar* contains the NEC abbreviation in front of code Q28.1, which means a more specific code cannot be assigned in the code book. When verifying code Q28.1 in the Tabular List of Diseases and Injuries, notice that the code description is *Other malformations of precerebral vessels* and that the NEC abbreviation does not appear in the code description. Code Q28.1 is assigned to *aberrant basilar artery* because the index's NEC abbreviation directs the coder to that code.

Example 2: ICD-10-CM TABULAR LIST OF DISEASES AND INJURIES—NEC ABBREVIATION: Locate code Q28.8 in the tabular list, and notice that the NEC abbreviation is included next to *Congenital aneurysm, specified site NEC* below the code description.

The ICD-10-CM index and tabular list contain the abbreviation **NOS (not otherwise specified)**, which is the equivalent of "unspecified." It identifies codes that are to be assigned when information needed to assign a more specific code cannot be obtained from the provider. Because selecting a code from the index based on limited documentation results in the coder being directed to an "unspecified" code in the tabular list, the coder should contact the physician to request that additional documentation be provided so that a more specific diagnosis or procedure code can be assigned. A review of the patient record to assign a more specific code is also an important part of the coding process (e.g., laboratory data, radiology reports, operative report, pathology report).

 NOTE:

It is appropriate to ask the physician for clarification about a diagnosis if the patient's record contains documentation (e.g., laboratory data) to support the assignment of a more specific code.

Example 1: ICD-10-CM INDEX TO DISEASES AND INJURIES—NOS ABBREVIATION: The index entry for *Bronchomycosis NOS B49 [J99]* directs the coder to B49, which is an *unspecified* code.

Example 2: ICD-10-CM TABULAR LIST OF DISEASES AND INJURIES—NOS ABBREVIATION: Locate code A03.9 in the tabular list, and notice the NOS abbreviation appears after *dysentery*.

Punctuation

ICD-10-CM includes the following **punctuation**:

- Brackets
- Parentheses
- Colons

Brackets are used to identify manifestation codes in the ICD-10-CM Index to Diseases and Injuries and abbreviations, alternate wording, explanatory phrases, or synonyms in the ICD-10-CM Tabular List of Diseases and Injuries. (Italicized brackets enclose manifestation codes in the ICD-10-CM index.) A **manifestation** is a condition that occurs as the result of another condition, and manifestation codes are always reported as secondary codes. The code and description may or may not appear in italics in the tabular list. When code descriptions are not italicized in the tabular list, make sure you sequence the codes according to the sequence in the index entry.

 NOTE:

When reporting manifestation codes, do not enclose them in brackets.

```
CORRECT:    E85.4
            I43
INCORRECT:  E85.4
            [I43]
```

Example: ICD-10-CM INDEX TO DISEASES AND INJURIES—BRACKETS: The index entry for *Amyloid heart (disease) E85.4 [I43]* indicates that two codes should be reported: E85.4 and I43. Because code I43 appears in brackets, it is reported as a secondary code. When verifying code I43 in the tabular list, notice that its description is italicized and a "*Code first underlying disease*, such as: amyloidosis (E85.-)" instruction is provided, prompting you to report code I43 as the second code.

Brackets are used in the ICD-10-CM index and tabular list to enclose abbreviations, synonyms, alternative wording, or explanatory phrases.

Example 1: ICD-10-CM INDEX TO DISEASES AND INJURIES—SQUARE BRACKETS: The index entry for *Abnormal, electrocardiogram [ECG] [EKG] R94.31* encloses abbreviations in square brackets.

Example 2: ICD-10-CM TABULAR LIST OF DISEASES AND INJURIES—SQUARE BRACKETS: Code I45.89 uses square brackets to enclose the abbreviation for *atrioventricular* as *[AV]*.

Parentheses are used in both the ICD-10-CM index and tabular list to enclose nonessential modifiers, which are supplementary words that may be present in or absent from the physician's statement of a disease or procedure without affecting the code to which it is assigned. The nonessential modifiers in the index apply to subterms that are located below a main term; *however, when a nonessential modifier and a subterm are mutually exclusive, the subterm takes precedence.*

Example 1: ICD-10-CM INDEX TO DISEASES AND INJURIES—PARENTHESES (supplementary terms): Index entry *abasia (-astasia) (hysterical) F44.4* contains two nonessential modifiers in parentheses, which means that the terms may be present or absent from the provider's diagnostic statement.

Example 2: ICD-10-CM INDEX TO DISEASES AND INJURIES—PARENTHESES (mutually exclusive modifiers): Index entry *Bronchiolitis* contains nonessential modifier *acute* in parentheses and essential modifier *chronic* as a subterm. Nonessential modifier *acute* does *not* have to be documented in the provider's diagnosis statement to report code J21.9; however, essential modifier *chronic* must be documented to report code J44.89.

Example 3: ICD-10-CM TABULAR LIST OF DISEASES AND INJURIES—PARENTHESES: Code I47.9 contains a nonessential modifier, (-*Hoffman*), in parentheses, which means that the term may be present or absent from the provider's diagnostic statement.

A **colon** is used after an incomplete term or phrase in the ICD-10-CM index and tabular list when one or more of the **modifiers** (additional terms) following the colon is needed to make the condition assignable to a given category.

Example 1: ICD-10-CM INDEX TO DISEASES AND INJURIES—COLON: The second qualifier *with retinal:* (located after index main term *Detachment* and subterm *retina (without retinal break) (serous) H33.2-*) requires the type of detachment (e.g., giant break H33.03-) to be documented in the patient record so that a specific code can be selected.

Example 2: ICD-10-CM TABULAR LIST OF DISEASES AND INJURIES—COLON: Underneath category *A40 Streptococcal sepsis*, a colon is used in the *Excludes1: neonatal (P36.0-P36.1)* instruction to indicate the excluded codes are never reported at the same time as code A40.

Other and Unspecified Codes

When **other** or **other specified** appears in a code description, the code is assigned when patient record documentation provides detail for which a specific code does not exist in ICD-10-CM. ICD-10-CM index entries that contain the abbreviation NEC are classified to "other" codes in the tabular list. These index entries represent specific disease entities for which no specific code exists in the tabular list, so the term is included within an "other" code.

Unspecified codes are assigned when patient record documentation is insufficient to assign a more specific code. When an ICD-10-CM tabular list category does not contain an "unspecified code," the "other specified" code may represent both "other and unspecified."

Before assigning an ICD-10-CM other, other specified, or unspecified code from the tabular list, review the patient record carefully or generate a physician query to determine whether a more specific code can be assigned. (Official coding conventions also direct coders to *See Section I.B.18. Use of Signs/Symptom/ Unspecified Codes*, covered in the General ICD-10-CM Diagnosis Coding Guidelines section of this chapter.)

Example:

- D64.89 is an *other specified* code.
- D64.9 is an *unspecified* code.
- I70.9- is an *other and unspecified* code.

 NOTE:

- Poisoning codes are reported *first*, followed by conditions that resulted from the poisoning (e.g., coma).
- Adverse effect codes are reported *after* conditions (e.g., rash) that resulted from taking medications as prescribed.
- Underdosing codes are reported *after* the condition (e.g., hypertension) for which the medication was originally prescribed *and* conditions that resulted from taking less than the prescribed medication.
- Tables appear in the ICD-10-CM Index to Diseases and Injuries, and their use is further discussed in Chapters 3–5 and 7 of this textbook.

Includes Note

An **includes note** appears in the ICD-10-CM tabular list below certain categories to further define, clarify, or provide examples about the content below a category.

Example: ICD-10-CM TABULAR LIST OF DISEASES AND INJURIES—INCLUDES NOTE: The includes note located below category code *H80 Otosclerosis* in the Tabular List of Diseases and Injuries indicates that *otospongiosis* is classified to that same category. This means that the provider could document *otosclerosis* or *otospongiosis*, and a code from category H80 would be assigned.

Inclusion Terms

Lists of inclusion terms are included below certain codes in the ICD-10-CM tabular list. The **inclusion terms** indicate some of the conditions for which that code may be assigned. They may be synonyms with the code title, or for "other specified" codes they may provide a list of various conditions included for a code. The ICD-10-CM index is an important supplement to the tabular list because it contains many terms that do not appear in the tabular list.

Example 1: ICD-10-CM TABULAR LIST OF DISEASES AND INJURIES—INCLUSION TERMS: The following inclusion terms are located in the Tabular List of Diseases and Injuries for diagnosis code M54.50, Low back pain, unspecified:

- Loin pain
- Lumbago NOS

Example 2: ICD-10-CM TABULAR LIST OF DISEASES AND INJURIES—INCLUSION TERMS (conditions classified to "other specified" subcategory codes): If the provider documents *polyalgia* as the patient's condition, assign code M79.89 even though the code description indicates it is an *other specified* code.

The inclusion terms listed below codes in the tabular list are not meant to be exhaustive, and additional terms found only in the index may also be assigned to a tabular list code. This concept is called **trust the index**, because when you locate a term and a code in the index, and that term is not repeated in the tabular list (as an inclusion term below a category or subcategory), that code can still be assigned. The tabular list would be too cumbersome to use if all index terms were listed below categories and subcategories.

> **Example:** ICD-10-CM INDEX TO DISEASES AND INJURIES AND TABULAR LIST OF DISEASES AND INJURIES—*TRUST THE INDEX*: Locate the index entry for *infection, fish tapeworm, larval B70.1*. Then, go to the tabular list to verify code B70.1, where you will notice that *infection due to fish tapeworm, larval* is not listed as an inclusion term. The coder has to *trust the index* and assign code B70.1 for the documented condition.

Excludes Notes

The ICD-10-CM Tabular List of Diseases and Injuries contains two types of excludes notes. Each note has a different definition for use. However, they are similar in that they both indicate that codes excluded from each other are independent of each other.

An **excludes1 note** is a pure excludes. It means "not coded here" and indicates mutually exclusive codes, in other words—two or more conditions that cannot be reported together.

> **Example 1:** ICD-10-CM TABULAR LIST OF DISEASES AND INJURIES—EXCLUDES1 NOTE: Locate ICD-10-CM code Q03 Congenital hydrocephalus in the tabular list, and find the Excludes1 note for *acquired hydrocephalus (G91.-)*. Hydrocephalus diagnosed in a newborn is assigned a code from Q03.0–Q03.9. For hydrocephalus that develops later in life, a code from G91.0 to G91.9 is assigned. A congenital form of a disease is not reported with an acquired form of the same condition. Thus, the excluded code is never reported with the code located above the Excludes1 note.

 Coding Tip

> An excludes1 note instructs you to assign one code or the other *except when documentation supports existence of both conditions.*

> **Example 2:** ICD-10-CM TABULAR LIST OF DISEASES AND INJURIES—EXCLUDES1 NOTE: Locate ICD-10-CM code E10 Type 1 diabetes mellitus in the tabular list, and find the Excludes1 note for *type 2 diabetes mellitus (E11.-)*. Type 1 diabetes mellitus is classified to a code from E10.10 to E10.9. Thus, a code for type 2 diabetes mellitus (E11.00–E11.9) would never be assigned with a code for type 1 diabetes mellitus.

An exception to the excludes1 definition is the circumstance when two or more documented conditions are unrelated to one another. If it is not clear whether the conditions for which an excludes1 note exists in ICD-10-CM are related or not, query the provider.

> **Example 1:** ICD-10-CM TABULAR LIST OF DISEASES AND INJURIES—EXCLUDES1 EXCEPTION: The Excludes1 note for code range R40–R46 in the tabular list states that symptoms and signs constituting part of a pattern of mental disorder (F01–F99) cannot be assigned with the R40–R46 codes. However, if dizziness (R42) is not a component of the mental health condition (e.g., dizziness is unrelated to bipolar disorder), then separate codes may be assigned for both dizziness and bipolar disorder.

> **Example 2:** ICD-10-CM TABULAR LIST OF DISEASES AND INJURIES—EXCLUDES1 EXCEPTION: Code range I60–I69 (Cerebrovascular Diseases) has an Excludes1 note for traumatic intracranial hemorrhage (S06.-). Codes in I60–I69 should not be used for a diagnosis of traumatic intracranial hemorrhage. However, if the patient has both a current traumatic intracranial hemorrhage and sequelae from a previous stroke, it would be appropriate to assign both a code from categories S06 and I69.

An **excludes2 note** means "not included here" and indicates that although the excluded condition is not classified as part of the condition it is excluded from, a patient may be diagnosed with all conditions at the same time. Therefore, when an excludes2 note appears under a code, it may be acceptable to assign both the code and the excluded code(s) together if supported by the medical documentation.

Coding Tip

An excludes2 note instructs you to assign more than one code when medical documentation supports all conditions.

Example: ICD-10-CM TABULAR LIST OF DISEASES AND INJURIES—EXCLUDES2 NOTE: ICD-10-CM subcategory M19.14 Post-traumatic osteoarthritis, hand in the tabular list contains an Excludes2 note for post-traumatic osteoarthritis of first carpometacarpal joint (M18.2-, M18.3-). The Excludes2 note means that because a patient can be diagnosed with both "post-traumatic osteoarthritis of the hand" and "post-traumatic osteoarthritis of the first carpometacarpal joint," it is acceptable to assign codes to both conditions if supported by medical documentation.

Etiology and Manifestation Convention

The **etiology and manifestation convention** includes the following notes in the ICD-10-CM Tabular List of Diseases and Injuries:

- Code first underlying disease
- Code, if applicable, any causal condition first
- Use additional code
- In diseases classified elsewhere

To classify certain conditions completely, codes must be assigned to the underlying *etiology* (cause or origin of disease) and multiple body system *manifestations* (resulting symptoms or conditions) due to the underlying etiology. For such conditions, the underlying condition is sequenced first, if applicable, followed by the manifestation.

Etiology/manifestation conditions are listed together in the ICD-10-CM Index to Diseases and Injuries; the etiology code is listed first, followed by the manifestation codes in brackets. (The manifestation code listed in brackets is always sequenced second.) (Official coding conventions also direct coders to *See Section I.B.7. Multiple coding for a single condition*, covered in the General ICD-10-CM Diagnosis Coding Guidelines section of this chapter.)

Example: ICD-10-CM INDEX TO DISEASES AND INJURIES AND TABULAR LIST OF DISEASES AND INJURIES— ETIOLOGY/MANIFESTATION CODES: Diagnostic statement idiopathic pulmonary hemosiderosis includes two codes in the ICD-10-CM index: E83.1- [*J84.03*]. Code J84.03 is enclosed in italicized brackets in the index, which indicates it is reported second because it is a manifestation code. In the ICD-10-CM tabular list, code J84.03 is in italics and contains a code first underlying disease note.

Wherever an etiology and manifestation combination of codes exists, the tabular list etiology code contains a **use additional code** note and the manifestation code contains a **code first underlying disease** note. These instructional notes assist coders in the proper sequencing of the codes: etiology code followed by manifestation code. In most cases, the manifestation code will have in its title an **in diseases classified elsewhere** note, which indicates that the manifestation codes are a component of the etiology/manifestation coding convention. A manifestation code that does not contain *in diseases classified elsewhere* in its title will contain a "use additional code" note. (Make sure to sequence the manifestation code *after* the etiology code.) *Code first underlying disease* and *use additional code* notes are also used as sequencing rules in ICD-10-CM for certain codes that are not part of an etiology/manifestation combination.

Example: ICD-10-CM TABULAR LIST OF DISEASES AND INJURIES—USE ADDITIONAL CODE: The patient is diagnosed with *benign hypertrophy of the prostate with urinary urgency*. Locate subcategory code N40.1 in the ICD-10-CM tabular list, and notice the *use additional code for associated symptoms, when specified* instruction... urinary urgency (R39.15). Therefore, assign codes N40.1 and R39.15.

NOTE:

Manifestation codes that include the instruction *code first underlying condition* are never reported first on health insurance claims. They must be reported in conjunction with an underlying condition (etiology) code, and they must be listed after the underlying condition code.

The instruction to **code, if applicable, any causal condition first** requires the causal condition to be sequenced first if present. A *causal condition* is a disease (e.g., diabetes mellitus) that manifests (or results in) another condition (e.g., diabetic cataracts). If no causal condition is documented, the code that contains the instruction (*code, if applicable, any causal condition first*) may be reported without the causal condition code. (This differs from the instruction to *code first underlying condition*, which does not allow for the code that contains the instruction to be reported without first sequencing the underlying condition.)

> **Example:** ICD-10-CM TABULAR LIST OF DISEASES AND INJURIES—CODE, IF APPLICABLE, ANY CAUSAL CONDITION FIRST: A patient with an alcohol dependence (F10.20) was seen in the office, complaining of urinary incontinence. The physician determined that the condition was nonorganic in origin and most likely the result of the patient being too inebriated to realize urination had occurred while unconscious. Code F98.0 is assigned to urinary incontinence that is of nonorganic origin. Code R32 is assigned to urinary incontinence that is organic in nature (e.g., due to urethritis, N34.2).

And

When the word **and** appears in category titles and code descriptions in the ICD-10-CM Tabular List of Diseases and Injuries, it is interpreted as meaning *and/or*.

> **Example:** ICD-10-CM TABULAR LIST OF DISEASES—AND: The word *and* in category code J04 (Acute laryngitis and tracheitis) means that codes are reported for conditions of the larynx, trachea, or larynx and trachea.

With

When the word **with** appears in the ICD-10-CM Index to Diseases and Injuries, it is located immediately below either the main term or a subterm, not in alphabetical order. To assign a code from the list of qualifiers below the word *with*, the physician must document the presence of both conditions in the patient's record.

The word "with" is interpreted to mean "associated with" or "due to" when it appears in a code title, the index, or an instructional note in the tabular list. Thus, ICD-10-CM presumes a causal relationship between the two conditions linked by the term "with" in the index or tabular list. Such conditions should be coded as related even in the absence of provider documentation explicitly linking them, *unless the documentation clearly states the conditions are unrelated or when another official coding guideline exists that specifically requires a documented linkage between two conditions* (e.g., sepsis guideline for "acute organ dysfunction that is not clearly associated with the sepsis"). For conditions not specifically linked by these relational terms in the classification or when an official coding guideline requires that a linkage between two conditions be explicitly documented, provider documentation must link the conditions in order to code them as related.

> **Example:** ICD-10-CM INDEX TO DISEASES AND INJURIES—WITH: Locate main term *Angina* in the index, and notice that the word *with* appears above a list of second qualifiers. To assign a code from the list, the physician must document both conditions, such as *angina with documented spasm* (I20.1). The physician could also document:
> - Angiospastic angina
> - Prinzmetal angina
> - Spasm-induced angina
> - Variant angina

Due To

The subterm **due to** is located in the ICD-10-CM Index to Diseases and Injuries in alphabetical order to indicate the presence of a cause-and-effect (or causal) relationship between two conditions. When the index includes *due to* as a subterm, the code is assigned only if the physician documented the causal relationship between two conditions, such as meningitis due to adenovirus. It is possible that a patient could have meningitis along with an unrelated adenovirus at the same time. (The *due to* phrase is included in tabular list code descriptions, but it is not a coding instruction.)

 NOTE:

The ICD-10-CM index also includes subterm *in* (*due to*) to indicate the presence of a cause-and-effect (or causal) relationship between two conditions.

ICD-10-CM occasionally presumes a causal relationship between two conditions. This means that the physician is not required to document *due to* in the diagnostic statement, such as when the patient has hypertension and chronic renal failure. This condition is coded as hypertensive renal failure, which is interpreted as hypertension due to chronic renal failure.

Example 1: ICD-10-CM INDEX TO DISEASES AND INJURIES—DUE TO: When the physician documents *pneumonitis due to inhalation of regurgitated food*, a causal relationship exists, and code J69.0 is assigned.

Example 2: ICD-10-CM INDEX TO DISEASES AND INJURIES—IN (DUE TO): When the physician documents *anemia in stage 3 (moderate) chronic kidney disease*, a causal relationship exists, and codes N18.30 and D63.1 are assigned.

In

When the word **in** appears in the ICD-10-CM index, it is located in alphabetical order below the main term. To assign a code from the list of qualifiers below the word *in*, the physician must document both conditions in the patient's record. The word "in" is interpreted to mean "associated with" or "due to" when it appears in a code title, the index, or an instructional note in the tabular list. Thus, ICD-10-CM classifies certain conditions as if there were a cause-and-effect relationship present because they occur together much of the time (e.g., pneumonia in Q fever).

Example: ICD-10-CM INDEX TO DISEASES AND INJURIES—IN: Locate main term *Pneumonia* in the index, and notice that the word *in* appears in alphabetical order above a list of second qualifiers. To assign a code from the list, the physician must document a relationship between both conditions, such as *pneumonia in measles* (or *postpneumonia measles*) to which combination code B05.2 is assigned. (Other conditions that occur together may require the assignment of multiple codes, one for the etiology and another for the manifestation.)

Cross References

The ICD-10-CM index includes **cross references**, which instruct the coder to assign the correct code by referring to another entry in the index (e.g., *see*) or, for ICD-10-CM, to the tabular list (e.g., *see* category).

- The *see* cross reference after a main term directs the coder to refer to another term in the ICD-10-CM index to locate the code. The coder must go to the referenced main term to locate the correct code.
- The *see also* cross reference is located after a main term or subterm in the ICD-10-CM index and directs the coder to another main term (or subterm) that may provide additional useful index entries. The *see also* instruction does not have to be followed if the original main term (or subterm) provides the correct code.

- The **see category** cross reference directs the coder to the ICD-10-CM tabular list, where a code can be selected from the options provided there.

- The **see condition** cross reference directs the coder to the main term for a condition, found in the ICD-10-CM index.

Example 1: ICD-10-CM INDEX TO DISEASES AND INJURIES—*SEE*: Locate main term *Laceration* and subterm *blood vessel* in the ICD-10-CM index. Notice that a cross-reference directs you to "*See* Injury, blood vessel," which is at a different location in the index where the code can be found.

Example 2: ICD-10-CM INDEX TO DISEASES AND INJURIES—*SEE ALSO*: The *see also* instruction is optional if the correct code can be located below the main term (e.g., laceration of lower back, S31.010). If the correct code cannot be located, the *see also* cross-reference directs the coder to a different location in the index where the code can be found.

Example 3: ICD-10-CM INDEX TO DISEASES AND INJURIES—*SEE* CATEGORY: Locate main term *Pyelitis*, subterm *with*, and second qualifier *calculus* in the ICD-10-CM index. Notice that a cross-reference directs you to *see* category N20. To assign the correct code, review category N20 in the tabular list to select the appropriate fourth character.

Example 4: ICD-10-CM INDEX TO DISEASES AND INJURIES—*SEE* CONDITION: Locate main term *Accidental* in the ICD-10-CM index, and notice that a cross-reference directs you to *see* condition, which means the patient record needs to be reviewed to determine the condition (e.g., fracture).

Code Also Note

A **code also** note in the ICD-10-CM tabular list provides instruction that two codes may be required to fully describe a condition, but this note does not provide sequencing direction. Code sequencing depends on the circumstances of the encounter.

Example: A patient is diagnosed with plasminogen deficiency and ligneous conjunctivitis. ICD-10-CM code E88.02 (Plasminogen deficiency) contains an instruction to "Code also, if applicable, ligneous conjunctivitis (H10.51). Because the patient was diagnosed with both conditions, both codes are assigned.

Default Codes

A code listed next to a main term in the ICD-10-CM index is referred to as a **default code**, which represents the condition that is most commonly associated with the main term or is the unspecified code for the condition. If a condition is documented in a medical record (e.g., appendicitis) without any additional information, such as acute or chronic, assign the default code (after verifying the code in the ICD-10-CM tabular list).

Exercise 2.6 – ICD-10-CM Coding Conventions

Instructions: Assign ICD-10-CM code(s) to each statement. Make sure you appropriately interpret ICD-10-CM coding conventions when assigning codes.

_____   **1.** Acariasis infestation

_____   **2.** Hashimoto's disease

_____   **3.** Aberrant abdominal artery

_____   **4.** Healed amputation stump

_____   **5.** Retinal detachment with single retinal break, right eye

Exercise 2.6 – continued

_____   6. Pharmacoresistant epilepsy

_____   7. Adenocarcinoma of urinary bladder neck as primary site

_____   8. Accidental overdose, Absinthe (beverage), initial encounter

_____   9. Hallucinosis due to Trazodone taken as prescribed (initial encounter)

_____   10. Underdosing of Aceclidine for glaucoma (initial encounter)

_____   11. Acute disseminated tuberculosis

_____   12. Extraintestinal yersiniosis

_____   13. Hypertension

_____   14. Acute recurrent maxillary antritis

_____   15. Pruritic dermatitis

_____   16. Ulcerative impetigo

_____   17. Bone hypoplasia

_____   18. Amyloid heart disease

_____   19. Acute laryngitis

_____   20. Lymphadenitis due to diphtheria

_____   21. Aseptic meningitis in leptospirosis

_____   22. Microdrepanocytosis with acute chest syndrome

_____   23. Abdominalgia, lower left quadrant

_____   24. Benign papilloma, urinary bladder

_____   25. Pyelitis with calculus

Code Assignment and Clinical Criteria

The assignment of a diagnosis code is based on the physician's diagnostic statement that the condition exists. The provider's statement that the patient has a particular condition is sufficient. Code assignment is *not* based on clinical criteria used by the provider to establish the diagnosis. If there is conflicting medical record documentation, query the provider.

Example: The physician documented "Alzheimer's disease with dementia and behavioral disturbances" (G30.9, F02.81-) as the discharge diagnoses. Clinical criteria (e.g., brain imaging study) are not documented in the hospital record. Codes G30.9 and F02.818 are reported because code assignment is based on the physician's diagnostic statement that the condition exists, not clinical criteria. In this case, the physician used *pattern recognition* to establish the discharge diagnoses. This involves the physician using experience to recognize a "pattern" of clinical characteristics; it is based on certain signs and/or symptoms typically associated with a disease process. The coder would *not* query the provider to question the discharge diagnosis.

Exercise 2.7 – Code Assignment and Clinical Criteria

Instructions: Assign an ICD-10-CM code to each statement. Make sure that you appropriately interpret the intent of the *code assignment and clinical criteria* coding convention.

_____   1. Patient admitted for difficulty breathing and fever. Physician's discharge diagnosis is pneumonia.

_____   2. Patient admitted with malaise. Physician's discharge diagnosis is depression.

(continues)

Exercise 2.7 – continued

_____ 3. Patient admitted with severe headache. Physician's discharge diagnosis is intractable migraine.

_____ 4. Patient admitted with abdominal pain and fever. Physician's discharge diagnosis is acute appendicitis.

_____ 5. Patient admitted with pain and swelling, left ankle. Physician's discharge diagnosis is sprain, left ankle.

General ICD-10-CM Diagnosis Coding Guidelines

The general coding guidelines are followed when assigning ICD-10-CM diagnosis codes for inpatient, outpatient, and physician office settings.

Locating a Code in ICD-10-CM—Use of Index and Tabular List

Use the index and the tabular list when locating and assigning codes because relying on just the index or tabular list results in coding errors and less specificity when selecting codes.

Locate Each Term in the Alphabetic Index

Locate each term in the ICD-10-CM index first, and verify the code selected in the tabular list. Make sure you read and are guided by coding conventions (e.g., excludes1, excludes2) that appear in either the index or the tabular list. (The ICD-10-CM index includes an alphabetic index of diseases and injuries, an index of external cause of injuries, a table of neoplasms, and a table of drugs and chemicals.)

 NOTE:

Use *both* the ICD-10-CM index and tabular list because the index does not always provide the complete code. Selection of the complete code, including laterality (e.g., bilateral, right side, left side) and any applicable seventh character is done using the tabular list. A dash (-) at the end of a code in the index indicates that additional character(s) are required. Even if a dash is *not* included at the index entry, refer to the tabular list to verify whether additional character(s) are required.

Example: The ICD-10-CM Index to Diseases and Injuries entry for *diabetes mellitus* lists code E11.9, as verified in the tabular list.

Level of Detail in Coding

Pay attention to the level of detail when assigning codes because diagnosis codes are to be reported using the highest number of digits or characters available and to the highest level of specificity documented in the medical record.

 NOTE:

ICD-10-CM codes contain three, four, five, six, or seven characters. Codes with three characters are called categories, and they may be further subdivided by assigning up to four additional characters to provide greater detail.

Codes with four, five, or six characters that require additional character(s) are subcategories. Codes that do *not* require additional character(s) are simply called *codes*. (It might be helpful to think of such *codes* as *complete codes* or *valid codes*.) A three-character code is reported only if it is not further subdivided. Where fourth through seventh characters are provided, they *must* be assigned. A code is invalid if the complete number of characters required for that code have not been assigned.

Example: ICD-10-CM category M1a (chronic gout) requires the assignment of a fourth, fifth, sixth, and seventh character to complete the code. It is incorrect to report a category M1a code without the fourth through seventh characters. Thus, you would assign code M1a.0110 to a patient diagnosed with idiopathic chronic gout of the right shoulder, without tophus.

Codes from A00.0–T88.9, Z00–Z99.8, U00–U85

Appropriate codes from ICD-10-CM (A00.0–T88.9, Z00–Z99.8, and U00–U85) are reported to identify diagnoses, symptoms, conditions, problems, complaints, or other reason(s) for the encounter. Codes from ICD-10-CM Chapter 22 (U codes) are temporary codes that are also reported to identify diagnoses.

 NOTE:

Codes V00 through Y99 are reported for external causes of morbidity.

Signs and Symptoms

For outpatient and physician office encounters, codes that describe symptoms and signs are reported when a related definitive diagnosis has not been established (or confirmed) by the provider. For inpatient hospital encounters, codes are assigned for uncertain diagnoses (e.g., possible, probable, rule out, suspicious conditions). (Official general coding guidelines also provide direction to *See Section I.B.18. Use of Signs/Symptom/ Unspecified Codes*, covered later in this section of the chapter.)

 NOTE:

ICD-10-CM Chapter 18 (Symptoms, Signs, and Abnormal Clinical and Laboratory Findings, Not Elsewhere Classified) contains many, but not all, codes for signs and symptoms. Some codes are found in other ICD-10-CM chapters (e.g., acute neoplasm-related pain, G89.3).

Example of Physician Office Encounter: The patient is seen at a physician's office for an initial visit, complaining of pain and limited range of motion (stiffness), right little finger. The physician examines the finger and notices a solid mass. The physician orders an x-ray to rule out ganglion. Upon the follow-up visit, the x-ray results reveal no arthritis. The diagnosis is ganglion cyst, right little finger joint. The patient is scheduled for outpatient surgery to remove the ganglion cyst.

For the initial visit, assign ICD-10-CM codes for pain (M79.644), stiffness (M25.641), and mass of the little finger (R22.31).

For the follow-up visit, assign ICD-10-CM code M67.441 for the ganglion cyst, right little finger. Code M67.441 is reported as a definitive diagnosis, which means signs and symptoms codes for pain, limited range of motion (stiffness), or mass of the little finger knuckle joint are *not* reported on the claim for the follow-up visit.

Example of Inpatient Hospital Encounter: An 85-year-old patient was admitted as a hospital inpatient with a suspicious solid mass, right little finger. The patient's advanced age, chronic conditions, and past history of bone cancer with surgical resection and follow-up chemotherapy necessitated inpatient hospitalization. The patient's chief complaint was pain and limited range of motion (stiffness), right little finger. During physical examination, the provider pressed on the mass, eliciting pain. When a a light was shined on it, the indication was a solid mass. X-ray results revealed no arthritis and were inconclusive regarding solid tumor. MRI confirmed a somewhat solid mass that appeared cyst like. An attempt at withdrawing possible fluid was unsuccessful. Surgical excision of the mass resulted in pathology results that ruled out cancer, and the patient was relieved to be diagnosed with a ganglion cyst, right little finger.

For the inpatient hospital encounter, assign ICD-10-CM code M67.441 for ganglion cyst, right little finger (along with ICD-10-CM codes for documented chronic conditions and past history of bone cancer and an ICD-10-PCS code for surgical excision of the mass). Do *not* assign codes for suspicious solid mass, pain, or limited range of motion (stiffness) of the right little finger because the definitive diagnosis was a ganglion cyst.

Conditions That Are an Integral Part of a Disease Process

Signs and symptoms that are associated with a disease process should *not* be assigned as additional codes (unless otherwise instructed by ICD-10-CM) because they are included in the disease process.

Example: The patient is seen at the hospital's emergency department (ED) with a complaint of shortness of breath. A chest x-ray reveals pneumonia, and the ED physician prescribes an antibiotic. Assign ICD-10-CM code J18.9 to the pneumonia, and do not assign a code for the shortness of breath because it is a symptom of pneumonia.

Conditions That Are *Not* an Integral Part of a Disease Process

Conditions that are not considered an integral part of a disease process, such as additional signs and symptoms that may not be associated routinely with a disease process, should be coded when present (e.g., severe headache for which treatment or medical management is provided is coded when the patient is diagnosed with pneumonia).

Example: The patient is seen at the physician's office for follow-up care of controlled hypertension and tells the physician about recent bouts of insomnia. The physician discusses possible reasons for the insomnia with the patient, who admits to being under extreme stress recently. The patient is reluctant to take over-the-counter or prescription medications for the insomnia, and the physician suggests alternative solutions. The physician also instructs the patient to return in two weeks for follow-up of the insomnia. Assign ICD-10-CM code I10 to the hypertension. In addition, assign ICD-10-CM code G47.00 to the insomnia because it is not a symptom of hypertension and it was medically managed during the visit.

Multiple Coding for a Single Condition

The etiology/manifestation coding convention requires that two codes be reported to completely describe a single condition that affects multiple body systems.

Example: The diagnosis amyloid polyneuropathy requires ICD-10-CM codes E85.1 and G63 be reported in that order. (Remember: italicized codes in the tabular list are never sequenced first.)

In addition, other single conditions require more than one code to be reported, such as those associated with "use additional code" notes found in the tabular list. These codes are not part of an etiology/manifestation pair where a secondary code is useful to describe a condition fully. The sequencing rule for "use additional code" is the same as the etiology/manifestation pair in that a secondary code should be reported, if known. A "use additional code" note will usually be found at the infectious disease code, indicating the need to report the organism code as a secondary code.

 NOTE:

Multiple codes also may need to be reported for ICD-10-CM *sequelae*, complications, and obstetrical cases to describe more fully the patient's conditions. (Refer to specific guidelines below for further instruction.)

Example: For a diagnosis of urinary tract infection due to *Escherichia coli*, report ICD-10-CM codes N39.0 and B96.20, in that order.

"Code first" notes are also located below certain ICD-10-CM codes in the tabular list that are not specifically manifestation codes but may be due to an underlying cause. When a "code first" note is present *and* an underlying condition is documented in the patient record, the underlying condition is reported first, if known.

Example: The physician documents rheumatic pneumonia in the patient's record. Upon review of the index and tabular list, assign ICD-10-CM codes I00 and J17 for the condition, in that order.

NOTE:

For bacterial infections not included in ICD-10-CM Chapter 2, a secondary code from category B96 (Other bacterial agents as the cause of diseases classified elsewhere) may be required to identify the bacterial organism causing the infection.

"Code, if applicable, any causal condition first" notes in the ICD-10-CM tabular list indicate that this code may be assigned as a first-listed or principal diagnosis when the causal condition is unknown or not applicable. If a causal condition is known, the code for that condition should be reported as the first-listed or principal diagnosis.

> **Example:** The patient is diagnosed with urinary incontinence and congenital ureterocele. Assign ICD-10-CM codes Q62.31 and R32 (although generating a physician query could result in a more specific urinary incontinence code), in that order.

Acute and Chronic Conditions

If the same condition is described as both acute (or subacute) and chronic and separate subentries exist in the ICD-10-CM index at the same indentation level, code both and sequence the acute (or subacute) code first.

> **Example:** The diagnoses acute gastritis and chronic gastritis are assigned ICD-10-CM codes K29.00 and K29.50, in that order.

Combination Code

Assign combination codes when available and multiple codes as needed. A **combination code** is a single code that is used to classify two diagnoses, a diagnosis with an associated secondary process (e.g., manifestation), or a diagnosis with an associated complication. Combination codes are located by referring to subterm entries in the ICD-10-CM index and by following "includes" and "excludes" notes in the ICD-10-CM tabular list. Assign two or more **multiple codes** to completely classify the elements of a complex diagnosis statement, which contain words or phrases such as *due to, incidental to, secondary to,* and *with.* Make sure you carefully review tabular list entries, which provide guidance regarding the assignment of multiple codes.

Make sure you assign only the combination code when that code fully identifies the diagnostic conditions involved or when the index so directs. Do not report multiple codes when ICD-10-CM provides a combination code that clearly identifies all of the elements documented in the diagnosis. When a combination code lacks necessary specificity in describing the manifestation or a complication, an additional code should be reported as a secondary code.

> **Example 1: Combination Code:** Assign ICD-10-CM combination code K80.00 to the diagnosis acute cholecystitis and cholelithiasis because the code description includes both conditions. (The fifth-character 0 is assigned to this code because there is no mention of obstruction in the diagnostic statement.)

> **Example 2: Multiple Codes:** The diagnosis trigonitis due to *Escherichia coli* is assigned ICD-10-CM codes N30.30 and B96.20, in that order.

Sequelae (Late Effects)

A **sequela** is the **residual effect** (condition produced) after the acute phase of an illness or injury has terminated. *There is no time limit on when a sequela code can be reported.* The residual may be apparent early (e.g., hemiparesis in cerebral infarction), or it may occur months or years later (e.g., scarring due to a previous burn).

Coding of a sequela generally requires two codes sequenced in the following order:

- Residual condition or nature of the sequela is sequenced first.
- Sequela code is sequenced second.

An exception to the above guidelines occurs when the sequela code has been expanded (at the fourth-, fifth-, or sixth-character levels) to include the manifestation(s). *The code for the acute phase of an illness or injury that led to the sequela is never used with a code for the late effect.*

In the ICD-10-CM Index to Diseases and Injuries, the main term is *Sequela (of)* and it includes a "–*see also* condition" instruction because in the tabular list the seventh-character "S" is added to condition codes for which sequelae (residual conditions) are treated. (Historically, ICD-9-CM referred to a sequela as a *late effect* of an illness or injury.) (Official general coding guidelines also provide direction to *See Section I.C.9. Sequelae of cerebrovascular disease*, covered in textbook Chapter 3, *See Section I.C.15. Sequelae of complication of pregnancy, childbirth and the puerperium*, and *See Section I.C.19. Application of 7th characters for Chapter 19*, covered in textbook Chapter 4.)

NOTE:

- The code for the acute phase of an illness or injury that led to the sequela is never reported with a code for the sequela (because treatment for the acute phase has ended).
- Do not confuse sequelae with complications that are associated with current acute illness or injuries and usually develop from problems that occur during the course of medical or surgical care (e.g., postoperative wound infection).
- Multiple codes are assigned to classify a sequela when no combination code exists, such as "headaches due to intracranial injury without loss of consciousness that occurred several years ago" for which ICD-10-CM codes G44.309 and S06.9X0S are both assigned. (In ICD-10-CM, the sequelae of injuries are classified by assigning an S as the seventh character of the injury code.)
- A combination code is assigned to classify a sequela when it exists, such as "nondominant left-sided paralysis due to previous CVA" for which ICD-10-CM I69.864 only is assigned.

Example: The patient was in an accident last year and sustained fractures of the left femur and right tibia, which healed without incident. The patient presents with stiffness of the left hip and numbness of the left leg. Assign codes to the stiffness of the left hip (M25.652); numbness of the left leg (R20.0); and sequela of fracture, femur (S72.92XS).

Impending or Threatened Condition

Code any condition described at the time of encounter/visit as "impending" or "threatened" as follows:

- If the condition did occur, code as confirmed diagnosis.
- If the condition did not occur, reference the index to determine if the condition has a subentry term for *impending* or *threatened* and also reference main term entries for *impending* and *threatened*.
- If subterms for *impending* or *threatened* are listed, assign the listed code.
- If subterms for *impending* or *threatened* are not listed, code the existing underlying condition(s), and *not* the condition described as *impending* or *threatened* (except for inpatient cases when impending/threatened conditions are coded).

Example: The patient is treated for impending myocardial infarction (MI) and is assigned ICD-10-CM code I20.0 because the MI diagnosis has not been confirmed.

Reporting Same Diagnosis Code More Than Once

Each unique ICD-10-CM diagnosis code is reported only once for an encounter. This applies to bilateral conditions *when there are no distinct ICD-10-CM codes identifying laterality* or two different conditions that are classified to the same ICD-10-CM diagnosis code.

Example: On March 14, the patient was diagnosed with bilateral lung abscesses. Even though both lungs contain abscesses, assign ICD-10-CM code J85.2 only once.

Laterality

ICD-10-CM codes that indicate **laterality** specifically classify conditions that occur on the left, right, or bilaterally. If a bilateral ICD-10-CM code is not provided *and the condition is bilateral*, assign separate codes for both the left and right sides.

> **Example:** *Bilateral contusion of fallopian tubes, initial encounter* is assigned ICD-10-CM code S37.522A.

When a patient has a bilateral condition *and each side is treated during separate encounters*, assign the "bilateral" code for the encounter during which the first side is treated (because the condition still exists on both sides). For the second encounter during which the other side is treated (and after the other side has been successfully treated and because the condition no longer exists on that side), assign the appropriate unilateral code for the side where the condition still exists. The bilateral code is not assigned for the subsequent encounter because the patient no longer has the condition at the previously treated site. However, if treatment for the first side did not completely resolve the condition, reporting the bilateral code would still be appropriate.

> **Example:** The patient was diagnosed with bilateral cataracts. On May 5, the patient successfully underwent cataract surgery of the left eye. The ICD-10-CM code for *cataracts, bilateral eyes*, is reported for the May 5 encounter. On July 5, the patient successfully underwent cataract surgery of the right eye. The ICD-10-CM code for *cataract, right eye*, is reported for the July 5 encounter.

When laterality is not documented by the patient's provider, code assignment for the affected side may be based on medical record documentation from other clinicians. If there is conflicting medical record documentation regarding the affected side, generate a physician query to obtain clarification. Codes for *unspecified* side should rarely be used, such as when documentation in the medical record is insufficient to determine the affected side and it is not possible to obtain clarification from the provider.

Documentation by Clinicians Other Than the Patient's Provider

Code assignment is based on the documentation by the patient's provider (e.g., physician or other qualified health care practitioner legally accountable for establishing the patient's diagnosis). There are exceptions when code assignment may be based on medical record documentation from clinicians who are not the patient's provider. In this context, *clinicians other than the patient's provider* refer to health care professionals permitted, based on regulatory or accreditation requirements or internal hospital policies, to document in a patient's official medical record. These exceptions include codes for

- Body mass index (BMI)
- Depth of non-pressure chronic ulcers
- Pressure ulcer stage
- Coma scale
- NIH stroke scale (NIHSS)
- Social determinants of health (SDOH) classified to ICD-10-CM Chapter 21
- Laterality
- Blood alcohol level
- Underimmunization status

This information is typically, or may be, documented by other clinicians involved in the care of the patient (e.g., dietitian documents BMI, nurse documents pressure ulcer stages, and emergency medical technician documents coma scale). However, the associated diagnosis (e.g., obesity, pressure ulcer, coma, or a condition classifiable to category F10, Alcohol related disorders) must be documented by the patient's provider. When there is conflicting medical record documentation, either from the same clinician or different clinicians, generate a physician query to obtain clarification.

ICD-10-CM codes for BMI, coma scale, NIHSS, blood alcohol level, social determinants of health, and underimmunization status should only be *reported as secondary diagnoses*. (Official general coding guidelines also provide direction to *See Section I.C.21.c.17. for additional information regarding coding social determinants of health*, covered in textbook Chapter 4.)

> **Example:** Patient's BMI of 40.4 was documented by the dietician, and patient has an established diagnosis of morbid obesity. Report ICD-10-CM codes E66.01 and Z68.41, in that order.

Syndromes

When assigning codes to syndromes, follow ICD-10-CM index guidance, such as locating main term Syndrome. In the absence of index guidance, assign codes for the documented manifestations (e.g., signs, symptoms) of the syndrome. Additional codes for manifestations that are *not an integral part of the disease process* (e.g., anxiety) may also be assigned when the condition does not have a unique code. A **syndrome** is a set of signs, symptoms, or conditions that occur together and suggest the presence of a certain disease or an increased chance of developing the disease.

> **Example 1:** Patient is diagnosed with Alagille syndrome, which is a congenital liver malformation. ICD-10-CM index main term *Syndrome* and subterm *Alagille (-Watson) Q44.71*.

> **Example 2:** Patient is diagnosed with Barlow's syndrome, which is defined as nonrheumatic mitral valve prolapse. ICD-10-CM index main term *Syndrome* does **not** contain a subterm for *Barlow's*. ICD-10-CM index main term *Prolapse* and subterm *mitral (valve)* I34.1 is described as nonrheumatic mitral (valve) prolapse in the ICD-10-CM tabular list. (Be sure to locate the definition of any syndrome, such as Barlow's syndrome, when it is not located as a subterm below main term *Syndrome* in the ICD-10-CM index.)

Documentation of Complications of Care

The assignment of codes for complications of care is based on the provider's documentation of a relationship between the condition and the procedure or service provided, unless otherwise instructed by ICD-10-CM. This guideline applies to any complications of care, regardless of the ICD-10-CM chapter in which the code is located. It is important to note that not all conditions that occur during or following medical care or surgery are classified as *complications*. There must be a cause-and-effect relationship between the procedure or service provided and the condition, and the documentation must support that the condition is clinically significant. It is not necessary for the provider to explicitly document the term *complication*. For example, if the condition alters the course of the surgery as documented in the operative report, then it would be appropriate to report a complication code. Query the provider for clarification if the documentation is not clear about the relationship between the condition and the care provided or procedure performed.

> **Example 1:** The patient is seen today for dehiscence of a surgical amputation stump, which means that the surgical incision separated. In the ICD-10-CM index, go to main term *Dehiscence (of)* and subterm *amputation stump*, which lists code T87.81 (described as *Dehiscence of amputation stump* in the ICD-10-CM tabular list). Another way to locate the code in the ICD-10-CM is to go to main term *Complication(s) (from) (of)*, subterm *amputation stump*, and second qualifier *dehiscence*, which lists code T87.81.

> **Example 2:** The patient underwent left knee replacement surgery last month and is seen today for an initial encounter to evaluate instability of the left knee joint prosthesis. It is determined that the joint prosthesis was recalled due to a mechanical defect. Surgical intervention to replace the joint prosthesis is scheduled. For this initial encounter, in the ICD-10-CM index, go to main term *Complication*, subterm *joint prosthesis*, second qualifier *mechanical*, and third qualifier *instability* where code T84.02- is listed. Review of the ICD-10-CM tabular list indicates that code T84.023A (Instability of internal left knee prosthesis, initial encounter) is to be reported.

Borderline Diagnosis

When the provider documents a *borderline diagnosis* at the time of discharge, code the diagnosis as confirmed unless ICD-10-CM provides a specific entry. If a borderline condition has a specific index entry in ICD-10-CM, it should be coded as such. Since borderline conditions are not uncertain diagnoses, no distinction is made between the health care setting (inpatient versus outpatient). Whenever the documentation is unclear regarding a borderline condition, coders are encouraged to query the provider for clarification.

> **Example:** The patient is diagnosed with borderline diabetes mellitus. In the ICD-10-CM index, go to main term *Borderline* and subterm *diabetes mellitus*, which lists code R73.03 (described as *Prediabetes* in the ICD-10-CM tabular list).

Use of Sign/Symptom/Unspecified Codes

Assigning codes to signs, symptoms, and unspecified conditions is acceptable, and it is sometimes even necessary. Specific diagnosis codes should be reported when supported by available patient record documentation and clinical knowledge of the patient's health condition. However, there are instances when signs, symptoms, or unspecified codes are the best choices for accurately reflecting the encounter. Each encounter should be coded to the level of certainty known.

A joint effort between the health care provider and the coder is essential to achieving complete and accurate documentation, code assignment, and reporting of diagnoses and procedures. The importance of consistent, complete documentation in the medical record cannot be overemphasized. Without such documentation accurate coding cannot be achieved. The entire record should be reviewed to determine the specific reason for the encounter and the conditions treated.

When a definitive diagnosis is *not* established during an encounter, report codes for signs and/or symptoms instead. When a specific code cannot be assigned because sufficient clinical information about a particular health condition is unknown or unavailable, report the appropriate unspecified code instead. Unspecified codes are reported when they most accurately reflect what is known about the patient's condition at the end of an encounter. It is inappropriate to assign a more specific code that is *not* supported by the patient record documentation. It is also inappropriate for a provider to order diagnostic testing that is medically *un*necessary to determine a more specific code.

> **Example:** The patient is diagnosed with pneumonia, and the specific type was not able to be determined by the end of an encounter. Report code J18.9 (Pneumonia, unspecified organism).

Coding for Health Care Encounters in Hurricane Aftermath

a. Use of External Cause of Morbidity Codes

An external cause of morbidity code should be assigned to identify the cause of the injury(ies) incurred as a result of the hurricane. The use of external cause of morbidity codes is supplemental to the application of ICD-10-CM codes. External cause of morbidity codes are never to be recorded as a principal diagnosis (first-listed in non-inpatient settings). The appropriate injury code should be sequenced before any external cause codes. The external cause of morbidity codes capture how the injury or health condition happened (cause), the intent (unintentional or accidental; or intentional, such as suicide or assault), the place where the event occurred, the activity of the patient at the time of the event, and the person's status (e.g., civilian, military). They should not be assigned for encounters to treat hurricane victims' medical conditions when no injury, adverse effect or poisoning is involved. External cause of morbidity codes should be assigned for each encounter for care and treatment of the injury. External cause of morbidity codes may be assigned in all health care settings. For the purpose of capturing complete and accurate ICD-10-CM data in the aftermath of the hurricane, a health care setting should be considered as any location where medical care is provided by licensed health care professionals.

b. Sequencing of External Causes of Morbidity Codes

Codes for cataclysmic events, such as a hurricane, take priority over all other external cause codes except child and adult abuse and terrorism and should be sequenced before other external cause of injury codes. Assign as many external cause of morbidity codes as necessary to fully explain each cause.

Example: If an injury occurs as a result of a building collapse during the hurricane, external cause codes for both the hurricane and the building collapse should be assigned, with the external cause code for hurricane being sequenced as the first external cause code.

For injuries incurred as a direct result of the hurricane, assign the appropriate code(s) for the injuries, followed by the code X37.0-, Hurricane (with the appropriate 7th character), and any other applicable external cause of injury codes. Code X37.0- also should be assigned when an injury is incurred as a result of flooding caused by a levee breaking related to the hurricane. Code X38.-, Flood (with the appropriate 7th character), should be assigned when an injury is from flooding resulting directly from the storm. Code X36.0.-, Collapse of dam or man-made structure, should not be assigned when the cause of the collapse is due to the hurricane. Use of code X36.0- is limited to collapses of man-made structures due to earth surface movements, not due to storm surges directly from a hurricane.

c. Other External Causes of Morbidity Code Issues

For injuries that are not a direct result of the hurricane, such as an evacuee that has incurred an injury as a result of a motor vehicle accident, assign the appropriate external cause of morbidity code(s) to describe the cause of the injury, but do not assign code X37.0-, Hurricane. If it is not clear whether the injury was a direct result of the hurricane, assume the injury is due to the hurricane and assign code X37.0-, Hurricane, as well as any other applicable external cause of morbidity codes. In addition to code X37.0-, Hurricane, other possible applicable external cause of morbidity codes include

X30-   Exposure to excessive natural heat

X31-   Exposure to excessive natural cold

X38-   Flood

d. Use of Z codes

Z codes (other reasons for health care encounters) may be assigned as appropriate to further explain the reasons for presenting for health care services, including transfers between health care facilities, or provide additional information relevant to a patient encounter. The *ICD-10-CM Official Guidelines for Coding and Reporting* identify which codes may be assigned as principal or first-listed diagnosis only, secondary diagnosis only, or principal/first-listed or secondary (depending on the circumstances). Possible applicable Z codes include

Z59.0-   Homelessness

Z59.1   Inadequate housing

Z59.5   Extreme poverty

Z75.1   Person awaiting admission to adequate facility elsewhere

Z75.3   Unavailability and inaccessibility of health care facilities

Z75.4   Unavailability and inaccessibility of other helping agencies

Z76.2   Encounter for health supervision and care of other healthy infant and child

Z99.12   Encounter for respirator [ventilator] dependence during power failure

The external cause of morbidity codes and the Z codes listed above are not an all-inclusive list. Other codes may be applicable to the encounter based upon the documentation. Assign as many codes as necessary to fully explain each health care encounter. Since patient history information may be very limited, use any available documentation to assign the appropriate external cause of morbidity and Z codes.

Exercise 2.8 – General ICD-10-CM Diagnosis Coding Guidelines

Instructions: Assign an ICD-10-CM code(s) to each statement. Make sure you appropriately interpret general ICD-10-CM diagnosis coding guidelines when assigning codes.

_____   **1.** Acute cholecystitis with nausea, vomiting and fever

_____   **2.** Chronic tonsillitis and adenoiditis

_____   **3.** Acute cystitis with hematuria due to _Escherichia coli_

_____   **4.** Multisystem inflammatory syndrome (MIS) as post-acute sequela of COVID-19

_____   **5.** Admission for adjustment of left partial artificial leg

Summary

The _International Classification of Diseases, 10th Revision, Clinical Modification_ (ICD-10-CM) replaced ICD-9-CM effective October 2015 and includes many more codes because it is designed to collect data on every type of health care encounter (e.g., inpatient, outpatient, hospice, home health care, and long-term care). ICD-10-CM disease and injury codes contain at least three characters, but most have three characters followed by a decimal point and between one and four additional characters. There are two main parts of the ICD-10-CM manual: the alphabetic index and the tabular list. ICD-10-CM Index to Diseases and Injuries entries are organized according to main terms, subterms, second qualifiers, third qualifiers, and fourth qualifiers. The ICD-10-CM Tabular List of Diseases and Injuries contains 22 chapters. It is a sequential list of codes contained within chapters based on body system or condition, and codes are then organized within major topic headings, categories, subcategories, and codes.

Medical necessity is the measure of whether a health care procedure or service is appropriate for the diagnosis or treatment of a condition. This decision-making process is based on the payer's contractual language and the treating provider's documentation. Generally, the following criteria are used to determine medical necessity: purpose, scope, evidence, and value. The DHHS agencies CMS and NCHS prepare guidelines for coding and reporting using ICD-10-CM, which are approved by the four organizations that comprise the cooperating parties for the ICD-10-CM/PCS and include the AHA, AHIMA, CMS, and NCHS, and are used as a companion document when assigning ICD-10-CM codes. The ICD-10-CM guidelines are rules that were developed to accompany and complement the official conventions and instructions provided in ICD-10-CM. They are based on coding and sequencing instructions in ICD-10-CM, but provide additional instruction.

A joint effort between the health care provider and the coder is essential to achieving complete and accurate documentation, code assignment, and reporting of diagnoses and procedures. Consistent, complete documentation in the patient record is crucial because without such documentation, accurate codes cannot be assigned. In addition, the entire patient record must be reviewed to determine the specific reason for the encounter and the conditions treated so that appropriate codes are assigned.

Upon implementation of ICD-10-CM (and ICD-10-PCS), ICD-9-CM became a _legacy coding system (or legacy classification system)_, which means it is used as archive data but is no longer supported or updated. _General equivalence mappings (GEMs)_ are translation dictionaries or crosswalks of codes that can be used to roughly identify ICD-10-CM codes for their ICD-9-CM equivalent codes (and vice versa).

Coding conventions are general rules used in the ICD-10-CM classification, independent of official coding guidelines. An indented format is used for ease in reference in the ICD-10-CM index. ICD-10-CM contains eponyms and abbreviations. Punctuation in ICD-10-CM includes parentheses, brackets, square brackets, and colons. Certain main terms in the ICD-10-CM index, including the Table of Neoplasms, are followed by boxed notes, which contain special instructions. The ICD-10-CM index contains a Table of Neoplasms and a Table of

Drugs and Chemicals. The ICD-10-CM tabular list contains includes notes, excludes1 and excludes2 notes, and inclusion terms.

"Other" and "other specified" codes are assigned when patient record documentation provides detail for which a specific code does not exist in ICD-10-CM. "Unspecified" codes are assigned because patient record documentation is insufficient for the assignment of a more specific code. Etiology and manifestation codes contain the following notes in the ICD-10-CM tabular list: code first underlying disease; code, if applicable, any causal condition first; use additional code; and in diseases classified elsewhere. When the word *and* appears in category titles and code descriptions in the ICD-10-CM index and tabular list, it is interpreted as meaning "and/or."

The instruction *due to* is located in ICD-10-CM as a subterm (in alphabetical order) to indicate the presence of a cause-and-effect relationship between two conditions. The word *in* as it appears in the ICD-10-CM index is located in alphabetical order below the main term. The word *with* appears in the ICD-10-CM and ICD-10-PCS indexes immediately below the main term, and it is not in alphabetical order. A causal relationship is presumed between two conditions linked by terms *in, with*, and *due to* in the index and tabular list; such conditions are coded as related even when physician documentation explicitly linking them is absent (unless the documentation clearly states the conditions are unrelated) or when another official coding guideline exists that specifically requires a documented linkage between two conditions. For conditions not specifically linked by the terms *with* and *due to* in ICD-10-CM or when an official coding guideline requires that a linkage between two conditions be explicitly documented, physician documentation must link the conditions to code them as related.

Cross-reference terms in the ICD-10-CM index instruct the coder to refer to another entry in the index or to go directly to the tabular list or table, respectively, to assign or build the correct code. The code assignment and clinical criteria coding convention bases the assignment of a diagnosis code on the physician's diagnostic statement that the condition exists, not clinical criteria used to establish the diagnosis. The general coding guidelines are followed when assigning ICD-10-CM diagnosis codes for inpatient, outpatient, and physician office settings.

Internet Links

AHA Coding Clinic Advisor: www.codingclinicadvisor.com

ICD-10-CM: Go to **www.cms.gov**, click on Medicare, click on ICD-10 under Coding, and click on links in the first column to locate coding manual PDF files, general equivalence mappings (GEMs), and more.

ICD-10-CM search tool: https://icd10cmtool.cdc.gov

ICD-10-CM updates: Go to **www.cms.gov**, click on the Medicare link, click on the ICD-10 link under Coding, and scroll down to click on this year's ICD-10-CM link.

JustCoding News free e-newsletter: Go to **www.justcoding.com**, and click on the eNewsletter Signup link at the top of the page.

Review

2.1 – Multiple Choice: Format of the ICD-10-CM Index to Diseases and Injuries

Instructions: Select the most appropriate response to indicate the format used in the ICD-10-CM Index to Diseases and Injuries.

ICD-10-CM Index to Diseases and Injuries
Abnormal, abnormality, abnormalities
–*see also* Anomaly
chromosome, chromosomal Q99.9
sex Q99.8
female phenotype Q97.9

1. Which ICD-10-CM Index to Diseases and Injuries entry uses the *continuation line* format?
    a. Abnormal, abnormality, abnormalities
    b. *–see also* Anomaly
    c. chromosome, chromosomal Q99.9
    d. sex Q99.8
    e. female phenotype Q97.9

2. Which ICD-10-CM Index to Diseases and Injuries entry uses the *main term* format?
    a. Abnormal, abnormality, abnormalities
    b. *–see also* Anomaly
    c. chromosome, chromosomal Q99.9
    d. sex Q99.8
    e. female phenotype Q97.9

3. Which ICD-10-CM Index to Diseases and Injuries entry uses the *second qualifier* format?
    a. Abnormal, abnormality, abnormalities
    b. *–see also* Anomaly
    c. chromosome, chromosomal Q99.9
    d. sex Q99.8
    e. female phenotype Q97.9

4. Which ICD-10-CM Index to Diseases and Injuries entry uses the *subterm* format?
    a. Abnormal, abnormality, abnormalities
    b. *–see also* Anomaly
    c. chromosome, chromosomal Q99.9
    d. sex Q99.8
    e. female phenotype Q97.9

5. Which ICD-10-CM Index to Diseases and Injuries entry uses the *third qualifier* format?
    a. Abnormal, abnormality, abnormalities
    b. *–see also* Anomaly
    c. chromosome, chromosomal Q99.9
    d. sex Q99.8
    e. female phenotype Q97.9

2.2 – Multiple Choice: ICD-10-CM Tabular List of Diseases and Injuries

Instructions: Select the most appropriate response to indicate the format used in the ICD-10-CM Tabular List of Diseases and Injuries.

ICD-10-CM Tabular List of Diseases and Injuries
DISEASES OF THE NERVOUS SYSTEM (G00-G99)
EPISODIC AND PAROXYSMAL DISORDERS (G40-G47)
G43 Migraine
G43.C Periodic headache syndromes in child or adult
G43.C0 Periodic headache syndromes in child or adult, not intractable

1. Which ICD-10-CM Tabular List of Diseases and Injuries entry uses the *category* format?
    a. DISEASES OF THE NERVOUS SYSTEM (G00-G99)
    b. EPISODIC AND PAROXYSMAL DISORDERS (G40-G47)
    c. G43 Migraine
    d. G43.C Periodic headache syndromes in child or adult
    e. G43.C0 Periodic headache syndromes in child or adult, not intractable

2. Which ICD-10-CM Tabular List of Diseases and Injuries entry uses the *chapter title* format?
   a. DISEASES OF THE NERVOUS SYSTEM (G00-G99)
   b. EPISODIC AND PAROXYSMAL DISORDERS (G40-G47)
   c. G43 Migraine
   d. G43.C Periodic headache syndromes in child or adult
   e. G43.C0 Periodic headache syndromes in child or adult, not intractable

3. Which ICD-10-CM Tabular List of Diseases and Injuries entry uses the (valid) *code* format?
   a. DISEASES OF THE NERVOUS SYSTEM (G00-G99)
   b. EPISODIC AND PAROXYSMAL DISORDERS (G40-G47)
   c. G43 Migraine
   d. G43.C Periodic headache syndromes in child or adult
   e. G43.C0 Periodic headache syndromes in child or adult, not intractable

4. Which ICD-10-CM Tabular List of Diseases and Injuries entry uses the *section title* format?
   a. DISEASES OF THE NERVOUS SYSTEM (G00-G99)
   b. EPISODIC AND PAROXYSMAL DISORDERS (G40-G47)
   c. G43 Migraine
   d. G43.C Periodic headache syndromes in child or adult
   e. G43.C0 Periodic headache syndromes in child or adult, not intractable

5. Which ICD-10-CM Tabular List of Diseases and Injuries entry uses the *subcategory* format?
   a. DISEASES OF THE NERVOUS SYSTEM (G00-G99)
   b. EPISODIC AND PAROXYSMAL DISORDERS (G40-G47)
   c. G43 Migraine
   d. G43.C Periodic headache syndromes in child or adult
   e. G43.C0 Periodic headache syndromes in child or adult, not intractable

2.3 – Multiple Choice: Introduction to ICD-10-CM Coding and Conventions

Instructions: Select the most appropriate response.

1. ICD-10-CM was developed to classify _____ data from inpatient and outpatient records, including physician office records.
   a. morbidity
   b. mortality
   c. procedure
   d. service

2. During a physician office encounter, a patient underwent T3–T4 and blood glucose laboratory test, bone density scan, and chest x-ray. The provider documented hypothyroidism, diabetes mellitus, osteoporosis, and chest pain due to possible hiatal hernia. Which diagnosis justifies medical necessity for the T3–T4 blood test?
   a. chest pain
   b. diabetes mellitus
   c. hypothyroidism
   d. osteoporosis

3. General equivalence mappings are translation dictionaries or _____ of codes.
   a. appendices
   b. crosswalks
   c. indexes
   d. tabular lists

4. Outcome of delivery, follow-up, history, and vaccination are examples of ICD-10-CM
     a. external causes of morbidity.
     b. factors influencing health status.
     c. conditions originating in the perinatal period.
     d. symptoms, signs, and abnormal findings.

5. The Table of Neoplasms is located in the ICD-10-CM
     a. Addendum to the coding manual.
     b. Index to Diseases and Injuries.
     c. Official Guidelines for Coding and Reporting.
     d. Tabular List of Disease and Injuries.

6. Review the ICD-10-CM Index to Diseases and Injuries entry for main term *Contusion* and locate subterm "arm" indented below it. Which ICD-10-CM code appears next to the subterm?
     a. S40
     b. S40.0
     c. S40.02
     d. S40.02-

7. A patient is diagnosed with "tactile agnosia involving body image and other senses." Referring to the ICD-10-CM Index to Diseases and Injuries, which is the main term for this condition?
     a. agnosia
     b. body image
     c. other sense
     d. tactile

8. A patient is diagnosed with "traumatic hematoma with intact skin surface". Referring to the ICD-10-CM Index to Diseases and Injuries, which is the main term for this condition?
     a. hematoma
     b. intact
     c. skin surface
     d. traumatic

9. ICD-10-CM _____ codes are reported by all health care settings.
     a. disease
     b. medical equipment
     c. procedure
     d. service

10. Adhering to official coding guidelines is
     a. at the discretion of a health care facility's operating procedures.
     b. mandated by the Cooperating Parties for the ICD-10-CM/PCS.
     c. not necessary if the facility has a 90 percent or higher coding accuracy rate.
     d. required by the Health Insurance Portability and Accountability Act.

11. Which organization approves the *ICD-10-CM Official Guidelines for Coding and Reporting?*
     a. American Medical Association (AMA)
     b. Cooperating Parties for the ICD-10-CM/PCS
     c. Centers for Medicare and Medicaid Services (CMS)
     d. National Center for Health Statistics (NCHS)

12. If an index entry is too lengthy to fit on one line, additional text is
     a. edited so that the content fits onto just one line.
     b. located on the next line, flush with the preceding line.
     c. moved to the second line and indented two spaces.
     d. printed on the next line and indented five spaces.

13. When an entry in the ICD-10-CM index contains the abbreviation NEC and verification of the code in the tabular list validates the assignment of code, which coding convention explains this code assignment?
    a. Information needed to assign a more specific code has not been obtained from the provider.
    b. The coder is directed to an "other specified" code by the index when a specific code is not available in the tabular list.
    c. Use of a more general code is indicated when the coder is unsure about information contained in documentation.
    d. Whenever a specific code is not available in the index for a condition, the coder is directed to the "other specified" code in the tabular list.

14. When the ICD-10-CM tabular list contains the abbreviation NOS, which coding convention is followed to determine code assignment?
    a. A coder should assign the three-character category code when unsure about the information contained in documentation.
    b. If information to assign a more specific code was not documented by the provider, the coder assigns an "unspecified" code.
    c. The coder is directed to an "other specified" code by the index when a specific code is not available in the tabular list.
    d. Whenever a specific code is not available in the index for a condition, the coder is directed to the "other specified" code in the tabular list.

15. The use of a colon in the ICD-10-CM tabular list indicates
    a. assignment of etiology and manifestation codes, with the manifestation code listed second.
    b. one or more additional terms are needed in the diagnostic statement to classify a condition.
    c. terms following the colon may be present or absent from the provider's diagnostic statement.
    d. the use of synonyms, alternative wording, or explanatory phrases in the coding manual.

16. *Includes* notes appear
    a. below an ICD-10-CM category in the tabular list.
    b. after main terms in the ICD-10-CM index.
    c. above an ICD-10-CM code in the tabular list.
    d. underneath essential modifiers in the ICD-10-CM index.

17. *Excludes1* and *Excludes2* notes appear in the
    a. ICD-10-CM index and tables.
    b. ICD-10-CM index and tabular list.
    c. ICD-10-CM tabular list only.
    d. ICD-10-CM index only.

18. *Trust the index* is an ICD-10-CM concept that is used when
    a. a subterm located in the index is not listed in the tabular list.
    b. additional information was not obtained from the provider.
    c. insufficient documentation prevents the assignment of a more specific code.
    d. the coder is directed to the "other specified" code in the tabular list.

19. Unspecified codes
    a. are classified as "other" codes in the ICD-10-CM tabular list.
    b. contain the NEC abbreviation in the ICD-10-CM index.
    c. result when a code is not found in the ICD-10-CM index for a specified condition.
    d. often contain a fourth or fifth character of 8 or 9.

20. Etiology codes
    a. are designated in the ICD-10-CM index by brackets.
    b. classify a condition that occurs as the result of another condition.
    c. contain a *use additional code* instruction in the ICD-10-CM tabular list.
    d. must be sequenced second as the underlying condition code.

21. The *see also* instruction in the ICD-10-CM index follows a main term, subterm, or qualifier, and it refers the coder to another main term that

    a. allows for assignment of a secondary code.

    b. contains the code that is to be assigned.

    c. may provide additional useful index entries.

    d. must be followed to assign the correct code.

22. Upon review of the ICD-10-CM Index to Diseases and Injuries entry below, the coder locates main term *Retching* and notes the *–see* Vomiting instruction, which means the coder should

ICD-10-CM Index to Diseases and Injuries
Retching *–see* Vomiting
Vomiting R11.10
with nausea R11.2
asphyxia *–see* Foreign body, by site, causing asphyxia, gastric contents

    a. generate a physician query to ask the physician to document a specific diagnosis.

    b. go to main term *Vomiting* in the ICD-10-CM index to begin locating the code.

    c. locate the main term in the ICD-9-CM index and use the GEM to assign the code.

    d. review the ICD-10-CM Tabular List of Diseases and Injuries to locate the code.

23. A patient was using a nail gun and accidentally nailed the fleshy skin between the left thumb and fore-finger to the roof of his home. The patient was able to pull the flesh free, but the nail remained embedded in the skin of the left hand. The patient received treatment for *puncture, left hand, with retention of foreign body*. After reviewing the ICD-10-CM index entries below and following the *–see* cross-reference for main term *Foreign body* and subterm *in*, the coder should

ICD-10-CM Index to Diseases and Injuries
Foreign body
in
puncture wound *–see* Puncture, by site, with foreign body
soft tissue (residual) M79.5
Puncture
hand S61.439
with
foreign body S61.449
finger *–see* Puncture, finger
left S61.432
with
foreign body S61.442

    a. assign code M79.5 after verifying it in the tabular list.

    b. locate code S61.439 in the tabular list, adding seventh character A.

    c. look up code S61.449 in the tabular list, adding seventh character A.

    d. verify code S61.442 in the tabular list, adding seventh character A.

24. Upon review of the ICD-10-CM tabular list entry below, which code would be assigned for a patient who was struck in the right eye with a plastic straw three months ago and is being seen today for pain and swelling, right eye, due to a tiny piece of plastic embedded in the soft tissue?

ICD-10-CM Tabular List of Diseases and Injuries
H05.5 **Retained (old) foreign body following penetrating wound of orbit**
Retrobulbar foreign body
Use additional code to identify the type of retained foreign body (Z18.-)
EXCLUDES1 *current penetrating wound of orbit (S05.4-)*
EXCLUDES2 *retained foreign body of eyelid (H02.81-)*
retained intraocular foreign body (H44.6-, H44.7-)
H05.50 **Retained (old) foreign body following penetrating wound of unspecified orbit**
H05.51 **Retained (old) foreign body following penetrating wound of right orbit**
H05.52 **Retained (old) foreign body following penetrating wound of left orbit**
H05.53 **Retained (old) foreign body following penetrating wound of bilateral orbits**

    a. H02.81-   c. H05.51
    b. H05.50   d. S05.4-

25. Upon review of the ICD-10-CM index entry below, which code would be selected for a patient diagnosed with *hypotension due to hemodialysis*?

ICD-10-CM Index to Diseases and Injuries
Hypotension (arterial) (constitutional) I95.9
chronic I95.89
due to (of) hemodialysis I95.3
drug-induced I95.2
iatrogenic I95.89
idiopathic (permanent) I95.0

    a. I95.0   c. I95.3
    b. I95.2   d. I95.89

26. Upon review of the ICD-10-CM index entry below, which action should the coder take to locate the code for *strangulated hernia*?

ICD-10-CM Index to Diseases and Injuries
Strangulation, strangulated *–see also* Asphyxia, traumatic
appendix K38.8
bladder-neck N32.0
bowel or colon K56.2
food or foreign body *–see* Foreign body, by site
hemorrhoids *–see* Hemorrhoids, with complication
hernia *–see also* Hernia, by site, with obstruction
with gangrene *–see* Hernia, by site, with gangrene
intestine (large) (small) K56.2
with hernia *–see* also Hernia, by site, with obstruction
with gangrene *–see* Hernia, by site, with gangrene

    a. Follow the *see also* instruction, and go to Asphyxia, traumatic.
    b. Follow the *see also* instruction, and locate Hernia, by site, with obstruction.
    c. Locate code K56.2 in the ICD-10-CM Tabular List of Diseases and Injuries.
    d. Report code K56.2 in addition to the strangulated hernia code.

27. Using both the ICD-10-CM index and tabular list when assigning codes results in
    a. accurate code assignment.
    b. coding errors.
    c. less specificity when selecting codes.
    d. selection of laterality for all codes.

28. When a related definitive diagnosis has not been established (or confirmed) by the provider for an outpatient or physician office encounter, codes are assigned to
    a. canceled procedures.
    b. hierarchical conditions.
    c. ruled out diagnoses.
    d. signs and symptoms.

29. When the provider documents the same condition as acute (or subacute) and chronic during an encounter, and the ICD-10-CM index contains subentries for each,
    a. assign a code to the acute (or subacute) condition only.
    b. generate a physician query to determine code sequencing.
    c. code both, and sequence the acute (or subacute) code first.
    d. report codes for both, and sequence the chronic condition first.

30. When a residual effect is documented after the acute phase of injury or illness has ended, a code for the _____ condition is sequenced first.
    a. acute
    b. diagnostic
    c. qualified
    d. residual

2.4 – Coding Practice: General ICD-10-CM Coding Guidelines and Coding Conventions

Instructions: Use the ICD-10-CM index and tabular list to assign the appropriate code to each diagnostic statement. Refer to general ICD-10-CM coding guidelines and coding conventions when assigning codes.

1. Borderline hypertension _____

2. Postoperative incisional hernia (following open cholecystectomy three months ago) _____

3. Acute abdominal syndrome _____

4. Adjustment disorder with anxiety _____

5. Anorexia nervosa, restricting type _____

6. Parkinsonism with neurogenic orthostatic hypotension _____

7. Hyperthyroidism due to ectopic thyroid tissue with thyroid storm _____

8. Alzheimer's disease, early onset with behavioral disturbance _____

9. Bone hypoplasia _____

10. Iatrogenic hypopituitarism _____

Chapter-Specific Coding Guidelines: ICD-10-CM Chapters 1–10

Chapter Outline

ICD-10-CM Chapter-Specific Coding Guidelines

ICD-10-CM Chapter 1: Certain Infectious and Parasitic Diseases (A00–B99), U07.1, U09.9

ICD-10-CM Chapter 2: Neoplasms (C00–D49)

ICD-10-CM Chapter 3: Diseases of the Blood and Blood-Forming Organs and Certain Disorders Involving the Immune Mechanism (D50–D89)

ICD-10-CM Chapter 4: Endocrine, Nutritional, and Metabolic Diseases (E00–E89)

ICD-10-CM Chapter 5: Mental, Behavioral, and Neurodevelopmental Disorders (F01–F99)

ICD-10-CM Chapter 6: Diseases of the Nervous System (G00–G99)

ICD-10-CM Chapter 7: Diseases of the Eye and Adnexa (H00–H59)

ICD-10-CM Chapter 8: Diseases of the Ear and Mastoid Process (H60–H95)

ICD-10-CM Chapter 9: Diseases of the Circulatory System (I00–I99)

ICD-10-CM Chapter 10: Diseases of the Respiratory System (J00–J99), U07.0

Chapter Objectives

At the conclusion of this chapter, the student should be able to:

1. Define key terms related to chapter-specific coding guidelines for ICD-10-CM Chapters 1 through 10.
2. Assign ICD-10-CM codes to certain infectious and parasitic diseases according to chapter-specific coding guidelines.
3. Assign ICD-10-CM codes to neoplasms according to chapter-specific coding guidelines.
4. Assign ICD-10-CM codes to diseases of the blood and blood-forming organs and certain disorders involving the immune mechanism according to chapter-specific coding guidelines.
5. Assign ICD-10-CM codes to endocrine, nutritional, and metabolic diseases according to chapter-specific coding guidelines.
6. Assign ICD-10-CM codes to mental, behavioral, and neurodevelopmental disorders according to chapter-specific coding guidelines.
7. Assign ICD-10-CM codes to diseases of the nervous system according to chapter-specific coding guidelines.

8. Assign ICD-10-CM codes to diseases of the eye and adnexa according to chapter-specific coding guidelines.

9. Assign ICD-10-CM codes to diseases of the ear and mastoid process according to chapter-specific coding guidelines.

10. Assign ICD-10-CM codes to diseases of the circulatory system according to chapter-specific coding guidelines.

11. Assign ICD-10-CM codes to diseases of the respiratory system according to chapter-specific coding guidelines.

Key Terms

benign	metastatic cancer	secondary malignancy	uncertain behavior
carcinoma (Ca) *in situ*	neoplasm	type 1 diabetes mellitus	unspecified behavior
contiguous sites	overlapping sites	type 2 diabetes mellitus	
malignant	primary malignancy		

Introduction

This chapter includes content about the following chapter-specific coding guidelines for ICD-10-CM Chapters 1 through 10. Chapter-specific coding guidelines are used as a companion to the ICD-10-CM coding manual, which contains coding conventions to ensure accurate coding.

- Certain Infectious and Parasitic Diseases (A00–B99), U07.1, U09.9
- Neoplasms (C00–D49)
- Diseases of the Blood and Blood-forming Organs and Certain Disorders Involving the Immune Mechanism (D50–D89)
- Endocrine, Nutritional, and Metabolic Diseases (E00–E89)
- Mental, Behavioral, and Neurodevelopmental Disorders (F01–F99)
- Diseases of the Nervous System (G00–G99)
- Diseases of the Eye and Adnexa (H00–H59)
- Diseases of the Ear and Mastoid Process (H60–H95)
- Diseases of the Circulatory System (I00–I99)
- Diseases of the Respiratory System (J00–J99), U07.0, U09.9

The *ICD-10-CM Official Guidelines for Coding and Reporting* (and the *ICD-10-PCS Official Guidelines for Coding and Reporting*) are rules that were developed to accompany and complement the official conventions and instructions located in the classification system. They are based on coding and sequencing instructions in the classification system but provide additional instruction. Adherence to these guidelines when assigning diagnosis and procedure codes is required under HIPAA. ICD-10-CM diagnosis codes were adopted for all health care settings. (ICD-10-PCS procedure codes were adopted for inpatient hospital procedures.) A joint effort between the health care provider and the coder is essential to achieve complete and accurate documentation.

NOTE:

- ICD-10-PCS procedure coding is located in Chapters 6 and 7 because it impacts inpatient hospital coding only.
- When reviewing examples and completing exercises and review questions in this chapter, use your ICD-10-CM coding manual to locate index entries and to verify codes in the tabular list.

ICD-10-CM codes assigned to patient encounters must be supported by documentation in the patient's record. Third-party payers require submitted claims to demonstrate medical necessity for treatment, which means that a diagnosis code must be reported for each procedure or service code included on the claim. (ICD-10-PCS procedure codes are reported for inpatient hospital procedures, and its codes and coding guidelines are discussed in Chapters 6 and 7. HCPCS Level II and CPT codes are reported on outpatient claims and are discussed in Chapters 8–19.)

ICD-10-CM Chapter-Specific Coding Guidelines

In addition to coding conventions and general coding guidelines, the *ICD-10-CM Official Guidelines for Coding and Reporting* contain chapter-specific coding guidelines that clarify the assignment of disease codes. Unless otherwise indicated, chapter-specific coding guidelines apply to all health care settings. Some coding guidelines include the following terms, which apply to the reporting of outpatient (and physician office) diagnoses (Chapter 5) and inpatient hospital diagnoses and procedures (Chapters 6 and 7). The terms are briefly defined below to clarify their use in the chapter-specific coding guidelines.

- *Principal diagnosis* is reported for inpatient hospital care *only*, and it is "that condition established after study to be chiefly responsible for occasioning the admission of the patient to the hospital for care."

- *Secondary diagnoses* are additional conditions that affect patient care (in any health care setting), requiring clinical evaluation, therapeutic treatment and diagnostic procedures, extended lengths of hospital stay, increased nursing care, or monitoring in inpatient hospitals.

- *First-listed diagnosis* is reported for outpatient and physician office care *only* (instead of the principal diagnosis), and it is the diagnosis, condition, problem, or other reason for an encounter or visit documented in the medical record to be chiefly responsible for the services provided. (The first-listed diagnosis was previously called the *primary diagnosis*. Some third-party payers, government health plans, and vendors continue to refer to *primary diagnosis*, which is interpreted as *first-listed diagnosis*. CPT also refers to *primary procedure* in its coding system, which is a concept that requires assignment of a CPT primary procedure code before a CPT add-on or additional code is assigned.)

ICD-10-CM Chapter-Specific Coding Guidelines

To locate the ICD-10-CM chapter-specific coding guidelines online, go to **cms.gov**, click on the Medicare link, scroll down to the Coding heading and click on the ICD-10 link; then, click on the current year's ICD-10-CM link and click on the current year's Coding Guidelines (PDF) link, which will open as an Adobe PDF file.

The *ICD-10-CM Official Guidelines for Coding and Reporting* publication includes a table of contents that organizes chapter-specific coding guidelines according to chapters in the ICD-10-CM classification system (Table 3-1). Although chapter-specific coding guidelines have not been created for every ICD-10-CM chapter, the title of each ICD-10-CM chapter is included in the table of contents with the statement "Reserved for future guideline expansion." Refer to chapter-specific coding guidelines when assigning ICD-10-CM diagnosis codes.

TABLE 3-1 Portion of Chapter-Specific Coding Guidelines Table of Contents from *ICD-10-CM Official Guidelines for Coding and Reporting*

Courtesy of the Centers for Medicare & Medicaid Services, www.cms.gov

ICD-10-CM Chapter 1: Certain Infectious and Parasitic Diseases (A00–B99), U07.1, U09.9

NOTE:

Infections are also classified in other ICD-10-CM chapters, such as Chapter 10, Diseases of the Respiratory System.

This ICD-10-CM chapter classifies the following infectious and parasitic diseases (Table 3-2):

- Intestinal infectious diseases
- Tuberculosis
- Certain zoonotic bacterial diseases
- Other bacterial diseases
- Infections with a predominantly sexual mode of transmission
- Other spirochetal diseases
- Other diseases caused by chlamydiae
- Rickettsioses
- Viral and prion infections of the central nervous system
- Arthropod-borne viral fevers and viral hemorrhagic fevers
- Viral infections characterized by skin and mucous membrane lesions
- Other human herpesviruses
- Viral hepatitis
- Human immunodeficiency virus (HIV) disease
- Other viral diseases (e.g., coronavirus)
- Mycoses
- Protozoal diseases
- Helminthiases
- Pediculosis, acariasis, and other infestations
- Sequelae of infectious and parasitic diseases
- Bacterial and viral infectious agents
- Other infectious diseases

TABLE 3-2 Organisms

Organism	Definition
Bacteria	• Single-celled organisms that in certain conditions cause illnesses such as strep throat, most ear infections, and bacterial pneumonia • Some bacteria are considered helpful (e.g., intestinal *Escherichia coli*)
Chlamydia	• Infection caused by a parasitic bacteria called *Chlamydia trachomatis* • Affects male and female genitals
Fungi	• Opportunistic pathogens such as *Aspergillus, Candida*, and *Cryptococcus* that cause infections in immunocompromised people such as cancer patients, transplant recipients, and people with AIDS • Pathogens such as endemic mycoses, histoplasmosis, coccidioidomycosis, and superficial mycoses that cause infections in healthy people
Helminths	• Parasitic worms that usually lodge in the intestines • Include roundworm, pinworm, *Trichinella spiralis* (causes trichinosis), tapeworm, and fluke
Mycoplasmas	• Surface parasites of the human respiratory and urogenital tracts • Mainly affect children aged 5 to 9 years • Spread by close personal contact • Have a long incubation period

Protozoans	• Single-celled organisms (e.g., amoeba) that cause parasitic diseases in people with AIDS
	  ○ Toxoplasmosis
	  ○ Cryptosporidiosis
	• *Pneumocystis jirovecii* pneumonia (PJP) is caused by fungi
	  ○ Does not respond to antifungal treatment
	  ○ Formerly known as *Pneumocystis carinii pneumonia* (PCP)

Rickettsiae	• Intracellular parasites that grow and reproduce only in living cells of their host • Named for U.S. pathologist Howard T. Ricketts, who died of typhus in 1910 while investigating the spread of the disease • Typhus fever is caused by *Rickettsia prowazekii* when transmitted to humans by lice • Rocky Mountain spotted fever is a rickettsial disease transmitted to humans by ticks
Viruses	• Submicroscopic parasites that cause disease • Contain DNA or RNA, are surrounded by protein, and use host cells to replicate • Include varicella (chickenpox virus), cold viruses, coronaviruses, hepatitis viruses, herpesviruses, and human immunodeficiency virus (HIV)

ICD-10-CM Chapter-Specific Coding Guidelines

Chapter 1: Certain Infectious and Parasitic Diseases (A00–B99), U07.1, U09.9

a. Human Immunodeficiency Virus (HIV) infections

   1) Code only confirmed cases

   Code only confirmed cases of HIV infection/illness. This is an exception to the hospital inpatient guideline Section II, H (Uncertain Diagnosis).

   In this context, "confirmation" does not require documentation of positive serology or culture for HIV; the provider's diagnostic statement that the patient is HIV positive or has an HIV-related illness is sufficient.

Example: A 38-year-old patient with symptomatic HIV disease is seen in follow-up at the office. The patient was discharged from the hospital last week after inpatient treatment of *Pneumocystis jirovecii* pneumonia (PJP), which is an opportunistic infection for an HIV-positive patient. Lab tests today reveal CBC hemoglobin of 9.0, hematocrit 27, and normal WBC differential and platelets. Hepatitis A, B, and C tests negative. Cytomegalovirus (CMV) test negative. Rapid plasma reagin test negative. Decreased reticulocytes of 0.3 noted. Normal peripheral smear. Parvovirus B19 antibody test negative. Comprehensive metabolic panel was normal. CD4 test revealed somewhat depressed T helper cell level of 460. Viral load is 22,000. Erythropoietin level elevated at 120 milliunits per milliliter. Patient was started on medications of nevirapine plus Combivir.

In this example, the provider's statement of a "symptomatic HIV-positive patient" is sufficient to assign ICD-10-CM code B20 for HIV infection. Because the PJP is resolved, code B59 is not assigned.

2) Selection and sequencing of HIV codes

(a) Patient admitted for HIV-related condition

If a patient is admitted for an HIV-related condition, the principal diagnosis should be B20, Human immunodeficiency virus [HIV] disease, followed by additional diagnosis codes for all reported HIV-related conditions.

An exception to this guideline is if the reason for admission is hemolytic-uremic syndrome associated with HIV disease. Assign code D59.31, Infection-associated hemolytic-uremic syndrome, followed by code B20, Human immunodeficiency virus [HIV] disease.

Example: A 42-year-old symptomatic HIV-positive patient undergoes treatment for septic arthritis of the left shoulder. Culture and sensitivity lab test reveals *Klebsiella pneumoniae* as the bacterial agent. Because septic arthritis is considered an opportunistic infection in an HIV-positive patient, sequence the HIV code (B20) first and then the opportunistic infection codes (M00.812 and B96.1).

(b) Patient with HIV disease admitted for unrelated condition

If a patient with HIV disease is admitted for an unrelated condition (such as a traumatic injury), the code for the unrelated condition (e.g., the nature of injury code) should be the principal diagnosis. Other diagnoses would be B20 followed by additional diagnosis codes for all reported HIV-related conditions.

Example: A 53-year-old patient with symptomatic HIV disease undergoes treatment for a closed left wrist fracture. In this example, a fracture is not considered an opportunistic infection or disease in an HIV-positive patient, and it is considered a condition unrelated to HIV status. Therefore, sequence the closed left wrist fracture code (S62.102A) and then the HIV code (B20).

(c) Whether the patient is newly diagnosed

Whether the patient is newly diagnosed or has had previous admissions/encounters for HIV conditions is irrelevant to the sequencing decision.

(d) Asymptomatic human immunodeficiency virus

Z21, Asymptomatic human immunodeficiency virus [HIV] infection status, is to be applied when the patient without any documentation of symptoms is listed as being "HIV positive," "known HIV," "HIV test positive," or similar terminology. Do not use this code if the term *AIDS* or *HIV disease* is used or if the patient is treated for any HIV-related illness or is described as having any condition(s) resulting from their HIV-positive status; use B20 in these cases.

Example: A 42-year-old HIV-positive asymptomatic patient undergoes routine CD4 testing to determine current levels. In this example, even though the patient is HIV-positive, the patient is also asymptomatic, which means that there are no documented symptoms. Therefore, assign code Z21 for asymptomatic HIV status. *Do not assign code B20, which is assigned to patients diagnosed as HIV positive who are treated for HIV-related illness(es) or to patients described as having AIDS.*

(continues)

ICD-10-CM Chapter-Specific Coding Guidelines (*continued*)

(e) Patients with inconclusive HIV serology

Patients with inconclusive HIV serology, but no definitive diagnosis or manifestations of the illness, may be assigned code R75, Inconclusive laboratory evidence of human immunodeficiency virus [HIV].

Example: A 52-year-old asymptomatic patient was seen in the office after having undergone HIV testing, the results of which proved inconclusive. Patient is scheduled for repeat HIV test. In this example, assign code R75 for an inconclusive laboratory evidence of HIV and code Z11.4 for "screening for HIV status" because the patient is being seen to determine HIV status. If HIV counseling was provided during the encounter, code Z71.7 would also be assigned. If the patient was determined to be in a high-risk group for HIV, such as *high risk bisexual behavior*, code Z72.53 would also be assigned.

(f) Previously diagnosed HIV-related illness

Patients with any known prior diagnosis of an HIV-related illness should be coded to B20. Once a patient has developed an HIV-related illness, the patient should always be assigned code B20 on every subsequent admission/encounter. Patients previously diagnosed with any HIV illness (B20) should never be assigned to R75 (inconclusive laboratory evidence of human immunodeficiency virus [HIV]) or Z21 (asymptomatic human immunodeficiency virus [HIV] infection status).

Example: A 29-year-old HIV-positive patient is seen in the office to undergo routine CD4 testing. The patient has a past history of being treated for HIV wasting syndrome and Hodgkin disease and is currently asymptomatic. In this example, because the patient has known prior diagnoses of HIV-related illnesses, assign code B20 for HIV disease. *Although the patient is currently asymptomatic, according to official coding guidelines, it is incorrect to assign code R75 for inconclusive HIV test or code Z21 for asymptomatic HIV status.*

(g) HIV infection in pregnancy, childbirth, and the puerperium

During pregnancy, childbirth or the puerperium, a patient admitted (or presenting for a health care encounter) because of an HIV-related illness should receive a principal diagnosis code of O98.7-, Human immunodeficiency [HIV] disease complicating pregnancy, childbirth and the puerperium, followed by B20 and the code(s) for the HIV-related illness(es). Codes from Chapter 15 (of ICD-10-CM) always take sequencing priority. Patients with asymptomatic HIV infection status admitted (or presenting for a health care encounter) during pregnancy, childbirth, or the puerperium should be assigned codes O98.7- and Z21.

Example: A 33-year-old HIV-positive patient in the second trimester of pregnancy received inpatient treatment for cytomegalovirus (CMV) disease, which is an HIV-related illness. The patient was discharged to follow up with Dr. Jones regarding the CMV and will continue to receive prenatal care from Dr. Miller. When a pregnant patient is admitted for an HIV-related illness, assign code O98.712, Human immunodeficiency virus [HIV] disease complicating pregnancy, second trimester. Then, assign code B20 for HIV disease and code B25.9 for the HIV-related condition of CMV.

When this patient is admitted for delivery, even if an asymptomatic HIV infection status is documented upon admission, assign code O98.72 for the delivery and code B20 for HIV disease (because the patient was admitted during the antepartum period for treatment of an HIV-related condition). (In the case of an HIV-positive patient who delivers and who has *not* been treated for an HIV-related condition in the past, assign codes O98.72 and Z21.) (An outcome of delivery code is also assigned.)

(h) Encounters for testing for HIV

If a patient is being seen to determine his/her HIV status, use code Z11.4, Encounter for screening for human immunodeficiency virus [HIV]. Use additional codes for any associated high-risk behavior, if applicable. If a patient with signs or symptoms is being seen for HIV testing, code the signs and symptoms. An additional counseling code Z71.7, Human immunodeficiency virus [HIV] counseling, may be used if counseling is provided during the encounter for the test.

When a patient returns to be informed of his/her HIV test results and the test result is negative, use code Z71.7, Human immunodeficiency virus [HIV] counseling. If the results are positive see previous guidelines and assign codes as appropriate.

(i) HIV managed by antiretroviral medication

If a patient with documented HIV disease, HIV-related illness, or AIDS is currently managed on antiretroviral medications, assign code B20, Human immunodeficiency virus [HIV] disease. Code Z79.899, Other long term (current) drug therapy, may be assigned as an additional code to identify the long-term (current) use of antiretroviral medications.

Example: Patient with HIV disease is seen in the office today for management of long-term antiretroviral medications. Assign codes B20 and Z79.899, in that order.

(j) Encounter for HIV prophylaxis measures

When a patient is seen for administration of pre-exposure prophylaxis medication for HIV, assign code Z29.81, Encounter for HIV pre-exposure prophylaxis. Pre-exposure prophylaxis (PrEP) is intended to prevent infection in people who are at risk for getting HIV through sex or injection drug use. Any risk factors for HIV should also be coded.

b. Infectious agents as the cause of diseases classified to other chapters

Certain infections are classified in chapters other than Chapter 1 and no organism is identified as part of the infection code. In these instances, it is necessary to use an additional code from ICD-10-CM Chapter 1 to identify the organism. A code from category B95, *Streptococcus*, *Staphylococcus*, and *Enterococcus* as the cause of diseases classified to other chapters, B96, Other bacterial agents as the cause of diseases classified to other chapters, or B97, Viral agents as the cause of diseases classified to other chapters, is to be used as an additional code to identify the organism. An instructional note will be found at the infection code advising that an additional organism code is required.

Example: A patient is diagnosed with urinary tract infection due to *Escherichia coli*. Assign codes N39.0 (Urinary tract infection, site unspecified) and B96.20 (Unspecified *Escherichia coli* [*E. coli*] as the cause of diseases classified elsewhere), in that order. (An instruction note below code N39.0 in the ICD-10-CM tabular list directs the coder to use an additional code to identify the infectious agent.)

c. Infections resistant to antibiotics

Many bacterial infections are resistant to current antibiotics. It is necessary to identify all infections documented as antibiotic resistant. Assign a code from category Z16, Resistance to antimicrobial drugs following the infection code only if the infection code does not identify drug resistance.

Example: Antibiotics, antimicrobials, and antimycobacterials are generally classified according to chemical structure, with some classes destroying microorganisms and others preventing them from multiplying. *Antibiotics* destroy or slow the growth of bacteria. *Antimicrobials* destroy or slow the spread of microorganisms in general (e.g., bacteria, fungi, helminths, protozoans, viruses) without damaging the host using a process called *selective toxicity*. *Antimycobacterials* inhibit growth or destroy mycobacteria that cause tuberculosis and leprosy. The ICD-10-CM Index to Diseases and Injuries provides direction to code assignment for patient resistance to individual drugs and multiple drug groupings. In the ICD-10-CM index, go to main term *Resistance, resistant (to)*, subterm *organism(s)*, second qualifier *to*, and third qualifier *drug* to review fourth and fifth qualifiers that include individual drugs (e.g., amoxicillin) and multiple drug groupings (e.g., antibiotics, antimicrobials, and antimycobacterials).

- For a patient with resistance to the amoxicillin antibiotic, assign code Z16.11 (Resistance to penicillins). The ICD-10-CM index provides direction to the code, and the drug is listed as an inclusion term below the code description. *Penicillin* is a drug class that destroys bacteria by preventing formation of the bacterial cell wall. The term *beta-lactam* is used in the category description, and it is a drug class that prevents penicillin (and cephalosporin) drugs from being destroyed by an enzyme produced by some bacteria, increasing the drugs' effectiveness. (Penicillins can be administered orally as well as via injection or infusion.) (When a patient is resistant to multiple antibiotic drugs, code Z16.24, Resistance to multiple antibiotics, is reported.)

(continues)

ICD-10-CM Chapter-Specific Coding Guidelines (*continued*)

Example (*continued*)

- For a patient with resistance to both the vancomycin antibiotic *and* the quinine antimicrobial, assign codes Z16.21 (Resistance to vancomycin) *and* Z16.31 (Resistance to antiparasitic drugs) because the drugs are classed differently. Vancomycin is a *glycopeptide* (drug class), which destroys bacteria, is administered by injection or infusion, and is classified to ICD-10-CM subcategory Z16.2- (Resistance to other antibiotics). Quinine is an *antiparasitic* (drug class), which destroys parasites (e.g., parasite that causes malaria) and is classified to ICD-10-CM subcategory Z16.3- (Resistance to other antimicrobial drugs).

d. Sepsis, Severe Sepsis, and Septic Shock Infections resistant to antibiotics

   1) Coding of Sepsis and Severe Sepsis

      (a) Sepsis

For a diagnosis of sepsis, assign the appropriate code for the underlying systemic infection. If the type of infection or causal organism is not further specified, assign code A41.9, Sepsis, unspecified organism. A code from subcategory R65.2, Severe sepsis, should not be assigned unless severe sepsis or an associated acute organ dysfunction is documented.

Example 1: Patient is diagnosed with sepsis due to gonococcus, and code A54.86 (Gonococcal sepsis) is reported because the infection is specified. Do not report A41.9 (Sepsis, unspecified organism).

Example 2: Patient is diagnosed with gram-negative sepsis with acute respiratory failure. Report codes A41.50 (Gram-negative sepsis, unspecified), R65.20 (Sepsis without septic shock), and J96.00 (Acute respiratory failure, unspecified whether with hypoxia or hypercapnia), in that order.

(i) Negative or inconclusive blood cultures and sepsis

Negative or inconclusive blood cultures do *not* preclude a diagnosis of sepsis in patients with clinical evidence of the condition; however, the provider should be queried.

(ii) Urosepsis

The term *urosepsis* is a nonspecific term. It is not to be considered synonymous with sepsis. It has no default code in the [ICD-10-CM Index to Diseases and Injuries] Alphabetic Index. Should a provider use this term, he/she must be queried for clarification.

(iii) Sepsis with organ dysfunction

If a patient has sepsis and associated acute organ dysfunction or multiple organ dysfunction (MOD), follow the instructions for coding severe sepsis.

(iv) Acute organ dysfunction that is not clearly associated with the sepsis

If a patient has sepsis and an acute organ dysfunction, but the medical record documentation indicates that the acute organ dysfunction is related to a medical condition other than the sepsis, do not assign a code from subcategory R65.2, Severe sepsis. An acute organ dysfunction must be associated with the sepsis in order to assign the severe sepsis code. If the documentation is not clear as to whether an acute organ dysfunction is related to the sepsis or another medical condition, query the provider.

      (b) Severe sepsis

The coding of severe sepsis requires a minimum of two codes: a code for the underlying systemic infection, followed by a code from subcategory R65.2, Severe sepsis. If the causal organism is not documented, assign code A41.9, Sepsis, unspecified organism, for the infection. Additional code(s) for the associated acute organ dysfunction are also required. Due to the complex nature of severe sepsis, some cases may require querying the provider prior to assignment of the codes.

2) Septic shock

Septic shock generally refers to circulatory failure associated with severe sepsis, and therefore, it represents a type of acute organ dysfunction.

For cases of septic shock, the code for the systemic infection should be sequenced first, followed by code R65.21, Severe sepsis with septic shock or code T81.12, Postprocedural septic shock. Any additional codes for the other acute organ dysfunctions should also be assigned. As noted in the sequencing instructions in the ICD-10-CM tabular list, the code for septic shock *cannot* be assigned as a principal diagnosis.

Example: Patient is diagnosed with septic shock due to *Enterococcus*; acute respiratory failure. Report codes A41.81 (Sepsis due to *Enterococcus*), R65.21 (Severe sepsis with septic shock), and J96.01 (Acute respiratory failure with hypoxia), in that order.

3) Sequencing of severe sepsis

If severe sepsis is present on admission, and meets the definition of principal diagnosis, the underlying systemic infection should be assigned as principal diagnosis followed by the appropriate code from subcategory R65.2 as required by the sequencing rules in the ICD-10-CM tabular list. A code from subcategory R65.2 can never be assigned as a principal diagnosis.

When severe sepsis develops during an encounter (it was not present on admission), the underlying systemic infection and the appropriate code from subcategory R65.2 should be assigned as secondary diagnoses.

Severe sepsis may be present on admission but the diagnosis may not be confirmed until sometime after admission. If the documentation is not clear whether severe sepsis was present on admission, the provider should be queried.

For infection-associated hemolytic-uremic syndrome with severe sepsis, see guideline I.C.1.d.9.

4) Sepsis or severe sepsis with a localized infection

If the reason for admission is sepsis or severe sepsis and a localized infection, such as pneumonia or cellulitis, a code(s) for the underlying systemic infection should be assigned first and the code for the localized infection should be assigned as a secondary diagnosis. If the patient has severe sepsis, a code from subcategory R65.2 should also be assigned as a secondary diagnosis. If the patient is admitted with a localized infection, such as pneumonia, and sepsis/severe sepsis doesn't develop until after admission, the localized infection should be assigned first, followed by the appropriate sepsis/severe sepsis codes.

For hemolytic-uremic syndrome associated with severe sepsis, see guideline I.C.1.d.9.

Example: Patient is diagnosed with acute liver failure due to severe sepsis from Pseudomonas. Report codes A41.52 (Sepsis due to pseudomonas), R65.20 (Severe sepsis without septic shock), and K72.00 (Acute and subacute hepatic failure without coma), in that order.

- For code A41.5, go to ICD-10-CM index main term Sepsis (generalized) (unspecified organism) and subterm *Pseudomonas (pseudomonas aeroginosa)* A41.52. Verify the code in the tabular list.

- For R65.20, to go main term Sepsis (generalized) (unspecified organism), subterm with, and second qualifier organ dysfunction (acute) (multiple) R65.20. Verify the code in the tabular list.

- For code K72.00, go to index main term Shock and subterm liver K72.00. Verify the code in the tabular list.

5) Sepsis due to a postprocedural infection

(a) Documentation of causal relationship

As with all postprocedural complications, code assignment is based on the provider's documentation of the relationship between the infection and the procedure.

(b) Sepsis due to a postprocedural infection

For sepsis following a postprocedural wound (surgical site) infection, a code from T81.41 to T81.43, Infection following a procedure, or a code from O86.00 to O86.03, Infection of obstetric surgical wound, that identifies the site of the infection should be sequenced first, if known. Assign an additional code

(continues)

ICD-10-CM Chapter-Specific Coding Guidelines (*continued*)

for sepsis following a procedure (T81.44) or sepsis following an obstetrical procedure (O86.04). Use an additional code to identify the infectious agent. If the patient has severe sepsis, the appropriate code from subcategory R65.2 should also be assigned with the additional code(s) for any acute organ dysfunction.

For infections following infusion, transfusion, therapeutic injection, or immunization, a code from subcategory T80.2, Infections following infusion, transfusion, and therapeutic injection, or code T88.0-, Infection following immunization, should be coded first, followed by the code for the specific infection. If the patient has severe sepsis, the appropriate code from subcategory R65.2 should also be assigned, with the additional codes(s) for any acute organ dysfunction.

(c) **Postprocedural infection and postprocedural septic shock**

If a postprocedural infection has resulted in postprocedural septic shock, assign the codes indicated above for sepsis due to a postprocedural infection, followed by code T81.12-, Postprocedural septic shock. Do not assign code R65.21, Severe sepsis with septic shock. Additional code(s) should be assigned for any acute organ dysfunction.

6) **Sepsis and severe sepsis associated with a noninfectious process (condition)**

In some cases, a noninfectious process (condition) such as trauma, may lead to an infection which can result in sepsis or severe sepsis. If sepsis or severe sepsis is documented as associated with a noninfectious condition, such as a burn or serious injury, and this condition meets the definition for principal diagnosis, the code for the noninfectious condition should be sequenced first, followed by the code for the resulting infection. If severe sepsis is present a code from subcategory R65.2 should also be assigned with any associated organ dysfunction(s) codes. It is not necessary to assign a code from subcategory R65.1, Systemic inflammatory response syndrome (SIRS) of non-infectious origin, for these cases.

If the infection meets the definition of principal diagnosis it should be sequenced before the non-infectious condition. When both the associated non-infectious condition and the infection meet the definition of principal diagnosis either may be assigned as principal diagnosis.

Only one code from category R65, Symptoms and signs specifically associated with systemic inflammation and infection, should be assigned. Therefore, when a non-infectious condition leads to an infection resulting in severe sepsis, assign the appropriate code from subcategory R65.2, Severe sepsis. Do not additionally assign a code from subcategory R65.1, Systemic inflammatory response syndrome (SIRS) of non-infectious origin.

See Section I.C.18. SIRS due to non-infectious process.

Example: Patient experienced an abrasion to the left inner thigh, after playing soccer. The area developed into a boil that ruptured, and the patient presented to the emergency department with fever, headache, muscle aches, fatigue, shivering, and a generalized sick feeling. Patient was admitted as a hospital inpatient, and skin culture grew methicillin-resistant *Staphylococcus aureus* (MRSA). Inpatient diagnoses included abrasion, left inner thigh, and sepsis due to MRSA. Report code A41.02 for the sepsis and code S70.312A for the abrasion, in that order because sepsis is the reason, after study, for inpatient hospitalization.

For a patient who received initial treatment at the physician's office for the abrasion of left inner thigh, code S70.312A is reported first for that office encounter. If a skin culture was positive for MRSA, code A49.02 for the MRSA infection would also be reported.

7) **Sepsis and septic shock complicating abortion, pregnancy, childbirth, and the puerperium**

See Section I.C.15. Sepsis and septic shock complicating abortion, pregnancy, childbirth and the puerperium.

8) **Newborn sepsis**

See Section I.C.16. f. Bacterial sepsis of NEWBORN.

9) **Hemolytic-uremic syndrome associated with sepsis**

If the reason for admission is hemolytic-uremic syndrome that is associated with sepsis, assign code D59.31, Infection-associated hemolytic-uremic syndrome, as the principal diagnosis. Codes for the underlying systemic infection and any other conditions (such as severe sepsis) should be assigned as secondary diagnoses.

e. Methicillin-Resistant *Staphylococcus aureus* (MRSA) conditions

1) Selection and sequencing of MRSA codes

(a) Combination codes for MRSA infection

When a patient is diagnosed with an infection that is due to methicillin-resistant *Staphylococcus aureus* (MRSA), and that infection has a combination code that includes the causal organism (e.g., sepsis, pneumonia) assign the appropriate combination code for the condition (e.g., code A41.02, Sepsis due to Methicillin-resistant *Staphylococcus aureus*, or code J15.212, Pneumonia due to Methicillin-resistant *Staphylococcus aureus*). Do not assign code B95.62, Methicillin-resistant *Staphylococcus aureus* infection as the cause of diseases classified elsewhere, as an additional code because the combination code includes the type of infection and the MRSA organism. Do not assign a code from subcategory Z16.11, Resistance to penicillins, as an additional diagnosis.

See Section C.1. for instructions on coding and sequencing of sepsis and severe sepsis.

(b) Other codes for MRSA infection

When there is documentation of a current infection (e.g., wound infection, stitch abscess, urinary tract infection) due to MRSA, and that infection does not have a combination code that includes the causal organism, assign the appropriate code to identify the condition along with code B95.62, Methicillin-resistant *Staphylococcus aureus* infection as the cause of diseases classified elsewhere, for the MRSA infection. Do not assign a code from subcategory Z16.11, Resistance to penicillins.

(c) Methicillin-susceptible *Staphylococcus aureus* (MSSA) and MRSA colonization

The condition or state of being colonized or carrying MSSA or MRSA is called colonization or carriage, while an individual person is described as being colonized or being a carrier.

Colonization means that MSSA or MSRA is present on or in the body without necessarily causing illness. A positive MRSA colonization test might be documented by the provider as "MRSA screen positive" or "MRSA nasal swab positive."

Assign code Z22.322, Carrier or suspected carrier of Methicillin-resistant *Staphylococcus aureus*, for patients documented as having MRSA colonization. Assign code Z22.321, Carrier or suspected carrier of Methicillin-susceptible *Staphylococcus aureus*, for patients documented as having MSSA colonization. Colonization is not necessarily indicative of a disease process or as the cause of a specific condition the patient may have unless documented as such by the provider.

(d) MRSA colonization and infection

If a patient is documented as having both MRSA colonization and infection during a hospital admission, code Z22.322, Carrier or suspected carrier of Methicillin-resistant *Staphylococcus aureus*, and a code for the MRSA infection may both be assigned.

f. Zika virus infections

1) Code only confirmed cases

Code only a confirmed diagnosis of Zika virus (A92.5, Zika virus disease) as documented by the provider. This is an exception to the hospital inpatient guideline Section II, H. In that context, "confirmation" does not require documentation of the type of test performed; the provider's diagnostic statement that the condition is confirmed is sufficient.) The Zika virus code should be assigned regardless of the stated mode of transmission. If the provider documents "suspected," "possible," or "probable" Zika, do *not* assign code A92.5. Instead, assign code(s) explaining the reason for encounter (e.g., fever, rash, joint pain) or code Z20.821, Contact with and (suspected) exposure to Zika virus.

Example 1: After testing, the patient is diagnosed with the Zika virus. Report code A92.5 (Zika virus disease).

Example 2: Patient is diagnosed with congenital Zika virus disease. Report code P35.4 (congenital Zika virus disease).

(continues)

ICD-10-CM Chapter-Specific Coding Guidelines (*continued*)

Example 3: Patient reports symptoms of headache, right shoulder joint pain, and fever. Temperature in the office is not elevated. Patient just returned from a tropical vacation and is concerned about the Zika virus because of numerous mosquito bites on both lower legs. Examination reveals the bites to be well healed. Zika test is negative. Patient is instructed to take ibuprofen as directed and to follow up with the office if symptoms worsen. Report code Z20.821 (Contact with and [suspected] exposure to Zika virus) **or** codes R51.9 (Headache) and M25.511 (Pain in right shoulder).

g. Coronavirus infections

1) COVID-19 infection (infection due to SARS-CoV-2)

(a) Code only confirmed cases

Code only a confirmed diagnosis of the 2019 novel coronavirus disease (COVID-19) as documented by the provider, or [as the result of] documentation of a positive COVID-19 test result.

For a confirmed diagnosis, assign code U07.1, COVID-19. This is an exception to the hospital inpatient guideline Section II, H. In this context, "confirmation" does not require documentation of a positive test result for COVID-19; the provider's documentation that the individual has COVID-19 is sufficient. If the provider documents "suspected," "possible," "probable," or "inconclusive" COVID-19, do not assign code U07.1. Instead, code the signs and symptoms reported. *See guideline I.C.1.g.1.g.*

(b) Sequencing of codes

When COVID-19 meets the definition of principal diagnosis, code U07.1, COVID-19, should be sequenced first, followed by the appropriate codes for associated manifestations, except when another guideline requires that certain codes be sequenced first, such as obstetrics, sepsis, or transplant complications.

For a COVID-19 infection that progresses to sepsis, see Section I.C.1.d. Sepsis, Severe Sepsis, and Septic Shock.
See Section I.C.15.s. for COVID-19 infection in pregnancy, childbirth, and the puerperium.
See Section I.C.16.h. for COVID-19 infection in newborn.

For a COVID-19 infection in a lung transplant patient, see Section I.C.19.g.3.a. Transplant complications other than kidney.

(c) Acute respiratory manifestations of COVID-19

When the reason for the encounter/admission is a respiratory manifestation of COVID-19, assign code U07.1, COVID-19, as the principal/first-listed diagnosis and assign code(s) for the respiratory manifestation(s) as additional diagnoses. The following conditions are examples of common respiratory manifestations of COVID-19.

(i) Pneumonia

For a patient with pneumonia confirmed as due to COVID-19, assign codes U07.1, COVID-19, and J12.82, Pneumonia due to coronavirus disease 2019.

(ii) Acute bronchitis

For a patient with acute bronchitis confirmed as due to COVID-19, assign codes U07.1, and J20.8, Acute bronchitis due to other specified organisms. Bronchitis not otherwise specified (NOS) due to COVID-19 should be coded using codes U07.1 and J40, Bronchitis, not specified as acute or chronic.

(iii) Lower respiratory infection

If the COVID-19 is documented as being associated with a lower respiratory infection, not otherwise specified (NOS), or an acute respiratory infection, NOS, codes U07.1 and J22, Unspecified acute lower respiratory infection, should be assigned. If the COVID-19 is documented as being associated with a respiratory infection, NOS, codes U07.1 and J98.8, Other specified respiratory disorders, should be assigned.

(iv) Acute respiratory distress syndrome

For acute respiratory distress syndrome (ARDS) due to COVID-19, assign codes U07.1, and J80, Acute respiratory distress syndrome.

(v) Acute respiratory failure

> For acute respiratory failure due to COVID-19, assign code U07.1, and code J96.0-, Acute respiratory failure.

(d) Non-respiratory manifestations of COVID-19

> When the reason for the encounter/admission is a non-respiratory manifestation (e.g., viral enteritis) of COVID-19, assign code U07.1, COVID-19, as the principal/first-listed diagnosis and assign code(s) for the manifestation(s) as additional diagnoses.

(e) Exposure to COVID-19

> For asymptomatic individuals with actual or suspected exposure to COVID-19, assign code Z20.822, Contact with and (suspected) exposure to COVID-19.

> For symptomatic individuals with actual or suspected exposure to COVID-19 and the infection has been ruled out, or test results are inconclusive or unknown, assign code Z20.822, Contact with and (suspected) exposure to COVID-19. See guideline I.C.21.c.1, Contact/Exposure, for additional guidance regarding the use of category Z20 codes.

> If COVID-19 is confirmed, see guideline I.C.1.g.1.a.

(f) Screening for COVID-19

> For screening for COVID-19, including preoperative testing, assign code Z11.52, Encounter for screening for COVID-19.

(g) Signs and symptoms without definitive diagnosis of COVID-19

> For patients presenting with any signs/symptoms associated with COVID-19 (such as fever, etc.) but a definitive diagnosis has not been established, assign the appropriate code(s) for each of the presenting signs and symptoms such as:

- R05.1 Acute cough, or R05.9 Cough, unspecified
- R06.02 Shortness of breath
- R50.9 Fever, unspecified

> If a patient with signs/symptoms associated with COVID-19 also has an actual or suspected contact with or exposure to COVID-19, assign Z20.822, Contact with and (suspected) exposure to COVID-19, as an additional code.

(h) Asymptomatic individuals who test positive for COVID-19

> For asymptomatic individuals who test positive for COVID-19, see guideline I.C.1.g.1.a. Although the individual is asymptomatic, the individual has tested positive and is considered to have the COVID-19 infection.

(i) Personal history of COVID-19

> For patients with a history of COVID-19, assign code Z86.16, Personal history of COVID-19.

(j) Follow-up visits after COVID-19 infection has resolved

> For individuals who previously had COVID-19, without residual symptom(s) or condition(s), and are being seen for follow-up evaluation, and COVID-19 test results are negative, assign codes Z09, Encounter for follow-up examination after completed treatment for conditions other than malignant neoplasm, and Z86.16, Personal history of COVID-19. For follow-up visits for individuals with symptom(s) or condition(s) related to a previous COVID-19 infection, *see guideline I.C.1.g.1.m.*

> *See Section I.C.21.c.8, Factors influencing health states and contact with health services, Follow-up.*

(k) Encounter for antibody testing

> For an encounter for antibody testing that is not being performed to confirm a current COVID-19 infection, nor is a follow-up test after resolution of COVID-19, assign Z01.84, Encounter for antibody response examination.

> Follow the applicable guidelines above if the individual is being tested to confirm a current COVID-19 infection.

> *For follow-up testing after a COVID-19 infection, see guideline I.C.1.g.1.j.*

(continues)

ICD-10-CM Chapter-Specific Coding Guidelines (*continued*)

(l) **Multisystem Inflammatory Syndrome**

For individuals with multisystem inflammatory syndrome (MIS) and COVID-19, assign code U07.1, COVID-19, as the principal/first-listed diagnosis and assign code M35.81, Multisystem inflammatory syndrome, as an additional diagnosis.

If an individual with a history of COVID-19 develops MIS, assign codes M35.81, Multisystem inflammatory syndrome, and U09.9, Post COVID-19 condition, unspecified.

If an individual with a known or suspected exposure to COVID-19, and no current COVID-19 infection or history of COVID-19, develops MIS, assign codes M35.81, Multisystem inflammatory syndrome, and Z20.822, Contact with and (suspected) exposure to COVID-19.

Additional codes should be assigned for any associated complications of MIS.

(m) **Post COVID-19 condition**

For sequela of COVID-19, or associated symptoms or conditions that develop following a previous COVID-19 infection, assign a code(s) for the specific symptom(s) or condition(s) related to the previous COVID-19 infection, if known, and code U09.9, Post COVID-19 condition, unspecified. Code U09.9 should not be assigned for manifestations of an active (current) COVID-19 infection.

If a patient has a condition(s) associated with a previous COVID-19 infection and develops a new active (current) COVID-19 infection, code U09.9 may be assigned in conjunction with code U07.1, COVID-19, to identify that the patient also has a condition(s) associated with a previous COVID-19 infection. Code(s) for the specific condition(s) associated with the previous COVID-19 infection and code(s) for manifestation(s) of the new active (current) COVID-19 infection should also be assigned.

(n) **Underimmunization for COVID-19 Status**

Code Z28.310, Unvaccinated for COVID-19, may be assigned when the patient has not received at least one dose of any COVID-19 vaccine. Code Z28.311, Partially vaccinated for COVID-19, may be assigned when the patient has received at least one dose of a multi-dose COVID-19 vaccine regimen, but has not received the full set of doses necessary to meet the Centers for Disease Control and Prevention (CDC) definition of "fully vaccinated" in place at the time of the encounter. For information, visit the CDC's website **https://www.cdc.gov/coronavirus/2019ncov/vaccines/**.

See Section I.B.14. for underimmunization documentation by clinicians other than patient's provider.

Exercise 3.1 – Certain Infectious and Parasitic Diseases

Instructions: Assign the appropriate ICD-10-CM code(s).

_____ 1. Human immunodeficiency disease

_____ 2. Asymptomatic human immunodeficiency virus

_____ 3. Urinary tract infection due to *Enterococcus* complicated by vancomycin-resistant *Enterococci* (VRE) infection

_____ 4. Severe sepsis due to *Staphylococcus aureus* with septic shock and hepatorenal failure

_____ 5. Pneumonia due to COVID-19

ICD-10-CM Chapter 2: Neoplasms (C00–D49)

This ICD-10-CM chapter classifies malignant and benign neoplasms according to anatomical site (e.g., breast) and body system (e.g., urinary tract). Neoplasms are classified in the ICD-10-CM index according to malignant primary, malignant secondary, ca *in situ*, benign, uncertain behavior, and unspecified behavior. Official coding guidelines are extensive and include admissions/encounters for treatment of primary site and secondary site, coding/sequencing of complications, primary malignancy previously excised, admissions/encounters involving chemotherapy/immunotherapy/radiation therapy, signs/symptoms/abnormal findings associated with neoplasms, and more.

 NOTE:

Functionally active malignant neoplasms behave like their surrounding tissue, such as a thyroid tumor that secretes thyroxine and causes hyperthyroidism.

Neoplasms are new growths or tumors in which cell reproduction is out of control, and they are classified according to appearance and growth pattern (Figure 3-1). For coding purposes, the provider should specify whether the tumor is benign (noncancerous, nonmalignant, or noninvasive) or **malignant** (cancerous, invasive, or capable of spreading to other parts of the body).

Another term associated with neoplasms is *lesion*, which is defined as "any discontinuity of tissue (e.g., skin or organ) that may or may not be malignant." Index entries for *lesion* contain subterms according to anatomical site (e.g., organs or tissue), and the term *lesion* should be referenced if the diagnostic statement does not confirm a malignancy. In addition, conditions that are examples of benign lesions and are listed as separate index entries include adenosis, cyst, dysplasia, mass (unless the word neoplasm is included in the diagnostic statement), and polyp.

Do not first reference the neoplasm table to assign codes for benign conditions. Instead, locate the specific term in the disease index, and then locate the subterm for the specific organ or body area. When the specific organ or body area is *not* listed as a subterm, follow the instructions provided (e.g., *see, see also,* or *see category*).

> **Example:** The provider documents "liver mass" as the final diagnosis because the pathology report of examined tissue is not yet available. A "mass" is not a "neoplasm." In the ICD-10-CM index, locate main term *Mass* and subterm *liver* to assign R16.0 (after verifying it in the tabular list). (When pathology reports are available, assign a more appropriate code.)

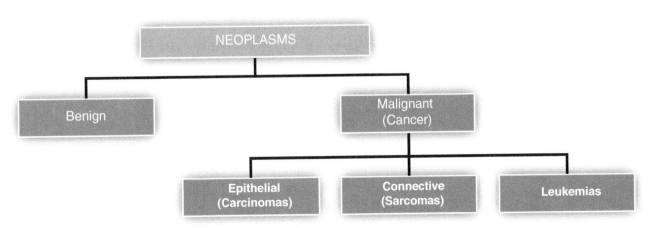

FIGURE 3-1 Classification of neoplasms

The ICD-10-CM Table of Neoplasms (Figure 3-2) is indexed by anatomical site and contains four cellular classifications: malignant, benign, uncertain behavior, and unspecified nature. The malignant classification is subdivided into three divisions: primary, secondary, and carcinoma *in situ*. The six neoplasm classifications are defined as follows:

- **Primary malignancy**: Original tumor site.

 NOTE:

Malignant tumors are considered primary unless otherwise documented as metastatic or secondary.

- **Secondary malignancy** (or **metastatic cancer**): Tumor that has metastasized, or spread, to a secondary site either adjacent to the primary site or to a remote region of the body.
- **Carcinoma (Ca) *in situ***: Malignant tumor that is localized, circumscribed, encapsulated, and noninvasive, but has not spread to deeper or adjacent tissues or organs.
- **Benign**: Noninvasive, nonspreading, nonmalignant tumor.
- **Uncertain behavior**: Subsequent morphology or behavior that cannot be predicted based on the submitted specimen; the tissue appears to be in transition, and the pathologist cannot establish a definitive diagnosis. (To assign a code from this column, the pathology report must specify "uncertain behavior" of the neoplasm.)
- **Unspecified behavior**: A neoplasm is identified, but the results of pathology examination are not available; thus, there is no indication as to histology or nature of the tumor. (Assign a code from the unspecified behavior column when pathology results are pending.)

	Malignant Primary	Malignant Secondary	Ca *in situ*	Benign	Uncertain Behavior	Unspecified Behavior
Note: The list below gives the code number for neoplasms by anatomical site. For each site there are six possible code numbers according to whether the neoplasm in question is malignant, benign, *in situ*, of uncertain behavior, or of unspecified nature. The description of the neoplasm will often indicate which of the six columns is appropriate; e.g., malignant melanoma of skin, benign fibroadenoma of breast, carcinoma in situ of cervix uteri.						
Where such descriptors are not present, the remainder of the Index should be consulted where guidance is given to the appropriate column for each morphological (histological) variety listed; e.g., Mesonephroma *–see* Neoplasm, malignant; Embryoma *–see also* Neoplasm, uncertain behavior; Disease, Bowen's *–see* Neoplasm, skin, *in situ*. However, the guidance in the Index can be overridden if one of the descriptors mentioned above is present; e.g., malignant adenoma of colon is coded to C18.9 and not to D12.6 as the adjective "malignant" overrides the Index entry "Adenoma *–see also* Neoplasm, benign."						
Codes listed with a dash (–), following the code have a required additional character for laterality. The Tabular must be reviewed for the complete code.						
Neoplasm, neoplastic	C80.1	C79.9	D09.9	D36.9	D48.9	D49.9
abdomen, abdominal	C76.2	C79.8-	D09.8	D36.7	D48.7	D49.89
cavity	C76.2	C79.8-	D09.8	D36.7	D48.7	D49.89
organ	C76.2	C79.8-	D09.8	D36.7	D48.7	D49.89
viscera	C76.2	C79.8-	D09.8	D36.7	D48.7	D49.89
wall–*see also* Neoplasm, abdomen, wall, skin	C44.509	C79.2-	D04.5	D23.5	D48.5	D49.2
connective tissue	C49.4	C79.8-	—	D21.4	D48.1	D49.2
skin	C44.509					
basal cell carcinoma	C44.519	—	—	—	—	—
specified type NEC	C44.599	—	—	—	—	—
squamous cell carcinoma	C44.529	—	—	—	—	—

FIGURE 3-2 ICD-10-CM Table of Neoplasms (partial)

To use the Table of Neoplasms, first identify the classification (e.g., malignant), and then locate the site of the neoplasm. Some diagnostic statements specifically document "neoplasm" classification, while others do not provide a clue. If the diagnostic statement classifies the neoplasm, the coder can refer directly to the neoplasm table to assign the proper code (after verifying the code in the tabular list).

When the diagnostic statement does not classify the neoplasm, the coder must refer to the disease index entry for the condition documented (instead of the neoplasm table) (e.g., lipoma). That entry either will contain a code number that can be verified in the tabular list or will refer the coder to the proper neoplasm table entry under which the code can be located.

Example 1: For non-Hodgkin lymphoma, go to main term *Lymphoma* in the ICD-10-CM index, subterm *non-Hodgkin*, and verify code C85.9 in the tabular list to assign the fifth character for the anatomical site.

Example 2: For adrenal gland adenolymphoma, go to main term *Adenolymphoma* in the ICD-10-CM index, and follow the instruction to *see Neoplasm, benign.* In the ICD-10-CM neoplasm table, go to index main term *Neoplasm, neoplastic,* subterm *adrenal,* and the *Benign* column to locate code D35.0-. Then, locate the code in the tabular list to assign fifth character 0 for unspecified adrenal gland, assigning code D35.00.

 Coding Tip

Assigning codes from the neoplasm table is a two-step process. First, classify the neoplasm by its behavior (e.g., malignant or benign); then classify the neoplasm by its anatomical site (e.g., acoustic nerve). To classify the neoplasm's behavior, review the provider's diagnostic statement (e.g., carcinoma of the throat) and locate the term *carcinoma* in the disease index. The entry will classify the behavior, directing you to the proper column in the Table of Neoplasms. (If the neoplasm is malignant, you still need to determine primary, secondary, or *in situ* based on documentation in the patient's record.)

Primary and Secondary Malignancies

A malignancy is coded as a primary site if the diagnostic statement documents

- Metastatic *from* a site
- Spread *from* a site
- *Primary neoplasm* of a site
- A malignancy for which there is no specific classification
- A *recurrent* tumor

Example: For "carcinoma of cervical lymph nodes, metastatic from the breast," the primary site is female breast and the secondary site is cervical lymph nodes.

Secondary malignancies are metastatic and indicate that a primary cancer has spread (metastasized) to another part of the body. Cancer described as *metastatic from* a site is *primary of* that site. Assign one code to the primary neoplasm and a second code to the secondary neoplasm of the specified site (if secondary site is known) or unspecified site (if secondary site is unknown). (Remember that sequencing of codes depends on which site is being treated.)

Example 1: For "metastatic carcinoma from left female breast to lung," assign two codes.

- Primary malignant neoplasm of left female breast (C50.912)
- Secondary neoplasm of lung (C78.00)

Example 2: For "metastatic carcinoma from left female breast," assign two codes.

- Primary malignant neoplasm of left female breast (C50.912)
- Secondary neoplasm of unspecified site (C79.9)

Cancer described as *metastatic to* a site is considered *secondary of* that site. Assign one code to the secondary site and a second code to the specified primary site (if primary site is known) or unspecified site (if primary site is unknown).

Example: For "metastatic carcinoma to right lung," assign two codes.

- Primary malignant neoplasm of unspecified site (C80.1)
- Secondary neoplasm of right lung (C78.01)

When anatomical sites are documented as *metastatic*, assign *secondary* neoplasm code(s) to those sites and assign a code to the primary malignant neoplasm described in the statement.

Example: For "metastatic renal carcinoma, right kidney, with spread to right lung," assign two codes.

- Primary renal carcinoma, right kidney (C64.1)
- Secondary neoplasm of right lung (C78.01)

Anatomical Site Is Not Documented

If the cancer diagnosis does not contain documentation of the anatomical site but the term *metastatic* is documented, assign codes for "unspecified site" for both the primary and secondary sites.

Example: For "metastatic chromophobe adenocarcinoma," assign two codes.

- Secondary neoplasm of unspecified site (C79.9)
- Primary adenocarcinoma of unspecified site (C80.1)

Inoperable Primary Site with Metastasis

When the primary neoplasm site is considered inoperable and is not treated, assign a code for the metastatic site first.

Example: For "carcinoma of fundus of stomach (inoperable) with metastasis to liver," assign two codes.

- Secondary malignant neoplasm of liver (C78.7)
- Primary malignant neoplasm of fundus of stomach (C16.1)

Reexcision of Tumors

A reexcision of a tumor occurs when the pathology report recommends that the surgeon perform a second excision to widen the margins of the original tumor site. The reexcision is performed to ensure that all tumor cells have been removed and that a clear border (margin) of normal tissue surrounds the excised specimen. Use the diagnostic statement found in the report of the original excision to code the reason for the reexcision. The pathology report for the reexcision may not specify a malignancy at that time, but the patient is still under treatment for the original neoplasm.

Coding Tip

1. Read all notes in the neoplasm table that apply to the condition you are coding.
2. Never assign a code directly from the neoplasm table (or index).
3. Report only those codes that represent the current status of the neoplasm.
4. Assign a neoplasm code if the tumor has been excised and the patient is still undergoing radiation or chemotherapy treatment.
5. Assign an ICD-10-CM Z code if the tumor is no longer present or if the patient is not receiving treatment but is returning for follow-up care (e.g., personal history of a malignancy).
6. The classification documented on a pathology report overrides the morphology classification entry in the index.

Morphology of Neoplasms

The World Health Organization (WHO) has published an adaptation of the International Classification of Diseases for Oncology (ICD-O) that contains a coded nomenclature for the morphology of neoplasms. The morphology codes consist of five characters, and these codes are reported to state cancer registries and other entities for cancer research purposes. The first four characters identify the histological type of the neoplasm, and the fifth character indicates behavior of the neoplasm (e.g., M8000/0). The one-character behavior codes include:

/0 Benign

/1 Uncertain whether benign or malignant

     Borderline malignancy

/2 Carcinoma *in situ*

     Intraepithelial

     Noninfiltrating

     Noninvasive

/3 Malignant, primary site

/6 Malignant, metastatic site

     Secondary site

/9 Malignant, uncertain whether primary or metastatic site

Example: Malignant chordoma is assigned morphology code M9370/3. However, benign chordoma is assigned morphology code M9370/0.

When a morphological diagnosis contains two qualifying adjectives that result in more than one morphology code, the higher morphology code is assigned.

> **Example:** Transitional cell epidermoid carcinoma is assigned morphology code M8120/3 (Transitional cell carcinoma NOS), while epidermoid carcinoma is assigned morphology code M8070/3 (Epidermoid carcinoma NOS). In this situation, the higher morphology code (M8120/3) is used because it is usually more specific.

ICD-10-CM Chapter-Specific Coding Guidelines

Chapter 2: Neoplasms (C00-D49)

General Guidelines

Chapter 2 of the ICD-10-CM contains the codes for most benign and all malignant neoplasms. Certain benign neoplasms, such as prostatic adenomas, may be found in the specific body system chapters. To properly code a neoplasm, it is necessary to determine from the record if the neoplasm is benign, *in situ*, malignant, or of uncertain histologic behavior. If malignant, any secondary (metastatic) sites should also be determined.

Primary malignant neoplasms overlapping site boundaries

A primary malignant neoplasm that overlaps two or more contiguous (next to each other) sites should be classified to the subcategory/code .8 ('overlapping lesion'), unless the combination is specifically indexed elsewhere. For multiple neoplasms of the same site that are not contiguous, such as tumors in different quadrants of the same breast, codes for each site should be assigned.

> **Example: Contiguous sites** (or **overlapping sites**) occur when the origin of the tumor (primary site) involves two adjacent sites. For a female patient who is diagnosed with a single primary malignant neoplasm of the right breast that extends from the lower-outer quadrant into the adjacent axillary tail, report code C50.811 (Malignant neoplasm of overlapping sites of right female breast) because the sites are contiguous.
>
> For a male patient who is diagnosed with two malignant neoplasms of left breast, one at the upper-outer quadrant and another at the lower-outer quadrant, report codes C50.422 (Malignant neoplasm of upper-outer quadrant of left male breast) and C50.522 (Malignant neoplasm of lower-outer quadrant of left male breast) because the sites are **not** contiguous.

Malignant neoplasm of ectopic tissue

Malignant neoplasms of ectopic tissue are to be coded to the site of origin mentioned; e.g., ectopic pancreatic malignant neoplasms involving the stomach are coded to malignant neoplasm of pancreas, unspecified (C25.9).

The neoplasm table in the ICD-10-CM Alphabetic Index should be referenced first. However, if the histological term is documented, that term should be referenced first, rather than going immediately to the neoplasm table, in order to determine which column in the neoplasm table is appropriate. For example, if the documentation indicates "adenoma," refer to the term in the ICD-10-CM Alphabetic Index to review the entries under this term and the instructional note to "see also neoplasm, by site, benign." The table provides the proper code based on the type of neoplasm and the site. It is important to select the proper column in the table that corresponds to the type of neoplasm. The ICD-10-CM tabular list should then be referenced to verify that the correct code has been selected from the table and that a more specific site code does not exist.

See Section I.C.21. Factors influencing health status and contact with health services, Status, for information regarding Z15.0, codes for genetic susceptibility to cancer.

a. **Admission/Encounter for treatment of primary site**

If the malignancy is chiefly responsible for occasioning the patient admission/encounter and treatment is directed at the primary site, designate the primary malignancy as the principal/first-listed diagnosis.

The only exception to this guideline is if the administration of chemotherapy, immunotherapy or external beam radiation therapy is chiefly responsible for occasioning the admission/encounter. In that case, assign the appropriate Z51.-- code as the first-listed or principal diagnosis, and the underlying diagnosis or problem for which the service is being performed as the secondary diagnosis.

b. **Admission/Encounter for treatment of secondary site**

When a patient is admitted because of a primary neoplasm with metastasis and treatment is directed toward the secondary site only, the secondary neoplasm is designated as the principal diagnosis even though the primary malignancy is still present.

Example: Patient with primary uterine adnexal cancer (that has not resolved) receives treatment today for metastatic (secondary) cancer of the liver. Report code C78.7 for liver cancer and C57.4 for uterine cancer, in that order.

c. **Coding and sequencing of complications**

Coding and sequencing of complications associated with the malignancies or with the therapy thereof are subject to the following guidelines:

1) **Anemia associated with malignancy**

When admission/encounter is for management of an anemia associated with the malignancy, and the treatment is only for anemia, the appropriate code for the malignancy is sequenced as the principal or first-listed diagnosis followed by the appropriate code for the anemia (such as code D63.0, Anemia in neoplastic disease).

Example: Patient is diagnosed with anemia due to malignant neoplasm of the mandible. Report code C41.1 for mandible cancer and code D63.0 for anemia in neoplastic disease. (The ICD-10-CM tabular list instruction states to "code first neoplasm.")

2) **Anemia associated with chemotherapy, immunotherapy, and radiation therapy**

When the admission/encounter is for management of an anemia associated with an adverse effect of the administration of chemotherapy or immunotherapy and the only treatment is for the anemia, the anemia code is sequenced first followed by the appropriate codes for the neoplasm and the adverse effect (T45.1X5-, Adverse effect of antineoplastic and immunosuppressive drugs).

Example: Patient with Burkitt-type mature B-cell leukemia, in relapse, is admitted today for treatment of anemia due to antineoplastic chemotherapy. Report codes D64.81 for anemia, C91.A2 for leukemia, and T45.1x5A for adverse effect, in that order.

When the admission/encounter is for management of an anemia associated with an adverse effect of radiotherapy, the anemia code should be sequenced first, followed by the appropriate neoplasm code and code Y84.2, Radiological procedure and radiotherapy as the cause of abnormal reaction of the patient, or of later complication, without mention of misadventure at the time of the procedure.

Example: Patient with Burkitt-type mature B-cell leukemia, in relapse, is admitted today for treatment of anemia related to radiation therapy. Report codes D64.89 for anemia, C91.A2 for leukemia, and Y84.2 for radiotherapy as cause of abnormal reaction, in that order.

(continues)

ICD-10-CM Chapter-Specific Coding Guidelines (*continued*)

3) Management of dehydration due to the malignancy

When the admission/encounter is for management of dehydration due to the malignancy and only the dehydration is being treated (e.g., intravenous rehydration), the dehydration is sequenced first, followed by the code(s) for the malignancy.

4) Treatment of a complication resulting from a surgical procedure

When the admission/encounter is for treatment of a complication resulting from a surgical procedure, designate the complication as the principal or first-listed diagnosis if treatment is directed at resolving the complication.

d. Primary malignancy previously excised

When a primary malignancy has been previously excised or eradicated from its site and there is no further treatment directed to that site and there is no evidence of any existing primary malignancy at that site, a code from category Z85, Personal history of malignant neoplasm, should be used to indicate the former site of the malignancy. Any mention of extension, invasion, or metastasis to another site is coded as a secondary malignant neoplasm to that site. The secondary site may be the principal or first-listed diagnosis, with the Z85 code used as a secondary code.

See section I.C.2.t. Secondary malignant neoplasm of lymphoid tissue.

Example: Patient underwent right radical mastectomy last year, and is seen today for metastatic carcinoma to the right lung. Report codes C78.01 (Secondary neoplasm of right lung), Z85.3 (Personal history of malignant neoplasm of right female breast), and Z90.11 (Acquired absence of right breast and nipple), in that order. Code Z90.11 is typically due to status post right mastectomy.

e. Admissions/Encounters involving chemotherapy, immunotherapy, and radiation therapy

1) Episode of care involves surgical removal of neoplasm

When an episode of care involves the surgical removal of a neoplasm, primary or secondary site, followed by adjunct chemotherapy or radiation treatment during the same episode of care, the code for the neoplasm should be assigned as principal or first-listed diagnosis.

2) Patient admission/encounter chiefly for administration of chemotherapy, immunotherapy, and radiation therapy

If a patient admission/encounter is chiefly for the administration of chemotherapy, immunotherapy, or external beam radiation therapy, assign code Z51.0, Encounter for antineoplastic radiation therapy, or Z51.11, Encounter for antineoplastic chemotherapy, or Z51.12, Encounter for antineoplastic immunotherapy as the first-listed or principal diagnosis. If a patient receives more than one of these therapies during the same admission, more than one of these codes may be assigned, in any sequence.

The malignancy for which the therapy is being administered should be assigned as a secondary diagnosis.

If a patient admission/encounter is for the insertion or implantation of radioactive elements (e.g., brachytherapy) the appropriate code for the malignancy is sequenced as the principal or first-listed diagnosis. Code Z51.0 should not be assigned.

3) Patient admitted for radiation therapy, chemotherapy or immunotherapy and develops complications

When a patient is admitted for the purpose of external beam radiotherapy, immunotherapy, or chemotherapy and develops complications such as uncontrolled nausea and vomiting or dehydration, the principal or first-listed diagnosis is Z51.0, Encounter for antineoplastic radiation therapy, or Z51.11, Encounter for antineoplastic chemotherapy, or Z51.12, Encounter for antineoplastic immunotherapy, followed by any codes for the complications.

When a patient is admitted for the purpose of insertion or implantation of radioactive elements (e.g., brachytherapy) and develops complications such as uncontrolled nausea and vomiting or dehydration, the principal or first-listed diagnosis is the appropriate code for the malignancy followed by any codes for the complications.

f. **Admission/encounter to determine extent of malignancy**

When the reason for admission/encounter is to determine the extent of the malignancy, or for a procedure such as paracentesis or thoracentesis, the primary malignancy or appropriate metastatic site is designated as the principal or first-listed diagnosis, even though chemotherapy or radiotherapy is administered.

g. **Symptoms, signs, and ill-defined conditions listed in [ICD-10-CM] Chapter 18 associated with neoplasms**

Symptoms, signs, and ill-defined conditions listed in [ICD-10-CM] Chapter 18 characteristic of, or associated with, an existing primary or secondary site malignancy cannot be used to replace the malignancy as principal or first-listed diagnosis, regardless of the number of admissions or encounters for treatment and care of the neoplasm.

See section I.C.21. Factors influencing health status and contact with health services, Encounter for prophylactic organ removal.

h. **Admission/encounter for pain control/management**

See Section I.C.6. for information on coding admission/encounter for pain control/management.

i. **Malignancy in two or more noncontiguous sites**

A patient may have more than one malignant tumor in the same organ. These tumors may represent different primaries or metastatic disease, depending on the site. Should the documentation be unclear, the provider should be queried as to the status of each tumor so that the correct codes can be assigned.

j. **Disseminated malignant neoplasm, unspecified**

Code C80.0, Disseminated malignant neoplasm, unspecified, is for use only in those cases where the patient has advanced metastatic disease and no known primary or secondary sites are specified. It should not be used in place of assigning codes for the primary site and all known secondary sites.

k. **Malignant neoplasm without specification of site**

Code C80.1, Malignant (primary) neoplasm, unspecified, equates to Cancer, unspecified. This code should only be used when no determination can be made as to the primary site of a malignancy. This code should rarely be used in the inpatient setting.

l. **Sequencing of neoplasm codes**

1) **Encounter for treatment of primary malignancy**

If the reason for the encounter is for treatment of a primary malignancy, assign the malignancy as the principal/first-listed diagnosis. The primary site is to be sequenced first, followed by any metastatic sites.

Example: Patient is admitted for treatment of "oat cell carcinoma of the lung with spread to the brain." The primary site is lung, and the secondary site is brain.

2) **Encounter for treatment of secondary malignancy**

When an encounter is for a primary malignancy with metastasis and treatment is directed toward the metastatic (secondary) site(s) only, the metastatic site(s) is designated as the principal/first-listed diagnosis. The primary malignancy is coded as an additional code.

Example: A female patient is admitted for treatment of "metastatic carcinoma from right breast to right lung." The primary site is the right breast and continues to display evidence of cancer. Report codes C78.01 (Secondary neoplasm of right lung) and C50.911 (Malignant neoplasm of unspecified site of right breast), in that order.

3) **Malignant neoplasm in a pregnant patient**

When a pregnant patient has a malignant neoplasm, a code from subcategory O9A.1-, Malignant neoplasm complicating pregnancy, childbirth, and the puerperium, should be sequenced first, followed by the appropriate code from Chapter 2 to indicate the type of neoplasm.

(continues)

ICD-10-CM Chapter-Specific Coding Guidelines (*continued*)

4) Encounter for complication associated with a neoplasm

When an encounter is for management of a complication associated with a neoplasm, such as dehydration, and the treatment is only for the complication, the complication is coded first, followed by the appropriate code(s) for the neoplasm.

The exception to this guideline is anemia. When the admission/encounter is for management of an anemia associated with the malignancy, and the treatment is only for anemia, the appropriate code for the malignancy is sequenced as the principal or first-listed diagnosis followed by code D63.0, Anemia in neoplastic disease.

5) Complication from surgical procedure for treatment of a neoplasm

When an encounter is for treatment of a complication resulting from a surgical procedure performed for the treatment of the neoplasm, designate the complication as the principal/first-listed diagnosis. See the guideline regarding the coding of a current malignancy versus personal history to determine if the code for the neoplasm should also be assigned.

6) Pathologic fracture due to a neoplasm

When an encounter is for a pathological fracture due to a neoplasm, and the focus of treatment is the fracture, a code from subcategory M84.5, Pathological fracture in neoplastic disease, should be sequenced first, followed by the code for the neoplasm.

If the focus of treatment is the neoplasm with an associated pathological fracture, the neoplasm code should be sequenced first, followed by a code from M84.5 for the pathological fracture.

m. Current malignancy versus personal history of malignancy

When a primary malignancy has been excised but further treatment, such as an additional surgery for the malignancy, radiation therapy or chemotherapy is directed to that site, the primary malignancy code should be used until treatment is completed.

When a primary malignancy has been previously excised or eradicated from its site, there is no further treatment (of the malignancy) directed to that site, and there is no evidence of any existing primary malignancy at that site, a code from category Z85, Personal history of malignant neoplasm, should be used to indicate the former site of the malignancy.

Codes from subcategories Z85.0–Z85.85 should only be assigned for the former site of a primary malignancy, not the site of a secondary malignancy. Code Z85.89 may be assigned for the former site(s) of either a primary or secondary malignancy.

See Section I.C.21. Factors influencing health status and contact with health services, History (of)

n. Leukemia, multiple myeloma, and malignant plasma cell neoplasms in remission versus personal history

The categories for leukemia, and category C90, Multiple myeloma and malignant plasma cell neoplasms, have codes indicating whether or not the leukemia has achieved remission. There are also codes Z85.6, Personal history of leukemia, and Z85.79, Personal history of other malignant neoplasms of lymphoid, hematopoietic and related tissues. If the documentation is unclear as to whether the leukemia has achieved remission, the provider should be queried.

See Section I.C.21. Factors influencing health status and contact with health services, History (of)

o. Aftercare following surgery for neoplasm

See Section I.C.21. Factors influencing health status and contact with health services, Aftercare

p. Follow-up care for completed treatment of a malignancy

See Section I.C.21. Factors influencing health status and contact with health services, Follow-up

q. Prophylactic organ removal for prevention of malignancy

See Section I.C.21. Factors influencing health status and contact with health services, Prophylactic organ removal

r. Malignant neoplasm associated with transplanted organ

A malignant neoplasm of a transplanted organ should be coded as a transplant complication. Assign first the appropriate code from category T86.-, Complications of transplanted organs and tissue, followed by code C80.2, Malignant neoplasm associated with transplanted organ. Use an additional code for the specific malignancy.

s. **Breast implant associated anaplastic large cell lymphoma**

Breast implant associated anaplastic large cell lymphoma (BIA-ALCL) is a type of lymphoma that can develop around breast implants. Assign code C84.7A, Anaplastic large cell lymphoma, ALK-negative, breast, for BIA-ALCL. Do not assign a complication code from chapter 19.

t. **Secondary malignant neoplasm of lymphoid tissue**

When a malignant neoplasm of lymphoid tissue metastasizes beyond the lymph nodes, a code from categories C81-C85 with a final character "9" should be assigned identifying "extranodal and solid organ sites" rather than a code for the secondary neoplasm of the affected solid organ. For example, for metastasis of diffuse large B-cell lymphoma to the lung, brain and left adrenal gland, assign code C83.39, Diffuse large B-cell lymphoma, extranodal and solid organ sites.

Exercise 3.2 – Neoplasms

Instructions: Assign the appropriate ICD-10-CM code(s).

_____ **1.** Carcinoma *in situ*, cervix uteri

_____ **2.** Adenocarcinoma, left breast (male patient), extending from lower-outer quadrant into adjacent axillary tail

_____ **3.** Treatment of secondary liver cancer due to metastatic colorectal cancer

_____ **4.** Anemia due to primary brain cancer involving the basal ganglia

_____ **5.** Personal history of malignant melanoma

ICD-10-CM Chapter 3: Diseases of the Blood and Blood-Forming Organs and Certain Disorders Involving the Immune Mechanism (D50–D89)

This ICD-10-CM chapter classifies the following:

- Nutritional anemias
- Hemolytic anemias
- Aplastic and other anemias and other bone marrow failure syndromes
- Coagulation defects, purpura, and other hemorrhagic conditions
- Other disorders of blood and blood-forming organs
- Intraoperative and postprocedural complications of the spleen
- Certain disorders involving the immune mechanism

Bone marrow is the principal site for hemopoietic cell proliferation and differentiation. One of the largest organs in the human body, hemopoietic tissue is responsible for producing erythrocytes (red blood cells), neutrophils, eosinophils, basophils, monocytes, platelets, and lymphocytes.

Anemia refers to a lower-than-normal erythrocyte count or level of hemoglobin in the circulating blood. A clinical sign rather than a diagnostic entity, anemia can be classified by three morphological variations of the erythrocyte: size (volume), hemoglobin content, and shape. These variations give clinicians clues to the specific type of anemia. In laboratory blood tests, erythrocyte size is gauged by estimating the volume of red cells in the circulating blood.

- Red cell volume (or mean corpuscular volume) is estimated by dividing the patient's hematocrit (percentage of red blood cells in whole blood) by the red blood cell count (RBC). Normal values are normocytic, abnormally low values are microcytic, and abnormally high values are macrocytic.

- Hemoglobin content refers to the average amount of hemoglobin in each red blood cell. This value, called the mean cell hemoglobin, is calculated by dividing the patient's hemoglobin by the number of red blood cells. Normal values are normochromic, less-than-normal values are hypochromic, and greater-than-normal values are hyperchromic.

- Shape is determined by microscopy. Normally, red blood cells have a smooth, concave shape. Erythrocytes with irregular shapes are called poikilocytes, a general term meaning "abnormally shaped." Terms referring to specific abnormal cell shapes include *acanthocytes, leptocytes, nucleated erythrocytes, macro-ovalocytes, schistocytes, helmet cells, teardrop cells, sickle cells*, and *target cells*.

Once the cell morphology is determined, the anemia can be further classified based on certain physiological and pathological criteria.

Example: Constitutional aplastic anemia (D61.09) is classified physiologically as an anemia of hypoproliferation and pathologically as inborn error of heredity.

The term *coagulation defect* refers to deficiencies or disorders of hemostasis. A complicated process involving substances in the injured tissues, formed elements of blood (platelets and monocytes), and the coagulation proteins, coagulation requires the production of thrombin, a substance that stabilizes the platelet plug and forms the fibrin clot. Together they mechanically block the extravasation of blood from ruptured vessels. The coagulation process can be interrupted by a genetic or disease-caused protein deficiency, by an increase in the catabolism of coagulation proteins, or by antibodies directed against the coagulation proteins. Many proteins are involved in coagulation, many of which are identified by the term *factor* followed by a Roman numeral. The appropriate Roman numeral followed by the suffix *a* indicates the activated form of a coagulation factor.

Example: When protein factor II (prothrombin) is activated by the enzyme thrombin, it is designated factor IIa.

The term *purpura* refers to a condition characterized by hemorrhage, or extravasation of blood, into the tissues, producing bruises and small red patches on the skin. Purpura may be associated with thrombocytopenia or can occur in a nonthrombocytopenic form. Thrombocytopenia is a decrease of the number of platelets in the circulating blood and may be primary (hereditary or idiopathic) or secondary to a known cause.

Diseases of white blood cells refer to increases, decreases, or genetic or idiopathic anomalies of white blood cells not associated with malignant disease classified to categories C81–C96, *Malignant neoplasms of lymphoid, hematopoietic and related tissue.*

ICD-10-CM Chapter-Specific Coding Guidelines

Chapter 3: Diseases of the Blood and Blood-Forming Organs and Certain Disorders Involving the Immune Mechanism (D50–D89)

Reserved for future guideline expansion.

Exercise 3.3 – Diseases of the Blood and Blood-Forming Organs and Certain Disorders Involving the Immune Mechanism

Instructions: Assign the appropriate ICD-10-CM code(s).

_____ 1. Acquired polycythemia

_____ 2. Acute posthemorrhagic anemia

_____ 3. Secondary agranulocytosis

_____ 4. Chronic simple anemia

_____ 5. Chronic congestive splenomegaly

ICD-10-CM Chapter 4: Endocrine, Nutritional, and Metabolic Diseases (E00–E89)

This ICD-10-CM chapter classifies the following:

- Disorders of the thyroid gland
- Diabetes mellitus
- Other disorders of glucose regulation and pancreatic internal secretion
- Disorders of other endocrine glands
- Intraoperative complications of the endocrine system
- Malnutrition
- Other nutritional deficiencies
- Overweight, obesity, and other hyperalimentation
- Metabolic disorders
- Postprocedural endocrine and metabolic complications and disorders, not elsewhere classified

The endocrine system includes specialized organs and body tissues that produce, secrete, and store hormones. Hormones regulate the body's development, control the function of various tissues, support reproduction, and regulate metabolism. Hormones from the endocrine system are secreted into the blood, where proteins keep them intact and regulate their release. Other changes in the body also influence hormone secretions.

Example: The normal hormone function of the parathyroid hormone causes the body to increase the level of calcium in blood. As calcium levels rise, the secretion of parathyroid hormone decreases.

Nutritional deficiencies in ICD-10-CM Chapter 4 cover deficiencies in vitamins, minerals, and protein-calorie malnutrition. Metabolic diseases in ICD-10-CM Chapter 4 cover a wide range of diseases, including problems with amino acid and carbohydrate transport; lipoid metabolism; plasma protein metabolism; gout; mineral metabolism; and fluid, electrolyte, and acid-base imbalances. Cystic fibrosis, porphyrin, purine and pyrimidine metabolism, and obesity are also classified.

ICD-10-CM Chapter-Specific Coding Guidelines

Chapter 4: Endocrine, Nutritional, and Metabolic Diseases E00–E89

a. Diabetes mellitus

The diabetes mellitus codes are combination codes that include the type of diabetes mellitus, the body system affected, and the complications affecting that body system. As many codes within a particular category as are necessary to describe all of the complications of the disease may be used. They should be sequenced based on the reason for a particular encounter. Assign as many codes from categories E08–E13 as needed to identify all of the associated conditions that the patient has.

1) Type of diabetes

The age of a patient is not the sole determining factor, though most type 1 diabetics develop the condition before reaching puberty. For this reason, type 1 diabetes mellitus is also referred to as juvenile diabetes.

Example: For **type 1 diabetes mellitus**, the patient's body is *unable to produce insulin*, and code E10.9 (Type 1 diabetes mellitus without complications) is reported if there are no complications.

2) Type of diabetes mellitus not documented

If the type of diabetes mellitus is not documented in the patient record, the default is E11.-, Type 2 diabetes mellitus.

Example: For **type 2 diabetes mellitus**, the patient's body is *unable to properly use insulin produced*, and code E11.9 (Type 2 diabetes mellitus without complications) is reported if there are no complications.

3) Diabetes mellitus and the use of insulin, oral hypoglycemics, and injectable non-insulin drugs

If the documentation in a medical record does not indicate the type of diabetes but does indicate that the patient uses insulin, code E11-, Type 2 diabetes mellitus, should be assigned. Additional code(s) should be assigned from category Z79 to identify the long-term (current) use of insulin, oral hypoglycemic drugs, or injectable non-insulin antidiabetic [drugs], as follows:

If the patient is treated with both oral hypoglycemic drugs and insulin, both code Z79.4, Long term (current) use of insulin, and code Z79.84, Long term (current) use of oral hypoglycemic drugs, should be assigned.

If the patient is treated with both insulin and an injectable non-insulin antidiabetic drug, assign codes Z79.4, Long term (current) use of insulin, and Z79.85, Long-term (current) use of injectable non-insulin antidiabetic drugs.

If the patient is treated with both oral hypoglycemic drugs and an injectable non-insulin antidiabetic drug, assign codes Z79.84, Long term (current) use of oral hypoglycemic drugs, and Z79.85, Long-term (current) use of injectable non-insulin antidiabetic drugs.

Code Z79.4 should not be assigned if insulin is given temporarily to bring a type 2 patient's blood sugar under control during an encounter.

Example: Patient has type 2 diabetes mellitus without complications and has used insulin for long-term management. Report code E11.9 for diabetes and Z79.4 for use of insulin.

4) Diabetes mellitus in pregnancy and gestational diabetes

See Section I.C.15. Diabetes mellitus in pregnancy.

See Section I.C.15. Gestational (pregnancy induced) diabetes.

5) Complications due to insulin pump malfunction

(a) Underdose of insulin due to insulin pump failure

An underdose of insulin due to an insulin pump failure should be assigned to a code from subcategory T85.6, Mechanical complication of other specified internal and external prosthetic devices, implants and grafts, that specifies the type of pump malfunction, as the principal or first-listed code, followed by code

T38.3X6-, Underdosing of insulin and oral hypoglycemic [antidiabetic] drugs. Additional codes for the type of diabetes mellitus and any associated complications due to the underdosing should also be assigned.

Example: Type 1 diabetic patient is seen for an elevated blood sugar level due to a malfunctioning insulin pump. Report codes T85.615A for mechanical breakdown of insulin pump, T38.3X6A for underdosing of insulin, and E10.65 for type 1 diabetes with hyperglycemia, in that order.

(b) Overdose of insulin due to insulin pump failure

The principal or first-listed code for an encounter due to an insulin pump malfunction resulting in an overdose of insulin should also be T85.6-, Mechanical complication of other specified internal and external prosthetic devices, implants and grafts, followed by code T38.3X1-, Poisoning by insulin and oral hypoglycemic [antidiabetic] drugs, accidental (unintentional).

Example: Type 1 diabetic patient is treated for hypoglycemia due to malfunctioning insulin pump. Report code T85.614A for mechanical breakdown of insulin pump, T38.3X1A for poisoning by insulin (accidental), and E10.649 for diabetes with hypoglycemia (without coma).

6) Secondary diabetes mellitus

Codes under category E08, Diabetes mellitus due to underlying condition, E09, Drug or chemical induced diabetes mellitus, and E13, Other specified diabetes mellitus, identify complications/manifestations associated with secondary diabetes mellitus. Secondary diabetes is always caused by another condition or event (e.g., cystic fibrosis, malignant neoplasm of pancreas, pancreatectomy, adverse effect of drug, or poisoning).

(a) Secondary diabetes mellitus and the use of insulin, oral hypoglycemic drugs, or injectable non-insulin drugs

For patients with secondary diabetes mellitus who routinely use insulin, oral hypoglycemic drugs, or injectable non-insulin drugs, additional code(s) from category Z79 should be assigned to identify the long term (current) use of insulin, oral hypoglycemic drugs, or non-injectable non-insulin drugs as follows:

If the patient is treated with both oral hypoglycemic drugs and insulin, both code Z79.4, Long term (current) use of insulin, and code Z79.84, Long term (current) use of oral hypoglycemic drugs, should be assigned.

If the patient is treated with both insulin and an injectable non-insulin antidiabetic drug, assign codes Z79.4, Longterm (current) use of insulin, and Z79.85, Long-term (current) use of injectable non-insulin antidiabetic drugs.

If the patient is treated with both oral hypoglycemic drugs and an injectable non-insulin antidiabetic drug, assign codes Z79.84, Long term (current) use of oral hypoglycemic drugs, and Z79.85, Long-term (current) use of injectable non-insulin antidiabetic drugs.

Code Z79.4 should not be assigned if insulin is given temporarily to bring a secondary diabetic patient's blood sugar under control during an encounter.

(b) Assigning and sequencing secondary diabetes codes and its causes

The sequencing of the secondary diabetes codes in relationship to codes for the cause of the diabetes is based on the Tabular List instructions for categories E08, E09 and E13.

(i) Secondary diabetes mellitus due to pancreatectomy

For postpancreatectomy diabetes mellitus (lack of insulin due to the surgical removal of all or part of the pancreas), assign code E89.1, Postsurgical hypoinsulinemia. Assign a code from category E13 and a code from subcategory Z90.41, Acquired absence of pancreas, as additional codes.

(continues)

Courtesy of the Centers for Medicare & Medicaid Services, www.cms.gov.

ICD-10-CM Chapter-Specific Coding Guidelines (*continued*)

(ii) Secondary diabetes due to drugs

Secondary diabetes may be caused by an adverse effect of correctly administered medications, poisoning, or sequela of poisoning.

See Section I.C.19.e. for coding of adverse effects and poisoning, and section I.C.20. for external code reporting.

Exercise 3.4 – Endocrine, Nutritional, and Metabolic Diseases

Instructions: Assign the appropriate ICD-10-CM code(s).

_____ 1. Diabetes mellitus, type 1, with hyperglycemia

_____ 2. Diabetes mellitus with amyotrophy

_____ 3. Type 2 diabetes mellitus with long term (current) use of insulin

_____ 4. Postpancreatectomy hypoinsulinemia (total), diabetes mellitus with hyperglycemia, requiring long term (current) insulin use, and status post pancreatectomy

_____ 5. Streptococcal acute thyroiditis

ICD-10-CM Chapter 5: Mental, Behavioral, and Neurodevelopmental Disorders (F01–F99)

This ICD-10-CM chapter classifies the following:

- Mental disorders due to known physiological conditions
- Mental and behavioral disorders due to psychoactive substance use
- Schizophrenia, schizotypal, delusional, and other non-mood psychotic disorders
- Mood [affective] disorders
- Anxiety, dissociative, stress-related, somatoform, and other nonpsychotic mental disorders
- Behavioral syndromes associated with physiological disturbances and physical factors
- Disorders of adult personality and behavior
- Intellectual disabilities
- Pervasive and specific developmental disorders
- Behavioral and emotional disorders with onset usually occurring in childhood and adolescence
- Unspecified mental disorders

ICD-10-CM Chapter-Specific Coding Guidelines

Chapter 5: Mental, Behavioral, and Neurodevelopmental Disorders (F01–F99)

a. Pain disorders related to psychological factors

Assign code F45.41, for pain that is exclusively related to psychological disorders. As indicated by the Excludes1 note under category G89, a code from category G89 should not be assigned with code F45.41.

Code F45.42, Pain disorders with related psychological factors, should be used with a code from category G89, Pain, not elsewhere classified, if there is documentation of a psychological component for a patient with acute or chronic pain.

See Section I.C.6. Pain.

b. **Mental and behavioral disorders due to psychoactive substance use**

1) In remission

Selection of codes describing "in remission" for categories F10–F19, Mental and behavioral disorders due to psychoactive substance use (categories F10–F19 with -.11, -.21, -.91) requires the provider's clinical judgment and are assigned only on the basis of provider documentation (as defined in the *ICD-10-CM Official Guidelines for Coding and Reporting*) unless otherwise instructed by the classification.

Mild substance use disorders in early or sustained remission are classified to the appropriate codes for substance abuse in remission, and moderate or severe substance use disorders in early or sustained remission are classified to the appropriate codes for substance dependence in remission.

2) Psychoactive substance use, abuse and dependence

When the provider documentation refers to use, abuse and dependence of the same substance (e.g. alcohol, opioid, cannabis, etc.), only one code should be assigned to identify the pattern of use based on the following hierarchy:

- If both use and abuse are documented, assign only the code for abuse.
- If both abuse and dependence are documented, assign only the code for dependence.
- If use, abuse and dependence are all documented, assign only the code for dependence.
- If both use and dependence are documented, assign only the code for dependence.

Example 1: Patient is diagnosed with cannabis use, abuse, and dependence. Report code F12.20 for cannabis dependence only.

Example 2: For a patient who is diagnosed with both cannabis-related disorders and nicotine-related disorders, report a code from each of categories F12 (Cannabis related disorders) and F17 (Nicotine dependence). More than one code is assigned when the patient is diagnosed with use, abuse, and dependence of multiple substances.

Example 3: For a patient who is diagnosed with vaping of nicotine, report a code from subcategory F17.29 (Nicotine dependence, other tobacco product). Electronic nicotine delivery systems [ENDS] are noncombustible tobacco products.

3) Psychoactive substance use, unspecified

As with all other unspecified diagnoses, the codes for unspecified psychoactive substance use (F10.9-, F11.9-, F12.9-, F13.9-, F14.9-, F15.9-, F16.9-, F18.9-, F19.9-) should only be assigned based on provider documentation and when they meet the definition of a reportable diagnosis (*see Section III, Reporting Additional Diagnoses*). These codes are to be used only when the psychoactive substance use is associated with a substance-related disorder included in (ICD-10-CM chapter 5 disorders such as sexual dysfunction, sleep disorder, or a mental or behavioral disorder) or medical condition, and such a relationship is documented by the provider.

Example: At a friend's party, the patient became intoxicated with alcohol, fell, and sprained their left ankle. Provider's diagnoses are left ankle sprain and alcohol use with intoxication. Report codes S93.402A for the sprained ankle and F10.929 for the alcohol use with intoxication.

 NOTE:

See Section I.C.15.I.3, Drug use during pregnancy, childbirth and the puerperium.

4) Medical conditions due to psychoactive substance use, abuse and dependence

Medical conditions due to substance use, abuse, and dependence are not classified as substance-induced disorders. Assign the diagnosis code for the medical condition as directed by the Alphabetical Index along with the appropriate psychoactive substance use, abuse or dependence code. For example, for alcoholic pancreatitis due

(continues)

ICD-10-CM Chapter-Specific Coding Guidelines (*continued*)

to alcohol dependence, assign the appropriate code from subcategory K85.2, Alcohol induced acute pancreatitis, and the appropriate code from subcategory F10.2, such as code F10.20, Alcohol dependence, uncomplicated. It would not be appropriate to assign code F10.288, Alcohol dependence with other alcohol-induced disorder.

5) Blood alcohol level

A code from category Y90, Evidence of alcohol involvement determined by blood alcohol level, may be assigned when this information is documented and the patient's provider has documented a condition classifiable to category F10, Alcohol related disorders. The blood alcohol level does not need to be documented by the patient's provider in order for it to be coded.

See Section I.B.14. for blood alcohol level documentation by clinicians other than patient's provider.

c. Factitious Disorder

Factitious disorder imposed on self or Munchausen's syndrome is a disorder in which a person falsely reports or causes his or her own physical or psychological signs or symptoms. For patients with documented factitious disorder on self or Munchausen's syndrome, assign the appropriate code from subcategory F68.1-, Factitious disorder imposed on self.

Munchausen's syndrome by proxy (MSBP) is a disorder in which a caregiver (perpetrator) falsely reports or causes an illness or injury in another person (victim) under his or her care, such as a child, an elderly adult, or a person who has a disability. The condition is also referred to as "factitious disorder imposed on another" or "factitious disorder by proxy." The perpetrator, not the victim, receives this diagnosis. Assign code F68.A, Factitious disorder imposed on another, to the perpetrator's record. For the victim of a patient suffering from MSBP, assign the appropriate code from categories T74, Adult and child abuse, neglect and other maltreatment, confirmed, or T76, Adult and child abuse, neglect and other maltreatment, suspected.

See Section I.C.19.f. Adult and child abuse, neglect and other maltreatment.

d. Dementia

The ICD-10-CM classifies dementia (categories F01, F02, and F03) on the basis of the etiology and severity (unspecified, mild, moderate or severe). Selection of the appropriate severity level requires the provider's clinical judgment and codes should be assigned only on the basis of provider documentation (as defined in the *ICD-10-CM Official Guidelines for Coding and Reporting*), unless otherwise instructed by the classification. If the documentation does not provide information about the severity of the dementia, assign the appropriate code for unspecified severity.

If a patient is admitted to an inpatient acute care hospital or other inpatient facility setting with dementia at one severity level and it progresses to a higher severity level, assign one code for the highest severity level reported during the stay.

Exercise 3.5 – Mental, Behavioral, and Neurodevelopmental Disorders

Instructions: Assign the appropriate ICD-10-CM code(s).

_____ 1. Opioid use, abuse, and dependence with intoxication and delirium

_____ 2. Paranoid schizophrenia

_____ 3. Alcoholic delirium tremens

_____ 4. Factitious disorder, imposed on self, with predominantly physical signs and symptoms

_____ 5. Major depressive disorder, recurrent, with psychotic features

ICD-10-CM Chapter 6: Diseases of the Nervous System (G00–G99)

This ICD-10-CM chapter classifies the following:

- Inflammatory diseases of the central nervous system
- Systemic atrophies primarily affecting the central nervous system
- Extrapyramidal and movement disorders
- Other degenerative diseases of the nervous system
- Demyelinating diseases of the central nervous system
- Episodic and paroxysmal disorders
- Nerve, nerve root, and plexus disorders
- Polyneuropathies and other disorders of the peripheral nervous system
- Diseases of the myoneural junction and muscle
- Cerebral palsy and other paralytic syndromes
- Other disorders of the nervous system

ICD-10-CM Chapter-Specific Coding Guidelines

Chapter 6: Diseases of the Nervous System (G00–G99)

a. **Dominant/nondominant side**

Codes from category G81, Hemiplegia and hemiparesis, and subcategories, G83.1, *Monoplegia of lower limb*, G83.2, *Monoplegia of upper limb*, and G83.3, *Monoplegia, unspecified*, identify whether the dominant or nondominant side is affected. Should the affected side be documented, but not specified as dominant or nondominant, and the classification system does not indicate a default, code selection is as follows:

- For ambidextrous patients, the default should be dominant.
- If the left side is affected, the default is non-dominant.
- If the right side is affected, the default is dominant.

Example: Patient is diagnosed with spastic hemiplegia, right side. Patient is left-handed. Report code G81.13 (Spastic hemiplegia affecting right nondominant side).

b. **Pain – Category G89**

1) **General coding information**

Codes in category G89, Pain, not elsewhere classified, may be used in conjunction with codes from other categories and chapters to provide more detail about acute or chronic pain and neoplasm-related pain, unless otherwise indicated below.

If the pain is not specified as acute or chronic, post-thoracotomy, postprocedural, or neoplasm-related, do not assign codes from category G89.

A code from category G89 should not be assigned if the underlying (definitive) diagnosis is known, unless the reason for the encounter is pain control/management and *not* management of the underlying condition.

When an admission or encounter is for a procedure aimed at treating the underlying condition (e.g., spinal fusion, kyphoplasty), a code for the underlying condition (e.g., vertebral fracture, spinal stenosis) should be assigned as the principal diagnosis. No code from category G89 should be assigned.

(continues)

ICD-10-CM Chapter-Specific Coding Guidelines (*continued*)

(a) Category G89 codes as principal or first-listed diagnosis

Category G89 codes are acceptable as principal diagnosis or the first-listed code:

- When pain control or pain management is the reason for the admission/encounter (e.g., a patient with displaced intervertebral disc, nerve impingement, and severe back pain presents for injection of steroid into the spinal canal). The underlying cause of the pain should be reported as an additional diagnosis, if known.

- When a patient is admitted for the insertion of a neurostimulator for pain control, assign the appropriate pain code as the principal or first-listed diagnosis. When an admission or encounter is for a procedure aimed at treating the underlying condition and a neurostimulator is inserted for pain control during the same admission/encounter, a code for the underlying condition should be assigned as the principal diagnosis and the appropriate pain code should be assigned as a secondary diagnosis.

(b) Use of category G89 codes in conjunction with site-specific pain codes

(i) Assigning category G89 codes and site-specific pain codes

Codes from category G89 may be used in conjunction with codes that identify the site of pain (including codes from Chapter 18) if the category G89 code provides additional information. For example, if the code describes the site of the pain but does not fully describe whether the pain is acute or chronic, both codes should be assigned.

(ii) Sequencing of category G89 codes with site-specific pain codes

The sequencing of category G89 codes with site-specific pain codes (including Chapter 18 codes), is dependent on the circumstances of the encounter/admission as follows:

- If the encounter is for pain control or pain management, assign the code from category G89 followed by the code identifying the specific site of pain (e.g., encounter for pain management for acute neck pain from trauma is assigned code G89.11, Acute pain due to trauma, followed by code M54.2, Cervicalgia, to identify the site of pain).

- If the encounter is for any other reason except pain control or pain management, and a related definitive diagnosis has not been established (confirmed) by the provider, assign the code for the specific site of pain first, followed by the appropriate code from category G89.

2) Pain due to devices, implants, and grafts

See Section I.C.19. Pain due to medical devices.

3) Postoperative pain

The provider's documentation should be used to guide the coding of postoperative pain, as well as *Section III. Reporting Additional Diagnoses* and *Section IV. Diagnostic Coding and Reporting in the Outpatient Setting*. The default for post-thoracotomy and other postoperative pain not specified as acute or chronic is the code for the acute form.

Routine or expected postoperative pain immediately after surgery should not be coded.

(a) Postoperative pain not associated with specific postoperative complication

Postoperative pain not associated with a specific postoperative complication is assigned to the appropriate postoperative pain code in category G89.

(b) Postoperative pain associated with specific postoperative complication

Postoperative pain associated with a specific postoperative complication (such as painful wire sutures) is assigned to the appropriate code(s) found in Chapter 19, Injury, Poisoning, and Certain Other Consequences of External Causes. If appropriate, use additional code(s) from category G89 to identify acute or chronic pain (G89.18 or G89.28).

4) Chronic pain

Chronic pain is classified to subcategory G89.2. There is no time frame defining when pain becomes chronic pain. The provider's documentation should be used to guide the use of these codes.

5) Neoplasm-related pain

Code G89.3 is assigned to pain documented as being related, associated with or due to cancer, primary or secondary malignancy, or tumor. This code is assigned regardless of whether the pain is acute or chronic.

This code may be assigned as the principal or first-listed code when the stated reason for the admission/encounter is documented as pain control/pain management. The underlying neoplasm should be reported as an additional diagnosis.

When the reason for the admission/encounter is management of the neoplasm and the pain associated with the neoplasm is also documented, code G89.3 may be assigned as an additional diagnosis. It is not necessary to assign an additional code for the site of the pain.

See Section I.C.2. for instructions on the sequencing of neoplasms for all other stated reasons for the admission/encounter (except pain control/pain management).

Example: Patient with metastatic bone cancer has related chronic pain and is seen today for management of pain medication. Report codes G89.3 for neoplasm-related pain and C79.51 for secondary malignant neoplasm of bone.

6) Chronic pain syndrome

Central pain syndrome (G89.0) and chronic pain syndrome (G89.4) are different than the term "chronic pain," and therefore codes should only be used when the provider has specifically documented this condition.

See Section I.C.5. Pain disorders related to psychological factors.

Courtesy of the Centers for Medicare & Medicaid Services, www.cms.gov.

Exercise 3.6 – Diseases of the Nervous System

Instructions: Assign the appropriate ICD-10-CM code(s).

1. _____ Flaccid hemiplegia, left dominant side
2. _____ Chronic pain syndrome (admission for pain management)
3. _____ Acute pain due to trauma; cervicalgia (admission for pain control)
4. _____ Acute transverse myelopathy
5. _____ Obstructive sleep apnea with hypopnea; morbid obesity with 51.4 BMI (adult patient)

ICD-10-CM Chapter 7: Diseases of the Eye and Adnexa (H00–H59)

This ICD-10-CM chapter classifies the following:

- Disorders of eyelid, lacrimal system, and orbit
- Disorders of conjunctiva
- Disorders of sclera, cornea, iris, and ciliary body
- Disorders of lens
- Disorders of choroid and retina
- Glaucoma
- Disorders of vitreous body and globe
- Disorders of optic nerve and visual pathways
- Disorders of ocular muscles, binocular movement, accommodation, and refraction
- Visual disturbances and blindness

- Other disorders of eye and adnexa
- Intraoperative and postprocedural complications and disorders of eye and adnexa, not elsewhere classified

ICD-10-CM Chapter-Specific Coding Guidelines

Chapter 7: Diseases of the Eye and Adnexa (H00-H59)

a. Glaucoma

1) Assigning glaucoma codes

Assign as many codes from category H40, Glaucoma, as needed to identify the type of glaucoma, the affected eye, and the glaucoma stage.

2) Bilateral glaucoma with same type and stage

When a patient has bilateral glaucoma and both eyes are documented as being the same type and stage, and there is a code for bilateral glaucoma, report only the code for the type of glaucoma, bilateral, with the seventh character for the stage.

When a patient has bilateral glaucoma and both eyes are documented as being the same type and stage, and the classification does not provide a code for bilateral glaucoma (e.g., subcategories H40.10 and H40.20) report only one code for the type of glaucoma with the appropriate seventh character for the stage.

3) Bilateral glaucoma stage with different types or stages

When a patient has bilateral glaucoma and each eye is documented as having a different type or stage, and the classification distinguishes laterality, assign the appropriate code for each eye rather than the code for bilateral glaucoma. When a patient has bilateral glaucoma and each eye is documented as having a different type, and the classification does not distinguish laterality (i.e., subcategories H40.10 and H40.20), assign one code for each type of glaucoma with the appropriate seventh character for the stage.

When a patient has bilateral glaucoma and each eye is documented as having the same type, but different stage, and the classification does not distinguish laterality (i.e., subcategories H40.10 and H40.20), assign a code for the type of glaucoma for each eye with the seventh character for the specific glaucoma stage documented for each eye.

4) Patient admitted with glaucoma and stage evolves during the admission

If a patient is admitted with glaucoma and the stage progresses during the admission, assign the code for highest stage documented.

Example: Patient is admitted for treatment of primary open-angle glaucoma, left eye, with progression from mild to moderate. Report code H40.1122 for the higher stage of moderate glaucoma.

5) Indeterminate stage glaucoma

Assignment of the seventh character "4" for "indeterminate stage" should be based on the clinical documentation. The seventh character "4" is used for glaucomas whose stage cannot be clinically determined. This seventh character should not be confused with the seventh character "0," unspecified, which should be assigned when there is no documentation regarding the stage of the glaucoma.

b. Blindness

If "blindness" or "low vision" of both eyes is documented but the visual impairment category is not documented, assign code H54.3, Unqualified visual loss, both eyes. If "blindness" or "low vision" in one eye is documented but the visual impairment category is not documented, assign a code from H54.6-, Unqualified visual loss, one eye. If "blindness" or "visual loss" is documented without any information about whether one or both eyes are affected, assign code H54.7, Unspecified visual loss.

Example: For a patient diagnosed with low vision right eye, category 1, and normal vision left eye, report code H54.511A.

Courtesy of the Centers for Medicare & Medicaid Services, www.cms.gov.

Exercise 3.7 – Diseases of the Eye and Adnexa

Instructions: Assign the appropriate ICD-10-CM code(s).

_____   1. Primary open-angle glaucoma, right eye, with progression from mild to moderate stage during hospitalization, right eye

_____   2. Blindness, left eye, category 5; right eye normal

_____   3. Degenerative myopia, bilateral eyes

_____   4. Alternating exotropia

_____   5. Cystoid macular degeneration, bilateral eyes

ICD-10-CM Chapter 8: Diseases of the Ear and Mastoid Process (H60–H95)

This ICD-10-CM chapter classifies the following:

- Diseases of external ear
- Diseases of middle ear and mastoid
- Diseases of inner ear
- Other disorders of the ear
- Intraoperative and postprocedural complications and disorders of the ear and mastoid process, not elsewhere classified

ICD-10-CM Chapter-Specific Coding Guidelines

Chapter 8: Diseases of the Ear and Mastoid Process (H60–H95)

Reserved for future guideline expansion.

Courtesy of the Centers for Medicare & Medicaid Services, www.cms.gov.

Exercise 3.8 – Diseases of the Ear and Mastoid Process

Instructions: Assign the appropriate ICD-10-CM code(s).

_____   1. Swimmer's ear, right ear

_____   2. Acute serous otitis media, left ear

_____   3. Central perforation of tympanic membrane, left ear

_____   4. Vertigo of central origin

_____   5. Granulation of postmastoidectomy cavity, left ear

ICD-10-CM Chapter 9: Diseases of the Circulatory System (I00–I99)

This ICD-10-CM chapter classifies the following:

- Acute rheumatic fever
- Chronic rheumatic heart diseases
- Hypertensive diseases
- Ischemic heart diseases
- Pulmonary heart disease and diseases of pulmonary circulation
- Other forms of heart disease
- Cerebrovascular diseases
- Diseases of arteries, arterioles, and capillaries
- Diseases of veins, lymphatic vessels, and lymph nodes, not elsewhere classified
- Other and unspecified disorders of the circulatory system

ICD-10-CM Chapter-Specific Coding Guidelines

Chapter 9: Diseases of the Circulatory System (I00–I99)

a. Hypertension

The classification presumes a causal relationship between hypertension and heart involvement and between hypertension and kidney involvement, as the two conditions are linked by the term "with" in the Alphabetic Index. These conditions should be coded as related even in the absence of provider documentation explicitly linking them, unless the documentation clearly states the conditions are unrelated. For hypertension and conditions not specifically linked by relational terms such as "with," "associated with" or "due to" in the classification, provider documentation must link the conditions in order to code them as related.

1) Hypertension with heart disease

Hypertension with heart conditions classified to I50.- or I51.4–I51.7, I51.89, I51.9, are assigned to a code from category I11, Hypertensive heart disease. Use an additional code from category I50, Heart failure, to identify the type of heart failure in those patients with heart failure. The same heart conditions (I50.-, I51.4–I51.7, I51.89, I51.9) with hypertension are coded separately if the provider has specifically documented that they are unrelated to the hypertension. Sequence according to the circumstances of the admission/encounter.

Example: Patient is diagnosed with acute right heart failure and has hypertension, which is managed by medication. Report codes I11.0 for hypertensive heart failure and I50.811 for acute right heart failure, in that order.

2) Hypertensive chronic kidney disease

Assign codes from category I12, Hypertensive chronic kidney disease, when both hypertension and a condition classifiable to category N18, Chronic kidney disease (CKD), are present. CKD should not be coded as hypertensive if the provider indicates the CKD is not related to the hypertension.

The appropriate code from category N18 should be used as a secondary code with a code from category I12 to identify the stage of chronic kidney disease.

See Section I.C.14. Chronic kidney disease.

If a patient has hypertensive chronic kidney disease and acute renal failure, the acute renal failure should also be coded. Sequence according to the circumstances of the admission/encounter.

Example 1: Patient is hospitalized for hypertensive end-stage renal disease (ESRD). Report codes I12.0 for hypertensive ESRD and N18.6 for ESRD.

Example 2: Patient treated for ESRD and also has hypertension due to hyperthyroidism. Report codes N18.6 for ESRD, I10 for hypertension, and E05.90 for hyperthyroidism.

3) Hypertensive heart and chronic kidney disease

Assign codes from combination category I13, Hypertensive heart and chronic kidney disease, when there is hypertension with both heart and kidney involvement. If heart failure is present, assign an additional code from category I50 to identify the type of heart failure.

The appropriate code from category N18, Chronic kidney disease, should be used as a secondary code with a code from category I13 to identify the stage of chronic kidney disease.

See Section I.C.14. Chronic kidney disease.

The codes in category I13, Hypertensive heart and chronic kidney disease, are combination codes that include hypertension, heart disease and chronic kidney disease. The Includes note at I13 specifies that the conditions included at I11 and I12 are included together in I13. If a patient has hypertension, heart disease and chronic kidney disease, then a code from I13 should be used, not individual codes for hypertension, heart disease and chronic kidney disease, or codes from I11 or I12.

For patients with both acute renal failure and chronic kidney disease, the acute renal failure should also be coded. Sequence according to the circumstances of the admission/encounter.

4) Hypertensive cerebrovascular disease

For hypertensive cerebrovascular disease, first assign the appropriate code from categories I60-I69, followed by the appropriate hypertension code.

5) Hypertensive retinopathy

Subcategory H35.0, Background retinopathy and retinal vascular changes, should be used along with a code from categories I10–I15, in the Hypertensive diseases section, to include systemic hypertension. The sequencing is based on the reason for the encounter.

6) Hypertension, secondary

Secondary hypertension is due to an underlying condition. Two codes are required: one to identify the underlying etiology and one from category I15 to identify the hypertension. Sequencing of codes is determined by the reason for admission/encounter.

7) Hypertension, transient

Assign code R03.0, Elevated blood pressure reading without diagnosis of hypertension, unless patient has an established diagnosis of hypertension. Assign code O13.-, Gestational [pregnancy-induced] hypertension without significant proteinuria, or O14.-, Pre-eclampsia, for transient hypertension of pregnancy.

8) Hypertension, controlled

This diagnostic statement usually refers to an existing state of hypertension under control by therapy. Assign the appropriate code from categories I10–I15, Hypertensive diseases.

9) Hypertension, uncontrolled

Uncontrolled hypertension may refer to untreated hypertension or hypertension not responding to current therapeutic regimen. In either case, assign the appropriate code from categories I10–I15, Hypertensive diseases.

10) Hypertensive crisis

Assign a code from category I16, Hypertensive crisis, for documented hypertensive urgency, hypertensive emergency or unspecified hypertensive crisis. Code also any identified hypertensive disease (I10–I15). The sequencing is based on the reason for the encounter.

11) Pulmonary Hypertension

Pulmonary hypertension is classified to category I27, Other pulmonary heart diseases. For secondary pulmonary hypertension (I27.1, I27.2-), code also any associated conditions or adverse effects of drugs or toxins. The sequencing is based on the reason for the encounter, except for adverse effects of drugs (See Section I.C.19.e.).

(continues)

ICD-10-CM Chapter-Specific Coding Guidelines (*continued*)

12) Hypertension, Resistant

Resistant hypertension refers to blood pressure of a patient with hypertension that remains above goal in spite of the use of antihypertensive medications. Assign code I1A.0, Resistant hypertension, as an additional code when apparent treatment resistant hypertension, treatment resistant hypertension, or true resistant hypertension is documented by the provider. A code for the specific type of existing hypertension is sequenced first, if known.

b. Atherosclerotic coronary artery disease and angina

ICD-10-CM has combination codes for atherosclerotic heart disease with angina pectoris. The subcategories for these codes are I25.11, Atherosclerotic heart disease of native coronary artery with angina pectoris and I25.7, Atherosclerosis of coronary artery bypass graft(s) and coronary artery of transplanted heart with angina pectoris.

When using one of these combination codes it is not necessary to use an additional code for angina pectoris. A causal relationship can be assumed in a patient with both atherosclerosis and angina pectoris, unless the documentation indicates the angina is due to something other than the atherosclerosis.

If a patient with coronary artery disease is admitted due to an acute myocardial infarction (AMI), the AMI should be sequenced before the coronary artery disease.

See Section I.C.9. Acute myocardial infarction (AMI)

c. Intraoperative and postprocedural cerebrovascular accident

Medical record documentation should clearly specify the cause-and-effect relationship between the medical intervention and the cerebrovascular accident in order to assign a code for intraoperative or postprocedural cerebrovascular accident.

Proper code assignment depends on whether it was an infarction or hemorrhage and whether it occurred intraoperatively or postoperatively. If it was a cerebral hemorrhage, code assignment depends on the type of procedure performed.

d. Sequelae of cerebrovascular disease

1) Category I69, sequelae of cerebrovascular disease

Category I69 is used to indicate conditions classifiable to categories I60–I67 as the causes of sequela (neurologic deficits), themselves classified elsewhere. These "late effects" include neurologic deficits that persist after initial onset of conditions classifiable to categories I60–I67. The neurologic deficits caused by cerebrovascular disease may be present from the onset or may arise at any time after the onset of the condition classifiable to categories I60–I67.

Codes from category I69, Sequelae of cerebrovascular disease, that specify hemiplegia, hemiparesis and monoplegia identify whether the dominant or nondominant side is affected. Should the affected side be documented, but not specified as dominant or nondominant, and the classification system does not indicate a default, code selection is as follows:

- For ambidextrous patients, the default should be dominant.

- If the left side is affected, the default is non-dominant.

- If the right side is affected, the default is dominant.

2) Codes from category I69 with codes from I60–I67

Codes from category I69 may be assigned on a health care record with codes from I60–I67, if the patient has a current cerebrovascular disease and deficits from an old cerebrovascular disease.

3) Codes from category I69 and PERSONAL history of transient ischemic attack (TIA) and cerebral infarction (Z86.73)

Codes from category I69 should not be assigned if the patient does not have neurologic deficits.

See Section I.C.21.4. History (of) for use of personal history codes.

e. Acute myocardial infarction (AMI)

1) Type 1 ST elevation myocardial infarction (STEMI) and non-ST elevation myocardial infarction (NSTEMI)

The ICD-10-CM codes for type 1 acute myocardial infarction (AMI) identify the site, such as anterolateral wall or true posterior wall. Subcategories I21.0–I21.2 and code I21.3 are used for type 1 ST elevation myocardial infarction (STEMI). Code I21.4, Non-ST elevation (NSTEMI) myocardial infarction, is used for type 1 non-ST elevation myocardial infarction (NSTEMI) and nontransmural MIs.

If a type 1 NSTEMI evolves to STEMI, assign the STEMI code. If a type 1 STEMI converts to NSTEMI due to thrombolytic therapy, it is still coded as STEMI.

For encounters occurring while the myocardial infarction is equal to, or less than, four weeks old, including transfers to another acute setting or a postacute setting, and the myocardial infarction meets the definition for "other diagnoses" (*see Section III, Reporting Additional Diagnoses*), codes from category I21 may continue to be reported. For encounters after the 4-week time frame and the patient is still receiving care related to the myocardial infarction, the appropriate aftercare code should be assigned, rather than a code from category I21. For old or healed myocardial infarctions not requiring further care, code I25.2, Old myocardial infarction, may be assigned.

2) Acute myocardial infarction, unspecified

Code I21.9, Acute myocardial infarction, unspecified, is the default for unspecified acute myocardial infarction or unspecified site. If only type 1 STEMI or transmural MI without the site is documented, assign code I21.3, ST (STEMI) elevation myocardial infarction of unspecified site.

3) AMI documented as nontransmural or subendocardial but site provided

If an AMI is documented as nontransmural or subendocardial, but the site is provided, it is still coded as a subendocardial AMI.

See Section I.C.21.3. for information on coding status post administration of tPA in a different facility within the last 24 hrs.

4) Subsequent acute myocardial infarction

A code from category I22, Subsequent ST elevation (STEMI) and non-ST elevation (NSTEMI) myocardial infarction, is to be used when a patient who has suffered a type 1 or unspecified AMI has a new AMI within the 4 week time frame of the initial AMI. A code from category I22 must be used in conjunction with a code from category I21. The sequencing of the I22 and I21 codes depends on the circumstances of the encounter.

Do not assign code I22 for subsequent myocardial infarctions other than type 1 or unspecified. For subsequent type 2 AMI assign only code I21.A1. For subsequent type 4 or type 5 AMI, assign only code I21.A9.

If a subsequent myocardial infarction of one type occurs within 4 weeks of a myocardial infarction of a different type, assign the appropriate codes from category I21 to identify each type. Do not assign a code from I22. Codes from category I22 should only be assigned if both the initial and subsequent myocardial infarctions are type 1 or unspecified.

5) Other types of myocardial infarction

The ICD-10-CM provides codes for different types of myocardial infarction. Type 1 myocardial infarctions are assigned to codes I21.0–I21.4.

Type 2 myocardial infarction (myocardial infarction due to demand ischemia or secondary to ischemic imbalance) is assigned to code I21.A1, Myocardial infarction type 2 with the underlying cause coded first. Do not assign code I24.89, Other forms of acute ischemic heart disease, for the demand ischemia. Sequencing of type 2 AMI or the underlying cause is dependent on the circumstances of admission. If a type 2 AMI is described as NSTEMI or STEMI, only assign code I21.A1. Codes I21.01–I21.4 should only be assigned for type 1 AMIs.

Acute myocardial infarctions type 3, 4a, 4b, 4c and 5 are assigned to code I21.A9, Other myocardial infarction type.

The "Code also" and "Code first" notes should be followed related to complications, and for coding of postprocedural myocardial infarctions during or following cardiac surgery.

(continues)

ICD-10-CM Chapter-Specific Coding Guidelines (*continued*)

6) Myocardial Infarction with Coronary Microvascular Dysfunction

Coronary microvascular dysfunction (CMD) is a condition that impacts the microvasculature by restricting microvascular flow and increasing microvascular resistance. Code I21.B, Myocardial infarction with coronary microvascular dysfunction, is assigned for myocardial infarction with coronary microvascular disease, myocardial infarction with coronary microvascular dysfunction, and myocardial infarction with non-obstructive coronary arteries (MINOCA) with microvascular disease.

Exercise 3.9 – Diseases of the Circulatory System

Instructions: Assign the appropriate ICD-10-CM code(s).

_____ 1. Non-ST elevation myocardial infarction (NSTEMI), inferolateral wall, initial episode of care

_____ 2. Type 1 acute inferoposterior transmural ST elevation myocardial infarction (STEMI), and subsequent type 1 acute inferior STEMI three days later (during same inpatient admission)

_____ 3. Aphasia as sequela of cerebral infarction

_____ 4. Hypertension and stage 4 chronic kidney disease

_____ 5. Atherosclerotic heart disease of native coronary artery with unstable angina pectoris

ICD-10-CM Chapter 10: Diseases of the Respiratory System (J00–J99), U07.0

This ICD-10-CM chapter classifies the following:

- Acute upper respiratory infections
- Influenza and pneumonia
- Other acute lower respiratory infections
- Other diseases of upper respiratory tract
- Chronic lower respiratory diseases
- Lung diseases due to external agents
- Other respiratory diseases principally affecting the interstitium
- Suppurative and necrotic conditions of the lower respiratory tract
- Other diseases of the pleura
- Intraoperative and postprocedural complications and disorders of respiratory system, not elsewhere classified
- Other diseases of the respiratory system

The respiratory system is responsible for pulmonary ventilation and the exchange of oxygen and carbon dioxide between the lungs and ambient air. The organs of the respiratory system also perform non-respiratory functions such as warming and moisturizing the air passing into the lungs, providing airflow for the larynx and vocal cords for speech, and releasing excess body heat in the process of thermoregulation for homeostasis. The lungs also perform important metabolic and embolic filtering functions.

ICD-10-CM Chapter-Specific Coding Guidelines

Chapter 10: Diseases of the Respiratory System (J00–J99), U07.0

a. Chronic obstructive pulmonary disease [COPD] and asthma

1) Acute exacerbation of chronic obstructive bronchitis and asthma

The codes in categories J44 and J45 distinguish between uncomplicated cases and those in acute exacerbation. An acute exacerbation is a worsening or a decompensation of a chronic condition. An acute exacerbation is not equivalent to an infection superimposed on a chronic condition, though an exacerbation may be triggered by an infection.

Example: Patient is diagnosed with COPD with acute exacerbation. Report code J44.1.

b. Acute respiratory failure

1) Acute respiratory failure as principal diagnosis

A code from subcategory J96.0, Acute respiratory failure, or subcategory J96.2, Acute and chronic respiratory failure, may be assigned as a principal diagnosis when it is the condition established after study to be chiefly responsible for occasioning the admission to the hospital, and the selection is supported by the Alphabetic Index and Tabular List. However, chapter-specific coding guidelines (such as obstetrics, poisoning, HIV, newborn) that provide sequencing direction take precedence.

Example: Patient is diagnosed with acute and chronic respiratory failure for which code J96.20 is reported.

2) Acute respiratory failure as secondary diagnosis

Respiratory failure may be listed as a secondary diagnosis if it occurs after admission, or if it is present on admission but does not meet the definition of principal diagnosis.

3) Sequencing of acute respiratory failure and another acute condition

When a patient is admitted with respiratory failure and another acute condition (e.g., myocardial infarction, cerebrovascular accident, aspiration pneumonia), the principal diagnosis will not be the same in every situation. This applies whether the other acute condition is a respiratory or nonrespiratory condition. Selection of the principal diagnosis will be dependent on the circumstances of admission. If both the respiratory failure and the other acute condition are equally responsible for occasioning the admission to the hospital and there are no chapter-specific sequencing rules, the guideline regarding two or more diagnoses that equally meet the definition for principal diagnosis (*Section II, C.*) may be applied in these situations.

If the documentation is not clear as to whether acute respiratory failure and another condition are equally responsible for occasioning the admission, query the provider for clarification.

c. Influenza due to certain identified influenza viruses

Code only confirmed cases of influenza due to certain identified influenza viruses (category J09), and due to other identified influenza virus (category J10). This is an exception to the hospital inpatient guideline Section II, H. (Uncertain Diagnosis).

In this context, "confirmation" does not require documentation of positive laboratory testing specific for avian or other novel influenza A or other identified influenza virus. However, coding should be based on the provider's diagnostic statement that the patient has avian influenza, or other novel influenza A, for category J09, or has another particular identified strain of influenza, such as H1N1 or H3N2, but not identified as novel or variant, for category J10.

If the provider records "suspected" or "possible" or "probable" avian influenza, or novel influenza, or other identified influenza, then the appropriate influenza code from category J11, Influenza due to unidentified influenza virus, should be assigned. A code from category J09, Influenza due to certain identified influenza viruses, should not be assigned nor should a code from category J10, Influenza due to other identified influenza virus.

(continues)

ICD-10-CM Chapter-Specific Coding Guidelines (*continued*)

d. Ventilator associated pneumonia

1) Documentation of ventilator associated pneumonia

As with all procedural or postprocedural complications, code assignment is based on the provider's documentation of the relationship between the condition and the procedure.

Code J95.851, Ventilator associated pneumonia, should be assigned only when the provider has documented ventilator associated pneumonia (VAP). An additional code to identify the organism (e.g., *Pseudomonas aeruginosa,* code B96.5) should also be assigned. Do not assign an additional code from categories J12–J18 to identify the type of pneumonia.

Code J95.851 should not be assigned for cases where the patient has pneumonia and is on a mechanical ventilator and the provider has not specifically stated that the pneumonia is ventilator-associated pneumonia. If the documentation is unclear as to whether the patient has a pneumonia that is a complication attributable to the mechanical ventilator, query the provider.

2) Ventilator associated pneumonia [VAP] develops after admission

A patient may be admitted with one type of pneumonia (e.g., code J13, Pneumonia due to Streptococcus pneumonia) and subsequently develop VAP. In this instance, the principal diagnosis would be the appropriate code from categories J12–J18 for the pneumonia diagnosed at the time of admission.

Code J95.851, Ventilator associated pneumonia, would be assigned as an additional diagnosis when the provider has also documented the presence of ventilator associated pneumonia.

e. Vaping-related disorders

For patients presenting with condition(s) related to vaping, assign code U07.0, Vaping-related disorder, as the principal diagnosis. For lung injury due to vaping, assign only code U07.0. Assign additional codes for other manifestations, such as acute respiratory failure (subcategory J96.0-) or pneumonitis (code J68.0).

Associated respiratory signs and symptoms due to vaping, such as cough, shortness of breath, etc., are not coded separately, when a definitive diagnosis has been established. However, it would be appropriate to code separately any gastrointestinal symptoms, such as diarrhea and abdominal pain.

See Section I.C.1.g.1.c.i. for Pneumonia confirmed as due to COVID-19.

Courtesy of the Centers for Medicare & Medicaid Services, www.cms.gov.

Exercise 3.10 – Diseases of the Respiratory System

Instructions: Assign the appropriate ICD-10-CM code(s).

_____   1. Acute exacerbation of chronic obstructive pulmonary disease (COPD)

_____   2. Human immunodeficiency virus disease and subsequent acute respiratory failure with hypoxia

_____   3. Influenza due to identified novel influenza A virus

_____   4. Acute adenoviral pneumonia with development of ventilator-associated pneumonia after admission

_____   5. Lung damage due to vaping; acute respiratory distress syndrome

Summary

Chapter-specific coding guidelines clarify the assignment of ICD-10-CM disease codes. Unless otherwise indicated, the ICD-10-CM chapter-specific coding guidelines apply to all health care settings.

Internet Links

ICD-10-CM Official Guidelines for Coding and Reporting: **Go to cms.gov,** click on Medicare, click on Coding & billing, and click on ICD-10 codes.

MedLine Plus Interactive Tutorials (for diseases and procedures): Go to **www.nlm.nih.gov.** Click on the Site Map, and scroll to Videos & Tools where health videos, health check tools, and games can be selected.

Review

3.1 – Multiple Choice

Instructions: Select the most appropriate response.

1. Sepsis due to *E. coli.*
   - a. A41.4
   - b. A41.50
   - c. A41.51
   - d. A41.9

2. Metastatic carcinoma from the lung.
   - a. C34.90, C79.9
   - b. C79.9, D49.1
   - c. D49.9, C34.90
   - d. D49.9, C80.1

3. Type 2 diabetes mellitus with diabetic macular edema and retinopathy, right eye, resolved following treatment.
   - a. E08.371
   - b. E09.371
   - c. E10.371
   - d. E11.371

4. Anemia, neutropenia, and thrombocytopenia.
   - a. D61.09
   - b. D61.9
   - c. D64.9, D70.9, D69.6
   - d. P61.4, D70.4, D69.3

5. Alcohol dependence with withdrawal delirium.
   - a. F10.121, F10.20
   - b. F10.231
   - c. F10.96, F10.26
   - d. G25.1, F10.20

6. Flaccid hemiplegia affecting right dominant side due to old spinal cord injury, lumbar region.
   - a. G81.01, S34.01XS
   - b. G81.01, S30.9XXS
   - c. G81.01, S34.109S
   - d. G81.01, S34.119S

7. Bilateral anterior cerebral artery thrombosis.
   - a. I66.03
   - b. I66.13
   - c. I66.23
   - d. I66.8

8. Asymptomatic human immunodeficiency virus disease.
   - a. B20
   - b. R75
   - c. Z20.6
   - d. Z21

9. Primary open-angle glaucoma, right eye, mild stage.
   - a. H40.1111
   - b. H44.511
   - c. P15.3
   - d. Q15.0

10. Acute nasopharyngitis.
    a. J00
    b. J02.9
    c. J31.1
    d. J31.2

11. Acute suppurative otitis media, left ear, with central perforated eardrum.
    a. H65.02, S09.22XA
    b. H66.012
    c. H66.012, H72.02
    d. H67.2, S09.22XA

12. Central pain syndrome.
    a. F45.41
    b. G89.0
    c. G89.4
    d. R52

13. Spastic hemiplegia affecting left dominant side.
    a. G80.9
    b. G81.02
    c. G81.12
    d. G81.92

14. Factitious disorder by proxy.
    a. F45.9
    b. F54
    c. F68.A
    d. Z76.5

15. Type 2 diabetes mellitus with ketoacidosis and coma, requiring long term (current) insulin use.
    a. E08.11, T38.3X6A, Z79.4
    b. E09.11, T38.3X5A, Z79.4
    c. E10.11, Z79.4
    d. E11.11, Z79.4

3.2 – Coding Practice – Diseases

Instructions: Assign the appropriate ICD-10-CM code(s) to each disease.

1. Classical hemophilia _____

2. Adenocarcinoma, lower-outer quadrant of right breast (male) _____

3. Multiple personality disorder _____

4. Pneumonia due to *Streptococcus*, group B _____

5. Postsurgical hypothyroidism _____

6. Pulmonary arteriosclerosis _____

7. Sandflea infestation _____

8. Cholera due to *Vibrio cholerae* 01, biovar eltor _____

9. Arachnoid cyst (acquired) _____

10. Hypertensive emergency due to uncontrolled hypertension _____

11. Day blindness _____

12. Chronic nonsuppurative mucoid otitis media, left ear _____

13. Chronic hypertensive systolic (congestive) heart failure _____

14. Hypertensive end-stage renal disease _____

15. Acute respiratory failure with hypercapnia _____

Chapter-Specific Coding Guidelines: ICD-10-CM Chapters 11–22

Chapter Outline

ICD-10-CM Chapter 11: Diseases of the Digestive System (K00–K95)

ICD-10-CM Chapter 12: Diseases of the Skin and Subcutaneous Tissue (L00–L99)

ICD-10-CM Chapter 13: Diseases of the Musculoskeletal System and Connective Tissue (M00–M99)

ICD-10-CM Chapter 14: Diseases of the Genitourinary System (N00–N99)

ICD-10-CM Chapter 15: Pregnancy, Childbirth, and the Puerperium (O00–O9A)

ICD-10-CM Chapter 16: Certain Conditions Originating in the Perinatal Period (P00–P96)

ICD-10-CM Chapter 17: Congenital Malformations, Deformations, and Chromosomal Abnormalities (Q00–Q99)

ICD-10-CM Chapter 18: Symptoms, Signs, and Abnormal Clinical and Laboratory Findings, Not Elsewhere Classified (R00–R99)

ICD-10-CM Chapter 19: Injury, Poisoning, and Certain Other Consequences of External Causes (S00–T88)

ICD-10-CM Chapter 20: External Causes of Morbidity (V00–Y99)

ICD-10-CM Chapter 21: Factors Influencing Health Status and Contact with Health Services (Z00–Z99)

ICD-10-CM Chapter 22: Codes for Special Purposes (U00–U85)

Chapter Objectives

At the conclusion of this chapter, the student should be able to:

1. Define key terms related to chapter-specific coding guidelines for ICD-10-CM Chapters 11 through 22.
2. Assign codes to diseases of the digestive system according to chapter-specific guidelines.
3. Assign codes to diseases of the skin and subcutaneous tissue according to chapter-specific guidelines.
4. Assign codes to diseases of the musculoskeletal system and connective tissue according to chapter-specific guidelines.
5. Assign codes to diseases of the genitourinary system according to chapter-specific guidelines.
6. Assign codes to pregnancy, childbirth, and the puerperium according to chapter-specific guidelines.

7. Assign codes to certain conditions originating in the perinatal period according to chapter-specific guidelines.
8. Assign codes to congenital malformations, deformations, and chromosomal abnormalities according to chapter-specific guidelines.
9. Assign codes to symptoms, signs, and abnormal clinical and laboratory findings, not elsewhere classified, according to chapter-specific guidelines.
10. Assign codes to injury, poisoning, and certain other consequences of external causes according to chapter-specific guidelines.
11. Assign codes to external causes of morbidity according to chapter-specific guidelines.
12. Assign codes to factors influencing health status and contact with health services according to chapter-specific guidelines.
13. Assign codes to coding for special purposes according to chapter-specific guidelines.

Key Terms

closed fracture	fracture	nonunion	perinatal period
compound fracture	malunion	open fracture	simple fracture

Introduction

This chapter includes content about chapter-specific coding guidelines for ICD-10-CM Chapters 11 through 22. Chapter-specific coding guidelines are used as a companion to the ICD-10-CM coding manual, which contains coding conventions to ensure accurate coding.

- Diseases of the Digestive System (K00–K95)
- Diseases of the Skin and Subcutaneous Tissue (L00–L99)
- Diseases of the Musculoskeletal System and Connective Tissue (M00–M99)
- Diseases of the Genitourinary System (N00–N99)
- Pregnancy, Childbirth, and the Puerperium (O00–O9A)
- Certain Conditions Originating in the Perinatal Period (P00–P96)
- Congenital Malformations, Deformations, and Chromosomal Abnormalities (Q00–Q99)
- Symptoms, Signs, and Abnormal Clinical and Laboratory Findings, Not Elsewhere Classified (R00–R99)
- Injury, Poisoning, and Certain Other Consequences of External Causes (S00–T88)
- External Causes of Morbidity (V00–Y99)
- Factors Influencing Health Status and Contact with Health Services (Z00–Z99)
- Codes for Special Purposes (U00–U85)

ICD-10-CM Chapter 11: Diseases of the Digestive System (K00–K95)

This ICD-10-CM chapter classifies the following:

- Diseases of oral cavity and salivary glands
- Diseases of esophagus, stomach, and duodenum
- Diseases of appendix
- Hernia

- Noninfective enteritis and colitis
- Other diseases of intestines
- Diseases of peritoneum and retroperitoneum
- Diseases of liver
- Disorders of gallbladder, biliary tract, and pancreas
- Other diseases of the digestive system

The alimentary tract (or digestive tract) is the long, muscular tube that begins at the mouth and ends at the anus. Major digestive organs include the pharynx, esophagus, stomach, and intestines. Accessory, or secondary, organs include the salivary and parotid glands, jaw, teeth, and supporting structures of the teeth, tongue, liver, gallbladder and biliary tract, pancreas, and peritoneum. Structures that support the digestive process from outside this continuous tube are also included in this system: gallbladder, pancreas, and liver. (These organs provide secretions that are critical to food absorption and use by the body.)

Example: The following are examples of diseases that interfere with the digestive function, and they are classified in ICD-10-CM Chapter 11:

- Dental caries (tooth decay), assigned ICD-10-CM code K02.9, has a direct effect on digestion because the disease process interferes with mastication, the mechanical breakdown of food by chewing.
- Portal hypertension, assigned ICD-10-CM code K76.6, is high blood pressure in the liver's portal circulatory system. Although it does not directly affect digestion, portal hypertension is included because it represents a disease of a digestive system organ. Portal hypertension has no apparent effect on the digestive process until the disease has progressed to the point that the liver can no longer perform its function as a digestive organ. (Portal hypertension can be caused by cirrhosis of the liver and other conditions that cause obstruction to the portal vein, such as cancer.)

ICD-10-CM Chapter-Specific Coding Guidelines

Chapter 11: Diseases of the Digestive System (K00–K95)

Reserved for future guideline expansion.

Courtesy of the Centers for Medicare & Medicaid Services, www.cms.gov.

Exercise 4.1 – Diseases of the Digestive System

Instructions: Assign the appropriate ICD-10-CM code(s).

_____ **1.** Crohn's disease
_____ **2.** Canker sore
_____ **3.** Acute gastrojejunal ulcer, with perforation
_____ **4.** Gastroesophageal reflux
_____ **5.** Unilateral inguinal hernia

ICD-10-CM Chapter 12: Diseases of the Skin and Subcutaneous Tissue (L00–L99)

This ICD-10-CM chapter classifies the following:

- Infections of the skin and subcutaneous tissue
- Bullous disorders
- Dermatitis and eczema

- Papulosquamous disorders
- Urticaria and erythema
- Radiation-related disorders of the skin and subcutaneous tissue
- Disorders of skin appendages
- Intraoperative and postprocedural complications of skin and subcutaneous tissue
- Other disorders of the skin and subcutaneous tissue

ICD-10-CM Chapter-Specific Coding Guidelines

Chapter 12: Diseases of the Skin and Subcutaneous Tissue (L00–L99)

a. Pressure ulcer stage codes

1) Pressure ulcer stages

Codes in category L89, Pressure ulcer, identify the site and stage of the pressure ulcer.

The ICD-10-CM classifies pressure ulcer stages based on severity, which is designated by stages 1–4, deep tissue pressure injury, unspecified stage, and unstageable.

Assign as many codes from category L89 as needed to identify all the pressure ulcers the patient has, if applicable.

See Section I.B.14 for pressure ulcer stage documentation by clinicians other than patient's provider.

Example: Patient is diagnosed with stage 4 pressure ulcer, right elbow, and stage 2 pressure ulcer, left elbow. Report codes L89.014 for the right elbow pressure ulcer and L89.022 for the left elbow pressure ulcer.

2) Unstageable pressure ulcers

Assignment of the code for unstageable pressure ulcer (L89.--0) should be based on the clinical documentation. These codes are used for pressure ulcers whose stage cannot be clinically determined (e.g., the ulcer is covered by eschar or has been treated with a skin or muscle graft). This code should not be confused with the codes for unspecified stage (L89.--9). When there is no documentation regarding the stage of the pressure ulcer, assign the appropriate code for unspecified stage (L89.--9). If during an encounter, the stage of an unstageable pressure ulcer is revealed after debridement, assign only the code for the stage revealed following debridement.

Example 1: Patient is diagnosed with pressure ulcer, right elbow, which cannot be staged due to presence of skin graft. Report code L89.010 (Pressure ulcer of right elbow, unstageable).

Example 2: Patient is diagnosed with pressure ulcer, right upper back. Report code L89.119 (Pressure ulcer of right upper back, unspecified stage) because the provider did not document the stage. (A physician query should be generated to request staging information.)

3) Documented pressure ulcer stage

Assignment of the pressure ulcer stage code should be guided by clinical documentation of the stage or documentation of the terms found in the Alphabetic Index. For clinical terms describing the stage that are not found in the Alphabetic Index, and there is no documentation of the stage, the provider should be queried.

4) Patients admitted with pressure ulcers documented as healed

No code is assigned if the documentation states that the pressure ulcer is completely healed at the time of admission.

5) Pressure ulcers documented as healing

Pressure ulcers described as healing should be assigned the appropriate pressure ulcer stage code based on the documentation in the medical record. If the documentation does not provide information about the stage of the healing pressure ulcer, assign the appropriate code for unspecified stage.

If the documentation is unclear as to whether the patient has a current (new) pressure ulcer or if the patient is being treated for a healing pressure ulcer, query the provider.

For ulcers that were present on admission but healed at the time of discharge, assign the code for the site and stage of the pressure ulcer at the time of admission.

6) **Patient admitted with pressure ulcer evolving into another stage during the admission**

If a patient is admitted to an inpatient hospital with a pressure ulcer at one stage and it progresses to a higher stage, two separate codes should be assigned: one code for the site and stage of the ulcer on admission and a second code for the same ulcer site and the highest stage reported during the stay.

7) **Pressure-induced deep tissue damage**

For pressure-induced deep tissue damage or deep tissue pressure injury, assign only the appropriate code for pressure-induced deep tissue damage (L89.--6).

b. **Non-pressure chronic ulcers**

1) **Patients admitted with non-pressure ulcers documented as healed**

No code is assigned if the documentation states that the non-pressure ulcer is completely healed at the time of admission.

2) **Non-pressure ulcers documented as healing**

Non-pressure ulcers described as healing should be assigned the appropriate non-pressure ulcer code based on the documentation in the medical record. If the documentation does not provide information about the severity of the healing non-pressure ulcer, assign the appropriate code for unspecified severity.

If the documentation is unclear as to whether the patient has a current (new) non-pressure ulcer or if the patient is being treated for a healing non-pressure ulcer, query the provider.

For ulcers that were present on admission but healed at the time of discharge, assign the code for the site and severity of the non-pressure ulcer at the time of admission.

3) **Patient admitted with non-pressure ulcer that progresses to another severity level during the admission**

If a patient is admitted to an inpatient hospital with a non-pressure ulcer at one severity level and it progresses to a higher severity level, two separate codes should be assigned: one code for the site and severity level of the ulcer on admission and a second code for the same ulcer site and the highest severity level reported during the stay.

See Section I.B.14 for pressure ulcer stage documentation by clinicians other than patient's provider.

Exercise 4.2 – Diseases of the Skin and Subcutaneous Tissue

Instructions: Assign the appropriate ICD-10-CM code(s).

_____ 1. Alopecia areata

_____ 2. Carbuncle, left foot, due to methicillin-resistant *Staphylococcus*

_____ 3. Decubitus ulcer, left buttock, stage 3

_____ 4. Chronic ulcer, right heel, with skin breakdown only due to postthrombotic syndrome

_____ 5. Keloid

ICD-10-CM Chapter 13: Diseases of the Musculoskeletal System and Connective Tissue (M00–M99)

This ICD-10-CM chapter classifies the following:

- Infectious arthropathies
- Autoinflammatory syndromes
- Inflammatory polyarthropathies
- Osteoarthritis
- Other joint disorders
- Dentofacial anomalies [including malocclusion] and other disorders of jaw
- Systemic connective tissue disorders
- Deforming dorsopathies
- Spondylopathies
- Other dorsopathies
- Disorders of muscles
- Disorders of synovium and tendon
- Other soft tissue disorders
- Disorders of bone density and structure
- Other osteopathies
- Chondropathies
- Other disorders of the musculoskeletal system and connective tissue
- Intraoperative and postprocedural complications and disorders of musculoskeletal system, not elsewhere classified
- Periprosthetic fracture around internal prosthetic
- Biomechanical lesions, not elsewhere classified

Localized osteoarthritis is classified as primary or secondary. Primary osteoarthritis (or polyarticular degenerative arthritis) has an unknown etiology (cause), which means it is idiopathic. It affects apophyseal joints (joints with nodular or bony eminence) of the hips, knees, spine, and small joints of the hands and feet. Secondary osteoarthritis (or monoarticular arthritis) is caused by external or internal injuries (acute or chronic trauma) or disease processes and is confined to the joints of one area. Disease processes include endocrine, infectious, metabolic, and neuropathic diseases, as well as disease processes that alter the normal structure and function of hyaline cartilage (e.g., chondrocalcinosis, gout, and Paget's disease).

> **Example:** A patient is diagnosed with degenerative joint disease, bilateral knees. Assign ICD-10-CM code M17.0 (Bilateral primary osteoarthritis of knee).

ICD-10-CM Chapter-Specific Coding Guidelines

Chapter 13: Diseases of Musculoskeletal and Connective Tissue (M00–M99)

a. Site and laterality

Most of the codes within Chapter 13 have site and laterality designations. The site represents the bone, joint or the muscle involved. For some conditions where more than one bone, joint or muscle is usually involved, such as osteoarthritis, there is a "multiple sites" code available. For categories where no multiple site code is provided and more than one bone, joint or muscle is involved, multiple codes should be used to indicate the different sites involved.

Example: Patient is diagnosed with enteropathic arthropathies of the left knee, ankle, and foot. Report code M07.69 for enteropathic arthropathies of multiple sites.

1) Bone versus joint

For certain conditions, the bone may be affected at the upper or lower end (e.g., avascular necrosis of bone, M87, Osteoporosis, M80, M81). Though the portion of the bone affected may be at the joint, the site designation will be the bone, not the joint.

Example: Patient is diagnosed with avascular necrosis of bone (osteonecrosis), right index finger joint. Report code M87.844, Other osteonecrosis, right finger(s).

b. Acute traumatic versus chronic or recurrent musculoskeletal conditions

Many musculoskeletal conditions are a result of previous injury or trauma to a site, or are recurrent conditions. Bone, joint or muscle conditions that are the result of a healed injury are usually found in ICD-10-CM Chapter 13. Recurrent bone, joint or muscle conditions are also usually found in ICD-10-CM Chapter 13. Any current, acute injury should be coded to the appropriate injury code from ICD-10-CM Chapter 19. Chronic or recurrent conditions should generally be coded with a code from ICD-10-CM Chapter 13. If it is difficult to determine from the documentation in the record which code is best to describe a condition, query the provider.

c. Coding of Pathologic Fractures

7th character A is for use as long as the patient is receiving active treatment for the fracture. While the patient may be seen by a new or different provider over the course of treatment for a pathological fracture, assignment of the 7th character is based on whether the patient is undergoing active treatment and not whether the provider is seeing the patient for the first time.

7th character D is to be used for encounters after the patient has completed active treatment and is receiving routine care for the fracture during the healing or recovery phase. The other 7th characters, listed under each subcategory in the Tabular List, are to be used for subsequent encounters for treatment of problems associated with the healing, such as malunions, nonunions, and sequelae.

Care for complications of surgical treatment for fracture repairs during the healing or recovery phase should be coded with the appropriate complication codes.

See Section I.C.19. Coding of traumatic fractures.

d. Osteoporosis

Osteoporosis is a systemic condition, meaning that all bones of the musculoskeletal system are affected. Therefore, site is not a component of the codes under category M81, Osteoporosis without current pathological fracture. The site codes under category M80, Osteoporosis with current pathological fracture, identify the site of the fracture, not the osteoporosis.

1) Osteoporosis without pathological fracture

Category M81, Osteoporosis without current pathological fracture, is for use for patients with osteoporosis who do not currently have a pathologic fracture due to the osteoporosis, even if they have had a fracture in the past. For patients with a history of osteoporosis fractures, status code Z87.310, Personal history of (healed) osteoporosis fracture, should follow the code from M81.

2) Osteoporosis with current pathological fracture

Category M80, Osteoporosis with current pathological fracture, is for patients who have a current pathologic fracture at the time of an encounter. The codes under M80 identify the site of the fracture. A code from category M80, not a traumatic fracture code, should be used for any patient with known osteoporosis who suffers a fracture, even if the patient had a minor fall or trauma, if that fall or trauma would not usually break a normal, healthy bone.

e. Multisystem Inflammatory Syndrome

See Section I.C.1.g.1.l for Multisystem Inflammatory Syndrome.

Exercise 4.3 – Diseases of the Musculoskeletal System and Connective Tissue

Instructions: Assign the appropriate ICD-10-CM code(s).

_____   1. Arthralgia, left ankle

_____   2. Osteonecrosis, right humerus, due to long-term prescribed steroid use (sequela)

_____   3. Contracture, left hip joint

_____   4. Recurrent atlantoaxial subluxation with myelopathy

_____   5. Pathological fracture, left humerus, due to postmenopausal osteoporosis (initial encounter for fracture)

ICD-10-CM Chapter 14: Diseases of the Genitourinary System (N00–N99)

This ICD-10-CM chapter classifies the following:

- Glomerular diseases
- Renal tubulo-interstitial diseases
- Acute kidney failure and chronic kidney disease
- Urolithiasis
- Other disorders of kidney and ureter
- Other diseases of the urinary system
- Diseases of male genital organs
- Disorders of breast
- Inflammatory diseases of female pelvic organs
- Noninflammatory disorders of female genital tract
- Intraoperative and postprocedural complications and disorders of genitourinary system, not elsewhere classified

ICD-10-CM Chapter-Specific Coding Guidelines

Chapter 14: Diseases of the Genitourinary System (N00–N99)

a. Chronic kidney disease

1) Stages of chronic kidney disease (CKD)

The ICD-10-CM classifies CKD based on severity. The severity of CKD is designated by stages 1–5. Stage 2, code N18.2, equates to mild CKD; stage 3, codes N18.30–N18.32, equate to moderate CKD; and stage 4, code N18.4, equates to severe CKD. Code N18.6, End stage renal disease (ESRD), is assigned when the provider has documented end-stage renal disease (ESRD).

If both a stage of CKD and ESRD are documented, assign code N18.6 only.

Example: Patient is diagnosed with stage 2 CKD, for which code N18.2 is reported.

2) Chronic kidney disease and kidney transplant status

Patients who have undergone kidney transplant may still have some form of CKD because the kidney transplant may not fully restore kidney function. Therefore, the presence of CKD alone does not constitute a transplant complication. Assign the appropriate N18 code for the patient's stage of CKD and code Z94.0, Kidney transplant status. If a transplant complication such as failure or rejection or other transplant complication is documented, see Section I.C.19.g. for information on coding complications of a kidney transplant. If the documentation is unclear as to whether the patient has a complication of the transplant, query the provider.

Example: Patient is diagnosed with stage 1 chronic kidney disease (CKD) of transplanted kidneys. Report codes N18.1 for CKD and Z94.0 for kidney transplant status.

3) Chronic kidney disease (CKD) with other conditions

Patients with CKD may also suffer from other serious conditions, most commonly diabetes mellitus and hypertension. The sequencing of the CKD code in relationship to codes for other contributing conditions is based on the conventions in the Tabular List.

Example: Patient is diagnosed with diabetes mellitus due to chronic kidney disease (CKD), stage 1. Report codes E08.22 for diabetes mellitus due to CKD and N18.1 for stage 1 CKD, in that order.

See I.C.9. Hypertensive chronic kidney disease.

See I.C.19. Chronic kidney disease and kidney transplant complications.

Exercise 4.4 – Diseases of the Genitourinary System

Instructions: Assign the appropriate ICD-10-CM code(s).

_____ **1.** Chronic kidney disease, stage 2

_____ **2.** Stage 1 chronic kidney disease of transplanted kidneys

_____ **3.** Type 2 diabetic chronic kidney disease, stage 3

_____ **4.** Hypertensive chronic kidney disease, stage 2

_____ **5.** Diabetes mellitus due to stage 1 chronic kidney disease

---

ICD-10-CM Chapter 15: Pregnancy, Childbirth, and the Puerperium (O00–O9A)

This ICD-10-CM chapter classifies the following, which occur during pregnancy, childbirth, and the six weeks immediately following childbirth:

- Pregnancy with abortive outcome
- Supervision of high-risk pregnancy
- Edema, proteinuria, and hypertensive disorders in pregnancy, childbirth, and the puerperium
- Other maternal disorders predominantly related to pregnancy

- Maternal care related to the fetus and amniotic cavity and possible delivery problems
- Complications of labor and delivery
- Encounter for delivery
- Complications predominantly related to the puerperium
- Other obstetric conditions, not elsewhere classified

Obstetrical Discharges

All obstetrical discharges require a code from ICD-10-CM Chapter 15, and these codes are *never* reported on the baby's record.

- When the pregnancy is incidental to the encounter, assign code Z33.1 (Pregnant state, incidental).
- When an obstetrical patient's encounter is related to the pregnancy, report a code from O00–O9A first, followed by codes for secondary conditions.
- When the obstetrical patient delivers, assign an outcome of delivery code from category Z37 as a secondary code.

ICD-10-CM Chapter-Specific Coding Guidelines

Chapter 15: Pregnancy, Childbirth, and the Puerperium (O00–O9A)

a. General rules for obstetric cases

1) Codes from Chapter 15 and sequencing priority

Obstetric cases require codes from Chapter 15, codes in the range O00–O9A, Pregnancy, Childbirth, and the Puerperium. Chapter 15 codes have sequencing priority over codes from other chapters. Additional codes from other chapters may be used in conjunction with Chapter 15 codes to further specify conditions. Should the provider document that the pregnancy is incidental to the encounter, code Z33.1, Pregnant state, incidental, should be used in place of any Chapter 15 codes. It is the provider's responsibility to state that the condition being treated is not affecting the pregnancy.

Example: Patient is at 30 weeks gestation and is treated for urinary tract infection (UTI) due to *Escherichia coli* (*E. coli*). Report codes O23.43 for third trimester UTI, B96.20 for *E. coli*, and Z3A.30 for 30 weeks of gestation of pregnancy.

2) Chapter 15 codes used only on the maternal record

Chapter 15 codes are to be used only on the maternal record, never on the record of the newborn.

3) Final character for trimester

The majority of codes in Chapter 15 have a final character indicating the trimester of pregnancy. The time frames for the trimesters are indicated at the beginning of the chapter. If trimester is not a component of a code it is because the condition always occurs in a specific trimester, or the concept of trimester of pregnancy is not applicable. Certain codes have characters for only certain trimesters because the condition does not occur in all trimesters, but it may occur in more than just one.

Assignment of the final character for trimester should be based on the provider's documentation of the trimester (or number of weeks) for the current admission/encounter. This applies to the assignment of trimester for pre-existing conditions as well as those that develop during or are due to the pregnancy. The provider's documentation of the number of weeks may be used to assign the appropriate code identifying the trimester.

Whenever delivery occurs during the current admission, and there is an "in childbirth" option for the obstetric complication being coded, the "in childbirth" code should be assigned. When the classification does not provide an obstetric code with an "in childbirth" option, it is appropriate to assign a code describing the current trimester.

Example: Patient is treated for malnutrition in pregnancy during the third trimester at 37 weeks. Report codes O25.13 for the pregnancy and Z3A.37 for the weeks of gestation.

4) Selection of trimester for inpatient admissions that encompass more than one trimester

In instances when a patient is admitted to a hospital for complications of pregnancy during one trimester and remains in the hospital into a subsequent trimester, the trimester character for the antepartum complication code should be assigned on the basis of the trimester when the complication developed, not the trimester of the discharge. If the condition developed prior to the current admission/encounter or represents a pre-existing condition, the trimester character for the trimester at the time of the admission/encounter should be assigned.

5) Unspecified trimester

Each category that includes codes for trimester has a code for "unspecified trimester." The "unspecified trimester" code should rarely be used, such as when the documentation in the record is insufficient to determine the trimester and it is not possible to obtain clarification.

6) 7th character for fetus identification

Where applicable, a 7th character is to be assigned for certain categories (O31, O32, O33.3–O33.6, O35, O36, O40, O41, O60.1, O60.2, O64, and O69) to identify the fetus for which the complication code applies.

Assign 7th character "0":

- For single gestations
- When the documentation in the record is insufficient to determine the fetus affected and it is not possible to obtain clarification.
- When it is not possible to clinically determine which fetus is affected.

7) Completed weeks of gestation

In ICD-10-CM, "completed" weeks of gestation refers to full weeks. For example, if the provider documents gestation at 39 weeks and 6 days, the code for 39 weeks of gestation should be assigned, as the patient has not yet reached 40 completed weeks.

b. Selection of OB principal or first-listed diagnosis

1) Routine outpatient prenatal visits

For routine outpatient prenatal visits when no complications are present, a code from category Z34, Encounter for supervision of normal pregnancy, should be used as the first-listed diagnosis. These codes should not be used in conjunction with Chapter 15 codes.

2) Supervision of high-risk pregnancy

Codes from category O09, Supervision of high-risk pregnancy, are intended for use only during the prenatal period. For complications during the labor or delivery episode as a result of a high-risk pregnancy, assign the applicable complication codes from Chapter 15. If there are no complications during the labor or delivery episode, assign code O80, Encounter for full-term uncomplicated delivery.

For routine prenatal outpatient visits for patients with high-risk pregnancies, a code from category O09, Supervision of high-risk pregnancy, should be used as the first-listed diagnosis. Secondary [ICD-10-CM] Chapter 15 codes may be used in conjunction with these codes if appropriate.

3) Episodes when no delivery occurs

In episodes when no delivery occurs, the principal diagnosis should correspond to the principal complication of the pregnancy, which necessitated the encounter. Should more than one complication exist, all of which are treated or monitored, any of the complication codes may be sequenced first.

4) When a delivery occurs

When an obstetric patient is admitted and delivers during that admission, the condition that prompted the admission should be sequenced as the principal diagnosis. If multiple conditions prompted the admission, sequence the one most related to the delivery as the principal diagnosis. A code for any complication of the

(continues)

ICD-10-CM Chapter-Specific Coding Guidelines (*continued*)

delivery should be assigned as an additional diagnosis. In cases of cesarean delivery, if the patient was admitted with a condition that resulted in the performance of a cesarean procedure, that condition should be selected as the principal diagnosis. If the reason for the admission was unrelated to the condition resulting in the cesarean delivery, the condition related to the reason for the admission should be selected as the principal diagnosis.

5) Outcome of delivery

A code from category Z37, Outcome of delivery, should be included on every maternal record when a delivery has occurred. These codes are not to be used on subsequent records or on the newborn record.

c. Pre-existing conditions versus conditions due to the pregnancy

Certain categories in Chapter 15 distinguish between conditions of the mother that existed prior to pregnancy (pre-existing) and those that are a direct result of pregnancy. When assigning codes from Chapter 15, it is important to assess if a condition was pre-existing prior to pregnancy or developed during or due to the pregnancy in order to assign the correct code.

Categories that do not distinguish between pre-existing and pregnancy-related conditions may be used for either. It is acceptable to use codes specifically for the puerperium with codes complicating pregnancy and childbirth if a condition arises postpartum during the delivery encounter.

d. Pre-existing hypertension in pregnancy

Category O10, Pre-existing hypertension complicating pregnancy, childbirth and the puerperium, includes codes for hypertensive heart and hypertensive chronic kidney disease. When assigning one of the O10 codes that includes hypertensive heart disease or hypertensive chronic kidney disease, it is necessary to add a secondary code from the appropriate hypertension category to specify the type of heart failure or chronic kidney disease.

See Section I.C.9. Hypertension.

e. Fetal conditions affecting the management of the mother

1) Codes from categories O35 and O36

Codes from categories O35, Maternal care for known or suspected fetal abnormality and damage, and O36, Maternal care for other fetal problems, are assigned only when the fetal condition is actually responsible for modifying the management of the mother, i.e., by requiring diagnostic studies, additional observation, special care, or termination of pregnancy. The fact that the fetal condition exists does not justify assigning a code from this series to the mother's record.

2) *In utero* surgery

In cases when surgery is performed on the fetus, a diagnosis code from category O35, Maternal care for known or suspected fetal abnormality and damage, should be assigned identifying the fetal condition. Assign the appropriate procedure code for the procedure performed.

No code from Chapter 16, the perinatal codes, should be used on the mother's record to identify fetal conditions. Surgery performed *in utero* on a fetus is still to be coded as an obstetric encounter.

f. HIV infection in pregnancy, childbirth, and the puerperium

During pregnancy, childbirth, or the puerperium, a patient admitted because of an HIV-related illness should receive a principal diagnosis from subcategory O98.7-, Human immunodeficiency [HIV] disease complicating pregnancy, childbirth and the puerperium, followed by the code(s) for the HIV-related illness(es).

Patients with asymptomatic HIV-infection status admitted during pregnancy, childbirth, or the puerperium should receive codes of O98.7- and Z21, Asymptomatic human immunodeficiency virus [HIV] infection status.

g. Diabetes mellitus in pregnancy

Diabetes mellitus is a significant complicating factor in pregnancy. Pregnant patients who are diabetic should be assigned a code from category O24, Diabetes mellitus in pregnancy, childbirth, and the puerperium, first, followed by the appropriate diabetes code(s) (E08-E13) from Chapter 4.

h. Long-term use of insulin and oral hypoglycemics

See section I.C.4.a.3 for information on the long-term use of insulin and oral hypoglycemics.

i. **Gestational (pregnancy-induced) diabetes**

Gestational (pregnancy-induced) diabetes can occur during the second and third trimesters of pregnancy in patients who were not diabetic prior to pregnancy. Gestational diabetes can cause complications in the pregnancy similar to those of pre-existing diabetes mellitus. It also puts the patient at greater risk of developing diabetes after the pregnancy.

Codes for gestational diabetes are in subcategory O24.4, Gestational diabetes mellitus. No other code from category O24, Diabetes mellitus in pregnancy, childbirth, and the puerperium, should be used with a code from O24.4.

The codes under subcategory O24.4 include diet controlled, insulin controlled, and controlled by oral hypoglycemic drugs. If a patient with gestational diabetes is treated with both diet and insulin, only the code for insulin-controlled is required. If a patient with gestational diabetes is treated with both diet and oral hypoglycemic medications, only the code for "controlled by oral hypoglycemic drugs" is required. Codes Z79.4, Long-term (current) use of insulin, or Z79.84, Long-term (current) use of oral hypoglycemic drugs, and Z79.85, Long-term (current) use of injectable non-insulin antidiabetic drugs, should not be assigned with codes from subcategory O24.4.

An abnormal glucose tolerance in pregnancy is assigned a code from subcategory O99.81, Abnormal glucose complicating pregnancy, childbirth, and the puerperium.

j. **Sepsis and septic shock complicating abortion, pregnancy, childbirth and the puerperium**

When assigning a Chapter 15 code for sepsis complicating abortion, pregnancy, childbirth, and the puerperium, a code for the specific type of infection should be assigned as an additional diagnosis. If severe sepsis is present, a code from subcategory R65.2, Severe sepsis, and code(s) for associated organ dysfunction(s) should also be assigned as additional diagnoses.

Example: For a patient diagnosed as right tubal pregnancy with pelvic sepsis due to *Enterococcus*, report codes O00.101 (Right tubal pregnancy without intrauterine pregnancy), O08.82 (Sepsis following ectopic and molar pregnancy), and B95.2 (*Enterococcus*).

k. **Puerperal sepsis**

Code O85, Puerperal sepsis, should be assigned with a secondary code to identify the causal organism (e.g., for a bacterial infection, assign a code from category B95–B96, Bacterial infections in conditions classified elsewhere). A code from category A40, Streptococcal sepsis, or A41, Other sepsis, should not be used for puerperal sepsis. If applicable, use additional codes to identify severe sepsis (R65.2-) and any associated acute organ dysfunction. Code O85 should not be assigned for sepsis following an obstetrical procedure (*See Section I.C.1.d.5.b., Sepsis due to a postprocedural infection*).

l. **Alcohol, tobacco, and drug use during pregnancy, childbirth, and the puerperium**

1) **Alcohol use during pregnancy, childbirth, and the puerperium**

Codes under subcategory O99.31, Alcohol use complicating pregnancy, childbirth, and the puerperium, should be assigned for any pregnancy case when a patient uses alcohol during the pregnancy or postpartum. A secondary code from category F10, Alcohol related disorders, should also be assigned to identify manifestations of the alcohol use.

2) **Tobacco use during pregnancy, childbirth, and the puerperium**

Codes under subcategory O99.33, Smoking (tobacco) complicating pregnancy, childbirth, and the puerperium, should be assigned for any pregnancy case when a patient uses any type of tobacco product during the pregnancy or postpartum. A secondary code from category F17, Nicotine dependence, should also be assigned to identify the type of nicotine dependence.

3) **Drug use during pregnancy, childbirth, and the puerperium**

Codes under subcategory O99.32, Drug use complicating pregnancy, childbirth, and the puerperium, should be assigned for any pregnancy case when a patient uses drugs during the pregnancy or postpartum. This can involve illegal drugs, or inappropriate use or abuse of prescription drugs. Secondary code(s) from categories F11–F16 and F18–F19 should also be assigned to identify manifestations of the drug use.

m. **Poisoning, toxic effects, adverse effects and underdosing in a pregnant patient**

A code from subcategory O9A.2, Injury, poisoning and certain other consequences of external causes complicating pregnancy, childbirth, and the puerperium, should be sequenced first, followed by the

(continues)

ICD-10-CM Chapter-Specific Coding Guidelines (*continued*)

appropriate injury, poisoning, toxic effect, adverse effect or underdosing code, and then the additional code(s) that specifies the condition caused by the poisoning, toxic effect, adverse effect or underdosing.

See Section I.C.19. Adverse effects, poisoning, underdosing and toxic effects.

n. Normal delivery, code O80

1) Encounter for full term uncomplicated delivery

Code O80 should be assigned when a patient is admitted for a full-term normal delivery and delivers a single, healthy infant without any complications antepartum, during the delivery, or postpartum during the delivery episode. Code O80 is always a principal diagnosis. It is not to be used if any other code from Chapter 15 is needed to describe a current complication of the antenatal, delivery, or postnatal period. Additional codes from other chapters may be used with code O80 if they are not related to or are in any way complicating the pregnancy.

2) Uncomplicated delivery with resolved antepartum complication

Code O80 may be used if the patient had a complication at some point during the pregnancy, but the complication is not present at the time of the admission for delivery.

3) Outcome of delivery for O80

Z37.0, Single live birth, is the only outcome of delivery code appropriate for use with O80.

Example: Patient was admitted to the hospital and delivered a liveborn infant. Report codes O80 (Encounter for full-term uncomplicated delivery) and Z37.0 (Single live birth).

 NOTE:

A multigestational pregnancy (e.g., twins, triplets, and so on) is never classified as code O80 (normal delivery). Instead, go to ICD-10-CM index main term Pregnancy and the appropriate subterm for twin, triplet, quadruplet to locate the code. Review the ICD-10-CM tabular list for assignment of the documented trimester of the pregnancy. (Multiple gestation pregnancies greater than quadruplets are classified as *other* when the number of fetuses is documented or *unspecified* when the number of fetuses is not documented.) Code also any complications specific to multiple gestation (e.g., preterm labor).

o. The peripartum and postpartum periods

1) Peripartum and postpartum periods

The postpartum period begins immediately after delivery and continues for six weeks following delivery. The peripartum period is defined as the last month of pregnancy to five months postpartum.

2) Peripartum and postpartum complication

A postpartum complication is any complication occurring within the six-week period.

Example: Patient is discharged from the hospital after third-trimester delivery of a single live female. Complications occurred during delivery, including "ablatio placenta" and "delayed postpartum bleed." Report codes O45.93 (Premature separation of placenta, unspecified, third trimester), O72.2 (Delayed and secondary postpartum hemorrhage), and Z37.0 (Single live birth).

3) Pregnancy-related complications after 6-week period

Chapter 15 codes may also be used to describe pregnancy-related complications after peripartum or postpartum period if the provider documents that a condition is pregnancy related.

4) Admission for routine postpartum care following delivery outside hospital

When the mother delivers outside the hospital prior to admission and is admitted for routine postpartum care and no complications are noted, code Z39.0, Encounter for care and examination of mother immediately after delivery, should be assigned as the principal diagnosis.

5) Pregnancy associated cardiomyopathy

Pregnancy associated cardiomyopathy, code O90.3, is unique in that it may be diagnosed in the third trimester of pregnancy but may continue to progress months after delivery. For this reason, it is referred to as peripartum cardiomyopathy. Code O90.3 is only for use when the cardiomyopathy develops as a result of pregnancy in a patient who did not have pre-existing heart disease.

p. **Code O94, Sequelae of complication of pregnancy, childbirth, and the puerperium**

1) **Code O94**

Code O94, Sequelae of complication of pregnancy, childbirth, and the puerperium, is for use in those cases when an initial complication of a pregnancy develops a sequela or sequelae requiring care or treatment at a future date.

2) **After the initial postpartum period**

This code may be used at any time after the initial postpartum period.

3) **Sequencing of code O94**

This code, like all late effect codes, is to be sequenced following the code describing the sequelae of the complication.

q. **Termination of pregnancy and spontaneous abortions**

1) **Abortion with liveborn fetus**

When an attempted termination of pregnancy results in a liveborn fetus, assign code Z33.2, Encounter for elective termination of pregnancy and a code from category Z37, Outcome of Delivery.

2) **Retained products of conception following an abortion**

Subsequent encounters for retained products of conception following a spontaneous abortion or elective termination of pregnancy, without complications, are assigned O03.4, Incomplete spontaneous abortion without complication, or code O07.4, Failed attempted termination of pregnancy without complication. This advice is appropriate even when the patient was discharged previously with a discharge diagnosis of complete abortion.

If the patient has a specific complication associated with the spontaneous abortion or elective termination of pregnancy in addition to retained products of conception, assign the appropriate complication code (e.g., O03.-, O04.-, O07.-) instead of code O03.4 or O07.4.

3) **Complications leading to abortion**

Codes from Chapter 15 may be used as additional codes to identify any documented complications of the pregnancy in conjunction with codes in categories in O04, O07 and O08.

Example: For a patient diagnosed with embolism following failed attempted termination of pregnancy, report code O07.0 (Genital tract and pelvic infection following failed attempted termination of pregnancy).

4) **Hemorrhage following elective abortion**

For hemorrhage post elective abortion, assign code O04.6, Delayed or excessive hemorrhage following (induced) termination of pregnancy. Do not assign code O72.1, Other immediate postpartum hemorrhage, as this code should not be assigned for post abortion conditions.

r. **Abuse in a pregnant patient**

For suspected or confirmed cases of abuse of a pregnant patient, a code(s) from subcategories O9A.3, Physical abuse complicating pregnancy, childbirth, and the puerperium, O9A.4, Sexual abuse complicating pregnancy, childbirth, and the puerperium, and O9A.5, Psychological abuse complicating pregnancy, childbirth, and the puerperium, should be sequenced first, followed by the appropriate codes (if applicable) to identify any associated current injury due to physical abuse, sexual abuse, and the perpetrator of abuse.

See Section 1.C.19 Adult and child abuse, neglect and other maltreatment.

s. **COVID-19 infection in pregnancy, childbirth, and the puerperium**

During pregnancy, childbirth or the puerperium, when COVID-19 is the reason for admission/encounter, code O98.5-, Other viral diseases complicating pregnancy, childbirth and the puerperium, should be sequenced as the principal/first-listed diagnosis, and code U07.1, COVID-19, and the appropriate codes for associated manifestation(s) should be assigned as additional diagnoses. Codes from Chapter 15 always take sequencing priority.

(continues)

Courtesy of the Centers for Medicare & Medicaid Services, www.cms.gov.

ICD-10-CM Chapter-Specific Coding Guidelines (*continued*)

If the reason for admission/encounter is unrelated to COVID-19 but the patient tests positive for COVID-19 during the admission/encounter, the appropriate code for the reason for admission/encounter should be sequenced as the principal/first-listed diagnosis, and codes O98.5-and U07.1, as well as the appropriate codes for associated COVID-19 manifestations, should be assigned as additional diagnoses.

Exercise 4.5 – Pregnancy, Childbirth, and the Puerperium

Instructions: Assign the appropriate ICD-10-CM code(s).

_____ 1. Amnionitis, third trimester

_____ 2. Engorgement of female breasts (postpartum)

_____ 3. Gestational diabetes mellitus, controlled by diet, week 33 of pregnancy

_____ 4. Supervision of high-risk pregnancy due to elderly primigravida and pre-existing essential hypertension, third trimester

_____ 5. Full-term vaginal delivery of single liveborn infant

---

ICD-10-CM Chapter 16: Certain Conditions Originating in the Perinatal Period (P00–P96)

This ICD-10-CM chapter classifies the following:

- Newborn affected by maternal factors and by complications of pregnancy, labor, and delivery
- Disorders of newborn related to length of gestation and fetal growth
- Abnormal findings on neonatal screening

 NOTE:

Codes from ICD-10-CM Chapter 16 are reported for the newborn's encounter *only*.

- Birth trauma
- Respiratory and cardiovascular disorders specific to the perinatal period
- Infections specific to the perinatal period
- Hemorrhagic and hematological disorders of newborn
- Transitory endocrine and metabolic disorders specific to newborn
- Digestive system disorders of newborn
- Conditions involving the integument and temperature regulation of newborn
- Other problems with newborn
- Other disorders originating in the perinatal period

This chapter classifies conditions that begin during the perinatal period even if death or morbidity occurs later. The **perinatal period** is the interval of time occurring before, during, and up to 28 days following birth. These codes classify causes of morbidity and mortality in the fetus or newborn. Additional codes can be assigned from other ICD-10-CM chapters to further specify the newborn's condition.

ICD-10-CM Chapter-Specific Coding Guidelines

Chapter 16: Certain Conditions Originating in the Perinatal Period (P00–P96)

For coding and reporting purposes, the perinatal period is defined as "before birth through the 28th day following birth." The following guidelines are provided for reporting purposes.

a. General perinatal rules

1) Use of Chapter 16 codes

Codes in this chapter are *never* for use on the maternal record. Codes from Chapter 15, the obstetrics chapter, are never permitted on the newborn record. Chapter 16 codes may be used throughout the life of the patient if the condition is still present.

2) Principal diagnosis for birth record

When coding the birth episode in a newborn record, assign a code from category Z38, Liveborn infants according to place of birth and type of delivery, as the principal diagnosis. A code from category Z38 is assigned only once, to a newborn at the time of birth. If a newborn is transferred to another institution, a code from category Z38 should not be used at the receiving hospital.

A code from category Z38 is used only on the newborn record, not on the mother's record.

Example: Single liveborn infant via vaginal delivery was diagnosed with Down syndrome. Report codes Z38.00 (single liveborn via vaginal delivery) and Q90.9 (Down syndrome).

3) Use of codes from other chapters with codes from Chapter 16

Codes from other chapters may be used with codes from Chapter 16 if the codes from the other chapters provide more specific detail. Codes for signs and symptoms may be assigned when a definitive diagnosis has not been established. If the reason for the encounter is a perinatal condition, the code from Chapter 16 should be sequenced first.

Example: The patient is a one-day-old single liveborn infant, delivered vaginally, who is diagnosed with transient tachypnea of newborn and cradle cap. Report codes Z38.00 for the single liveborn infant status, P22.1 for tachypnea, and L21.0 for cradle cap (seborrhea capitis).

4) Use of Chapter 16 codes after the perinatal period

Should a condition originate in the perinatal period, and continue throughout the life of the patient, the perinatal code should continue to be used regardless of the patient's age.

5) Birth process or community-acquired conditions

If a newborn has a condition that may be either due to the birth process or community-acquired and the documentation does not indicate which it is, the default is "due to the birth process" and the code from Chapter 16 should be used. If the condition is "community-acquired," a code from Chapter 16 should not be assigned.

For COVID-19 infection in a newborn, see guideline I.C.16.h.

6) Code all clinically significant conditions

All clinically significant conditions noted on routine newborn examination should be coded. A condition is clinically significant if it requires:

- Clinical evaluation
- Therapeutic treatment
- Diagnostic procedures

- Extended length of hospital stay
- Increased nursing care and/or monitoring
- Implications for future health care needs

(continues)

ICD-10-CM Chapter-Specific Coding Guidelines (*continued*)

Note: The perinatal guidelines listed above are the same as the general coding guidelines for "additional diagnoses," except for the final point regarding implications for future health care needs. Codes should be assigned for conditions that have been specified by the provider as having implications for future health care needs.

b. **Observation and evaluation of newborns for suspected conditions not found**

1) **Use of Z05 codes**

Assign a code from category Z05, Observation and evaluation of newborn for suspected diseases and conditions ruled out, to identify those instances when a healthy newborn is evaluated for a suspected condition/disease that is determined after study not to be present. Do not use a code from category Z05 when the patient is documented to have signs or symptoms of a suspected problem; in such cases code the sign or symptom.

2) **Z05 on other than the birth record**

A code from category Z05 may also be assigned as a principal or first-listed code for readmissions or encounters when the code from category Z38 code no longer applies. Codes from category Z05 are for use only for healthy newborns and infants for which no condition after study is found to be present.

3) **Z05 on a birth record**

A code from category Z05 is to be used as a secondary code after the code from category Z38, Liveborn infants according to place of birth and type of delivery.

c. **Coding additional perinatal diagnoses**

1) **Assigning codes for conditions that require treatment**

Assign codes for conditions that require treatment or further investigation, prolong the length of stay, or require resource utilization.

2) **Codes for conditions specified as having implications for future health care needs**

Assign codes for conditions that have been specified by the provider as having implications for future health care needs.

Note: This guideline should not be used for adult patients.

d. **Prematurity and fetal growth retardation**

Providers utilize different criteria in determining prematurity. A code for prematurity should not be assigned unless it is documented. Assignment of codes in categories P05, Disorders of newborn related to slow fetal growth and fetal malnutrition, and P07, Disorders of newborn related to short gestation and low birth weight, not elsewhere classified, should be based on the recorded birth weight and estimated gestational age.

When both birth weight and gestational age are available, two codes from category P07 should be assigned, with the code for birth weight sequenced before the code for gestational age.

e. **Low birth weight and immaturity status**

Codes from category P07, Disorders of newborn related to short gestation and low birth weight, not elsewhere classified, are for use for a child or adult who was premature or had a low birth weight as a newborn and this is affecting the patient's current health status.

See Section I.C.21. Factors influencing health status and contact with health services, Status.

f. **Bacterial sepsis of newborn**

Category P36, Bacterial sepsis of newborn, includes congenital sepsis. If a perinate is documented as having sepsis without documentation of congenital or community acquired, the default is congenital and a code from category P36 should be assigned. If the P36 code includes the causal organism, an additional code from category B95, Streptococcus, Staphylococcus, and Enterococcus as the cause of diseases classified elsewhere, or B96, Other bacterial agents as the cause of diseases classified elsewhere, should not be assigned. If the P36 code does not include the causal organism, assign an additional code from category B96. If applicable, use additional codes to identify severe sepsis (R65.2-) and any associated acute organ dysfunction.

g. Stillbirth

Code P95, Stillbirth, is only for use in institutions that maintain separate records for stillbirths. No other code should be used with P95. Code P95 should not be used on the mother's record.

h. COVID-19 Infection in Newborn

For a newborn that tests positive for COVID-19, assign code U07.1, COVID-19, and the appropriate codes for associated manifestation(s) in neonates/newborns in the absence of documentation indicating a specific type of transmission. For a newborn that tests positive for COVID-19 and the provider documents the condition was contracted in utero or during the birth process, assign codes P35.8, Other congenital viral diseases, and U07.1, COVID-19. When coding the birth episode in a newborn record, the appropriate code from category Z38, Liveborn infants according to place of birth and type of delivery, should be assigned as the principal diagnosis.

Courtesy of the Centers for Medicare & Medicaid Services, www.cms.gov.

Exercise 4.6 – Certain Conditions Originating in the Perinatal Period

Instructions: Assign the appropriate ICD-10-CM code(s).

_____ 1. Liveborn infant born in hospital, delivered vaginally, with cyanotic attacks of newborn

_____ 2. Exceptionally large single liveborn infant, born in hospital and delivered by cesarean, with birthweight of 4675 grams and seborrheic infantile dermatitis

_____ 3. Outpatient encounter for facial palsy due to birth injury, which began as infant and continues to present as toddler

_____ 4. Observation of single liveborn infant, born in hospital vaginally, for suspected cardiac condition, ruled out; newborn presented without signs or symptoms

_____ 5. Congenital sepsis of newborn due to *Escherichia coli*

ICD-10-CM Chapter 17: Congenital Malformations, Deformations, and Chromosomal Abnormalities (Q00–Q99)

This ICD-10-CM chapter classifies the following congenital malformations (and deformations) according to body system (e.g., nervous system), along with cleft lip and cleft palate, and chromosomal abnormalities. Congenital malformations may be the result of genetic factors (chromosomes), teratogens (agents causing physical defects in the embryo), or both. The malformations may be apparent at birth or hidden and identified sometime after birth. Regardless of origin, dysmorphology (clinical structural abnormality) is generally the primary indication of a congenital anomaly; in many cases, a syndrome may be classified according to a single anatomical anomaly rather than a complex of symptoms.

ICD-10-CM does not differentiate between intrinsic abnormalities (defects related to the fetus) or extrinsic abnormalities (defects that are the result of intrauterine problems). ICD-10-CM also does make a distinction in the classification of an anomaly as compared to a deformity. An anomaly is a malformation caused by abnormal fetal development (e.g., transposition of great vessels, or spina bifida). A deformity is an alteration in structure caused by an extrinsic force, such as intrauterine compression. The force may cause a disruption in a normal fetal structure, including congenital amputations from amniotic bands. In some cases, assigning two codes is necessary to describe the condition.

ICD-10-CM Chapter-Specific Coding Guidelines

Chapter 17: Congenital Malformations, Deformations, and Chromosomal Abnormalities (Q00–Q99)

Assign an appropriate code(s) from categories Q00–Q99, Congenital malformations, deformations, and chromosomal abnormalities, when a malformation/deformation or chromosomal abnormality is documented. A malformation/deformation or chromosomal abnormality may be the principal/first-listed diagnosis on a record or a secondary diagnosis.

When a malformation/deformation or chromosomal abnormality does not have a unique code assignment, assign additional code(s) for any manifestations that may be present.

When the code assignment specifically identifies the malformation/deformation or chromosomal abnormality, manifestations that are an inherent component of the anomaly should not be coded separately. Additional codes should be assigned for manifestations that are not an inherent component.

Codes from Chapter 17 may be used throughout the life of the patient. If a congenital malformation or deformity has been corrected, a personal history code should be used to identify the history of the malformation or deformity. Although present at birth, a malformation/deformation/chromosomal abnormality may not be identified until later in life. Whenever the condition is diagnosed by the provider, it is appropriate to assign a code from codes Q00–Q99.

For the birth admission, the appropriate code from category Z38, Liveborn infants, according to place of birth and type of delivery, should be sequenced as the principal diagnosis, followed by any congenital anomaly codes, Q00–Q99.

Example 1: Patient is diagnosed with Apert's syndrome (or acrocephalosyndactyly), which is a group of congenital syndromes that include peaking at the head due to premature closure of skull sutures and fusion or webbing of digits. Apert's syndrome is a single anatomical anomaly of a multicomplex syndrome, which can include fusion in the hands and facial anomalies. Report Q87.0 for Apert's syndrome.

Example 2: Thalidomide phocomelia results from influence of the drug thalidomide on the developing fetus during the perinatal period. It is a congenital birth defect in which the hands and feet are attached to abbreviated arms and legs, respectively. To classify this condition, multiple codes are reported, including:

- Q71.13, Congenital absence of upper arm and forearm with hand present, bilateral
- Q72.13, Congenital absence of thigh and lower leg with foot present, bilateral
- P04.18, Newborn affected by other maternal medication

Codes Q71.13 and Q72.13 classify the limb deformities. Code P04.18 classifies the transmission of the drug across the placenta, which in this case resulted in the limb deformities.

Exercise 4.7 – Congenital Malformations, Deformations, and Chromosomal Abnormalities

Instructions: Assign the appropriate ICD-10-CM code(s).

_____   **1.** Anomalies of aortic arch (tortuous)

_____   **2.** Congenital heart block; patient admitted for surgery at age 24

_____   **3.** History of congenital hydrocephalus (corrected)

_____   **4.** Cystic eyeball, congenital

_____   **5.** Single liveborn infant, vaginally delivered in hospital; congenital fissure of tongue

ICD-10-CM Chapter 18: Symptoms, Signs, and Abnormal Clinical and Laboratory Findings, Not Elsewhere Classified (R00–R99)

This ICD-10-CM chapter classifies symptoms, signs, and abnormal clinical and laboratory findings, abnormal tumor markers, and ill-defined and unknown causes of mortality. In general, codes from this chapter are used to report symptoms, signs, and ill-defined conditions that point with equal suspicion to two or more diagnoses or represent important problems in medical care that may affect management of the patient. In addition, this chapter classifies abnormal findings that are reported without a corresponding definitive diagnosis. Codes for such findings can be located in the alphabetic index under the following terms:

- Abnormal, abnormality, abnormalities
- Decrease, decreased
- Elevation
- Findings, abnormal, without diagnosis

Codes from this chapter are used to report symptoms and signs that existed on initial encounter but proved to be transient and without a specified cause. Also included are provisional diagnoses for patients who fail to return for further investigation, cases referred elsewhere for further investigation before being diagnosed, and cases in which a more definitive diagnosis was not available for other reasons. Do not assign a code from ICD-10-CM categories R00–R99 when the symptoms, signs, and abnormal findings pertain to a definitive diagnosis.

> **Example:** A patient presents with dyspnea (shortness of breath), and the provider has not documented a definitive diagnosis for the encounter. Report code R06.00 (Dyspnea, unspecified).

ICD-10-CM Chapter-Specific Coding Guidelines

Chapter 18: Symptoms, Signs, and Abnormal Clinical and Laboratory Findings, Not Elsewhere Classified (R00–R99)

Chapter 18 includes symptoms, signs, abnormal results of clinical or other investigative procedures, and ill-defined conditions regarding which no diagnosis classifiable elsewhere is recorded. Signs and symptoms that point to a specific diagnosis have been assigned to a category in other chapters of the classification.

a. **Use of symptom codes**

Codes that describe symptoms and signs are acceptable for reporting purposes when a related definitive diagnosis has not been established (confirmed) by the provider.

> **Example 1:** The patient is seen in the office for severe headaches, which occur daily, and fatigue. Report codes R51.9 (headache) and R53.83 (fatigue).

> **Example 2:** The patient complains of abdominal pain, the physical examination reveals abdominal rigidity, and after workup the patient is diagnosed with acute appendicitis. Report code K35.80 (acute appendicitis). Do **not** assign symptom code R10.9 (abdominal pain) or sign code R19.30 (abdominal rigidity).

b. **Use of a symptom code with a definitive diagnosis code**

Codes for signs and symptoms may be reported in addition to a related definitive diagnosis when the sign or symptom is not routinely associated with that diagnosis, such as the various signs and symptoms associated with complex syndromes. The definitive diagnosis code should be sequenced before the symptom code.

Signs or symptoms that are associated routinely with a disease process should not be assigned as additional codes, unless otherwise instructed by the classification.

(continues)

ICD-10-CM Chapter-Specific Coding Guidelines (*continued*)

Example: The patient is diagnosed with adenoviral pneumonia and epistaxis. Report codes J12.0 (adenoviral pneumonia) and R04.0 (epistaxis). (Epistaxis is not routinely associated with pneumonia and is coded separately.)

c. Combination codes that include symptoms

ICD-10-CM contains a number of combination codes that identify both the definitive diagnosis and common symptoms of that diagnosis. When using one of these combination codes, an additional code should not be assigned for the symptom.

d. Repeated falls

Code R29.6, Repeated falls, is for use for encounters when a patient has recently fallen and the reason for the fall is being investigated. Code Z91.81, History of falling, is for use when a patient has fallen in the past and is at risk for future falls. When appropriate, both codes R29.6 and Z91.81 may be assigned together.

e. Coma

Code R40.20, Unspecified coma, should be assigned when the underlying cause of the coma is not known, or the cause is a traumatic brain injury and the coma scale is not documented in the medical record. *Do not report codes for unspecified coma, individual or total Glasgow coma scale scores for a patient with a medically induced coma or a sedated patient.*

1) Coma Scale

The coma scale codes (R40.21- to R40.24-) can be used in conjunction with traumatic brain injury codes. These codes cannot be used with code R40.2A, Nontraumatic coma due to underlying condition. They are primarily for use by trauma registries, but they may be used in any setting where this information is collected. The coma scale codes should be sequenced after the diagnosis code(s).

These codes, one from each subcategory, are needed to complete the scale. The 7th character indicates when the scale was recorded. The 7th character should match for all three codes.

At a minimum, report the initial score documented on presentation at your facility. This may be a score from the emergency medicine technician (EMT) or in the emergency department. If desired, a facility may choose to capture multiple Glasgow coma scale scores.

Assign R40.24-, Glasgow coma scale, total score, when only the total score is documented in the medical record and not the individual score(s).

If multiple coma scores are captured within the first 24 hours after hospital admission, assign only the code for the score at the time of admission. ICD-10-CM does not classify coma scores that are reported after admission but less than 24 hours later.

See Section I.B.14. for coma scale documentation by clinicians other than patient's provider.

f. Functional quadriplegia

GUIDELINE HAS BEEN DELETED EFFECTIVE OCTOBER 1, 2017.

g. SIRS due to non-infectious process

The systemic inflammatory response syndrome (SIRS) can develop as a result of certain non-infectious disease processes, such as trauma, malignant neoplasm, or pancreatitis. When SIRS is documented with a non-infectious condition, and no subsequent infection is documented, the code for the underlying condition, such as an injury, should be assigned, followed by code R65.10, Systemic inflammatory response syndrome (SIRS) of non-infectious origin without acute organ dysfunction, or code R65.11, Systemic inflammatory response syndrome (SIRS) of non-infectious origin with acute organ dysfunction. If an associated acute organ dysfunction is documented, the appropriate code(s) for the specific type of organ dysfunction(s) should be assigned in addition to code R65.11. If acute organ dysfunction is documented, but it cannot be determined if the acute organ dysfunction is associated with SIRS or due to another condition (e.g., directly due to the trauma), the provider should be queried.

h. Death NOS

Code R99, Ill-defined and unknown cause of mortality, is only for use in the very limited circumstance when a patient who has already died is brought into an emergency department or other health care facility and is pronounced dead upon arrival. It does not represent the discharge disposition of death.

i. **NIHSS Stroke Scale**

The NIH stroke scale (NIHSS) codes (R29.7--) can be used in conjunction with acute stroke codes (I60–I63) to identify the patient's neurological status and the severity of the stroke. The stroke scale codes should be sequenced after the acute stroke diagnosis code(s).

At a minimum, report the initial score documented. If desired, a facility may choose to capture multiple stroke scale scores.

See Section I.B.14. for NIHSS stroke scale documentation by clinicians other than patient's provider.

Exercise 4.8 – Symptoms, Signs, and Abnormal Clinical and Laboratory Findings, Not Elsewhere Classified

Instructions: Assign the appropriate ICD-10-CM code(s).

_____   1. Abnormal reflex

_____   2. Adnexa pain

_____   3. Generalized anxiety with headaches

_____   4. Ascites due to alcoholic cirrhosis; alcohol abuse in remission

_____   5. Heatstroke (initial encounter) with systemic inflammatory response syndrome

---

ICD-10-CM Chapter 19: Injury, Poisoning, and Certain Other Consequences of External Causes (S00–T88)

This ICD-10-CM chapter classifies the following:

- Injuries
- Effects of foreign body entering through natural orifice
- Burns and corrosions
- Frostbite
- Poisonings by, adverse effects of, and underdosing of drugs, medicaments, and biological substances
- Toxic effects of substances chiefly nonmedicinal as to source
- Other and unspecified effects of external causes
- Certain early complications of trauma
- Complications of surgical and medical care, not elsewhere classified

NOTE:

Injury and poisoning codes are not assigned for complications of surgical wounds (e.g., postoperative infection). (For such conditions, refer to main term *Complication* in the ICD-10-CM index.)

Separate codes are assigned for each injury except when a combination code is provided in ICD-10-CM. When multiple codes are assigned, the code for the most serious injury is sequenced first (as determined by the provider and based on treatment provided).

Fractures

A **fracture** is a break in a bone resulting from two possible causes.

- Direct or indirect application of undue force against the bone (injury)
- Pathological changes resulting in spontaneous fractures (disease process)

The provider always determines whether a fracture is open or closed, which is one of the first determinations made. A **closed fracture** (or **simple fracture**) is contained beneath the skin and has intact ligaments and skin, while an **open fracture** (or **compound fracture**) indicates an associated open wound.

 NOTE:

ICD-10-CM Chapter 19 classifies **malunion** (or **nonunion**) of fractured bones, which is the failure of the ends of a fractured bone to heal (unite) by adding a seventh character (e.g., S72.001K, S72.001P).

The following terms typically describe closed fractures:

- *Comminuted fracture:* A splintering of the fractured bone
- *Depressed fracture:* Portion of the skull broken and driven inward from a forceful blow
- *Fissured fracture:* Fracture that does not split the bone
- *Greenstick fracture:* Occurs in children; the bone is somewhat bent and partially broken
- *Impacted fracture:* One fractured bone end wedged into another
- *Linear fracture:* Fracture that is in a straight line
- *Slipped epiphysis:* Separation of the growth plate, which is the growing end of the bone, or epiphysis, from the shaft of the bone; occurs in children and young adults who still have active epiphyses
- *Spiral fracture:* Fracture resembles a helix or has a corkscrew shape

 Coding Tip

If there is no documentation whether a fracture is open or closed, the fracture is coded as closed.

An open fracture is classified as a compound fracture because it contains a wound that leads to the fracture or has broken bone ends protruding through the skin. There is a very high risk of infection with open fractures because the tissues are exposed to contaminants (toxins). There may be foreign bodies (or missiles) embedded in the tissues that must be removed during surgery, and puncture wounds may also be present.

Open and closed fractures may both be described as "complicated," which means a bone fragment has injured an internal organ.

Example: Fractured ribs that injure internal organs is a complicated fracture.

Burns

Burns (ICD-10-CM categories T20–T32) are classified according to the following:

- Depth
  - First-degree (erythema)
  - Second-degree (blistering)

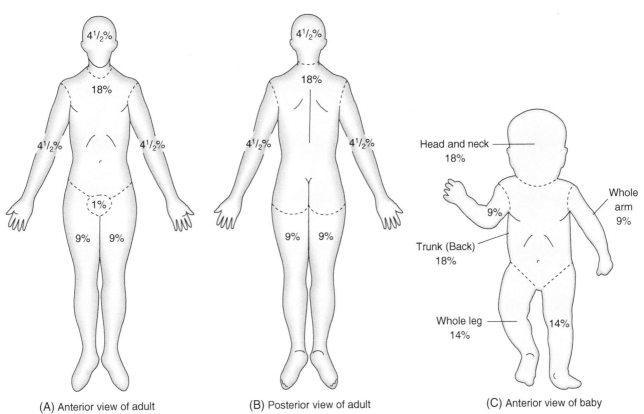

(A) Anterior view of adult (B) Posterior view of adult (C) Anterior view of baby

FIGURE 4-1 The rule of nines is used to calculate the percentage of body surface affected by burns (ICD-10-CM category T32). (Percentage assignments are modified to accommodate infants and children who have proportionately larger heads than adults or for patients who have large buttocks, thighs, or abdomen.)

- Third-degree (full-thickness involvement)
- Extent (percentage of body surface involved) (Figure 4-1)
- Agent (e.g., chemicals, fire, sun) (assigned an external cause code)

Adverse Effects, Poisonings, Underdosings, and Toxic Effects

Certain drugs, medicinal substances, and biological substances (or combinations of them) may cause toxic reactions. Such drug toxicity is classified in ICD-10-CM as

- *Adverse effects* (or adverse reaction): Appearance of a pathological condition caused by ingestion or exposure to a chemical substance properly administered or taken
- *Poisonings:* Occur as the result of an overdose; wrong substance administered or taken; or intoxication, which involves combining prescribed drugs with nonprescribed drugs or (ethyl) alcohol
- *Underdosings:* Taking less of a medication than is prescribed by a provider or a manufacturer's instruction
- *Toxic effects:* When a harmful substance is ingested or comes in contact with a person

 Coding Tip

To locate the code for an adverse effect, go to main term *Effect, adverse* in the ICD-10-CM Index to Diseases and Injuries, and locate the appropriate subterm (e.g., drugs and medicinals). Or, go to main term *Reaction*, and locate the appropriate subterm(s) (e.g., *drug NEC*). Then, assign the appropriate code from the Table of Drugs and Chemicals, Therapeutic Use column.

Substance	Poisoning, Accidental (unintentional)	Poisoning, Intentional Self-harm	Poisoning, Assault	Poisoning, Undetermined	Adverse Effect	Underdosing
1-propanol	T51.3X1	T51.3X2	T51.3X3	T51.3X4	—	—
2-propanol	T51.2X1	T51.2X2	T51.2X3	T51.2X4	—	—
2, 4-D (dichloro-phenoxyacetic acid)	T60.3X1	T60.3X2	T60.3X3	T60.3X4	—	—
2, 4-toluene diisocyanate	T65.0X1	T65.0X2	T65.0X3	T65.0X4	—	—
2, 4, 5-T (trichloro-phenoxyacetic acid)	T60.1X1	T60.1X2	T60.1X3	T60.1X4	—	—
3,4-methylenedioxymethamphetamine	T43.641	T43.642	T43.643	T43.644	—	—
14-hydroxydihydromorphinone	T40.2X1	T40.2X2	T40.2X3	T40.2X4	T40.2X5	T40.2X6
ABOB	T37.5X1	T37.5X2	T37.5X3	T37.5X4	T37.5X5	T37.5X6
Abrine	T62.2X1	T62.2X2	T62.2X3	T62.2X4	—	—
Abrus (seed)	T62.2X1	T62.2X2	T62.2X3	T62.2X4	—	—
Absinthe	T51.0X1	T51.0X2	T51.0X3	T51.0X4	—	—
beverage	T51.0X1	T51.0X2	T51.0X3	T51.0X4	—	—
Acaricide	T60.8X1	T60.8X2	T60.8X3	T60.8X4	—	—
Acebutolol	T44.7X1	T44.7X2	T44.7X3	T44.7X4	T44.7X5	T44.7X6
Acecarbromal	T42.6X1	T42.6X2	T42.6X3	T42.6X4	T42.6X5	T42.6X6
Aceclidine	T44.1X1	T44.1X2	T44.1X3	T44.1X4	T44.1X5	T44.1X6
Acedapsone	T37.0X1	T37.0X2	T37.0X3	T37.0X4	T37.0X5	T37.0X6
Acefylline piperazinef	T48.6X1	T48.6X2	T48.6X3	T48.6X4	T48.6X5	T48.6X6

Courtesy of the Centers for Medicare & Medicaid Services, www.cms.gov

FIGURE 4-2 ICD-10-CM Table of Drugs and Chemicals (partial)

Coding Tip

To locate the code for a poisoning or toxic effect, go to the Table of Drugs and Chemicals, determine the circumstances for the poisoning (e.g., accidental, intentional self-harm, assault, undetermined), and assign the code from the appropriate Poisoning column. If more than one substance is documented as causing the poisoning, assign codes from the Table of Drugs and Chemicals for *each* substance. Verify each code in the ICD-10-CM Tabular List of Diseases and Injuries.

Coding Tip

- The term *intoxication* often indicates that ethyl alcohol (e.g., beer, wine) was involved (e.g., alcohol intoxication) or that an accumulation effect of a medication in the patient's bloodstream occurred (e.g., Coumadin intoxication). When this occurs, assign a code from the appropriate Poisoning column of the ICD-10-CM Table of Drugs and Chemicals. In this situation, intoxication means "poisoning."

- When an accumulation effect of a medication occurs, assign the manifestation code first (e.g., dizziness) and a code from the ICD-10-CM Adverse Effect column in the Table of Drugs and Chemicals.

- When less of a medication than is prescribed by a provider or a manufacturer's instruction is taken, first code the medical condition for which the (*underdosing*) drug was prescribed by referring to the appropriate entry in the ICD-10-CM index. Then, code the medication by referring to the Underdosing column in the Table of Drugs and Chemicals (highlighted in yellow in Figure 4-2).

Refer to the Table of Drugs and Chemicals in the ICD-10-CM index (Figure 4-2) when assigning codes for adverse effects, poisonings, and toxic effects.

Coding Tip

The ICD-10-CM Table of Drugs and Chemicals contains a listing of the generic names of the drugs or chemicals. (Some publishers add brand names to the table.)

For adverse effects, first code the nature of the adverse effect (e.g., rash), followed by the chemical substance by referring to the Therapeutic Use column of the Table of Drugs and Chemicals. If more than one substance is documented as causing the adverse effect, assign codes from the Table of Drugs and Chemicals for *each* substance.

Example: Gastritis due to prescribed tetracycline. In this statement, gastritis is the adverse effect (or manifestation) of the properly administered drug tetracycline. ICD-10-CM codes are reported as K29.70 (gastritis) and T36.4X5A (adverse effect of tetracycline), in that order.

For poisonings and toxic effects in ICD-10-CM, go to the appropriate Poisoning column of the Table of Drugs and Chemicals to assign the code. If more than one substance is documented as causing the poisoning or toxic effect, assign codes from the Table of Drugs and Chemicals for *each* substance. Next code the result or manifestation of the poisoning or toxic effect (e.g., coma).

Example 1: Accidental (unintentional) overdose of tetracycline resulting in severe vomiting, initial encounter. ICD-10-CM codes reported are T36.4X1A (unintentional accidental poisoning by tetracycline) and R11.2 (vomiting), in that order.

Example 2: Acute nicotine exposure can be toxic, and children and adults have been poisoned by swallowing, breathing, or absorbing e-cigarette liquid through their skin or eyes. For these patients assign a code from subcategory T65.291- (Toxic effect of other nicotine and tobacco, accidental [unintentional]; includes toxic effect of other tobacco and nicotine NOS). For a patient with acute tetrahydrocannabinol (THC) toxicity, assign a code from subcategory T40.711- (Poisoning by cannabis [derivatives], accidental [unintentional]). Also report codes for results or manifestations of the toxic effect, such as agitation, confusion, diarrhea, vomiting, and so on.

ICD-10-CM Chapter-Specific Coding Guidelines

Chapter 19: Injury, Poisoning, and Certain Other Consequences of External Causes (S00–T88)

a. Application of 7th Characters in Chapter 19

Most categories in Chapter 19 have a 7th character requirement for each applicable code. Most categories in this chapter have three 7th character values (with the exception of fractures): A, initial encounter, D, subsequent encounter and S, sequela. Categories for traumatic fractures have additional 7th character values. While the patient may be seen by a new or different provider over the course of treatment for an injury, assignment of the 7th character is based on whether the patient is undergoing active treatment and not whether the provider is seeing the patient for the first time.

For complication codes, active treatment refers to treatment for the condition described by the code, even though it may be related to an earlier precipitating problem. For example, code T84.50XA, Infection and inflammatory reaction due to unspecified internal joint prosthesis, initial encounter, is used when active treatment is provided for the infection, even though the condition relates to the prosthetic device, implant, or graft that was placed at a previous encounter.

7th character "A", initial encounter is used for each encounter where the patient is receiving active treatment for the condition. (Examples of active treatment are: surgical treatment, emergency department encounter, and continuing treatment by the same or a different physician.)

7th character "D" subsequent encounter is used for encounters after the patient has completed active treatment of the condition and is receiving routine care for the condition during the healing or recovery phase. (Examples of subsequent care are: cast change or removal, an x-ray to check healing status of fracture, removal of external or internal fixation device, medication adjustment, other aftercare and follow up visits following treatment of the injury or condition.)

Example: Patient whose right maxillary fracture was initially treated eight weeks ago returns again today for routine follow-up care; x-ray was performed to check the fracture's healing status, and results indicate the fracture is healing well. Report code S02.40CD (Maxillary fracture, right side, subsequent encounter for fracture with routine healing). (External cause of injury codes would also be reported to classify activity and place of occurrence.)

The aftercare Z codes should not be used for aftercare for conditions such as injuries or poisonings, where 7th characters are provided to identify subsequent care. (For example, for aftercare of an injury, assign the acute injury code with the 7th character "D" for subsequent encounter.)

(continues)

ICD-10-CM Chapter-Specific Coding Guidelines (*continued*)

7th character "S", sequela, is for use for complications or conditions that arise as a direct result of a condition, such as scar formation after a burn. The scars are sequelae of the burn. When using 7th character "S", it is necessary to use both the injury code that precipitated the sequela and the code for the sequela itself. The "S" is added only to the injury code, not the sequela code. The 7th character "S" identifies the injury responsible for the sequela. The specific type of sequela (e.g. scar) is sequenced first, followed by the injury code.

See Section I.B.10. Sequelae, (Late Effects).

b. Coding of injuries

When coding injuries, assign separate codes for each injury unless a combination code is provided, in which case the combination code is assigned. Codes from category T07, Unspecified multiple injuries should not be assigned in the inpatient setting unless information for a more specific code is not available. Traumatic injury codes (S00–T14.9) are not to be used for normal, healing surgical wounds or to identify complications of surgical wounds.

The code for the most serious injury, as determined by the provider and the focus of treatment, is sequenced first.

1) Superficial injuries

Superficial injuries such as abrasions or contusions are not coded when associated with more severe injuries of the same site.

Example: Patient is diagnosed with abrasions and contusions of the upper right arm and closed greenstick fracture of shaft, right humerus. Report code S42.311A (Greenstick fracture of shaft of humerus, right arm, initial encounter for closed fracture) with external cause of injury codes for activity and place of occurrence. Do not assign codes to the abrasions and contusions.

2) Primary injury with damage to nerves/blood vessels

When a primary injury results in minor damage to peripheral nerves or blood vessels, the primary injury is sequenced first with additional code(s) for injuries to nerves and spinal cord (such as category S04), and/or injury to blood vessels (such as category S15). When the primary injury is to the blood vessels or nerves, that injury should be sequenced first.

3) Iatrogenic injuries

Injury codes from Chapter 19 should not be assigned for injuries that occur during, or as a result of, a medical intervention. Assign the appropriate complication code(s).

c. Coding of traumatic fractures

The principles of multiple coding of injuries should be followed in coding fractures. Fractures of specified sites are coded individually by site in accordance with both the provisions within categories S02, S12, S22, S32, S42, S49, S52, S59, S62, S72, S79, S82, S89, S92 and the level of detail furnished by medical record content. A fracture not indicated as open or closed should be coded to closed. A fracture not indicated whether displaced or not displaced should be coded to displaced.

More specific guidelines are as follows:

1) Initial vs. subsequent encounter for fractures

Traumatic fractures are coded using the appropriate 7th character extension for initial encounter (A, B, C) for each encounter where the patient is receiving active treatment for the fracture. The appropriate 7th character for initial encounter should also be assigned for a patient who delayed seeking treatment for the fracture or nonunion.

Example: Active treatment of fractures includes emergency department encounters, evaluation and management as continuing (ongoing) treatment, and surgery.

Fractures are coded using the appropriate 7th character for subsequent care for encounters after the patient has completed active treatment of the fracture and is receiving routine care for the fracture during the healing or recovery phase.

Care for complications of surgical treatment for fracture repairs during the healing or recovery phase should be coded with the appropriate complication codes.

Care of complications of fractures, such as malunion and nonunion, should be reported with the appropriate 7th character for subsequent care with nonunion (K, M, N) or subsequent care with malunion (P, Q, R).

Malunion/nonunion: The appropriate 7th character for initial encounter should also be assigned for a patient who delayed seeking treatment for the fracture or nonunion.

The open fracture designations in the assignment of the 7th character for fractures of the forearm, femur and lower leg, including ankle are based on the Gustilo open fracture classification. When the Gustilo classification type is not specified for an open fracture, the 7th character for open fracture type I or II should be assigned (B, E, H, M, Q).

A code from category M80, not a traumatic fracture code, should be used for any patient with known osteoporosis who suffers a fracture, even if the patient had a minor fall or trauma, if that fall or trauma would not usually break a normal, healthy bone.

See Section I.C.13. Osteoporosis.

The aftercare Z codes should not be used for aftercare for traumatic fractures. For aftercare of a traumatic fracture, assign the acute fracture code with the appropriate 7th character.

2) Multiple fractures sequencing

Multiple fractures are sequenced in accordance with the severity of the fracture.

3) Physeal fractures

For physeal fractures, assign only the code identifying the type of physeal fracture. Do not assign a separate code to identify the specific bone that is fractured. (A *physeal fracture* is a growth-plate fracture.)

d. Coding of burns and corrosions

The ICD-10-CM makes a distinction between burns and corrosions. The burn codes are for thermal burns, except sunburns, that come from a heat source, such as a fire or hot appliance. The burn codes are also for burns resulting from electricity and radiation. Corrosions are burns due to chemicals. The guidelines are the same for burns and corrosions.

Current burns (T20–T25) are classified by depth, extent and by agent (X code). Burns are classified by depth as first degree (erythema), second degree (blistering), and third degree (full-thickness involvement). Burns of the eye and internal organs (T26–T28) are classified by site, but not by degree.

1) Sequencing of burn and related condition codes

Sequence first the code that reflects the highest degree of burn when more than one burn is present.

(a) When the reason for the admission or encounter is for treatment of external multiple burns, sequence first the code that reflects the burn of the highest degree.

(b) When a patient has both internal and external burns, the circumstances of admission govern the selection of the principal diagnosis or first-listed diagnosis.

(c) When a patient is admitted for burn injuries and other related conditions such as smoke inhalation and/or respiratory failure, the circumstances of admission govern the selection of the principal or first-listed diagnosis.

2) Burns of the same anatomic site

Classify burns of the same anatomic site and on the same side but of different degrees to the subcategory identifying the highest degree recorded in the diagnosis (i.e., for second and third degree burns of right thigh, assign only code T24.311-).

3) Nonhealing burns

Nonhealing burns are coded as acute burns.

Necrosis of burned skin should be coded as a nonhealed burn.

4) Infected burn

For any documented infected burn site, use an additional code for the infection.

(continues)

ICD-10-CM Chapter-Specific Coding Guidelines (*continued*)

5) Assign separate codes for each burn site

When coding burns, assign separate codes for each burn site. Category T30, Burn and corrosion, body region, unspecified, is extremely vague and should rarely be used.

Codes for burns of "multiple sites" should only be assigned when the medical record documentation does not specify the individual sites.

6) Burns and corrosions classified according to extent of body surface involved

Assign codes from category T31, Burns classified according to extent of body surface involved, or T32, Corrosions classified according to extent of body surface involved, for acute burns or corrosions when the site of the burn or corrosion is not specified or when there is a need for additional data. It is advisable to use category T31 as additional coding when needed to provide data for evaluating burn mortality, such as that needed by burn units. It is also advisable to use category T31 as an additional code for reporting purposes when there is mention of a third-degree burn involving 20 percent or more of the body surface. Codes from categories T31 and T32 should *not* be used for sequelae of burns or corrosions.

Categories T31 and T32 are based on the classic "rule of nines" in estimating body surface involved: head and neck are assigned nine percent, each arm nine percent, each leg 18 percent, the anterior trunk 18 percent, posterior trunk 18 percent, and genitalia one percent. Providers may change these percentage assignments where necessary to accommodate infants and children who have proportionately larger heads than adults, and patients who have large buttocks, thighs, or abdomen that involve burns.

7) Encounters for treatment of sequela of burns

Encounters for the treatment of the late effects (sequelae) of burns or corrosions (i.e., scars or joint contractures) should be coded with a burn or corrosion code with the 7th character "S" for sequela.

8) Sequelae with a late effect code and current burn

When appropriate, both a code for a current burn or corrosion with 7th character "A" or "D" and a burn or corrosion code with 7th character "S" may be assigned on the same record (when both a current burn and sequelae of an old burn exist). Burns and corrosions do not heal at the same rate and a current healing wound may still exist with sequela of a healed burn or corrosion.

See Section 1.B.10. Sequela (Late Effect).

9) Use of an external cause code with burns and corrosions

An external cause code should be used with burns and corrosions to identify the source and intent of the burn, as well as the place where it occurred.

e. Adverse effects, poisoning, underdosing, and toxic effects

Codes in categories T36–T65 are combination codes that include the substance that was taken as well as the intent. No additional external cause code is required for poisonings, toxic effects, adverse effects and underdosing codes.

1) Do not code directly from the Table of Drugs and Chemicals

Do not code directly from the Table of Drugs and Chemicals. Always refer back to the Tabular List.

2) Use as many codes as necessary to describe

Use as many codes as necessary to describe completely all drugs, medicinal or biological substances.

3) If the same code would describe the causative agent

If the same code would describe the causative agent for more than one adverse reaction, poisoning, toxic effect or underdosing, assign the code only once.

4) If two or more drugs, medicinal or biological substances

If two or more drugs, medicinal or biological substances are taken, code each individually unless a combination code is listed in the Table of Drugs and Chemicals.

If multiple unspecified drugs, medicinal or biological substances were taken, assign the appropriate code from subcategory T50.91, Poisoning by, adverse effect of and underdosing of multiple unspecified drugs, medicaments and biological substances.

5) The occurrence of drug toxicity is classified in ICD-10-CM as follows:

(a) Adverse effect

When coding an adverse effect of a drug that has been correctly prescribed and properly administered, assign the appropriate code for the nature of the adverse effect followed by the appropriate code for the adverse effect of the drug (T36–T50). The code for the drug should have a 5th or 6th character "5" (for example T36.0X5-). Examples of the nature of an adverse effect are tachycardia, delirium, gastrointestinal hemorrhaging, vomiting, hypokalemia, hepatitis, renal failure, or respiratory failure.

(b) Poisoning

When coding a poisoning or reaction to the improper use of a medication (e.g., overdose, wrong substance given or taken in error, wrong route of administration), first assign the appropriate code from categories T36–T50. The poisoning codes have an associated intent as their 5th or 6th character (accidental, intentional self-harm, assault and undetermined). If the intent of the poisoning is unknown or unspecified, code the intent as accidental intent. The undetermined intent is only for use if the documentation in the record specifies that the intent cannot be determined. Use additional code(s) for all manifestations of poisonings.

If there is also a diagnosis of abuse or dependence of the substance, the abuse or dependence is assigned as an additional code.

Examples of poisoning include:

(i) Error was made in drug prescription

Errors made in drug prescription or in the administration of the drug by provider, nurse, patient, or other person.

(ii) Overdose of a drug intentionally taken

If an overdose of a drug was intentionally taken or administered and resulted in drug toxicity, it would be coded as a poisoning.

(iii) Nonprescribed drug taken with correctly prescribed and properly administered drug

If a nonprescribed drug or medicinal agent was taken in combination with a correctly prescribed and properly administered drug, any drug toxicity or other reaction resulting from the interaction of the two drugs would be classified as a poisoning.

(iv) Interaction of drug(s) and alcohol

When a reaction results from the interaction of a drug(s) and alcohol, this would be classified as poisoning.

See Section I.C.4. if poisoning is the result of insulin pump malfunctions.

For Sequela (Late Effects), see Section I.B.10.

(c) Underdosing

Underdosing refers to taking less of a medication than is prescribed by a provider or a manufacturer's instruction. Discontinuing the use of a prescribed medication on the patient's own initiative (not directed by the patient's provider) is also classified as an underdosing. For underdosing, assign the code from categories T36–T50 (fifth or sixth character "6"). Documentation of a change in the patient's condition is not required in order to assign an underdosing code. Documentation that the patient is taking less of a medication than is prescribed or discontinued the prescribed medication is sufficient for code assignment.

Codes for underdosing should never be assigned as principal or first-listed codes. If a patient has a relapse or exacerbation of the medical condition for which the drug is prescribed because of the reduction in dose, then the medical condition itself should be coded.

Noncompliance (Z91.12-, Z91.13-, Z91.14- and Z91.A4-) or complication of care (Y63.6–Y63.9) codes are to be used with an underdosing code to indicate intent, if known.

(d) Toxic effects

When a harmful substance is ingested or comes in contact with a person, this is classified as a toxic effect. The toxic effect codes are in categories T51–T65. When coding a toxic effect, assign the toxic effect code first, followed by codes for all associated manifestations of the toxic effect.

(continues)

ICD-10-CM Chapter-Specific Coding Guidelines (*continued*)

Toxic effect codes have an associated intent: accidental, intentional self-harm, assault and undetermined.

For Sequela (Late Effects), see Section I.B.10. Sequela.

f. Adult and child abuse, neglect and other maltreatment

Sequence first the appropriate code from categories T74 (Adult and child abuse, neglect and other maltreatment, confirmed) or T76 (Adult and child abuse, neglect and other maltreatment, suspected) for abuse, neglect and other maltreatment, followed by any accompanying mental health or injury code(s).

If the documentation in the medical record states abuse or neglect, it is coded as confirmed (T74.-). It is coded as suspected if it is documented as suspected (T76.-).

For cases of confirmed abuse or neglect an external cause code from the assault section (X92–Y09) should be added to identify the cause of any physical injuries. A perpetrator code (Y07) should be added when the perpetrator of the abuse is known. For suspected cases of abuse or neglect, do not report external cause or perpetrator code.

If a suspected case of abuse, neglect or mistreatment is ruled out during an encounter code Z04.71, Encounter for examination and observation following alleged physical adult abuse, ruled out, or code Z04.72, Encounter for examination and observation following alleged child physical abuse, ruled out, should be used, not a code from T76.

If a suspected case of alleged rape or sexual abuse is ruled out during an encounter, code Z04.41, Encounter for examination and observation following alleged adult rape, or code Z04.42, Encounter for examination and observation following alleged child rape, should be used, not a code from T76.

If a suspected case of forced sexual exploitation or forced labor exploitation is ruled out during an encounter, code Z04.81, Encounter for examination and observation of victim following forced sexual exploitation, or code Z04.82, Encounter for examination and observation of victim following forced labor exploitation, should be used, not a code from T76.

See Section I.C.15. Abuse in a pregnant patient.

g. Complications of care

1) General guidelines for complications of care

(a) Documentation of complications of care

See Section I.B.16. for information on documentation of complications of care.

2) Pain due to medical devices

Pain associated with devices, implants or grafts left in a surgical site (for example painful hip prosthesis) is assigned to the appropriate code(s) found in Chapter 19, Injury, poisoning, and certain other consequences of external causes. Specific codes for pain due to medical devices are found in the T code section of the ICD-10-CM. Use additional code(s) from category G89 to identify acute or chronic pain due to presence of the device, implant or graft (G89.18 or G89.28).

3) Transplant complications

(a) Transplant complications other than kidney

Codes under category T86, Complications of transplanted organs and tissues, are for use for both complications and rejection of transplanted organs. A transplant complication code is only assigned if the complication affects the function of the transplanted organ. Two codes are required to fully describe a transplant complication: the appropriate code from category T86 and a secondary code that identifies the complication.

Pre-existing conditions or conditions that develop after the transplant are not coded as complications unless they affect the function of the transplanted organs.

See I.C.21. for transplant organ removal status.

See I.C.2. for malignant neoplasm associated with transplanted organ.

See I.C.1.d.4. for sequencing of sepsis due to infection in transplanted organ.

(b) Kidney transplant complications

Patients who have undergone kidney transplant may still have some form of chronic kidney disease (CKD) because the kidney transplant may not fully restore kidney function. Code T86.1- should be assigned for documented complications of a kidney transplant, such as transplant failure or rejection or other transplant complication. Code T86.1- should not be assigned for post kidney transplant patients who have chronic kidney disease (CKD) unless a transplant complication such as transplant failure or rejection is documented. If the documentation is unclear as to whether the patient has a complication of the transplant, query the provider.

Conditions that affect the function of the transplanted kidney, other than CKD, should be assigned from subcategory T86.1, Complications of transplanted organ, Kidney, and a secondary code that identifies the complication.

For patients with CKD following a kidney transplant, but who do not have a complication such as failure or rejection, *see section I.C.14. Chronic kidney disease and kidney transplant status.*

See I.C.1.d.4. for sequencing of sepsis due to infection in transplanted organ.

4) Complication codes that include the external cause

As with certain other T codes, some of the complications of care codes have the external cause included in the code. The code includes the nature of the complication as well as the type of procedure that caused the complication. No external cause code indicating the type of procedure is necessary for these codes.

5) Complications of care codes within the body system chapters

Intraoperative and postprocedural complication codes are found within the body system chapters with codes specific to the organs and structures of that body system. These codes should be sequenced first, followed by a code(s) for the specific complication, if applicable.

Complication codes from the body system chapters should be assigned for intraoperative and postprocedural complications (e.g., the appropriate complication code from Chapter 9 would be assigned for a vascular intraoperative or postprocedural complication) unless the complication is specifically indexed to a T code in Chapter 19.

Courtesy of the Centers for Medicare & Medicaid Services, www.cms.gov.

Exercise 4.9 – Injury, Poisoning, and Certain Other Consequences of External Causes

Instructions: Assign the appropriate ICD-10-CM code(s). (Do *not* enter codes for external cause of diseases and injuries.)

_____   1. Closed fracture of mandible, subcondylar, right (initial encounter for closed fracture)

_____   2. Wedge compression fracture of first thoracic vertebra (initial encounter)

_____   3. Concussion with loss of consciousness (30 minutes) (initial encounter)

_____   4. Foot burn, left, blisters, epidermal loss (second-degree) (initial encounter)

_____   5. Heart laceration with hemopericardium due to open wound laceration, left frontal wall of thorax, with diaphragmatic contusions (initial encounter)

_____   6. Hives resulting from penicillin taken as prescribed (initial encounter)

_____   7. Coma due to overdose of barbiturates during an attempted suicide (initial encounter)

_____   8. Thrombophlebitis, left tibial vein, due to underdosing of Coumadin; patient could not afford to purchase medication (initial encounter)

_____   9. Ventricular flutter due to accidental interaction of prescribed ephedrine and ethyl alcohol intoxication (accident) (initial encounter)

_____   10. Painful left knee prosthesis (initial encounter)

ICD-10-CM Chapter 20: External Causes of Morbidity (V00–Y99)

This ICD-10-CM chapter classifies the reporting of *external causes of morbidity* codes, which are reported as secondary codes for use in any health care setting.

ICD-10-CM Chapter 20 headings include the following:

- Accidents
- Transport accidents
- Pedestrian injured in transport accident
- Pedal cycle rider injured in transport accident
- Motorcycle rider injured in transport accident
- Occupant of three-wheeled motor vehicle injured in transport accident
- Car occupant injured in transport accident
- Occupant of pick-up truck or van injured in transport accident
- Occupant of heavy transport vehicle injured in transport accident
- Bus occupant injured in transport accident
- Other land transport accidents
- Water transport accidents
- Air and space transport accidents
- Other and unspecified transport accidents
- Other external causes of accidental injury
- Slipping, tripping, stumbling, and falls
- Exposure to inanimate mechanical forces
- Exposure to animate mechanical forces
- Accidental non-transport drowning and submersion
- Exposure to electric current, radiation, and extreme ambient air temperature and pressure
- Exposure to smoke, fire, and flames
- Contact with heat and hot substances
- Exposure to forces of nature
- Overexertion and strenuous or repetitive movements
- Accidental exposure to other specified factors
- Intentional self-harm
- Assault
- Event of undetermined intent
- Legal intervention, operations of war, military operations, and terrorism
- Complications of medical and surgical care
- Misadventures to patients during surgical and medical care
- Medical devices associated with adverse incidents in diagnostic and therapeutic use
- Surgical and other medical procedures as the cause of abnormal reaction of the patient, or of later complication, without mention of misadventure at the time of the procedure
- Supplementary factors related to causes of morbidity classified elsewhere

External Causes of Morbidities codes are reported as secondary codes for use in any health care setting because they provide data for injury research and evaluation of injury prevention strategies. These codes are assigned to capture the following:

- *Cause of injury* ("how" the injury occurred, such as abuse, accident, assault, burn, collision, and so on)

- *Activity being performed* ("what" the patient was doing at the time of injury, such as playing a sport, gardening, sleeping, using a cell phone, and so on)

- *Place of occurrence* ("where" the patient was when the injury occurred, such as at home or work, in a post office, on a highway, and so on)

- *Status at the time of injury* (indicates if injury is related to leisure, military, student, volunteer, and so on, as applicable)

Example: A patient fell off the toilet in the downstairs bathroom of their single-family house during an attempt to coax the cat to come down from the top of a cabinet. It apparently worked because the cat jumped off the cabinet and landed on the patient. However, the patient was so surprised that they screamed and fell off the toilet onto the floor. The patient landed on the left arm due to the fall and experienced extremely sharp pain. Patient was evaluated in the emergency department and diagnosed with a closed nondisplaced comminuted fracture of the shaft of the humerus, left. Patient received treatment for this initial encounter and was discharged home to follow-up with the primary care physician in the office.

For ICD-10-CM, report the injury (fracture) (S42.355A), cause of injury (fall) (W18.11XA), and place of occurrence (bathroom of patient's home) (Y92.012). ICD-10-CM's level of specificity results in different codes for other locations in the patient's home (e.g., bathroom). (Seventh-character A is reported for the initial encounter during which the patient receives active treatment.)

The ICD-10-CM place of injury codes for this case indicate that the patient's health insurance policy should be billed, not a liability or workers' compensation policy. If the place of occurrence had been at a grocery store or other place of business, the business's liability insurance would be billed (instead of the patient's health insurance). If the place of occurrence had been at the patient's employment setting, workers' compensation would be billed.

ICD-10-CM Chapter-Specific Coding Guidelines

Chapter 20: External Causes of Morbidity (V00–Y99)

The external causes of morbidity codes should never be sequenced as the first-listed or principal diagnosis.

External cause codes are intended to provide data for injury research and evaluation of injury prevention strategies. These codes capture how the injury or health condition happened (cause), the intent (unintentional or accidental; or intentional, such as suicide or assault), the place where the event occurred, the activity of the patient at the time of the event, and the person's status (e.g., civilian, military).

There is no national requirement for mandatory ICD-10-CM external cause code reporting. Unless a provider is subject to a state-based external cause code reporting mandate or these codes are required by a particular payer, reporting of ICD-10-CM codes in Chapter 20, External Causes of Morbidity, is not required. In the absence of a mandatory reporting requirement, providers are encouraged to voluntarily report external cause codes, as they provide valuable data for injury research and evaluation of injury prevention strategies.

a. General external cause coding guidelines

   1) Used with any code in the range of A00.0–T88.9, Z00–Z99

   An external cause code may be used with any code in the range of A00.0–T88.9, Z00–Z99, classification that represents a health condition due to an external cause. Though they are most applicable to injuries, they are also valid for use with such things as infections or diseases due to an external source, and other health conditions, such as a heart attack that occurs during strenuous physical activity.

Example: Patient got out of bed to walk to the bathroom and tripped on a wooden bed post in the bedroom but did not fall. Diagnosis is sprained great toe, right. Report codes S93.501A (sprain, initial encounter), W18.49XA (tripping, initial encounter), Y93.01 (walking), and Y92.003 (home).

   2) External cause code used for length of treatment

   Assign the external cause code, with the appropriate 7th character (initial encounter, subsequent encounter, or sequela) for each encounter for which the injury or condition is being treated.

(continues)

ICD-10-CM Chapter-Specific Coding Guidelines (*continued*)

Most categories in Chapter 20 have a 7th character requirement for each applicable code. Most categories in this chapter have three 7th character values: A, initial encounter, D, subsequent encounter, and S, sequela. While the patient may be seen by a new or different provider over the course of treatment for an injury or condition, assignment of the 7th character for external cause should match the 7th character of the code assigned for the associated injury or condition for the encounter.

Example: Patient returned to the office for routine follow-up care of sprained great toe, right; patient had tripped at home and stubbed the right toe. Report codes S93.501D (sprain, subsequent encounter) and W18.49XD (tripping, subsequent encounter).

3) Use the full range of external cause codes

Use the full range of external cause codes to completely describe the cause, the intent, the place of occurrence, and if applicable, the activity of the patient at the time of the event, and the patient's status, for all injuries, and other health conditions due to an external cause.

4) Assign as many external cause codes as necessary

Assign as many external cause codes as necessary to fully explain each cause. If only one external code can be recorded, assign the code most related to the principal diagnosis.

5) The selection of the appropriate external cause code

The selection of the appropriate external cause code is guided by the Alphabetic Index of External Causes and by Inclusion and Exclusion notes in the Tabular List.

6) External cause code can never be a principal diagnosis

An external cause code can never be a principal (first-listed) diagnosis.

7) Combination external cause codes

Certain of the external cause codes are combination codes that identify sequential events that result in an injury, such as a fall which results in striking against an object. The injury may be due to either event or both. The combination external cause code used should correspond to the sequence of events regardless of which caused the most serious injury.

8) No external cause code needed in certain circumstances

No external cause code from Chapter 20 is needed if the external cause and intent are included in a code from another chapter (e.g., T36.0X1-Poisoning by penicillins, accidental (unintentional)).

b. Place of occurrence guideline

Codes from category Y92, Place of occurrence of the external cause, are secondary codes for use after other external cause codes to identify the location of the patient at the time of injury or other condition.

Generally, a place of occurrence code is assigned only once, at the initial encounter for treatment. However, in the rare instance that a new injury occurs during hospitalization, an additional place of occurrence code may be assigned. No 7th characters are used for Y92.

Do not use place of occurrence code Y92.9 if the place is not stated or is not applicable.

c. Activity code

Assign a code from category Y93, Activity code, to describe the activity of the patient at the time the injury or other health condition occurred.

An activity code is used only once, at the initial encounter for treatment. Only one code from Y93 should be recorded on a medical record.

The activity codes are not applicable to poisonings, adverse effects, misadventures, or sequelae.

Do not assign Y93.9, Unspecified activity, if the activity is not stated.

A code from category Y93 is appropriate for use with external cause and intent codes if identifying the activity provides additional information about the event.

d. **Place of occurrence, activity, and status codes used with other external cause code**

When applicable, place of occurrence, activity, and external cause status codes are sequenced after the main external cause code(s). Regardless of the number of external cause codes assigned, generally there should be only one place of occurrence code, one activity code, and one external cause status code assigned to an encounter. However, in the rare instance that a new injury occurs during hospitalization, an additional place of occurrence code may be assigned.

e. **If the reporting format limits the number of external cause codes**

If the reporting format limits the number of external cause codes that can be used in reporting clinical data, report the code for the cause/intent most related to the principal diagnosis. If the format permits capture of additional external cause codes, the cause/intent, including medical misadventures, of the additional events should be reported rather than the codes for place, activity, or external status.

f. **Multiple external cause coding guidelines**

More than one external cause code is required to fully describe the external cause of an illness or injury. The assignment of external cause codes should be sequenced in the following priority:

If two or more events cause separate injuries, an external cause code should be assigned for each cause. The first-listed external cause code will be selected in the following order:

External codes for child and adult abuse take priority over all other external cause codes.

See Section I.C.19., Child and Adult abuse guidelines.

External cause codes for terrorism events take priority over all other external cause codes except child and adult abuse.

External cause codes for cataclysmic events take priority over all other external cause codes except child and adult abuse and terrorism.

External cause codes for transport accidents take priority over all other external cause codes except cataclysmic events, child and adult abuse, and terrorism.

Activity and external cause status codes are assigned following all causal (intent) external cause codes.

The first-listed external cause code should correspond to the cause of the most serious diagnosis due to an assault, accident, or self-harm, following the order of hierarchy listed above.

g. **Child and adult abuse guideline**

Adult and child abuse, neglect and maltreatment are classified as assault. Any of the assault codes may be used to indicate the external cause of any injury resulting from the confirmed abuse.

For confirmed cases of abuse, neglect and maltreatment, when the perpetrator is known, a code from Y07, Perpetrator of maltreatment and neglect, should accompany any other assault codes.

See Section I.C.19. Adult and child abuse, neglect and other maltreatment.

h. **Unknown or undetermined intent guideline**

If the intent (accident, self-harm, assault) of the cause of an injury or other condition is unknown or unspecified, code the intent as accidental intent. All transport accident categories assume accidental intent.

1) **Use of undetermined intent**

External cause codes for events of undetermined intent are only for use if the documentation in the record specifies that the intent cannot be determined.

i. **Sequelae (Late Effects) of external cause guidelines**

1) **Sequelae external cause codes**

Sequelae are reported using the external cause code with the 7th character "S" for sequela. These codes should be used with any report of a late effect or sequela resulting from a previous injury.

See Section I.B.10. Sequela (Late Effects).

2) **Sequela external cause code with a related current injury**

A sequela external cause code should never be used with a related current nature of injury code.

(continues)

ICD-10-CM Chapter-Specific Coding Guidelines (*continued*)

3) Use of sequela external cause codes for subsequent visits

Use a late effect external cause code for subsequent visits when a late effect of the initial injury is being treated. Do not use a late effect external cause code for subsequent visits for follow-up care (e.g., to assess healing, to receive rehabilitative therapy) of the injury when no late effect of the injury has been documented.

j. Terrorism guidelines

1) Cause of injury identified by the Federal Government (FBI) as terrorism

When the cause of an injury is identified by the Federal Government (FBI) as terrorism, the first-listed external cause code should be a code from category Y38, Terrorism. The definition of terrorism employed by the FBI is found at the inclusion note at the beginning of category Y38. Use additional code for place of occurrence (Y92.-). More than one Y38 code may be assigned if the injury is the result of more than one mechanism of terrorism.

2) Cause of an injury is suspected to be the result of terrorism

When the cause of an injury is suspected to be the result of terrorism, a code from category Y38 should not be assigned.

Suspected cases should be classified as assault.

3) Code Y38.9, terrorism, secondary effects

Assign code Y38.9, Terrorism, secondary effects, for conditions occurring subsequent to the terrorist event. This code should not be assigned for conditions that are due to the initial terrorist act.

It is acceptable to assign code Y38.9 with another code from Y38 if there is an injury due to the initial terrorist event and an injury that is a subsequent result of the terrorist event.

k. External cause status

A code from category Y99, External cause status, should be assigned whenever any other external cause code is assigned for an encounter, including an Activity code, except for the events noted below. Assign a code from category Y99, External cause status, to indicate the work status of the person at the time the event occurred. The status code indicates whether the event occurred during military activity, whether a non-military person was at work or whether an individual, including a student or volunteer, was involved in a non-work activity at the time of the causal event.

A code from Y99, External cause status, should be assigned, when applicable, with other external cause codes, such as transport accidents and falls. The external cause status codes are not applicable to poisonings, adverse effects, misadventures or late effects.

Do not assign a code from category Y99 if no other external cause codes (cause, activity) are applicable for the encounter.

An external cause status code is used only once, at the initial encounter for treatment. Only one code from Y99 should be recorded on a medical record.

Do not assign code Y99.9, Unspecified external cause status, if the status is not stated.

Exercise 4.10 – External Causes of Morbidity

Instructions: Assign the appropriate ICD-10-CM external cause V through Y code(s).

_____	**1.** Fall from skateboard at public park (initial encounter)
_____	**2.** Burning pajamas (nightwear) resulting from cooking in kitchen of mobile home (initial encounter)
_____	**3.** Explosion in powered watercraft (initial encounter)
_____	**4.** Fall from ladder (initial encounter)
_____	**5.** Accidental fall down a ramp at baseball field

ICD-10-CM Chapter 21: Factors Influencing Health Status and Contact with Health Services (Z00–Z99)

This ICD-10-CM chapter classifies circumstances other than a disease, injury or external cause classifiable to categories A00–Y89, which are recorded as "diagnoses" or "problems." Certain Z codes in ICD-10-CM can be reported as a first-listed or additional diagnosis for outpatient care. The chapter classifies the following:

- Persons encountering health services for examinations
- Genetic carrier and genetic susceptibility to disease
- Resistance to antimicrobial drugs
- Estrogen receptor status
- Retained foreign body fragments
- Hormone sensitivity malignancy status
- Persons with potential health hazards related to communicable diseases
- Persons encountering health services in circumstances related to reproduction
- Encounters for other specific health care
- Persons with potential health hazards related to socioeconomic and psychosocial circumstances
- Do not resuscitate status
- Blood type
- Body mass index (BMI)
- Persons encountering health services in other circumstances
- Persons with potential health hazards related to family and personal history and certain conditions influencing health status

 NOTE:

Verify history of codes in the tabular list before reporting. Also do not confuse personal history of with family history of codes.

Reporting Z Codes

Such circumstances can arise when the following occurs, for which reporting a Z code is appropriate:

- A person who may or may not be sick encounters the health services for some specific purpose.
  - Limited care or service for a current condition
  - Donation of an organ or tissue
  - Prophylactic vaccination (immunization)
  - Discussion of a problem which is in itself not a disease or injury
- A situation or problem is present that influences the person's health status but is not in itself a current illness or injury.
- A person with a known disease or injury, whether it is current or resolving, encounters the health care system for a specific treatment of that disease or injury (e.g., dialysis for renal disease, chemotherapy for malignancy, or a cast change).
- Some circumstance or problem is present that influences the person's health status but is not in itself a current illness or injury. Such factors may be elicited during population surveys, when the person may or may not be currently sick, or may be recorded as an additional factor to be borne in mind when the person is receiving care for some current illness or injury classifiable to ICD-10-CM categories A00–Y99.

  In this situation, the ICD-10-CM Z code should be assigned as an other (additional) code and is not selected as the principal diagnosis for inpatient cases or the first-listed diagnosis for outpatient cases.

For example, such circumstances include personal history of certain diseases or a person with an artificial heart valve *in situ*.

Coding Tip

Refer to ICD-10-CM index main terms to begin assigning a Z code. Common main terms include:

Admission	Donor	Outcome of delivery
Aftercare	Encounter for	Pregnancy
Attention to	Examination	Procedure (surgical) not done
Carrier (suspected) of	Exposure	Prophylactic
Checking	Fitting	Removal
Checkup	Follow-up	Resistance, resistant
Closure	History, family	Routine postpartum follow-up
Contact	History (personal) of	Screening
Contraception, contraceptive	Maladjustment	Status
Counseling	Newborn	Test(s)
Dialysis	Observation	Vaccination

ICD-10-CM Chapter-Specific Coding Guidelines

Chapter 21: Factors Influencing Health Status and Contact with Health Services (Z00–Z99)

Note: The chapter-specific guidelines provide additional information about the use of Z codes for specified encounters.

a. **Use of Z codes in any healthcare setting**

Z codes are for use in any healthcare setting. Z codes may be used as either a first-listed (principal diagnosis code in the inpatient setting) or secondary code, depending on the circumstances of the encounter. Certain Z codes may only be used as first-listed or principal diagnosis.

b. **Z Codes indicate a reason for an encounter *or provide additional information about a patient encounter***

Z codes are not procedure codes. A corresponding procedure code must accompany a Z code to describe any procedure performed.

c. **Categories of Z codes**

1) **Contact/Exposure**

Category Z20 indicates contact with, and suspected exposure to, communicable diseases. These codes are for patients who are suspected to have been exposed to a disease by close personal contact with an infected individual or are in an area where a disease is epidemic.

Category Z77, Other contact with and (suspected) exposures hazardous to health, indicates contact with and suspected exposures hazardous to health.

Contact/exposure codes may be used as a first-listed code to explain an encounter for testing, or, more commonly, as a secondary code to identify a potential risk.

2) **Inoculations and vaccinations**

Code Z23 is for encounters for inoculations and vaccinations. It indicates that a patient is being seen to receive a prophylactic inoculation against a disease. Procedure codes are required to identify the actual administration of the injection and the type(s) of immunizations given. Code Z23 may be used as a secondary code if the inoculation is given as a routine part of preventive health care, such as a well-baby visit.

Example: Five-year-old patient seen for annual well-child visit during which provider planned to administer a flu vaccine. The parent refused to allow the vaccine to be administered. Report codes Z00.129 (Routine infant or child health check) and Z28.82 (Vaccination not carried out because of caregiver refusal). (If the vaccine had been administered, code Z23 would be reported.)

3) Status

Status codes indicate that a patient is either a carrier of a disease or has the sequela or residual of a past disease or condition. This includes things such as the presence of prosthetic or mechanical devices resulting from past treatment. A status code is informative because the status may affect the course of treatment and its outcome. A status code is distinct from a history code. The history code indicates that the patient no longer has the condition.

A status code should not be used with a diagnosis code from one of the body system chapters *if the diagnosis code includes the information provided by the status code*. For example, code Z94.1, Heart transplant status, should not be used with code T86.2, Complications of heart. The complication code indicates that the patient is a heart transplant patient.

For encounters for weaning from a mechanical ventilator, assign a code from subcategory J96.1, Chronic respiratory failure, followed by code Z99.11, Dependence on respirator [ventilator] status.

The status Z codes/categories are:

Z14   Genetic carrier

Genetic carrier status indicates that a person carries a gene, associated with a particular disease, which may be passed to offspring who may develop that disease. The person does not have the disease and is not at risk of developing the disease.

Z15   Genetic susceptibility to disease

Genetic susceptibility indicates that a person has a gene that increases the risk of that person developing the disease.

Codes from category Z15 should not be used as principal or first-listed codes. If the patient has the condition to which he/she is susceptible, and that condition is the reason for the encounter, the code for the current condition should be sequenced first. If the patient is being seen for follow-up after completed treatment for this condition, and the condition no longer exists, a follow-up code should be sequenced first, followed by the appropriate personal history and genetic susceptibility codes. If the purpose of the encounter is genetic counseling associated with procreative management, code Z31.5, Encounter for genetic counseling, should be assigned as the first-listed code, followed by a code from category Z15.

Additional codes should be assigned for any applicable family or personal history.

Z16   Resistance to antimicrobial drugs

This code indicates that a patient has a condition that is resistant to antimicrobial drug treatment. Sequence the infection code first.

Z17   Estrogen receptor status

Z18   Retained foreign body fragments

Z19   Hormone sensitivity malignancy status

Z21   Asymptomatic HIV infection status

This code indicates that a patient has tested positive for HIV but has manifested no signs or symptoms of the disease.

(continues)

ICD-10-CM Chapter-Specific Coding Guidelines (*continued*)

Z22   Carrier of infectious disease

Carrier status indicates that a person harbors the specific organisms of a disease without manifest symptoms and is capable of transmitting the infection.

Z28.3   Underimmunization status

See Section I.B.14. for underimmunization documentation by clinicians other than the patient's provider.

Z33.1   Pregnant state, incidental

This code is a secondary code only for use when the pregnancy is in no way complicating the reason for visit.

Otherwise, a code from the obstetrics chapter is required.

Z66   Do not resuscitate

This code may be used when it is documented by the provider that a patient is on do not resuscitate status at any time during the stay.

Z67   Blood type

Z68   Body mass index (BMI)

BMI codes should only be assigned when there is an associated, reportable diagnosis (such as obesity). Do not assign BMI codes during pregnancy.

See Section I.B.14. for BMI documentation by clinicians other than the patient's provider.

Z74.01   Bed confinement status

Z76.82   Awaiting organ transplant status

Z78   Other specified health status

Code Z78.1, Physical restraint status, may be used when it is documented by the provider that a patient has been put in restraints during the current encounter.

Please note that this code should not be reported when it is documented by the provider that a patient is temporarily restrained during a procedure.

Z79   Long-term (current) drug therapy

Codes from this category indicate a patient's continuous use of a prescribed drug (including such things as aspirin therapy) for the long-term treatment of a condition or for prophylactic use. It is not for use for patients who have addictions to drugs. This subcategory is not for use of medications for detoxification or maintenance programs to prevent withdrawal symptoms (e.g., methadone maintenance for opiate dependence). Assign the appropriate code for the drug use, abuse, or dependence instead.

Assign a code from Z79 if the patient is receiving a medication for an extended period as a prophylactic measure (such as for the prevention of deep vein thrombosis) or as treatment of a chronic condition (such as arthritis) or a disease requiring a lengthy course of treatment (such as cancer). Do not assign a code from category Z79 for medication being administered for a brief period of time to treat an acute illness or injury (such as a course of antibiotics to treat acute bronchitis).

Z88   Allergy status to drugs, medicaments and biological substances

Except: Z88.9, Allergy status to unspecified drugs, medications and biological substances status

Z89   Acquired absence of limb

Z90   Acquired absence of organs, not elsewhere classified

Z91.0-   Allergy status, other than to drugs and biological substances

Z92.82   Status post administration of tissue plasminogen activator (tPA) (recombinant [rtPA]) in a different facility within the last 24 hours prior to admission to a current facility.

Assign code Z92.82, Status post administration of tPA (rtPA) in a different facility within the last 24 hours prior to admission to current facility, as a secondary diagnosis when a patient is received by transfer into a facility and documentation indicates they were administered tPA within the last 24 hours prior to admission to the current facility.

This guideline applies even if the patient is still receiving the tPA at the time they are received into the current facility.

The appropriate code for the condition for which the tPA was administered (such as cerebrovascular disease or myocardial infarction) should be assigned first.

Code Z92.82 is only applicable to the receiving facility record and not to the transferring facility record.

Z93   Artificial opening status

Z94   Transplanted organ and tissue status

Z95   Presence of cardiac and vascular implants and grafts

Z96   Presence of other functional implants

Z97   Presence of other devices

Z98   Other postprocedural states

Assign code Z98.85, Transplanted organ removal status, to indicate that a transplanted organ has been previously removed. This code should not be assigned for the encounter in which the transplanted organ is removed. The complication necessitating removal of the transplant organ should be assigned for that encounter.

See section I.C.19. for information on the coding of organ transplant complications.

Z99   Dependence on enabling machines and devices, not elsewhere classified

Note: Categories Z89–Z90 and Z93–Z99 are for use only if there are no complications or malfunctions of the organ or tissue replaced, the amputation site or the equipment on which the patient is dependent.

4) History (of)

There are two types of history Z codes, personal and family. Personal history codes explain a patient's past medical condition that no longer exists and is not receiving any treatment but that has the potential for recurrence and, therefore, may require continued monitoring.

Family history codes are for use when a patient has a family member(s) who has had a particular disease that causes the patient to be at higher risk of also contracting the disease.

Personal history codes may be used in conjunction with follow-up codes, and family history codes may be used in conjunction with screening codes to explain the need for a test or procedure. History codes are also acceptable on any medical record regardless of the reason for visit. A history of an illness, even if no longer present, is important information that may alter the type of treatment ordered.

The reason for the encounter (for example, screening or counseling) should be sequenced first and the appropriate personal and/or family history code(s) should be assigned as additional diagnos(es).

Example 1: Patient with a history of colon cancer, removed two years ago, is seen for follow-up examination to determine whether there is recurrence. Report codes Z08 (Encounter for follow-up examination after completed treatment for malignant neoplasm) and Z85.038 (Personal history of other malignant neoplasm of large intestine).

(continues)

ICD-10-CM Chapter-Specific Coding Guidelines (*continued*)

Example 2: Patient has extensive family history of ovarian cancer (e.g., mother, aunts, and sisters) and elects to undergo screening as a preventive measure. Report codes Z12.73 (Encounter for screening for malignant neoplasm of ovary) and Z80.41 (Family history of malignant neoplasm of ovary).

The history Z code categories are:

Z80	Family history of primary malignant neoplasm
Z81	Family history of mental and behavioral disorders
Z82	Family history of certain disabilities and chronic diseases (leading to disablement)
Z83	Family history of other specific disorders
Z84	Family history of other conditions
Z85	Personal history of malignant neoplasm
Z86	Personal history of certain other diseases
Z87	Personal history of other diseases and conditions
Z91.4-	Personal history of psychological trauma, not elsewhere classified
Z91.5-	Personal history of self-harm
Z91.81	History of falling
Z91.82	Personal history of military deployment
Z91.85	Personal history of military service
Z92	Personal history of medical treatment

> Except: Z92.0, Personal history of contraception
>
> Except: Z92.82, Status post administration of tPA (rtPA) in a different facility within the last 24 hours prior to admission to a current facility

5) Screening

Screening is the testing for disease or disease precursors in seemingly well individuals so that early detection and treatment can be provided for those who test positive for the disease (e.g., screening mammogram).

The testing of a person to rule out or confirm a suspected diagnosis because the patient has some sign or symptom is a diagnostic examination, not a screening. In these cases, the sign or symptom is used to explain the reason for the test.

A screening code may be a first-listed code if the reason for the visit is specifically the screening exam. It may also be used as an additional code if the screening is done during an office visit for other health problems. A screening code is not necessary if the screening is inherent to a routine examination, such as a Pap smear done during a routine pelvic examination.

Should a condition be discovered during the screening, then the code for the condition may be assigned as an additional diagnosis.

The Z code indicates that a screening exam is planned. A procedure code is required to confirm that the screening was performed.

The screening Z code categories are:

Z11	Encounter for screening for infectious and parasitic diseases
Z12	Encounter for screening for malignant neoplasms
Z13	Encounter for screening for other diseases and disorders

Except: Z13.9, Encounter for screening, unspecified

Z36   Encounter for antenatal screening for mother

6) Observation

There are three observation Z code categories. They are for use in very limited circumstances when a person is being observed for a suspected condition that is ruled out. The observation codes are not for use if an injury or illness or any signs or symptoms related to the suspected condition are present. In such cases, the diagnosis/symptom code is used with the corresponding external cause code.

The observation codes are primarily to be used as principal/first-listed diagnosis. An observation code may be assigned as a secondary diagnosis code when the patient is being observed for a condition that is ruled out and is unrelated to the principal/first-listed diagnosis. Also, when the principal diagnosis is required to be a code from category Z38, Liveborn infants according to place of birth and type of delivery, then a code from category Z05, Encounter for observation and evaluation of newborn for suspected diseases and conditions ruled out, is sequenced after the Z38 code. Additional codes may be used in addition to the observation code but only if they are unrelated to the suspected condition being observed.

Codes from subcategory Z03.7, Encounter for suspected maternal and fetal conditions ruled out, may be used either as a first listed or as an additional code assignment depending on the case. They are for use in very limited circumstances on a maternal record when an encounter is for a suspected maternal or fetal condition that is ruled out during that encounter (for example, a maternal or fetal condition may be suspected due to an abnormal test result). These codes should not be used when the condition is confirmed. In those cases, the confirmed condition should be coded. In addition, these codes are not for use if an illness or any signs or symptoms related to the suspected condition or problem are present. In such cases, the diagnosis/symptom code is used.

Additional codes may be used in addition to the code from subcategory Z03.7, but only if they are unrelated to the suspected condition being evaluated.

Codes from subcategory Z03.7 may not be used for encounters for antenatal screening of mother. *See Section I.C.21. Screening.*

For encounters for suspected fetal condition that are inconclusive following testing and evaluation, assign the appropriate code from category O35, O36, O40, or O41.

The observation Z code categories are:

Z03   Encounter for medical observation for suspected diseases and conditions ruled out

Z04   Encounter for examination and observation for other reasons

>   Except: Z04.9, Encounter for examination and observation for unspecified reason

Z05   Encounter for observation and evaluation of newborn for suspected diseases and conditions ruled out

7) Aftercare

Aftercare visit codes cover situations when the initial treatment of a disease has been performed and the patient requires continued care during the healing or recovery phase, or for the long-term consequences of the disease. The aftercare Z code should not be used if treatment is directed at a current, acute disease. The diagnosis code is to be used in these cases. Exceptions to this rule are codes Z51.0, Encounter for antineoplastic radiation therapy, and codes from subcategory Z51.1, Encounter for antineoplastic chemotherapy and immunotherapy. These codes are to be first listed, followed by the diagnosis code when a patient's encounter is solely to receive radiation therapy, chemotherapy or immunotherapy for the treatment of a neoplasm. If the reason for the encounter is more than one type of antineoplastic therapy, code Z51.0 and a code from subcategory Z51.1 may be assigned together, in which case one of these codes would be reported as a secondary diagnosis.

ICD-10-CM Chapter-Specific Coding Guidelines (*continued*)

The aftercare Z codes should also not be used for aftercare for injuries. For aftercare of an injury, assign the acute injury code with the appropriate 7th character (for subsequent encounter).

The aftercare codes are generally first listed to explain the specific reason for the encounter. An aftercare code may be used as an additional code when some type of aftercare is provided in addition to the reason for admission and no diagnosis code is applicable. An example of this would be the closure of a colostomy during an encounter for treatment of another condition.

Aftercare codes should be used in conjunction with other aftercare codes or diagnosis codes to provide better detail on the specifics of an aftercare encounter visit, unless otherwise directed by the classification. The sequencing of multiple aftercare codes depends on the circumstances of the encounter.

Certain aftercare Z code categories need a secondary diagnosis code to describe the resolving condition or sequela. For others, the condition is included in the code title.

Additional Z code aftercare category terms include fitting and adjustment, and attention to artificial openings.

Status Z codes may be used with aftercare Z codes to indicate the nature of the aftercare. For example, code Z95.1, Presence of aortocoronary bypass graft, may be used with code Z48.812, Encounter for surgical aftercare following surgery on the circulatory system, to indicate the surgery for which the aftercare is being performed. A status code should not be used when the aftercare code indicates the type of status, such as using Z43.0, Encounter for attention to tracheostomy, with Z93.0, Tracheostomy status.

The aftercare Z category/codes are:

Z42   Encounter for plastic and reconstructive surgery following medical procedure or healed injury

Z43   Encounter for attention to artificial openings

Z44   Encounter for fitting and adjustment of external prosthetic device

Z45   Encounter for adjustment and management of implanted device

Z46   Encounter for fitting and adjustment of other devices

Z47   Orthopedic aftercare

Z48   Encounter for other postprocedural aftercare

Z49   Encounter for care involving renal dialysis

Z51   Encounter for other aftercare and medical care

Example: Patient is diagnosed with right breast cancer, undergoes mastectomy, and is admitted today for chemotherapy. Report codes Z51.11 (Encounter for antineoplastic chemotherapy) and C50.911 (Malignant neoplasm of unspecified site of right female breast), in that order.

8) Follow-up

The follow-up codes are used to explain continuing surveillance following completed treatment of a disease, condition, or injury. They imply that the condition has been fully treated and no longer exists. They should not be confused with aftercare codes, or injury codes with a seventh character for subsequent encounter, that explain current treatment for a healing condition or its sequela. Follow-up codes may be used in conjunction with history codes to provide the full picture of the healed condition and its treatment. The follow-up code is sequenced first, followed by the history code.

A follow-up code may be used to explain multiple visits. Should a condition be found to have recurred on the follow-up visit, then the diagnosis code for the condition should be assigned in place of the follow-up code.

The follow-up Z codes/categories are:

| Z08 | Encounter for follow-up examination after completed treatment for malignant neoplasm |
| Z09 | Encounter for follow-up examination after completed treatment for conditions other than malignant neoplasm. |

Codes Z08, Encounter for follow-up examination after completed treatment for malignant neoplasm, and Z09, Encounter for follow up examination after completed treatment for conditions other than malignant neoplasm, may be assigned following any type of completed treatment modality (including both medical and surgical treatments).

| Z39 | Encounter for maternal postpartum care and examination |

9) Donor

Codes in category Z52, Donors of organs and tissues, are used for living individuals who are donating blood or other body tissue. These codes are only for individuals donating for others, as well as for self-donations. They are not used to identify cadaveric donations.

10) Counseling

Counseling Z codes are used when a patient or family member receives assistance in the aftermath of an illness or injury, or when support is required in coping with family or social problems.

The counseling Z codes/categories are:

Z30.0-	Encounter for general counseling and advice on contraception
Z31.5	Encounter for procreative genetic counseling
Z31.6-	Encounter for general counseling and advice on procreation
Z32.2	Encounter for childbirth instruction
Z32.3	Encounter for childcare instruction
Z69	Encounter for mental health services for victim and perpetrator of abuse
Z70	Counseling related to sexual attitude, behavior and orientation
Z71	Persons encountering health services for other counseling and medical advice, not elsewhere classified

Note: Code Z71.84, Encounter for health counseling related to travel, is to be used for health risk and safety counseling for future travel purposes.

Code Z71.85, Encounter for immunization safety counseling, is to be used for counseling of the patient or caregiver regarding the safety of a vaccine. This code should not be used for the provision of general information regarding risks and potential side effects during routine encounters for the administration of vaccines.

Code Z71.87, Encounter for pediatric-to-adult transition counseling, should be assigned when pediatric-to-adult transition counseling is the sole reason for the encounter or when this counseling is provided in addition to other services, such as treatment of a chronic condition. If both transition counseling and treatment of a medical condition are provided during the same encounter, the code(s) for the medical condition(s) treated and code Z71.87 should be assigned, with sequencing depending on the circumstances of the encounter.

| Z76.81 | Expectant mother prebirth pediatrician visit |

11) Encounters for obstetrical and reproductive services

See Section I.C.15. Pregnancy, Childbirth, and the Puerperium, for further instruction on the use of these codes.

Z codes for pregnancy are for use in those circumstances when none of the problems or complications included in the codes from the Obstetrics chapter exist (a routine prenatal visit or postpartum care). Codes in category Z34, Encounter for supervision of normal pregnancy, are always first listed and are not to be used with any other code from the OB chapter.

(continues)

ICD-10-CM Chapter-Specific Coding Guidelines (*continued*)

Codes in category Z3A, Weeks of gestation, may be assigned to provide additional information about the pregnancy. Category Z3A codes should not be assigned for pregnancies with abortive outcomes (categories O00–O08), elective termination of pregnancy (code Z33.2), nor for postpartum conditions, as category Z3A is not applicable to these conditions. The date of the admission should be used to determine weeks of gestation for inpatient admissions that encompass more than one gestational week.

The outcome of delivery, category Z37, should be included on all maternal delivery records. It is always a secondary code. Codes in category Z37 should not be used on the newborn record.

Z codes for family planning (contraceptive) or procreative management and counseling should be included on an obstetrical record either during the pregnancy or the postpartum stage, if applicable.

Z codes/categories for obstetrical and reproductive services are:

Z30	Encounter for contraceptive management
Z31	Encounter for procreative management
Z32.2	Encounter for childbirth instruction
Z32.3	Encounter for childcare instruction
Z33	Pregnant state
Z34	Encounter for supervision of normal pregnancy
Z36	Encounter for antenatal screening of mother
Z3A	Weeks of gestation
Z37	Outcome of delivery
Z39	Encounter for maternal postpartum care and examination
Z76.81	Expectant mother prebirth pediatrician visit

12) Newborns and infants

See Section I.C.16. Newborn (Perinatal) Guidelines, for further instruction on the use of these codes.
Newborn Z codes/categories are:

Z76.1	Encounter for health supervision and care of foundling
Z00.1-	Encounter for routine child health examination
Z38	Liveborn infants according to place of birth and type of delivery

13) Routine and administrative examinations

The Z codes allow for the description of encounters for routine examinations, such as a general check-up, or examinations for administrative purposes, such as a preemployment physical. The codes are not to be used if the examination is for diagnosis of a suspected condition or for treatment purposes. In such cases, the diagnosis code is used. During a routine exam, should a diagnosis or condition be discovered, it should be coded as an additional code. Pre-existing and chronic conditions and history codes may also be included as additional codes as long as the examination is for administrative purposes and not focused on any particular condition.

Some of the codes for routine health examinations distinguish between "with" and "without" abnormal findings. Code assignment depends on the information that is known at the time the encounter is being coded. For example, if no abnormal findings were found during the examination, but the encounter is being coded before test results are back, it is acceptable to assign the code for "without abnormal findings." When assigning a code for "with abnormal findings," additional code(s) should be assigned to identify the specific abnormal finding(s).

Preoperative examination and preprocedural laboratory examination Z codes are for use only in those situations when a patient is being cleared for a procedure or surgery and no treatment is given.

Example: Patient undergoes outpatient chest x-ray the day after routine physical examination. The patient has no signs or symptoms, and the physician orders the x-ray. Report code Z01.89 (Encounter for other specified special examinations) as the first-listed diagnosis.

The Z codes/categories for routine and administrative examinations are:

Z00	Encounter for general examination without complaint, suspected or reported diagnosis
Z01	Encounter for other special examination without complaint, suspected or reported diagnosis
Z02	Encounter for administrative examination
	Except: Z02.9, Encounter for administrative examinations, unspecified
Z32.0-	Encounter for pregnancy test

14) Miscellaneous Z codes

The miscellaneous Z codes capture a number of other health care encounters that do not fall into one of the other categories. Some of these codes identify the reason for the encounter, others are for use as additional codes that provide useful information on circumstances that may affect a patient's care and treatment.

Prophylactic organ removal

For encounters specifically for prophylactic removal of an organ (such as prophylactic removal of breasts due to a genetic susceptibility to cancer or a family history of cancer), the principal or first-listed code should be a code from category Z40, Encounter for prophylactic surgery, followed by the appropriate codes to identify the associated risk factor (such as genetic susceptibility or family history).

If the patient has a malignancy of one site and is having prophylactic removal at another site to prevent either a new primary malignancy or metastatic disease, a code for the malignancy should also be assigned in addition to a code from subcategory Z40.0, Encounter for prophylactic surgery for risk factors related to malignant neoplasms. A Z40.0 code should not be assigned if the patient is having organ removal for treatment of a malignancy, such as the removal of the testes for the treatment of prostate cancer.

Miscellaneous Z codes/categories are:

Z28	Immunization not carried out
	Except: Z28.3-, Underimmunization status
Z29	Encounter for other prophylactic measures
Z40	Encounter for prophylactic surgery
Z41	Encounter for procedures for purposes other than remedying health state
	Except: Z41.9, Encounter for procedure for purposes other than remedying health state, unspecified
Z53	Persons encountering health services for specific procedures and treatment, not carried out
Z72	Problems related to lifestyle
	N o t e : These codes should be assigned only when the documentation specifies that the patient has an associated problem.
Z73	Problems related to life management difficulty
	N o t e : These codes should be assigned only when the documentation specifies that the patient has an associated problem.

(continues)

ICD-10-CM Chapter-Specific Coding Guidelines (*continued*)

Z74   Problems related to care provider dependency
        Except: Z74.01, Bed confinement status

Z75   Problems related to medical facilities and other health care

Z76.0   Encounter for issue of repeat prescription

Z76.3   Healthy person accompanying sick person

Z76.4   Other boarder to healthcare facility

Z76.5   Malingerer [conscious simulation]

Z91.1-   Patient's noncompliance with medical treatment and regimen

Z91.A-   Caregiver's noncompliance with patient's medical treatment and regimen

Z91.83   Wandering in diseases classified elsewhere

Z91.84-   Oral health risk factors

Z91.89   Other specified personal risk factors, not elsewhere classified

See Section I.B.14. for Z55-Z65 Persons with potential health hazards related to socioeconomic and psychosocial circumstances, documentation by clinicians other than the patient's provider.

15) Nonspecific Z codes

Certain Z codes are so nonspecific, or potentially redundant with other codes in the classification, that there can be little justification for their use in the inpatient setting. Their use in the outpatient setting should be limited to those instances when there is no further documentation to permit more precise coding. Otherwise, any sign or symptom or any other reason for visit that is captured in another code should be used.

Nonspecific Z codes/categories are:

Z02.9   Encounter for administrative examinations, unspecified

Z04.9   Encounter for examination and observation for unspecified reason

Z13.9   Encounter for screening, unspecified

Z41.9   Encounter for procedure for purposes other than remedying health state, unspecified

Z52.9   Donor of unspecified organ or tissue

Z86.59   Personal history of other mental and behavioral disorders

Z88.9   Allergy status to unspecified drugs, medicaments and biological substances status

Z92.0   Personal history of contraception

16) Z codes that may only be principal/first-listed diagnosis

The following Z codes/categories may only be reported as the principal/first-listed diagnosis, except when there are multiple encounters on the same day and the medical records for the encounters are combined:

Z00   Encounter for general examination without complaint, suspected or reported diagnosis
        Except: Z00.6

Z01   Encounter for other special examination without complaint, suspected or reported diagnosis

Z02   Encounter for administrative examination

Z04   Encounter for examination and observation for other reasons

Z31.81   Encounter for male factor infertility in female patient

Z31.83   Encounter for assisted reproductive fertility procedure cycle

Z31.84	Encounter for fertility preservation procedure
Z33.2	Encounter for elective termination of pregnancy
Z34	Encounter for supervision of normal pregnancy
Z38	Liveborn infants according to place of birth and type of delivery
Z39	Encounter for maternal postpartum care and examination
Z40	Encounter for prophylactic surgery
Z42	Encounter for plastic and reconstructive surgery following medical procedure or healed injury
Z51.0	Encounter for antineoplastic radiation therapy
Z51.1-	Encounter for antineoplastic chemotherapy and immunotherapy
Z52	Donors of organs and tissues
	Except: Z52.9, Donor of unspecified organ or tissue
Z76.1	Encounter for health supervision and care of foundling
Z76.2	Encounter for health supervision and care of other healthy infant and child
Z99.12	Encounter for respirator [ventilator] dependence during power failure

17) Social Determinants of Health

Social determinants of health (SDOH) codes describing social problems, conditions, or risk factors that influence a patient's health should be assigned when this information is documented in the patient's medical record. Assign as many SDOH codes as are necessary to describe all of the social problems, conditions, or risk factors documented during the current episode of care.

Example: A patient who lives alone may suffer an acute injury temporarily impacting their ability to perform routine activities of daily living. When documented as such, this would support assignment of code Z60.2, Problems related to living alone. However, merely living alone, without documentation of a risk or unmet need for assistance at home, would not support assignment of code Z60.2.

Documentation by a clinician (or patient-reported information that is signed off by a clinician) that the patient expressed concerns with access and availability of food would support assignment of code Z59.41, Food insecurity. Similarly, medical record documentation indicating the patient is homeless would support assignment of a code from subcategory Z59.0-, Homelessness.

For social determinants of health classified to chapter 21, such as information found in categories Z55-Z65, Persons with potential health hazards related to socioeconomic and psychosocial circumstances, code assignment may be based on medical record documentation from clinicians involved in the care of the patient who are not the patient's provider since this information represents social information, rather than medical diagnoses. For example, coding professionals may utilize documentation of social information from social workers, community health workers, case managers, or nurses, if their documentation is included in the official medical record.

Patient self-reported documentation may be used to assign codes for social determinants of health, as long as the patient self-reported information is signed-off by and incorporated into the medical record by either a clinician or provider.

Social determinants of health codes are located primarily in these Z code categories:

Z55	Problems related to education and literacy
Z56	Problems related to employment and unemployment
Z57	Occupational exposure to risk factors

(continues)

ICD-10-CM Chapter-Specific Coding Guidelines (*continued*)

Z58	Problems related to physical environment
Z59	Problems related to housing and economic circumstances
Z60	Problems related to social environment
Z62	Problems related to upbringing
Z63	Other problems related to primary support group, including family circumstances
Z64	Problems related to certain psychosocial circumstances
Z65	Problems related to other psychosocial circumstances

See Section I.B.14. Documentation by Clinicians Other than the Patient's Provider.

Exercise 4.11 – Factors Influencing Health Status and Contact with Health Services

Instructions: Assign the appropriate ICD-10-CM code(s).

_____   **1.** Bone marrow donor

_____   **2.** Chemotherapy encounter for left female breast cancer

_____   **3.** Examination for summer camp

_____   **4.** Exposure to smallpox

_____   **5.** Family history of stroke

ICD-10-CM Chapter 22: Codes for Special Purposes (U00–U85)

This ICD-10-CM chapter is used for the *provisional* assignment of codes for emerging diseases and new diseases of uncertain etiology or for emergency use. The World Health Organization (WHO) is responsible for the initial assignment of the provisional codes (e.g., vaping-related disorder, COVID-19, Post COVID-19 condition, unspecified). Official chapter-specific coding guidelines about codes for special purposes are located in the appropriate ICD-10-CM chapter, such as Chapter 1: Certain Infectious and Parasitic Diseases (A00-B99), where guidance can be found about the use of code U07 (COVID-19). Because U codes are temporary, new permanent codes may be assigned by the WHO and published in a future ICD-10-CM. CMS will publish updated official coding guidelines.

Example 1: In 2016, code U06.9 was created by WHO to classify *Zika virus disease, unspecified.* Effective 2017, the ICD-10 Coordination and Maintenance Committee created new code A92.5 to classify Zika virus disease in Chapter 1 of ICD-10-CM. (Code U06.9 was deleted from ICD-10-CM 2021.)

Example 2: In 2020, category U07 (Emergency Use of U07) was established, and subcategory codes U07.0 (Vaping-related disorder) and U07.1 (COVID-19) were created. Codes U07.0 and U07.1 appeared in ICD-10-CM encoder software as of April 1, 2020. Official coding guidelines for these conditions are located in Chapter 1 of the chapter-specific coding guidelines in the *ICD-10-CM Official Guidelines for Coding and Reporting,* covered in Chapter 4 of this textbook.

Example 3: In 2021, category U09 (Post COVID-19 condition) was established, and subcategory code U09.9 (Post COVID-19 condition, unspecified) was created, and the code includes post-acute sequela of COVID-19. ICD-10-CM coding instructions below the code description state, "This code enables establishment of a link with COVID-19. This code is not to be used in cases that are still presenting with active COVID-19. However, an exception is made in cases of re-infection with COVID-19 occurring with a condition related to prior COVID-19." In addition, a list of conditions that should be reported first (if known) when code U09.9 is assigned are listed below the code description (e.g., pulmonary fibrosis, J84.10)

ICD-10-CM Chapter-Specific Coding Guidelines

Chapter 22: Codes for Special Purposes (U00–U85)

U07.0	Vaping-related disorder *(see Section I.C.10.e., Vaping-related disorders)*
U07.1	COVID-19 *(see Section I.C.1.g.1., COVID-19 infection)*
U09.9	Post COVID-19 condition, unspecified *(see Section I.C.1.g.1.m.)*

Courtesy of the Centers for Medicare & Medicaid Services. www.cms.gov.

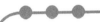

Exercise 4.12 Coding for Special Purposes

Instructions: Enter a response for each statement.

1. The international organization that initially creates codes to classify emerging diseases is called the _____.

2. The U.S. organization that creates new codes to classify emerging diseases (e.g., COVID-19) is called the _____.

3. Official coding guidelines about codes created for coding for special purposes, such as COVID-19, are located in the appropriate ICD-10-CM _____.

4. In 2020, category U07 (Emergency Use of U07) was created, and subcategory code _____ classifies COVID-19.

5. In 2021, category U09 (Post COVID-19 condition) was created, and subcategory code _____ classifies Post COVID-19 condition, unspecified.

Summary

Chapter-specific coding guidelines clarify the assignment of ICD-10-CM disease codes. Unless otherwise indicated in an individual chapter-specific guideline, the ICD-10-CM chapter-specific guidelines apply to all health care settings.

Internet Links

ICD-10-CM Official Guidelines for Coding and Reporting: Go to **cms.gov**, click on Medicare, click on Coding & billing, and click on ICD-10 codes.

MedLine Plus Interactive Tutorials (for diseases and procedures): Go to **www.nlm.nih.gov**. Click on the Site Map, and scroll to Videos & Tools where health videos, health check tools, and games can be selected.

Review

4.1 – Multiple Choice

Instructions: Select the most appropriate response.

1. Patient admitted for ligation of vas deferens sterilization procedure.
   - **a.** Z30.2
   - **b.** Z31.0
   - **c.** Z31.42
   - **d.** Z31.89

2. Diverticulitis of the colon with hemorrhage.
   - **a.** K57.20
   - **b.** K57.21
   - **c.** K57.32
   - **d.** K57.33

3. Acute prostatitis due to streptococci.
   - **a.** N41.0
   - **b.** N41.0, A40.9
   - **c.** N41.0, B95.5
   - **d.** N41.0, Z22.338

4. Spontaneous delivery of full-term pregnancy (single liveborn).
   - **a.** O80, Z37.0
   - **b.** O82, Z37.0
   - **c.** Z34.00, Z37.0
   - **d.** Z34.90, Z38.00

5. Hard corn of right little toe.
   - **a.** L84
   - **b.** M20.5X1
   - **c.** M20.61
   - **d.** M21.271

6. Herniated cervical intervertebral disc. No evidence of myelopathy.
   - **a.** M50.00
   - **b.** M50.10
   - **c.** M50.20
   - **d.** M50.30

7. Congenital partial dislocation of the right hip.
   - **a.** Q65.01
   - **b.** Q65.2
   - **c.** Q65.31
   - **d.** Q65.5

8. Liveborn infant, born in taxi cab, and then admitted for evaluation. Newborn discharged in excellent condition after treatment of transitory tachypnea.
   - **a.** Z38.00, P22.1
   - **b.** Z38.01, P22.1
   - **c.** Z38.1, P22.1
   - **d.** Z38.2, P22.1

9. Abnormal mammogram.
   - **a.** R92.0
   - **b.** R92.1
   - **c.** R92.2
   - **d.** R92.8

10. First- and second-degree burns of right forearm, initial encounter.
    - **a.** T22.019A, T31.0
    - **b.** T22.011A, T31.0
    - **c.** T22.111A, T22.211A, T31.0
    - **d.** T22.211A, T31.0

11. Chronic kidney disease (CKD) with end-stage renal disease (ESRD) admitted for renal dialysis.
    - **a.** N18.4, Z99.2
    - **b.** N18.4, N18.6, Z99.2
    - **c.** N18.5, Z99.2
    - **d.** N18.6, Z99.2

12. Family history of sudden cardiac death (SCD).
    - **a.** Z82.41
    - **b.** Z82.49
    - **c.** Z86.74
    - **d.** Z87.898

13. Which code is reported for COVID-19?
    - **a.** U07.1
    - **b.** U09.9
    - **c.** Z11.52
    - **d.** Z20.882

14. Patient injured while swimming. Select the activity code.
    - **a.** Y92.016
    - **b.** Y92.026
    - **c.** Y93.11
    - **d.** Y93.14

15. Patient fell while at a bank. Select the place of occurrence code.
    - **a.** Y92.214
    - **b.** Y92.510
    - **c.** Y92.513
    - **d.** Y92.61

4.2 – Coding Practice: Diseases

Instructions: Assign the appropriate ICD-10-CM code(s) to each disease, injury, or reason for treatment.

1. Fitting of cardiac pacemaker _____

2. Grey syndrome as adverse reaction to chloramphenicol administration in newborn as prescribed (initial encounter) _____

3. Injury by shotgun, undetermined whether accidental or intentional (shooting) (initial encounter) _____

4. Irritable bowel syndrome _____

5. Medial dislocation of right tibia, proximal end (initial encounter) _____

6. Motor vehicle traffic accident involving a collision with a pedestrian (initial encounter) _____

7. Nausea with vomiting _____

8. Personal history of penicillin allergy _____

9. Pauciarticular juvenile rheumatoid arthritis, right shoulder _____

10. Polycystic kidney, autosomal recessive _____

11. Complete spontaneous abortion, complicated by excessive hemorrhage _____

12. Preterm labor with preterm delivery of liveborn twins, third trimester _____

13. Uterine prolapse, first degree _____

14. Staphylococcal scalded skin syndrome _____

15. Infective myositis, right shoulder, *Streptococcus* _____

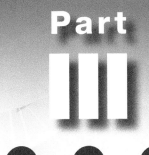

Part III

ICD-10-CM Outpatient and Physician Office Coding

ICD-10-CM Outpatient and Physician Office Coding

Chapter Outline

Outpatient Care

Outpatient Diagnostic Coding and Reporting Guidelines

Chapter Objectives

At the conclusion of this chapter, the student should be able to:

1. Define key terms related to ICD-10-CM outpatient and physician office coding.
2. Explain the differences among outpatient and physician office health care settings.
3. Assign ICD-10-CM diagnosis codes according to outpatient coding and reporting guidelines.

Key Terms

ambulatory care

ambulatory patient

ambulatory surgery patient

clinic outpatient

Data Elements for Emergency Department Systems (DEEDS)

Diagnostic Coding and Reporting Guidelines for Outpatient Services

emergency patient

first-listed diagnosis

inconclusive diagnosis

observation patient

Outcome and Assessment Information Set (OASIS)

outpatient

outpatient care

preadmission testing (PAT)

primary care

primary care provider (PCP)

qualified diagnosis

referred outpatient

triage

Uniform Ambulatory Care Data Set (UACDS)

Introduction

This chapter defines outpatient care settings and interprets the *Diagnostic Coding and Reporting Guidelines for Outpatient Services*, published in the Centers for Medicare and Medicaid Services (CMS) *ICD-10-CM Official Guidelines for Coding and Reporting*.

It is important to remember that coding guidelines are to be used as a companion to the official version of the *International Classification of Diseases, Tenth Revision, Clinical Modification* (ICD-10-CM), which contains coding conventions and instructions to ensure accurate coding.

ICD-10-CM codes are assigned to outpatient and physician office diagnoses for health care financial planning, reimbursement, and statistical purposes. (Outpatient reimbursement systems are discussed in Chapter 20 after students have learned how to assign HCPCS Level II and CPT codes to procedures and services.) Patient demographic data and codes are reported to third-party payers on the CMS-1500 claim to generate reimbursement.

 NOTE:

Outpatient health care settings, such as home health care and hospice, use the UB-04 claim instead of the CMS-1500 claim.

Coders review patient records to locate conditions and diseases to which ICD-10-CM codes are assigned. Coders also assign HCPCS Level II and CPT codes to procedures and services (discussed in Chapters 8–19). Similar to the inpatient coding process, outpatient coders may not assign codes to conditions and diseases when the provider does not specifically document the diagnoses or procedures/services. Such *assumption coding* is considered fraud, and the coder should query the physician to determine whether the documented diagnosis should be edited so a more specific code can be assigned. (Refer to Chapter 1 for more information about the physician query process.)

 NOTE:

The **Uniform Ambulatory Care Data Set (UACDS)** was established by the federal government as a standard data set for ambulatory care facility records. Its goal is to improve data comparison for ambulatory and outpatient care settings.

Home health agencies (HHAs) report data according to the **Outcome and Assessment Information Set (OASIS)**, which is a core set of comprehensive assessments for adult home care patients that is used to

* Measure patient outcomes for Outcome-Based Quality Improvement (OBQI)
* Conduct patient assessment, patient care planning, and internal HHA performance improvements
* Generate agency-level case mix reports that contain aggregate statistics about various patient characteristics such as demographic, health, or functional status at start of care

HHAs use Home Assessment and Validation and Entry (HAVEN) data entry software to report OASIS data.

Hospital-based emergency departments report **Data Elements for Emergency Department Systems (DEEDS)** for uniform collection of data to reduce incompatibility in emergency department records.

Outpatient Care

Outpatient care (or **ambulatory care**) includes any health care service provided to a patient who is not admitted as an inpatient to a facility. Such care may be provided in a physician's office, a stand-alone health care facility, a hospital outpatient or emergency department (ED), or the patient's home. Regardless of health care setting, official coding guidelines classify all of these visits as *encounters*. Claims submitted to third-party payers for encounters contain diagnosis and procedure/service codes. When a payer conducts a record review and requests clarification about documented diagnoses and procedures/services, the health care provider is the individual authorized to clarify diagnoses and procedures/services. (Coders edit submitted codes when payers deny claims due to incomplete or inaccurate coding.)

Primary Care Services

Primary care includes both preventive and acute care services, which are often provided as outpatient care and are referred to as the *point of first contact*. Services are usually provided by a general practitioner or another health professional (e.g., nurse practitioner) who has first contact with a patient seeking medical treatment, including general dental, ophthalmic, and pharmaceutical services. These services are usually provided in an office setting where the care is continuous (e.g., quarterly office visits for a chronic condition) and comprehensive (e.g., preventive and medical care). The **primary care provider (PCP)** manages and coordinates the patient's care, including referring the patient to a medical specialist (Table 5-1) for consultation and a second opinion. Primary care services include the following:

- Annual physical examinations
- Early detection of disease
- Family planning
- Health education

- Immunizations
- Treatment of minor illnesses and injuries
- Vision and hearing screening

Hospital Outpatient Services

Hospital outpatients include ambulatory patients, ambulatory surgery patients, emergency patients, and observation care patients. The maximum length of stay of an outpatient is 23 hours, 59 minutes, and 59 seconds. **Ambulatory patients** (or **outpatients**) are treated and usually released the same day and do not stay overnight in the hospital. **Ambulatory surgery patients** undergo certain procedures that can be performed on an outpatient basis, with the patient treated and released the same day. An ambulatory surgery patient who requires a longer stay must be admitted to the facility as an inpatient. **Emergency patients** are treated for urgent problems (e.g., trauma) and are either released the same day or admitted to the hospital as inpatients. **Observation patients** receive services furnished on a hospital's premises that are ordered by a physician (or another authorized individual), including use of a bed and periodic monitoring by nursing or other staff, and that are reasonable and necessary to evaluate the outpatient's condition or determine the need for possible admission as an inpatient.

Outpatient care allows patients to receive care in one day without the need for inpatient hospitalization. Care is provided in a freestanding center or facility (Table 5-2), hospital-based department or program (Table 5-3), or hospital-owned facility (Table 5-4)

TABLE 5-1 Medical Specialties

Medical Specialty	Description
Allergy & Immunology	Evaluation and treatment of immune system disorders (e.g., asthma, anaphylaxis, eczema, rhinitis, and adverse reactions to drugs/foods/insect stings)
Anesthesiology	Assessment of patient risks for undergoing surgery, management of pain relief, monitoring of patients during and after surgery (postanesthesia recovery), and resuscitative care of patients with cardiac or respiratory emergencies (assessment of need for artificial ventilation)
Colon & Rectal Surgery	Diagnosis and medical/surgical treatment of diseases in the intestinal tract, colon, rectum, anal canal, perianal region, and related organs and tissues (e.g., liver)
Dermatology	Diagnosis and treatment of skin disorders (e.g., contact dermatitis and benign and malignant lesions, or growths) and cosmetic disorders of the skin (e.g., scars)
Family Practice	Management of an individual's or family's total health care, including geriatrics, gynecology, internal medicine, obstetrics, pediatrics, and psychiatry, with an emphasis on preventive and primary care

TABLE 5-1 *(continued)*

Medical Specialty	Description
General Surgery	Management of conditions for which general surgery is warranted (e.g., appendectomy, tonsillectomy, and hernia repair), including diagnosis and preoperative, intraoperative, and postoperative care to surgical patients
Gynecology	Diagnosis and treatment (includes preventive management) of female reproductive and urinary system disorders
Internal Medicine	Management of common and complex illnesses of patients of all ages (e.g., cancer; infections; and diseases of blood, digestive system, heart, joints, kidneys, and respiratory and vascular systems). Primary care internal medicine includes disease prevention, mental health, substance abuse, and wellness. Subspecialties include the following: • Adolescent medicine • Cardiovascular medicine • Critical care medicine • Electrophysiology • Endocrinology • Gastroenterology • Geriatrics • Hematology • Immunology • Infectious disease • Nephrology • Oncology • Pulmonary medicine • Rheumatology • Sports medicine
Medical Genetics	Diagnosis and treatment of patients with genetically linked diseases
Neurology	Diagnosis and treatment of disorders of the nervous system
Obstetrics	Management of pregnancy, from prenatal to puerperium
Ophthalmology	Diagnosis and treatment of eye disorders
Orthopedics	Diagnosis and treatment of musculoskeletal disease and injury
Otorhinolaryngology	Diagnosis and treatment of ear, nose, and throat diseases
Plastic & Reconstructive Surgery	Surgery for the purpose of reconstructing, repairing, or restoring body structures
Psychiatry	Diagnosis and treatment of behavioral health diseases
Radiology	Diagnosis of diseases and injuries, using radiological methods (e.g., electromagnetic radiation, x-ray, radionuclides, and ultrasound). Treatment of diseases (e.g., cancer), using radiant energy (e.g., radiation oncologist)
Thoracic Surgery	Surgical management of disease within the chest (e.g., coronary artery disease and lung cancer)
Urology	Diagnosis and treatment of disorders of the genitourinary system and the adrenal gland

TABLE 5-2 Freestanding Centers and Facilities

Type of Center/ Facility	Characteristics
Ambulatory surgery center	• Surgery is performed on an outpatient basis. • Patients arrive on the day of procedure, undergo surgery in an operating room, and recover under the care of nursing staff.
Cardiovascular center	• Provides ambulatory cardiovascular services to include diagnosis and treatment, disease prevention, research, education, and cardiac rehabilitation. • Diagnostic and treatment services include cardiac catheterization, Coumadin care, echocardiography, enhanced external counterpulsation (EECP), heart scans, pacemaker care, and percutaneous transluminal coronary angioplasty (PTCA).

(continues)

TABLE 5-2 *(continued)*

Type of Center/Facility	Characteristics
Clinical laboratory	• Performs diagnostic testing in microbiology, clinical chemistry, and toxicology, which are ordered by physicians on samples of body fluids, tissues, and wastes. • Information obtained from tests helps physicians diagnose illness, monitor treatment, and check general health. Results from tests are reported to physicians, who interpret them and explain them to patients. • Directed by a pathologist; testing is performed by certified professional technologists and technicians.
Imaging center	• Provides radiographic (e.g., x-rays) and other imaging services (e.g., magnetic resonance imaging) to ambulatory patients. • May also provide training and participate in national research projects.
Industrial health clinic	• Located in a business setting (e.g., factory). • Emphasis is on employee health and safety.
Infusion center	• Dispenses and administers prescribed medications by continuous or intermittent infusion to ambulatory patients. • Infusion is supervised by a licensed health care professional (e.g., registered nurse). • Also called ambulatory infusion centers (AICs).
Neighborhood health center	• Health care is provided to economically disadvantaged and treatment is family-centered because illnesses may result indirectly from crowded living conditions, unsanitary facilities, and other socioeconomic factors. • Family care team consisting of a physician, nurse, and social worker provides continuity of care to families.
Pain management center	• Specializes in treatment of acute and chronic pain syndromes, using proven medications and procedures. • Usually uses a multidisciplinary approach involving participating specialists such as physiatrists, psychiatrists, neurologists, neurosurgeons, internists, and physical and occupational therapists.
Physician's office	• Solo physicians' practices do not have physician partners or employment affiliations with other practice organizations. • Single-specialty group physician practices consist of two or more physicians who provide patients with one specific type of care (e.g., primary care). • Multispecialty group physician practices offer various types of medical specialty care in one organization, and they may be located in more than one location.
Primary care center	• Offers adult and family care medicine in internal medicine, pediatrics, and family practice. • Internal medicine physicians specialize in the care of adults. • Pediatricians provide comprehensive services for infants, children, and adolescents. • Family practitioners provide care for the entire family and focus on general medicine, obstetrics, pediatrics, and geriatrics.
Public health department	• Provides preventive medicine services such as well-baby clinics. • Care includes immunizations and routine checkups.

Radiology center	• Provides image-guided procedures, as follows:
	  ○ Computed tomography (CT scan), in which the source of x-ray beams rotates around the patient, the beams are detected by sensors, and information from sensors is computer-processed and displayed as an image on a video screen.
	  ○ Magnetic resonance imaging (MRI), which uses a large magnet that surrounds the patient, along with radiowaves and a computer, to produce images.
	  ○ Mammography, which is a method for detecting early-stage breast abnormalities.
	  ○ Nuclear medicine, which uses very small amounts of radioactive materials or radiopharmaceuticals to study organ function and structure and to treat disease. (Radiopharmaceuticals are substances that are attracted to specific organs, bones, or tissues.)

TABLE 5-2 *(continued)*

Type of Center/ Facility	Characteristics
	○ Positron emission tomography (PET), which measures radioactive tracers (e.g., radioactive glucose) injected into the body.
	○ Radiography (x-ray), which detects disease or injury in the body when an image (x-ray film) is produced as the result of passing a small amount of radiation through the body to expose sensitive film on the other side.
	○ Ultrasonography, which uses high-frequency sound waves to study parts of the body, including the heart and vessels, to generate an image of the area being studied.
	• Directed by a radiologist and staffed by registered x-ray technicians.
Rehabilitation facility	• Provides occupational, physical, and speech therapy to patients with orthopedic injuries, work-related injuries, sports-related injuries, and various neurologic and neuromuscular conditions.
	• Occupational therapy provides services to patients who have experienced loss of function resulting from injury or disease. Physical therapy uses physical agents of exercise, massage, and other modalities. Speech/language pathology provides services to evaluate, diagnose, plan, and provide therapy to patients with speech, language, and swallowing difficulties.
Staff model health maintenance organization (HMO)	• Similar to large, multispecialty group practices.
	• May be partially owned by physician employees, with the physicians typically functioning as employees of either the physician group owning the practice or the insurer.
	• Most physicians are paid a salary.
Student health center	• Provides health care to full- and part-time students who become ill or injured.
	• Services usually include allergy injections, contraception and counseling, health education, immunizations, HIV testing, laboratory services, routine medications, primary care and preventive medicine, screening for sexually transmitted diseases (STDs), smoking cessation, and women's health care.
Urgent care center (or emergency care center)	• Immediate care is provided by an on-duty physician (usually salaried).
	• May be owned by private corporations (e.g., Humana) in states where they are permitted or by nonprofit facilities (e.g., municipal hospital).

TABLE 5-3 Hospital-Based Departments and Programs

Type of Department/ Program	Characteristics
Ambulatory surgery	• Elective surgery is performed on patients who are admitted and discharged the same day (e.g., biopsy); both general and local anesthesia are administered.
	• Also called short-stay or day surgery
	• Patients undergo **preadmission testing (PAT)** prior to registering for ambulatory surgery, undergoing a preoperative nursing assessment, and receiving preanesthesia evaluation by an anesthesiologist. As part of PAT, phlebotomists draw blood samples for preoperative testing and electrocardiograms and chest x-rays are performed if ordered. PAT results are documented in the patient's record and are available to the patient care team prior to the patient's surgery.
Emergency department	• Crisis care is provided 24 hours per day by an on-duty physician to patients who have sustained trauma or have urgent problems (e.g., heart attack).
	• Patients initially undergo **triage**, which is an organized method of identifying and treating patients according to urgency of care required.
Outpatient department	• **Clinic outpatients** receive scheduled diagnostic and therapeutic care (e.g., chemotherapy, kidney dialysis).
	• **Referred outpatients** receive diagnostic (e.g., laboratory tests) or therapeutic care (e.g., physical therapy) because such care is unavailable in the primary care provider's office; follow-up is done at the primary care provider's office.

(continues)

TABLE 5-3 *(continued)*

Type of Department/ Program	Characteristics
Partial hospitalization program	• Program for hospital patients who regularly use the hospital facilities for a substantial number of daytime or nighttime hours (e.g., behavioral health, geriatric, and rehabilitative care).

TABLE 5-4 Hospital-Owned Facilities

Facility	Characteristics
Hospital-owned physician practice	• Hospital-owned practices are at least partially owned by the hospital. • Physicians participate in a compensation plan provided by the hospital.
Satellite clinics	• Ambulatory care centers that are established remotely from the hospital. • Primary care is provided by an on-duty physician (usually salaried).

Exercise 5.1 – Outpatient Care

Instructions: Complete each statement.

1. Care provided in a physician's office, a stand-alone health care facility, a hospital outpatient or emergency department, or the patient's home is classified as _____ or outpatient care.

2. Preventive and acute care is often provided on an outpatient basis, is referred to as the point of first contact, and is categorized as _____ care.

3. The primary care provider manages and coordinates patient care, and provides _____ to a medical specialist for consultation and a second opinion.

4. Patients treated and released the same day and who do not stay overnight in the hospital are called ambulatory patients or _____.

5. Patients who undergo certain procedures that can be performed on an outpatient basis, with the patient treated and released the same day, are called ambulatory _____ patients or outpatients.

6. Patients who are treated for urgent problems (e.g., trauma) and are either released the same day or admitted to the hospital as inpatients are called _____ department (ED) patients.

7. Patients who receive services furnished on a hospital's premises as ordered by a physician, including use of a bed and periodic monitoring by nursing or other staff, and that are reasonable and necessary to evaluate the outpatients' conditions or determine the need for possible admission as inpatients (and who are in the unit no longer than 23 hours, 59 minutes, and 59 seconds), are called _____ patients.

8. An organized method of identifying and treating patients according to urgency of care required is called _____.

9. Patients who receive scheduled diagnostic and therapeutic care are called _____ outpatients.

10. Patients who receive diagnostic or therapeutic care because such care is unavailable in the primary care provider's office are called _____ outpatients.

Outpatient Diagnostic Coding and Reporting Guidelines

The *Diagnostic Coding and Reporting Guidelines for Outpatient Services* were developed by CMS and approved for use by hospitals and providers for coding and reporting hospital-based outpatient services and provider-based office visits. Although the guidelines were originally developed for use in submitting government program claims, health insurance companies have also adopted them (sometimes with variation).

 NOTE:

Because variations may contradict official coding guidelines, review health insurance company's coding guidelines when employed.

Selection of First-Listed Condition

In the outpatient setting, the **first-listed diagnosis** is reported (instead of the inpatient setting's *principal diagnosis*); it is the diagnosis, condition, problem, or other reason for encounter/visit documented in the patient record to be chiefly responsible for the services provided. It is determined in accordance with ICD-10-CM *coding conventions* (or rules) as well as general and disease-specific coding guidelines. It reflects the reason for the encounter, which often is a sign or symptom. Because diagnoses are often not established at the time of the patient's initial encounter or visit, two or more visits may be required before a diagnosis is confirmed.

 NOTE:

When reviewing the coding guidelines, the terms *encounter* and *visit* are used interchangeably in coding guidelines when describing outpatient and physician office services.

Coding guidelines for inconclusive or qualified diagnoses (e.g., probable, suspected, rule out) were developed for inpatient reporting only; they do not apply to outpatients.

An outpatient is a person treated in one of four settings.

- *Ambulatory surgery center*: Patient is released prior to a 24-hour stay and length of stay must be 23 hours, 59 minutes, and 59 seconds or less
- *Health care provider's office* (e.g., physician's office)
- *Hospital clinic, emergency department, outpatient department, same-day surgery unit*: Length of stay must be 23 hours, 59 minutes, and 59 seconds or less
- *Hospital observation status or hospital observation unit*: Patient's length of stay is 23 hours, 59 minutes, and 59 seconds or less unless documentation for additional observation is medically justified

 NOTE:

- *Outpatient Surgery*: When a patient presents for outpatient surgery, code the reason for the surgery as the first-listed diagnosis (reason for the encounter) even if the surgery is canceled due to a contraindication (e.g., patient's blood pressure increases unexpectedly upon administration of anesthesia).
- *Observation Stay*: When a patient is admitted for observation for a medical condition, assign a code for the medical condition as the first-listed diagnosis.

When a patient presents for outpatient surgery and develops complications requiring admission to observation, code the reason for the surgery as the first-listed diagnosis (reason for the encounter) followed by codes for the complications (e.g., respiratory distress) as secondary diagnoses.

Example: A patient underwent outpatient laparoscopic cholecystectomy for acute cholecystitis. During recovery from surgery, the patient's temperature spiked at 101 degrees, and patient was admitted for observation care and administered intravenous antibiotics. Wound culture grew *Escherichia coli* (*E. coli*). The first-listed diagnosis is acute cholecystitis (K81.0), and the secondary diagnosis is postoperative infection of superficial incisional surgical site (T81.41XA) due to *E. coli* (B96.20), which is a complication of surgery.

Example 1: The patient was seen in the physician's office with a complaint of chest pain over the past few days. Patient explained that when lying in bed is when they really notice the pain, especially if they snacked later at night. EKG was negative. Cardiac enzyme lab test and chest x-ray were ordered. The physician suspects gastroesophageal reflux disease. The first-listed ICD-10-CM code reported for this case is chest pain (R07.9).

The patient returned to the physician's office for follow-up on the complaint of chest pain and was told cardiac enzyme lab test and chest x-ray were negative. The physician documented gastroesophageal reflux disease (GERD) as the patient's diagnosis. The first-listed ICD-10-CM code reported for this case is GERD (K21.9).

Example 2: A patient received ED care for an injury to the right arm, which upon x-ray revealed closed displaced oblique fracture of the shaft of the right humerus (S42.331A). While receiving treatment for the fracture, the physician also medically managed the patient's chronic obstructive asthma (J44.9).

The first-listed diagnosis code is S42.331A and the secondary diagnosis code is J44.9.

Codes from A00.0–T88.9, Z00–Z99, U00–U85

The appropriate code or codes from the ICD-10-CM Tabular List of Diseases (A00.0–T88.9, Z00–Z99, U00–U85) must be used to identify diagnoses, symptoms, conditions, problems, complaints, or other reason(s) for the encounter/visit.

Accurate Reporting of ICD-10-CM Diagnosis Codes

For accurate reporting of ICD-10-CM diagnosis codes, the documentation should describe the patient's condition, using terminology that includes specific diagnoses as well as symptoms, problems, or reasons for the encounter. There are ICD-10-CM codes to describe all of these.

Codes That Describe Signs and Symptoms

Codes that describe signs and symptoms, as opposed to definitive diagnoses, are acceptable for reporting purposes when a diagnosis has not been established (confirmed) by the provider.

In ICD-10-CM, Chapter 18 (Symptoms, Signs, and Abnormal Clinical and Laboratory Findings Not Elsewhere Classified) (R00–R99) contains many, but not all, codes for symptoms.

Some signs and symptoms codes are located in other ICD-10-CM chapters, which can be found by properly using the ICD-10-CM Index to Diseases and Injuries.

Example: A 52-year-old patient presents with feeling flushed off and on, headaches, difficulty falling asleep and remaining asleep, and some confusion. Last menstruation was eight months ago. The physician's diagnosis is symptomatic menopause (N95.1), which contains a "use additional code" directing the coder to also assign codes for associated symptoms, in this case feeling flushed (R23.2), headaches (R51.9), sleeplessness (G47.01), and confusion (R41.0).

Encounters for Circumstances Other Than a Disease or Injury

ICD-10-CM provides codes to deal with encounters for circumstances other than a disease or an injury.

Factors Influencing Health Status and Contact with Health Services (Z00–Z99) are provided so that codes can be assigned for occasions when circumstances other than a disease or injury are documented as diagnoses or problems. (Additional guidance about factors influencing health status and contact with health services is located in Chapter 4.)

Example: A patient is seen in the office due to concerns about exposure to someone who was diagnosed with the Zika virus. The physician determines that the patient presents no signs or symptoms of the Zika virus. ICD-10-CM code Z20.821, Contact with and (suspected) exposure to Zika virus, is reported as the first-listed diagnosis.

Level of Detail in Coding

ICD-10-CM diagnosis codes contain 3, 4, 5, 6, or 7 characters.

1. *ICD-10-CM codes with 3, 4, 5, 6, or 7 characters*: Disease codes with three characters are included in ICD-10-CM as the heading of a category of codes that may be further subdivided by the use of fourth, fifth, sixth, or seventh characters to provide greater specificity.

2. *Use of full number of characters required for a code*: A three-character code is to be assigned only if it cannot be further subdivided. A code is invalid if it has not been coded to the full number of characters required for that code, including the seventh character extension, if applicable (with appropriate use of placeholder X).

3. *Highest level of specificity*: Code to the highest level of specificity when supported by the medical record documentation.

> **Example:** A patient was diagnosed with a crushing injury of the skull (initial encounter). ICD-10-CM category S07 (Crushing injury of head) and subcategory code S07.1 requires "X" placeholders to be entered in front of seventh-character A to report a valid code, S07.1XXA.
>
> **S07 Crushing injury of head**
> > **Use additional** code for all associated injuries, such as:
> > > intracranial injuries (S06.-)
> > >
> > > skull fractures (S02.-)
> >
> > The appropriate 7th character is to be added to each code from category S07
> > > A initial encounter
> > >
> > > D subsequent encounter
> > >
> > > S sequela
> >
> > **S07.0 Crushing injury of face**
> > **S07.1 Crushing injury of skull**
> > **S07.8 Crushing injury of other parts of head**
> > **S07.9 Crushing injury of head, part unspecified**

ICD-10-CM Code for the Diagnosis, Condition, Problem, or Other Reason for Encounter/Visit

Report first the ICD-10-CM code for the diagnosis, condition, problem, or other reason for encounter documented in the patient record as chiefly responsible for the services provided. Then report additional codes that describe any coexisting conditions treated or medically managed or that influenced the treatment of the patient during the encounter, which are called comorbidities. In some cases, the first-listed diagnosis may be a sign or symptom when a diagnosis has not been established (confirmed) by the provider.

> **Example:** During a physician's office encounter, the patient's severe headaches were evaluated. The patient explained that the onset of the headaches was sudden, and they could be due to stress. Patient had recently changed jobs. The patient's hypertension was also medically managed during the encounter. The first-listed ICD-10-CM code is R51.9 (headache), and I10 (hypertension) is reported as a secondary code.

Uncertain Diagnoses

For outpatient and physician office encounters, do *not* code diagnoses documented as probable, suspected, questionable, rule out, or working diagnosis, compatible with, consistent with, or other similar terms indicating uncertainty, all of which are considered **inconclusive diagnoses** or **qualified diagnoses**. Instead, code condition(s) to the highest degree of certainty for that outpatient encounter, such as symptoms, signs, abnormal test results, or other reasons for the encounter.

NOTE:

According to *ICD-10-CM Official Guidelines for Coding and Reporting*, short-term, acute care, long-term, and psychiatric hospitals assign ICD-10-CM codes to uncertain diagnoses for inpatient admissions. Codes for signs and symptoms are also reported for inpatient admissions when relevant, such as for comparative diagnoses.

Example: During the first half of 2021 before the COVID-19 diagnosis was confirmed, some inpatient hospital records documented final diagnoses of "influenza versus viral pneumonia" and the patient's signs and symptoms, all of which were assigned ICD-10-CM codes. The uncertain diagnosis was documented because patients presented with severe signs and symptoms that were beyond the scope of those associated with typical influenza and viral pneumonia inpatient cases. Reporting uncertain (or qualified) diagnosis codes with signs/symptoms codes facilitated the research of a severe (and often fatal) illness that was later determined to be COVID-19.

Example:

For Qualified Diagnosis:	Code the Following Documented Sign or Symptom:
Suspected pneumonia	Shortness of breath, wheezing
Questionable Raynaud's	Numbness of hands
Possible wrist fracture	Wrist pain and swelling
Rule out pneumonia	Chest pain and fever

Uncertain diagnoses are a necessary part of the hospital and office chart until a specific diagnosis can be determined. Although uncertain diagnoses are routinely coded for hospital inpatient admissions and reported on the UB-04 claim, CMS *specifically prohibits the reporting of uncertain diagnoses on the CMS-1500 claim submitted for outpatient care*. CMS regulations permit the reporting of patients' signs and/or symptoms instead of the qualified diagnoses.

An additional incentive for not coding uncertain diagnoses resulted from the Missouri case of *Stafford v. Neurological Medicine Inc.*, 811 F. 2d 470 (8th Cir., 1987). In this case, the diagnosis stated in the physician's office chart was *rule out brain tumor*. The claim submitted by the office listed the diagnosis code for *rule out brain tumor*, although test results were available that proved a brain tumor did not exist. The physician assured the patient that although there was a diagnosis of lung cancer, there was no metastasis to the brain. Some time after the insurance company received the provider's claim, it was inadvertently sent to the patient. When the patient received the claim, she was so devastated by the diagnosis that she took her own life. The spouse sued and was awarded $200,000 on the basis of *negligent paperwork* because the physician's office had reported a *qualified or uncertain diagnosis*.

Chronic Diseases

Chronic diseases treated on an ongoing basis may be coded and reported as many times as the patient receives treatment and care for the condition(s).

Example: The patient is seen for a physician office encounter, which is a six-month follow-up encounter for hypertension and diabetes mellitus. Examination is negative, and the patient states they feel well. Blood pressure is 120/75 and blood glucose is 95. Because hypertension (I10) and diabetes mellitus (E11.9) are chronic conditions, a code for each condition is reported for this encounter (even though the patient's blood pressure and glucose level are normal).

Code All Documented Conditions That Coexist

Code all documented conditions that coexist at the time of the encounter/visit and that require or affect patient care, treatment, or management. Do not code conditions that were previously treated and no longer exist. However, history codes ICD-10-CM categories Z80–Z87 may be reported as secondary codes if the historical condition or family history has an impact on current care or influences treatment.

Example: The patient was seen for an outpatient encounter in follow-up for acute bronchitis due to rhinovirus. Past history of chronic asthma has resolved. Report acute bronchitis (J20.6) as the first-listed diagnosis and personal history of chronic asthma (Z87.09) as the secondary diagnosis.

 NOTE:

Third-party payers review claims for "family history of" codes to determine reimbursement eligibility. Some plans reimburse for conditions that may not normally be eligible for payment when family history of a related condition is documented in the patient's record and reported on the claim.

Patients Receiving Diagnostic Services Only

For patients receiving *diagnostic services only* during an encounter, report first the diagnosis, condition, problem, or other reason for encounter that is documented as being chiefly responsible for the outpatient services provided during the encounter. (This is the *first-listed diagnosis*.) Codes for other diagnoses (e.g., chronic conditions) may be reported as additional diagnoses.

For encounters for routine laboratory/radiology testing in the absence of any signs, symptoms, or associated diagnosis, assign Z01.89 (Encounter for other specified special examinations). If routine testing is performed during the same encounter as a non-routine test to evaluate a sign, symptom, or diagnosis, it is appropriate to assign both the Z code and the code describing the reason for the nonroutine test.

For outpatient encounters for diagnostic tests that have been interpreted by a physician and for which the final report is available at the time of coding, code any confirmed or definitive diagnoses documented in the interpretation. *Do not code related signs and symptoms as additional diagnoses.*

Example: A patient diagnosed with probable anemia is seen in follow-up to discuss positive Ferritin laboratory test results. The physician's diagnosis is familial erythroblastic anemia (D56.1).

Patients Receiving Therapeutic Services Only

For patients receiving *therapeutic services only* during an outpatient encounter, sequence first the diagnosis, condition, problem, or other reason for encounter chiefly responsible for the outpatient services provided during the encounter.

Assign codes to other diagnoses (e.g., chronic conditions) that are treated or medically managed or that would affect the patient's receipt of therapeutic services during this encounter.

The only exception to this rule is when the reason for encounter is for chemotherapy, radiation therapy, or rehabilitation. For these services, the appropriate ICD-10-CM Z code for the service is listed first and the diagnosis or problem for which the service is being performed is reported second.

Example: The patient was diagnosed with thyroid cancer last month and today underwent the first in a series of radiation therapy treatments as an outpatient. Encounter for antineoplastic radiation therapy (Z51.0) is the first-listed diagnosis, and malignant neoplasm of thyroid gland (C73) is the secondary diagnosis.

Patients Receiving Preoperative Evaluations Only

For patients receiving *preoperative evaluations only*, assign and report first the appropriate code from ICD-10-CM subcategory Z01.81- (Encounter for preprocedural examinations) to describe the preoperative consultations.

Assign an additional code for the condition that describes the reason for the surgery. Also assign additional code(s) to any findings discovered during the preoperative evaluation.

Example: A patient scheduled for reduction mammoplasty due to massive hypertrophy of the right and left breasts underwent preoperative evaluation during today's outpatient encounter. Findings were negative, and the patient was cleared for surgery. Report codes Z01.818 (Encounter for pre-procedural examination) and N62 (Hypertrophy of breast).

NOTE:

Preadmission testing (PAT) is routinely completed prior to an inpatient admission or outpatient surgery to facilitate patient treatment and reduce length of stay. As an incentive, some payers provide higher reimbursement for PAT, making it important to assign codes properly.

Ambulatory Surgery (or Outpatient Surgery)

For *ambulatory surgery* (or *outpatient surgery*), assign a code to the diagnosis for which the surgery was performed. If the postoperative diagnosis is different from the preoperative diagnosis when the diagnosis is confirmed, assign a code to the postoperative diagnosis instead (because it is more definitive).

> **Example:** A patient diagnosed with uterine polyps and dysfunctional uterine bleeding underwent outpatient laparoscopic hysterectomy surgery. Pathology report results confirmed benign polyps and revealed adenocarcinoma, uterine endometrium. Adenocarcinoma, uterine endometrium, which is a primary malignancy (C54.1), is reported as the first-listed diagnosis, followed by polyp of corpus uteri (N84.0).

Routine Outpatient Prenatal Visits

For routine outpatient prenatal visits when no complications are present, report a code from ICD-10-CM category Z34 (Encounter for supervision of normal pregnancy) as the first-listed diagnosis. *Do not report this code in combination with ICD-10-CM Chapter 15 codes.*

For routine prenatal outpatient visits for patients with high-risk pregnancies, report an ICD-10-CM code from category O09 (supervision of high-risk pregnancy) as the first-listed diagnosis. A code from ICD-10-CM Chapter 15 may also be reported as a secondary diagnosis, if appropriate.

Encounters for General Medical Examinations with Abnormal Findings

The subcategories for encounters for general adult medical examinations (Z00.0-) and encounters for routine child health examinations (Z00.12-) provide codes for *with* and *without* abnormal findings. Should a general medical examination result in an abnormal finding, the code for general medical examination with abnormal finding should be assigned as the first-listed diagnosis. An *examination with abnormal findings* refers to a condition or diagnosis that is newly identified or a change in severity of a chronic condition (e.g., uncontrolled hypertension, acute exacerbation of COPD) during a routine physical examination. A secondary code for the abnormal finding should also be assigned.

> **Example:** During this 72-year-old patient's annual health examination, the physician noted an abnormally high blood pressure of 145/95. The blood pressure was taken again at the conclusion of the examination, and it was still abnormally high (143/97). All other findings during examination were negative. The physician prescribed Hyzaar and scheduled the patient for a follow-up office visit within one month. Encounter for general adult medical examination with abnormal findings (Z00.01) is reported as the first-listed diagnosis, and code hypertension (I10) is reported as the secondary diagnosis.

Encounters for Routine Health Screenings

Screening is the testing for disease or disease precursors in seemingly well individuals so that early detection and treatment can be provided for those who test positive for the disease (e.g., screening mammogram).

The testing of a person to rule out or confirm a suspected diagnosis because the patient has some sign or symptom is a diagnostic examination, not a screening. In these cases, the sign or symptom is used to explain the reason for the test.

A screening code may be a first-listed code if the reason for the visit is specifically the screening exam. It may also be used as an additional code if the screening is done during an office visit for other health problems. A screening code is not necessary if the screening is inherent to a routine examination, such as a Pap smear done during a routine pelvic examination.

Should a condition be discovered during the screening, the code for the condition may be assigned as an additional diagnosis.

The Z code indicates that a screening exam is planned. A procedure code is required to confirm that the screening was performed.

The screening Z codes/categories include the following:

- Z11   Encounter for screening for infectious and parasitic diseases
- Z12   Encounter for screening for malignant neoplasms
- Z13   Encounter for screening for other diseases and disorders

    Except: Z13.9, Encounter for screening, unspecified

- Z36   Encounter for antenatal screening for mother

Example: The patient undergoes screening for alcoholism during an outpatient encounter. There is a family history of chronic alcoholism on both sides of the family. Patient does not drink to excess, and clarifies that they do enjoy a glass of wine most evenings. Screening for alcoholism (Z13.39) is reported as the first-listed code, and family history of alcohol abuse and dependence (Z81.1) is reported as the secondary diagnosis.

Exercise 5.2 – Diagnostic Coding and Reporting Guidelines for Outpatient Services: Hospital-Based and Physician Office

Instructions: Select the first-listed diagnosis for each case scenario.

1. The patient underwent office treatment for the removal of a skin lesion from the face. The patient also received a renewed prescription for chronic asthma.

   a. chronic asthma

   b. skin lesion

2. The physician ordered a chest x-ray to rule out pneumonia and also documented shortness of breath in the record.

   a. rule out pneumonia

   b. shortness of breath

3. The patient fell out of a tree and sustained a fractured humerus, left, which was treated in the emergency department (ED). While in the ED, the physician noted severe swelling of the arm.

   a. fractured humerus, left

   b. swelling of the arm

4. The patient was seen in the office, complaining of severe stomach pain and vomiting. The physician diagnosed gastroenteritis.

   a. gastroenteritis

   b. stomach pain and vomiting

5. The patient was treated in the outpatient department for urinary frequency. The physician documented probable cystitis in the record.

   a. probable cystitis

   b. urinary frequency

6. The patient was treated on an outpatient basis for both acute and chronic bronchitis, for which each was assigned an ICD-10-CM diagnosis code.

   a. acute bronchitis

   b. chronic bronchitis

7. The patient was treated for back pain in the physician's office. The physician documented that the patient's previously diagnosed influenza had completely resolved.

   a. back pain

   b. influenza

(continues)

Exercise 5.2 – continued

8. The patient was seen for complaints of dizziness, shakiness, and fainting spells; blood was drawn and sent to the lab to have a blood glucose level performed. Lab results revealed a blood glucose level of 325, patient was placed on oral insulin, and the physician documented diabetes mellitus in the record.

   a. diabetes mellitus, type 2

   b. dizziness, fainting spells, and shakiness

9. The patient had an encounter for outpatient chemotherapy for the treatment of breast cancer.

   a. breast cancer

   b. encounter for outpatient chemotherapy

10. The patient's preoperative diagnosis was cholelithiasis, and a laparoscopic cholecystectomy was performed. The postoperative diagnosis was acute cholecystitis with cholelithiasis.

    a. acute cholecystitis with cholelithiasis

    b. cholelithiasis

Summary

Outpatient care includes any health care service provided to a patient who is not admitted to a facility. Such care may be provided in a physician's office, a stand-alone health care facility, a hospital outpatient or emergency department, or the patient's home. The CMS *Diagnostic Coding and Reporting Guidelines for Outpatient Services: Hospital-Based and Physician Office* were developed by the federal government and have been approved for use by hospitals and providers for coding and reporting hospital-based outpatient services and provider-based office visits. Although the guidelines were originally developed for use in submitting government claims, insurance companies have also adopted them (sometimes with variation). The CMS Coding Guidelines for Outpatient Diagnostic Tests includes instructions and examples that are to be used when assigning ICD-10-CM codes for diagnostic test results. The instructions and examples provide guidance regarding the appropriate assignment of ICD-10-CM diagnosis codes to simplify coding for diagnostic tests, consistent with the CMS *Diagnostic Coding and Reporting Guidelines for Outpatient Services: Hospital-Based and Physician Office.*

Internet Links

EncoderPro.com: **www.EncoderPro.com**

Find-A-Code: **www.findacode.com**

HCPro, Inc.: Go to **www.hcmarketplace.com**, and click on the "Sign up for our FREE e-Newsletters" link. Enter your contact information, and click on the box located in front of *JustCoding News: Outpatient* (along with other e-Newsletters that interest you) subscribe.

Medical Information Bureau (MIB): www.mib.com

National Practitioner Data Bank (NPDB) and the Healthcare Integrity and Protection Data Bank (HIPDB): www.npdb-hipdb.com

Web-based training courses (free from CMS): Go to **cms.gov**, click on Outreach & Education, click on Get Training under the Learn heading, click on CMS National Training Program, and click each type of training.

Review

5.1 — Multiple Choice

Instructions: Select the most appropriate response.

1. A patient was seen on an outpatient basis to have lab tests performed. The next day the patient underwent an outpatient procedure. Due to complications, the patient was admitted to the hospital. One week after discharge from the hospital, the patient was seen in the physician's office for a follow-up visit. Coding guidelines classify all of these visits as

   a. admissions.　　　　**b.** appointments.　　　　**c.** claims.　　　　**d.** encounters.

2. A patient's record underwent review because the outpatient diagnosis about multiple injuries was unclear. Who is authorized to clarify the diagnosis?

   a. Health care provider　　　　　　　**c.** Insurance company

   b. HIM supervisor　　　　　　　　　　**d.** Outpatient coder

3. A patient is diagnosed with osteoarthritis, and the encounter is assigned code M19.90. When referring to the ICD-10-CM index and following tabular list entries, the code assignment of M19.90 was

---

INDEX TO DISEASES

`Osteoarthritis M19.90`

TABULAR LIST OF DISEASES

`M19  Other and unspecified osteoarthritis`

　　　　EXCLUDES1 `polyarthritis (M15.-)`

　　　　EXCLUDES2 `arthrosis of spine (M47.-)`

　　　　　　　　　`hallux rigidus (M20.2)`

　　　　　　　　　`osteoarthritis of spine (M47.-)`

`    M19.9 Osteoarthritis, unspecified site`

`        M19.90 Unspecified osteoarthritis, unspecified site`

　　　　　　　　`Arthrosis NOS`

　　　　　　　　`Arthritis NOS`

　　　　　　　　`Osteoarthritis NOS`

`        M19.91 Primary osteoarthritis, unspecified site`

　　　　　　　　`Primary osteoarthritis NOS`

`        M19.92 Post-traumatic osteoarthritis, unspecified site`

　　　　　　　　`Post-traumatic osteoarthritis NOS`

`        M19.93 Secondary osteoarthritis, unspecified site`

　　　　　　　　`Secondary osteoarthritis NOS`

---

   a. correct because M19.9 is listed in the index as the code for osteoarthritis.
   b. correct because no further information was available in the patient record to assign a more specific code.
   c. invalid because upon verifying M19.90 in the tabular list, the coder should have assigned a sixth digit.
   d. incorrect because the tabular list's excludes1 note directs the coder to assign a code for polyarthritis (M15.-)

4. In ICD-10-CM, code Z85.020 (personal history of malignant carcinoid tumor of stomach) is reported as a _____ code.
   - **a.** complication
   - **b.** first-listed
   - **c.** primary
   - **d.** secondary

5. When a definitive diagnosis has not been established or confirmed by the provider, which should be reported?
   - **a.** Codes that describe symptoms and signs
   - **b.** None because code assignment must wait until a diagnosis is confirmed
   - **c.** Office visit only
   - **d.** Qualified diagnosis, such as rule out, possible, or suspected

Use these tabular list entries to answer the question that follows.

6. When referring to the ICD-10-CM index and following tabular list entries, duodenitis with bleeding (K29.81) is an example of a _____ code.

> **INDEX TO DISEASES AND INJURIES**
>
> `Duodenitis` (nonspecific) (peptic) K29.80
>   with bleeding K29.81

> **TABULAR LIST OF DISEASES AND INJURIES**
>
> `K29.8 Duodenitis`
>   `K29.80 Duodenitis without bleeding`
>   `K29.81 Duodenitis with bleeding`

   - **a.** combination
   - **b.** history
   - **c.** late effect
   - **d.** multiple

7. When a bacterial organism is documented as the cause of a condition (e.g., ear infection), it is
   - **a.** coded as either a first-listed or a secondary code.
   - **b.** coded as a first-listed diagnosis only.
   - **c.** reported as a secondary code, below the code for the condition.
   - **d.** not coded because bacterial organisms are always classified in the disease code.

8. When determining the first-listed diagnosis, the ICD-10-CM coding conventions and _____ guidelines, except the Uncertain Diagnosis guideline, take precedence over the official outpatient guidelines.
   - **a.** drugs and adverse effects
   - **b.** eponyms and procedure/surgical
   - **c.** external cause of injury and poisoning
   - **d.** general and chapter-specific

9. For accurate reporting of ICD-10-CM diagnosis codes
   - **a.** a definitive diagnosis must be documented by the physician who provides care to the patient.
   - **b.** all diagnosis and condition codes must contain seven characters.
   - **c.** A00.0 through T88.9, Z00–Z99, and U00-U85 are used to classify the encounter.
   - **d.** definitive diagnoses in addition to all signs and symptoms are classified.

10. Codes that describe symptoms and signs are acceptable for outpatient reporting purposes when the physician has documented an
    - **a.** encounter for circumstances other than disease or injury.
    - **b.** established diagnosis or confirmed condition.
    - **c.** ongoing chronic condition.
    - **d.** uncertain diagnosis.

11. An encounter is reported with codes for symptoms listed first, followed by an unrelated secondary condition code. Thus, the reason for the visit has
    a. been confirmed, and a coexisting condition was treated or medically managed during the same encounter.
    b. been confirmed, and the patient also exhibited unrelated signs and symptoms during the same encounter.
    c. not been confirmed at the time of coding, and a coexisting condition was treated or medically managed during the same encounter.
    d. not been confirmed at the time of coding, and the patient also exhibited unrelated signs and symptoms during the same encounter.

12. A woman is examined for a routine prenatal visit. Which would be the reason for this encounter?
    a. Complications of pregnancy and childbirth
    b. Encounter for pregnancy test, result positive
    c. Personal history of complications of pregnancy
    d. Supervision of normal uncomplicated pregnancy

13. Which is assigned when the provider documents a reason for a patient seeking health care that is not a disorder or disease?
    a. Conditions that are ruled out
    b. Diagnoses that are qualified
    c. External causes of morbidity
    d. Factors influencing health status

14. The X character in an ICD-10-CM code is called a(n) _____.
    a. eponym
    b. modifier
    c. placeholder
    d. qualifier

15. Which ICD-10-CM Index to Diseases and Injuries entry (below) identifies the second qualifier?

    Stricture *–see also* Stenosis
       aqueduct of Sylvius (congenital) Q03.0
          with spina bifida *–see* Spina bifida, by site, with hydrocephalus

    a. Aqueduct of Sylvius
    b. Stenosis
    c. Stricture
    d. With spina bifida

16. The patient is seen in the office because of chronic asthma. Coding guidelines for chronic conditions state that such codes
    a. are not to be reported if the condition is already being medically managed.
    b. may be reported as additional diagnosis only if medically managed.
    c. may be reported as first-listed if medically managed during the encounter.
    d. should never be reported on an outpatient claim.

17. A hospital outpatient complains of nausea and abdominal pain and undergoes an endoscopy for suspected hiatal hernia. The test results were negative, so the physician instructed the patient to return next week to be tested for possible gastroesophageal reflux disease. To code the endoscopy encounter to the highest degree of accuracy and completeness, which would be reported?
    a. Gastroesophageal reflux disease
    b. Hiatal hernia
    c. Nausea and abdominal pain
    d. Nausea and vomiting and gastroesophageal reflux disease

18. Urinary tract infection due to *E. coli* is coded as _____.
    a. B96.20
    b. B96.20, N39.0
    c. N39.0
    d. N39.0, B96.20

19. Routine child health examination (age 2) is coded as _____.
    a. Z00.00
    b. Z00.129
    c. Z00.2
    d. Z01.89

20. Pneumonia due to *Pseudomonas* is coded as _____.

    a. A24.0   c. J15.1

    b. B96.5   d. J17, A24.0

5.2 — Coding Practice

5.2A — Coding Practice — Ambulatory Surgery Center (ASC)

Instructions: Review each case scenario, and assign and properly sequence ICD-10-CM diagnosis codes.

1. SUBJECTIVE: This 20-year-old patient with a past medical history significant for asthma underwent a total thyroidectomy due to feelings of fatigue and weight gain for the past six months.

    OBJECTIVE: Thyroid function tests revealed that the patient was hypothyroid with a thyroid-stimulating hormone level of 110.2, free thyroxine index of 0.9, and total T3 of 0.41. The patient also has a palpable mass in the left lobe of the thyroid, and thyroid ultrasound revealed a nodule in the thyroid gland. Thyroid lobes were biopsied bilaterally; based on those results, the patient underwent total thyroidectomy.

    DIAGNOSES:

    _____ Nodule, thyroid gland

    _____ Hypothyroidism

    _____ History of asthma

2. SUBJECTIVE: 42-year-old patient with past family history of gastric polyposis underwent upper gastrointestinal endoscopy, which revealed multiple gastric polyps in the fundus and body of the stomach.

    OBJECTIVE: Biopsies of the gastric polyps were submitted for pathological examination.

    DIAGNOSES:

    _____ Multiple gastric polyps

    _____ Family history of gastric polyposis

3. This 35-year-old states that her menstrual periods have been regular, and she had been taking birth control pills until January of this year. Since that time, she has been using other methods of birth control that are unsatisfactory to her. She and her partner also desire tubal ligation for prevention of further pregnancies.

    PHYSICAL EXAMINATION reveals a morbidly obese female in no obvious distress; heart and lungs normal to auscultation; abdomen flat; on pressure, the cervix protrudes to the opening of the vaginal os; otherwise, the uterus was average size. Patient was taken to surgery and underwent laparoscopic bilateral tubal ligation. She was discharged in stable condition to be seen by Dr. Baker for follow-up care next week.

    DIAGNOSES:

    _____ Elective sterilization

    _____ Morbid obesity

4. A 53-year-old patient is admitted with a right inguinal hernia. Laboratory results were within normal limits. Right inguinal herniorrhaphy was performed, and the patient did well; there were no complications. Patient was discharged to be seen in the office in several days for suture removal. No specific diet or medication was prescribed. The patient was advised to avoid any strenuous activities.

    DIAGNOSIS:

    _____ Right inguinal hernia

5. This 31-year-old female is admitted to the ambulatory surgery unit with chief complaint of multiparity. She states that she wants to undergo a sterilization procedure. She underwent laparoscopic tubal fulguration, bilateral. There are no familial diseases such as epilepsy, diabetes, bleeding tendency, tuberculosis, or heart

attacks. She smokes a pack of cigarettes a day and takes no alcohol. She is married, but now separated. She has been in good health and has had no other problems. Her menses are every 28 days and last 4 days. No clots or pains. Her last period was January 1. She has two children living and well, ages 11 and 5.

DIAGNOSES:

_____ Elective sterilization

_____ Multiparity

_____ Nicotine dependence, cigarettes

5.2B — Coding Practice — Chiropractic Office

Instructions: Review each case scenario, and assign and properly sequence ICD-10-CM diagnosis codes, including ICD-10-CM external cause codes for any applicable activity performed, external cause status, place of occurrence, and/or type of accident.

1. A 37-year-old male civilian contractor was hired by a home owner. While lifting boards from his truck on the job in the private driveway at a single-family private house, he began to experience acute burning pain in his neck from this sudden strenuous movement. His symptoms persisted, and he was seen by his chiropractor who checked the range of motion in his neck and noted restriction in lateral bending and rotation. Neurologic screening revealed decreased sensation at the left thumb and first finger. Reflexes were normal (intact), but there was some muscle weakness in the left arm. Patient underwent magnetic resonance imaging (MRI), which was negative, and received chiropractic treatment.

   DIAGNOSES:

   _____ Cervical disc syndrome

   _____ Building and construction (external cause activity)

   _____ Private driveway at single-family private house (external cause place of occurrence)

   _____ Civilian activity done for income (external cause status)

2. A 15-year-old male high school student was playing in a basketball game one evening. On the basketball court when he went up for a rebound, he felt his neck "wrench" backward and experienced immediate pain in both sides of his neck. That evening he felt pain and stiffness in his neck, and he had trouble turning his head.

   DIAGNOSES:

   _____ Acute cervical sprain (initial encounter)

   _____ Basketball (external cause activity)

   _____ Basketball court (external cause place of occurrence)

   _____ Student activity (external cause status)

3. A 48-year-old female online college professor who sits at a computer, keyboarding all day in her office at the college, has been experiencing neck pain accompanied by soreness and stiffness in her upper back. She became concerned when numbness and tingling started in her left arm, especially at night. History reveals no weakness in her arms and minor arm pain. All neurologic signs are normal, and the patient has full range of motion in her neck except for some restriction when she bends her head to the left. Tight and very tender muscles in the upper back and along both side of the neck are palpated. There are also joint restrictions in the middle back. Chiropractic treatment was provided.

   DIAGNOSES:

   _____ Cervical neck strain (initial encounter)

   _____ Myalgia, upper back

   _____ Computer keyboarding (external cause activity)

   _____ College (external cause place of occurrence)

   _____ Civilian activity done for income (external cause status)

4. A 77-year-old individual experiences neck pain and seeks chiropractic treatment. Upon examination, all neurologic signs are normal. There is restricted joint motion and tight muscles along both sides of the neck and into the upper and midback. Previous x-ray of the neck revealed osteoarthritis. The patient undergoes chiropractic treatment.

DIAGNOSIS:

_____ Osteoarthritis, cervical spine

5. A 25-year-old college student is seen for chiropractic treatment. The patient complains of neck stiffness and headaches. Neck x-rays are negative. Chiropractic treatment included adjustment and heat therapy.

DIAGNOSIS:

_____ Neck sprain (initial encounter)

5.2C — Coding Practice — Hospital Emergency Department

Instructions: Review each case scenario, and assign and properly sequence ICD-10-CM diagnosis codes, including ICD-10-CM external cause codes for any applicable activity performed, external cause status, place of occurrence, and/or type of accident.

1. SUBJECTIVE: 15-year-old male patient with previous diagnoses of congenital cataracts and retinal detachments had experienced an episode of orbital hemorrhage, which was treated in the past. He arrived in the ED today after developing pain behind his right eye yesterday.

OBJECTIVE: Physical examination revealed no redness of the eye. The left pupil is deviated medially with a steamy anterior chamber. This is the normal appearance, according to the mother. There was no sight in that eye. Funduscopic examination shows a pigmented retina in the right eye, but no evidence of hemorrhage or optic disc cupping. Schiotz tonometry showed a right orbital pressure of 21 and left orbital pressure of 0. There was no cervical lymphadenopathy. Tympanic membranes were clear. Chest was clear, and heart is regular rate and rhythm. There is full range of motion of the neck. No palpable temporal arteries; no abrasions or swelling. There has been no fever.

ASSESSMENT: Headache, etiology unknown.

PLAN: I called his primary care physician, who explained that this has been a problem in the past and that neurologically, the patient has been evaluated for this type of problem but nothing was ever found. He believed that the pressure of 21 was okay and that the patient could be discharged on some sort of analgesic. The patient is scheduled to be seen by him in two weeks.

DIAGNOSIS:

_____ Headache

2. SUBJECTIVE: 25-year-old male was working with a heavy sledgehammer in the garden of a single-family house as part of a landscaping project, which is a hobby, when he noted pain in his right shoulder area. The pain developed suddenly as he was swinging the hammer rather vigorously. The pain has persisted over the past three weeks. At certain times, it was somewhat better, but it became painful once again. The patient has continued working, which involves swinging this sledgehammer.

OBJECTIVE: Physical examination reveals tenderness over the anterior joint line; there is no swelling or abnormal mass present. The rotator cuff does not seem involved, as the patient can tolerate extreme downward pressure on his elbows without any pain whatsoever. What really causes the patient's pain is bringing the arms apart when they are in the midline in front of his chest. Distal neurovascular status is intact. X-ray of the shoulder was negative.

TREATMENT: The patient was given a prescription for Motrin 600 milligrams three times daily and advised to apply heat to the area once or twice each day. He is also to rest the arm as much as possible; however, he says he must work and will not take time off. He was told that this pain may last for a number of weeks before it resolves completely. He is to return to see Dr. Callus if there are any problems.

DIAGNOSES:

_____ Pain, right shoulder

_____ Gardening and landscaping (external cause activity)

_____ Garden in single-family (private) house (external cause place of occurrence)

_____ Hobby (external cause status)

3. SUBJECTIVE: This 48-year-old man is a patient of mine who complains of midsternal chest pain but no radiation. This has occurred intermittently today since 10 P.M. and did not occur reliably with exertion. He has not been exerting himself too much as a pastor at a Baptist church. He complains of feeling quite warm, but has had no diaphoresis or shortness of breath. He previously had his gallbladder removed. He has been taking Inderal 40 milligrams four times each day, and he took Isordil sublingually with mixed results during the day today. He says that Tylenol will help somewhat with the pain in the midsternal area.

OBJECTIVE: Physical examination reveals a mildly anxious middle-aged male in little distress. The neck is supple; carotids are two plus without bruits. Chest is symmetrical in expansion, and lungs show few abnormal sounds and some rales in the right base. Heart is regular rate and rhythm; S1 and S2 and 2/4; no murmurs, clicks, heaves, gallops, or rubs were appreciated. The abdomen is soft and nontender. There is a right upper quadrant surgical scar; no masses or organomegaly noted. EKG was done and read as normal. Chest x-ray shows slightly increased density at right lower lobe. He was given Mylanta without any change in his pain.

DIAGNOSES:

_____ Bronchitis

_____ Pneumonia, right side

4. SUBJECTIVE: This 22-year-old female twisted her left ankle yesterday while playing softball at a local baseball field as a leisure activity. She states that she developed pain in that ankle subsequent to this injury and has been on crutches prior to her arrival in the ED this morning. She denies any previous significant injuries to the ankle.

OBJECTIVE: Physical examination reveals a healthy, cooperative 22-year-old female in no acute distress. There is tenderness about the left ankle. There is no ecchymoses or swelling present. There is tenderness beneath both malleoli and anteriorly across the ankle. X-rays of the ankle show no evidence of fracture.

PLAN: The patient was instructed to use crutches for seven days and to avoid any weight-bearing and then begin partial weight-bearing. If she is uncomfortable, she is to return to using crutches for several more days before attempting weight-bearing. She is to elevate the leg and use ice compresses, and she was advised to be reevaluated if she is not able to walk comfortably in 7 to 10 days.

DIAGNOSES:

_____ Sprain, left ankle (initial encounter)

_____ Softball (external cause activity)

_____ Baseball field (external cause place of occurrence)

_____ Leisure activity (external cause status)

5. SUBJECTIVE: This is a 28-year-old female who was handed a knife by her spouse, blade first, while cooking in the kitchen of their apartment, which is a leisure activity for her; she accidentally punctured her left ring finger on the blade.

    OBJECTIVE: Patient has a superficial puncture wound over the lateral aspect of the left fourth finger. The area has been cleansed well, and a bandage was applied.

    ASSESSMENT: Puncture wound, left ring finger. (Initial encounter.)

    PLAN: Patient is to watch for any signs of infection and follow up with her primary care physician.

    DIAGNOSES:

    _____ Puncture wound, left ring finger (initial encounter)

    _____ Accidental contact with knife (initial encounter) (external cause accidental contact)

    _____ Cooking (external cause activity)

    _____ Kitchen of apartment (external cause place of occurrence)

    _____ Leisure activity (external cause status)

5.2D — Coding Practice — Hospital Outpatient Department

Instructions: Review each case scenario, and assign and properly sequence ICD-10-CM diagnosis codes.

1. A 39-year-old female patient undergoes a screening electrocardiogram (EKG) as an outpatient. She has a family history of cardiovascular disease. EKG results were negative. The nonspecific T-wave changes illustrated on the EKG were explained to the patient as probably due to anxiety and positional changes.

    DIAGNOSES:

    _____ Encounter for screening for cardiovascular disorders

    _____ Family history of cardiovascular disease

2. A 42-year-old patient diagnosed with systemic lupus erythematosus received a scheduled transfusion of erythrocytes and platelets in the ambulatory transfusion clinic.

    DIAGNOSIS:

    _____ Systemic lupus erythematosus

3. A 54-year-old patient previously diagnosed with atherosclerotic heart disease of native coronary artery with unstable angina pectoris underwent scheduled right and left cardiac catheterization as an outpatient. The patient has no past history of previous coronary artery bypass graft (CABG) surgery. Cardiac catheterization results revealed 40 percent blockage of the right coronary artery, 70 percent blockage of the left main coronary artery, and 80 percent blockage of the left anterior descending coronary artery. Surgical intervention options to treat the blockages were discussed with the patient, and the patient will be admitted in two days to undergo triple CABG.

    DIAGNOSIS:

    _____ Arteriosclerotic heart disease of native coronary artery with unstable angina pectoris

4. A 62-year-old patient with known congestive heart failure registered for outpatient services at the heart failure clinic and receives lifestyle modification counseling about his diet and activities. Patient received instruction from the dietician about following a low-sodium, low-fat diet, and he was also counseled to avoid tobacco and heavy alcohol use. Current medications were reviewed, and diuretic dosage was adjusted.

DIAGNOSES:

_____ Congestive heart failure

_____ Dietary counseling

5. A 45-year-old patient registered as an outpatient to undergo scheduled hemodialysis. The patient was born with just one kidney, which failed at age 30. Patient previously underwent a kidney transplant, which also failed. Currently, dialysis is the only option for end-stage renal failure as patient awaits the availability of another kidney for transplant. The hemodialysis takes three hours and is uneventful.

DIAGNOSES:

_____ Kidney transplant failure

_____ Renal agenesis, unilateral

_____ End-stage renal failure

_____ Dependence on renal dialysis

_____ Awaiting organ transplant

_____ Complication following kidney transplant (external cause surgical complication)

5.2E — Coding Practice — Hospital Same Day Surgery

Instructions: Review each case scenario, and assign and properly sequence ICD-10-CM diagnosis codes.

1. This 5-year-old patient is admitted with the chief complaint of recurrent bouts of tonsillitis and tonsils so large that food gets stuck in them and patient chokes on it. Patient has had a sore throat now for four to five weeks, and this is the second time this year that this has happened. Patient has consulted Dr. Blair who advised that the patient undergo tonsillectomy and adenoidectomy (T&A). The patient has no ear problems and has not had strep throat that the patient knows of.

PAST MEDICAL HISTORY: No operations, serious illnesses, or injuries.

FAMILY HISTORY: No familial diseases such as cancer, tuberculosis, epilepsy, diabetes, bleeding tendency, or heart attacks.

SOCIAL HISTORY: The patient is in kindergarten and lives with their parents and has no social problems.

SYSTEMIC REVIEW: The parent states that their son has been in good health and has had no other problems.

PHYSICAL EXAMINATION: Reveals tonsils to be huge. There is evidence that he had an anterior lymphadenopathy.

LABORATORY STUDIES: Urinalysis negative. Bleeding time 1 minute 30 seconds. Partial prothrombin time 30 seconds. Hemoglobin 12.3 grams, hematocrit 37 volume percent, white blood count 6500 with 34 polys. Chest x-ray normal. The patient was prepared for surgery and taken to the operating room where, under satisfactory general intratracheal anesthesia, T&A was performed. Following the operation, patient had an uncomplicated postoperative recovery. Patient had no bleeding, was afebrile, tonsillar fossa are clean, and has had no anesthetic complications.

DIAGNOSIS:

_____ Greatly hypertrophied tonsils and adenoids

2. This is an 89-year-old patient who was apparently in good health except for pneumonia in 1938 and had never had any serious medical problems since then. For about a month prior to outpatient surgery, patient developed urgency and frequency upon urination and marked nocturia every hour, followed finally by the passing of blood in the urine. Patient was seen in the emergency room (ER) last week due to passing blood in the urine every day for several days and having a great deal of difficulty voiding. ER treatment involved inserting a Foley catheter, from which 400 cc of grossly bloody urine was evacuated.

PHYSICAL EXAMINATION: Reveals a degree of blindness due to cataracts. The testes are atrophic. Prostate is a grade II benign, enlarged gland.

LABORATORY AND X-RAY FINDINGS: BUN 62, blood sugar 155, CO_2 14, creatinine 3.6. Urinalysis reveals many red blood cells per high-power field and WBC 4–6. Urine culture reveals innumerable *Enterococci*. Complete blood count reveals hemoglobin of 11.9 grams, hematocrit of 35. Blood gases reveal pH of 7.38, pCO_2 of 22.9, PO_2 of 91, HCO of 313. WBC of 12,200. EKG was negative. Drip infusion IVP revealed poorly functioning kidneys and one bladder diverticulum with elevation of the bladder floor consistent with a large prostate gland. Chest x-ray showed bilateral basal pulmonary infiltration and calcification of the thoracic aorta. Upper gastrointestinal and gallbladder series and small bowel series revealed small active ulcer crater of the lesser curvature of the pyloric canal. Patient underwent cystoscopy and retropubic prostatectomy.

DIAGNOSES:

_____ Benign prostatic hypertrophy

_____ Chronic renal insufficiency

_____ Urinary tract infection (UTI)

_____ *Enterococci* (as cause of UTI)

_____ Urinary frequency

_____ Nocturia

_____ Urgency

3. This 48-year-old patient has had an anal fissure for several months and is complaining of pain and bleeding. This has not responded to conservative measures, and patient is scheduled to undergo outpatient fissurectomy and hemorrhoidectomy.

PHYSICAL EXAMINATION: Reveals no other pertinent positive findings except the presence of obesity, anal fissure, and hemorrhoids. X-ray of the chest was unremarkable. Barium enema studies were unremarkable. EKG showed no abnormality. Lab results revealed blood sugar 92, BUN 14, normal electrolytes, and normal enzymes. CBC and differential were normal. Urinalysis was essentially unremarkable. After adequate workup, the patient was taken to surgery; under endotracheal anesthesia, a fissurectomy, hemorrhoidectomy, and sphincterotomy were performed. Post-op, the patient was voiding and comfortable. The patient was pre-scribed Tylenol with Codeine, Metamucil, sitz baths, and limited activity. The patient will be followed in my office.

DIAGNOSES:

_____ Anal fissure

_____ First-degree bleeding hemorrhoids

4. This 51-year-old patient has noticed a steady enlargement on the left side of the neck for the past year. A thyroid scan revealed a cold nodule in the right lobe, and carcinoma is to be ruled out. The patient also complains of some difficulty with pain in the neck and on swallowing.

PHYSICAL EXAMINATION: Reveals a large mass in the left lobe of the thyroid and a questionable mass on the right side. The patient was taken to surgery, where at the time of exploration, both lobes of the thyroid were markedly enlarged and revealed multiple nodules. A total thyroidectomy was performed after identifying the parathyroid glands and protecting them. The patient was discharged and instructed to return for follow-up examination within two weeks. Patient was placed on Synthroid 0.15 mcg daily.

DIAGNOSES:

_____ Diffuse (colloid) nontoxic goiter, left and right lobes of thyroid

_____ Degenerating follicular adenoma, right lobe of thyroid

5. Patient was diagnosed as missed abortion at 20 weeks' gestation. The patient was noted to have grown appreciably in the last month of prenatal care, and it was noted that bleeding had begun three days before being seen in the office yesterday. At the time of the office visit, the patient was passing clots. The cervix was dilated, and a foul-smelling discharge was noted but no morbidity. The patient was scheduled for outpatient surgery, during which pregnancy was removed with curettage of the uterus. The patient was discharged in satisfactory condition. Hemoglobin was 13.8 grams, and white blood cell count was normal differential. Pathology revealed products of conception and degenerated decidual and placental tissue.

DIAGNOSIS:

_____ Missed abortion

5.2F — Coding Practice — Physician Office

Instructions: Review each case scenario, and assign and properly sequence ICD-10-CM diagnosis codes, including ICD-10-CM external cause codes for any applicable activity performed, external cause status, place of occurrence, and/or type of accident.

1. This 38-year-old man was accidentally poked in his left eye by his nine-month-old little girl yesterday when she came to visit him in his office on a college campus, where he teaches. He says that her finger accidentally poked him in the left eye, and her fingernail scratched his eyeball. Patient states, "My eye is killing me!" Since that time, he has pain in his left eye and a lot of watering. He has had no changes in vision, no blurriness noted, and he is otherwise well. Physical examination shows the conjunctiva to be inflamed. Funduscopic examination is normal, and extraocular movements are intact. Stain with fluorescein shows positive corneal abrasion. I administered an ophthalmic topical analgesic to relieve his discomfort and Chloromycetin ointment to the eye to prevent infection. He was fitted with an eye patch and is to see me tomorrow for a recheck.

DIAGNOSES:

_____ Corneal laceration, left eye (initial encounter)

_____ Accidental scratch by child (initial encounter) (external cause accident)

_____ College (external cause place of occurrence)

2. This 15-year-old patient was struck on the left leg by a stick yesterday, which created a puncture wound in the skin. The patient presents today with swelling and localized redness around the wound. Physical exam reveals a healthy and cooperative 15-year-old patient in no acute distress with a small puncture-type wound approximately 5 millimeters in length on the anterior aspect of the left leg, just proximal to the knee. The wound is noted to have a small amount of induration, approximately 2 centimeters in diameter around the area with localized redness. There is no discomfort to motion of the knee.

PLAN: The patient was instructed to use warm soaks to that knee several times each day and have it rechecked if it becomes worse. Patient will return or be seen sooner if the knee does not appear to improve. Patient was started on Keflex 500 milligrams four times daily.

DIAGNOSES:

_____ Puncture wound, left knee (initial encounter)

_____ Struck by a stick (initial encounter) (external cause striking)

3. This 34-year-old patient who has had a hydrocele in the past and had been seen and treated by Dr. Wise, returns now for continued pain and swelling in the hydrocele, which is causing poor sleep habits. Apparently, the patient has been given some kind of "fluid pill" for the discomfort.

   OBJECTIVE: Patient has a tender, swelling right scrotal region about the size of a grapefruit, which is very tense.

   ASSESSMENT: Right-sided hydrocele.

   PLAN: The patient is to wear tight, supportive underwear; take Tylenol #3 for pain; and see Dr. Wise for evaluation.

   DIAGNOSIS:

   _____ Right-sided hydrocele

4. This patient cut the left thumbnail and thumb with a powered hand saw today, which flapped back the lateral aspect of the thumb. The thumb was cleansed, numbed, and one stitch put through the nail, fixing the flap in place. Patient is current on tetanus immunizations and will return to the office to have the stitch removed in six to eight days unless symptoms are noted, in which case patient is to call the office to be seen.

   DIAGNOSES:

   _____ Laceration, thumbnail and thumb, left (initial encounter)

   _____ Contact with powered hand saw (initial encounter) (external cause contact)

5. This 1-year-old little girl injured her hand while "playing the drum" by banging away at pots and pans on the floor of the kitchen at a single-family house while her mother was nearby preparing last evening's meal. The child slept fitfully last night, and this morning her left hand is somewhat swollen and painful to touch. X-ray was taken and is negative for fracture. I treated her with a sling, ice, and elevation, which will continue at home. She will be rechecked as needed. She left the office in good condition.

   DIAGNOSES:

   _____ Swelling, left hand

   _____ Pain, left hand

   _____ Striking pots and pans (initial encounter) (external cause striking against)

   _____ Kitchen of single-family house (external cause place of occurrence)

   _____ Leisure activity (external cause status)

5.2G — Coding Practice — Stand-Alone Radiology Center

Instructions: Review each case scenario, and assign and properly sequence ICD-10-CM diagnosis codes.

1. A 50-year-old patient underwent ultrasound of neck and ultrasound-guided placement of internal jugular dialysis catheter. Indication for radiographic procedures is chronic renal failure and obstructed dialysis brachial vascular access graft. Real-time ultrasound examination was done of the neck and showed patency of both internal jugular veins. Following sterile prep and drape and infiltration with local anesthetic, puncture was done of the lower aspect of the right internal jugular vein using a 21-gauge needle. Using Seldinger technique, the tract was dilated and a 14-French dialysis catheter was introduced and positioned within the right atrium. The catheter was secured with a silk suture and irrigated, and the patient sent for dialysis.

   DIAGNOSES:

   _____ Chronic renal failure

   _____ Complication, brachial vascular graft, mechanical obstruction (initial encounter)

2. Gallbladder cholecystogram shows moderate concentration of dye in the gallbladder, no evidence of stone, and moderate hypertrophic change of the gallbladder. Small intestinal pattern is normal below the level of the duodenum. Impression is hypertrophic gallbladder with no diagnostic evidence of stones.

   DIAGNOSIS:

   _____ Gallbladder hypertrophy

3. Patient underwent upper gastrointestinal study due to severe stomach pain. Study reveals esophagus and stomach to be normal in appearance, and first portion of duodenum is normal. There is moderate deformity of the medial aspect of the second portion of the duodenum with moderate flattening of the mucosal pattern in this area, but without any definite evidence of ulceration. The duodenal loop is not significantly widened, but there does appear to be slight extrinsic pressure and probable stiffening of the medial wall of the second portion of the duodenum.

   IMPRESSION: Second portion of duodenum is consistent with residues of recurrent pancreatitis with probable exacerbation of the pancreatitis at this time. The possibility of neoplasm arising in the head of the pancreas is not excluded.

   DIAGNOSIS:

   _____ Recurrent chronic pancreatitis

4. Patient underwent excretory urogram for complaints of urinary incontinence. Urogram revealed that both kidneys appear to concentrate Renografin media in a satisfactory manner. Renal collecting system on the left appears grossly normal. Visualized lateral contour of right kidney appears normal. Renal pelvis and ureters are of normal caliber. Urinary bladder is moderately distended, normal in contour, and shows some indentation on its dome, probably due to the adjacent uterus. There is moderate post voiding residual. Impression is normal right and left calices, small post voiding residual with indentation on dome of urinary bladder, possibly due to an enlarged uterus.

   DIAGNOSIS:

   _____ Urinary incontinence

5. Patient underwent opaque right knee arthrogram for severe pain and limited mobility. Following shaving and scrubbing of the knee in the usual manner, local anesthetic was infiltrated along the lateral approach to the patellofemoral joint. A needle was directed through the anesthetized tissue and into the joint with subsequent removal of 30 cc of pink-colored joint fluid. Then, 11 cc of Renografin 76 was injected and films taken in various projections. Fissures are demonstrated in the posterior segment of the medial meniscus. Cruciate ligaments and lateral meniscus appear intact. Impression is knee joint effusion and rupture of posterior segment of right medial meniscus.

   DIAGNOSES:

   _____ Effusion, right knee

   _____ Complex rupture of posterior segment, right medial meniscus (initial encounter)

5.2H — Coding Practice — Stand-Alone Urgent Care Center

Instructions: Review each case scenario, and assign and properly sequence ICD-10-CM diagnosis codes, including ICD-10-CM external cause codes for any applicable activity performed, external cause status, place of occurrence, and/or type of accident.

1. SUBJECTIVE: A 45-year-old female was seen complaining of right leg abrasions and severe pain of the right knee and ankle after having been in a motorcycle accident earlier today in the driveway of her home. She was a passenger on the motorcycle. She has difficulty bearing weight on her right leg.

   OBJECTIVE: She has a sprain of the right knee. X-rays of the right knee were negative. Multiple views revealed no bony abnormality. There was slight soft tissue swelling over the lateral malleolus.

   TREATMENT: The right lower leg abrasions were cleansed. She was given a tetanus toxoid booster, and a sterile dressing was applied. The patient was told to elevate her right leg, and she is to be rechecked by her primary care physician in 48 hours. She left in good condition.

   DIAGNOSES:

   _____ Sprain, right knee (initial encounter)

   _____ Abrasions, right lower leg (initial encounter)

   _____ Motorcycle passenger (initial encounter) (external cause nontraffic accident)

   _____ Driveway of single-family house (external cause place of occurrence)

2. The patient is a 41-year-old male seen for treatment of cellulitis of his right hand that he noticed about a week ago. It did not seem to bother the patient too much. The patient became quite concerned today because he has had blood poisoning once before due to an infected hair follicle on that hand. The patient was instructed to come to the urgent care center for evaluation. The patient does have swelling and induration around the area of the original scratch. It is red and warm, but there is no streaking that I can see in the lymphatic channels. I think the patient is developing an infection there, or cellulitis.

    DISPOSITION: Hot soaks three or four times each day. Amoxil 250 milligrams three times each day for a week. If it should progressively worsen and become more swollen, the patient should call and have it checked again to be sure he isn't developing an abscess; otherwise, we'll give the patient a few days. If it hasn't cleared within five to seven days, patient is to let me know.

    DIAGNOSIS:

    _____ Cellulitis, right hand (initial encounter)

3. This 44-year-old male presents with a chief complaint of back pain. HPI: 44-year-old gentleman states that he went fishing Wednesday. He did not fall or injure himself, but Thursday he was feeling quite bad with right flank pain radiating into the back of his leg and into the testicle. He stated that he had no change in the color of urine and that the pain actually started to subside. Friday, he had another recurrence of pain, and it gradually worsened and stayed with him. Today, it was much worse, he was unable to work, and he came to the urgent care center for evaluation and treatment. The patient walks leaning to the right where his pain is. He has a significant amount of difficulty in hyperextension and also forward bending. It does not hurt too much to bend to the right, but it hurts quite a bit to bend to the left. He has a lot of tenderness in the sacroiliac region and also in the superior rim of the ilium and the sacrum. X-rays of the area appear normal to my eye. The radiology report is not back at this time.

    PLAN: We will treat him with Tylenol with Codeine, two tablets every four hours as needed, and Flexeril 10 milligrams three times a day. He should not work tomorrow or Monday, and perhaps he will be able to return to work on Tuesday. He was instructed to call the urgent care center if he gets any worse. He is instructed to schedule a follow-up visit in one week. He left the urgency care center in satisfactory condition.

    DIAGNOSIS:

    _____ Sacroiliac inflammation

4. This 15-year-old male presents to the urgent care center with the complaint of a cyst on his right cheek. Over the past two days, the patient has developed a reddened, tender mass on the right cheek, just lateral to the nose. Physical exam reveals an erythematous, tender mass approximately 7 millimeters in diameter on the right cheek. It is hard and tender, but does not seem to be fluctuant at this time.

    PLAN: The patient was instructed to use warm soaks frequently and was given a prescription for tetracycline 250 milligrams four times daily. He was instructed to see Dr. Smith in two days. He is to return sooner if he has further difficulty.

    DIAGNOSIS:

    _____ Sebaceous cyst, right cheek

5. This young lady has had intermittent nosebleeds and was brought to the urgent care center and examined. There was moderate swelling in the nose and quite a bit of edema and swelling in the nasal mucosa, but there is no active bleeding noted at the present time. No treatment was given other than Dimetapp one every 12 hours, and the patient was told to avoid taking aspirin. She is to take Tylenol and apply ice to her nose. The detention center staff person who accompanied the patient to the urgent care center was told to call if the patient experienced further problems.

    DIAGNOSIS:

    _____ Epistaxis

ICD-10-PCS Coding System

Part IV of *3-2-1 Code It!* contains the following chapter, which covers an introduction to ICD-10-PCS and its coding conventions and section coding guidelines. All ICD-10-PCS sections are included in the chapter, and they are organized according to the official ICD-10-PCS coding manual.

Introduction to ICD-10-PCS Coding, Conventions, and Guidelines

Chapter Outline

Overview of ICD-10-PCS Coding

ICD-10-PCS Index

ICD-10-PCS Tables

ICD-10-PCS Official Guidelines for Coding and Reporting

ICD-10-PCS Coding Conventions

ICD-10-PCS Sections and Coding Guidelines

Chapter Objectives

At the conclusion of this chapter, the student should be able to:

1. Define key terms related to the introduction of ICD-10-PCS coding, conventions, and guidelines.
2. Explain an overview of the ICD-10-PCS classification system.
3. Locate main terms for procedure statements using the ICD-10-PCS index.
4. Construct procedure codes using ICD-10-PCS tables.
5. Explain the intent of *ICD-10-PCS Official Guidelines for Coding and Reporting*.
6. Interpret ICD-10-PCS coding conventions to assign codes.
7. Interpret ICD-10-PCS section coding guidelines to assign codes.

Key Terms

axis of classification	*see*	multiaxial structure	root operation
coding conventions (ICD-10-PCS)	*use*	*ICD-10-PCS Official Guidelines for Coding and Reporting*	root type
	Index		Tables
cross references	modality		values

Introduction

The *International Classification of Diseases, 10th Revision, Procedure Classification System* (ICD-10-PCS) was developed by the Centers for Medicare and Medicaid Services (CMS) for reporting inpatient hospital procedures and services *only. ICD-10-PCS Official Guidelines for Coding and Reporting* are used as a companion to the official version of ICD-10-PCS to ensure accurate coding. This chapter includes an overview of ICD-10-PCS, content about the ICD-10-PCS index, tables, and the official guidelines for coding and reporting, and descriptions of coding conventions and section coding guidelines.

Overview of ICD-10-PCS Coding

The *International Classification of Diseases, 10th Revision, Procedure Classification System* (ICD-10-PCS) was developed by the Centers for Medicare and Medicaid Services (CMS) for use in the United States. ICD-10-PCS is used to report codes for inpatient hospital settings *only,* and structurally it contains an alphabetical index and tables, which are used to construct procedure codes. The ICD-10-PCS classification contains the following major attributes:

- Completeness
- Expandability
- Multiaxial structure
- Standardized terminology

ICD-10-PCS contains unique codes for all substantially different procedures to create a *complete* classification. As new procedures are developed, additional unique codes are easily incorporated, which facilitates *expandability.* (ICD-10-PCS contains more than 87,000 seven-character alphanumeric procedure codes.) ICD-10-PCS codes use a **multiaxial structure** (or **axis of classification**), which requires the selection of a character from each of seven axes, also called hierarchies or positions, to construct a valid seven-character alphanumeric code (e.g., 047K04Z).

Example: The seven axes (or positions) for the ICD-10-PCS Medical and Surgical Section are similar to those associated with the Imaging Section, but they are not identical. In this example, review the highlighted axes to notice how they differ.

Comparison of Medical and Surgical Section and Imaging Section		
Axis (Position)	**Medical and Surgical Section**	**Imaging Section**
1	Section (medical and surgical)	Section (imaging)
2	Body system (e.g., heart and great vessels)	Body system (e.g., respiratory system)
3	Operation (e.g., dilation)	Type (e.g., plain radiology scan)
4	Body part (e.g., skin)	Body part (e.g., lungs)
5	Approach (e.g., open)	Contrast (e.g., low osmolar)
6	Device (e.g., drainage device)	Qualifier (e.g., laser)
7	Qualifier (e.g., anterior)	Qualifier (e.g., intraoperative)

- The third axis is *Operation* for the Medical and Surgical section, while it is *Type* for the Imaging section.
- The fifth axis is *Approach* for the Medical and Surgical section, while it is *Contrast* for the Imaging section.
- The sixth axis is *Device* for the Medical and Surgical section, while it is *Qualifier* for the Imaging section.

 NOTE:

There is no decimal used in ICD-10-PCS codes, and letters I and O are never used because they are too easily confused with the numbers 1 and 0.

Standardized terminology is a unique vocabulary developed for ICD-10-PCS, and the coding manual contains appendices of definitions and a body part key, device key, substance key, and device aggregation table. While meanings of specific words vary in common usage, ICD-10-PCS does *not* include multiple meanings for the same term.

- Each term in ICD-10-PCS is assigned a specific meaning.
- Because providers are *not* required to use ICD-10-PCS terminology when documenting procedures, coders use ICD-10-PCS appendices to learn how to interpret provider documentation for accurate code assignment.

Example: When a provider documents *partial gastric resection* as the procedure performed during an inpatient hospital admission, coders do not locate *resection* in the ICD-10-PCS index. Instead, *excision* is located as the main term because its ICD-10-PCS definition is *cutting out or off, without replacement, a* portion *of a body part.* (*Resection* is defined as *cutting out or off, without replacement,* all *of a body part.*) Thus, a *partial gastric resection* is an *excision*, not a resection (while a *total gastric resection* would be considered a *resection*).

The development of ICD-10-PCS followed these general principles:

- *Diagnostic information is* not *included in procedure code descriptions.* Instead, ICD-10-CM codes classify diseases and injuries.
- *Level of specificity is enhanced.* All procedures currently performed can be assigned a specific code in ICD-10-PCS. The frequency (or infrequency) with which a procedure is performed is not a consideration. Thus, a unique code is classified for each variation of a procedure performed.
- *Not elsewhere classified (NEC) is* not *used in ICD-10-PCS.* All significant components of a procedure are required to create the seven-character ICD-10-PCS code. Where necessary ICD-10-PCS does include some nonspecific language, such as "other device" because new devices are frequently developed and the specific name of a device might not be included in the coding manual until a subsequent revision year.
- *Not otherwise specified (NOS) is* not *used in ICD-10-PCS.* A minimal level of specificity is required for each component of the procedure so that the seven-character ICD-10-PCS code is created.

 NOTE:

Not otherwise specified (NOS) and *not elsewhere classified (NEC)* are ICD-10-CM coding conventions (rules). They are *not* used in ICD-10-PCS.

ICD-10-PCS Format and Structure

The ICD-10-PCS index uses an indented format for ease in reference. ICD-10-PCS also makes use of the boldface and italic typeface for ease in reference. Boldface type is used for main term entries in the ICD-10-PCS index and characters in ICD-10-PCS tables, including its three-character heading. Italicized type is used for cross references *see* and *use* in the ICD-10-PCS index and row and column headings in ICD-10-PCS tables.

Example 1: ICD-10-PCS INDEX—INDENTED FORMAT, BOLDFACE, AND ITALICS: Main term Laparotomy in the ICD-10-PCS index is boldfaced, subterm Drainage is indented two spaces below the "L" of Laparotomy, and *see* is italicized.

ICD-10-PCS Index
Laparotomy
Drainage *see* Drainage, Peritoneal Cavity 0W9G
Exploratory *see* Inspection, Peritoneal Cavity 0WJG

Example 2: ICD-10-PCS TABLES—BOLDFACE AND ITALICS: In ICD-10-PCS Table 001, row headings and column headings are in italics, and the characters are boldfaced.

ICD-10-PCS Table (portion)			
001			
Section	**0** Medical and Surgical		
Body System	**0** Central Nervous System and Cranial Nerves		
Operation	**1** Bypass: Altering the route of passage of the contents of a tubular body part		
Body Part	*Approach*	*Device*	*Qualifier*
6 Cerebral Ventricle	**0** Open **3** Percutaneous **4** Percutaneous Endoscopic	**Z** No Device	**B** Cerebral Cisterns

ICD-10-PCS Codes Contain Independent Values

ICD-10-PCS codes contain independent values (characters and terms), and each axis retains its meaning across broad ranges of codes (to the extent possible). Thus, unique codes are constructed for all substantially different procedures. Its multiaxial structure allows new procedures to be easily incorporated as new ICD-10-PCS codes.

- Within a defined code range, a character specifies the same type of information for that axis of classification.
- All seven characters that comprise the ICD-10-PCS code must be specified to construct a valid code.
- If documentation is incomplete for coding purposes, query the physician for the necessary information to construct a valid code.

Updating ICD-10-PCS

The National Center for Health Statistics (NCHS) and the Centers for Medicare & Medicaid Services (CMS) are the U.S. Department of Health & Human Services (DHHS) agencies that comprise the ICD-10 Coordination and Maintenance Committee, which is responsible for overseeing all changes and modifications to ICD-10-PCS. CMS is responsible for annually updating the ICD-10-PCS classification.

The Medicare Prescription Drug, Improvement, and Modernization Act (MMA) requires all code sets (e.g., ICD-10-CM, ICD-10-PCS) to be valid at the time services are provided. New code releases publish on April 1 and October 1 (and include deleted, new, and revised ICD-10-PCS codes). Coding updates for ICD-10-CM/PCS must be implemented immediately so accurate codes are reported on claims. (HIPAA legislation requires the reporting of codes on health insurance claims, such as the UB-04 for hospital inpatient and outpatient health care services.)

CMS also publishes the following reference addenda:

- Edits made to the current year's definitions (of terms), index, and tables
- ICD-10-PCS conversion table (to assist with data retrieval)
- ICD-10-PCS codes file (text file with valid codes and full and abbreviated code descriptions)
- General equivalence mappings (of ICD-10-PCS to ICD-9-CM, and vice versa)
- *ICD-10-PCS Official Guidelines for Coding and Reporting*

Reporting ICD-10-PCS Codes

ICD-10-PCS codes are reported on the UB-04 (or CMS-1450) claim for inpatient hospital procedures. The *UB-04 claim* is a uniform institutional provider claim submitted by hospitals for inpatient and outpatient health care services to third-party payers. It is designated as the CMS-1450 by CMS and uses ANSI ASC X12N 837I as the standard format for submission of electronic claims by institutional health care services.

 NOTE:

> Institutional providers that submit the UB-04 claim include hospitals, skilled nursing facilities, end-stage renal disease providers, home health agencies, hospices, outpatient rehabilitation clinics, comprehensive outpatient rehabilitation facilities, community mental health centers, critical access hospitals, federally qualified health centers, histocompatibility laboratories, Indian Health Service facilities, organ procurement organizations, religious non-medical health care institutions, and rural health clinics. *However, ICD-10-PCS codes are reported for inpatient hospital procedures only.*

Data elements in the UB-04 for uniform electronic billing specifications are consistent with the hard copy data set. Patient data from an institution's electronic health record populates the UB-04 claim, which is electronically transmitted to the payer, a clearinghouse, or a third-party administrator for processing. An exception allows certain institutions to submit paper UB-04 claims, such as health care facilities with fewer than 25 full-time equivalent (FTE) employees.

Valid ICD-10-PCS codes are reported on UB-04 claims (Figure 6-1) for reimbursement purposes. The principal procedure code is reported in form locator 74, and other procedure codes are reported in form locators 74a-e. (ICD-10-CM codes are also reported on UB-04 claims *without the decimal* in form locators 66, 67, 69, and 70.)

66	K8012	Y				

69 ADMIT DX	K8012	70 PATIENT REASON DX	K8012		I10	
74	PRINCIPAL PROCEDURE CODE DATE		a.	OTHER PROCEDURE CODE DATE		
	0FT40ZZ	1313YY				
c.	OTHER PROCEDURE CODE DATE		d.	OTHER PROCEDURE CODE DATE		

Courtesy of the Centers for Medicare & Medicaid Services, www.cms.gov; claim data created by author.

FIGURE 6-1 Portion of UB-04 claim with completed form locators 66, 67, 69, 70, and 74

Exercise 6.1 – Overview of ICD-10-PCS

Instructions: Complete each statement.

1. ICD-10-PCS was developed by CMS for use in _____ hospital settings *only*.
2. ICD-10-PCS codes are reported for surgical _____.
3. ICD-10-PCS contains unique codes for all substantially different procedures, which is a major attribute that results in a _____ (or comprehensive) classification.
4. As new procedures are developed, additional unique ICD-10-PCS codes are easily added and incorporated to facilitate _____ as a major attribute.
5. A valid 7-character ICD-10-PCS alphanumeric code is constructed using a _____ structure (or axis of classification) as a major attribute.
6. A unique vocabulary was developed for ICD-10-PCS as a major attribute, using _____ terminology.
7. Diagnostic information is *not* included in ICD-10-PCS code descriptions; instead, diseases and injuries are assigned _____ codes.
8. The ICD-10-PCS classification's level of specificity includes codes for all procedures currently performed, resulting in construction of _____ and valid codes.
9. Each April 1 and October 1, ICD-10-CM and _____ codes are updated immediately so that accurate codes are reported on submitted inpatient hospital claims.
10. ICD-10-PCS codes are reported on the _____ (or CMS-1450) claim.

ICD-10-PCS Index

The ICD-10-PCS **Index** (Figure 6-2) is an alphabetical listing of procedures that includes the first 3–5 characters (and sometimes all 7 characters) of a 7-character ICD-10-PCS procedure code. When the ICD-10-PCS index provides the first three or four characters of a code, the table is used to construct the 7-character code. When the index provides a 7-character code for an entry, the appropriate ICD-10-PCS table is consulted to verify that the code contains valid characters. Cross references provide direction to root operations in the index and tables *(see)* and standardized terminology in tables *(use)*, and they are covered later in this section of the chapter.

Purpose of ICD-10-PCS Index

The purpose of the ICD-10-PCS index is to locate the appropriate table that contains all information necessary to construct a procedure code. The ICD-10-PCS tables must always be consulted to construct the most appropriate valid code. It is not possible to construct a procedure code by using just the alphabetic index.

ICD-10-PCS Index

A

Abdominal aortic plexus *use* Abdominal Sympathetic Nerve
Abdominal cavity *use* Peritoneal Cavity
Abdominal esophagus *use* Esophagus, Lower
Abdominohysterectomy *see* Resection, Uterus 0UT9
Abdominoplasty
> *see* Alteration, Abdominal Wall 0W0F
> *see* Repair, Abdominal Wall 0WQF
> *see* Supplement, Abdominal Wall 0WUF

Abductor hallucis muscle
> *use* Foot Muscle, Right
> *use* Foot Muscle, Left

ABECMA® *use* Idecabtagene Vicleucel Immunotherapy
AbioCor® Total Replacement Heart *use* Synthetic Substitute
Ablation
> *see* Control bleeding in
> *see* Destruction

Abortion
> Products of Conception 10A0
> Abortifacient 10A07ZX
> Laminaria 10A07ZW
> Vacuum 10A07Z6

Abrasion *see* Extraction
Absolute Pro Vascular (OTW) Self-Expanding Stent System
> *use* Intraluminal Device

Accelerate PhenoTest(tm) BC XXE5XN6
Accessory cephalic vein
> *use* Cephalic Vein, Right
> *use* Cephalic Vein, Left

Accessory obturator nerve *use* Lumbar Plexus
Accessory phrenic nerve *use* Phrenic Nerve

FIGURE 6-2 ICD-10-PCS Index (partial)

Main Terms and Subterms

The ICD-10-PCS index reflects the structure of the ICD-10-PCS tables, and its standardized terminology is used in the index to provide direction to tables where valid codes are constructed. This ensures a consistent pattern of organization and a multiaxial structure (hierarchies). Typically, just the first 3–5 characters of a 7-character procedure code are listed after an ICD-10-PCS index main term or subterm, and the appropriate table is used to construct a complete and valid 7-character code.

The ICD-10-PCS index is organized as an alphabetical lookup, and it is based on the standardized terminology located in the classification's tables. (In ICD-10-PCS tables, terms associated with characters are called **values**.) Usually, index terms are based on the third or fourth character of a code. *Main terms* include root operations, root (procedure) types, modalities, and common procedure terms.

Subterms are indented below main terms, and they include anatomical sites and other terms. In the ICD-10-PCS index, the word *with* appears in the main term or indented in alphabetical order below the main term or a subterm. To assign a code from the list of qualifiers below the word *with*, the physician must document the presence of both procedures in the patient's record.

Example: ICD-10-PCS INDEX—WITH: Locate main term *Phacoemulsification, lens* in the index, and notice the terms with (and without) appear as subterms. The subterm entries refer coders to ICD-10-PCS Tables 08R or 08D, depending on the procedure performed.

ICD-10-PCS Index (portion)
Phacoemulsification, lens
With IOL implant see Replacement, Eye 08R
Without IOL implant see Extraction, Eye 08D

Main terms in the ICD-10-PCS index often provide direction to tables for construction of valid codes, such as:

- Beam radiation (modality)
- Fluoroscopy (root type)
- Prostatectomy (common procedure term)
- Resection (root operation)

Other main terms provide direction to corresponding terms used in ICD-10-PCS tables for the purpose of constructing valid codes after the coder has first identified the appropriate table for the root operation, root procedure type, or modality, such as:

- Bard® Dulex™ mesh (device)
- Brachiocephalic artery (anatomical site)

There are a variety of ways to locate main terms in the ICD-10-PCS index, depending on the procedure performed.

Common Procedure Terms

Common procedure terms may appear as main terms in the ICD-10-PCS index. After locating a common procedure term (e.g., appendectomy) as the main term, coders are directed to the appropriate root operation main term in the ICD-10-PCS index or table.

Example 1: The patient underwent an *appendectomy* procedure, which was located as an ICD-10-PCS index main term with direction to cross reference (or *see*) root operations *excision or resection*.

- *Appendectomy* is a common procedure term, which is listed as a main term in the ICD-10-PCS index.
- *Excision* involves cutting out or off, without replacement, a <u>portion</u> of a body part. An emergency excision of the appendix might be performed prior to a CT scan (where the entire organ is depicted). A subsequent excision (of the appendix) procedure may be required when an infection of the appendix stump is diagnosed.
- *Resection* involves cutting out or off, without replacement, *all* of a body part. Most appendectomies involve resection of the entire appendix.

Because the operative report documented that the appendix was resected, the coder locates main term *Resection* and subterm *Appendix 0DTJ* in the ICD-10-PCS index. The coder can also go directly to ICD-10-PCS table 00BJ or 0DTJ to construct the appropriate code.

ICD-10-PCS Index (portion)
Appendectomy
see Excision, Appendix 0DBJ
see Resection, Appendix 0DTJ
Excision
Appendix 0DBJ
Resection
Appendix 0DTJ

(continues)

Example 1 (continued): Reviewing the operative report also determines the procedure method used (e.g., open). In this case, an open appendectomy was performed to resect the entire appendix. Table 0DT is located in the ICD-10-PCS coding manual, and fourth character J (appendix), fifth character 0 (open), sixth character Z (no device), and seventh character Z (no qualifier) are selected. As a result, ICD-10-PCS code 0DTJ0ZZ is constructed.

ICD-10-PCS Table			
0DT			
Section	**0**	Medical and Surgical	
Body System	**D**	Gastrointestinal System	
Operation	**T**	Resection: Cutting out or off, without replacement, all of a body part	
Body Part	*Approach*	*Device*	*Qualifier*
1 Esophagus, Upper **2** Esophagus, Middle **3** Esophagus, Lower **4** Esophagogastric Junction **5** Esophagus **6** Stomach **7** Stomach, Pylorus **8** Small Intestine **9** Duodenum **A** Jejunum **B** Ileum **C** Ileocecal Valve **E** Large Intestine **F** Large Intestine, Right **H** Cecum **J** Appendix **K** Ascending Colon **P** Rectum **Q** Anus	**0** Open **4** Percutaneous Endoscopic **7** Via Natural or Artificial Opening **8** Via Natural or Artificial Opening Endoscopic	**Z** No Device	**Z** No Qualifier

Example 2: The patient underwent a *cauterization procedure, adenoids, open.* Cauterization is a common procedure name, and the coder located it as a main term in the ICD-10-PCS index. A cross reference provided direction to *see* Destruction or Repair. Because the operative report documented that the adenoids were removed using cauterization, the coder locates main term *Destruction* and subterm *Adenoids 0C5Q* in the ICD-10-PCS index.

ICD-10-PCS Index (portion)
Cauterization
see Destruction
see Repair
Destruction
Acetabulum
Left 0Q55
Right 0Q54
Adenoids 0C5Q
Ampulla of Vater 0F5C

(continues)

Example 2 (continued): Table 0C5 is located in the ICD-10-PCS coding manual, and fourth character Q (adenoids), fifth character 0 (open), sixth character Z (no device), and seventh character Z (no qualifier) are selected. As a result, ICD-10-PCS code 0C5Q0ZZ is constructed.

ICD-10-PCS Table		
0C5		

Section	**0**	Medical and Surgical
Body System	**C**	Mouth and Throat
Operation	**5**	Destruction: Physical eradication of all or a portion of a body part by the direct use of energy, force, or a destructive agent

Body Part	Approach	Device	Qualifier
0 Upper Lip **1** Lower Lip **2** Hard Palate **3** Soft Palate **4** Buccal Mucosa **5** Upper Gingiva **6** Lower Gingiva **7** Tongue **N** Uvula **P** Tonsils **Q** Adenoids	**0** Open **3** Percutaneous **X** External	**Z** No Device	**Z** No Qualifier

Root Operations

Locate *root operations* (or *common procedure names*) in the ICD-10-PCS index for direction to tables (other than ancillary tables).

Root operations are associated with the third character in the following ICD-10-PCS sections. The **root operation** describes the intent or objective of the procedure.

- Medical and Surgical (e.g., resection, such as appendectomy)
- Obstetrics (e.g., delivery)
- Placement (e.g., compression)
- Administration (e.g., transfusion)
- Measurement and Monitoring (e.g., measurement, such as an electrocardiogram)
- Extracorporeal or Systemic Assistance and Performance (e.g., performance, such as extracorporeal circulation)
- Extracorporeal or Systemic Therapies (e.g., decompression, such as hyperbaric oxygenation)
- Osteopathic (e.g., treatment, such as osteopathic treatment)
- Other Procedures (e.g., other procedures, such as external examination of female reproductive system)
- Chiropractic (e.g., manipulation, such as chiropractic)
- New Technology (e.g., dilation, replacement)

Example: The patient underwent a manually-assisted delivery of a single liveborn infant. Delivery is the root operation, which is located as the main term in the ICD-10-PCS index. For this main term index entry, the seven-character code is listed as 10E0XZZ. (Verification in ICD-10-PCS Table 10E is required to ensure code validity.)

ICD-10-PCS Index (portion)
Delivery
Cesarean see Extraction, Products of Conception 10D0
Forceps see Extraction, Products of Conception 10D0
Manually assisted 10E0XZZ
Products of Conception 10E0XZZ
Vacuum assisted see Extraction, Products of Conception 10D0

Table 10E is located in the ICD-10-PCS coding manual, and fourth character 0 (products of conception), fifth character X (external), sixth character Z (no device), and seventh character Z (no qualifier) are selected. As a result, ICD-10-PCS code 10E0XZZ is constructed.

ICD-10-PCS Table			
10E			
Section	**1**	Obstetrics	
Body System	**0**	Pregnancy	
Operation	**E**	Delivery: Assisting the passage of the products of conception from the genital canal	
Body Part	*Approach*	*Device*	*Qualifier*
0 Products of Conception	**X** External	**Z** No Device	**Z** No Qualifier

NOTE:

If the patient had undergone a Cesarean section, ICD-10-PCS index common procedure name, Cesarean section, directs the coder to see Extraction, Products of Conception 10D0. Thus, ICD-10-PCS Table 10D is referenced for that procedure.

Root Types

Locate *root types* (*instead of* root operations) in the ICD-10-PCS index for direction to appropriate ancillary section tables.

Root types are associated with the third character in the following ICD-10-PCS sections. The **root type** describes the intent or purpose of the procedure or service.

- Imaging (e.g., plain radiography)
- Nuclear Medicine (e.g., PET imaging)
- Physical Rehabilitation and Diagnostic Audiology (e.g., speech assessment)
- Mental Health (e.g., psychological tests)
- Substance Abuse Treatment (e.g., detoxification services)

Example: A patient underwent a planar nuclear medicine imaging procedure of the abdomen to introduce radioactive materials and create a single plane display of images that are developed from capturing radioactive emissions. *Planar Nuclear Medicine Imaging* is the root (procedure) type, which is located as a main term in the ICD-10-PCS index. Subterm *Abdomen CW10* directs the coder to ICD-10-PCS Table CW1.

ICD-10-PCS Index (portion)
Planar Nuclear Medicine Imaging
Abdomen CW10
Abdomen and Chest CW14
Abdomen and Pelvis CW11

Table CW1 is located in the ICD-10-PCS coding manual, and the nuclear medicine procedure report documents planar nuclear medicine imaging using Technetium 99m (Tc-99m) as the radionuclide. Fourth character 0 (abdomen), fifth character 1 (Technetium 99m [Tc-99m]), sixth character Z (no qualifier), and seventh character Z (no qualifier) are selected. As a result, ICD-10-PCS code CW101ZZ is constructed.

ICD-10-PCS Table				
CW1				
Section	**C**	Nuclear Medicine		
Body System	**W**	Anatomical Regions		
Type	**1**	Planar Nuclear Medicine Imaging: Introduction of radioactive materials into the body for single plane display of images developed from the capture of radioactive emissions		
Body Part		*Radionuclide*	*Qualifier*	*Qualifier*
0 Abdomen **1** Abdomen and Pelvis **4** Chest and Abdomen **6** Chest and Neck **B** Head and Neck **D** Lower Extremity **J** Pelvic Region **M** Upper Extremity **N** Whole Body		**1** Technetium 99m (Tc-99m) **D** Indium 111 (In-111) **F** Iodine 123 (I-123) **G** Iodine 131 (I-131) **L** Gallium 67 (Ga-67) **S** Thallium 201 (Tl-201) **Y** Other Radionuclide	**Z** None	**Z** None

Modalities

Modalities are associated with the third character in Radiation Therapy section tables. The **modality** describes a method of treatment.

- Beam radiation
- Brachytherapy
- Stereotactic radiosurgery
- Other radiation

Example: A patient underwent brachytherapy of the brain. (During *brachytherapy*, sealed radioactive material is inserted inside the body in preparation for delivery of high doses of radiation to specific body areas.)

ICD-10-PCS Index (portion)
Brachytherapy
Bone Marrow D710
Brain D010
Brain Stem D011

(continues)

Example (continued): Table D01 is located in the ICD-10-PCS coding manual, and the brachytherapy report documents placement of low dose rate (LDR) Palladium 103 (Pd-103) as the unidirectional source in the brain. Fourth character 0 (brain), fifth character B (low dose rate), sixth character B Palladium 103 (Pd-103), and seventh character 1 (unidirectional source) are selected. As a result, ICD-10-PCS code D010BB1 is constructed.

ICD-10-PCS Table			
D01			
Section	**D**	Radiation Therapy	
Body System	**0**	Central and Peripheral Nervous System	
Type	**1**	Brachytherapy	
Treatment Site	*Modality Qualifier*	*Isotope*	*Qualifier*
0 Brain **1** Brain Stem **6** Spinal Cord **7** Peripheral Nerve	**9** High Dose Rate (HDR)	**7** Cesium 137 (Cs-137) **8** Iridium 192 (Ir-192) **9** Iodine 125 (I-125) **B** Palladium 103 (Pd-103) **C** Californium 252 (Cf-252) **Y** Other Isotope	**Z** None
0 Brain **1** Brain Stem **6** Spinal Cord **7** Peripheral Nerve	**B** Low Dose Rate (LDR)	**6** Cesium 131 (Cs-131) **7** Cesium 137 (Cs-137) **8** Iridium 192 (Ir-192) **9** Iodine 125 (I-125) **C** Californium 252 (Cf-252) **Y** Other Isotope	**Z** None
0 Brain **1** Brain Stem **6** Spinal Cord **7** Peripheral Nerve	**B** Low Dose Rate (LDR)	**B** Palladium 103 (Pd-103)	**1** Unidirectional Source **Z** None

Cross References

Cross references *see* and *use* in the ICD-10-PCS index provide direction to alternate terms in the index or tables for proper code assignment.

See

- Located after common procedure names and other terms
- Directs coders to an ICD-10-PCS *root operation*, *root procedure type*, or *modality* as the main term in the index, or
- Provides direction to specific ICD-10-PCS tables instead of another main term in the index

Example 1: Tendonectomy is a *common procedure name*, which is listed as a main term in the ICD-10-PCS index. It contains a *see* cross reference, which directs coders to *root operation* Excision or Resection as the main term. (According to ICD-10-PCS, *excision* is the cutting out or off, without replacement, a portion of a body part. *Resection* is the cutting out or off, without replacement, all of a body part.) When the coder locates Excision or Resection as the main term for the root operation in the index, anatomical site subterms Tendons 0LB and Tendons 0LT are indented below each main term. The cross reference also provides direction to Medical and Surgical Table 0LB or 0LT for construction of a valid ICD-10-PCS code for the root operation.

ICD-10-PCS Index (portion)
Tendonectomy
see Excision, Tendons 0LB   *see* Resection, Tendons 0LT

Example 2: Acetabuloplasty is a *common procedure name*, which is listed as a main term in the ICD-10-PCS index. It contains a *see* cross reference, which directs coders to an ICD-10-PCS table *and not another index subterm.* ICD-10-PCS Table 0QQ contains a list of body parts for lower bones (e.g., acetabulum, patella, tibia).

Notice that for index main term Repair, there is no subterm for Lower Bones 0QQ between main terms Liver 0FQ0 and Lung. (Subterms for specific lower bones, such as acetabulum, are located below main term Repair.)

ICD-10-PCS Index (portion)
Acetabuloplasty
see Repair, Lower Bones 0QQ
see Replacement, Lower Bones 0QR
see Supplement, Lower Bones 0QU
Repair
Acetabulum
Left 0QQ5
Right 0QQ4

ICD-10-PCS Index (portion)
Repair
Liver 0FQ0
Left Lobe 0FQ2
Right Lobe 0FQ1
Lung
Bilateral 0BQM
Left 0BQL
Lower Lobe
Left 0BQJ

Use

- Located after anatomical sites, devices, and other terms
- Directs coders to anatomic sites form the ICD-10-PCS Body Part Key *or* device terms from the ICD-10-PCS Device Key, so that the appropriate value for a site or term in an ICD-10-PCS table can be selected
- Direction is *not* provided to a specific ICD-10-PCS table. The appropriate table has already been selected, based on the procedure performed.
- Direction is *not* provided to an alternate main term in the index. Guidance is provided about alternate terms in an ICD-10-PCS table so that values (and their characters) can be selected.

Example: The patient underwent an *endoscopic dilation procedure, right lacrimal duct canaliculus.* Main term *dilation,* and subterms *duct, lacrimal,* and *right* direct the coder to ICD-10-PCS Table 087.

ICD-10-PCS Index (portion)
Dilation
Duct
Lacrimal
Left 087Y
Right 087X
Lacrimal canaliculus
use Lacrimal Duct, Right
use Lacrimal Duct, Left

Upon review of Table 087, because the coder notices that there is no body part value for *right lacrimal canaliculus,* the ICD-10-PCS index is referenced again. Main term *right lacrimal canaliculus* directs the coder to use *Lacrimal Duct, Right* in the table. Thus, fourth character X (right) is selected. In addition, fifth character 8 (via natural or artificial opening endoscopic), sixth character Z (no device), and seventh character Z (no device) are selected. As a result, ICD-10-PCS code 087X8ZZ is constructed.

(continues)

Example (continued):

ICD-10-PCS Table				
087				
Section	**0**	Medical and Surgical		
Body System	**8**	Eye		
Operation	**7**	Dilation: Expanding an orifice or the lumen of a tubular body part		
Body Part	*Approach*		*Device*	*Qualifier*
X Lacrimal Duct, Right **Y** Lacrimal Duct, Left	**0** Open **3** Percutaneous **7** Via Natural or Artificial Opening **8** Via Natural or Artificial Opening Endoscopic		**D** Intraluminal Device **Z** No Device	**Z** No qualifier

NOTE:

- The ICD-10-PCS index contains a hierarchical alphabetical lookup for locating a table that includes supplemental procedure terms (e.g., appendectomy) that correspond to root operation options. (The hierarchy includes boldfaced main terms, indented subterms, and indented qualifiers.)
- It is not possible to construct an ICD-10-PCS procedure code from the index. The purpose of the index is to locate the appropriate table that contains all information necessary to construct a procedure code.
- Coders are not required to consult the index before proceeding to the tables to construct an ICD-10-PCS code. A valid code can be constructed directly from the tables (by locating the appropriate section, body system, and root operation table). However, the index provides guidance to the appropriate table.

Exercise 6.2 – ICD-10-PCS Index

6.2A – Completion

Instructions: Complete each statement.

1. The ICD-10-PCS index is an alphabetical listing of procedures that usually includes the first 3–6 (and sometimes all 7) _____ of the procedure code.

2. When the index provides a seven-character code, the coder should always consult the appropriate ICD-10-PCS _____ to verify that the code is valid.

3. It is not possible to construct a procedure code by using just the ICD-10-PCS _____.

4. The Medical and Surgical section tables are referenced by locating _____ operations as main terms in the ICD-10-PCS index.

5. Coders are directed to the appropriate root operation as the main term in the ICD-10-PCS index for surgical procedures such as *Appendectomy*, which is considered a _____ procedure term.

6. The ICD-10-PCS Ancillary section tables (except for Radiation Therapy) contain root _____ as the third character.

7. ICD-10-PCS Radiation Therapy section tables contain _____ as the third character.

8. ICD-10-PCS index terms *see* and *use*, which direct coders to alternate terms in the index or tables, are considered _____.

(continues)

Exercise 6.2 – continued

9. Refer to Figure 6-2, and locate common procedure name *Abdominohysterectomy* and its cross reference. The coder is directed to *see* _____ as the root operation in the ICD-10-PCS index or table.

10. Refer to Figure 6-2, and locate *Accessory phrenic nerve* and its cross reference. The coder is directed to *use* _____ as the anatomic site in the ICD-10-PCS tables.

6.2B – Using the ICD-10-PCS Index

Instructions: Use the ICD-10-PCS index *only* to enter the portion of the code for each procedure. Answers may be less than seven characters in length.

_____ 1. Manually assisted delivery

_____ 2. Magnetic resonance imaging (MRI), left breast

_____ 3. Termination of pregnancy, dilation and curettage

_____ 4. Heart transplantation

_____ 5. Ultrasonography, abdomen

6.2C – ICD-10-PCS Index *With*

Instructions: Use the ICD-10-PCS index *only* to enter the portion of the code for each procedure. Answers may be less than seven characters in length.

_____ 1. Computer-assisted procedure of the lower extremity with computerized tomography

_____ 2. Herniorrhaphy, abdominal wall, with synthetic substitute

_____ 3. Interrogation, cardiac rhythm-related device, with cardiac function testing

_____ 4. Phacoemulsification of right lens, with intraocular lens implant

_____ 5. Vasotomy with ligation, bilateral vas deferens, percutaneous approach

6.2D – ICD-10-PCS Index *Cross References*

Instructions: Use the ICD-10-PCS index *only* to enter the cross reference for each procedure. For example, *see* Extraction is the answer for index entry "Abrasion *see* Extraction," and *use* Brain is the answer for index entry "Cerebrum *use* Brain."

_____ 1. Abrasion

_____ 2. Achillorrhaphy

_____ 3. Canthorrhaphy

_____ 4. Accessory obturator nerve

_____ 5. Cardiac event recorder

ICD-10-PCS Tables

ICD-10-PCS **Tables** are used to construct a complete and valid code (using a *build-a-code approach*) using characters from a table's rows and columns (Figure 6-3). Each character has an associated *value* (term), which is selected to construct a valid seven-character ICD-10-PCS code.

- The top three rows of each table include values for the first three characters of a code, including definitions of root operations, root procedure types, and modalities.

- The next row includes headings for the fourth through seventh characters and values, with the characters and values appearing in columns below each heading.

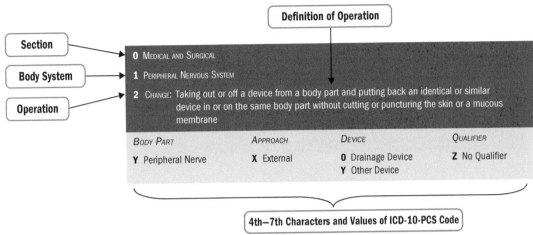

FIGURE 6-3 ICD-10-PCS Table 012 with rows and columns that contain characters and values

 NOTE:

- Some ICD-10-PCS tables are extensive, and coders must continue on to the next page of the coding manual to build an accurate code. (Coders say "a table bleeds onto the next page" to describe this.)
- In ICD-10-PCS, the term "procedure" refers to the complete specification of the seven characters that comprise a complete code. The first character of the seven-character code always specifies the section. Then, depending on the ICD-10-PCS section in which a procedure is classified, the values of characters 2–7 may vary. *However, the values of characters 2–7 within a particular section remain the same.*

Sections of ICD-10-PCS Tables

ICD-10-PCS tables are organized in sections (Figure 6-4) that identify the general type of procedure, and each of the seven characters in a table has a specific meaning. Within a section, all character meanings remain constant, and the first character of an ICD-10-PCS procedure code *always* specifies the section. The Medical and Surgical section and its related sections begin with characters 0–9 and X. Ancillary sections begin with characters B, C, D, F, G, and H.

ICD-10-PCS SECTIONS	
0	Medical and Surgical
1	Obstetrics
2	Placement
3	Administration
4	Measurement and Monitoring
5	Extracorporeal or Systemic Assistance and Performance
6	Extracorporeal or Systemic Therapies
7	Osteopathic
8	Other Procedures
9	Chiropractic
B	Imaging
C	Nuclear Medicine
D	Radiation Therapy
F	Physical Rehabilitation and Diagnostic Audiology
G	Mental Health
H	Substance Abuse Treatment
X	New Technology

FIGURE 6-4 ICD-10-PCS sections

Each value in an ICD-10-PCS table represents a specific option for the general character definition.

Example: The character in position two *usually* represents the body system. The Administration section of ICD-10-PCS contains just three values, only one of which is actually a body system.

0	Circulatory
C	Indwelling Device
E	Physiological Systems and Anatomical Regions

There are just four tables in the Administration section

302	Administration (section), Circulatory (body system), Transfusion (operation)
3C1	Administration (section), Indwelling Device (body system), Irrigation (operation)
3E0	Administration (section), Physiological Systems and Anatomical Regions (body system), Introduction (operation)
3E1	Administration (section), Physiological Systems and Anatomical Regions (body system), Irrigation (operation)

Build-a-Code Approach

ICD-10-PCS uses a *build-a-code approach* to classify procedures, which means one character is assigned to each of 7 axes (*multiaxial structure*). For example, code 02700ZZ is created using ICD-10-PCS Table 027 for open dilation of one coronary artery. A detailed knowledge of medical terminology, anatomy and physiology, and ICD-10-PCS's unique vocabulary associated with root operations, root types, and modalities requires mastery when building codes.

The ICD-10-PCS code assigned is the result of a *build-a-code approach* after locating the procedure term in an index and a table. The 10 digits 0–9 and the 24 letters A–H, J–N, and P–Z may be used in each of the 7 characters, depending on the documented procedure. Letters I and O are not used so as to avoid confusion with numerical digits 0 and 1.

A code is built by selecting a specific value for each of the 7 characters (Figure 6-5). ICD-10-PCS procedures are first divided into sections (Figure 6-5, column 1), which identify the general type of procedure (e.g., medical and surgical, obstetrics, imaging).

- The first character of the 7-character procedure code always specifies the section.
- While characters 2–7 have the same meaning within a section, they may have different meanings in different sections (Figure 6-5, columns 2–7).
- Within all sections, the third character specifies either the operation, type (of procedure performed), or modality.
- Characters 4–7 provide additional information (e.g., body part, approach) to build the procedure code.
- Then, depending on the ICD-10-PCS section in which a procedure is classified, the values of characters 2–7 may vary (Figure 6-5, columns 2–7). *However, the values of characters 2–7 within a particular section remain the same.*

Meaning of Each Character Within a Section						
Section (1st)	2nd	3rd	4th	5th	6th	7th
Medical and Surgical	Body system	Operation	Body part	Approach	Device	Qualifier
Obstetrics	Body system	Operation	Body part	Approach	Device	Qualifier
Placement	Body system	Operation	Body region	Approach	Device	Qualifier
Administration	Body system	Operation	Body system/ region	Approach	Substance	Qualifier
Measurement and Monitoring	Body system	Operation	Body system	Approach	Function/ Device	Qualifier
Extracorporeal or Systemic Assistance and Performance	Physiological system	Operation	Body system	Duration	Function	Qualifier
Extracorporeal or Systemic Therapies	Physiological system	Operation	Body system	Duration	Qualifier	Qualifier
Osteopathic	Body system	Operation	Body region	Approach	Method	Qualifier
Other Procedures	Body system	Operation	Body region	Approach	Method	Qualifier
Chiropractic	Body system	Operation	Body region	Approach	Method	Qualifier
Imaging	Body system	Type	Body part	Contrast	Qualifier	Qualifier
Nuclear Medicine	Body system	Type	Body part	Radionuclide	Qualifier	Qualifier
Radiation Therapy	Body system	Modality	Treatment site	Modality qualifier	Isotope	Qualifier
Physical Rehabilitation and Diagnostic Audiology	Section qualifier	Type	Body system/ region	Type qualifier	Equipment	Qualifier
Mental Health	Body system	Type	Qualifier	Qualifier	Qualifier	Qualifier
Substance Abuse Treatment	Body system	Type	Qualifier	Qualifier	Qualifier	Qualifier
New Technology	Body system	Operation	Body part	Approach	Device/ Substance/ Technology	Qualifier

FIGURE 6-5 Value assigned to each character in a 7-character ICD-10-PCS code

Valid Characters

All seven characters of an ICD-10-PCS code must contain valid characters (selected from the appropriate table) to construct a valid code. If documentation is incomplete for coding purposes, query the physician for the necessary information. According to ICD-10-PCS coding guidelines, the coder is *not* required to query the physician when the correlation between documentation and defined ICD-10-PCS terms is clear (e.g., surgeon documents *partial resection* and coder determines that root operation *excision* applies).

Within an ICD-10-PCS table, valid characters include all combinations of choices for the fourth through seventh characters that are contained in the same row of a table. Columns in ICD-10-PCS tables contain values for characters 4 through 7. Rows in ICD-10-PCS tables contain valid combinations of characters. Any combination of characters *not* contained in a single row of an ICD-10-PCS table is invalid (and results in construction of an invalid code if used).

When the fourth character of the ICD-10-PCS codes indicates an *anatomical site* or *body part* that cannot be found in the table, locate them in the index. Follow the *use* cross reference in the index, which provides direction to an alternate term for the anatomical site or body part in an ICD-10-PCS table and select an appropriate value.

When the sixth character of an ICD-10-PCS code indicates a *device*, a character is assigned only when a device is inserted (e.g., pacemaker, drain). In many cases, ICD-10-PCS tables include just one option for a device, the letter Z (no device). When the name of the documented device cannot be found in the ICD-10-PCS table, refer to the index to locate the device name. Then, follow the *use* cross reference for direction to an alternate term located in the table and select an appropriate value.

Example: In this portion of a Medical and Surgical section table, notice that 0JHT3VZ is a valid code; however, 0JHW3VZ is *not* a valid code. The "V" in code 0JHW3VZ is *not* valid for the sixth character device character because it is associated with the *subcutaneous tissue and fascia, trunk* body part, not the *subcutaneous tissue and fascia, lower extremity* body part.

Section	0	Medical and Surgical
Body System	J	Subcutaneous Tissue and Fascia
Operation	H	Insertion: Putting in a nonbiological appliance that monitors, assists, performs, or prevents a physiological function but does not physically take the place of a body part

Body Part	Approach	Device	Qualifier
S Subcutaneous Tissue and Fascia, Head and Neck V Subcutaneous Tissue and Fascia, Upper Extremity W Subcutaneous Tissue and Fascia, Lower Extremity	0 Open 3 Percutaneous	1 Radioactive Element 3 Infusion Device Y Other Device	Z No Qualifier
T Subcutaneous Tissue and Fascia, Trunk	0 Open 3 Percutaneous	1 Radioactive Element 3 Infusion Device V Infusion Pump Y Other Device	Z No Qualifier

 NOTE:

Cross-reference *use* does not provide direction to a specific ICD-10-PCS table. Coders have already located the appropriate table based on the procedure performed. The *use* cross reference indicates the value to be selected from the table.

Step-by-Step Approach to Constructing a Valid ICD-10-PCS Code

A step-by-step approach is used to construct an ICD-10-PCS code, as follows:

Step 1   After identifying the name of the procedure performed in the operative report, locate the main term in the ICD-10-PCS Index.

Step 2   After following any instructional notes (e.g., *see*, *use*) present after a main term, locate the appropriate main term and subterm(s) to identify the first 3 (or 4–5) values of a 7-character code.

Example: When a physician creates a shunt for the spinal canal, ICD-10-PCS index main term *Shunt creation* includes a cross reference to *see* Bypass. The coder goes to ICD-10-PCS main term *Bypass* and subterm *Spinal Canal 001U*. Table 001 in ICD-10-PCS is referenced where the remainder of the code is selected.

ICD-10-PCS Index
S
Shortening
see Excision
see Repair
see Reposition
Shunt creation *see* Bypass

ICD-10-PCS Index
B
Bypass
Spinal Canal 001U
Stomach 0D16
Trachea 0B11
Ureter

Step 3   Locate the ICD-10-PCS table that corresponds to the first 3 values of a seven-character code, and review the procedure performed to assign a character to each position in the complete seven-character code.

Example: The patient underwent an *open bypass from the spinal canal to the peritoneal cavity using synthetic substitute* procedure to decrease cerebrospinal fluid levels. Use the step-by-step approach to constructing an ICD-10-PCS code, and review the yellow-highlighted content in Table 001 to *build-a-code*.

- Table 001 is selected to construct the code because the documented procedure is located in the Medical and Surgical section (character 0), Central Nervous System body system (character 0), and Bypass root operation (character 1). (*Bypass* is defined in the table to help ensure the accuracy of creating the code).
- To construct the code, the fourth through seventh character values need to be selected from the columns based on documentation of the procedure included in the example.
  - Character U is selected as the fourth character value for spinal canal as the body part.
  - Character 0 is selected as the fifth character value for open as the approach.
  - Character J is selected as the sixth character value for synthetic substitute as the device.
  - Character 6 is selected as the seventh character value for peritoneal cavity as the qualifier.

Section	0	Medical and Surgical		
Body System	0	Central Nervous System		
Operation	1	Bypass: Altering the route of passage of the contents of a tubular body part		

Body Part	Approach	Device	Qualifier
6 Cerebral Ventricle	0 Open 3 Percutaneous 4 Percutaneous Endoscopic	7 Autologous Tissue Substitute J Synthetic Substitute K Nonautologous Tissue Substitute	0 Nasopharynx 1 Mastoid Sinus 2 Atrium 3 Blood Vessel 4 Pleural Cavity 5 Intestine 6 Peritoneal Cavity 7 Urinary Tract 8 Bone Marrow A Subgaleal Space B Cerebral Cisterns
6 Cerebral Ventricle	0 Open 3 Percutaneous 4 Percutaneous Endoscopic	Z No Device	B Cerebral Cisterns
U Spinal Canal	0 Open 3 Percutaneous 4 Percutaneous Endoscopic	7 Autologous Tissue Substitute J Synthetic Substitute K Nonautologous Tissue Substitute	2 Atrium 4 Pleural Cavity 6 Peritoneal Cavity 7 Urinary Tract 9 Fallopian Tube

Exercise 6.3 – ICD-10-PCS Tables

6.3A – Completion

Instructions: Complete each statement.

1. ICD-10-PCS tables are used to _____ (or build) a complete and valid code using a *build-a-code approach*.

2. The rows and columns of ICD-10-PCS tables include characters and terms, called _____, which are selected to build the seven-character code.

(continues)

Exercise 6.3 – continued

3. The ICD-10-PCS tables are organized in _____ that identify the general type of procedure, and each of the seven characters in a table has a specific meaning.

4. Refer to Figure 6-3. New Technology section codes begin with the letter _____.

5. The letters I and _____ are never used in ICD-10-PCS codes.

6. Refer to Figure 6-5. The value (term) associated with character 5 of the Medical and Surgical section is the _____.

7. According to ICD-10-PCS coding guidelines, the coder is not required to _____ (or ask a question of) the physician when the correlation between documentation and defined ICD-10-PCS terms is clear.

8. Any combination of characters *not* contained in a single row of an ICD-10-PCS table is _____ (or inaccurate).

9. Refer to Figure 6-3. ICD-10-PCS code 012YX0Z is a valid code. The one other valid code that can be constructed using ICD-10-PCS Table 012 is _____.

10. Use the step-by-step approach to construct an ICD-10-PCS code for an *open procedure of the spinal canal to insert a subarachnoid-pleural shunt using autologous tissue substitute for the purpose of decreasing cerebrospinal fluid levels via bypass (using the shunt) to the peritoneal cavity*. The ICD-10-PCS code is _____.

6.3B – Using ICD-10-PCS Tables

Instructions: Refer to Table 0JH, and construct an ICD-10-PCS code for each procedure. (The first three characters of each code will be 0JH.)

ICD-10-PCS Table				
0JH				
Section	**0**	Medical and Surgical		
Body System	**J**	Subcutaneous Tissue and Fascia		
Operation	**H**	Insertion: Putting in a nonbiological appliance that monitors, assists, performs, or prevents a physiological function but does not physically take the place of a body part		
Body Part		*Approach*	*Device*	*Device*
S Subcutaneous Tissue and Fascia, Head and Neck **V** Subcutaneous Tissue and Fascia, Upper Extremity **W** Subcutaneous Tissue and Fascia, Lower Extremity		**0** Open **3** Percutaneous	**1** Radioactive Element **3** Infusion Device **Y** Other Device	**Z** No Qualifier
T Subcutaneous Tissue and Fascia, Trunk		**0** Open **3** Percutaneous	**1** Radioactive Element **3** Infusion Device **V** Infusion Device, Pump **Y** Other Device	**Z** No Qualifier

_____ 1. Insertion of radioactive element, subcutaneous tissue of neck, open approach

_____ 2. Insertion of infusion device, subcutaneous tissue and fascia, trunk, percutaneous approach

_____ 3. Insertion of radioactive element, subcutaneous tissue of lower leg, percutaneous approach

Exercise 6.3 – continued

_____   4. Insertion of wound vacuum device, fascia of upper extremity, open approach

_____   5. Insertion of infusion pump into subcutaneous tissue, trunk, open approach

6.3C – Using the ICD-10-PCS Coding Manual: Index and Tables

Instructions: Use the ICD-10-PCS index and tables to assign an appropriate code for each procedure.

Remember! The ICD-10-PCS index entry usually contains just the first three or four characters of a code, which provides direction to the appropriate table to "build a code." When the entire seven-character code is provided in the index, verify its accuracy in the appropriate ICD-10-PCS table.

_____   1. Diagnostic open biopsy, left axillary lymph nodes

_____   2. Open cholecystectomy, total

_____   3. Cystoscopy

_____   4. Exploratory laparotomy, open

_____   5. Intravenous right pyelogram (using fluoroscopy)

_____   6. Total appendectomy (open)

_____   7. Open biopsy of left frontal nasal sinus

_____   8. Percutaneous biopsy of prostate

_____   9. Right frontal craniotomy, open

_____   10. Transurethral biopsy of bladder

ICD-10-PCS Official Guidelines for Coding and Reporting

The _ICD-10-PCS Official Guidelines for Coding and Reporting_, as approved by the Cooperating Parties for the ICD-10-PCS (that include the AMA, AHIMA, CMS, and NCHS), are a set of rules that have been developed to accompany and complement coding conventions and instructions provided within ICD-10-PCS. (NCHS is an agency of the CDC.) They provide direction that is applicable in most circumstances; however, there may be unique circumstances where exceptions apply. (The instructions and conventions of the classification take precedence over the guidelines.)

The guidelines are based on the coding and sequencing instructions in the ICD-10-PCS definitions, index, and tables, but provide additional instruction. Adherence to the guidelines when assigning ICD-10-PCS procedure codes is required under the Health Insurance Portability and Accountability Act (HIPAA), which also requires the adoption of the codes for hospital inpatient health care settings.

A joint effort between the health care provider and the coder is essential to achieve complete and accurate documentation, code assignment, and reporting of (diagnoses and) procedures. The guidelines were developed to assist both the health care provider and the coder in identifying procedures to be reported. Consistent, complete documentation in the patient record is crucial to accurate coding.

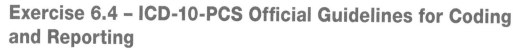

Exercise 6.4 – ICD-10-PCS Official Guidelines for Coding and Reporting

Instructions: Complete each statement.

1. The *ICD-10-PCS Official Guidelines for Coding and Reporting* were approved by the four organizations that make up the _____ Parties for the ICD-10-PCS.

2. Official coding guidelines are a set of _____ developed to accompany and complement coding conventions and instructions provided within ICD-10-PCS.

3. A joint effort between the health care provider and the coder is essential to achieve complete and accurate _____, code assignment, and reporting of (diagnoses and) procedures.

4. Official coding guidelines were developed to assist both the health care provider and the coder in identifying procedures to be _____.

5. Consistent, complete documentation in the patient record is crucial to _____ coding.

ICD-10-PCS Coding Conventions

ICD-10-PCS **coding conventions** are general rules used in the ICD-10-PCS classification system that are independent of coding guidelines and provide for coding consistency. The coding conventions in CMS's *ICD-10-PCS Official Guidelines for Coding and Reporting* are labeled A1 through A11. (To facilitate student learning, a title for each coding convention, A1–A11, was created for this chapter.)

A1 – Structure of Codes

ICD-10-PCS codes are composed of seven characters. Each character is an axis of classification that specifies information about the procedure performed. Within a defined code range, a character specifies the same type of information in that axis of classification.

Example: The fifth axis of classification specifies the *approach* in section values 0 through 4, 7 through 9, and X. Because each Medical and Surgical table begins with first-character 0, the fifth character is always the *approach*.

ICD-10-PCS Table			
OKH			
Section	**0**	Medical and Surgical	
Body System	**K**	Muscles	
Operation	**H**	Insertion: Putting in a nonbiological appliance that monitors, assists, performs, or prevents a physiological function but does not physically take the place of a body part	
Body Part	*Approach*	*Device*	*Qualifier*
X Upper Muscle **Y** Lower Muscle	**0** Open **3** Percutaneous **4** Percutaneous Endoscopic	**M** Stimulator Lead **Y** Other Device	**Z** No Qualifier

A2 – Unique Values

One of 34 possible values can be assigned to each axis of classification in the seven-character code. They are the numbers 0 through 9 and the alphabet *(except letters I and O because they are easily confused with numbers 1 and 0)*. The number of unique values used in an axis of classification differs as needed.

Example: Where the fifth axis of classification is an approach, different values are used to specify the type of approach.

ICD-10-PCS Table				
095				
Section	**0**	Medical and Surgical		
Body System	**9**	Ear, Nose, Sinus		
Operation	**5**	Destruction: Physical eradication of all or a portion of a body part by the direct use of energy, force, or a destructive agent		
Body Part	*Approach*		*Device*	*Qualifier*
3 External Auditory Canal, Right **4** External Auditory Canal, Left	**0** Open **3** Percutaneous **4** Percutaneous Endoscopic **7** Via Natural or Artificial Opening **8** Via Natural or Artificial Opening Endoscopic **X** External		**Z** No Device	**Z** No Qualifier

A3 – Expanding Values

The valid values for an axis of classification can be added as needed [by CMS].

Example: If a significantly distinct type of device is used in a new procedure, a new device value can be added to ICD-10-PCS tables.

Surgical glue is commonly used during procedures. However, there are currently no *device* values for surgical glue listed in the *Skin and Breast body system* and the *Revision root operation* for the *Medical and Surgical section*. Thus, value Y (other device) is selected to classify surgical glue, creating code 0HWPXYZ.

ICD-10-PCS Table				
0HW				
Section	**0**	Medical and Surgical		
Body System	**H**	Skin and Breast		
Operation	**W**	Revision: Correcting, to the extent possible, a portion of a malfunctioning device or the position of a displaced device		
Body Part	*Approach*	*Device*		*Qualifier*
P Skin	**X** External	**0** Drainage Device **7** Autologous Tissue Substitute **J** Synthetic Substitute **K** Nonautologous Tissue Substitute **Y** Other Device		**Z** No Qualifier

A4 – Meaning of a Single Value

As with words in their context, the meaning of any single value is a combination of its axis of classification and any preceding values on which it may be dependent.

Example: The meaning of a body part value in the Medical and Surgical section is always dependent on the body system value. The body part value 1 in the Central Nervous System and Cranial Nerves body system specifies Cerebral Meninges, and body part character 1 in the Peripheral Nervous body system specifies Cervical Nerve.

ICD-10-PCS Table			
00U			
Section	**0**	Medical and Surgical	
Body System	**0**	Central Nervous System and Cranial Nerves	
Operation	**U**	Supplement: Putting in or on biological or synthetic material that physically reinforces and/or augments the function of a portion of a body part	
Body Part	**Approach**	**Device**	**Qualifier**
1 Cerebral Meninges 2 Dura Mater 6 Cerebral Ventricle F Olfactory Nerve G Optic Nerve H Oculomotor Nerve J Trochlear Nerve K Trigeminal Nerve L Abducens Nerve M Facial Nerve N Acoustic Nerve P Glossopharyngeal Nerve Q Vagus Nerve R Accessory Nerve S Hypoglossal Nerve T Spinal Meninges	0 Open 3 Percutaneous 4 Percutaneous Endoscopic	7 Autologous Tissue Substitute J Synthetic Substitute K Nonautologous Tissue Substitute	Z No Qualifier

ICD-10-PCS Table			
01U			
Section	**0**	Medical and Surgical	
Body System	**1**	Peripheral Nervous System	
Operation	**U**	Supplement: Putting in or on biological or synthetic material that physically reinforces and/or augments the function of a portion of a body part	
Body Part	**Approach**	**Device**	**Qualifier**
1 Cervical Nerve 2 Phrenic Nerve 4 Ulnar Nerve 5 Median Nerve 6 Radial Nerve 8 Thoracic Nerve B Lumbar Nerve C Pudendal Nerve D Femoral Nerve F Sciatic Nerve G Tibial Nerve H Peroneal Nerve R Sacral Nerve	0 Open 3 Percutaneous 4 Percutaneous Endoscopic	7 Autologous Tissue Substitute J Synthetic Substitute K Nonautologous Tissue Substitute	Z No Qualifier

A5 – Increasing Detail in ICD-10-PCS Codes

As ICD-10-PCS is expanded to become increasingly detailed, over time more values will depend on preceding values for their meaning.

Example: In the Lower Joints body system, device value 3 in the root operation Insertion specifies Infusion Device, while device value 3 in the root operation Replacement specifies Ceramic Synthetic Substitute.

ICD-10-PCS Table (portion)			
0SH			
Section	**0**	Medical and Surgical	
Body System	**S**	Lower Joints	
Operation	**H**	Insertion: Putting in a nonbiological appliance that monitors, assists, performs, or prevents a physiological function but does not physically take the place of a body part	
Body Part	*Approach*	*Device*	*Qualifier*
2 Lumbar Vertebral Disc **4** Lumbosacral Disc	**0** Open **3** Percutaneous **4** Percutaneous Endoscopic	**3** Infusion Device **8** Spacer	**Z** No Qualifier

ICD-10-PCS Table (portion)			
0SR			
Section	**0**	*Medical and Surgical*	
Body System	**S**	Lower Joints	
Operation	**R**	Replacement: Putting in or on biological or synthetic material that physically takes the place and/or function of all or a portion of a body part	
Body Part	*Approach*	*Device*	*Qualifier*
R Hip Joint, Femoral Surface, Right **S** Hip Joint, Femoral Surface, Left	**0** Open	**1** Synthetic Substitute, Metal **3** Synthetic Substitute, Ceramic **J** Synthetic Substitute	**9** Cemented **A** Uncemented **Z** No Qualifier

A6 – Index and Tables

The purpose of the ICD-10-PCS alphabetic index is to locate the appropriate table(s) that contains all information necessary to construct a procedure code. The ICD-10-PCS table(s) should always be consulted to find the most appropriate valid code.

 NOTE:

Content about the ICD-10-PCS index and its tables was previously covered in this chapter.

A7 – Coding Directly From Tables

It is not required to consult the ICD-10-PCS index first before proceeding to its tables to complete the code. A valid code may be chosen directly from the ICD-10-PCS tables.

Example: There is just one Chiropractic Section table, which means a coder who assigns inpatient procedure codes for chiropractic services may go directly to ICD-10-PCS Table 9WB to construct the code(s).

ICD-10-PCS Table			
9WB			
Section	**9**	Chiropractic	
Body System	**W**	Anatomical Regions	
Operation	**B**	Manipulation: Manual procedure that involves a directed thrust to move a joint past the physiological range of motion, without exceeding the anatomical limit	
Body Region	*Approach*	*Method*	*Qualifier*
0 Head **1** Cervical **2** Thoracic **3** Lumbar **4** Sacrum **5** Pelvis **6** Lower Extremities **7** Upper Extremities **8** Rib Cage **9** Abdomen	**E** External	**B** Non-Manual **C** Indirect Visceral **D** Extra-Articular **F** Direct Visceral **G** Long Lever Specific Contact **H** Short Lever Specific Contact **J** Long and Short Lever Specific Contact **K** Mechanically Assisted **L** Other Method	**Z** No Qualifier

A8 – Valid Codes: Seven Alphanumeric Characters

All seven alphanumeric characters must be specified to be a valid code. If the documentation is incomplete for coding purposes, the physician should be queried for the necessary information.

Example: Code HZ2ZZZZ is reported for detoxication, which is classified in the Substance Treatment section of ICD-10-PCS.

ICD-10-PCS Table			
HZ2			
Section	**H**	Substance Abuse Treatment	
Body System	**Z**	None	
Operation	**2**	Detoxification Services: Detoxification from alcohol and/or drugs	
Qualifier	*Qualifier*	*Qualifier*	*Qualifier*
Z None	**Z** None	**Z** None	**Z** None

A9 – Valid Codes: Selecting Characters 4–7 in the Same Row of a Table

Within an ICD-10-PCS table, valid codes include all combinations of choices for characters 4 through 7, contained in the same row of the table.

Example: For Table 0JH, code 0JHT3VZ is valid. Code 0JHW3VZ is not a valid code because character V is not included in the Device column for character W (Subcutaneous Tissue and Fascia, Lower Extremity).

- A border line separates Body Part characters S, V, and W from Body Part character T.
- Device characters 1, 3, and Y only are to be selected for body part characters S, V, and W.

ICD-10-PCS Table			
0JH			
Section	**0**	Medical and Surgical	
Body System	**J**	Subcutaneous Tissue and Fascia	
Operation	**H**	Insertion: Putting in a nonbiological appliance that monitors, assists, performs, or prevents a physiological function but does not physically take the place of a body part	
Body Part		*Approach*	*Device*	*Device*
S Subcutaneous Tissue and Fascia, Head and Neck **V** Subcutaneous Tissue and Fascia, Upper Extremity **W** Subcutaneous Tissue and Fascia, Lower Extremity		**0** Open **3** Percutaneous	**1** Radioactive Element **3** Infusion Device **Y** Other Device	**Z** No Qualifier
T Subcutaneous Tissue and Fascia, Trunk		**0** Open **3** Percutaneous	**1** Radioactive Element **3** Infusion Device **V** Infusion Device, Pump **Y** Other Device	**Z** No Qualifier

A10 – And

"And," when used in a code description, means "and/or" except when used to describe a combination of multiple body parts for which separate values exist for each body part (e.g., *Skin and Subcutaneous Tissue* used as a qualifier, where there are separate body part values for *Skin* and *Subcutaneous Tissue*).

Example: In ICD-10-PCS Table 3E0, the *and* in the Body System title means procedures performed on Physiological Systems *or* Anatomical Regions are classified in the body systems. The *and* in the Body System/Region column for Skin and Mucous Membranes means procedures performed on skin *or* mucous membranes are classified.

- The external administration of monoclonal antibodies into *skin* as an antineoplastic treatment is assigned code 3E00X0M.
- The external administration of monoclonal antibodies into *mucous membranes* as an antineoplastic treatment is also assigned code 3E00X0M.

ICD-10-PCS Table (portion)			
3E0			
Section	**3**	Administration	
Body System	**E**	Physiological Systems and Anatomical Regions	
Operation	**0**	Introduction: Putting in or on a therapeutic, diagnostic, nutritional, physiological, or prophylactic substance except blood or blood products	
Body System / Region	*Approach*	*Substance*	*Qualifier*
0 Skin and Mucous Membranes	**X** External	**0** Antineoplastic	**5** Other Antineoplastic **M** Monoclonal Antibody
0 Skin and Mucous Membranes	**X** External	**2** Anti-infective	**8** Oxazolidinones **9** Other Anti-infective

A11 – Definition of ICD-10-PCS Terms

Many of the terms used to construct ICD-10-PCS codes are defined within its tables and their addenda. It is the coder's responsibility to review the patient record to locate documentation that matches ICD-10-PCS code terms. *The physician is not expected to use ICD-10-PCS code description terms, and the coder is not required to query the physician when a correlation between documentation and defined ICD-10-PCS terms is clear.*

> **Example:** When the physician documents "partial resection," the coder can independently go to root operation Excision in the ICD-10-PCS index *without querying the physician for clarification.* (Excision is the cutting out or off, without replacement, a *portion* of a body part. Thus, a partial resection is an excision and not a resection.)

Exercise 6.5 – ICD-10-PCS Coding Conventions

6.5A – Completion

Instructions: Complete each statement.

1. The general rules used in the ICD-10-PCS classification system that are independent of coding guidelines and provide for coding consistency are called coding _____.

2. Within a defined ICD-10-PCS code range, a _____ and its value specify the same type of information in that axis of classification.

3. ICD-10-PCS codes are constructed using a build-a-code process, and each character has up to 34 possible _____.

4. ICD-10-PCS codes contain independent characters and values, and each axis retains its meaning across broad ranges of codes, which allows for construction of _____ seven-character codes for all substantially different procedures.

5. The meaning of any single ICD-10-PCS value is a combination of its axis of classification and any preceding values on which it may be _____ (or based).

6. As ICD-10-PCS is expanded to become increasingly detailed, over time more characters and values will depend on preceding values for their _____.

7. To construct a seven-character ICD-10-PCS code, coders can refer first to the alphabetic index; however, the tables must always be used to construct a _____ and accurate code.

8. When documentation is incomplete for coding purposes, the coder must _____ the physician to obtain necessary information.

9. When the word "and" appears in a code description, it means _____ except when used to describe a combination of multiple body parts for which separate characters and values exist for each body part.

10. Many of the terms, such as root operations, used to construct codes are defined within ICD-10-PCS _____ and the ICD-10-PCS addenda.

6.5B – Assigning ICD-10-PCS Codes Using Coding Conventions

Instructions: Use the ICD-10-PCS index and tables to construct a code for each procedure, and refer to coding conventions in this chapter to obtain clarification about constructing the code.

_____ 1. Ultrasonography of head

_____ 2. Insertion of oropharyngeal intraluminal airway device

_____ 3. Open division of muscle, left upper arm

_____ 4. Change of laryngeal drainage tube

_____ 5. Open biopsy, tonsils

ICD-10-PCS Sections and Coding Guidelines

ICD-10-PCS section coding guidelines provide direction about constructing codes, as follows:

- Medical and surgical section guidelines
  - Body system
  - Root operation
  - Body part
  - Approach
  - Device
- Obstetrics section guidelines
- Radiation therapy guidelines
- New technology section guidelines

The remaining ICD-10-PCS sections (e.g., Placement, Administration) do not currently have associated coding guidelines. However, they are included in this chapter as organized in the official ICD-10-PCS coding manual to provide important content (e.g., terms, definitions) and to allow for future expansion of official coding guidelines. (To facilitate student learning, official guideline titles are included for this chapter.)

Medical and Surgical Section Coding Guidelines

Coding guidelines associated with the *Medical and Surgical* section of ICD-10-PCS include the following topics:

- Body system
- Root operation
- Body part
- Approach
- Device

NOTE:

The official CMS coding guidelines indicator (e.g., B2.1a.) is entered at the beginning of each new guideline. This allows you to easily reference each official coding guideline within the *ICD-10-PCS Official Guidelines for Coding and Reporting.*

Body System

Official coding guidelines for Body System include general coding guidelines only.

Body System—General Guidelines

B2.1a. The procedure codes in the *Anatomical Regions, General; Anatomical Regions, Upper Extremities; and Anatomical Regions, Lower Extremities* body systems can be used *when*

- The procedure is performed on an anatomical region rather than a specific body part.
- Insufficient information is available to support the assignment of a value to a specific body part.

Example: Chest tube drainage of the pleural cavity is coded to root operation Drainage, and the pleural cavity is located in body system Anatomical Regions, General. Suture repair of the abdominal wall is coded to root operation Repair in body system Anatomical Regions, General. Amputation of the foot is coded to root operation Detachment in body system Anatomical Regions, Lower Extremities.

B2.1b. Where general body part values "upper" and "lower" are provided as an option in the Upper Arteries, Lower Arteries, Upper Veins, Lower Veins, Muscles and Tendons body systems, "upper" or "lower" *specifies body parts located above or below the diaphragm*, respectively.

> **Example:** The jugular veins are located above the diaphragm (in the neck), and they are assigned values from the *Upper Veins* body system in the *Medical and Surgical* section. The saphenous veins are located below the diaphragm (in the legs), and they are assigned values from the *Medical and Surgical* section and *Lower Veins* body system.

Root Operation

Official coding guidelines for Root Operation include the following:

- General guidelines
- Multiple procedures
- Discontinued or incomplete procedures
- Biopsy procedures
- Biopsy followed by more definitive procedure
- Overlapping body layers
- Bypass procedures
- Control vs. more specific root operations
- Excision vs. resection
- Excision for graft
- Fusion procedures of the spine

- Inspection procedures
- Occlusion vs. restriction for vessel embolization procedures
- Release procedures
- Release vs. division
- Reposition for fracture treatment
- Transplantation vs. administration
- Transfer procedures using multiple tissue layers
- Excision/Resection followed by replacement
- Detachment procedures of extremities

Root Operation—General Guidelines

B3.1a. To determine the appropriate root operation, apply the *complete* definition and explanation of the root operation (located in the ICD-10-PCS tables).

The root operation is specified in the third character, and in the *Medical and Surgical* section of ICD-10-PCS, there are 31 different root operations. The root operation identifies the objective of the procedure, and each root operation has a precise definition (Table 6-1), created specifically for ICD-10-PCS and may differ from those found in medical dictionaries and other resources.

B3.1b. Components of a procedure that are included in the root operation's definition or explanation as integral to that root operation are *not* coded separately. Procedural steps necessary to reach the operative site *and* to close the operative site, including anastomosis of a tubular body part, are also *not* coded separately.

> **Example 1:** *Resection of a joint as part of a joint replacement procedure is included in the root operation definition for Replacement and is not coded separately.* During an *open left knee joint replacement procedure using a synthetic substitute*, the original knee joint was resected. Index main term *Replacement*, subterm *Joint*, second qualifier *Knee*, third qualifier *Left* list values 0SRD. Go to ICD-10-PCS Table 0SR to construct code 0SRD0JZ for the joint replacement procedure *only*. (The resection of the original joint is *not* assigned a separate code.)

> **Example 2:** *Laparotomy performed to reach the site of an open liver biopsy is not coded separately.* A laparotomy is performed to reach the site where an open liver biopsy (diagnostic) is carried out. Index main term *Biopsy* and its subterm provide a cross reference to *see Excision with qualifier Diagnostic*. Index main term *Excision* and subterm *Liver* list values 0FB0. Go to ICD-10-PCS Table 0FB to construct code 0FB00ZX for the open liver biopsy *only*.
>
> - The index cross reference for main term *Biopsy* includes the term *Diagnostic*, which means seventh qualifier value X is assigned instead of Z.
> - The laparotomy is *not* coded separately.

TABLE 6-1 Medical and Surgical Section Root Operations and Definitions

Root Operation	Definition
Alteration	Modifying the natural anatomical structure of a body part without affecting the function of the body part
Bypass	Altering the route of passage of the contents of a tubular body part
Change	Taking out or off a device from a body part and putting back an identical or similar device in or on the same body part without cutting or puncturing the skin or a mucous membrane
Control	Stopping, or attempting to stop, postprocedural or other acute bleeding
Creation	Putting in or on biological or synthetic material to form a new body part that to the extent possible replicates the anatomic structure or function of an absent body part
Destruction	Physical eradication of all or a portion of a body part by the direct use of energy, force, or a destructive agent
Detachment	Cutting off all or a portion of the upper or lower extremities
Dilation	Expanding an orifice or the lumen of a tubular body part
Division	Cutting into a body part without draining fluids and gases from the body part in order to separate or transect a body part
Drainage	Taking or letting out fluids and gases from a body part
Excision	Cutting out or off, without replacement, a portion of a body part
Extirpation	Taking or cutting out solid matter from a body part
Extraction	Pulling or stripping out or off all or a portion of a body part by the use of force
Fragmentation	Breaking solid matter in a body part into pieces
Fusion	Joining together portions of an articular body part rendering the articular body part immobile
Insertion	Putting in a nonbiological appliance that monitors, assists, performs, or prevents a physiological function but does not physically take the place of a body part
Inspection	Visually or manually exploring a body part
Map	Locating the route of passage of electrical impulses and locating functional areas in a body part
Occlusion	Completely closing an orifice or lumen of a tubular body part
Reattachment	Putting back in or on all or a portion of a separated body part to its normal location or other suitable location
Release	Freeing a body part from an abnormal physical constraint by cutting or by the use of force
Removal	Taking out or off a device from a body part
Repair	Restoring, to the extent possible, a body part to its normal anatomical structure and function
Replacement	Putting in or on biological or synthetic material that physically takes the place and/or function of all or a portion of a body part
Reposition	Moving to its normal location or other suitable location all or a portion of a body part
Resection	Cutting out or off, without replacement, all of a body part
Restriction	Partially closing an orifice or lumen of a tubular body part
Revision	Correcting, to the extent possible, a portion of a malfunctioning device or the position of a displaced device
Supplement	Putting in or on biological or synthetic material that physically reinforces and/or augments the function of a portion of a body part
Transfer	Moving, without taking out, all or a portion of a body part to another location to take over the function of all or a portion of a body part
Transplantation	Putting in or on all or a portion of a living body part taken from another individual or animal to physically take the place and/or function of all or a portion of a similar body part

Root Operation—Multiple Procedures

B3.2. During the same operative episode, multiple procedures are coded *if* the

- Same root operation (e.g., excision, replacement) is performed on different body parts, as defined by distinct values of the body part axis of classification.

> **Example:** Two different ICD-10-PCS codes are constructed for diagnostic excision (e.g., biopsy) of the liver and of the pancreas.
>
> - Index main term *Biopsy* and its subterm provide a cross reference to *see Excision with qualifier Diagnostic*. Index main term *Excision* and subterm *Liver* list values 0FB0. Go to ICD-10-PCS Table 0FB to construct code 0FB00ZX for the liver biopsy.
> - Index main term *Excision* and subterm *Pancreas* list values 0FBG. Return to ICD-10-PCS Table 0FB to construct code 0FBG0ZX for the pancreatic biopsy.
> - The index cross reference for main term *Biopsy* includes the term *Diagnostic*, which means seventh qualifier value X is assigned (instead of Z).

- Same root operation is repeated at different body sites that are included in the same body part axis of classification.

> **Example:** Two ICD-10-PCS codes are constructed for *biopsies of the right sartorius muscle and right gracilis muscle*, both of which are classified to the *Upper Leg Muscle, Right* body part.
>
> - Index main term *Biopsy* and its subterm provide a cross reference to *see Excision with qualifier Diagnostic*. Index main term *Excision*, subterm *Muscle*, second qualifier *Upper Leg*, and third qualifier *Right* list values 0KBQ. Go to ICD-10-PCS Table 0KB to construct both codes 0KBQ3ZX (right sartorius muscle) and 0KBQ3ZX (right gracilis muscle).
> - The codes are identical (and both are reported) because the biopsy was performed on two different muscles, which are considered two different body sites within the same *Upper Leg Muscle, Right*, body part axis of classification.
> - The index cross reference for main term *Biopsy* includes the term *Diagnostic*, which means seventh qualifier value X is assigned (instead of Z).

 NOTE:

> Root operation names and definitions were created specifically for ICD-10-PCS and may differ from those found in medical dictionaries and other resources.

- Multiple root operations with distinct objectives are performed on the same body part.

> **Example:** Two codes are constructed for *Endoscopic destruction of lesion, sigmoid colon*, and *bypass of sigmoid colon, open*.
>
> - Index main term *Destruction*, subterm *Colon*, and second qualifier *Sigmoid* list values 0D5N. Go to ICD-10-PCS Table 0D5 to construct code 0D5N8ZZ.
> - Index main term *Bypass*, subterm *Colon*, and second qualifier *Sigmoid* list values 0D1N. Go to ICD-10-PCS Table 0D1 to construct code 0D1N0ZN.

- Intended root operation is attempted using one approach, but it is converted to a different approach.

> **Example:** *Laparoscopic cholecystectomy converted to an open cholecystectomy* is assigned two codes: one for the percutaneous endoscopic *Inspection* root operation and a different code for the open *Resection* root operation.
>
> - Index main term *Inspection* and subterm *Gallbladder* list values 0FJ4. Go to ICD-10-PCS Table 0FJ to construct code 0FJ44ZZ.
> - Index main term *Resection* and subterm *Gallbladder* list values 0FT4. Go to ICD-10-PCS Table 0FT to construct code 0FT40ZZ.

Root Operation—Discontinued or Incomplete Procedures

B3.3. When the intended procedure is discontinued or otherwise not completed, code the procedure to the root operation performed.

> **Example:** A planned *total abdominal hysterectomy was discontinued after resecting just the uterus, leaving the ovaries and fallopian tubes intact* because there was no evidence of dysplasia. Index main term *Hysterectomy* and subterm *total* provide a cross reference to *see Resection, Uterus OUT9*. Go to ICD-10-PCS Table OUT to construct code OUT90ZZ. (If bilateral ovaries and fallopian tubes had also been resected, codes OUT20ZZ and OUT70ZZ would also be constructed.)

When a procedure is discontinued before any other root operation is performed, assign a code to the *Inspection* root operation of the body part or anatomical region inspected.

> **Example:** A planned *aortic valve replacement procedure was discontinued after initial thoracotomy, but before any incision was made into the heart muscle*, due to the patient becoming hemodynamically unstable. Index main term *Inspection* and subterm *Mediastinum* list values OWJC. Go to ICD-10-PCS Table OWJ to construct code OWJCOZZ.
>
> - Do not go to index main term *Thoracotomy* because its cross reference is to *see Drainage, Anatomical Regions, General OW9*, which was not the procedure performed.
> - The coding guideline provides direction to locate index main term *Inspection*, and the subterm is the body part or anatomical region that was inspected.

Root Operation—Biopsy Procedures

B3.4a. Biopsy procedures are coded using the root operations Excision, Extraction, or Drainage and the qualifier Diagnostic.

> **Example 1:** Fine needle aspiration biopsy of lung is coded to the root operation Drainage with qualifier Diagnostic.

> **Example 2:** Biopsy of bone marrow is coded to the root operation Extraction with qualifier Diagnostic.

> **Example 3:** Lymph node sampling for biopsy is coded to the root operation Excision with qualifier Diagnostic.

Root Operation—Biopsy Followed by More Definitive Treatment

B3.4b. If a diagnostic excision, extraction, or drainage procedure (biopsy) is followed by a more definitive procedure (e.g., destruction, excision, resection) *at the same procedure site*, assign separate codes for the biopsy and the more definitive treatment.

> **Example:** For *open biopsy of left breast with open left partial mastectomy*, assign a code for the biopsy *and* a separate code for the partial mastectomy.
>
> - Index main term *Biopsy* provides a cross reference to *see Excision with qualifier Diagnostic*. Index main term *Excision*, subterm *Breast*, and second qualifier *Left* list values OHBU. Go to ICD-10-PCS Table OHB to construct code OHBUOZX. (The index cross reference for main term *Biopsy* includes the term *Diagnostic*, which means seventh qualifier value X is assigned instead of Z.)
> - Index main term *Mastectomy* includes a cross reference to *see Excision, Skin and Breast OHB*. Go to ICD-10-PCS Table OHB to construct code OHBUOZZ.

Root Operation—Overlapping Body Layers

B3.5. When root operations Excision, Extraction, Repair, or Inspection are performed on overlapping layers of the musculoskeletal system, the body part specifying the *deepest layer* is coded.

Example: For an *open excisional debridement of the skin, subcutaneous tissue, and muscle, left foot*, assign just one code for the procedure performed on the *Muscle* body part (because muscle is the deepest layer). Index main term *Debridement* and subterm *Excisional* include cross reference *see Excision*. Thus, index main term *Excision*, subterm *Muscle*, second qualifier *Foot*, and third qualifier *Left* list values 0KBW. Go to ICD-10-PCS Table 0KB to construct code 0KBW0ZZ.

Root Operation—Bypass Procedures

B3.6a. Bypass procedures are coded by identifying the body part bypassed *from* and the body part bypassed *to*.

- The fourth character (body part) specifies the body part bypassed *from*.
- The seventh character qualifier specifies the body part bypassed *to*.

Example: For an *open bypass from stomach to jejunum*, stomach is the body part (fourth character) and jejunum is the qualifier (seventh character). Index main term *Bypass*, subterm *Stomach* list values 0D16. Go to ICD-10-PCS Table 0D1 to construct code 0D160ZA.

B3.6b. Coronary artery bypass procedures are coded differently than other bypass procedures that are described in the previous guideline. Rather than identifying the body part bypassed from, the *body part identifies the number of coronary arteries bypassed to*, and the *qualifier specifies the vessel bypassed from*.

- The fourth character (body part) value classifies the number of coronary arteries bypassed *to*.
- The seventh character qualifier classifies the vessel bypassed *from*.

 Coding Tip

Coronary artery bypass procedures are classified the *opposite* of other bypass procedures (as explained in the above *Root Operation—Bypass Procedures* coding guideline) because the fourth character body part classifies the number of coronary arteries bypassed *to*, and the seventh character qualifier classifies the vessel bypassed *from*.

Example: For an *open aortocoronary artery bypass of left anterior descending coronary artery and obtuse marginal coronary artery, using synthetic substitute for each bypass*, the two coronary arteries are the body part (fourth character) and aorta is the qualifier (seventh character). Index main term *Bypass*, subterm *Artery*, second qualifier *Coronary*, third qualifier *Two Arteries* list values 0211. Go to ICD-10-PCS Table 021 to construct code 02110JW.

B3.6c. When multiple coronary arteries are bypassed, a separate procedure code is assigned for each coronary artery *that uses a different device and/or qualifier*.

Example: For an *open aortocoronary artery bypass and open right internal mammary coronary artery bypass using synthetic substitute for each bypass*, assign two codes because there are different seventh character qualifier values for the aorta and for the right internal mammary artery. Index main term *Bypass*, subterm *Artery*, second qualifier *Coronary*, and third qualifier *One Artery* list values 0210. Go to ICD-10-PCS Table 021 to construct both codes 02100JW and 02100J8. (Index third qualifier *Two Arteries* is *not* used because the seventh character qualifiers differ for each code.)

Root Operation—Control vs. More Specific Root Operations

B3.7. Root operation *Control* is defined as *stopping, or attempting to stop, postprocedural or other acute bleeding*. *Control* is the root operation coded when the procedure performed to achieve hemostasis, beyond what would be considered integral to a procedure, utilizes techniques (e.g. cautery, application of substances or pressure, suturing or ligation or clipping of bleeding points at the site) that are not described by a more specific root operation definition, such as *Bypass, Detachment, Excision, Extraction, Reposition, Replacement,* or *Resection.* If a more specific root operation definition applies to the procedure performed, then the more specific root operation is coded *instead of Control.*

Example 1: Use of silver nitrate cautery to treat acute nasal bleeding is coded to the root operation *Control.* Index main term *Control bleeding in* and subterm *Nasal Mucosa and Soft Tissue 093K* provide direction to ICD-10-PCS Table 093, where code 093K7ZZ is constructed. (There is no mention of endoscopic approach in the statement.)

Example 2: Liquid embolization of the right internal iliac artery, percutaneous approach, to treat acute hematoma by stopping blood flow is coded to the root operation *Occlusion.* Index main term *Embolization* contains a cross reference to *see Occlusion* (and to *see* Restriction). (Embolization procedures involve placing medications or synthetic materials through a catheter into blood vessels to block or prevent blood flow to an area.) Index main term Occlusion and subterms Artery, Internal Iliac, and Right 04LE provide direction to ICD-10-PCS Table 04L, where code 04LE3ZZ is constructed. (No intraluminal or extraluminal device was used because a liquid embolic agent was performed, such as *N*-BCA glue.)

Example 3: The suctioning of residual blood to achieve hemostasis during a transbronchial cryobiopsy is considered integral to the cryobiopsy procedure *and is not coded separately.*

Example 4: The ICD-10-PCS code for *open splenectomy to stop bleeding* is constructed using the *Medical and Surgical* section, *Lymphatic and Hemic Systems* body system, and *Resection* root operation *(instead of root operation Control* because an open splenectomy involves resecting the organ and not just stopping the bleeding). Index main term *Splenectomy* contains a subterm cross reference to *see Resection, Lymphatic and Hemic Systems,* which list values 07T. Go to ICD-10-PCS Table 07T to construct code 07TP0ZZ.

- Although the objective of the procedure was to *stop postprocedural bleeding,* the *Control* root operation is not used because the spleen was resected.

- If surgical cautery or sutures had been performed to stop postprocedural bleeding, the code would have been constructed using the *Control* root operation in the *Anatomical Regions, General* body system and *Medical and Surgical* system.

Root Operation—Excision vs. Resection

B3.8. ICD-10-PCS contains specific body parts for anatomical subdivisions of a body part (e.g., lobes of the lungs or liver, regions of the intestine). The resection of a specific body part is coded whenever all of that body part is cut out or off (instead of coding an excision of a less specific body part).

Example: For a *total open left upper lung lobectomy, Resection* is the root operation and *Upper Lung Lobe, Left* is the body part (instead of the *Excision* root operation and *Lung, Left* body part). Index main term *Resection,* subterm *Lung,* second qualifier *Upper Lobe,* and third qualifier *Left* list values 0BTG. Go to ICD-10-PCS Table 0BT to construct code 0BTG0ZZ.

Root Operation—Excision for Graft

B3.9. When an autograft is obtained from a different body part in order to complete the objective of the procedure, a separate procedure is coded *except when the seventh character qualifier value in the ICD-10-PCS table fully specifies the site from which the autograft was obtained.*

Example 1: For an *open aortocoronary bypass with open excision of right greater saphenous vein (for use as aortocoronary bypass graft material),* the *excision of saphenous vein* is assigned a separate code.

- Index main term *Bypass,* subterm *Artery,* second qualifier *Coronary,* and third qualifier *One Artery* list values 0210. Go to ICD-10-PCS Table 021 to construct code 021009W.

- Index main term *Excision,* subterm *Vein,* second qualifier *Saphenous,* and third qualifier *Right* list values 06BP. Go to ICD-10-PCS Table 06B to construct code 06BP0ZZ.

> **Example 2:** For a *replacement of breast with autologous deep inferior epigastric artery perforator (DIEP) flap*, the excision of the DIEP flap is *not* coded separately because seventh qualifier Deep Inferior Epigastric Artery Perforator Flap in the Replacement table specifies the site of the autograft harvest.

Root Operation—Fusion Procedures of the Spine

B3.10a. The body part coded for a *spinal vertebral joint(s) rendered immobile by a spinal fusion procedure* is classified according to the level of the spine (e.g., thoracic). There are distinct body part values for a single vertebral joint and for multiple vertebral joints at each spinal level.

> **Example:** Go to ICD-10-PCS Table 0RG, and locate values 1, 2, and 4 for body parts *Cervical Vertebral Joint, Cervical Vertebral Joints, 2 or more*, and *Cervicothoracic Vertebral Joint*, respectively.

B3.10b. When multiple vertebral joints are fused, a separate procedure code is assigned for *each vertebral joint that uses a different device and/or qualifier*.

> **Example:** *Open fusion of lumbar vertebral joint, posterior approach, anterior column, synthetic substitute* and *open fusion of lumbar vertebral joint, posterior approach, posterior column, synthetic substitute* are each assigned separate codes. Index main term *Fusion* and subterm *Lumbar Vertebral* list values 0SG0. Go to ICD-10-PCS Table 0SG to construct codes 0SG00JJ and 0SG00J1.

B3.10c. Combinations of devices and materials are often used on a vertebral joint to render the joint immobile. When combinations of devices are used on the *same* vertebral joint, the device value assigned to the procedure code is as follows:

- If an interbody fusion device is used to render the joint immobile (containing bone graft or bone graft substitute), refer to device value *Interbody Fusion Device*.

> **Example:** *Open fusion of lumbar vertebral joint, posterior approach, anterior column, using a cage style interbody internal fusion device containing morselized bone graft* is assigned a device value for *Interbody Internal Fusion Device*. Index main term *Fusion*, and subterm *Lumbar Vertebral* 0SG0. Go to ICD-10-PCS Table 0SG to construct code 0SG00AJ.

- If bone graft is the *only* device used to render the joint immobile, refer to device value *Nonautologous Tissue Substitute* or *Autologous Tissue Substitute*.

> **Example:** *Open fusion of the right elbow joint using bone graft material from a bone bank* is assigned a device value for *Nonautologous Tissue Substitute*. Index main term *Fusion*, subterm *Elbow*, and second qualifier *Right* list values 0RGL. Go to ICD-10-PCS Table 0RG to construct code 0RGL0KZ.

- If a mixture of autologous and nonautologous bone graft (with or without biological or synthetic extenders or binders) is used to render the joint immobile, refer to device value *Autologous Tissue Substitute*.

> **Example:** *Open fusion of the left temporomandibular joint using both autologous bone graft and bone bank bone graft* is assigned a device value for *Autologous Tissue Substitute*. Index main term *Fusion*, subterm *Temporomandibular*, and second qualifier *Left* list values 0RGD. Go to ICD-10-PCS Table 0RG to construct code 0RGD07Z.

Root Operation—Inspection Procedures

B3.11a. Inspection of a body part(s) that is performed to achieve the objective of a procedure is *not* coded separately.

Example: For *fiberoptic bronchoscopy with irrigation of bronchus*, code only the *irrigation of bronchus* procedure. Index main term *Irrigation* and subterm *Respiratory Tract, Irrigating Substance* list values 3E1F. Go to ICD-10-PCS Table 3E1 to construct code 3E1F88Z.

- The bronchus is a part of the respiratory tract.
- Do *not* assign a code for the bronchoscopy.

B3.11b. When *multiple tubular body parts are inspected*, the most distal body part inspected is assigned a body part value.

Example: For *cystoureteroscopy with inspection of urethra, urinary bladder and ureters*, code only the inspection of the ureter (ureteroscopy) because it is distal to both the urethra and the urinary bladder. Index main term *Ureteroscopy* lists code 0TJ98ZZ. Go to ICD-10-PCS Table 0TJ to construct code 0TJ98ZZ (to verify its accuracy).

When *multiple nontubular body parts in a region are inspected*, the body part that specifies the entire area inspected is assigned a body part value.

Example: Exploratory laparotomy with percutaneous endoscopic inspection of abdominal contents is assigned the *Peritoneal Cavity* body part value. Index main term *Laparotomy* provides a cross reference for *Exploratory* to *see Inspection, Peritoneal Cavity 0WJG*. Go to ICD-10-PCS Table 0WJ to construct code 0WJG4ZZ.

B3.11c. When both an inspection procedure and another procedure are performed on the same body part during the same operative episode, if the inspection procedure is performed using a different approach than the other procedure, the inspection procedure is coded separately.

Example: For *percutaneous endoscopic inspection of the duodenum and open biopsy of the duodenum*, two codes are assigned. (The duodenum is part of the lower intestinal tract.)

- Index main term *Inspection*, subterm *Intestinal Tract*, and second qualifier *Lower* list values 0DJD. Go to ICD-10-PCS Table 0DJ to construct code 0DJD4ZZ.
- Index main term *Biopsy* contains a cross reference to *see Excision with qualifier Diagnostic*. Index main term *Excision* and subterm *Duodenum* list values 0DB9. Go to ICD-10-PCS Table 0DB to construct code 0DB90ZX. (The index cross reference for main term *Biopsy* includes the term *Diagnostic*, which means seventh qualifier value X is assigned instead of Z.)

Root Operation—Occlusion vs. Restriction for Vessel Embolization Procedures

B3.12. When the objective of an embolization procedure is to completely close a vessel, a value for root operation *Occlusion* is assigned. Embolization procedures are performed by placing medications or synthetic materials through a catheter into blood vessels to block or prevent blood flow to an area.

Example: *Percutaneous tumor embolization, left axillary artery*, is assigned a value for root operation *Occlusion* because the objective of the procedure is to block or prevent the blood supply to the vessel. Index main term *Embolization* includes a cross reference to *see Occlusion*. Index main term *Occlusion*, subterm *Artery*, second qualifier *Axillary*, and third qualifier *Left* list values 03L6. Go to ICD-10-PCS Table 03L to construct code 03L63ZZ.

When the objective of an embolization procedure is to narrow the lumen of a vessel, a value for root operation *Restriction* is assigned.

Example: *Clipping of right popliteal artery with intraluminal device, open*, is assigned a value for root operation *Restriction* because the objective of the procedure is to narrow the lumen of the vessel at the site of the aneurysm where it is abnormally wide (not to close off the vessel entirely). Index main term *Clipping, aneurysm* includes a cross reference to *see Restriction using Extraluminal Device*. Index main term *Restriction*, subterm *Artery*, second qualifier *Popliteal*, and third qualifier *Right* list values 04VM. Go to ICD-10-PCS Table 04V to construct code 04VM0DZ.

Root Operation—Release Procedures

B3.13. In root operation *Release*, a value is assigned to the body part being freed, *not* to the tissue being manipulated or cut to free the body part.

> **Example:** *Open lysis of ascending colon adhesions* is assigned a value for the *Ascending Colon* body part. Index main term *Lysis* includes a cross reference to *see Release*. Index main term *Release*, subterm *Colon*, and second qualifier *Ascending* list values 0DNK. Go to ICD-10-PCS Table 0DN to construct code 0DNK0ZZ.

Root Operation—Release vs. Division

B3.14. When the sole objective of the procedure is to free a body part *without cutting into the body part*, a value is assigned to root operation *Release*.

> **Example:** *Freeing of vagus nerve root from surrounding scar tissue via open approach to relieve pain* is coded to root operation *Release*. Index main term *Release*, subterm *Nerve*, and second qualifier *Vagus* list values 00NQ. Go to ICD-10-PCS Table 00N to construct code 00NQ0ZZ.

When the sole objective of the procedure is to separate or transect a body part, a value is assigned to root operation *Division*.

> **Example:** *Severing a vagus nerve root via open approach* to stop hiccups is coded to the root operation *Division*. Index main term *Division*, subterm *Nerve*, and second qualifier *Vagus* list values 008Q. Go to ICD-10-PCS Table 008 to construct code 008Q0ZZ.

Root Operation—Reposition for Fracture Treatment

B3.15. The reduction of a displaced fracture is coded to root operation *Reposition*, and the application of a cast or splint in conjunction with the reposition procedure is *not* coded separately. Treatment of a nondisplaced fracture is coded to the procedure performed.

> **Example 1:** *Open insertion of pin as an internal fixation device in a nondisplaced fracture of left fibula* is coded to root operation *Insertion of device in*. Index main term *Insertion of device in*, subterm *Fibula*, second qualifier *Left* list values 0QHK. Go to ICD-10-PCS Table 0QH to construct code 0QHK04Z.

> **Example 2:** *Applying a cast to a nondisplaced right radial fracture* is coded to root operation *Immobilization* in the *Placement* section. Index main term *Casting* includes a cross reference to *see Immobilization*. Index main term *Immobilization*, subterm *Arm*, second qualifier *Lower,* and third qualifier *Right* list values 2W3CX. Go to ICD-10-PCS Table 2W3 to construct code 2W3CX2Z.

Root Operation—Transplantation vs. Administration

B3.16. Putting in a mature and functioning living body part taken from another individual or animal is coded to root operation *Transplantation*.

> **Example:** For *left kidney transplant, allogeneic*, Index main term *Transplantation*, subterm *Kidney*, and second qualifier *Left* list values 0TY10Z. Go to ICD-10-PCS Table 0TY to construct code 0TY10Z0.

Inserting autologous or nonautologous cells is coded to the *Administration* section (and root operation *Transfusion*).

> **Example:** *Percutaneous autologous bone marrow transplant via central venous line* is coded to the *Administration* section and root operation Transfusion. Go to index main term *Transfusion* and subterms *Vein, Central,* and *Bone Marrow* 30243G. Go to ICD-10-PCS Table 302 to construct code 30243G0.

Root Operation—Transfer Procedures Using Multiple Tissue Layers

B3.17. The root operation *Transfer* contains qualifiers that can be used to specify when a transfer flap is composed of more than one tissue layer, such as a musculocutaneous flap (or a myocutaneous flap). For the transfer of multiple tissue layers including skin, subcutaneous tissue, fascia, or muscle, *the procedure is coded to the body part value that describes the deepest tissue layer in the flap, and the qualifier describes the other tissue layer(s) in the transfer flap.*

> **Example:** A musculocutaneous flap transfer is coded to the appropriate body part value in body system *Muscles*, and the qualifier describes additional tissue layers from the transfer flap, such as 0KXG0Z5 (open *latissimus dorsi* myocutaneous flap transfer to trunk muscle, left).

Excision/Resection Followed by Replacement

B3.18. When an excision or resection of a body part procedure is followed by a replacement procedure, report codes for both procedures to identify each distinct objective (of the procedure), *except when the excision or resection is considered integral and preparatory for the replacement procedure.*

> **Example 1:** For a mastectomy followed by reconstruction (of the breast) procedure, report codes for both the resection (mastectomy) and replacement (reconstruction) of the breast to fully capture the distinct objectives of the procedures performed.

> **Example 2:** For a maxillectomy with obturator reconstruction procedure, report codes for both the excision (maxillectomy) and replacement (obturator reconstruction) of the maxilla to fully capture the distinct objectives of the procedures performed.

> **Example 3:** For an excisional debridement of a tendon with skin graft procedure, report codes for both excision of the tendon and replacement with a skin graft to fully capture the distinct objectives of the procedures performed.

> **Example 4:** For an esophagectomy followed by reconstruction with colonic interposition procedure, report codes for both the resection (esophagectomy) and the transfer of the large intestine to function as the esophagus (reconstruction) to fully capture the distinct objectives of the procedures performed.

> **Example 5:** For resection of a joint as part of a joint replacement procedure, the resection of the joint is considered integral and preparatory for the replacement procedure. Thus, the resection is not coded separately.

> **Example 6:** For resection of a valve as part of a valve replacement procedure, the resection is considered integral and preparatory for the valve replacement procedure. Thus, the resection is not coded separately.

Detachment Procedures of Extremities

B3.19. The root operation Detachment contains qualifiers that can be used to specify the level where the extremity was amputated. These qualifiers are dependent on the body part value in the "upper extremities" and "lower extremities" body systems. For procedures involving the detachment of all or part of the upper or lower extremities, the procedure is coded to the body part value that describes the site of the detachment.

> **Example:** An amputation at the proximal portion of the shaft of the tibia and fibula is coded to the Lower leg body part value in the body system Anatomical Regions, Lower Extremities, and the qualifier High is used to specify the level where the extremity was detached.

The following definitions were developed for the Detachment qualifiers

Body Part	Qualifier	Definition
Upper arm and upper leg	1	High: Amputation at the proximal portion of the shaft of the humerus or femur
	2	Mid: Amputation at the middle portion of the shaft of the humerus or femur
	3	Low: Amputation at the distal portion of the shaft of the humerus or femur
Lower arm and lower leg	1	High: Amputation at the proximal portion of the shaft of the radius/ulna or tibia/fibula
	2	Mid: Amputation at the middle portion of the shaft of the radius/ulna or tibia/fibula
	3	Low: Amputation at the distal portion of the shaft of the radius/ulna or tibia/fibula
Hand and foot	0	Complete*
	4	Complete 1st Ray
	5	Complete 2nd Ray
	6	Complete 3rd Ray
	7	Complete 4th Ray
	8	Complete 5th Ray
	9	Partial 1st Ray
	B	Partial 2nd Ray
	C	Partial 3rd Ray
	D	Partial 4th Ray
	F	Partial 5th Ray
Thumb, finger, or toe	0	Complete: Amputation at the metacarpophalangeal/metatarsal-phalangeal joint
	1	High: Amputation anywhere along the proximal phalanx
	2	Mid: Amputation through the proximal interphalangeal joint or anywhere along the middle phalanx
	3	Low: Amputation through the distal interphalangeal joint or anywhere along the distal phalanx

*When coding amputation of Hand and Foot, the following definitions are followed
- *Complete*: Amputation through the carpometacarpal joint of the hand, or through the tarsal-metatarsal joint of the foot.
- *Partial*: Amputation anywhere along the shaft or head of the metacarpal bone of the hand, or of the metatarsal bone of the foot.

Body Part

Official coding guidelines for Body Part include the following:

- General guidelines
- Branches of body parts
- Bilateral body part values
- Coronary arteries

- Tendons, ligaments, bursae, and fascia near a joint
- Skin, subcutaneous tissue, and fascia overlying a joint
- Fingers and toes
- Upper and lower intestinal tract

Body Part—General Guidelines

B4.1a. When a procedure is performed on a portion of a body part that does not have a separate body part value, code the body part value corresponding to the whole body part.

> **Example:** A procedure performed on the alveolar process of the mandible is assigned a value for body part *Mandible*. Index main term *Alveolar process of mandible* includes a cross reference to *use Mandible, Left* or *use Mandible, Right*.

B4.1b. If the prefix *peri* is combined with a body part to identify the site of the procedure, and the site of the procedure is not further specified, the procedure is coded to the body part named. However, for a procedure site described as periurethral where documentation indicates vulvar tissue (not urethral tissue) as the procedure site, vulva is selected as the body part (instead of urethra). In addition, a procedure site documented as *involving the periosteum* is coded to the documented bone as the body part.

> **Example:** A procedure site identified as *perirenal* is assigned a value for the body part *Kidney*.

B4.1c. If a single vascular procedure is performed on a continuous section of an arterial or venous body part, code the body part value corresponding to the anatomically most proximal (closest to the heart) portion of the arterial or venous body part.

> **Example:** A procedure performed on a continuous section of artery from the femoral artery to the external iliac artery, with the point of entry at the *femoral artery*, is coded to the *External Iliac Artery* body part. When that procedure is performed on a continuous section of artery from the femoral artery to the external iliac artery has the point of entry at the *external iliac artery* (instead of the femoral artery), *it is also coded to the External Iliac Artery body part.*

Body Part—Branches of Body Parts

B4.2. Where a specific branch of a body part does not have its own body part value in ICD-10-PCS, the body part is typically coded to the closest proximal branch that has a specific body part value. In the cardiovascular body systems, if a general body part is available in the correct root operation table, and coding to a proximal branch would require assigning a code in a different body system, the procedure is coded using the general body part value.

> **Example 1:** A procedure performed on the *mandibular branch of the trigeminal nerve* is assigned a value for body part *Trigeminal Nerve*.

> **Example 2:** Occlusion of the bronchial artery is coded to body part value Upper Artery in body system Upper Arteries, *not to body part value Thoracic Aorta, Descending in body system Heart and Great Vessels.*

Body Part—Bilateral Body Part Values

B4.3. Bilateral body part values are available for a limited number of body parts. If the identical procedure is performed on contralateral body parts, and a bilateral body part value exists for that body part, just one code is assigned using the bilateral body part value. If no bilateral body part value exists, each procedure is assigned a separate code using the appropriate body part value.

> **Example 1:** An identical procedure performed on both fallopian tubes is assigned a value for body part *Fallopian Tube, Bilateral.*

> **Example 2:** An identical procedure performed on both knee joints is assigned two different codes, which means assigning values for body part *Knee Joint, Right* and *Knee Joint, Left* to each code.

Body Part—Coronary Arteries

B4.4. The coronary arteries are classified as a single body part that is further specified by number of arteries treated. One procedure code specifying multiple arteries is used when the same procedure is performed, including the same device and qualifier values.

> **Example 1:** An angioplasty of two distinct coronary arteries with placement of two stents is assigned a code as *Dilation of Coronary Arteries, Two Arteries, with two Intraluminal Devices*.

> **Example 2:** An angioplasty of two distinct coronary arteries, one with stent placement and one without, is assigned two separate codes as *Dilation of Coronary Artery, One Artery with Intraluminal Device*, and *Dilation of Coronary Artery, One Artery with No Device*.

Body Part—Tendons, Ligaments, Bursae, and Fascia Near a Joint

B4.5. Procedures performed on tendons, ligaments, bursae, and fascia supporting a joint are coded to the body part in the respective body system that is the focus of the procedure. Procedures performed on joint structures themselves are coded to the body part in the joint body systems.

> **Example 1:** *Repair of anterior cruciate ligament, left knee* is assigned a value from body part *Knee Bursae and Ligament* in the body system *Bursae and Ligaments*.

> **Example 2:** A *knee arthroscopy with shaving of articular cartilage* is assigned a value from body part *Knee Joint* in body system *Lower Joints*.

Body Part—Skin, Subcutaneous Tissue, and Fascia Overlying a Joint

B4.6. When a procedure is performed on skin, subcutaneous tissue, or fascia overlying a joint, assign a value to body parts as indicated below:

- Shoulder is assigned a value for body part *Upper Arm*.
- Elbow is assigned a value for body part *Lower Arm*.
- Wrist is assigned a value for body part *Lower Arm*.
- Hip is assigned a value for body part *Upper Leg*.
- Knee is assigned a value for body part *Lower Leg*.
- Ankle is assigned a value for body part *Foot*.

Body Part—Fingers and Toes

B4.7. When a body system does not contain a separate body part value for the fingers, procedures performed on the fingers are assigned value(s) for body part *Hand*. If a body system does not contain a separate body part value for the toes, procedures performed on the toes are assigned value(s) for body part *Foot*.

> **Example:** *Excision of finger muscle* is assigned a value for body part *Hand Muscle* in body system *Muscles*.

Body Part—Upper and Lower Intestinal Tract

B4.8. For the gastrointestinal body system, general body part values *Upper Intestinal Tract* and *Lower Intestinal Tract* are provided as an option for root operations such as *Change, Insertion, Inspection, Removal,* and *Revision.* The upper intestinal tract includes the portion of the gastrointestinal tract from the esophagus down to and including the duodenum. The lower intestinal tract includes the portion of the gastrointestinal tract from the jejunum down to and including the rectum and anus.

Example: Change of a device in the jejunum is coded as 0D2DXUZ, using body part *lower intestinal tract.*

Approach

Official coding guidelines for Approach include the following:

- Open approach with percutaneous endoscopic assistance
- Percutaneous endoscopic approach with extension of incision
- External approach
- Percutaneous procedure via device

The technique used to reach the site of the procedure is called the *approach*, and there are seven different approaches.

- *Open*: Cutting through the skin or mucous membrane and any other body layers necessary to expose the site of the procedure
- *Percutaneous*: Entry, by puncture or minor incision, of instrumentation through the skin or mucous membrane and any other body layers necessary to reach the site of the procedure
- *Percutaneous Endoscopic*: Entry, by puncture or minor incision, of instrumentation through the skin or mucous membrane and any other body layers necessary to reach and visualize the site of the procedure
- *Via Natural or Artificial Opening*: Entry of instrumentation through a natural or artificial external opening to reach the site of the procedure
- *Via Natural or Artificial Opening Endoscopic*: Entry of instrumentation through a natural or artificial external opening to reach and visualize the site of the procedure
- *Via Natural or Artificial Opening Endoscopic with Percutaneous Endoscopic Assistance*: Entry of instrumentation through a natural or artificial external opening to reach and visualize the site of the procedure, and entry, by puncture or minor incision, of instrumentation through the skin or mucous membrane and any other body layers necessary to aid in the performance of the procedure
- *External*: Procedures performed directly on the skin or mucous membrane and procedures performed indirectly by the application of external force through the skin or mucous membrane

An approach also includes the following three components:

- *Access Location*: For procedures performed on an internal body part, the access location specifies the external site through which the site of the procedure is reached. There are two general types of access locations.
  - Skin or mucous membranes, which can be cut or punctured to reach the procedure site
  - External openings, which are natural (e.g., mouth) or artificial (e.g., colostomy stoma)
- *Method*: For procedures performed on an internal body part, the method specifies how the external access location is entered, including:
  - Open method, which specifies cutting through skin or mucous membrane and any other intervening body layers necessary to expose the site of the procedure

NOTE:

Punctures and minor incisions are not considered open approaches because they do not expose the site of the procedure.

  - Instrumentation method, which specifies the entry of instrumentation through an access location (e.g., puncture, minor incision, external opening) to the internal procedure site
- *Type of Instrumentation*: For procedures performed on an internal body part, instrumentation refers to specialized equipment used to perform the procedure (e.g., sigmoidoscope)

Approach—Open Approach with Percutaneous Endoscopic Assistance

B5.2a. Procedures performed using the open approach with percutaneous endoscopic assistance are coded to the approach *Open.*

Example: *Laparoscopic-assisted sigmoidectomy* is assigned a value for approach *Open*.

Approach—Percutaneous Endoscopic Approach with Hand-Assistance or Extension of Incision

B5.2b. Procedures performed using the percutaneous endoscopic approach with hand-assistance, or with an incision or extension of an incision to assist in the removal of all or a portion of a body part, or to anastomose a tubular body part with or without the temporary exteriorization of a body structure, are coded to the approach value *Percutaneous Endoscopic*.

Example 1: A hand-assisted laparoscopic sigmoid colon resection with exteriorization of a segment of the colon to remove a specimen and return the colon back into the abdominal cavity is assigned a value for approach *Percutaneous Endoscopic*.

Example 2: A laparoscopic sigmoid colectomy with extension of stapling port for removal of specimen and direct anastomosis is assigned a value for approach *Percutaneous Endoscopic*.

Example 3: A laparoscopic nephrectomy with midline incision for removing the resected kidney is assigned a value for approach *Percutaneous Endoscopic*.

Example 4: A robotic-assisted laparoscopic prostatectomy with extension of incision for removal of the resected prostate is assigned a value for approach *Percutaneous Endoscopic*.

Approach—External Approach

B5.3a. Procedures performed within an orifice on structures that are visible without the aid of any instrumentation are coded to the approach *External*.

Example: *Resection of tonsils* is assigned a value for approach *External*.

B5.3b. Procedures performed indirectly by the application of external force through the intervening body layers are coded to the approach *External*.

Example: Closed reduction of fracture is assigned a value for approach *External*.

Approach—Percutaneous Procedure via Device

B5.4. Procedures performed percutaneously via a device placed for the procedure are coded to the approach *Percutaneous*.

Example: *Fragmentation of kidney stone performed via percutaneous nephrostomy* is assigned a value for approach *Percutaneous*.

Device

Official coding guidelines for Device include the following:

- General guidelines
- Drainage device

The sixth character device value is assigned for devices that remain after the procedure is completed. There are four general types of devices.

- Biological or synthetic material that takes the place of all or a portion of a body part (e.g., skin grafts and joint prosthesis)
- Biological or synthetic material that assists or prevents a physiological function (e.g., IUD)
- Therapeutic material that is not absorbed by, eliminated by, or incorporated into a body part (e.g., radioactive implant)
- Mechanical or electronic appliances used to assist, monitor, take the place of, or prevent a physiological function (e.g., cardiac pacemaker, orthopedic pins)

Device—General Guidelines

B6.1a. A device value is assigned *only if a device remains after the procedure is completed*. If no device remains, the *No Device* device value is assigned. In limited root operations, the classification provides qualifier values *Temporary and Intraoperative* to be used for specific procedures that involve clinically significant devices where the purpose of the device is to be utilized for a brief duration during the procedure or current inpatient stay.

When a device (that is intended to remain after the procedure is completed) requires removal before the end of the operative episode during which it was inserted (e.g., inadequate device size, event documented as a surgical complication), both the insertion and removal of the device are coded.

> **Example:** Patient underwent right hip replacement, open. During the operative episode, the surgeon determined that the inserted internal fixation device was too small, and it was removed. A larger device was inserted, and the surgeon determined that it was stable. Report codes 0SH904Z and 0SP904Z.

B6.1b. Materials such as sutures, ligatures, radiological markers, and temporary postoperative wound drains are considered integral to the performance of a procedure; thus, they are *not* coded as devices.

> **Example:** Patient underwent surgical excision of a sebaceous cyst, face. After successful removal skin layers were sutured. Report code 0HB1XZZ only. (Do **not** report a separate code for suture of skin layers.)

B6.1c. Procedures performed on a device only, and not on a body part, are classified to root operations *Change, Irrigation, Removal*, or *Revision*, and they are coded to the procedure performed.

> **Example:** *Irrigation of percutaneous nephrostomy tube* is classified to root operation *Irrigation, indwelling device* in the *Administration* section. Index main term *Irrigation*, subterm *Genitourinary Tract, Irrigating Substance* list values 3E1K. Go to ICD-10-PCS Table 3E1 to construct code 3E1K38Z.

Device—Drainage Device

B6.2. A separate procedure to insert a drainage device is assigned a value for root operation *Drainage* and a value for device *Drainage Device*.

> **Example:** *Percutaneous insertion of peritoneal cavity drainage device*. Index main term *Drainage*, subterm *Peritoneal Cavity* list values 0W9G. Go to ICD-10-PCS Table 0W9 to construct code 0W9G30Z.
>
> Notice that ICD-10-PCS Index main term *Insertion of device in* and subterm *Peritoneal Cavity* list values 0WHG, which directs you to ICD-10-PCS Table 0WH. However, Table 0WH is **not** used to construct the code because drainage devices are not classified in its column 3 *Device* column.

Obstetrics Section Coding Guidelines

Official coding guidelines for the Obstetrics Section include the following:

- Products of conception
- Procedures following delivery or abortion

The Obstetrics section includes the following root operations, all but two of which were defined in Table 6-1 (from the Medical and Surgery section coding guidelines previously covered): abortion, change, delivery, drainage, extraction, insertion, inspection, removal, repair, reposition, resection, and transplantation. The two additional root operations include:

- *Abortion*: Artificially terminating a pregnancy
- *Delivery*: Assisting the passage of the products of conception from the genital canal

A cesarean section is *not* a separate root operation because the underlying objective is *Extraction* (e.g., pulling out all or a portion of a body part).

Obstetrics Section—Products of Conception

C1. Procedures performed on the products of conception are coded to the *Obstetrics* section. Procedures performed on a pregnant individual, other than those performed on the products of conception, are coded to the appropriate root operation in the *Medical and Surgical* section.

> **Example 1:** *Amniocentesis* is assigned a value from body part *Products of Conception* in the *Obstetrics* section.

> **Example 2:** *Repair of obstetric urethral laceration* is assigned a value from body part *Urethra* in the *Medical and Surgical* section.

Obstetrics Section—Procedures Following Delivery or Abortion

C2. Procedures performed following a delivery or abortion for (1) curettage of the endometrium or (2) evacuation of retained products of conception are coded to the *Obstetrics* section, *Pregnancy* body system, *Extraction* root operation, and *Products of Conception, Retained* body part.

Diagnostic or therapeutic dilation and curettage performed during times *other than* the postpartum or post-abortion period are coded to the *Medical and Surgical* section, *Female Reproductive* body system, *Extraction* root operation, and *Endometrium* body part.

> **Example 1:** After delivery of a healthy term infant, the patient underwent endometrial dilation and curettage (D&C) to remove retained placenta. D&C code 10D17ZZ is constructed using values from the *Obstetrics* section, *Pregnancy* body system, *Extraction* root operation, and *Products of Conception, Retained* body part.

> **Example 2:** A 58-year-old patient underwent diagnostic D&C. Code 0UDB7ZX is constructed using values from the *Medical and Surgical* section, *Female Reproductive* body system, *Extraction* root operation, and *Endometrium* body part.

Placement Section

The Placement section includes seven root operations.

- *Change*: Taking out or off a device from a body part and putting back an identical or similar device in or on the same body part without cutting or puncturing the skin or a mucous membrane
- *Compression*: Putting pressure on a body region
- *Dressing*: Putting material on a body region for protection
- *Immobilization*: Limiting or preventing motion of an external body region
- *Packing*: Putting material in a body region or orifice
- *Removal*: Taking out or off a device from a body part
- *Traction*: Exerting a pulling force on a body region in a distal direction

Administration Section

The Administration section includes three root operations.

- *Introduction*: Putting in or on a therapeutic, diagnostic, nutritional, physiological, or prophylactic substance except blood or blood products
- *Irrigation*: Putting in or on a cleansing substance
- *Transfusion*: Putting in blood or blood products

Measurement and Monitoring Section

The Measurement and Monitoring section includes two root operations.

- *Measurement*: Determining the level of a physiological or physical function at a point in time
- *Monitoring*: Determining the level of a physiological or physical function repetitively over a period of time

Extracorporeal or Systemic Assistance and Performance Section

The Extracorporeal or Systemic Assistance and Performance section includes three root operations.

- *Assistance*: Taking over a portion of a physiological function by extracorporeal means
- *Performance*: Completely taking over a physiological function by extracorporeal means
- *Restoration*: Returning, or attempting to return, a physiological function to its natural state by extracorporeal means; this root operation contains a single procedure code that identifies *extracorporeal cardioversion*

Extracorporeal or Systemic Therapies Section

The Extracorporeal or Systemic Therapies section includes 11 root operations.

- *Atmospheric Control*: Extracorporeal control of atmospheric pressure and composition
- *Decompression*: Extracorporeal elimination of undissolved gas from body fluids; this root operation involves just one type of procedure, *treatment for decompression sickness* (or *the bends*) in a hyperbaric chamber
- *Electromagnetic Therapy*: Extracorporeal treatment by electromagnetic rays
- *Hyperthermia*: Extracorporeal raising of body temperature; *hyperthermia* describes both a temperature imbalance treatment and an adjunct radiation treatment for cancer. For temperature imbalance treatment, assign a code from the Extracorporeal Therapy section; for adjunct radiation treatment, assign a code from the Radiation Therapy section.
- *Hypothermia*: Extracorporeal lowering of body temperature
- *Perfusion*: Extracorporeal treatment by diffusion of therapeutic fluid
- *Pheresis*: Extracorporeal separation of blood products; *pheresis* has two main purposes: the treatment of diseases when too much of a blood component is produced (e.g., leukemia) and the removal of a blood product (e.g., platelets) from a donor for transfusion into another patient.
- *Phototherapy*: Extracorporeal treatment by light rays; *phototherapy* involves using a machine that exposes blood to light rays outside the body, recirculates it, and then returns it to the body.
- *Shock Wave Therapy*: Extracorporeal treatment by shock waves
- *Ultrasound Therapy*: Extracorporeal treatment by ultrasound
- *Ultraviolet Light Therapy*: Extracorporeal treatment by ultraviolet light

Osteopathic Section

The Osteopathic section includes just one root operation, *Treatment*, which is the manual treatment to eliminate or alleviate somatic dysfunction and related disorders. Osteopathic methods include:

- *Articulatory-Raising:* Passive joint and muscle stretching technique that uses palpation and movement
- *Fascial Release:* Direct or indirect forces (manipulations) that treat fascial restrictions
- *General Mobilization:* Massage that facilitates movement of fluid throughout body tissues
- *High Velocity-Low Amplitude:* Use of quick short thrusting techniques to overcome joint barriers, resulting in a popping noise as motion is restored to the joint
- *Indirect:* Indirect way of performing articulatory-raising, fascial release, general mobilization, or high velocity-low amplitude methods
- *Low Velocity-High Amplitude:* Use of slow thrusting techniques that are applied to specific body areas
- *Lymphatic Pump:* Manipulation of rib cage and thoracic region to improve lymphatic circulation in the chest
- *Muscle Energy-Isometric:* Resistance exercise that uses muscles in opposition with other muscles

- *Muscle Energy-Isotonic:* Resistance exercise that uses muscles in harmony with other muscles
- *Other Method:* Balanced tension (evaluation of manual motion in soft tissue to detect decreased or asymmetrical motion and follow that tissue in the direction opposite the restriction until the area feels balanced) or Percussion (use of *Foredom percussor*, also called the percussor or percussion hammer, which emits a tapping sensation on the body)

Other Procedures Section

The Other Procedures section has just one root operation, *other procedures*, which are methodologies that attempt to remediate or cure a disorder or disease. Other procedures methods include acupuncture; collection of fluids; computer-assisted, and fluorescence-guided, robotic-assisted procedures; near infrared spectroscopy; and therapeutic massage.

Chiropractic Section

The Chiropractic section has just one root operation, *manipulation*, which is a manual procedure that involves a directed thrust to move a joint past the physiological range of motion, without exceeding the anatomical limit. Chiropractic methods include:

- *Non-manual:* Use of a specialized chiropractic table that changes the patient's position using gravity
- *Indirect Visceral:* Manipulation performed on the abdomen using an indirect method
- *Extra-Articular:* Manipulation performed away from joints in the spine and other body parts
- *Direct Visceral:* Manipulation performed on the abdomen using a direct method
- *Indirect:* Extra-articular manipulation using an indirect method
- *Long Lever Specific Contact:* Manipulation of longer bones
- *Short Lever Specific Contact:* Manipulation of smaller, shorter bones
- *Long and Short Lever Specific Contact:* Manipulation of longer and shorter, smaller bones
- *Mechanically Assisted:* Use of the *Activator* adjusting instrument during manual manipulation of the back, neck, and extremities.
- *Other Method:* Use of the *Graston Technique*, which is soft-tissue instrument-assisted mobilization that helps break down scar tissue and fascial restrictions and stretches muscle and connective tissue

Imaging Section

The Imaging section includes five root types.

- *Computerized Tomography (CT Scan):* Computer-reformatted digital display of multiplanar images developed from the capture of multiple exposures of external ionizing radiation
- *Fluoroscopy:* Single plane or bi-plane real-time display of an image developed from the capture of external ionizing radiation on fluorescent screen. The image may also be stored by either digital or analog means.
- *Magnetic Resonance Imaging (MRI):* Computer reformatted digital display of multiplanar images developed from the capture of radiofrequency signals emitted by nuclei in a body site excited within a magnetic field
- *Plain Radiography:* Planar display of an image developed from the capture of external ionizing radiation on photographic or photoconductive plate
- *Ultrasonography:* Real-time display of images of anatomy or flow information developed from the capture of reflected and attenuated high-frequency sound waves

Nuclear Medicine Section

The Nuclear Medicine section includes seven root types.

- *Nonimaging Uptake*: Introduction of radioactive materials into the body for measurements of organ function, from the detection of radioactive emissions

- *Nonimaging Nuclear Medicine Probe*: Introduction of radioactive materials into the body for the study of distribution and fate of certain substances by the detection of radioactive emissions; alternatively, measurement of absorption of radioactive emissions from an external source

- *Nonimaging Assay*: Introduction of radioactive materials into the body for the study of body fluids and blood elements, by the detection of radioactive emissions

- *Planar Nuclear Medicine Imaging*: Introduction of radioactive materials into the body for single-plane display of images developed from the capture of radioactive emissions

- *Positron Emission Tomography (PET) Imaging*: Introduction of radioactive materials into the body for three-dimensional display of images developed from the simultaneous capture, 180 degrees apart, of radioactive emissions

- *Systemic Nuclear Medicine Therapy*: Introduction of unsealed radioactive materials into the body for treatment

- *Tomographic (Tomo) Nuclear Medicine Imaging*: Introduction of radioactive materials into the body for three-dimensional display of images developed from the capture of radioactive emissions

Radiation Therapy Section

Official coding guidelines for the Radiation Therapy Section include brachytherapy only. The Radiation Therapy section includes the following modalities: beam radiation, brachytherapy, stereotactic radiosurgery, and other radiation. *Beam radiation* is a radiation therapy modality that uses x-rays or gamma rays from a special machine (e.g., linear accelerator) that delivers the radiation dose at the surface of the body, directing it at the tumor through the body. The x-rays or gamma rays consist of tiny particles of photons, protons/ions, neutrons, or electrons.

Stereotactic radiosurgery (or *stereotaxic radiosurgery*) is an external radiation therapy that uses special equipment to position the patient and precisely administer a single large dose of radiation to a tumor. It is often used to treat brain tumors and other brain disorders that cannot be treated by regular surgery.

Other radiation modalities include contact radiation, hyperthermia, plaque radiation, and intraoperative radiation therapy (IORT).

- *Contact radiation* is a minimally invasive cancer therapy, such as for early-stage rectal cancer

- *Hyperthermia* is cancer therapy that exposes body tissue to high temperatures (up to 113°F) resulting in damage and destruction of cancer cells, usually with minimal injury to normal tissues.

- *Intraoperative radiation therapy (IORT)* includes intensive radiation treatment administered during surgery, which allows direct radiation to the target area while sparing normal surrounding tissue. IORT treats cancers that are difficult to remove and when microscopic amounts of cancer may remain.

- *Plaque radiation* involves positioning a sealed device onto the outside of the body part (e.g., eye) to deliver a continuous high dose of radiation to a tumor (until the plaque is removed). The plaque is a thin piece of metal (e.g., gold) that contains radioactive seeds on the side facing the tumor.

Brachytherapy

D1.a. *Brachytherapy* is a type of radiation therapy in which radioactive material (sealed in capsules, ribbons, and seeds) is inserted or placed directly into or near a tumor. Brachytherapy is also called implant radiation therapy, internal radiation therapy, and radiation brachytherapy, and it is coded to the modality Brachytherapy in the Radiation Therapy section. When a radioactive brachytherapy source is left in the body at the end of the procedure, it is coded separately to the root operation Insertion with the device value Radioactive Element.

Example: Brachytherapy with implantation of a low dose rate brachytherapy source left in the body at the end of the procedure is coded to the applicable treatment site in the Radiation Therapy section using modality Brachytherapy, modality qualifier Low Dose Rate, and the applicable isotope value and qualifier value. The implantation of the brachytherapy source is coded separately to device Radioactive Element in the appropriate Insertion table of the Medical and Surgical section. The Radiation Therapy section code identifies the specific modality and isotope of the brachytherapy, and root operation Insertion code identifies the implantation of the brachytherapy source that remains in the body at the end of the procedure.

An exception to the brachytherapy guideline is the implantation of Cesium-131 brachytherapy seeds embedded in a collagen matrix to the treatment site after resection of a brain tumor; the implantation is coded to root operation Insertion with device Radioactive Element, Cesium-131 Collagen Implant. This procedure is coded to root operation Insertion because the device identifies both the implantation of the radioactive element and a specific brachytherapy isotope that is not included in the Radiation Therapy section tables.

D1.b. A separate procedure to place a temporary applicator for delivering brachytherapy is coded to root operation Insertion and device Other Device.

Example: An intrauterine brachytherapy applicator placed during a separate procedure from the brachytherapy procedure is coded to Insertion of Other Device, and the brachytherapy is coded separately using modality Brachytherapy in the Radiation Therapy section.

An intrauterine brachytherapy applicator placed concomitantly with delivery of the brachytherapy dose is coded with a single code using modality Brachytherapy in the Radiation Therapy section.

Physical Rehabilitation and Diagnostic Audiology Section

The Physical Rehabilitation and Diagnostic Audiology section includes the following root types.

- *Activities of Daily Living Assessment*: Measurement of functional level for activities of daily living
- *Activities of Daily Living Treatment*: Exercise or activities to facilitate functional competence for activities of daily living
- *Caregiver Training*: Educating caregiver with the skills and knowledge used to interact with and assist the patient
- *Cochlear Implant Treatment*: Application of techniques to improve the communication abilities of individuals with cochlear implant
- *Device Fitting*: Fitting of a device designed to facilitate or support achievement of a higher level of function
- *Hearing Aid Assessment*: Measurement of the appropriateness and/or effectiveness of a hearing device
- *Hearing Assessment*: Measurement of hearing and related functions
- *Hearing Treatment*: Application of techniques to improve, augment, or compensate for hearing and related functional impairment
- *Motor and/or Nerve Function Assessment*: Measurement of motor, nerve, and related functions
- *Motor Treatment*: Exercise or activities to increase or facilitate motor function
- *Speech Assessment*: Measurement of speech and related functions
- *Speech Treatment*: Application of techniques to improve, augment, or compensate for speech and related functional impairment
- *Vestibular Assessment*: Measurement of the vestibular system and related functions
- *Vestibular Treatment*: Application of techniques to improve, augment, or compensate for vestibular and related functional impairment

Mental Health Section

The Mental Health section includes the following mental health procedures and services.

- *Biofeedback*: Provision of information from the monitoring and regulating of physiological processes in conjunction with cognitive-behavioral techniques to improve patient functioning or well-being

- *Counseling*: Application of psychological methods to treat an individual with normal developmental issues and psychological problems in order to increase function, improve well-being, alleviate distress, correct maladjustment, or resolve crises
- *Crisis Intervention*: Treatment of a traumatized, acutely disturbed, or distressed individual for the purpose of short-term stabilization
- *Electroconvulsive Therapy*: Application of controlled electrical voltages to treat a mental health disorder
- *Family Psychotherapy*: Treatment that includes one or more family members of an individual with a mental health disorder by behavioral, cognitive, psychoanalytic, psychodynamic, or psychophysiological means to improve functioning or well-being
- *Group Psychotherapy*: Treatment of two or more individuals with a mental health disorder by behavioral, cognitive, psychoanalytic, psychodynamic, or psychophysiological means to improve functioning or well-being
- *Hypnosis*: Induction of a state of heightened suggestibility by auditory, visual, and tactile techniques to elicit an emotional or behavioral response
- *Individual Psychotherapy*: Treatment of an individual with a mental health disorder by behavioral, cognitive, psychoanalytic, psychodynamic, or psychophysiological means to improve functioning or well-being
- *Light Therapy*: Application of specialized light treatments to improve functioning or well-being
- *Medication Management*: Monitoring and adjusting the use of medications for the treatment of a mental health disorder
- *Narcosynthesis*: Administration of intravenous barbiturates in order to release suppressed or repressed thoughts
- *Psychological Tests*: Administration and interpretation of standardized psychological tests and measurement instruments for the assessment of psychological function

Substance Abuse Treatment Section

The Substance Abuse Treatment section includes seven root types.

- *Detoxification Services*: Not a treatment modality but helps the patient stabilize physically and psychologically until the body becomes free of drugs and the effects of alcohol
- *Family Counseling*: Provides support and education for family members of addicted individuals. Family member participation is seen as critical to substance abuse treatment.
- *Group Counseling*: Provides structured group counseling sessions and healing power through the connection with others
- *Individual Counseling*: Comprising several techniques, which apply various strategies to address drug addiction
- *Individual Psychotherapy*: Includes behavior, cognitive/behavioral, cognitive, interactive, interpersonal, psychoanalysis, psychodynamic, psychophysiological, and supportive types
- *Medication Management*: Management of prescription drug dosages through laboratory testing and other evaluation and management services
- *Pharmacotherapy*: Management of mental disorders using pharmacological agents

New Technology Section

The New Technology section includes the following root operations: assistance, destruction, dilation, extirpation, fusion, introduction, measurement, monitoring, and replacement, all of which have been previously defined in this chapter. Official coding guidelines for the New Technology Section include general guidelines only. ICD-10-PCS Section X contains stand-alone codes to uniquely identify procedures that are requested as a result of the New Technology Application Process or that capture services not routinely classified in ICD-10-PCS.

After Section X codes have served their purpose, proposals to delete the codes and create new codes in the existing ICD-10-PCS tables will be addressed at ICD-10 Coordination and Maintenance meetings.

The structure of ICD-10-PCS Section X codes includes:

- First character – letter X
- Second character – body system value

- Third character – root operation value
- Fourth character – body part value
- Fifth character – approach value
- Sixth character – device/substance/technology value
- Seventh character – information indicating the year created (e.g., New Technology Group 3 codes were created for use in fiscal year 2018, beginning October 1, 2017)

General Guidelines

E1.a. Section X (New Technology) codes fully represent the specific procedure described in the code title, and they do not require additional codes from other sections of ICD-10-PCS. When section X contains a code title that fully describes a specific new technology procedure, and it is the only procedure performed, only the section X code is reported for the procedure. There is no need to report an additional code in another section of ICD-10-PCS.

> **Example:** Cefiderocol anti-infective was administered via a central vein. ICD-10-PCS code XW043A6 (Introduction of Cefiderocol Anti-infective into Central Vein, Percutaneous Approach, New Technology Group 6) is reported. A separate code from ICD-10-PCS Table 3E0 in the Administration section is *not* coded.

E1.b. When multiple procedures are performed, New Technology section X codes are reported by following the ICD-10-PCS multiple procedures guideline. (The *Root Operation—Multiple Procedures guideline* states that during the same operative episode, codes are constructed for multiple procedures performed if the same root operation, such as excision, is performed on different body parts, as defined by distinct values of the body part axis of classification.)

> **Example 1:** When dual filter cerebral embolic filtration is used during transcatheter aortic valve replacement (TAVR), code X2A5312 (Cerebral Embolic Filtration, Dual Filter in Innominate Artery and Left Common Carotid Artery, Percutaneous Approach, New Technology Group 2) is reported for the cerebral embolic filtration. A separate ICD-10-PCS code *is reported* for the TAVR procedure.

> **Example 2:** When a magnetically controlled growth rod (MCGR) is placed during a spinal fusion procedure, a code from Table XNS, Reposition of bones, is reported for the MCGR. A separate ICD-10-PCS code *is reported* for the spinal fusion procedure.

Exercise 6.6 – ICD-10-PCS Section Coding Guidelines

Instructions: Use ICD-10-PCS official coding guidelines to identify the name of the guideline that applies to each procedure statement. Then, use the ICD-10-PCS coding manual's index and tables to construct code(s).

1. Percutaneous chest tube insertion, right pleural cavity

   Guideline Name: _____

   ICD-10-PCS code(s): _____

2. Arterial vascular examination of right femoral artery, open

   Guideline Name: _____

   ICD-10-PCS code(s): _____

3. Open cholecystectomy after Kocher (right subcostal) incision

   Guideline Name: _____

   ICD-10-PCS code(s): _____

Exercise 6.6 – continued

4. Partial open resection of left lobe, liver; open cholecystectomy

    Guideline Name: _____

    ICD-10-PCS code(s): _____

5. Open right knee replacement procedure canceled due to uncontrolled hypertension during surgery; open right knee resection was completed

    Guideline Name: _____

    ICD-10-PCS code(s): _____

6. Open excisional biopsy, left axillary lymph nodes

    Guideline Name: _____

    ICD-10-PCS code(s): _____

7. Open excisional biopsy, left ovary; open oophorectomy, left ovary

    Guideline Name: _____

    ICD-10-PCS code(s): _____

8. Reattachment, right and left kidneys

    Guideline Name: _____

    ICD-10-PCS code(s): _____

9. Adenoidectomy via oral *os*

    Guideline Name: _____

    ICD-10-PCS code(s): _____

10. Open right knee replacement procedure using patellofemoral synthetic substitute and cement

    Guideline Name: _____

    ICD-10-PCS code(s): _____

11. Percutaneous endoscopic amnioscopy; therapeutic drainage of amniotic fluid via ultrasonic guidance

    Guideline Name: _____

    ICD-10-PCS code(s): _____

12. Manually-assisted delivery of healthy female term infant, and manual removal of retained placenta

    Guideline Name: _____

    ICD-10-PCS code(s): _____

13. High-dose rate (HDR) brachytherapy, uterus, Iridium 192, and insertion of intrauterine brachytherapy applicator via endoscopic approach

    Guideline Name: _____

    ICD-10-PCS code(s): _____

14. Subcutaneous injection of caplacizumab

    Guideline Name and Description: _____

    ICD-10-PCS code(s): _____

15. Placement of StrataGraft® on debrided skin, left forearm, followed by placement of a dressing to protect the site

    Guideline Name: _____

    ICD-10-PCS code(s): _____

Summary

The *International Classification of Diseases, 10th Revision, Procedure Coding System* (ICD-10-PCS) is a procedure classification system developed by the Centers for Medicare & Medicaid Services (CMS) for use in the United States for inpatient hospital settings only. It uses a multiaxial seven-character alphanumeric code structure that provides a unique code for all substantially different procedures. It also allows new procedures to be easily incorporated as new codes. ICD-10-PCS contains more than 87,000 seven-character alphanumeric procedure codes.

Two agencies within the Department of Health and Human Services, the Centers for Medicare and Medicaid Services (CMS) and the National Center for Health Statistics (NCHS), prepare guidelines for coding and reporting using ICD-10-PCS, which are used as a companion document when assigning ICD-10-PCS codes. A joint effort between the health care provider and the coder is crucial to achieving complete and accurate documentation, code assignment, and reporting of procedure codes. Coding conventions are general rules used in the ICD-10-PCS classification, and include the use of an indented format in the index, the use of *and* in the index and tables (and means and/or), and cross references (e.g., *see, use*) that instruct the coder to refer to another entry in the index or go directly to the table to build the correct code.

Internet Links

AHA Coding Clinic Advisor: www.codingclinicadvisor.com

ICD-10-PCS encoder (subscription-based): www.encoderpro.com (free trial available)

ICD-10-PCS updates: Go to **www.cms.gov**, click on the Medicare link, click on the ICD-10 link under Coding, and scroll down to click on this year's ICD-10-PCS link.

JustCoding News **free e-newsletter:** Go to **www.justcoding.com**, and click on the eNewsletter Signup link at the top of the page.

Review

6.1 – Multiple Choice

Instructions: Select the most appropriate response.

1. ICD-10-PCS codes are reported for
   a. emergency department services.
   b. hospital inpatient procedures.
   c. outpatient same day surgery.
   d. physician office encounters.

2. ICD-10-PCS uses a(n) _____ 7-character alphanumeric code structure that provides a unique code for all substantially different procedures.
   a. anatomic   b. complex   c. methodological   d. multiaxial

3. The ICD-10-PCS index is arranged
   a. alphabetically.
   b. anatomically.
   c. by service or procedure.
   d. numerically.

4. The development of ICD-10-PCS incorporates an attribute of completeness, which means there are _____ codes for all substantially different procedures.
   a. combination   b. independent   c. repetitive   d. unique

5. The development of ICD-10-PCS incorporates an attribute of standardized terminology, which means definitions of the terminology used are included, and while the meaning of specific words varies in common usage,
   a. as new procedures are developed, they are incorporated into existing codes.
   b. each term is assigned a specific meaning.
   c. codes consist of characters within the same individual axis.
   d. there are combination codes for all substantially different procedures.

6. The *ICD-10-PCS Official Guidelines for Coding and Reporting* are
   a. significant components of a surgical procedure so that codes are reported for substantially different procedures.
   b. diagnostic information that is incorporated into code descriptions for combination diagnosis/procedure codes reporting.
   c. requirements that documentation be at a minimal level of specificity for construction of a code for procedures.
   d. rules that were developed to accompany and complement coding conventions and instructions provided within ICD-10-PCS.

7. Which are *excluded* from use in ICD-10-PCS?
   a. alphanumeric characters
   b. capital letters I and O
   c. capital letters L and Z
   d. numbers 1 and 0

8. ICD-10-PCS codes
   a. contain decimals.
   b. do not contain decimals.
   c. have letters in position one only.
   d. include numbers in position seven only.

9. Which is an example of an ICD-10-PCS body system?
   a. anterior   b. lungs   c. osmolar   d. respiratory

10. Use ICD-10-PCS Table 001 to construct the code for a *percutaneous endoscopic bypass procedure from cerebral ventricle to cerebral cisterns*.

ICD-10-PCS Table (portion)			
001			
Section	**0** Medical and Surgical		
Body System	**0** Central Nervous System and Cranial Nerves		
Operation	**1** Bypass: Altering the route of passage of the contents of a tubular body part		
Body Part	*Approach*	*Device*	*Qualifier*
6 Cerebral Ventricle	**0** Open **3** Percutaneous **4** Percutaneous Endoscopic	**Z** No Device	**B** Cerebral Cisterns

   a. 00160ZB   b. 00163ZB   c. 001644B   d. 00164ZB

11. ICD-10-PCS coding conventions are general rules used in the classification that are
   a. dependent on coding guidelines.
   b. included in ICD-10-PCS as default codes and syndromes.
   c. incorporated into ICD-10-PCS as instructional notes.
   d. must be referenced in a written physician query.

12. In the ICD-10-PCS index, subterms are indented below
   a. code descriptions.   b. codes.   c. instructional notes.   d. main terms.

13. ICD-10-PCS makes use of boldface for
    a. code descriptions in the index.
    b. codes in the tabular list of procedures.
    c. instructional notes in tables.
    d. main term entries in the index.

14. The ICD-10-PCS index uses a(n) _____ for ease in reference when locating subterms.
    a. boxed note
    b. excludes instruction
    c. inclusion term
    d. indented format

15. ICD-10-PCS codes are constructed by using the
    a. appropriate table to build a code.
    b. drugs and chemicals table.
    c. neoplasms table.
    d. tabular list of procedures.

16. When the word *and* appears in category titles and code descriptions in the ICD-10-PCS Index and Tables, it is interpreted as meaning
    a. and/or.   b. due to.   c. in.   d. with.

17. In the ICD-10-PCS Index, the word *with* is located
    a. as an instructional notation to provide coding direction.
    b. in alphabetical order below the main term or a subterm.
    c. just below the main term or subterm, not in alphabetic order.
    d. within provider documentation as a requirement for coding.

18. The *see* cross reference located after a main term, or indented as a subterm, directs the coder to a root operation term in the ICD-10-PCS index or table, and the coder
    a. goes to the tabular list of procedures to locate the code.
    b. has the option to follow the cross reference or not to build the code.
    c. is directed to that referenced main term to construct the correct code.
    d. selects the incomplete code in the index for reporting purposes.

19. Which instruction directs the coder to a body part or a device in ICD-10-PCS tables?
    a. *see*   b. *see also*   c. *see category*   d. *use*

20. A patient underwent angiectomy of the left saphenous vein. Using the ICD-10-PCS index entry for main term Angiectomy, which cross reference should the coder follow?

ICD-10-PCS Index (partial)
Angiectomy
see Excision, Heart and Great Vessels 02B *see* Excision, Upper Arteries 03B *see* Excision, Lower Arteries 04B *see* Excision, Upper Veins 05B *see* Excision, Lower Veins 06B

    a. *see* Excision, Upper Arteries 03B
    b. *see* Excision, Lower Arteries 04B
    c. *see* Excision, Upper Veins 05B
    d. *see* Excision, Lower Veins 06B

21. A patient underwent *continuous cardiac assistance facilitated by use of an impeller pump*. Using the ICD-10-PCS index entry for main term Assistance, which code should be verified in the ICD-10-PCS tables?

ICD-10-PCS Index (partial)
Assistance
Cardiac
Continuous
Output
Balloon Pump 5A02210
Impeller Pump 5A0221D
Other Pump 5A02216
Pulsatile Compression 5A02215

    a. 5A02210   **b.** 5A0221D   **c.** 5A02216   **d.** 5A02215

22. The patient underwent *angiotripsy, right brachial artery*. Using the ICD-10-PCS index entry for main term Angiotripsy, which cross reference is followed?

ICD-10-PCS Index (partial)
Angiotripsy
See Occlusion, Upper Arteries 03L
See Occlusion, Lower Arteries 04L

    a. *See* Occlusion, Upper Arteries 03L
    b. *See* Occlusion, Lower Arteries 04L

23. The patient underwent *replacement of a spinal canal drainage device*. Using ICD-10-PCS Table 002, which code is constructed?

ICD-10-PCS Table			
002			
Section	**0**	Medical and Surgical	
Body System	**0**	Central Nervous System and Cranial Nerves	
Operation	**2**	Change: Taking out or off a device from a body part and putting back an identical or similar device in or on the same body part without cutting or puncturing the skin or a mucous membrane	
Body Part	*Approach*	*Device*	*Qualifier*
0 Brain **E** Cranial Nerve **U** Spinal Canal	**X** External	**0** Drainage Device **Y** Other Device	**Z** No Qualifier

    a. 0020X0Z   **b.** 002EX0Z   **c.** 002UX0Z   **d.** 002UXYZ

24. The patient underwent *stereotactic particulate radiosurgery, left eye*. Using ICD-10-PCS Table D82, which code is constructed?

ICD-10-PCS Table			
D82			
Section	**D**	Radiation Therapy	
Body System	**8**	Eye	
Modality	**2**	Stereotactic Radiosurgery	
Treatment Site	*Modality Qualifier*	*Isotope*	*Qualifier*
0 Eye	**D** Stereotactic Other Photon Radiosurgery **H** Stereotactic Particulate Radiosurgery **J** Stereotactic Gamma Beam Radiosurgery	**Z** None	**Z** None

    a. D820DZZ   **b.** D820HZZ   **c.** D820JJZ   **d.** D820JZZ

25. The patient underwent *chest x-ray* (plain radiography). Using ICD-10-PCS Table BB0, which code is constructed?

ICD-10-PCS Table		
BB0		
Section	**B**	Imaging
Body System	**B**	Respiratory System
Type	**0**	Plain Radiography: Planar display of an image developed from the capture of external ionizing radiation on photographic or photoconductive plate

Body Part	Contrast	Qualifier	Qualifier
7 Tracheobronchial Tree, Right **8** Tracheobronchial Tree, Left **9** Tracheobronchial Trees, Bilateral	**Y** Other Contrast	**Z** None	**Z** None
D Upper Airways	**Z** None	**Z** None	**Z** None

   a. BB07YZZ   **b.** BB08YZZ   **c.** BB09YZZ   **d.** BB0DZZZ

ICD-10-PCS Coding Practice

Instructions: Use the ICD-10-PCS coding manual's index and tables to construct appropriate code(s) for each procedure statement.

- The ICD-10-PCS index entry usually contains just the first three (or four) characters of a code, which direct coders to the appropriate table to "build a code."
- When the ICD-10-PCS index contains the seven-character code, verify its accuracy in the table.
- Refer to coding conventions and guidelines in this chapter for direction about constructing codes.

6.2 – Medical and Surgical Section

The Medical and Surgical Section root operations can be subdivided into groups that share similar attributes:

- *Take out some or all of a body part*: destruction, detachment, excision, extraction, and resection
- *Take out solids, fluids, and gases from a body part*: drainage, extirpation, and fragmentation
- *Involve cutting or separation only*: division and release
- *Put in, put back, or move some or all of a body part*: reattachment, reposition, transfer, and transplantation
- *Alter the diameter/route of a tubular body part*: bypass, dilation, occlusion, and restriction
- *Always involve a device*: change, insertion, removal, replacement, revision, and supplement
- *Involve examination only*: inspection and map
- *Involve repairs and other objectives:* alteration, control, creation, fusion, and repair

6.2A – Root Operations: Destruction, Detachment, Excision, Extraction, and Resection

1. _____ Percutaneous cryoablation of left breast lesion using ultrasound guidance
2. _____ Open disarticulation of fifth toe, right foot, complete
3. _____ Percutaneous endoscopic excisional biopsy, ascending colon
4. _____ Percutaneous endoscopic avulsion of abdominal sympathetic nerve
5. _____ Abdominohysterectomy, open

6.2B – Root Operations: Drainage, Extirpation, and Fragmentation

1. _____ Open myringotomy, right tympanic membrane, with placement of ventilation tube
2. _____ Percutaneous endoscopic ureterolithotomy, right ureter
3. _____ Extracorporeal shock wave lithotripsy, right kidney pelvis
4. _____ Percutaneous thrombectomy, left anterior tibial artery
5. _____ Percutaneous thoracentesis, right pleural cavity

6.2C – Root Operation: Division and Release

1. _____ Percutaneous cordotomy, thoracic spinal cord
2. _____ Percutaneous endoscopic lysis of peritoneal adhesions
3. _____ Open nephrolysis, left kidney
4. _____ Oophorotomy, left ovary, open
5. _____ Episiotomy

6.2D – Root Operations: Reattachment, Reposition, Transfer, and Transplantation

1. _____ Replantation, skin of scalp
2. _____ Open endoscopic transplant, left kidney (from organ donor)

> **⚠ Coding Tip**
>
> Transplantation procedures require selection of type of transplantation source, which includes allogeneic (e.g., organ donor), syngeneic (e.g., patient, patient's identical twin), and zooplastic (e.g., animal organ) sources.

3. _____ Pedicled transverse rectus abdominis myocutaneous (TRAM) flap reconstruction, right abdomen muscle, open
4. _____ Percutaneous endoscopic transfer of flexor hallucis longus tendon, right ankle
5. _____ Open liver transplant (from organ donor)

6.2E – Root Operations: Bypass, Dilation, Occlusion, and Restriction

1. _____ Open coronary artery bypass grafting (CABG) procedure using the patient's left internal mammary artery, which remained intact, with use of cardiopulmonary bypass (machine) for extracorporeal circulation

> **⚠ Coding Tip**
>
> CABG procedures require selection of type of grafting material, which includes autologous (e.g., patient's blood vessel, such as left internal mammary artery), nonautologous (e.g., donor artery or vein), synthetic substitute (e.g., manufactured product, such as *Regenerez® Poly[glycerol sebacate] Resin), and* zooplastic (e.g., animal artery or vein). The left internal mammary artery remained intact, which means it was *not* excised from its source. Instead, one end of the artery was freed up and grafted to bypass the occluded coronary artery. In addition to the CABG procedure code, construct a code for cardiopulmonary bypass (machine). Two codes are required to completely classify this CABG procedure.

2. _____ Percutaneous endoscopic transluminal coronary angioplasty (PTCA) of the left anterior descending and left circumflex arteries, with drug-eluting stent placement in both arteries
3. _____ Percutaneous occlusion of right lacrimal duct with placement of nasolacrimal stent as an intraluminal device

4. _____ Percutaneous endoscopic esophagogastric junction fundoplication with intraluminal device via natural opening

5. _____ Open Alfieri stitch valvuloplasty with use of cardiopulmonary bypass (machine) for extracorporeal circulation

6.2F – Root Operations: Change, Insertion, Removal, Replacement, Revision, and Supplement

1. _____ Change of nasogastric feeding tube

2. _____ Insertion of spinal cord stimulator generator between lower abdominal subcutaneous skin and fascia, open; percutaneous insertion of neurostimulator electrodes, spinal cord

3. _____ Open replacement of neurostimulator lead, epidural space of spinal cord

 Coding Tip

Replacement of a neurostimulator lead requires assignment of two ICD-10-PCS codes:

- Insertion of neurostimulator lead.
- Removal of ineffective neurostimulator lead.

4. _____ Percutaneous replacement of pacemaker lead in left atrium of heart

 Coding Tip

Assign two separate codes for this procedure.

- Insertion of pacemaker lead into left atrium. (A pacemaker lead is a cardiac lead.)
- Removal of broken pacemaker lead from left atrium.

5. _____ Open acetabuloplasty replacement procedure with metal prosthesis, right patella

6. _____ Open annuloplasty with annuloplasty ring as a supplement, aortic valve

7. _____ Change of endotracheal tube

8. _____ Abdominal aortoplasty replacement procedure using a fabric tube, open

9. _____ Gastric band revision, percutaneous laparoscopic approach

10. _____ Right breast mammoplasty using silicone implant as supplement, open

6.2G – Root Operations: Inspection and Map

1. _____ Percutaneous arterioscopy, right brachial artery

2. _____ Diagnostic laryngoscopy via natural opening

3. _____ Lesion-symptom mapping of cerebellum, open

4. _____ Open functional mapping, brain

5. _____ Exploratory laparotomy, open

6.2H – Root Operations: Alteration, Control, Creation, Fusion, and Repair

1. _____ Percutaneous endoscopic control of bleeding using through-the-scope hemostatic clips, upper gastrointestinal tract

2. _____ Percutaneous arthroscopic acetabuloplasty, right hip

3. _____ Rhinoplasty, external approach

4. _____ Gender reassignment surgery using amniotic membrane tissue (as autologous tissue substitute) to create a vagina in male patient

5. _____ Open arthrodesis of two cervical vertebral joints using interbody fusion device, posterior approach, anterior column

6.3 – Obstetrics Section

The Obstetrics Section includes root operations: abortion, change, delivery, drainage, extraction, insertion, inspection, removal, repair, reposition, resection, and transplantation.

1. _____ Manual suction curettage of retained placenta, post-Cesarean section

2. _____ Assisted vaginal delivery using vacuum extraction

3. _____ External cephalic version (repositioning) of breech infant at 36 weeks

4. _____ Open repair of heart defect, fetus (products of conception)

5. _____ Percutaneous endoscopic resection, ectopic products of conception

6.4 – Placement Section

The Placement Section includes root operations: change, compression, dressing, immobilization, packing, removal, and traction.

1. _____ Change of lower arm cast, right

2. _____ Nasal packing

3. _____ Removal of nasal packing

4. _____ Compression of abdominal wall with pressure dressing

5. _____ Placement of dressing, left hand

6.5 – Administration Section

The Administration Section of ICD-10-PCS includes root operations: introduction, irrigation, and transfusion.

1. _____ Percutaneous (peripheral) intravenous transfusion of autologous red blood cells

2. _____ Introduction of total parenteral nutrition via peripherally inserted central catheter (PICC) (percutaneous) line under ultrasound guidance

3. _____ External wound irrigation, skin of right hand

4. _____ Percutaneous intravenous transfusion of nonautologous 4-factor prothrombin complex concentrate

5. _____ Flushing, left eye

6.6 – Measurement and Monitoring Section

The Measurement and Monitoring Section includes root operations: measurement and monitoring.

1. _____ Blood pressure measurement, left arm

2. _____ Temperature monitoring, forehead

3. _____ Cardiac output monitoring via percutaneous pulmonary artery catheter

4. _____ Electromyogram

5. _____ Cardiac rhythm-related device interrogation of defibrillator functioning

6.7 – Extracorporeal or Systemic Assistance and Performance Section

The Extracorporeal or Systemic Assistance and Performance Section includes root operations: assistance, performance, and restoration.

1. _____ Cardiac assistance using continuous output balloon pump

2. _____ Cardioversion

3. _____ Continuous renal replacement therapy (CRRT)

4. _____ External cardiac massage

5. _____ Continuous positive airway pressure (CPAP) for respiratory assistance, 8 hours while sleeping

6.8 – Extracorporeal or Systemic Therapies Section

The Extracorporeal or Systemic Therapies Section includes root operations: atmospheric control, decompression, electromagnetic therapy, hyperthermia, hypothermia, perfusion, pheresis, phototherapy, ultrasound therapy, ultraviolet light therapy, and shock wave therapy.

1. _____ Hyperbaric oxygenation for decompression sickness, single treatment

2. _____ Electromagnetic therapy, central nervous system, single treatment

3. _____ Therapeutic hypothermia, single treatment, whole body

4. _____ Therapeutic leukopheresis, multiple treatments

5. _____ Donor heart perfusion preservation, single

6.9 – Osteopathic Section

The Osteopathic Section includes root operation: treatment.

1. _____ Indirect osteopathic treatment, rib cage

2. _____ General mobilization osteopathic treatment, cervical region

3. _____ Fascial release osteopathic treatment, lumbar region

4. _____ Low velocity-high amplitude osteopathic treatment, lower extremities

5. _____ Osteopathic treatment, abdomen, using a lymphatic pump

6.10 – Other Procedures Section

The Other Procedures Section includes root operation: other procedures.

1. _____ Blood specimen collection from indwelling device

2. _____ Cerebrospinal fluid collection from indwelling device

3. _____ Collection of breast milk (from patient's breasts)

4. _____ Collection of sperm sample

5. _____ *In vitro* fertilization

6.11 – Chiropractic Section

The Chiropractic Section includes root operation: manipulation.

1. _____ Chiropractic manipulation, cervical region, extra-articular method

2. _____ Chiropractic manipulation, thoracic region, mechanically assisted method

3. _____ Chiropractic manipulation, pelvis region, extra-articular method

4. _____ Chiropractic manipulation, abdominal region, indirect visceral method

5. _____ Chiropractic manipulation, lower extremities, long and short lever specific contact method

6.12 – Imaging Section

The Imaging Section includes root types: computerized tomography (CT scan), fluoroscopy, magnetic resonance imaging (MRI), plain radiography, and ultrasonography.

1. _____ Screening mammography, bilateral, with computer-aided detection

2. _____ Magnetic resonance imaging, lumbar spine

3. _____ CT scan, abdomen and pelvis, with contrast material

4. _____ Chest x-ray, 2 views

5. _____ Echocardiogram with contrast

6.13 – Nuclear Medicine Section

The Nuclear Medicine Section includes root types: nonimaging nuclear medicine assay, nonimaging nuclear medicine probe, planar nuclear medicine imaging, and tomographic (tomo) nuclear medicine imaging.

1. _____ PET scan, brain, using Carbon 11

2. _____ Planar nuclear medicine imaging, abdomen, using Technetium 99m

3. _____ Tomographic (tomo) nuclear medicine imaging, hepatobiliary system and pancreas, using a radionuclide

4. _____ Nonimaging nuclear medicine probe, brain, using Xenon 133

5. _____ Nonimaging nuclear medicine assay, blood, using Iodine 125

6.14 – Radiation Therapy Section

The Radiation Therapy Section includes root modalities: beam radiation, brachytherapy, other radiation, and stereotactic radiosurgery.

1. _____ Beam radiation, left breast, photons 10 MeV

2. _____ Brachytherapy, uterus, Iridium 192 (low-dose rate)

3. _____ Stereotactic radiosurgery, brain, using particulate radiosurgery

4. _____ Contact radiation, prostate

5. _____ Plaque radiation, right eye

6.15 – Physical Rehabilitation and Diagnostic Audiology Section

The Physical Rehabilitation and Diagnostic Audiology Section includes root types: activities of daily living assessment, activities of daily living treatment, caregiver training, cochlear implant treatment, device fitting, hearing aid assessment, hearing assessment, hearing treatment, motor and/or nerve function assessment, motor treatment, speech assessment, speech treatment, vestibular assessment, and vestibular treatment.

1. _____ Speech therapy treatment for aphasia using augmentative/alternate communication (hand movements, facial expressions, and gestures because patient is blind)

2. _____ Motor function assessment, upper back and extremities (musculoskeletal system), range of motion and joint integrity

3. _____ Activities of daily living treatment for bathing using assistive, adaptive, supportive, or protective equipment

4. _____ Vestibular treatment for postural control using an orthosis balance brace to stabilize posture, musculoskeletal system/whole body

5. _____ Hearing aid assessment for cochlear implant using audiometer equipment

6.16 – Mental Health Section

The Mental Health Section includes root types: biofeedback, counseling, crisis intervention, electroconvulsive therapy, family psychotherapy, group psychotherapy, hypnosis, individual psychotherapy, light therapy, medication management, narcosynthesis, and psychological tests.

1. _____ Determination of mental status

2. _____ Crisis intervention

3. _____ Medication management

4. _____ Individual cognitive-behavioral psychotherapy

5. _____ Electroconvulsive therapy, bilateral single seizure

6.17 – Substance Abuse Treatment Section

The Substance Abuse Treatment Section includes root types: detoxification services, family counseling, group counseling, individual counseling, individual psychotherapy, medication management, and pharmacotherapy.

1. _____ Detoxification services for alcohol abuse

2. _____ Antabuse pharmacotherapy for alcohol abuse

3. _____ Family counseling for substance abuse

4. _____ Group psychoeducation counseling for cocaine abuse

5. _____ Medication management for Methadone maintenance

6.18 – New Technology Section

The New Technology Section includes root operations: assistance, destruction, dilation, extirpation, fusion, introduction, measurement, monitoring, replacement, reposition, supplement, and transfusion.

1. _____ Percutaneous dilation, right anterior tibial artery, sustained release drug-eluting intraluminal device

2. _____ ENROUTE® Transcarotid Neuroprotection System, right common carotid artery, percutaneous approach, with placement of cerebral embolic filtration, extracorporeal flow reversal circuit

3. _____ Open fusion, thoracolumbar vertebral joint, with interbody fusion device, customizable

4. _____ Open insertion of tibial extension with motion sensors, right tibia

5. _____ Percutaneous nonautologous convalescent plasma transfusion, central vein

Part V

ICD-10-CM and ICD-10-PCS Inpatient Hospital Coding

Part V of *3-2-1 Code It!* contains the following chapter, which covers ICD-10-CM and ICD-10-PCS inpatient hospital coding.

 NOTE:

- Refer to Chapters 2 through 4 when assigning ICD-10-CM codes for inpatient hospital diagnoses.
- Refer to Chapter 6 when assigning ICD-10-PCS codes for inpatient hospital procedures and services.

Chapter 7: ICD-10-CM and ICD-10-PCS Inpatient Hospital Coding, 298

ICD-10-CM and ICD-10-PCS Inpatient Hospital Coding

Chapter Outline

Acute Care Facilities (Hospitals)

Inpatient Diagnosis Coding Guidelines

Inpatient Procedure Coding Guidelines

Coding Inpatient Diagnoses and Procedures

Chapter Objectives

At the conclusion of this chapter, the student should be able to:

1. Define key terms related to ICD-10-CM and ICD-10-PCS inpatient hospital coding.
2. Explain the differences among acute care inpatient settings.
3. Interpret inpatient diagnosis coding guidelines when assigning ICD-10-CM codes.
4. Interpret inpatient procedure coding guidelines when assigning ICD-10-PCS codes.
5. Assign ICD-10-CM and ICD-10-PCS codes for acute care inpatient hospital cases.

Key Terms

2-midnight rule

acute care facility (ACF)

acute care hospital

admitting diagnosis

ancillary service

bed count

bed size

behavioral health care
  hospital

comorbidity

complication

critical access hospital
  (CAH)

general hospital

hospital-acquired
  condition (HAC)

inpatient

long-term acute care
  hospital (LTACH)

long-term hospital

maximizing
  reimbursement

multihospital system

newborn patient

optimizing
  reimbursement

other (additional)
  diagnoses

other significant
  procedure

present on admission
  (POA)

present on admission
  (POA) indicator

principal diagnosis

principal procedure

rehabilitation hospital

secondary procedure

short-term hospital

single hospital

specialty hospital

subacute care patient

swing bed

Uniform Hospital
  Discharge Data Set
  (UHDDS)

Introduction

This chapter defines inpatient hospital acute care settings and includes an interpretation of the guidelines for sequencing diagnosis (and procedures, as required by some third-party payers) published in the Centers for Medicare and Medicaid Services (CMS) *ICD-10-CM Official Guidelines for Coding and Reporting* and *ICD-10-PCS Official Guidelines for Coding and Reporting*. When assigning ICD-10-CM and ICD-10-PCS codes for this chapter, refer to textbook Chapters 2–4 and 6 for coding guidance.

Coding guidelines discussed in this chapter (and in textbook Chapters 2 through 4 and 6) are to be used as a companion to the official version of the ICD-10-CM and ICD-10-PCS, which contain coding conventions to ensure accurate coding.

Acute Care Facilities (Hospitals)

An **acute care facility (ACF)** is a hospital that provides emergency department, inpatient, and outpatient health care services to patients who have serious, sudden, or acute illnesses or injuries and/or who need certain surgeries. ACFs provide a full range of health care services including ancillary services, emergency and critical care, surgery, and obstetrics (labor and delivery). **Ancillary services** are diagnostic and therapeutic services provided to inpatients and outpatients (e.g., laboratory, physical therapy). Most inpatient hospital stays are short (fewer than 30 days), although some patients may stay for a longer time if medically necessary. Because each inpatient hospital day is expensive, a utilization or case manager closely monitors patient care to determine whether acute health care services are required.

 NOTE:

This chapter focuses on inpatient hospital (acute care) ICD-10-CM and ICD-10-PCS coding.

Hospitals have an organized medical and professional staff, and inpatient beds are available 24 hours per day. The primary function of hospitals is to provide inpatient medical, nursing, and other health-related services to patients for surgical and nonsurgical conditions. (Hospitals usually provide emergency department and outpatient services as well, for which ICD-10-CM, CPT, and HCPCS Level II codes are assigned.) Hospitals are categorized as (1) **single hospitals** (hospitals are self-contained and not part of larger organizations) and (2) **multihospital systems** (where two or more hospitals are owned, managed, or leased by a single organization; these may include acute, long-term, pediatric, rehabilitation, or psychiatric care facilities).

Another consideration when discussing hospital organization is to identify the *population served by a health care facility*, which means that health care is provided to specific groups of people in that some hospitals specialize in the treatment of children (e.g., pediatric hospitals), while others have special units (e.g., burn unit). The hospital **bed size** (or **bed count**) is the total number of inpatient beds for which the facility is licensed by the state; the hospital must be equipped and staffed to care for these patient admissions. The hospital's average length of stay (LOS) determines classification as a

- **Short-term hospital** (or **acute care hospital**): Average LOS of 4–5 days and a total LOS of 25 days or less.
- **Long-term hospital** (or long-term acute care hospital or LTACH): Average LOS is more than 25 days.

> **Example:** Patient was admitted 4/5/YYYY and discharged on 4/10/YYYY. To calculate the LOS, count the day of admission but not the day of discharge. This patient's LOS is 5 days.

Hospitals are also categorized by type.

- **Critical access hospitals (CAHs)** are located more than 35 miles from any hospital or another CAH, or they are state-certified as being a necessary provider of health care to area residents. (The requirement is reduced to 15 miles in areas where only secondary roads are available or in mountainous terrains.) CAHs must provide emergency services 24 hours per day and maintain no more than 15 inpatient beds (except swing-bed facilities, which can have up to 25 inpatient beds if no more than 15 are used at any one time for acute care). Inpatients are restricted to 96-hour stays unless a longer period is required due to inclement weather or the development of another emergency condition. (A **swing bed** allows a rural hospital to admit a nonacute care patient.)
- **General hospitals** provide emergency care, perform general surgery, and admit patients for a range of problems from fractures to heart disease based on licensing by the state.
- **Long-term acute care hospitals (LTACH)** provide care designed specifically for patients who need functional restoration or rehabilitation and medical management for an average of 3 to 6 weeks.
- **Specialty hospitals** concentrate on a particular population of patients (e.g., children) or diseases (e.g., cancer).
- **Rehabilitation hospitals** admit patients who are diagnosed with trauma (e.g., car accident) or disease (e.g., stroke) and need to learn how to function.
- **Behavioral health care hospitals** specialize in treating individuals with mental health diagnoses.

   Hospital patients who receive care while residing in the facility are categorized as inpatients, newborn patients, and subacute care patients.

- **Inpatients** stay overnight in the facility for 24 or more hours and are provided with room and board and nursing services.
- **Newborn patients** receive infant care upon birth, and, if necessary, they receive neonatal intensive care (either within the hospital or as the result of transfer to another hospital).
- **Subacute care patients** receive specialized long-term acute care such as chemotherapy, injury rehabilitation, ventilator (breathing machine) support, wound care, and other types of health care services provided to seriously ill patients. Subacute care facilities look like *mini-intensive care units*, and they usually do not offer the full range of health care services available in acute care facilities (e.g., emergency departments [EDs], obstetrics, and surgery). Subacute care costs less than acute care, and patients are often transferred directly from an intensive care unit. Medicare will reimburse subacute care facilities if care provided is appropriate and medically necessary.

Medicare Part A Hospital Inpatient Order and Physician Certification

Coverage and reimbursement of Medicare Part A hospital inpatient services requires physician certification of *medical necessity* that such services be provided on an inpatient basis. A critical element of physician certification is the *practitioner order*, which is an inpatient admission order that must be documented by the provider in the patient record. In 2014, CMS issued a final rule (CMS-1599-F) called the **2-midnight rule**, which modified and clarified the policy about Medicare Administrative Contractor (MAC) review of inpatient hospital and critical access hospital (CAH) admissions for payment purposes. Under the final rule, surgical procedures, diagnostic tests, and other treatments (in addition to services designated as inpatient-only) are generally appropriate for inpatient hospital admission and payment under Medicare Part A *when the physician expects the beneficiary to require a stay that crosses at least two midnights and admits the beneficiary to the hospital based upon that expectation.* The rule was published as a response to facilities' and beneficiaries' concerns about increasingly long stays as outpatients (e.g., observation care) due to hospital uncertainties about payment.

Physician certification requires physician authentication of the practitioner order, documentation of a reason for inpatient services, estimated or actual length of time the beneficiary requires inpatient status, and plans for posthospital care.

For inpatient CAH services only, the physician must certify that the beneficiary may reasonably be expected to be discharged or transferred to a hospital within 96 hours after admission to the CAH. For inpatient rehabilitation facilities (IRF) services only, the documentation that IRFs are already required to complete to meet the IRF coverage requirements (e.g., preadmission screening physician review and concurrence, the post-admission physician evaluation, and the required admission orders) may be used to satisfy the certification and recertification statement requirements.

Exercise 7.1 – Acute Care Facilities (Hospitals)

Instructions: Complete each statement.

1. The type of hospital that provides health care services to patients who have serious, sudden, or acute illnesses or injuries and/or who need certain surgeries is called a(n) _____ care facility.

2. Diagnostic and therapeutic services provided to inpatients and outpatients (e.g., laboratory, physical therapy) are called _____ services.

3. Hospitals that are self-contained and not part of larger organizations are called _____ hospitals, while two or more hospitals owned, managed, or leased by a single organization are called multihospital systems.

4. The total number of inpatient beds for which a facility is licensed by the state is called the hospital _____ size or count.

5. A hospital's average length of stay (LOS) determines whether the hospital is classified as a(n) _____ hospital or acute-care hospital, which is characterized by an average LOS of 4–5 days and a total LOS of 25 days or less.

6. A _____ hospital has an average LOS of more than 25 days.

7. A patient was admitted on May 30 and discharged on June 3 of the same year. The LOS is calculated as _____ days.

8. A swing bed allows a rural hospital to admit a(n) _____ care patient.

9. Patients who are diagnosed with trauma or disease and who need to learn how to function are usually admitted to _____ hospitals.

10. A health care facility that concentrates on a particular population of patients (e.g., children) or disease (e.g., cancer) is called a(n) _____ hospital.

Inpatient Diagnosis Coding Guidelines

The circumstances of an inpatient admission govern the sequencing of diagnoses. The **Uniform Hospital Discharge Data Set (UHDDS)** was established by the federal government to define data collected for inpatient hospitalizations (e.g., age, sex, race, diagnoses, procedures, payment sources). UHDDS definitions have always been used by acute care hospitals to report inpatient data elements in a standardized manner. Since the creation of the UHDDS in 1985, the application of the UHDDS definitions has been expanded to include all non-outpatient settings (e.g., acute care, short-term, long-term, and psychiatric hospitals; home health agencies; rehabilitation facilities; and skilled nursing facilities and nursing homes).

Circumstances associated with an inpatient admission govern the following:

- Admitting diagnosis
- Principal diagnosis
- Additional diagnoses (e.g., comorbidities, complications)
- Hospital-Acquired Conditions and Present on Admission Indicator Reporting

Coding Tip

The ICD-10-CM *principal diagnosis* code is reported for inpatient hospital care, while the first-listed diagnosis code is reported for outpatient and physician office care. All health care settings report *secondary (or additional) diagnosis* codes.

ICD-10-PCS codes are reported for inpatient hospital care as *principal and secondary procedures* (instead of CPT and HCPCS Level II codes, which are reported as first-listed and secondary procedures and services for outpatient and physician office settings).

The attending physician does not document final diagnoses until an inpatient is discharged from the hospital; by that time, a definitive diagnosis has usually been established. Because inpatient coding guidelines prohibit the coding of signs and symptoms when a definitive diagnosis has been established, signs and symptoms are seldom documented as the principal diagnosis on inpatient charts. In addition, qualified (uncertain) diagnoses can be coded as principal and other diagnoses for hospital inpatients because physicians use hospital resources to treat the patient for these types of conditions and because hospital reimbursement is based on the utilization and consumption of resources. (In the outpatient setting, the physician usually does not have time to establish a definitive diagnosis during one encounter. Thus, signs and symptoms are often reported as the first-listed diagnosis for third-party payer reimbursement purposes.)

NOTE:

The attending physician is responsible for documenting the list of final diagnoses in the patient record.

Admitting Diagnosis

The **admitting diagnosis** is the provisional or tentative diagnosis upon which initial patient care is based. It is obtained from the patient's admitting or attending physician by patient registration staff who enter it on the inpatient face sheet. The admitting diagnosis may be a sign (e.g., fever, cough, rash) or symptom (e.g., chest pain, sore throat, numbness) instead of a definitive diagnosis. One admitting diagnosis ICD-10-CM code is reported on the UB-04.

Principal Diagnosis

The **principal diagnosis** is defined in the UHDDS as "that condition established after study to be chiefly responsible for occasioning the admission of the patient to the hospital for care." The application of this UHDDS definition was expanded to include *all non-outpatient settings* (e.g., acute-, short-term, long-term care, and psychiatric hospitals; home health agencies; rehabilitation facilities; nursing facilities.). The UHDDS definition also applies to hospice services (all levels of care).

The most important part of the definition is the phrase *after study*, which directs the coder to review all patient record documentation associated with an inpatient hospitalization to determine the clinical reason for the admission. The circumstances of admission that impact selection of the principal diagnosis include the chief complaint and the patient's signs and symptoms on admission, which are documented on the history and physical examination.

The entire patient record is reviewed to determine which condition was *established after study*. This requires the coder to review ancillary test results (e.g., laboratory, x-ray) and other reports (e.g., operative report, pathology report) to select the principal diagnosis. If selection of the principal diagnosis is unclear, a physician query is generated, and the outcome of the query corroborated with supporting documentation in the patient record. One principal diagnosis code is reported on the UB-04 claim.

NOTE:

When determining the principal diagnosis, ICD-10-CM coding conventions (discussed in textbook Chapter 2) take precedence over official coding guidelines.

HIPAA Alert!

HIPAA regulations for electronic transactions require providers and payers (including MACs) to adhere to the *Official Guidelines for Coding and Reporting*. Thus, a violation of the coding guidelines is a HIPAA violation. Unfortunately, some payers do not appear to be aware of or understand this HIPAA provision. Payers should be informed of the provision in the HIPAA regulation that references the use of coding guidelines. If payers deny claims because certain codes are reported as principal diagnosis, contact your regional CMS office or the HIPAA enforcement office (at CMS) to alert them about the HIPAA violation.

Example: A 51-year-old patient presented to the ED, complaining of ringing in both ears, dizziness, blurred vision, confusion, and difficulty walking. Upon evaluation by the ED physician, the patient stated that these symptoms started suddenly just two hours ago. Past history revealed that the patient takes medication for hypercholesterolemia and hypertension. The patient used to smoke two packs of cigarettes daily until five years ago. Physical examination revealed blood pressure of 175/110. When asked, the patient stated they had been taking the hypertension medication as prescribed.

Patient underwent bilateral carotid ultrasound to evaluate the blood flow of the carotid arteries, and results indicated the need for bilateral carotid angiogram to measure blockage of the carotid arteries. The ED physician transferred the case to a cardiologist, who performed a bilateral carotid angiogram that revealed 90% blockage of the right carotid artery and 50% blockage of the left carotid artery. The patient was admitted to the hospital and scheduled for bilateral carotid angioplasty with insertion of carotid stents in the morning, which was performed uneventfully. Final diagnoses were documented as bilateral carotid artery occlusion, hypertension, and hypercholesterolemia. Procedures performed included bilateral carotid ultrasound, bilateral carotid angiogram, and bilateral carotid angioplasty.

In this example, the principal diagnosis is bilateral carotid artery occlusion (I65.23). Other diagnoses (or secondary diagnoses) include hypertension (I10) and hypercholesterolemia (E78.00). Do not assign codes to the symptoms of ringing in both ears, dizziness, blurred vision, confusion, and difficulty walking because they are associated with bilateral carotid artery occlusion. Signs and symptoms are often documented in the patient's record, but they are not coded if they are considered part of an established diagnosis.

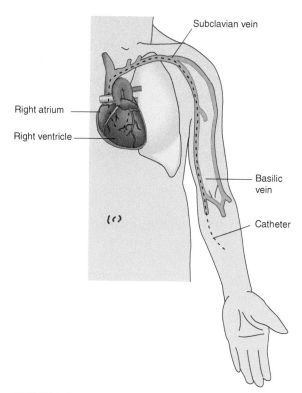

FIGURE 7-1 Cardiac catheterization

Codes for Symptoms, Signs, and Ill-Defined Conditions

Codes for symptoms, signs, and ill-defined conditions from ICD-10-CM Chapter 18 are *not* to be reported as the principal diagnosis when a related definitive diagnosis has been established.

> **Example:** The patient is admitted as a hospital inpatient after having been treated in the ED for chest pain and a positive electrocardiogram (EKG), which revealed anterolateral MI. The patient underwent cardiac catheterization (Figure 7-1) during hospitalization and subsequent quadruple coronary artery bypass graft surgery. The principal diagnosis for this case is acute anterolateral MI, first episode. The chest pain is not assigned a code because it is a symptom of the MI.

Two or More Interrelated Conditions, Each Potentially Meeting the Definition for Principal Diagnosis

When two or more interrelated *inpatient* conditions (e.g., diseases located in the same ICD-10-CM chapter, manifestations associated with a certain disease) potentially meet the definition of principal diagnosis, either condition may be sequenced first unless the circumstances of the admission, the therapy provided, or the ICD-10-CM index or tabular list indicates otherwise.

> **Example:** A patient is admitted as a hospital inpatient with chest pain, fever, and shortness of breath. Chest x-ray reveals exacerbated congestive heart failure (CHF). Physical examination reveals acute bronchitis. The patient's prior history and current EKG findings are consistent with unstable angina (Figure 7-2). All three conditions of CHF, acute bronchitis, and unstable angina are treated with medications, and all three diagnoses equally meet the criteria for the definition of principal diagnosis. The coder can code and sequence any one of the three diagnoses as the principal diagnosis.
>
> As an alternative scenario, this patient underwent coronary arteriography that revealed coronary artery disease and 95% blockage of two prominent arterial branches. Subsequently, the patient was taken to the operating room for percutaneous transluminal coronary angioplasty (PTCA). In this scenario, the coronary arteriography diagnostic workup and PTCA treatment criteria clearly distinguished coronary artery disease, identified as the etiology (cause) of the patient's unstable angina, as the principal diagnosis.

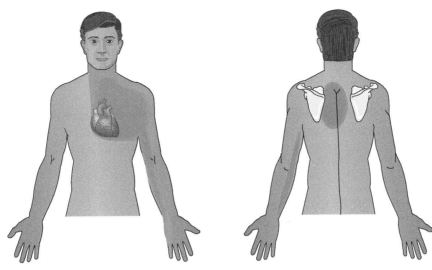

FIGURE 7-2 Patterns of angina

Two or More Diagnoses That Equally Meet the Definition for Principal Diagnosis

In the unusual instance when two or more *inpatient* diagnoses *equally* meet the criteria for principal diagnosis, *as determined by one or more of the following*, any one of the diagnoses may be reported as the principal diagnosis.

- Circumstances of admission
- Diagnostic workup and/or therapy provided
- ICD-10-CM index, tabular list, or other coding guidelines do not provide sequencing direction

Determining which of several diagnoses to report as the principal diagnosis when multiple diagnoses equally meet the criteria for selection as the principal diagnosis is called **optimizing reimbursement**, and it is permitted under the inpatient prospective payment system (IPPS), which uses diagnosis-related groups (DRGs). (DRGs are discussed in Chapter 20.) (Trauma cases often result in several diagnoses, any one of which could be selected and reported as the principal diagnosis.) **Maximizing reimbursement** is *not* permitted because it involves (1) selecting and reporting as principal diagnosis the code that results in the highest level of reimbursement for the facility, whether that diagnosis meets the criteria for selection or not, or (2) assigning a higher-paying code (upcoding) to a diagnosis (or ICD-10-PCS, CPT, or HCPCS Level II code to a procedure) even if patient record documentation does not support that code selection. (Under the IPPS, upcoding and maximizing reimbursement is called *DRG creep*.)

> **Example 1:** OPTIMIZING REIMBURSEMENT: The patient was admitted to the hospital after an automobile accident, initial evaluation was performed in the ED, and the patient was diagnosed with fractured left femur and fractured right humerus. Inpatient treatment included an open reduction internal fixation of the fractured left femur and open reduction internal fixation of the fractured right humerus. In this case, either the fractured left femur or the fractured right humerus could be reported as the principal diagnosis. The best practice would be to assign codes to each diagnosis and procedure, enter them into the diagnosis-related grouper, determine which would result in optimal reimbursement for the hospital, and report that code as the principal diagnosis.

> **Example 2:** MAXIMIZING REIMBURSEMENT AND UPCODING: The patient was admitted as a hospital inpatient for treatment of urosepsis, which is a urinary tract infection (UTI). (A secondary code is assigned to indicate the cause of the infection, such as *Escherichia coli*.) The DRG reimbursement rate is approximately $2,300. Using encoder and DRG grouper software, the coder may notice that the code for sepsis results in the higher DRG rate of approximately $6,400. If the code for sepsis is reported as principal diagnosis, this case would most likely be reviewed to verify accuracy of the reported code. Upon review, the error would be discovered and the hospital could be subject to sanctions (e.g., loss of Medicare participating provider status) and fines.

Two or More Comparative or Contrasting Conditions

In those rare instances when two or more *inpatient* contrasting or comparative diagnoses are documented as *either/or* (or similar terminology), they are coded as if the diagnoses were confirmed. The diagnoses are sequenced according to the circumstances of the admission. If no further determination can be made as to which diagnosis should be principal, either diagnosis may be sequenced first.

> **Example:** An older adult patient was treated for complaints of chest pain and shortness of breath, and the physician documented "acute asthma or acute pneumonia" on the patient's record. The patient died before diagnostic workup could be initiated, and the family declined to have the patient undergo an autopsy. Assign an ICD-10-CM code to both conditions, and either diagnosis may be sequenced as the principal diagnosis to optimize reimbursement.

Original Treatment Plan Not Carried Out

Even though treatment may not have been carried out during an inpatient stay due to unforeseen circumstances, the condition which, after study, occasioned the admission to the hospital is sequenced as the principal diagnosis.

> **Example:** The patient was scheduled for surgery due to severe ureteritis. After administration of anesthesia, the patient was prepped for an endoscopic biopsy of the right ureter. The endoscope passed easily into the urinary bladder but was unable to advance to the right ureter due to ureteral blockage. The surgeon removed the endoscope, and the patient was taken to the recovery room.
>
> In this example, the surgery was halted because after the cystourethroscope was advanced through the urinary bladder, it could not be advanced into the ureter. The principal diagnosis is ureteritis, and the significant other diagnosis is ureteral blockage.

Complications of Surgery and Other Medical Care

When an inpatient admission is for treatment of a complication resulting from surgery or other medical care, the complication code is sequenced as the principal diagnosis. If the complication is classified to the ICD-10-CM T80–T88 series and the code lacks the necessary specificity in describing the complication, an additional code for the specific complication should be assigned.

> **Example:** A 54-year-old patient was admitted to the hospital for severe stomach pain, nausea, vomiting, and fever of 102 degrees. The abdomen was rigid and distended. Past history revealed that two months ago, the patient had undergone open cholecystectomy for cholecystitis with cholelithiasis. Laboratory tests revealed elevated white blood cell count. Patient was scheduled for exploratory laparotomy, which revealed the presence of abscessed stitches. Cultures taken were positive for *Staphylococcus aureus*.
>
> In this example, the principal diagnosis is abscessed stitches, which is a complication of the open cholecystectomy. The significant other diagnoses include staphylococcal infection and postoperative status. The principal procedure is exploratory laparotomy, and the significant other procedure is reopening of recent laparotomy site.

Uncertain Diagnosis (or Qualified Diagnosis)

If the diagnosis documented at the time of discharge is uncertain or qualified with words such as *probable*, *suspected*, *likely*, *questionable*, *possible*, *still to be ruled out*, *compatible with*, *consistent with*, or other similar terms indicating uncertainty, code the diagnosis as if it existed or was established. The basis for this guideline is the diagnostic workup, arrangements for further workup or observation, and initial therapeutic approach that correspond most closely with the established diagnosis. Codes for signs and symptoms are also reported when relevant.

> **Example:** In 1980, before HIV was established as the cause of AIDS (and before AIDS was confirmed as a diagnosis), some hospital inpatients were documented as having "Viral pneumonia versus Sepsis" because patients presented with a combination of signs and symptoms not previously seen. Patients became ill so quickly and were unable to be treated; thus, in addition to codes for viral pneumonia and sepsis (or other uncertain/qualified diagnoses), codes for documented signs and symptoms were also reported due to the unique presentation of each patient. Providers had not previously seen patients present with a combination of cachexia, Kaposi's sarcoma lesions, oral thrush, *Pneumocystis carinii* (now named *Pneumocystis jirovecii*), and other signs and symptoms. Reporting uncertain (or qualified) diagnosis codes with signs/symptoms codes facilitated the research of what was then a confusing and fatal illness, later determined to be AIDS due to HIV.

NOTE:

Assigning *uncertain diagnosis* codes applies only to diagnoses reported for inpatient admissions to acute short-term, acute long-term, and psychiatric *hospitals*. Other non-outpatient health care settings (e.g., home health care, rehabilitation hospitals, skilled nursing facilities, nursing homes) and all outpatient health care settings do not assign codes to uncertain diagnoses. Instead, they assign codes to signs and symptoms when a provider has not documented a definitive diagnosis.

Example: A 24-year-old hospital inpatient was admitted due to fever of 102 degrees for a period of two days, as well as chills. The past history reveals a recent laparoscopic appendectomy, for which postoperative antibiotics were prescribed. Patient completed the prescription and then spiked a fever and started experiencing chills. Review of systems reveals complaints of painful urination for two days. The patient has a history of frequent urinary tract infections (UTIs). Although the urine culture was negative, it is likely that this patient has a UTI, which has to be treated aggressively given the patient's postoperative status.

Patient received intravenous ciprofloxacin and aminoglycoside for a period of 72 hours, improved, and was discharged for follow-up in the office. Patient was prescribed an oral antibiotic to be continued 10 days after discharge. Final diagnosis is possible UTI. In this example, although the final diagnosis of possible UTI is uncertain (or qualified), it is the principal diagnosis. The other significant diagnosis is postoperative surgical status.

Admission from Observation Unit

Admission Following Medical Observation. When a patient is admitted to an observation unit for a medical condition that either worsens or does not improve *and* is subsequently admitted as an inpatient to the same hospital for this same medical condition, the principal diagnosis would be the medical condition that led to the hospital inpatient admission.

Admission Following Postoperative Observation. When a patient is admitted to an observation unit to monitor a condition (or complication) that develops following outpatient surgery and is subsequently admitted as an inpatient of the same hospital, hospitals should apply the Uniform Hospital Discharge Data Set (UHDDS) definition of principal diagnosis as "that condition established after study to be chiefly responsible for occasioning the admission of the patient to the hospital for care."

Admission from Outpatient Surgery

When a patient undergoes surgery in the hospital's outpatient surgery department and is subsequently admitted for continuing inpatient care at the same hospital, the following guidelines should be followed in selecting the principal diagnosis for the inpatient admission:

- If the reason for the inpatient admission is a complication, assign the complication as the principal diagnosis.
- If no complication, or other condition, is documented as the reason for the inpatient admission, assign the reason for the outpatient surgery as the principal diagnosis.
- If the reason for the inpatient admission is another condition unrelated to the surgery, assign the unrelated condition as the principal diagnosis.

Admissions/Encounters for Rehabilitation

When the purpose for the admission or encounter is rehabilitation, sequence first the code for the condition for which the service is being performed. However, if the condition for which the rehabilitation service is being provided is no longer present, report the appropriate aftercare code as the first-listed or principal diagnosis unless the rehabilitation service is being provided following an injury. For rehabilitation services following active treatment of an injury, assign the injury code with the appropriate seventh character for subsequent encounter as the first-listed or principal diagnosis. (Official guidelines for coding and reporting also advise coders to (1) See Section I.C.21.c.7., Factors influencing health status and contact with health services, aftercare, and (2) See Section I.C.19.a., for additional information about the use of seventh characters for injury codes.)

Example 1: The patient is admitted for rehabilitation services for right-sided dominant hemiplegia following a cerebrovascular infarction. Report ICD-10-CM code I69.351 as the first-listed or principal diagnosis.

Example 2: The patient is admitted for rehabilitation services due to severe degenerative osteoarthritis of the hip. The patient previously underwent hip replacement surgery. Report aftercare code Z47.1 as the first-listed or principal diagnosis.

Example 3: A patient underwent initial rehabilitation following hip replacement for right intertrochanteric femur fracture, and code S72.141A (Displaced intertrochanteric fracture of right femur, initial encounter for closed fracture) was reported. The patient is admitted at a later date for additional rehabilitation, and code S72.141D (Displaced intertrochanteric fracture of right femur, subsequent encounter for closed fracture with routine healing) is reported as the principal diagnosis.

Reporting Additional Diagnoses

For reporting purposes, the definition for *other (additional) diagnoses* is interpreted as additional clinically significant conditions that affect patient care by requiring one or more of the following:

- Clinical evaluation
- Therapeutic treatment
- Diagnostic procedures
- Extended length of hospital stay
- Increased nursing care and/or monitoring

The UHDDS defines **other (additional) diagnoses** as "all [clinically significant] conditions that coexist at the time of admission, that develop subsequently, or that affect the treatment received and/or the length of stay." Diagnoses related to an earlier episode that have no bearing on the current hospital stay are not coded. The UHDDS definition applies to all non-outpatient settings (e.g., acute-care, short-term care, long-term care, and psychiatric hospitals; home health agencies; rehabilitation facilities; nursing facilities). The UHDDS definitions also apply to hospice services (all levels of care).

The Centers for Medicare & Medicaid Services (CMS) has developed a standard list of other (additional) diagnoses that are recognized as comorbidities and/or complications (CCs) or major comorbidities and/or complications (MCCs) for Medicare-severity diagnosis-related groups (MS-DRGs) (discussed in Chapter 20). When a CC or MCC is present as a secondary diagnosis, it can affect MS-DRG assignment. A **comorbidity** is a condition that coexists at the time of admission (e.g., diabetes mellitus, hypertension, asthma), and a **complication** is a condition that occurs during the course of the inpatient hospital episode (e.g., fractured hip resulting from fall while gait training, postoperative infection, hospital-acquired staphylococcal infection).

MS-DRGs with CC or MCC require a substantial increase in utilization of hospital resources, and the reimbursement for these DRGs reflects an increase in payment. While just one CC or MCC can change a *MS-DRG without CC or MCC* to an *MS-DRG with CC or MCC*, there are a number of stand-alone MS-DRGs that are not affected by the presence or absence of CCs. For stand-alone MS-DRGs, the MS-DRG (and reimbursement amount) will change (and increase) only if the principal diagnosis is changed or a significant surgical procedure is reported.

Example: An 86-year-old female was admitted to the hospital with complaints of severe shortness of breath, dyspnea, and chest pain. Upon evaluation, the attending physician determined that the patient has a history of intrinsic asthma and is currently experiencing acute exacerbation of that condition. The patient also has a past history of hypertension, for which she takes medication. Last year the patient was treated in the hospital's pain clinic on an outpatient basis for cluster headaches, which have not recurred. Patient received respiratory therapy and drug therapy for the asthma. The physician also ordered medications and patient education for the hypertension and blood pressure monitoring three times per nursing shift. The final diagnoses documented upon discharge include acute exacerbation of intrinsic asthma and hypertension.

In this example, the principal diagnosis is acute exacerbation of intrinsic asthma and the comorbidity (coexisting condition or other significant diagnosis) is hypertension. The hypertension increased nursing care and monitoring because medications were administered, patient teaching was performed, and the patient's blood pressure was taken three times per shift.

Coding Tip

> When other diagnoses are documented and no supporting documentation can be found in the patient record, query the physician to obtain clarification. For example, a patient is admitted for treatment of acute bronchitis; the provider also documents tendonitis, which is not treated. Code acute bronchitis but not the tendonitis.

The following guidelines apply when determining *other (additional) diagnoses* when neither the ICD-10-CM index nor tabular list provides direction. The documentation of diagnoses in the patient record is the responsibility of the provider.

- Previous conditions
- Abnormal findings
- Uncertain diagnoses

Previous Conditions

If the provider has documented a diagnosis in the list of diagnoses on the discharge summary or the face sheet in the patient record, it should ordinarily be coded. However, some providers document diagnoses for resolved conditions and chronic diagnoses from previous admissions that have no bearing on the current inpatient stay. Such conditions are usually *not* coded and reported for reimbursement purposes. However, family and personal history codes are reported as secondary codes *if* the historical condition or family history impacts current care or influences the patient's treatment.

> **Example:** A 92-year-old female patient was admitted as a hospital inpatient for acute MI of the anterolateral wall. The patient's history is negative for cardiovascular or respiratory complaints, and she states that she has not had an MI in the past. The patient does have a past history of localized uterine adenocarcinoma 20 years ago, for which she underwent vaginal hysterectomy. The final diagnosis is acute anterolateral wall MI, initial episode of care.
>
> In this example, the principal diagnosis is acute anterolateral wall MI, initial episode of care. The localized uterine adenocarcinoma is not assigned a neoplasm code from ICD-10-CM Chapter 2. Instead, it is appropriate to assign a code for history of uterine cancer.

Abnormal Findings

Abnormal findings (e.g., ancillary tests such as laboratory, x-ray, pathology, and other diagnostic results) are not coded and reported unless the provider documents their clinical significance. If the ancillary test findings are outside the normal range and the provider has ordered other tests to evaluate the condition or prescribed treatment, it is appropriate to ask the provider whether the abnormal finding should be added.

> **Example:** A 49-year-old patient was admitted as a hospital inpatient for acute pneumonia due to *Staphylococcus aureus*, which was evaluated and successfully treated. During hospitalization, the patient underwent an EKG that was interpreted by the cardiologist as being normal. The EKG report did document abnormal T-wave changes.
>
> In this example, the principal diagnosis is acute pneumonia due to *S. aureus*. The coder should query the physician to determine if a code should be assigned to "abnormal T-wave changes" as documented on the EKG. It is likely that the coder will be told by the physician that such changes are commonly associated with EKGs performed on anxious patients and that this patient was quite ill, which could cause anxiety.

NOTE:

In the outpatient setting, the provider interprets diagnostic test results, and codes are assigned for such encounters.

Uncertain Diagnosis (as Additional Diagnosis)

If the diagnosis documented at the time of discharge is qualified as "probable," "suspected," "likely," "questionable," "possible," "still to be ruled out," "compatible with," "consistent with," or other similar terms indicating uncertainty, code the condition as if it existed or was established. The bases for these guidelines are the diagnostic workup, arrangements for further workup or observation, and initial therapeutic approach that correspond most closely with the established diagnosis. Codes for signs and symptoms are also assigned when relevant (e.g., research for brand-new disease). (This is similar to the selection of principal diagnosis: uncertain diagnosis guideline.)

 NOTE:

The "uncertain diagnosis" guideline is applicable to inpatient admissions for short-term, acute, long-term care, and psychiatric hospitals. "Uncertain diagnosis" is also called "qualified diagnosis." (Uncertain diagnosis codes are *not* reported for outpatient encounters.)

Hospital-Acquired Conditions and Present on Admission Indicator Reporting

The Deficit Reduction Act (DRA) of 2005 requires the Secretary of the U.S. Department of Health and Human Services to identify hospital-acquired conditions (HACs) that (1) are high-cost, high-volume, or both; (2) result in higher claim payments to hospitals due to the presence of the HACs as a secondary diagnosis; and (3) could reasonably have been prevented through the application of evidence-based guidelines. The *DRA payment provision* was implemented to prevent hospitals from receiving additional payment for cases in which an identified HAC occurred but was not present on admission. Instead, such cases will be paid as though the HAC was not present. The goal is to establish a *pay-for-performance program* that links health care quality to inpatient hospital care and ensures patient safety.

Hospital-Acquired Conditions

Medicare implemented an *HAC Reduction Program* as a quality adjustment for Medicare-severity diagnosis-related group (MS-DRG) payments to prevent payment for *certain* **hospital-acquired conditions (HACs),** which are medical conditions that patients develop *during* an inpatient hospitalization, which were not present on admission. HACs include air embolism, blood incompatibility, falls and resulting trauma, foreign objects retained after surgery, hospital-acquired infections (or nosocomial infections).

> **Example:** The Medicare patient was admitted due to coronary artery disease and underwent coronary-artery bypass graft (CABG) surgery. During inpatient hospital recovery the patient fell out of bed and fractured the right hip, and subsequent surgery was performed during the same inpatient hospitalization to treat the fractured hip. When this case is submitted to Medicare for reimbursement, payment will be based on the surgical MS-DRG for the coronary artery disease and CABG surgery. The facility will not receive reimbursement for treatment of the hospital-acquired condition, fracture of right hip.

Present on admission (POA) includes conditions present at the time an order for inpatient hospital admission occurs, including conditions that develop during an outpatient hospital encounter that resulted in an inpatient hospitalization (including emergency department, observation care, or outpatient surgery). There is no required time frame for a provider to identify or document a condition as present on admission. In some clinical situations, it may not be possible for a provider to make a definitive diagnosis (or a condition may not be recognized or reported by the patient) for a period of time after admission. In some cases, it may be several days before the provider arrives at a definitive diagnosis. This does not mean that the condition was not present on admission. Determining that a condition was present on admission is based on applicable POA guidelines or the provider's best clinical judgment.

Present on Admission Indicator

Hospitals that receive reimbursement under the inpatient prospective payment system (IPPS) must submit present on admission (POA) indicators for the principal diagnosis and all secondary diagnoses for inpatient discharges.

The **present on admission (POA) indicator** is assigned by the coder to principal diagnosis, secondary diagnosis, and external cause of injury codes. The *POA indicator* is reported as the eighth character on the UB-04 (CMS-1450) in Field Locator 67 or on the 837 Institutional (837I) electronic claim in the appropriate health care information codes segment.

66 DX	I25119 Y I10 Y		
0			
69 ADMIT DX	I25119	70 PATIENT REASON DX	

- The coder reviews the patient record to determine whether a condition was present on admission or not.

- Issues related to inconsistent, missing, conflicting, or unclear documentation are resolved by the provider as a result of the "physical query" process.

Present on admission is considered *present at the time the order for inpatient admission occurs.* Thus, conditions that develop during an outpatient encounter, including emergency department, observation, or outpatient surgery, are considered as present on admission upon admission of the patient as a hospital inpatient. CMS reporting options and definitions include the following, and payment is made for "Y" and "W" indicators:

- Y = Yes (diagnosis was present at the time of inpatient admission)

- N = No (diagnosis was not present at the time of inpatient admission)

- U = Unknown (documentation is insufficient to determine if the condition was present at the time of inpatient admission) (Generate a *physician query* to determine a condition's POA status instead of reporting POA indicator U for unknown.)

- W = Clinically undetermined (provider is unable to clinically determine whether the condition was present at the time of inpatient admission)

- Blank = Unreported (exempt from POA reporting)

Assigning the POA Indicator

Present on admission (POA) indicator official guidelines are to be followed when assigning POA indicators.

- *Condition is on the "Exempt from Reporting" list.* Leave the *present on admission* field locator (on the UB-04 or 837I) blank if the condition is included on the *Exempt from Reporting* list of ICD-10-CM codes for which POA the field locator is not applicable. This is the only circumstance in which the field locator may be left blank.

- *POA explicitly documented.* Assign Y for any condition the provider explicitly documents as being present on admission. Assign N for any condition the provider explicitly documents as *not* present at the time of admission.

- *Conditions diagnosed prior to inpatient admission.* Assign Y for conditions that were diagnosed prior to admission (e.g., hypertension, diabetes mellitus, asthma).

- *Conditions diagnosed during the admission but clearly present before admission.* Assign Y for conditions diagnosed during the admission that were clearly present but not diagnosed until after admission occurred. Diagnoses subsequently confirmed after admission are considered present on admission if at the time of admission they are documented as suspected, possible, rule out, differential diagnosis, or constitute an underlying cause of a symptom that is present at the time of admission.

- *Condition develops during outpatient encounter prior to inpatient admission.* Assign Y for any condition that develops during an outpatient encounter prior to a written order for inpatient admission.

- *Documentation does not indicate whether condition was present on admission.* Assign U when documentation is unclear as to whether the condition was present on admission. Do *not* routinely assign

POA indicator U. It should be used in very limited circumstances, and coders are encouraged to query the providers when documentation is unclear.

- *Documentation states that it cannot be determined whether the condition was or was not present on admission.* Assign W when documentation indicates that it cannot be clinically determined whether or not the condition was present on admission.

- *Chronic condition with acute exacerbation during the admission.* If a single code identifies both the chronic condition and the acute exacerbation, refer to the *Codes that contain multiple clinical concepts* POA guideline. If a single code only identifies the chronic condition but not the acute exacerbation (e.g., acute exacerbation of chronic leukemia), assign Y to the chronic condition.

- *Conditions documented as possible, probable, suspected, or rule out at the time of discharge.* If the final diagnosis is a qualified or uncertain diagnosis (e.g., possible, probable, rule out, suspected) *and the final diagnosis is based on signs, symptoms, or clinical findings suspected at the time of inpatient admission*, assign Y. If the qualified or uncertain final diagnosis is based on signs, symptoms, or clinical findings *that were not present on admission*, assign N.

- *Conditions documented as impending or threatened at the time of discharge.* If the final diagnosis contains an impending or threatened diagnosis, and this diagnosis is based on symptoms or clinical findings that were present on admission, assign Y. If the final diagnosis contains an impending or threatened diagnosis, and this diagnosis is based on symptoms or clinical findings *that were not present on admission*, assign N.

- *Acute and chronic conditions.* Assign Y for acute conditions that are present at time of admission, and assign N for acute conditions that are *not* present at time of admission. Assign Y for chronic conditions, even though the condition may not be diagnosed until after admission. If a single code identifies both an acute and chronic condition, refer to the *Codes that contain multiple clinical concepts* POA guideline.

- *Codes that contain multiple clinical concepts.* Assign N if at least one of the clinical concepts included in the code *was not present on admission* (e.g., COPD with acute exacerbation but exacerbation was not present on admission, gastric ulcer that does not start bleeding until after admission, asthma patient who develops status asthmaticus after admission). Assign Y if *all* of the clinical concepts associated with a code were present on admission (e.g., duodenal ulcer that perforates prior to admission). For infection codes that include the causal organism, assign Y if the infection (or signs of the infection) were present on admission (even though culture results may not be known until after admission, such as a patient admitted with pneumonia, and the provider documents *Pseudomonas* as the causal organism a few days later).

- *Same diagnosis code for two or more conditions.* When the same ICD-10-CM diagnosis code applies to two or more conditions during the same encounter (e.g., two separate conditions classified to the same ICD-10-CM diagnosis code), assign Y if all conditions represented by the single ICD-10-CM code were present on admission (e.g., bilateral unspecified age-related cataracts). Assign N if any of the conditions represented by the single ICD-10-CM code *was not present on admission* (e.g., traumatic secondary and recurrent hemorrhage and seroma is assigned to a single ICD-10-CM code T79.2, but only one of the conditions was present on admission).

- *Obstetrical conditions.* Whether or not the patient delivers during the current hospitalization does not affect assignment of the POA indicator. The determining factor for POA assignment is whether the pregnancy complication or obstetrical condition described by the ICD-10-CM code was present at the time of admission or not.

  - If the pregnancy complication or obstetrical condition was present on admission (e.g., patient admitted in preterm labor), assign Y.

  - If the pregnancy complication or obstetrical condition was not present on admission (e.g., 2nd degree laceration during delivery, postpartum hemorrhage that occurred during current hospitalization, fetal distress develops after admission), assign N.

  - If the obstetrical code includes more than one diagnosis and any of the diagnoses identified by the code were not present on admission, assign N.

- *Perinatal conditions.* Newborns are not considered to be admitted until *after birth.* Therefore, any condition present at birth or that developed in utero *is considered present at admission* and should be assigned Y. This includes conditions that occur during delivery (e.g., injury during delivery, meconium aspiration, exposure to *Streptococcus* B in the vaginal canal).

- *Congenital conditions and anomalies.* Assign Y for congenital conditions and anomalies *except for categories Q00–Q99, Congenital anomalies*, which are on the *Exempt from Reporting* list. Congenital conditions are *always* considered present on admission.

- *External cause of injury codes.* Assign Y for any external cause ICD-10-CM code that represents an external cause of morbidity, which occurred prior to inpatient admission (e.g., patient fell out of bed at home, patient fell out of bed in emergency room prior to inpatient hospital admission). Assign N for any external cause ICD-10-CM code that presents an external cause of morbidity that occurred *during inpatient hospitalization* (e.g., patient fell out of hospital bed during hospital stay, patient experienced adverse reaction to medication properly administered after inpatient admission).

Exercise 7.2 – Inpatient Diagnosis Coding Guidelines

7.2A - Inpatient Diagnosis Coding Guidelines

Instructions: For each case scenario, select the most appropriate sequencing guideline.

1. The patient undergoes an appendectomy for acute appendicitis and develops a postoperative wound infection during inpatient hospitalization. Which sequencing guideline applies?

   a. Abnormal findings

   b. Complications of surgery and other medical care

   c. Other (additional) diagnoses reported

   d. Uncertain, or qualified, diagnosis

2. The patient is admitted with acute asthma and acute congestive heart failure, both of which were treated. Which sequencing guideline applies?

   a. Other (additional) diagnoses reported

   b. Two or more comparative or contrasting conditions coded as if the diagnosis is confirmed

   c. Two or more diagnoses equally meeting definition for principal diagnosis

   d. Two or more interrelated conditions equally meeting definition of principal diagnosis

3. The patient is admitted for rehabilitation services for left-sided dominant hemiplegia following a stroke. Which sequencing guideline applies?

   a. Complications of surgery and other medical care

   b. Other (additional) diagnoses reported

   c. Previous conditions stated as diagnoses

   d. Rehabilitation admission/encounter

4. A patient admitted and treated for acute gastroenteritis has an extremely low potassium level. A physician query was generated. Which sequencing guideline applies?

   a. Abnormal findings

   b. Complications of surgery and other medical care

   c. Other (additional) diagnoses reported

   d. Uncertain, or qualified, diagnosis

(continues)

Exercise 7.2 – continued

5. A patient is admitted with acute gastroenteritis versus acute gastric ulcer, and the patient is treated symptomatically. Which sequencing guideline applies?

   a. Complications of surgery and other medical care

   b. Two or more comparative or contrasting conditions coded as if the diagnosis is confirmed

   c. Two or more diagnoses equally meeting definition for principal diagnosis

   d. Two or more interrelated conditions equally meeting definition of principal diagnosis

6. An older patient was admitted with recent history of severe abdominal pain for which testing was performed. Final diagnoses are peritonitis and acute ulcerative colitis. Which sequencing guideline applies?

   a. Complications of surgery and other medical care

   b. Two or more comparative or contrasting conditions coded as if the diagnosis is confirmed

   c. Two or more diagnoses equally meeting definition for principal diagnosis

   d. Two or more interrelated conditions equally meeting definition of principal diagnosis

7. A patient is admitted for treatment of acute myocardial infarction and receives medication and patient education for previously diagnosed insulin-dependent type 2 diabetes mellitus. Which sequencing guideline applies?

   a. Abnormal findings

   b. Complications of surgery and other medical care

   c. Original treatment plan not carried out

   d. Other (additional) diagnoses reported

8. A patient is admitted as a hospital inpatient with right lower quadrant pain, elevated fever, possible ectopic pregnancy, and possible acute appendicitis. Which sequencing guideline applies?

   a. Complications of surgery and other medical care

   b. Original treatment plan not carried out

   c. Previous conditions stated as diagnoses

   d. Uncertain, or qualified, diagnosis

9. A patient admitted for treatment of fractured hip has a past history of cholecystitis with cholecystectomy one year ago. Which sequencing guideline applies?

   a. Abnormal findings

   b. Complications of surgery and other medical care

   c. Other (additional) diagnoses reported

   d. Previous conditions stated as diagnoses

10. A patient with multiparity is admitted for elective sterilization and was found to have an elevated temperature. Surgery was canceled. Which sequencing guideline applies?

    a. Complications of surgery and other medical care

    b. Original treatment plan not carried out

    c. Other (additional) diagnoses reported

    d. Uncertain, or qualified, diagnosis

7.2B - Present on Admission (POA) Indicators

Instructions: Select the most appropriate present on admission (POA) indicator for each case scenario.

1. A patient is admitted to the hospital for scheduled open cholecystectomy due to a diagnosis of acute cholecystitis with cholelithiasis. After 24 hours of intravenous antibiotic therapy, the surgery is successfully performed. What is the POA indicator for the acute cholecystitis with cholelithiasis?

   a. Y = Yes (diagnosis present at the time of inpatient admission)

   b. N = No (diagnosis was not present at the time of inpatient admission)

   c. U = Unknown (documentation is insufficient to determine if the condition was present at the time of inpatient admission)

   d. W = Clinically undetermined (provider is unable to clinically determine whether the condition was present at the time of inpatient admission)

2. A patient was admitted for inpatient hospitalization due to weakness and unsteady gait, and a diagnosis of cerebrovascular accident was established. During inpatient hospitalization the patient fell out of bed and fractured the left hip. What is the POA indicator for the fracture, left hip?

   a. Y = Yes (diagnosis present at the time of inpatient admission)

   b. N = No (diagnosis was not present at the time of inpatient admission)

   c. U = Unknown (documentation is insufficient to determine if the condition was present at the time of inpatient admission)

   d. W = Clinically undetermined (provider is unable to clinically determine whether the condition was present at the time of inpatient admission)

3. A hospital inpatient was treated for a persistent urinary tract infection due to *E. coli* during admission for COVID-19. What is the POA indicator for the urinary tract infection due to *E. coli*?

   a. Y = Yes (diagnosis present at the time of inpatient admission)

   b. N = No (diagnosis was not present at the time of inpatient admission)

   c. U = Unknown (documentation is insufficient to determine if the condition was present at the time of inpatient admission)

   d. W = Clinically undetermined (provider is unable to clinically determine whether the condition was present at the time of inpatient admission)

4. An 84-year-old patient is admitted for inpatient hospitalization due to fever with a temperature of 104 degrees, severe weakness, dehydration, and productive cough. The patient is diagnosed with viral pneumonia after admission. During hospitalization, the patient's condition rapidly deteriorates and admission to the intensive care unit is required. The physician documents severe sepsis as a secondary diagnosis. When queried as to whether the sepsis was present on admission, the physician stated that the patient went downhill so fast it is impossible to clinically determine whether the sepsis was present on admission. What is the POA indicator for the severe sepsis?

   a. Y = Yes (diagnosis present at the time of inpatient admission)

   b. N = No (diagnosis was not present at the time of inpatient admission)

   c. U = Unknown (documentation is insufficient to determine if the condition was present at the time of inpatient admission)

   d. W = Clinically undetermined (provider is unable to clinically determine whether the condition was present at the time of inpatient admission)

(continues)

Exercise 7.2 – continued

5. Twin liveborn infants are delivered via cesarean section in the hospital. The physician documents that Twin A has neonatal bradycardia. What is the POA indicator for Twin A's neonatal bradycardia?

   a. Y = Yes (diagnosis present at the time of inpatient admission)

   b. N = No (diagnosis was not present at the time of inpatient admission)

   c. U = Unknown (documentation is insufficient to determine if the condition was present at the time of inpatient admission)

   d. W = Clinically undetermined (provider is unable to clinically determine whether the condition was present at the time of inpatient admission)

Inpatient Procedure Coding Guidelines

Depending on state reporting requirements, when the circumstances of inpatient admission govern the sequencing of procedure codes, UHDDS definitions are used to report inpatient data elements in a standardized manner. Circumstances associated with an inpatient hospital admission govern the sequencing of

- Principal procedure
- Significant other procedures (or secondary procedures)

Example: New York State's (NYS) *Statewide Planning and Research Cooperative System (SPARCS)* is a comprehensive data reporting system that was established in 1979 in cooperation with the health care industry and state government. Initially created to collect information on discharges from hospitals, SPARCS now collects patient-level detail on patient characteristics, diagnoses and treatments, services, and charges for every NYS hospital discharge, ambulatory surgery patient, and emergency department admission. SPARCS created *output data dictionaries*, which include definitions, codes and values, and edit applications for inpatient and outpatient *output data elements*. For electronic claims purposes, SPARCS requires reporting of the principal procedure and significant other procedures. The SPARCS outpatient data dictionary's definition of these terms is based on the federal government's UHDDS definition.

 NOTE:

Inpatient hospital procedures are classified using ICD-10-PCS. Outpatient and physician office settings report CPT and HCPCS Level II codes for procedures/services (discussed in Chapters 8–19). CPT and HCPCS Level II codes are also assigned for physician professional services provided to hospital inpatients (e.g., subsequent hospital care).

 NOTE:

All operating room procedures performed that are surgical in nature, carry a procedural risk, carry an anesthetic risk, or require specialized training are assigned ICD-10-PCS codes and reported.

Principal Procedure

When required for reimbursement purposes, the principal procedure is sequenced first, followed by other significant procedure(s) (when more than one procedure is reported on an inpatient claim). The following instructions should be applied in the selection of **principal procedure**, and they provide clarification regarding the importance of the relation to the principal diagnosis when more than one procedure is performed:

1. When the procedure is performed for definitive treatment of both the principal diagnosis and secondary diagnosis, sequence the procedure performed for definitive treatment most related to the principal diagnosis as the principal procedure.

2. When the procedure is performed for definitive treatment and diagnostic procedures are performed for both the principal diagnosis and secondary diagnosis, sequence the procedure performed for definitive treatment most related to the principal diagnosis as the principal procedure.

3. When a diagnostic procedure is performed for the principal diagnosis, and a procedure is performed for definitive treatment of a secondary diagnosis, sequence the diagnostic procedure as the principal procedure because the procedure most related to the principal diagnosis takes precedence.

4. When procedures performed are not related to the principal diagnosis but are for the definitive treatment or diagnostic purpose related to a secondary diagnosis, sequence the procedure performed for definitive treatment of a secondary diagnosis as the principal procedure.

Significant Other Procedures (or Secondary Procedures)

Other significant procedures (or secondary procedures)

- Are surgical in nature (e.g., incision, excision, amputation)
- Carry a procedural (or operative) risk
- Carry an anesthetic risk
- Require highly trained personnel
- Require special facilities or equipment

Example: A 64-year-old patient presented to the ED complaining of ringing in both ears, dizziness, blurred vision, confusion, and difficulty walking. Upon evaluation by the ED physician, the patient stated that these symptoms started about 24 hours ago. Past history revealed that the patient takes medication for hypercholesterolemia and hypertension. Physical examination revealed blood pressure of 180/115. When asked, the patient stated that they had been taking the hypertension medication as prescribed. Patient underwent carotid ultrasound to evaluate the blood flow of the carotid arteries, and results indicated the need for carotid angiogram to measure blockage of the carotid arteries.

The ED physician transferred the case to a cardiologist, who admitted the patient to the hospital and performed a bilateral carotid angiogram. Angiogram revealed 92% blockage of the right carotid artery and 24% blockage of the left carotid artery. The patient was admitted to the hospital and scheduled for carotid angioplasty with insertion of carotid stent in the morning, which was performed uneventfully. Final diagnoses were documented as carotid artery occlusion, hypertension, and hypercholesterolemia. Procedures performed included carotid ultrasound, carotid angiogram, and carotid angioplasty.

In this example, the principal procedure is carotid angioplasty, Other significant procedures include insertion of carotid stent and carotid angiogram. (The carotid ultrasound is not categorized as an operating room procedure and is not reported.)

Exercise 7.3 – Inpatient Procedure Coding Guidelines

Instructions: Complete each statement.

1. Depending on state reporting requirements, when the circumstances of inpatient admission govern the sequencing of procedure codes, _____ definitions are used to report inpatient data elements in a standardized manner.

2. Inpatient procedures are classified using _____.

3. Upon implementation of MS-DRGs, CMS eliminated the requirement to _____ principal and secondary procedures.

4. When required for reimbursement purposes, the principal procedure is sequenced _____.

5. The principal procedure is defined as being performed for _____ treatment rather than for diagnostic or exploratory purposes, necessary to treat a complication, or most closely related to the principal diagnosis.

Coding Inpatient Diagnoses and Procedures

ICD-10-CM and ICD-10-PCS (abbreviated as ICD-10-CM/PCS) codes are assigned to inpatient cases to collect statistical data for education and research, determine third-party payer reimbursement, and facilitate health care financial planning. ICD-10-CM/PCS codes assigned to an inpatient case are entered into automated case abstracting software using a data entry screen (Figure 7-3) and diagnosis-related groups (DRGs) are assigned for reimbursement purposes. The ICD-10-CM/PCS codes are then transmitted to the facility's billing department where the inpatient UB-04 claim is generated for submission to third-party payers (to obtain reimbursement).

 NOTE:

As a result of data entry, the facility's information technology (IT) department has the capability of producing customized reports and summary data for education, quality management, research, and statistical purposes. Statistical data allow the facility to conduct financial planning to determine which facility services to expand or deactivate.

 NOTE:

Refer to textbook Chapter 20 for a discussion about the inpatient prospective payment system (IPPS), which includes DRGs, major diagnostic categories (MDCs), outliers, IPPS 3-day payment window (IPPS 72-hour rule), Medicare-severity DRGs (MS-DRGs), IPPS transfer rule, hospital-acquired conditions (HACs), and value-based purchasing (VBP).

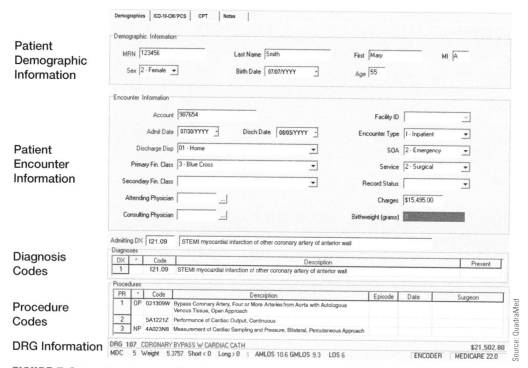

FIGURE 7-3 Inpatient abstracting data entry screen

When assigning ICD-10-CM/PCS codes, coders carefully review patient records to locate diagnoses and procedures to which codes are assigned.

NOTE:

Coders are prohibited from assigning codes to diagnoses and procedures that are not documented by the physician. This is called *assumption coding*, and it is considered fraudulent because the coder has mistakenly assumed certain facts about a patient's diagnosis or procedure even though documentation does not support codes assigned.

Consider the following when assigning ICD-10-CM/PCS to diagnoses and procedures.

- *Incomplete Documentation.* When patient record documentation is incomplete for coding purposes, generate a *physician query* to clarify documentation. (Refer to textbook Chapter 1 for more information about the physician query process.)

- *Coding Specificity.* When patient record documentation supports the assignment of a specific code, it is appropriate to assign that code. For example, when a physician documents *closed fracture of left femur* in the discharge summary, and review of the x-ray report identifies the fracture site (e.g., shaft of femur), the coder assigns the more specific code that includes "shaft" of the left femur in its code description. In addition, codes based on other physician (e.g., consultant) documentation may be assigned *as long as there is no conflicting documentation from the physician.*

- *Physician Documentation.* It is appropriate to base the assignment of codes on documentation by any physician involved in the care and treatment of a patient. A physician query is unnecessary if a physician involved in the care and treatment of the patient documents a diagnosis and no conflicting documentation by another physician exists. However, if documentation by two or more physicians conflicts, query the attending physician.

Hospital inpatient cases usually have multiple diagnoses and procedures documented. Once ICD-10-CM/PCS codes are assigned, (1) diagnoses are sequenced according to principal diagnosis and other (additional) diagnoses as defined by the UHDDS, and (2) procedures are sequenced according to principal procedure and secondary procedures as defined by the *ICD-10-PCS Official Guidelines for Coding and Reporting.* (Definitions of diagnoses and procedures related to sequencing were previously discussed in this chapter.)

Exercise 7.4 – Coding Inpatient Diagnoses and Procedures

Instructions: Review each case scenario, and assign and properly sequence the ICD-10-CM diagnosis and ICD-10-PCS procedure codes.

NOTE:

Do not assign procedure codes to ancillary tests (e.g., laboratory tests, x-rays) because they do not impact DRG assignment or the reimbursement amount for an inpatient case. (Some hospitals do assign codes to ancillary tests even though doing so does not impact the level of reimbursement received; therefore, you should be aware of this practice.)

1. Patient admitted for treatment of AIDS-related complex with associated *Pneumocystis jirovecii* and oral candidiasis. Patient underwent diagnostic fiberoptic bronchoscopy with bronchial cell washings for specimen collection.

   DISCHARGE DIAGNOSES:

   _____ AIDS-related complex

   _____ *Pneumocystis jirovecii* pneumonia

   _____ Oral candidiasis

   PROCEDURE:

   _____ Bronchial cell washings via fiberoptic bronchoscopy

   (continues)

Exercise 7.4 – continued

2. Patient admitted with slurred speech and weakness on the right side. Patient is right-handed. CT scan reveals left carotid artery occlusion with cerebral infarction. Patient discharged to inpatient rehabilitation facility for continued treatment of dysphasia and right hemiparesis.

DISCHARGE DIAGNOSES:

_____ Cerebral infarction due to left carotid occlusion

_____ Dysphasia

_____ Right hemiparesis (dominant side)

3. Patient was seen during an initial encounter after having sustained a closed fracture of the distal radius, left, due to a fall from the roof of their single-family house while cleaning gutters. X-ray of the left lower arm revealed nondisplaced fracture of distal radius with fracture fragments in good alignment. The physician determined that reduction was unnecessary, and a plaster splint was applied as a stabilizing device.

DISCHARGE DIAGNOSES:

_____ Closed fracture of distal radius, left (initial encounter)

_____ Fall from roof (initial encounter) (external cause injury)

_____ Single-family house roof (external cause place of occurrence)

_____ Cleaning gutters (external cause activity)

PROCEDURE:

_____ Plaster splint applied as stabilizing device, left lower arm

4. Patient admitted for treatment of type 2 diabetes mellitus due to chronic osteomyelitis, metatarsus bones, left ankle and foot. The patient has required long-term insulin use for many years. The patient underwent a complete left foot amputation, open approach, during this encounter.

DISCHARGE DIAGNOSES:

_____ Type 2 diabetes mellitus with osteomyelitis, left ankle and foot (bones)

_____ Chronic osteomyelitis, metatarsus bones, left ankle and foot

_____ Long-term insulin use

PROCEDURE:

_____ Complete left foot amputation, open approach

5. Patient admitted following repeated temporal lobe seizures. History revealed that the patient had had 18 seizures within the past 24 hours. Patient has had seizures since the age of 16, previously well controlled with long-term use of phenobarbital. Blood levels indicate an acceptable therapeutic level. During hospitalization, patient continued to seize at least hourly. Patient was immediately transferred to the neurology unit of tertiary care hospital due to localization-related intractable epilepsy with complex partial seizures.

DIAGNOSES:

_____ Localization-related symptomatic intractable epilepsy with complex partial seizures

_____ Long-term use of phenobarbital

Summary

Inpatient health care settings include acute care facilities (hospitals), behavioral health care facilities, hospice inpatient care, and long-term acute care hospitals (LTACHs). CMS publishes official ICD-10-CM and ICD-10-PCS guidelines for coding and reporting, which provide direction about assignment of diagnosis and procedure codes and the sequencing of diagnosis codes for reimbursement purposes. Depending on state reporting requirements, when the circumstances of inpatient admission govern the sequencing of procedure codes, UHDDS definitions are used to report inpatient data elements in a standardized manner, including sequencing of the principal diagnosis and other (additional) diagnoses. Circumstances associated with an inpatient admission also govern the sequencing of principal procedure and significant other procedures (or secondary procedures).

Internet Links

HCPro, Inc.: Go to **www.hcmarketplace.com**, and click on the Sign up for our FREE e-Newsletters link. Enter your contact information, and click on the box located in front of JustCoding News: Inpatient (along with other e-Newsletters that interest you) to subscribe.

NYS DOH SPARCS: Go to **www.health.ny.gov**, click on the Search link, and enter SPARCS in the search box to locate information about the Statewide Planning and Research Cooperative System (SPARCS).

Virtual Pediatric Hospital: www.virtualpediatrichospital.org

Review

7.1 – Multiple Choice (ICD-10-CM)

Instructions: Select the most appropriate response.

1. Fever of unknown origin. Rule out tuberculosis. (Final diagnosis at time of inpatient hospital discharge.)
   - **a.** A15.0
   - **b.** R50.9
   - **c.** R50.9, A15.0
   - **d.** Z03.818

2. Primary pancreatic cancer.
   - **a.** C25.1
   - **b.** C25.9
   - **c.** C77.2
   - **d.** C79.89

3. Graves, disease with thyroid storm.
   - **a.** E05.00
   - **b.** E05.00, E05.91
   - **c.** E05.01
   - **d.** E05.91

4. Acute posthemorrhagic anemia.
   - **a.** D50.0
   - **b.** D61.9
   - **c.** D62
   - **d.** D64.9, R58

5. Anorexia nervosa.
   - **a.** F50.00
   - **b.** F50.9
   - **c.** R63.0
   - **d.** R63.39

6. Hypertensive with CHF. Old MI, diagnosed on EKG (currently presenting no symptoms).
   - **a.** I50.9, I10
   - **b.** I11.0, I50.9, I25.2
   - **c.** I10, I11.9, I50.9
   - **d.** I50.9, I10, I25.2

7. Congenital hydrocephalus.
   - **a.** G91.0
   - **b.** G91.9
   - **c.** Q03.8
   - **d.** Q03.9

8. Respiratory distress syndrome (RDS) of newborn.
   - **a.** J80
   - **b.** P22.0
   - **c.** P27.8
   - **d.** P28.81

9. Stab wound injury into thoracic aorta due to knife assault (initial encounter).
   - **a.** S21.109A, X99.9XXA
   - **b.** S31.000A, X99.9XXA
   - **c.** S25.00XA, X99.1XXA
   - **d.** S29.001A, X99.8XXA

10. Neonatal cerebral ischemia.
    - **a.** G45.8
    - **b.** G45.9
    - **c.** I67.82
    - **d.** P91.0

7.2 – Multiple Choice (ICD-10-PCS)

Instructions: Select the most appropriate response.

1. Partial splenectomy, open.
   - **a.** 07BP3ZZ
   - **b.** 07BP4ZX
   - **c.** 07BP0ZZ
   - **d.** 07TP0ZZ

2. Needle biopsy of cerebral meninges.
   - **a.** 00B13ZX
   - **b.** 00B13ZZ
   - **c.** 00C13ZZ
   - **d.** 00D13ZZ

3. Complete substernal thyroidectomy, open approach.
   - **a.** 0GBG0ZX, 0GBH0ZX
   - **b.** 0GBH0ZZ
   - **c.** 0GPKX0Z
   - **d.** 0GTK0ZZ

4. Percutaneous myringotomy with placement of tube in right tympanic membrane.
   - **a.** 099700Z
   - **b.** 099730Z
   - **c.** 099740Z
   - **d.** 099770Z

5. Diagnostic lingula bronchial drainage via endoscopy.
   - **a.** 0BJ08ZZ
   - **b.** 0B998ZX
   - **c.** 3E1L38Z
   - **d.** 3E1F88Z

6. Repair of direct inguinal hernia, right side, via percutaneous endoscopic approach.
   - **a.** 0YQ50ZZ
   - **b.** 0YQ53ZZ
   - **c.** 0YQ54ZZ
   - **d.** 0YQ64ZZ

7. Extracorporeal shock wave lithotripsy of the right kidney pelvis (external approach).
   - **a.** 0TF3XZZ
   - **b.** 0TF6XZZ
   - **c.** 0TFDXZZ
   - **d.** 0WFRXZZ

8. Cesarean section, high, via open approach.
   - **a.** 10207YZ
   - **b.** 10900ZC
   - **c.** 10A00ZZ
   - **d.** 10D00Z0

9. Excision of pilonidal abscess.
   - **a.** 0H98X0Z
   - **b.** 0H90X0Z
   - **c.** 0HB8XZZ
   - **d.** 0HC0XZZ

10. Open temporomandibular joint (TMJ) repair, right.
    - **a.** 0RQC0ZZ
    - **b.** 0MM00ZZ
    - **c.** 0C00X7Z
    - **d.** 0KQ00ZZ

7.3 – Coding Practice: Inpatient Hospital Cases (ICD-10-CM)

Instructions: Review each case scenario, and assign and properly sequence the ICD-10-CM diagnosis codes.

1. A 70-year-old female presented to the hospital with fever, myalgia, arthralgia, tachycardia, and dehydration and was believed to be septic. This patient has a history of hypertension, CHF, and migraines. Routine medications include Lasix 40 milligrams by mouth each morning, if needed, for significant pedal edema and Isordil 20 milligrams by mouth four times a day.

   A variety of studies were obtained to further delineate the source of her problem. Urine cultures were negative. Blood cultures grew *Escherichia coli*. The blood urea nitrogen level was 22, and a random glucose was 149. An anterior-posterior film of the chest taken at the same time showed acute pulmonary edema.

   The patient received intravenous fluids. The patient's routine medications were continued, and she received intravenous antibiotics. On the fourth day of her hospital stay, it was believed that the patient had reached maximal hospital benefit and was therefore switched to oral antibiotics and was discharged. The patient left the hospital in good condition.

   DISCHARGE DIAGNOSES:

   _____ Sepsis due to *Escherichia coli*

   _____ Dehydration

_____ Hypertensive heart disease with

_____ Left ventricular failure

2. A 2-year-old patient presented with fever, vomiting, and abdominal pain. The patient was severely dehydrated with a blood urea nitrogen level of 54, indicating acute renal failure. Blood cultures obtained grew *Staphylococcus aureus*. The patient was treated with a 10-day course of intravenous vancomycin. The patient also received intravenous fluids and had improved renal function. Upon admission, the patient was noted to have a rash on the buttocks and was treated with topical ointment. The patient improved and was discharged.

DISCHARGE DIAGNOSES:

_____ Sepsis due to methicillin-susceptible *Staphylococcus aureus*

_____ Septic shock due to severe sepsis

_____ Acute kidney failure

_____ Dehydration

_____ Diaper rash

3. A 94-year-old patient was admitted to the hospital with a chief complaint of abdominal pain and loss of weight. The patient had a nebulizer at home for moderate persistent asthma. This medication was continued during the patient's stay. Physical examination revealed abdomen to be tender to palpation in the left mid and lower quadrants with some rebound. Bowel sounds were present, and there was no guarding. Blood pressure was normal. Pulse, respirations, and temperature were normal.

During hospitalization, sputum cytology was suggestive of adenocarcinoma. Chest x-ray showed metastatic lesions and chronic obstructive lung disease in the right lung field. Barium enema showed adenocarcinoma of proximal sigmoid colon. Abdominal series showed no evidence of obstruction, but moderate dilation of the transverse colon was evident. Patient was seen in consultation, and it was decided to do as little as possible at this time due to the patient's age and lung conditions. The patient agreed with this approach and requested discharge to home to receive hospice care.

DISCHARGE DIAGNOSES:

_____ Adenocarcinoma of sigmoid colon

_____ Probable metastatic adenocarcinoma, right lung

_____ Chronic obstructive lung disease

_____ Moderate persistent asthma

4. This patient is a 43-year-old female with a long history of joint pain. Lately she had been feeling very tired and weak. She also has had intermittent abdominal pain with nausea and vomiting. Her joint exam showed tenderness of the knees. She denied any problems suggestive of hypothyroidism. The patient's hematocrit was 27.6, serum iron was found to be decreased at 27, and thyroid functions were found to be markedly low. Upper GI series showed a 4-millimeter ulcer at the posterior wall of the duodenal bulb. The patient was transfused 2 units of packed red cells. She was started on ferrous sulfate 300 milligrams twice a day. She was also begun on Tagamet for the ulcer. Further questioning revealed that she had indeed been hypothyroid in the past and has been on thyroid medication until stopped by another physician. The patient was restarted on Synthroid 75 micrograms per day. She was discharged on the sixth hospital day.

DISCHARGE DIAGNOSES:

_____ Acute duodenal ulcer

_____ Anemia

_____ due to myxedema

5. This patient is a 14-year-old male who was admitted due to sickle-cell crisis and acute chest syndrome. His mother has sickle-cell anemia, and his father has the sickle-cell trait. Because of this, the patient was tested at birth; a blood sample was drawn, and it was sent to the laboratory for hemoglobin electrophoresis to obtain a definitive diagnosis. Unfortunately, the test was positive for sickle-cell disease. The patient was given intravenous fluids and was started on Darvocet for pain management. When the Darvocet failed to keep his pain at an acceptable level, he was switched to Vicodin. The patient is to be discharged with follow-up in the pediatrician's office tomorrow.

DISCHARGE DIAGNOSES:

_____ Sickle-cell crisis with acute chest syndrome

_____ Family history of sickle cell anemia

6. A 31-year-old male presented to the emergency room reportedly having mistakenly taken 8 to 10 naproxen at home during a four-hour period for a severe migraine, which he says is now gone but says "he feels like his heart is beating out of his chest." The patient is admitted to the telemetry unit due to paroxysmal ventricular tachycardia. The patient was started on intravenous metaraminol for the tachycardia. Fortunately, the patient seemed to sustain no other ill effects from the naproxen. The mental health service was consulted, and an appointment was made for outpatient services. He was discharged in good condition.

DISCHARGE DIAGNOSES:

_____ Accidental overdose with naproxen

_____ Paroxysmal ventricular tachycardia

7. A 52-year-old male bus driver is admitted to receive a course of electroconvulsive therapy for his depressive symptomatology. This patient was seen approximately one year ago in consultation; at that time, he was showing early evidence of moderate depressive reaction. He has had several admissions since that time, and on each occasion had been drinking excessively. It appears that he attempts to use alcohol as a tranquilizer. During the first two days of his admission, he continued to show marked depressive symptomatology and was started on unilateral-single seizure electroconvulsive therapy. After treatment, he showed a mitigation of his depressive symptomatology. He was discharged home on Pertofrane 25 milligrams twice a day and was instructed to call for follow-up care. Condition on discharge was improved.

DISCHARGE DIAGNOSIS:

_____ Moderate depressive reaction, recurrent

8. A 71-year-old patient presented to the hospital with the chief complaint of increasing confusion. The patient has been wandering away from home and has displayed aggressive behavior to family members. The patient is a known type 2 diabetic, which is controlled on Orinase 0.5 milligrams daily. The patient is thin and emaciated. During this period of hospitalization, the patient was uncooperative in all aspects, refusing food and medications. Patient was confused and seemed slightly paranoid. The family was consulted about the patient's worsening dementia, and the decision was made to transfer the patient to the state psychiatric hospital for care. The patient was transferred on the fifth hospital day.

DISCHARGE DIAGNOSES:

_____ Alzheimer's disease

_____   with senile dementia and aggressive behavior

_____ Diabetes mellitus, type 2

_____ Long-term use of oral anti-diabetic medication

_____ Wandering away from home

9. An 84-year-old female was admitted to the hospital because of severe dizziness and weakness. The patient has had previous brain stem transient ischemic attacks and also has completed radiation for what was assumed to be cancer of the endometrium. The patient is currently receiving short-term chemotherapy for the endometrial carcinoma on an outpatient basis, and she was administered her chemotherapy during this inpatient stay. The patient had 3+ hyperreflexia and rotary nystagmus on admission. The urinalysis showed white blood cells and bacteria. Her urine culture grew *Klebsiella pneumoniae*. The patient was started on Velosef. Over the next several days, the dizziness cleared, but the patient continued to be quite weak. Gait training physical therapy was started, and she was eventually able to walk with her walker without assistance. Her reflexia had come back down to 1+, which is her usual state. The patient had no more nystagmus and was switched from heparin to Persantine. The patient was discharged home and was to be seen as an outpatient in one month.

DISCHARGE DIAGNOSES:

_____ Brain stem transient ischemic attack

_____ Endometrial carcinoma

_____ Urinary tract infection

_____   due to *Klebsiella pneumoniae*

10. This patient is a practical nurse who presented to the hospital because her blood pressure was 240/140 at home. Her blood pressure at admission was 220/120. This patient has had multiple strokes, and her first stroke was 5 years ago. This patient has a history of hypertension and paroxysmal atrial fibrillation. She was started on intravenous Aldomet, Dyazide, Catapres, and Lanoxin. Her blood pressure lowered to 190/98. On admission, her radial, brachial, popliteal, and femoral pulses were 2–4. The next day, the femoral pulse was decreased to 1–4, and the posterior tibial pulses were not palpable. The leg on the left side was clammy and cold. There was minimal cyanosis over the heel of the left foot. Possible iliac artery embolism had to be ruled out, and it was decided to transfer the patient.

DISCHARGE DIAGNOSES:

_____ Hypertensive crisis

_____ Hypertension

_____ Possible bilateral iliac artery emboli

_____ Hemiplegia, nondominant left side, following previous cerebrovascular accident

_____ Aphasia, following previous cerebrovascular accident

_____ Paroxysmal atrial fibrillation

11. A 47-year-old male corrections officer presented to the emergency room with an acute onset of chest pain. The pain was described as a crushing pain and was accompanied with radiation of the pain into the jaw and diaphoresis. He does not have a history of previous myocardial infarction (MI). His risk factors include morbid obesity, hypertension, and hypercholesterolemia. The patient takes metoprolol and Lipitor. The cardiologist was consulted, and the patient was found to have an acute ST elevation anterior wall MI. The patient was admitted to the intensive care unit and was observed on telemetry. On the second day of hospitalization, the patient was thought to be stable for transfer. The patient was transferred for coronary angiography and possible angioplasty.

DISCHARGE DIAGNOSES:

_____ Acute ST elevation anterior wall myocardial infarction

_____ Hypertension

_____ Hypercholesterolemia

_____ Morbid obesity

12. A 16-month-old infant was admitted from the emergency room because of nausea and vomiting and some cough. She was felt to have acute bronchitis due to respiratory syncytial virus (RSV) with possible pneumonia. This child was hospitalized previously with meningitis but has had no other serious illnesses until the present time. She has no prior history of diabetes or tuberculosis. Her parents are alive and well. The physical examination revealed generalized sibilant rales. The patient's chest x-ray was normal. Pneumonia was ruled out. Her urinalysis was normal. Her hematocrit was 34. The low hematocrit was thought to be due to the persistent vomiting and lack of iron intake from her diet. The patient was given penicillin and Phenergan injections. She was also given nebulizer treatments every 6 hours on an as-needed basis. The patient was started on clear liquids, and she progressed to a general diet. After the first few days, the vomiting ceased. She was discharged with prescriptions for ferrous gluconate, ampicillin, and Phenergan.

DISCHARGE DIAGNOSES:

_____ Acute bronchitis due to RSV

_____ Nutritional anemia due to inadequate dietary iron intake

_____ Nausea and vomiting

13. The patient is a 77-year-old male admitted to the hospital due to shortness of breath and progressive chest pain. The patient has no past history of surgery. The patient has had evidence of acute bronchitis with discolored sputum for 5 days and, despite antibiotics, was not improving. With this, he developed an increasing need for nitroglycerin. During his hospitalization, the patient was treated with intravenous antibiotics, steroids, theophylline, and hand-held nebulizer with Alupent. The patient improved with the cough clearing nicely. Unfortunately, several days prior to discharge, he developed severe precordial chest pain typical of his angina. This required three nitroglycerin plus morphine to stop the pain. The EKG showed significant ischemic distress, which cleared over the next few hours, and there was no evidence of damage by isoenzyme study. The patient was monitored on telemetry and increased his activity slowly. The patient improved and was discharged to home on Procardia 10 milligrams every other day, nitroglycerin patch 5 milligrams daily, Isordil 10 milligrams every other day, Lasix 40 milligrams daily, Theo-Dur 300 milligrams twice a day, prednisone in a decreasing dose, and Velosef 500 milligrams twice a day and is to be seen in the office in one week.

DISCHARGE DIAGNOSES:

_____ Chronic obstructive pulmonary disease with acute bronchitis

_____ Arteriosclerotic cardiovascular disease, native coronary artery, with progressive unstable angina

_____ Mitral insufficiency

14. This patient was admitted to the hospital due to severe low back pain and a great amount of indigestion. She has had frequent episodes of abdominal pain in the past, but this is more severe and has failed to respond to therapy as an outpatient. She is known to have esophageal hiatus hernia and polyps of the gallbladder in addition to her osteoporosis and stenosis of the lumbar spine, all of which were medically managed during the inpatient stay. The physical examination revealed a 74-year-old woman who appeared to be acutely and chronically ill. She had epigastric tenderness with no masses palpable. The patient's EKG was normal. An upper gastrointestinal series showed a small sliding hiatal hernia and a duodenal ulcer with considerable evidence for an active ulcer. The gallbladder showed abnormal filling defects, which were consistent with polyps. The x-rays of the spine showed a great deal of osteoporosis and stenosis of the lumbar spine. The patient was given Demerol and Phenergan for the pain and was started on intravenous Prevacid. She was given Dalmane 30 milligrams at bedtime and a calcium supplement one time daily. She was started on a bland diet. The patient has slowly improved as far as the back pain. She is now up and about and is having less indigestion since therapy for the ulcer was begun. The patient is being discharged to be followed as an outpatient. She will continue on a bland diet and will be discharged on Prevacid, Carafate, a calcium substitute, and Darvocet.

DISCHARGE DIAGNOSES:

_____ Acute duodenal ulcer

_____ Sliding esophageal hiatus hernia

_____ Gallbladder polyps

_____ Osteoporosis

_____ Spinal stenosis of the lumbar region

15. This 84-year-old patient was admitted to the hospital because of extreme weakness and inability to eat. The patient had been a resident of a nursing home when she suddenly developed progression of her symptoms of weakness. She refused to eat. She has refused dialysis treatment. Several days later she was not responding well. Laboratory studies done at that time revealed the hemoglobin to be 8.4 and her white count to be 14,700. There were significant abnormalities of her blood work that included a blood urea nitrogen level of 181, a sodium level of 149, a potassium level of 5.1, and glucose of 232. The patient was admitted to the hospital and hydrated with intravenous fluids. With that, her hemoglobin dropped to a low of 6. The patient was administered 4 units of nonautologous packed red blood cells via peripheral vein, and this brought her blood count up to 14.3. With appropriate hydration, there was a continual decline of her blood urea nitrogen level and improvement of her electrolytes. Her blood urea nitrogen level was beginning to rise, and she was becoming less responsive. Her breathing began to slow, and she became completely unresponsive. At 1:10 A.M. of the next morning, she was pronounced dead.

DISCHARGE DIAGNOSES:

_____ Acute renal failure

_____ Dehydration

_____ End-stage renal disease

_____ Anemia in chronic kidney disease

7.4 – Coding Practice: Inpatient Hospital Cases (ICD-10-CM and ICD-10-PCS)

Instructions: Review each case scenario, and assign and properly sequence the ICD-10-CM diagnosis and ICD-10-PCS procedure codes, including appropriate ICD-10-CM external cause of injury codes.

1. This is a 62-year-old male patient seen in the office because of urinary difficulty. The patient noticed that he had to strain when he had to urinate. He has been having this problem off and on during the past year. Also, sometimes he has to move his bowels when he urinates because of the strain. His urinary stream is very slow. He has no history of dysuria or hematuria. His past history reveals that he has high blood pressure, and he is taking medication for that with occasional Valium. He also has been complaining of some pain in the lower back at the area of the coccyx bone. On his physical examination, the abdomen was soft with no tenderness or mass palpable. He has normal external genitalia with a rectally grade III smooth prostate gland. The patient's urological workup was done as an outpatient, and this showed an essentially normal upper urinary tract and enlarged prostate. He is admitted to the hospital for transurethral resection of the prostate (TURP). On the day of admission, under general anesthesia, transurethral resection of the prostate (via artificial opening) to trim away excess prostate tissue only was performed. Postoperatively, the patient did well. When his catheter was removed, he was able to void well without any difficulty. The pathology report revealed benign prostatic hyperplasia. Because of a tender coccyx bone, he did have several x-rays, which were negative. The pain was improved by injecting Aristocort and Novocain into this area. The patient's hypertension medication was continued. The patient was discharged and will be seen in the office in 3 weeks.

DISCHARGE DIAGNOSES:

_____ Benign hyperplasia of the prostate with urinary obstruction

_____ Straining to void

_____ Poor urinary stream

_____ Coccygodynia

_____ Hypertension

PROCEDURE:

_____ Transurethral resection of the prostate

2. The patient is a 23-year-old female, gravida 2, para 1, who has had no problems with her pregnancy until two days prior to admission. She began with some spotting, which progressed to heavier bleeding with cramping. The cramping became severe on the morning of admission; she began to bleed excessively then, and she presented herself to the emergency room. At that point, it was believed that she had had an incomplete abortion. At the time of admission, she was a well-developed, well-nourished female in no apparent distress. Her vital signs are stable. She is afebrile. Her pertinent physical findings included a negative abdominal exam and a pelvic exam that revealed blood, clots, and mucus in the external cervical canal and in the vaginal vault. The bimanual exam was deferred until the time of surgery when sterile conditions could be met. She was taken to the operating room after her complete blood count and urinalysis showed nothing unusual. In the operating room, a dilatation and curettage using a vaginal approach was done without problem. Postoperatively, she has done fine. She has had no unusual vaginal bleeding. She has had no problem with ambulation to the bathroom. Her abdomen is soft and nontender this morning. She feels fine. She is discharged to home in good condition.

    DISCHARGE DIAGNOSIS:

    _____ Incomplete spontaneous abortion with excessive vaginal bleeding

    PROCEDURE:

    _____ Dilatation and curettage to remove retained products of conception

3. The patient is a 25-year-old female, gravida 1, whose pregnancy has been benign. She had gone into spontaneous labor late in the evening and came to the obstetric unit at about 0230 hours. She was dilated a fingertip. She came to 50% effacement, and labor picked up every few minutes. By 8 o'clock in the morning, she was only 2 to 3 centimeters dilated. This continued until late in the afternoon. She was station minus 2 and had good contractions for several hours with no further progression of labor. Pelvimetry showed borderline cephalopelvic disproportion. It was finally decided to do a cesarean section. She was taken to the operating room and underwent a low transverse incision with delivery of a live female child. She had an essentially uneventful postoperative course. Her incision has been healing well, and her bowels have been moving. The abdomen is soft and nontender. The patient was anxious to go home and was discharged to home to be seen in the office for her 2-week postpartum check.

    DISCHARGE DIAGNOSES:

    _____ Obstructed labor due to fetopelvic disproportion

    _____ Failure to progress at labor

    _____ Single livebirth

    PROCEDURE:

    _____ Cesarean section, low

4. A 35-year-old male had a mass on his right wrist for quite some time. It had become tender and quite achy. It was, therefore, recommended that this be removed under axillary block anesthesia. Incidentally, he also had a lesion of the skin of the nose and requested removal of the lesion. The patient was admitted to undergo these surgeries under local anesthesia following removal of the ganglion cyst. His orthopedic examination at the time of admission revealed him to have a 1 × 2-centimeter fluctuant but fairly firm mass of the radial volar aspect of the right wrist, which was just proximal to the flexor crease. This was nonpulsatile. He also had what appeared to be a sebaceous cyst involving the skin on the tip of the nose. The patient's preoperative chest x-ray, complete blood count, and urinalysis were all within normal limits. An x-ray of the right wrist revealed no bony abnormality, but it did reveal a soft tissue mass on the lateral aspect of the wrist. The patient underwent the operative procedures described above, the first under axillary block and the other two under local anesthetic. The patient tolerated the procedures well and left the operating room in good condition. The pathology report revealed a ganglion cyst of the wrist and a sebaceous cyst of the nose. He was discharged the next day with instructions to return to the office for follow-up.

DISCHARGE DIAGNOSES:

_____ Ganglion cyst, right wrist

_____ Sebaceous cyst, nose

PROCEDURES:

_____ Open extirpation, ganglion cyst, right wrist

_____ Excision, lesion, skin of nose

5. This 62-year-old male patient has had a decubitus gangrenous ulcer on the dorsum of his left heel that had not improved and was, in fact, getting worse. He was given intensive medical treatment as an outpatient, but the entire foot became more swollen and redder, and he was brought to the hospital for more intensive therapy. Studies revealed a *Staphylococcus aureus* infection from the wound culture. He was treated for cellulitis with intravenous vancomycin and following surgery was placed on gentamicin and intravenous Vibramycin. These medications were effective in controlling his infection and improving the cellulitis. They were not, however, able to improve the ulcer. Whirlpool treatments for wound management and dressing changes also failed to improve the ulcer. It was ultimately decided that an above-the-knee amputation was necessary. After 5 days of intravenous antibiotics, the patient was taken to the operative suite, where it was determined that through-knee amputation of the left leg was appropriate, and that procedure was performed. He is now being transferred to a rehabilitation facility for continued care. His leg stump sutures will be removed as able, probably in about 2 weeks.

DISCHARGE DIAGNOSES:

_____ Gangrene, lower limb

_____ Decubitus ulcer, left heel, stage 4

_____ *Staphylococcus aureus* infection (as cause of gangrene)

PROCEDURE:

_____ Through-knee amputation, left leg

_____ Whirlpool physical therapy treatment

6. A 62-year-old female had been hospitalized 5 months previously with a subcapital fracture of the right hip. She underwent open reduction with internal fixation of the fracture. The fracture healed, but she continued to have difficulty with pain over the ends of the Gouffon pins. She was admitted for surgical removal of these pins. Postoperatively, her blood pressure dropped in the recovery room. This was treated with and responded to ephedrine. For the rest of her hospitalization, she had no further problems with her blood pressure. Her incision began to drain serous-type drainage. She was dangled on the side of her bed on her first postoperative day and was transferred out of bed and into the chair on her second postoperative day, and subsequently started on physical therapy for gait training with a walker. Serous drainage persisted from the hip, and a culture of the subcutaneous abscess wound from her right hip incision grew *Escherichia coli*. She was treated with cephalothin for this postoperative infection. She was ultimately discharged to home with care by the visiting nurse, who will do twice-a-week dressing changes.

DISCHARGE DIAGNOSES:

_____ Painful Gouffon pins of the right hip (initial encounter)

_____ Postoperative hypotension

_____ Postoperative wound infection, right hip (initial encounter)

_____ *Escherichia coli* (as cause of wound infection)

_____ Surgical complication (Gouffon pins)

PROCEDURE:

_____ Open removal of Gouffon pins, right hip

_____ Gait training using a walker

7. A 64-year-old male was admitted to the hospital, complaining of right knee pain. X-rays revealed that he had degenerative arthritis of the right knee. His options were discussed with him. He decided to undergo a right total knee replacement with insertion of a molded polyethylene synthetic knee implant. He underwent the procedure without incident. Postoperatively, he has done well. He began with physical therapy, ambulating with a walker. He was afebrile, and his wound was clean, dry, and intact upon discharge. He was stable upon discharge. He will have a home health nurse come to his house to remove his staples in 2 weeks' time. He should continue to work on range of motion and strengthening of his right leg. He should ambulate with the assistance of a walker. The patient should call immediately if he notices any redness, pain, or swelling around his incision.

DISCHARGE DIAGNOSIS:

_____ Degenerative primary osteoarthritis of right knee

PROCEDURE:

_____ Total knee replacement, right knee

_____ Gait training using a walker

8. The patient is a male infant who was born during this admission via cesarean section. The day after delivery, he appeared jaundiced. His blood was drawn and he was found to have an elevated bilirubin level. The patient was treated with single phototherapy directed at skin and was discharged the next day with great improvement of his bilirubin level. He is scheduled to see the pediatrician in 2 days for a repeat bilirubin test.

DISCHARGE DIAGNOSES:

_____ Term male, born by cesarean section

_____ Hyperbilirubinemia

PROCEDURE:

_____ Single phototherapy of a newborn directed at skin

9. A 22-year-old male was involved in a motorcycle-truck accident and was admitted with open comminuted type IIIA fracture of the shaft of the left fibula; a closed Colles' fracture of the distal radius on the right arm; and a laceration of the tongue, which was approximately 1 inch in length. He was the driver of the motorcycle, and lost control and hit a parked truck in a parking lot. The remainder of his physical and history was essentially noncontributory. He was started on lactated Ringer's and D5% dextrose and given 1 gram of Kefzol. His tetanus immunization was up-to-date. The laboratory studies included an EKG that was read as abnormal with nonspecific myocardial changes in the inferolateral region, not felt to be significant or warranting further follow-up. His chest x-ray was grossly normal on admission. The cervical spine was normal. He was taken to the operating room, where he underwent an open reduction and internal fixation of the fractured left fibula, upper extremity casting to immobilize the right radial fracture, and suturing of the tongue laceration. The patient was treated for a full 10 days with intravenous Keflex. His wounds looked good. His postreduction x-rays revealed good position of the right wrist and left leg fractures. He was discharged to follow-up in the office in 10 days. At that time, he will have an x-ray of the right wrist and left lower leg. He was given a prescription for Talwin 50 milligrams by mouth every four hours as needed for pain.

DISCHARGE DIAGNOSES:

_____ Traumatic open comminuted type IIIA fracture, left fibula

_____ Traumatic Colles' closed, distal radius, right (initial encounter)

_____ Laceration, tongue, approximately 1 inch in length (initial encounter)

_____ Motorcycle driver injured in collision (initial encounter)

_____ Parking lot (place of occurrence)

PROCEDURES:

_____ Open reduction, internal fixation device, left fibula

_____ Suture repair, tongue laceration

_____ Immobilization using cast, right upper extremity

10. A 70-year-old female with pancreatic head adenocarcinoma, confirmed by previous percutaneous fine needle aspiration and determined to be unresectable. The patient was also found to have probable metastasis to the lower lobe of the left lung, and she was admitted now for resection of the lower lobe of the left lung. The patient has a history of hypothyroidism and diet-controlled diabetes. During hospitalization, the patient was continued on Levoxyl, and a "no-concentrated-sweets diet" was ordered. The patient was taken to the operative suite, where a partial left lower lobe lung resection was performed. Pathology from this procedure revealed adenocarcinoma. The patient had an uneventful postoperative course and was discharged with an appointment to see the oncologist to discuss radiation and chemotherapy options.

DISCHARGE DIAGNOSES:

_____ Metastatic left lung cancer

_____ Pancreatic adenocarcinoma (as primary site)

_____ Hypothyroidism

_____ Diet-controlled type 2 diabetes mellitus

PROCEDURE:

_____ Left lower lung lobe resection (open)

Part VI

Health Care Procedure Coding System (HCPCS) Level II Coding System

HCPCS Level II Coding System

Chapter Outline

Overview of HCPCS

HCPCS Level II Codes

Assigning HCPCS Level II Codes

Determining Payer Responsibility

Chapter Objectives

At the conclusion of this chapter, the student should be able to:

1. Define key terms related to HCPCS Level II coding.
2. Provide an overview about the use of HCPCS codes.
3. List the HCPCS levels and their components.
4. Assign HCPCS Level II procedure and services codes for outpatient care.
5. Determine payer responsibility based on HCPCS Level II code assignment.

Key Terms

DME MAC medical
  review policies
durable medical
  equipment,
  prosthetics, orthotics,
  and supplies
  (DMEPOS)
durable medical
  equipment,
  prosthetics, orthotics,
  and supplies
  (DMEPOS) dealer

HCPCS Level I
HCPCS Level II
  miscellaneous codes
HCPCS Level II modifiers
HCPCS Level II
  permanent national
  codes
HCPCS Level II
  temporary codes

local coverage
  determinations (LCDs)
*Medicare Benefit Policy
  Manual*
*Medicare National
  Coverage
  Determinations Manual*
Medicare Pricing, Data
  Analysis, and Coding
  (PDAC) contractor

national coverage
  determinations (NCDs)
orthotics
prosthetics
transitional pass-through
  payment

Introduction

The HCPCS Level II coding system contains alphanumeric codes that were developed to complement the Current Procedural Terminology (CPT) coding system. It is also called the HCPCS (pronounced "hick-picks") national codes. HCPCS Level II was introduced in 1983 after Medicare found that its payers used more than 100 different coding systems, making it difficult to analyze claims data. HCPCS Level II furnishes health care providers and suppliers with a standardized language for reporting professional and nonphysician services, procedures, supplies, and equipment. (Most state Medicaid programs and many commercial payers also use the HCPCS Level II coding system.)

NOTE:

Optum's *HCPCS Level II* coding manual was used for chapter examples, exercises, and review questions.

NOTE:

Instruction about the HCPCS Level II coding system is sequenced prior to CPT Chapters 9–19 in this textbook to familiarize students with HCPCS Level II modifiers that must be added to CPT codes and HCPCS Level II codes that must be reported with CPT codes. Examples, exercises, and review questions in Chapters 9–19 of this textbook require students to report HCPCS Level II modifiers and codes, where appropriate. (Code ranges included in parentheses after section titles in the textbook chapters may differ from your HCPCS Level II coding manual.)

Overview of HCPCS

Two levels of codes are associated with HCPCS, commonly referred to as HCPCS Level I and II codes. Most of the procedures and services are reported using CPT (HCPCS Level I) codes. However, CPT does not describe durable medical equipment, prosthetics, orthotics, supplies (DMEPOS), and certain other services. Therefore, the Centers for Medicare & Medicaid Services (CMS) developed HCPCS Level II codes to report DMEPOS and other services.

HCPCS Level I

HCPCS Level I includes the CPT codes developed and published by the American Medical Association (AMA). The AMA is responsible for the annual update of this coding system and its two-digit modifiers. (CPT was defined in Chapter 1 of this textbook, and its content is covered in Chapters 9–19.)

HCPCS Level II

HCPCS Level II (or HCPCS national coding system) was created in 1983 to describe common medical services and supplies not classified in CPT. HCPCS Level II codes are five characters in length, and they begin with the letters *A–V* followed by four numbers. The codes identify services performed by physician and nonphysician providers (e.g., nurse practitioners, speech therapists), services provided by ambulance companies, and supplies and equipment provided by durable medical equipment (DME) companies, which are called durable medical equipment, prosthetics, orthotics, and supplies (DMEPOS) dealers. *Durable medical equipment (DME)* is defined by Medicare as equipment that is

- Durable (can withstand repeated use)
- Used for a medical reason
- Not usually useful to someone who isn't sick or injured
- Used in the patient's home
- Generally has an expected lifetime of at least three years

Durable medical equipment, prosthetics, orthotics, and supplies (DMEPOS) include artificial limbs, braces, medications, surgical dressings, and wheelchairs. **Durable medical equipment, prosthetics, orthotics, and supplies (DMEPOS) dealers** provide patients with DME (e.g., canes, crutches, walkers, commode chairs, and blood-glucose monitors). DMEPOS claims are submitted to DME Medicare administrative contractors (MACs) (previously called durable medical equipment regional carriers, or DMERCs) that were awarded contracts by CMS. Each DME MAC covers a specific geographic region of the country and is responsible for processing DMEPOS claims for its specific region.

 NOTE:

When claims are to be submitted to one of the four DME MACs, DMEPOS dealers that have coding questions should check with the **Medicare Pricing, Data Analysis, and Coding (PDAC) contractor** (formerly called the Statistical Analysis Durable Medical Equipment Regional Carrier, or SADMERC), which assists suppliers and manufacturers in determining HCPCS Level II codes to be used. The PDAC has a toll-free help line for this purpose at (877) 735-1326.

When people refer to HCPCS codes, they are most likely referring to HCPCS Level II codes. CMS is responsible for the annual updates to HCPCS Level II codes and the two-character alphanumeric modifiers. HCPCS Level II codes are further discussed in this chapter.

HCPCS Level III

Effective December 31, 2003, HCPCS Level III local codes were no longer required. They had the same structure as Level II codes, but were assigned by local Medicare carriers (LMCs) (now called Medicare administrative contractors or MACs), which process Medicare claims. HCPCS Level III codes began with the letters *W, X, Y,* or *Z*. (Some third-party payers continue to use the HCPCS Level III codes.)

Exercise 8.1 – Overview of HCPCS

Instructions: Complete each statement.

1. HCPCS Level II codes are also called _____ codes.
2. HCPCS Level II codes describe procedures; services; and *durable medical equipment, prosthetics, and orthotics supplies*, which is abbreviated as _____.
3. CPT codes are included as HCPCS Level _____ codes.
4. HCPCS Level II codes are _____ characters in length.
5. HCPCS Level II codes begin with the letters A through _____.

HCPCS Level II Codes

The HCPCS Level II coding system includes codes for similar medical products and services that facilitate efficient claims processing. Each code contains a description, and the codes are used primarily for billing purposes. The codes describe the following:

- DME devices, accessories, supplies, and repairs; prosthetics; orthotics; and medical and surgical supplies
- Medications
- Provider services

- Temporary Medicare codes
- Other items and services (e.g., ambulance services)

NOTE:

DMEPOS dealers report HCPCS Level II codes to identify equipment reported on claims submitted to private or public health insurers.

HCPCS is *not* a reimbursement methodology or payment system; it is important to understand that just because codes exist for certain products or services, coverage (e.g., payment) is not guaranteed. The HCPCS Level II coding system

- Ensures uniform reporting of medical products or services on claims
- Has code descriptors that identify similar products or services (instead of specific products or brand/trade names)
- Is not a reimbursement methodology for making coverage or payment determinations (Each payer makes determinations on coverage and payment outside this coding process.)

Responsibility for HCPCS Level II Codes

HCPCS Level II codes are developed and maintained by the *CMS HCPCS Workgroup*, which includes representatives of the major components of CMS, Medicaid state agencies, and the Pricing, Data Analysis and Coding (PDAC) contractors. HCPCS Level II codes are revised annually, and the revised codes are implemented each January. (The revision involves adding and deleting codes and revising code descriptors.)

NOTE:

HCPCS Level II temporary codes are maintained by CMS and other members of the CMS HCPCS Workgroup, independent of HCPCS Level II permanent codes. HCPCS Level II temporary codes allow payers the flexibility to add, delete, and revise codes on a quarterly basis throughout the year. HCPCS Level II permanent national codes are implemented once a year on January 1.

HCPCS Level II codes do not carry the copyright of a private organization; they are in the public domain, which allows many publishers to print annual coding manuals. Each publisher may elect to color-code the print or pages, include supplemental explanatory material, or provide reimbursement information from the *Medicare Benefit Policy Manual* for Part B or the *Medicare National Coverage Determinations Manual*. The ***Medicare Benefit Policy Manual*** provides direction about services and procedures to be reimbursed by the MAC. The ***Medicare National Coverage Determinations Manual*** indicates whether a service is covered or excluded under the Medicare program.

Some publishers include the following HCPCS Level II references in their version of the coding manual:

- General instructions or guidelines for each section
- Appendix that summarizes additions, deletions, and terminology revisions in HCPCS Level II codes
- Separate tables of drugs or deleted codes
- Symbols to identify codes excluded from Medicare coverage
- Codes for which payment is left to the discretion of the responsible MAC
- Codes with special coverage instructions
- Current HCPCS Level II modifiers

CMS has stated that it is not responsible for any errors that might occur in or from the use of these private printings of HCPCS Level II codes.

Types of HCPCS Level II Codes

HCPCS Level II codes are organized according to type depending on the purpose of the codes and the entity responsible for establishing and maintaining them. The four types are as follows:

- Permanent national codes
- Miscellaneous codes
- Temporary codes
- HCPCS Level II modifiers

 NOTE:

The American Dental Association publishes an annual *Current Dental Terminology (CDT)* coding manual, which contains D codes that are reported for dental procedures.

Permanent National Codes

HCPCS Level II permanent national codes are maintained by the CMS HCPCS Workgroup, which unanimously makes decisions about additions, revisions, and deletions. Because HCPCS Level II is a national coding system, none of the parties, including CMS, can make unilateral decisions regarding permanent national codes, which are intended for use by all private and public health insurers.

Miscellaneous Codes

HCPCS Level II miscellaneous codes include *miscellaneous/not otherwise classified* codes that are reported when a DMEPOS dealer submits a claim for a product or service for which there is no existing HCPCS Level II code. Miscellaneous codes allow DMEPOS dealers to submit a claim for a product or service as soon as it is approved by the Food and Drug Administration (FDA) even though there is no code that describes the product or service. The use of miscellaneous codes also helps avoid the inefficiency of assigning codes for items or services that are rarely furnished or for which MACs expect to receive few claims.

Claims that contain miscellaneous codes are manually reviewed by the payer, and the following must be provided for use in the review process:

- Complete description of product or service
- Pricing information for product or service
- Documentation to explain why the item or service is needed by the beneficiary

Before reporting a miscellaneous code on a claim, a DMEPOS dealer should check with the payer to determine if a specific code has been identified for use (instead of a miscellaneous code).

Temporary Codes

HCPCS Level II temporary codes (Table 8-1) are maintained by an internal subgroup of the CMS HCPCS Workgroup, independent of permanent HCPCS Level II codes. Permanent national codes are updated each January 1, but temporary codes allow payers the flexibility to add, delete, and revise codes on a quarterly basis throughout the year. Such codes are needed before the next January 1 annual update. Certain sections of the HCPCS Level II codes were set aside to allow CMS HCPCS Workgroup members to develop temporary codes, and decisions regarding the number and type of temporary codes and the way they are used are made independently by each CMS HCPCS Workgroup member. Temporary codes serve the purpose of meeting short time frame operational needs of a particular payer.

Although the CMS HCPCS Workgroup may decide to replace temporary codes with permanent codes, if permanent codes are not established, the temporary codes remain "temporary" indefinitely. When a permanent code replaces a temporary code, the temporary code is deleted.

HCPCS Level II Modifiers

HCPCS Level II modifiers are attached to any HCPCS Level I (CPT) or II (national) code to provide additional information regarding the product or service reported. Modifiers supplement the information provided by an HCPCS code descriptor to identify specific circumstances that may apply to an item or a service. HCPCS Level II modifiers (Figure 8-1) are added to five-character CPT or HCPCS Level II codes.

TABLE 8-1 Categories of HCPCS Level II Temporary Codes

Category	Descriptions
C codes	• Reported to Medicare administrative contractors (MACs) for hospital outpatient department procedures and services. • Include new and innovative drugs, biologicals, and devices that are eligible for transitional pass-through payments for the assignment of ambulatory payment classifications (APCs), associated with Medicare's outpatient prospective payment system (OPPS).
G codes	• Identify professional and outpatient health care procedures and services that are not assigned CPT codes. • G codes can be reported to all payers.
H codes	• Reported to state Medicaid agencies that are mandated by state law to establish separate codes for identifying mental health services (e.g., alcohol and drug treatment services).
K codes	• Reported to DME MACs when existing permanent national codes do not include codes needed to implement a medical review coverage policy.
Q codes	• Identify services that would not ordinarily be assigned a CPT code (e.g., drugs, biologicals, and other types of medical equipment or services). • Q codes can be reported to all payers.
S codes	• Used by private payers when no HCPCS Level II codes exist to report drugs, services, and supplies, but codes are needed to implement private payer policies and programs for claims processing. • S codes are reported to BCBS, Medicaid, and private third-party payers.
T codes	• Reported to state Medicaid agencies when no HCPCS Level II permanent codes exist, but codes are needed to administer the Medicaid program. • T codes are not reported to Medicare, but they can be reported to private third-party payers.

HCPCS Level II coding manuals often contain a list of modifiers inside the front and back covers or as a separate appendix. (CPT Appendix A includes a detailed list of CPT modifiers, and some HCPCS Level II modifiers are included inside its front cover.) Familiarity with all modifiers is crucial to reporting accurate CPT and HCPCS Level II codes for reimbursement purposes. A careful review of the patient record will help determine which modifier(s), if any, should be added to CPT and HCPCS Level II codes.

HCPCS Level II Modifiers	
AA	Anesthesia services performed personally by anesthesiologist
AB	Audiology service furnished personally by an audiologist...
AD	Medical supervision by a physician: more than 4 concurrent anesthesia procedures
AE	Registered dietician
AF	Specialty physician
AG	Primary physician
AH	Clinical psychologist

Permission to reprint granted by Optum360.

FIGURE 8-1 Sample listing of HCPCS Level II modifiers

NOTE:

Because modifiers are reported with HCPCS Level II codes, chapter content about modifiers precedes content about the assignment of HCPCS Level II codes.

Example: A clinical psychologist provides 45 minutes of group psychotherapy in a partial hospitalization setting. Report code G0410 AH.

Coding Tip

- HCPCS Level II alpha and alphanumeric modifiers may also be added to CPT codes to further define the procedure or service reported (e.g., 69436 RT for tympanostomy, right ear).
- Refer to HCPCS Level II and CPT coding manuals for a comprehensive list of modifiers.

General Guidelines for Modifier Use

Not all HCPCS Level I and II codes require modifiers, and the CMS has clarified the use of certain modifiers. (CPT modifiers are covered in textbook Chapter 9.)

- Modifiers GN, GO, and GP are reported with codes assigned for an outpatient plan of care.
  - Speech language therapy (GN)
  - Occupational therapy (GO)
  - Physical therapy (GP)
- The following are descriptive subset HCPCS Level II modifiers of CPT modifier 59, which means they are reported *instead of modifier 59 for Medicare claims:*
  - XE (Separate encounter, a service that is distinct because it occurred during a separate encounter)
  - XS (Separate structure, a service that is distinct because it was performed on a separate organ/structure)
  - XP (Separate practitioner, a service that is distinct because it was performed by a different practitioner)
  - XU (Unusual non-overlapping service, the use of a service that is distinct because it does not overlap usual components of the main service)

  While CMS continues to recognize modifier 59, it should not be reported when a more descriptive subset modifier is available.

- Modifiers are reported with codes for procedures and services when they
  - Add more information about the anatomical site of the procedure

Example: Cataract surgery on the right or left eye. Add modifier RT (right side) or LT (left side) to the CPT code reported for cataract surgery. (Modifiers LT and RT are used to identify procedures performed on the left or right side of the body, respectively.)

  - Help to eliminate duplicate billing

Example: Add modifier 76 (Repeat Procedure or Service by Same Physician or Other Qualified Health Care Professional) to the reported code when the same procedure is performed more than once by the same physician.

  - Help to eliminate unbundling of codes

Example: When codes Q0081 (Infusion therapy, using other than chemotherapeutic drugs, per visit) and 36000 (Introduction of needle or intracatheter, vein) are reported on the same claim, the payer will deny payment for one of the codes because they are duplicate services. Adding modifier 59 (distinct procedural service), *or its descriptive subset,* to code 36000, *if that procedure was performed for a reason other than as part of the IV infusion*, ensures appropriate processing of the claim and reimbursement for both procedures.

Laterality Modifiers

CPT and HCPCS Level II laterality modifiers are reported with procedures performed on one or both sides of a paired organ or body part.

- Report CPT modifier 50 (Bilateral procedure) with codes for procedures performed on *both sides* of a paired organ or body part.
  - Do *not* report modifier 50 when the code description contains unilateral or bilateral terminology.
  - Parenthetical notes, located below CPT code descriptions, sometimes provide guidance about reporting modifier 50.
- Report HCPCS Level II modifier LT (Left side) *or* RT (Right side) with codes for procedures performed on *one side* of a paired organ or body part.
  - Do *not* report modifiers LT and RT when modifier 50 is reported with a code.

> **Example:** Patient underwent outpatient hospital percutaneous breast biopsy procedures using magnetic resonance guidance, with placement of breast localization devices, right and left breast. Since this procedure was performed bilaterally (on the right and left breasts), report C7502 50. (*Do not report C7502 RT and C7502 LT.*)

- Report the following specific laterality modifiers *instead of LT (left) or RT (right)*, for eyelids, digits of hands and feet, and coronary arteries, when applicable. *Do not report modifiers 50, LT, or RT with specific laterality modifiers.*
  - E1–E4 (indicate upper or lower position and laterality of eyelids)
  - FA and F1–F9 (indicate digits and laterality of hands, such as FA for left hand, thumb)
  - LC (left circumflex coronary artery)
  - LD (left anterior descending coronary artery)
  - LM (left main coronary artery)
  - RC (right coronary artery)
  - RI (ramus intermedius coronary artery)
  - TA and T1–T9 (indicate digits and laterality of feet, such as T1 for left foot, 2nd digit)

> **Example:** Patient underwent outpatient hospital percutaneous transluminal coronary angioplasty procedure, left main coronary artery, with transcatheter placement of radiation delivery device for subsequent coronary intravascular brachytherapy. Report code C7533 LM. *Do not report C7533 LT.*

- Do not report laterality modifiers (e.g., 50, LT, RT) with CPT codes when a description includes *both* paired *and* nonpaired body parts or organs.
  - For example, CPT code 12031 describes "Repair, intermediate, wounds of scalp, axillae, trunk and/or extremities (excluding hands and feet); 2.5 cm or less."
  - The scalp and trunk are nonpaired body parts, and the axillae and extremities are paired body parts.
  - Thus, a laterality modifier cannot be assigned to CPT code 12031.

Reporting HCPCS Level II Modifiers on Claims

When more than one modifier applies, report the code on more than one line of the UB-04 claim with the appropriate modifier.

Example: Patient underwent simple drainage of a finger abscess, left-hand thumb and second finger (code 26010). On the UB-04, report the code on two lines as follows:

- 26010 FA

- 26010 F1

- Report modifiers on the hard copy UB-04 (CMS-1450) institutional insurance claim in Form Locator 44 (next to Form Locators where HCPCS codes are entered). (There is space for two modifiers on each hard copy UB-04.) For electronic claims, the UB-04 flat file allows entry of modifiers as record type 61, field numbers 6 and 7. (There is space for two modifiers, one in field 6 and one in field 7.)

Example: Modifier LT (left side) is reported as LT in form locator 44 of the UB-04.

42 REV. CD.	43 DESCRIPTION	44 HCPCS / RATE / HIPPS CODE	45 SERV. DATE	46 SERV. UNITS	47 TOTAL CHARGES	48 NON-COVERED CHARGES	49
0360	BREAST RECONSTRUCTION DIEP FLAP	S2068 LT	0505YY	1	4775 00	:	

Courtesy of the Centers for Medicare and Medicaid Services, www.cms.gov; claim data created by author.

- Report modifier(s) in Block 24D of the CMS-1500 claim professional services insurance claim, spacing once after the CPT or HCPCS Level II code. (Space once between modifiers when multiple modifiers are added to the same code.)

Example: Modifier AH (clinical psychologist) is reported as AH in form locator 24D of the CMS-1500.

24. A DATE(S) OF SERVICE From MM DD YY To MM DD YY	B Place of Service	C Type of Service	D PROCEDURES, SERVICES, OR SUPPLIES (Explain Unusual Circumstances) CPT/HCPCS | MODIFIER	E DIAGNOSIS POINTER	F $ CHARGES	G DAYS OR UNITS	H EPSDT Family Plan	I EMG	J COB	K RESERVED FOR LOCAL USE
1			G0410 AH							

Courtesy of the Centers for Medicare & Medicaid Services, www.cms.gov; claim data created by author.

NOTE:

On the CMS-1500, report the code and multiple modifiers on just one line of Block 24D, such as 26010 FA F1.

Modifiers for Ambulance and Nonemergency Transportation Services

Ambulance and nonemergency transportation services are reported with appropriate HCPCS Level II codes and modifiers that clarify the transport circumstances. When institutional-based providers deliver transportation services, one of the following modifiers is reported *first* for each HCPCS Level II ambulance and nonemergency transportation services code. According to CMS, institutional-based providers are hospitals, critical care facilities, rural emergency hospitals, skilled nursing facilities, and home health and hospice agencies. Modifiers QM and QN are *not* reported for non-institutional-based providers, such as a physician's office.

- QM (ambulance service provided under arrangement by a provider of services)
- QN (ambulance service furnished directly by a provider of services)

When more than one patient is transported in the vehicle at the same time, the following modifier is reported along with documentation that specifies the total number of patients and the Medicare beneficiary identifier for each patient.

- GM (multiple patients transported in same vehicle during one ambulance trip)

When the beneficiary was pronounced dead after the ambulance was called or dispatched *but before the ambulance arrived at the scene*, the appropriate HCPCS Level II code is reported with modifier QL.

- A0428 (ambulance service, basic life support, nonemergency transport [BLS])
- A0429 (ambulance service, basic life support, emergency transport [BLS], emergency)
- QL (Patient pronounced dead after ambulance called)

A modifier for the origin and destination of ambulance or nonemergency transportation services is created and reported with each ambulance and nonemergency transportation service. To create the modifier using the table, *first* select the origin character, and then select the destination character, such as HH when a patient is transported from one hospital to another. (When an institutional-based provider delivers transportation services, modifier QM or QN is reported first, followed by the origin/destination modifier.)

Character	Description of Origin and Destination
D	Diagnostic or therapeutic site[1] *other than P or H when used as origin character*
E	Residential, domiciliary, or custodial facility *other than 1819[2] (skilled nursing) facility*
G	Hospital-based end-stage renal disease (ESRD) facility
H	Hospital
I	Site of transfer (e.g., airport, helicopter pad) between modes of ambulance transport
J	Freestanding ESRD facility
N	Skilled nursing facility (SNF)
P	Physician's office
R	Residence (e.g., patient's home)
S	Scene of accident or acute event
X	Intermediate stop at physician's office on the way to hospital *as a destination character only*

[1]Diagnostic or therapeutic sites include community mental health centers, federally qualified health centers (FQHCs), rural health clinics (RHCs), urgent care facilities, non-provider-based ambulatory surgery centers (ASCs) or freestanding emergency centers, or any location furnishing dialysis services *that is not affiliated with an ESRD facility.*
[2]Section 1819 of the Social Security Act contains requirements for skilled nursing facilities that participate in the Medicare program.

Example: The patient arrived at the physician's office experiencing chest pain and difficulty breathing. The medical staff performed an EKG, determined that the patient was having an acute myocardial infarction, and called for an ambulance. The patient was transported to the hospital's emergency department while receiving level one advanced life support (ALS) services. Report code A0427 PH.

To create modifier PH, use the table of characters and description of origin and destination characters to first select P (physician's office), and then select H (hospital). (Do not report modifier QM or QN because a physician's office is *not* an institutional-based provider.)

Exercise 8.2 – HCPCS Level II Codes

Instructions: Complete each statement.

1. HCPCS Level II codes are developed and maintained by the CMS HCPCS _____.
2. Services and procedures that are reimbursed by a MAC can be found in the _____ Benefit Policy Manual.
3. Whether a service is covered or excluded under the Medicare program can be found in the Medicare National Coverage _____ Manual.

(continues)

Exercise 8.2 – continued

4. HCPCS Level II _____ are attached to any HCPCS Level I (CPT) or II (national) code to provide additional information regarding the product or service reported.

5. HCPCS Level II codes, CPT codes, and multiple modifiers are reported on the same line of Block 24D on the _____ claim.

6. HCPCS Level II miscellaneous codes are reported when a DMEPOS _____ submits a claim for a product or service for which there is no existing HCPCS Level II code.

7. HCPCS Level II _____ codes allow payers the flexibility to establish codes that are needed before the next January 1 update.

8. Refer to Figure 8-1, and enter the modifier that is added to a code when a procedure is performed by a registered dietician: _____.

9. CPT modifier _____ is added to codes for procedures that are performed on both sides during the same operative session.

10. When a radiology procedure is canceled, report a code to describe the _____ of the procedure performed.

Assigning HCPCS Level II Codes

Some services must be reported by assigning both a CPT and an HCPCS Level II code. The most common scenario uses the CPT code for the administration of an infusion or injection and the HCPCS Level II code to identify the medication. Most drugs have qualifying terms such as *dosage limits* that could alter the quantity reported (Figure 8-2).

- If a drug is administered in a 70-mg dose and the HCPCS Level II code description states "per 50 mg," the quantity billed is 2.

- If just 15 mg of a drug were administered and the HCPCS Level II code description stated "up to 20 mg," the quantity billed is 1.

 NOTE:

CMS developed HCPCS Level II codes for Medicare, but commercial payers also adopted them.

Imagine how much money providers lose by reporting only the CPT code for injections. Unless the payer or insurance plan advises the provider that it does not pay separately for the medication injected, always report this combination of codes. It is possible that a particular service would be assigned a CPT code and a HCPCS Level II code. Which one should you report? The answer is found in the instructions from the payer. Most commercial

DRUGS ADMINISTERED OTHER THAN ORAL METHOD	
J0475	Injection, baclofen, 10 mg
J0476	Injection, baclofen, 50 mcg for intrathecal trial
J0480	Injection, basiliximab, 20 mg
J0485	Injection, belatacept, 1 mg
J0490	Injection, belimumab, 10 mg
J0491	Injection, anifrolumab-fnia, 1 mg
J0500	Injection, dicyclomine HCl, up to 20 mg
J0515	Injection, benztropine mesylate, per 1 mg
J0517	Injection, benralizumab, 1 mg
J0520	Injection, bethanechol chloride, Mytonachol or Urecholine, up to 5 mg

FIGURE 8-2 Sample listing of HCPCS Level II J codes

payers require the CPT code. Medicare gives HCPCS Level II codes the highest priority if the CPT code is general and the HCPCS Level II code is more specific.

Most supplies are included in the charge for the office visit or the procedure. CPT provides code 99070 for all supplies and materials exceeding those usually included in the primary service or procedure performed. However, this CPT code may be too general to ensure correct payment. If the office provides additional supplies when performing a service, the HCPCS Level II codes may identify the supplies in sufficient detail to secure proper reimbursement.

Although CMS developed this system, some HCPCS Level I and II services are not payable by Medicare. Medicare may also place qualifications or conditions on payment for some services. As an example, an electrocardiogram (ECG) is a covered service for a cardiac problem but is not covered when performed as part of a routine examination. Also, the payment for some services may be left to the discretion of the MAC. Two CMS publications assist MACs in correctly processing claims: the *Medicare National Coverage Determinations Manual* advises the MAC as to whether a service is covered or excluded under Medicare regulations, and the *Medicare Claims Processing Manual* directs the MAC to pay or reject a service, using a specific "remark" or explanation code.

There are more than 7,000 HCPCS Level II codes, but you may find that no code exists for the procedure or service you need to report. Unlike CPT, HCPCS Level II does not have a consistent method of establishing codes for reporting "unlisted procedure" services. If the MAC does not provide special instructions for reporting these services in HCPCS, report them with the proper "unlisted procedure" code from CPT. Remember to submit documentation explaining the procedure or service when using the "unlisted procedure" codes.

HCPCS Level II Index

Because of the wide variety of services and procedures described in HCPCS Level II, the alphabetical index (Figure 8-3) is very helpful in finding the correct code. CMS has discontinued publication of an annual HCPCS Level II index; however, publishers (e.g., Optum) include an index that lists additional terms, making the search for codes easier and faster. The table of drugs and biologicals (Figure 8-4) lists codes assigned to medications, which include codes that begin with letters A, C, J, Q, and S. The table of drugs and biologicals also includes medication unit amounts (e.g., 10 mg) and routes of administration (e.g., IM). Some publishers print brand names beneath each generic description, and others provide a special expanded index of the drug codes.

It is important never to code directly from the index and always to verify the code in the appropriate code section of the coding manual. You may want to review the HCPCS Level II references from several publishers and select the one that best meets your needs and is easiest for you to use. If you have difficulty locating the service or procedure in the HCPCS Level II index, review the list of codes and descriptions in the appropriate section of the coding manual to locate the code.

Index

Abdomen/abdominal
    dressing holder/binder, A4461, A4463
    pad, low profile, L1270
Abduction
    control, each, L2624
    pillow, E1399
    rotation bar, foot, L3140-L3170
Ablation
    robotic, waterjet, C2596
    transbronchial, C9751
    ultrasound, C9734

FIGURE 8-3 Sample listing of HCPCS Level II index entries

Drug Name	Unit Per	Route	Code
ABATACEPT	10 mg	IV	J0129
ABCIXIMAB	10 mg	IV	J1030
ABELCET	10 mg	IV	J0287
ABILIFY	0.25 mg	IM	J0400
ABOBOTULINUMTOXINA	5 units	IM	J0586
ABRAXANE	1 mg	IV	J9264

FIGURE 8-4 Sample listing of HCPCS Level II table of drugs and biologicals

NOTE:

The Food and Drug Administration (FDA) publishes the *National Drug Code (NDC) directory*, which includes drug products that are identified and reported using a unique, three-segment number. Go to **www.fda.gov**, click on Menu, click on the Drugs link below the Products heading, scroll down and click on Drug Approvals and Databases, and scroll down and click on Drugs@FDA Search to locate information about FDA-approved drug products.

HCPCS Level II Code Sections

HCPCS Level II code sections are identified by an alphabetical first character (e.g., *B* for *enteral and parenteral therapy* and *C* for *outpatient PPS*). Some code sections are logical, such as *R* for *radiology*, whereas others, such as *J* for *drugs*, appear to be arbitrarily assigned.

Transportation Services Including Ambulance (A0000–A0999)

The Transportation Services Including Ambulance section of HCPCS Level II includes codes for ancillary transportation-related fees, ground and air ambulance, and nonemergency transportation (e.g., automobile, bus, taxi, and wheelchair van).

> **Example:** A Medicaid patient received emergency transport from home to the hospital emergency department in an ambulance that contained basic life support (BLS). Report code A0429 RH.

Medical and Surgical Supplies (A2000–A9999)

The Medical and Surgical Supplies section of HCPCS Level II includes codes for a wide variety of medical, surgical, some durable medical equipment-related (DME-related) supplies and accessories (e.g., syringes, replacement batteries, lancets, ostomy pouch), miscellaneous supplies, supplies for radiological procedures, and miscellaneous service components. DME-related supplies, accessories, maintenance, and repair ensure proper functioning of durable medical equipment (DME).

> **Example 1:** A 68-year-old patient who is undergoing treatment for unresected liver cancer was supplied with a refill kit for an implantable infusion pump. Report code A4220.

> **Example 2:** A 72-year-old patient was provided with artificial saliva, 30 milliliters. Report code A9155.

NOTE:

Some supplies are included during the administration of an evaluation and management (E/M) service, and separate HCPCS Level II codes are *not* assigned (e.g., sterile gauze). E/M services are assigned separate CPT codes, as discussed in textbook Chapter 10.

Enteral and Parenteral Therapy (B4000–B9999)

The Enteral and Parenteral Therapy section of HCPCS Level II includes codes for enteral and parenteral infusion pumps, enteral and parenteral supplies, enteral formulae, and parenteral nutritional solutions.

Example: The patient was supplied with a fiber additive for enteral formula. Report code B4104.

Outpatient PPS (C1000–C9999)

The Hospital Outpatient Prospective Payment System (Outpatient PPS) section of HCPCS Level II includes codes for biologicals, devices, and drugs eligible for transitional pass-through payments for hospitals, as well as items included in the new technology APCs under the OPPS. **Transitional pass-through payments** are temporary additional payments (over and above the OPPS payment) made for certain innovative medical devices, drugs, and biologicals provided to Medicare beneficiaries.

Example: Patient underwent insertion of a directional transluminal atherectomy catheter. Report code C1714.

 Coding Tip

The OPPS requires hospitals and ambulatory surgery centers to report product-specific HCPCS Level II "C codes" to obtain reimbursement for biologicals, devices, drugs, and other items associated with implantable device technologies. Reporting C codes in conjunction with CPT procedure codes greatly improves the quality of claims data Medicare uses to establish future APC payments. Outpatient coding edits (updated on a quarterly basis) identify C codes that should be billed with CPT procedure codes.

Applications are also submitted to CMS for "new" biologicals, devices, and drugs for consideration of "transitional pass-through payment status" and items for consideration of "new-technology APC designation." If certain criteria are met and CMS approves the "new" biologicals, devices, drugs, and items, C codes are assigned and published in program memorandums.

Durable Medical Equipment (E0100–E9999)

The Durable Medical Equipment section of HCPCS Level II includes codes for durable medical equipment, which can withstand repeated use, are used for a medical reason in the patient's home, and generally have an expected lifetime of at least 3 years (e.g., canes crutches, walkers, commodes, hospital beds).

Example: The patient was supplied with a pair of aluminum underarm crutches. Report code E0114.

Procedures/Professional Services (Temporary) (G0008–G9999)

The Procedures/Professional Services (Temporary) section of HCPCS Level II includes codes for professional health care procedures and services that either do not have codes identified in the CPT or require the reporting of G codes (instead of CPT codes).

Example: A patient became a Medicare beneficiary on March 1 and underwent an initial preventive physical examination (IPPE) and in-office electrocardiogram (ECG) on May 30. Report codes G0402 and G0403. (Make sure you report the appropriate ICD-10-CM Z code as the first-listed diagnosis.)

Alcohol and Drug Abuse Treatment Services (H0001–H9999)

The Alcohol and Drug Abuse Treatment Services section of HCPCS Level II includes codes used by state Medicaid agencies mandated by state law to establish separate codes for identifying mental health services that include alcohol and drug treatment services.

> **Example:** A patient underwent alcohol assessment prior to participating in psychotherapy. Report code H0001.

J Codes Drugs (J0100–J8500)

The Drugs section of HCPCS Level II includes codes for drugs that ordinarily cannot be self-administered, chemotherapy drugs, immunosuppressive drugs, inhalation solutions, and other miscellaneous drugs and solutions.

> **Example:** A home health patient received an injection of 10 mcg of teriparatide (brand name Forteo) for treatment of osteoporosis. Report code J3110.

Providers and suppliers report modifier JW (drug or biological amount discarded and not administered to any patient) on claims submitted for drugs and biologicals that are separately payable under Medicare Part B for unused and discarded amounts from single-dose containers or single-use packages. The patient's record must document the amount of discarded drugs or biologicals.

> **Example:** A provider documents the use of a single-dose container labeled as containing 100 units of a drug, administering 95 units to the Medicare Part B patient and discarding 5 units. Report the appropriate J code on the claim, entering 95 in the Units column. Then, report the same J code with modifier JW on the next line of the same claim, entering 5 in the Units column. Both line items of the claim are processed for payment, and the provider receives full reimbursement even though 5 units of the drug were discarded.

Providers and suppliers also report modifier JZ (zero drug or biological amount discarded and not administered to any patient) on claims submitted for drugs and biologicals from single-dose containers or single-use packages, which are separately payable under Medicare Part B *when there are no discarded amounts*.

> **Example:** A provider documents the use of a single-dose container labeled as containing 100 units of a drug, administering all 100 units to the Medicare Part B patient. Report the appropriate J code and modifier JZ on one line of the claim, entering 100 in the Units column. The provider receives full reimbursement because modifier JZ attests that no amount of the drug was discarded or administered to a different patient.

J Codes Chemotherapy Drugs (J8501–J9999)

The Chemotherapy Drugs section of HCPCS Level II includes codes reported for the administration of chemotherapy.

> **Example:** The patient was administered 5 milligrams of oral aprepitant. Report code J8501.

Temporary Codes (K0000–K9999)

The Temporary Codes section of HCPCS Level II includes codes for durable medical equipment (DME), as established by DME MACs (formerly DMERCs), when permanent national codes do not include codes needed to implement a DME MAC medical review policy.

> **Example:** The patient was supplied with a standard wheelchair. Report code K0001.

Orthotic Procedures and Devices (L0000–L4999)

The Orthotic Procedures and Devices section of HCPCS Level II includes codes for orthopedic shoes, orthotic devices and procedures, and scoliosis equipment. **Orthotics** is the branch of medicine that deals with the design and fitting of orthopedic (relating to bone disorders) devices (e.g., braces). Several orthotic procedures subsections include "addition" codes, which means they are reported in addition to base codes from the same subsection or a previous subsection.

> **Example:** Patient underwent a halo procedure during which the cervical halo was incorporated into a jacket vest. Patient also received a magnetic resonance image compatible system during the same encounter. Report codes L0810 and L0859.
>
> Because the description for code L0859 states "Addition to halo procedure, magnetic resonance image compatible system," it must be reported in addition to another HCPCS Level II code, such as L0810.

Prosthetic Procedures (L5000–L9999)

The Prosthetic Procedures section of HCPCS Level II includes codes for prosthetic devices, implants, and procedures. **Prosthetics** is the branch of medicine that deals with the design, production, and use of artificial body parts (e.g., artificial limbs). Several prosthetic procedures subsections include "addition" codes, meaning that they are reported in addition to base codes from the same subsection or from a previous subsection.

> **Example:** The patient received a below-knee PTB type socket, nonalignable system, pylon, no cover, SACH (solid ankle cushion heel) foot, plaster socket, direct-formed. The patient also received a test socket, below knee, during the same encounter. Report codes L5500 and L5620.
>
> Because the description for code L5620 states "Addition to lower extremity, test socket, below knee," it must be reported in addition to another HCPCS Level II code, such as L5500.

MIPS Value Pathways (M0001–M0005)

The *MIPS Value Pathways (MVPs)* section of HCPCS Levell II includes codes to fulfill MIPS reporting requirements, such as advancing cancer care, optimal care for kidney health, optimal care for patients with episodic neurological conditions, supportive care for neurodegenerative conditions, and promoting wellness.

> **Example:** Code M0005 is reported for promoting wellness MIPS value pathways.

Medical Services (M0075–M0301)

The Medical Services section of HCPCS Level II includes other medical services and cardiovascular services, including COVID-19 vaccine administration inside a patient's home, injections, intravenous infusion, and the following:

- *Cellular therapy* involves injecting processed tissue from animal embryos, fetuses, or organs for the purpose of rejuvenating diseased tissue; its therapeutic effect has not been established.
- *Fabric wrapping of an abdominal aneurysm* is performed to reinforce an aneurysm with a fabric-wrapped stent (a small, flexible mesh tube used to "patch" the blood vessel). This procedure has largely been replaced with other more effective treatment methods.
- *Intragastric hypothermia using gastric freezing* is performed for the treatment of chronic peptic ulcer disease; CMS considers this procedure obsolete.
- *IV chelation therapy* is also called chemical endarterectomy, and it is performed to treat arteriosclerosis; it is considered experimental in the United States.
- *Prolotherapy* is a form of nonsurgical ligament reconstruction as a treatment for chronic pain; its therapeutic effect has not yet been established.

> **Example:** The patient received cellular therapy services. Report code M0075.

Quality Measures (M1003–M1149)

The Quality Measures section of HCPCS Level II includes codes for tools that help quantify health care processes, outcomes, and patient perceptions associated with the ability to provide high-quality healthcare, such as tuberculosis screening, discharge/discontinuation of episode of care documented in medical record, female patients unable to bear children, aspirin or another antiplatelet therapy used, and more.

> **Example:** Code M1069 is reported for patients who are screened for future fall risk.

Pathology and Laboratory Services (P0000–P9999)

The Pathology and Laboratory Services section of HCPCS Level II includes codes for chemistry, microbiology, and toxicology tests; screening Papanicolaou smears; and miscellaneous blood tests.

> **Example:** The patient underwent screening cervical Papanicolaou smear, which was interpreted by the physician. Report code P3001.

Q Codes (Temporary) (Q0035–Q9999)

The Q Codes (Temporary) section of HCPCS Level II includes codes that are reported until permanent codes are available.

> **Example:** Effective 2001, casting supplies were removed from practice expenses for all HCPCS codes, including CPT codes for fracture management, casts, and splints. This means that when CPT codes are reported for services that include the provision of a cast or splint, codes Q4001–Q4051 are *also* reported to provide reimbursement to providers for the supplies used in creating casts.

Diagnostic Radiology Services (R0000–R9999)

The Diagnostic Radiology Services section of HCPCS Level II includes codes that are reported for the transportation of portable x-ray and/or EKG equipment, including testing.

> **Example:** The provider transported portable EKG equipment to the nursing facility for the purpose of testing patients. Report code R0076.
>
> When more than one patient undergoes EKG testing, report code R0076, but prorate the single allowed transportation cost among all patients. For example, if the single allowed transportation cost is $50 and five patients underwent EKG testing, the prorated cost for each patient is $10.

Temporary National Codes (Non-Medicare) (S0000–S9999)

The Temporary National Codes (Non-Medicare) section of HCPCS Level II are reported to BCBS and other private third-party payers for the provision of drugs, services, and supplies when national codes do not exist, but codes are needed by the private sector to implement policies, programs, or claims processing. Medicaid also uses these codes, but Medicare does not.

> **Example:** The patient was administered butorphanol tartrate (trade name Stadol NS), nasal spray, 25 mg. Report code S0012.

National T Codes Established for State Medicaid Agencies (T1000–T9999)

The National T Codes Established for State Medicaid Agencies section of HCPCS Level II are reported to Medicaid state agencies for behavioral health, home health, hospice, long-term care, nursing, and other services; substance abuse treatment; supplies; and certain training-related procedures that are not classified in CPT or another section of HCPCS Level II. Third-party payers also use these codes, but Medicare does not.

Example: The Medicaid patient required sign language services for 30 minutes. Report codes T1013 and T1013 (because the description of code T1013 states "per 15 minutes"). (On the CMS-1500 or UB-04 claim, T1013 is reported once and 2 is entered in the units column.)

Coronavirus Services (U0001–U0002)

The Coronavirus Services section of HCPCS Level II includes codes for diagnostic panel and infection agent detection of the 2019 novel coronavirus, also referred to as COVID-19, 2019-nCoV Coronavirus, and SARS-CoV-2/2019-nCoV. (SARS-CoV-2/2019-nCoV is the abbreviation for severe acute respiratory syndrome coronavirus 2, 2019 novel coronavirus.)

Example: The patient underwent CDC 2019 Novel Coronavirus (2019-nCoV) Real-Time RT-PCR Diagnostic Panel, which was negative. Report code U0001.

Vision Services (V0000–V2999)

The Vision Services section of HCPCS Level II includes codes for vision-related supplies (e.g., contact lenses, intraocular lenses, lenses, and spectacles).

Example: The patient was supplied with a custom plastic prosthetic eye. Report code V2623.

Hearing Services (V5000–V5999)

The Hearing Services section of HCPCS Level II includes codes that describe hearing tests and related supplies and equipment, speech-language pathology screenings, and repair of augmentative communicative systems.

Example: The audiologist dispenses a monaural, in-the-ear (ITE) hearing aid for a patient diagnosed with sensorineural hearing loss, combined types. Report codes V5050 and V5241.

Basic Steps for Using the HCPCS Level II Index and Sections

1. Review the patient record to determine the procedures performed or services provided.
2. Locate the main term in Optum's *HCPCS Level II* index. (CMS has discontinued the publication of an annual HCPCS Level II index.)
3. Identify the code next to the main term in the index. There may be one code or a range of codes listed.
4. Go to the appropriate HCPCS Level II section to locate the code(s), comparing code description(s) with documented procedures and services.
5. Review the list of modifiers to identify any that should be added to the code.
6. Assign the code (and any appropriate modifiers).

 NOTE:

When the main term for a procedure or service cannot be found in the index, go to HCPCS Level II sections to review code descriptions. Compare multiple code descriptions with documentation of procedures performed and services provided to select the proper code.

Exercise 8.3 – Assigning HCPCS Level II Codes

Instructions: Complete each statement.

1. Some services must be reported by assigning both a CPT and an HCPCS Level II code. The most common scenario uses a CPT code for administration of an infusion or injection and the HCPCS Level II code to identify the _____ (or drug).

2. If a drug is administered in a 100-mg dose and the HCPCS Level II code description states "per 50 mg," the quantity billed is _____.

3. If just 10 mg of a drug were administered and the HCPCS Level II code description states "up to 15 mg," the quantity billed is _____.

4. The charge for a physician office encounter usually includes _____ and materials needed to perform the procedure or service.

5. Although CMS developed the HCPCS Level II coding system, some of its procedures and services are not payable by _____.

6. Some HCPCS Level II coding manuals include a table of drugs and biologicals that lists J codes, which are assigned to _____ (or drugs).

7. When having difficulty locating a service or procedure in the HCPCS Level II _____, review the list of codes and descriptions in the appropriate section of the coding manual to locate the code.

8. HCPCS Level II codes sections are identified by an alphabetical first _____ (or letter).

9. CMS developed the HCPCS Level II codes for Medicare, but commercial third-party _____ (or commercial insurance companies) also adopted them.

10. If a code does not exist for a procedure or service, report the proper "unlisted procedure" code from _____ (also called HCPCS Level I), and submit documentation that explains the procedure or service provided.

Determining Payer Responsibility

The specific HCPCS Level II code determines whether the claim is sent to the primary MAC that processes provider claims or the DME MAC that processes DMEPOS dealer claims. A *Medicare administrative contractor (MAC)* is an organization (e.g., third-party payer) that contracts with CMS to process claims and perform program integrity tasks for Medicare Part A and Medicare Part B, home health care and hospice, and DMEPOS. Providers and DMEPOS dealers obtain annual lists of valid HCPCS Level II codes, which include billing instructions for services.

 NOTE:

The emphasis on keeping older adults in their own homes led to a rapid expansion in DME services and dealers, and many of the larger DME companies operated in several states and sent their claims to multiple Medicare administrative contractors (MACs). Unfortunately, a few DME companies formed for the sole purpose of collecting as much money as possible from the Medicare program and then closed down. When CMS began to investigate and pursue fraudulent claims, it became apparent that DME billings were out of control. CMS decided to have all DME claims processed by only four DME MACs to reduce fraudulent claims.

When the doctor treats a Medicare patient for a broken ankle and supplies the patient with crutches, two claims are generated. The claim for the fracture care, or professional service, is sent to the primary MAC; the claim for the crutches is sent to the DME MAC. The physician must register with both, review billing rules, comply with claims instructions, and forward claims correctly to secure payment for both services. If the physician is not registered with the DME MAC to provide medical equipment and supplies, the patient is given a prescription for crutches to take to a local DMEPOS dealer.

Some services, such as cosmetic procedures, are excluded as Medicare benefits by law and will not be covered by either MAC. Splints and casts for traumatic injuries have CPT numbers that are used to report these supplies or services to the primary MAC. Because the review procedure for adding new codes to HCPCS Level II is a much shorter process, new medical and surgical services may first be assigned an HCPCS Level II code and then incorporated into CPT at a later date.

Patient Record Documentation

The patient record includes documentation that justifies the medical necessity of procedures, services, and supplies coded and reported on an insurance claim. This means that the diagnoses reported on the claim must justify diagnostic and therapeutic procedures, services, and supplies provided. The patient's record should include documentation of the following:

- Site of service
- Medical necessity of equipment, services, and supplies provided
- Accurate reporting of items provided
- History, physical examination, and diagnoses, including duration (e.g., acute or chronic) and comorbidities that impact care
- Patient's clinical course, functional limitations, past experience with related items, and prognosis, including potential for rehabilitation

When DMEPOS items are reported on a claim, the DMEPOS dealer must keep the following documents on file:

- Standard written order (SWO) for DMEPOS item, which is completed, signed, and dated by the patient's physician
- Signed beneficiary notice of noncoverage if medical necessity for an item cannot be established

DMEPOS Claims

Providers, suppliers, and vendors submit claims to DME MACs to request reimbursement for services and supplies provided to Medicare patients.

 NOTE:

CMS discontinued the submission of certificate of medical necessity (CMN) and DME information form (DIF) documents, which were previously attached to DMEPOS claims. Improvements in claims processing and medical records management led to their discontinuation because the information was found either on the claim or documented in the medical record. The CMN and DIF originally documented medical necessity and other coverage criteria for selected DMEPOS items. Discontinuing the documents reduces administrative burdens, modernizes processes to ensure a reduction in improper payments, and increases customer satisfaction.

DME MAC medical review policies include **local coverage determinations (LCDs)** and **national coverage determinations (NCDs)**, both of which define coverage criteria, payment rules, and documentation required as applied to DMEPOS claims processed by DME MACs for frequently ordered DMEPOS equipment, services, and supplies. (National policies are included in the *Medicare Benefit Policy Manual, Medicare Program Integrity Manual*, and *Medicare National Coverage Determinations Manual*.) If DMEPOS equipment, services, or supplies do not have medical review policies established for coverage, the general coverage criteria apply. The DMEPOS equipment, services, or supplies must

- Fall within a benefit category
- Not be excluded by statute or by national CMS policy
- Be reasonable and necessary to diagnose and/or treat an illness or injury or to improve the functioning of a malformed body

DME MACs are required to follow national CMS policy when it exists; when there is no national CMS policy on a subject, DME MACs have the authority and responsibility to establish local policies. Because many DMEPOS dealers operate nationally, the CMS requires that medical review policies published by the DME MACs be identical in all four regions.

Exercise 8.4 – Determining Payer Responsibility

Instructions: Complete each statement below.

1. The specific HCPCS Level II _____ determines whether the claim is sent to the primary MAC that processes provider claims or the DME MAC that processes DMEPOS dealer claims.

2. Providers and DMEPOS dealers obtain annual lists of valid HCPCS Level II codes, which include _____ instructions for services.

3. CMS decided to have all DME claims processed by only four DME MACs to reduce _____ claims.

4. When a physician treats a Medicare patient for a fractured femur and supplies the patient with crutches, two claims are generated. The physician's claim for the fracture care, which is the professional service, is sent to the primary MAC. The claim for the supply of crutches is sent to the durable medical equipment MAC, which is abbreviated as the _____ MAC.

5. Providers, suppliers, and vendors submit _____ to DME MACs to obtain reimbursement for services and supplies provided to Medicare patients.

Summary

Three levels of codes are associated with HCPCS, commonly referred to as HCPCS Level I, II, and III codes. HCPCS Level I includes the five-character Current Procedural Terminology (CPT) codes developed and published by the American Medical Association (AMA). HCPCS Level II codes (or HCPCS national codes) were created in 1983 to describe common medical services and supplies not classified in CPT. (Effective December 31, 2003, HCPCS Level III local codes were no longer required; however, some third-party payers continue to use them.)

The HCPCS Level II coding system includes codes for similar medical products and services and facilitates efficient claims processing. Each code contains a description, and the codes are used primarily for billing purposes. The codes describe DME devices, accessories, supplies, and repairs; prosthetics; orthotics; medical and surgical supplies; medications; provider services; temporary Medicare codes (e.g., Q codes); and other items and services (e.g., ambulance services). Some services must be reported by assigning both a CPT and an HCPCS Level II code. The most common scenario uses the CPT code for the administration of an injection and the HCPCS code to identify the medication.

The specific HCPCS Level II code determines whether the claim is sent to the primary Medicare administrative contractor (MAC) that processes provider claims or the DME MAC that processes DMEPOS dealer claims. Providers and DMEPOS dealers obtain annual lists of valid HCPCS Level II codes, which include billing instructions for services.

Internet Links

CMS Online Manual System: Go to **www.cms.gov** and click on the Regulations & Guidance link, then click on the Manuals link below the Guidance heading.

HCPCS coding system: Go to **www.cms.gov** and click on the Medicare link, then scroll down to the Coding heading, and click on the HCPCS – General Information link.

Noridian Medicare Durable Medical Equipment: Go to **med.noridianmedicare.com** and click on the Durable Medical Equipment, Orthotics and Supplies link below the Jurisdiction A or Jurisdiction D heading.

Review

8.1 – Multiple Choice

Instructions: Select the most appropriate response.

1. Which would be assigned to report DMEPOS charges on insurance claims?
   - **a.** CPT codes
   - **b.** HCPCS Level I codes
   - **c.** HCPCS Level II codes
   - **d.** HCPCS Level III codes

2. Which provides suppliers and manufacturers with assistance in determining HCPCS Level II codes to be reported?
   - **a.** AMA
   - **b.** DME MAC
   - **c.** DMEPOS
   - **d.** PDAC

3. Which HCPCS Level II temporary codes can be reported to all payers?
   - **a.** G codes and Q codes
   - **b.** H codes and K codes
   - **c.** H codes, S codes, and T codes
   - **d.** S codes and T codes

4. Which is an example of assigning both CPT and HCPCS Level II codes to report a service?
   - **a.** administration of intramuscular injection and medication administered
   - **b.** ambulance and transportation services for emergency purposes
   - **c.** medical and surgical supplies provided in the physician office setting
   - **d.** miscellaneous services performed for investigational purposes

5. Which are HCPCS Level II codes reported to generate transitional pass-through payments under the Outpatient Prospective Payment System?
   - **a.** C codes
   - **b.** G codes
   - **c.** Q codes
   - **d.** S codes

6. HCPCS Level II orthotic procedures and devices and prosthetic procedures include "addition" codes that are reported
   - **a.** in addition to base codes from the same subsection or a previous subsection.
   - **b.** instead of other codes in the same HCPCS Level II section.
   - **c.** using HCPCS Level II modifiers to clarify the code description.
   - **d.** with CPT codes from a similar section in that coding manual.

7. HCPCS Level II modifiers
   - **a.** contain alphanumeric characters only.
   - **b.** contain numeric characters only.
   - **c.** may also be added to CPT codes.
   - **d.** modify HCPCS Level II codes only.

8. Which processes claims for providers?
   - **a.** DME MAC
   - **b.** DMEPOS dealer
   - **c.** DMERC
   - **d.** primary MAC

9. Which processes claims for DMEPOS dealers?
   - **a.** DME MAC
   - **b.** LMC
   - **c.** primary MAC
   - **d.** SADMERC

10. Which is submitted when Medicare requires proof of medical necessity for a submitted DMEPOS claim?
    a. advance beneficiary notice signed by the patient
    b. certificate of medical necessity
    c. DME information form
    d. medical record documentation

11. A patient was supplied with an air pressure mattress. Report code _____.
    a. E0181   b. E0184   c. E0185   d. E0186

12. Magnetic resonance imaging without contrast followed by with contrast, left breast. Report code _____.
    a. C8903 LT   b. C8905 LT   c. C8906 LT   d. C8908 LT

13. A patient received an injection of hydrocortisone acetate, 15 mg, for contact dermatitis. Report code(s) _____.
    a. J1700   c. J1720
    b. J1700, J1700   d. J1720, J1720

14. A patient received a gradient compression stocking, full length/chap style 30–40 mmHg. Report code _____.
    a. A6531   b. A6534   c. A6537   d. A6539

15. A patient required catheterization for the collection of a specimen. Report code _____.
    a. A4300   b. A4305   c. P9612   d. P9615

16. A patient received 2 mg IM injection of leuprolide acetate for treatment of prostate cancer. Report code(s) _____.
    a. J1950   b. J9217   c. J9218, J9218   d. J9219

17. A patient received behavioral health supportive treatment in the form of drug services, including methadone administration by a licensed physician. Report code _____.
    a. H0020   b. H0029   c. H0033   d. J1230

18. An eight-year-old boy is fitted with a long-arm plaster cast. Service is performed in part by a resident under the direction of a teaching physician. Report code _____.
    a. Q4007   b. Q4007 GC   c. Q4008 GC   d. Q4010

19. The patient's family received 30 minutes of family training and counseling, which was provided for the purpose of child development. Report code(s) _____.
    a. T1025   c. T1027
    b. T1026   d. T1027, T1027

20. A patient received a hand-held low-vision aid. Report code _____.
    a. V2020   b. V2510   c. V2600   d. V2610

8.2 – Coding Practice I

Instructions: Assign HCPCS Level II code(s) to each statement.

8.2A – Transport Services Including Ambulance (A0000–A0999)

_____ 1. Ambulance transport of patient from physician's office to hospital emergency department, including advanced life support, level 2.

_____ 2. Ambulance transport of newborn from rural hospital to a children's specialty hospital.

_____ 3. Patient received basic life support (BLS) during emergency transport from the patient's home to the hospital via ambulance.

_____   4. Patient received life-sustaining oxygen in an ambulance during transport to the hospital from a skilled nursing facility.

_____   5. Patient transported in wheelchair van from residential assisted living facility to physician's office.

8.2B – Medical and Surgical Supplies (A2000–A9999)

_____   1. RN swabbed the patient's upper torso with one pint of pHisoHex solution in preparation for an office procedure.

_____   2. Physician inserted a cervical cap for contraceptive use.

_____   3. Patient purchased a brand-new replacement adapter for breast pump from a local DMEPOS dealer.

_____   4. Patient was supplied with a sterile eye pad.

_____   5. Patient was administered a 2-millicurie I-131 sodium iodide capsule as the radiopharmaceutical diagnostic agent prior to a diagnostic radiology procedure.

8.2C – Enteral and Parenteral Therapy (B4000–B9999)

_____   1. Patient was provided with parenteral nutrition administration kits for two days of care.

_____   2. Patient received 1 unit of nutritionally incomplete/modular nutrients enteral formula via enteral feeding tube.

_____   3. A new enteral infusion pump with alarm was attached to the patient's enteral feeding tube system.

_____   4. Patient was provided with a new gravity-fed enteral feeding supply kit, one day.

_____   5. A Levine-type stomach tube was used during the procedure.

8.2D – Outpatient PPS (C1000–C9999)

_____   1. One brachytherapy source of high-dose-rate Iridium-192 was inserted into the patient by the radiation oncologist.

_____   2. A cardiac event recorder was implanted in the patient as a medically necessary service/supply.

_____   3. Implantable breast prosthesis was provided during surgery.

_____   4. Patient underwent MRA, abdomen.

_____   5. A short-term hemodialysis catheter was inserted in the patient's right forearm (patient is left-handed).

8.2E – Durable Medical Equipment (E0100–E9999)

_____   1. "Patient helper" trapeze bars and a grab bar were attached to the patient's bed.

_____   2. An adult oxygen tent was supplied to the patient.

_____   3. A bilirubin light with photometer was used to treat the patient.

_____   4. Provider reported a dispensing fee for use of a DME nebulizer with compressor (covered drug).

_____   5. Patient purchased a new folding walker, which has adjustable and fixed-height features.

8.2F – Procedures/Professional Services (Temporary) (G0000–G9999)

_____ 1. A complete CBC, automated, was performed.

_____ 2. Trimming of five dystrophic nails.

_____ 3. Patient received 20 minutes of individual smoking cessation counseling as part of a demonstration project.

_____ 4. Patient underwent colorectal cancer screening via flexible sigmoidoscopy.

_____ 5. Patient underwent full positron emission tomography (PET) imaging for initial diagnosis of breast cancer.

8-2G – Alcohol and Drug Abuse Treatment Services (H0001–H9999)

_____ 1. Patient received 30 minutes of behavioral health counseling and therapy as provided through an employee assistance program.

_____ 2. Patient received 18 hours of partial hospitalization care for mental health crisis.

_____ 3. One day of psychiatric/behavioral health care facility services was provided to the patient.

_____ 4. Three days of respite care services were provided to the patient in the hospice unit of the hospital.

_____ 5. Patient received 30 minutes of activity therapy delivered as part of outpatient physical therapy plan of care.

8.2H – J Codes Drugs (J0100–J8500) and J Codes Chemotherapy Drugs (J8501–J9999)

_____ 1. Injection, caffeine citrate, 5 mg.

_____ 2. Injection, gamma globulin, intramuscular, 1 cc.

_____ 3. Injection, paricalcitol, 1 mcg.

_____ 4. Injection, torsemide, 10 mg/mL.

_____ 5. Injection, doxorubicin HCl, 10 mg.

8.2I – Temporary Codes (K0000–K9999)

_____ 1. Repair service of 10-year-old DMEPOS device required supply of complete front caster assembly for wheelchair with two semipneumatic tires.

_____ 2. Patient was supplied with one IV hanger.

_____ 3. Patient was supplied with two leg straps for use with wheelchair.

_____ 4. Patient rented a prescribed lightweight portable motorized wheelchair.

_____ 5. A replacement alkaline battery, 1.5 volt, was provided for the patient-owned external infusion pump.

8.2J – Orthotic Procedures and Devices (L0000–L4999)

_____ 1. Patient was provided with a cervical wire frame, semirigid, for occipital/mandibular support.

_____ 2. Patient purchased a prescribed custom-fabricated thoracic rib belt.

_____ 3. Patient underwent halo procedure (cervical halo incorporated into Milwaukee orthosis).

_____ 4. Patient purchased a prescribed 2-inch neoprene heel and sole elevation lift.

_____ 5. Patient was supplied with an Orthomerica plastic foot drop brace, which is an ankle-foot orthosis (AFO), posterior solid ankle, plastic, custom fabricated.

8.2K – Prosthetic Procedures (L5000–L9999)

_____ 1. Patient was fitted with a knee disarticulation prosthesis that contained a molded socket, external knee joint, shin, and solid ankle cushion heel (SACH) foot.

_____ 2. Patient (adult) was fitted with an Otto Bock electric hand, myoelectrically controlled.

_____ 3. Patient was fitted with a partial foot prosthesis that contained a shoe insert with longitudinal arch, toe filler.

_____ 4. Patient was provided with an Offobock cosmetic glove (for terminal device), hand prosthesis.

_____ 5. During breast reconstruction surgery, a silicone breast prosthesis was inserted.

8.2L – MIPS Value Pathways (M0001-M0005), Medical Services (M0075–M0301), and Quality Measures (M1003–M1149)

_____ 1. Promoting wellness MIPS value pathways.

_____ 2. Cellular therapy.

_____ 3. Chemical endarterectomy via intravenous (IV) chelation therapy.

_____ 4. Fabric wrapping of abdominal aneurysm.

_____ 5. Prolotherapy.

8.2M – Pathology and Laboratory Services (P0000–P9999)

_____ 1. Catheterization for collection of specimen was performed for one patient.

_____ 2. Screening Pap smear, cervical, by technician under physician supervision.

_____ 3. Infusion of 250 mL of 5% albumin (human).

_____ 4. Two units of platelets were infused.

_____ 5. Two units of whole blood were used during transfusion.

8.2N – Q Codes (Temporary) (Q0000–Q9999)

_____ 1. Patient received chemotherapy administration, push technique (hospital reporting).

_____ 2. Patient underwent a collagen skin test.

_____ 3. Patient injected with 50 mg of teniposide.

_____ 4. As part of fracture treatment, 10-year-old patient received short-arm plaster splint.

_____ 5. Potassium hydroxide (KOH) preparation included as part of patient's treatment.

8.2O – Diagnostic Radiology Services (R0000–R9999)

_____ 1. Transportation of portable chest x-ray and radiology technician to nursing home; 20 patients underwent x-rays.

_____ 2. Transportation of portable EKG equipment to nursing facility; one patient underwent EKG.

_____ 3. Transportation of portable x-ray equipment and radiology technician to patients' home; husband and wife underwent x-rays.

_____ 4. Transportation of portable x-ray equipment and radiology technician to a patient's home; one patient underwent x-ray.

_____ 5. Transportation of portable x-ray equipment and radiology technician to boarding home; five patients underwent x-rays.

8.2P – Temporary National Codes (Non-Medicare) (S0000–S9999)

_____ 1. Allogenic cord blood-derived stem cell transplantation.

_____ 2. Echosclerotherapy.

_____ 3. Gastrointestinal fat absorption study.

_____ 4. Global fee for extracorporeal shock wave lithotripsy (ESWL) treatment of kidney stone.

_____ 5. Harvesting of multivisceral organs from cadaver donor with preparation and maintenance of allografts.

8.2Q – National T Codes Established for State Medicaid Agencies (T1000–T9999)

_____ 1. Patient underwent 15 minutes of family training and counseling for child development.

_____ 2. Human breast milk processing, storage, and distribution.

_____ 3. Intramuscular medication administration by home health licensed practical nurse (LPN).

_____ 4. Patient received 30 minutes of private-duty nursing from a registered nurse (RN).

_____ 5. Waiver of utility services to support medical equipment and assistive technology/devices.

8.2R – Coronavirus Services (U0001–U0002)

_____ 1. Patient underwent CDC 2019 novel coronavirus real-time RT-PCR diagnostic panel laboratory test.

_____ 2. Patient underwent 2019-nCoV Coronavirus, SARS-CoV-2/2019-nCoV (COVID-19), any technique, multiple types or subtypes (includes all targets), non-CDC [test].

8.2S – Vision Services (V0000–V2999)

_____ 1. Bifocal lenses, bilateral, 5.25 sphere, 2.12 cylinder, two lenses.

_____ 2. Deluxe frame.

_____ 3. Photochromatic tinting of two lenses.

_____ 4. Processing, preserving, and transporting corneal tissue.

_____ 5. Reduction of ocular prosthesis.

8.2T – Hearing Services (V5000–V5999)

_____ 1. Patient underwent repair of a hearing aid.

_____ 2. Provision of binaural, behind-the-ear hearing aid.

_____ 3. Provision of digitally programmable monaural hearing aid, analog, in the canal (ITC).

_____ 4. Dispensing fee, binaural contralateral routing of signals (BICROS).

_____ 5. Patient purchased prescribed telephone amplifier assistive listening device.

Part

VII

Current Procedural Terminology (CPT) Coding System

Introduction to CPT Coding

Chapter Outline

History of CPT

Overview of CPT

Organization of CPT

CPT Index

CPT Appendices

CPT Symbols

CPT Sections, Subsections, Categories, and Subcategories

CPT Modifiers

National Correct Coding Initiative (NCCI)

Chapter Objectives

At the conclusion of this chapter, the student should be able to:

1. Define key terms related to the introduction of CPT coding.
2. Identify key dates and events in the history of CPT.
3. Provide an overview about CPT.
4. Explain the organization of CPT.
5. Apply CPT index rules and conventions to identify main terms, subterms, cross-references, and code ranges.
6. Describe the types of codes included in each of the CPT appendices.
7. Interpret CPT symbols.
8. Summarize the contents of CPT sections, subsections, categories, and subcategories.
9. Add CPT modifiers to codes.
10. Describe how the National Correct Coding Initiative impacts CPT code assignment.

Key Terms

add-on code	CPT instructional notes	+	⊃
category I code	CPT symbols	⊘	★
category II code	●	⁄	◀
category III code	▲	#	⋈
CPT appendices	▶◀	⊃	↑↓
	;	⊃	descriptive qualifier

functional modifier	National Correct Coding Initiative (NCCI) program	payment modifier	statistical modifier
guidelines		pricing modifier	telemedicine
inferred words		range of codes	unlisted procedure
informational modifier	Notice of Exclusions from Medicare Benefits (NEMB)	single code	unlisted service
		special report	

Introduction

This chapter introduces the *Current Procedural Terminology* (CPT) coding system (or HCPCS Level I), a proprietary coding system published annually by the American Medical Association (AMA). (Exceptions to the January 1 annual release of CPT codes include (1) Medicine section vaccine product codes that are also released on July 1, and (2) category II codes that are released three times each year.) CPT contains a list of codes and descriptions for reporting outpatient procedures and services on claims. For *professional billing*, CPT codes are assigned to inpatient hospital professional services and procedures provided by physicians and other qualified health care professionals. For *institutional billing*, ICD-10-PCS codes are assigned to inpatient hospital services and procedures provided by the hospital. (ICD-10-CM codes are assigned to all diagnoses and conditions in all health care settings.)

 NOTE:

When reviewing examples and completing exercises and review questions in this chapter (and in Chapters 11–19), use your CPT coding manual to locate index entries and to verify codes in the appropriate section.

History of CPT

The AMA first published CPT in 1966, and subsequent editions expanded its descriptive terms and codes for diagnostic and therapeutic procedures. Five-digit codes were introduced in 1970, replacing the four-digit classification. In 1983, CPT was adopted as part of the Healthcare Common Procedure Coding System (HCPCS) (as HCPCS Level I) and its use was mandated for reporting Medicare Part B physician services. In 1986, HCPCS was required for reporting to Medicaid agencies, and the Omnibus Budget Reconciliation Act (OBRA) of 1986 mandated that CPT codes be reported for Medicare outpatient hospital surgical procedures. Today, CPT contains five-character codes.

The Health Insurance Portability and Accountability Act of 1996 (HIPAA) named CPT and HCPCS Level II as the procedure code sets for physician services, physical and occupational therapy services, radiological procedures, clinical laboratory tests, other medical diagnostic procedures, hearing and vision services, and transportation services including ambulance. (Also named are ICD-10-CM as the code set for all diagnoses, ICD-10-PCS for inpatient procedures, CDT for dental services, and NDC for drugs.) (HCPCS Level III local codes were eliminated effective December 2003; however, some private health insurance companies continue to use the codes.)

CMS enforced regulations resulting from the Medicare Prescription Drug, Improvement, and Modernization Act (MMA) in October 2004, which required that new, revised, and deleted CPT codes be implemented each January 1 (with CPT vaccine codes also released on July 1). (Molecular Pathology Tier 2 Administrative MAAA and PLA codes are released quarterly at the AMA CPT public website.) It is important to purchase updated coding manuals to avoid billing delays and claims rejections. If outdated codes are submitted on claims, providers and health care facilities will incur administrative costs associated with resubmitting corrected claims and delayed reimbursement for services provided.

Exercise 9.1 – History of CPT

Instructions: Complete each statement by entering the appropriate year.

1. The AMA first published CPT in the year _____, and subsequent editions expanded its descriptive terms and codes for diagnostic and therapeutic procedures.

2. Five-digit CPT codes were introduced in the year _____, replacing the four-digit classification.

3. CPT was adopted as part of the Healthcare Common Procedure Coding System (HCPCS) (as HCPCS Level I) in the year _____, and its use was mandated for reporting Medicare Part B physician services.

4. HCPCS was required for reporting to Medicaid agencies in the year _____ as a result of the Omnibus Budget Reconciliation Act (OBRA), which mandated that CPT codes be reported for outpatient hospital surgical procedures.

5. CMS enforced regulations resulting from the Medicare Prescription Drug, Improvement, and Modernization Act (MMA) in October _____, which required that new, revised, and deleted CPT codes be implemented each January 1.

Overview of CPT

CPT codes are used to report services and procedures performed on patients by physicians and other qualified health care professionals (e.g., nurse practitioner, physician assistant). CPT codes and descriptions are based on consistency with contemporary medical practice as performed by clinical providers throughout the country. The assignment of CPT codes simplifies reporting and assists in the accurate identification of procedures and services for third-party payer consideration. For *medical necessity* purposes, which requires justifying procedures and services provided to patients, ICD-10-CM code(s) are linked to CPT (and HCPCS Level II) codes reported on claims. When reporting CPT codes, some procedures and services are considered integral to the standard of practice, which means they are not assigned separate CPT codes.

> **Example:** The patient underwent an office procedure to remove a suspicious lesion, and the physician cleansed and prepped the skin prior to performing the procedure. A CPT code for excision of the lesion is reported; however, codes for cleansing and prepping skin are *not* reported because those services are integral to the excision procedure.

CPT Categories

CPT is compatible with electronic data interchange (EDI), the electronic health record (EHR), and reference/research databases. CPT is also used to track new technology and performance measures.

There are three categories of CPT codes.

- **Category I codes**: Procedures and services identified by five-character CPT codes and descriptions, which are traditionally associated with CPT and organized into six sections. Each section contains subsections and anatomic, procedural, condition, or descriptor categories and subcategories. Codes are presented in numerical order except for the Evaluation and Management (E/M) section, which appears as the first section because they are used by most physicians to report services. E/M codes are organized into categories and subcategories (instead of subsections and categories). Alphanumeric proprietary laboratory analyses (PLA) codes located in the Pathology and Laboratory section are covered in textbook Chapter 18.

- **Category II codes**: Optional "performance measurements" tracking codes are assigned an alphanumeric identifier with a letter in the last field. These codes are located after the Medicine section and eliminate the need to abstract patient records for the purpose of identifying services that impact positive health care outcomes and high-quality patient care.

> **Example:** A physician counsels a patient who smokes during an evaluation and management (E/M) service. Report CPT category II code 4000F (tobacco use cessation intervention, counseling). If the physician also prescribes a smoking cessation medication, report code 4001F (tobacco use cessation intervention, pharmacologic therapy). (CPT category II codes are reported in addition to the CPT E/M service and other procedure and service codes.)

- **Category III codes**: "Emerging technology" temporary codes are assigned an alphanumeric identifier with a letter in the last field. These codes are located after the category II codes and are reported until a permanent code is included in category I of CPT. If not accepted for placement within a category I section of CPT, the codes are archived after five years. Modifiers are reported with category III codes.

> **Example:** Prior to 2005, category III code 0012T was reported for a surgical arthroscopy of the knee with osteochondral autograft(s). In 2005, code 0012T was deleted and category I code 29866 was created with a description of "arthroscopy, knee, surgical; osteochondral autograft(s) (eg mosaicplasty) (including harvesting of the autograft[s])."

CPT "Early Release" Codes

The CPT Editorial Panel also approves the early release of new CPT codes. All changes provided as an early release take effect on the implementation date, which is six months after the early release of the codes. This means that codes included in an early release in January are implemented for use in July (and codes included in an early release in July are implemented the following January). To assist users in reporting the most recently approved codes, the AMA's CPT website will feature updates of the CPT Editorial Panel's actions and early release of the codes in July and January during a given CPT cycle. These dates for early release correspond with the CPT Editorial Panel's meetings for each CPT cycle.

Exercise 9.2 – Overview of CPT

Instructions: Complete each statement.

1. CPT codes and descriptions are based on consistency with contemporary medical practice as performed by clinical _____ (e.g., physicians) throughout the United States.
2. The assignment of CPT codes simplifies reporting and assists in the accurate identification of procedures and services for third-party _____ consideration.
3. CPT codes for procedures and services that are reported on a claim must be linked to the ICD-10-CM code that justifies the need for the service or procedure, which demonstrates medical _____ for the service or procedure provided.
4. Optional "performance measurements" tracking codes are assigned an alphanumeric identifier with a letter in the last field, and they are considered CPT category _____ codes.
5. Emerging technology temporary codes are assigned for data collection purposes, contain an alphanumeric identifier with a letter in the last field, and are considered CPT category _____ codes.

Organization of CPT

To accurately assign codes, it is necessary to become familiar with CPT's organizational characteristics.

- CPT categories and sections
- CPT code format
- Boldfaced type
- Italicized type
- Cross-reference term
- Single codes and code ranges
- Inferred words
- Guidelines
- Unlisted procedures and services
- Notes
- Descriptive qualifiers

CPT Category I Codes

CPT organizes category I procedures and services into six sections.

- Evaluation and Management (E/M)
- Anesthesia
- Surgery
- Radiology (including Nuclear Medicine and Diagnostic Ultrasound)
- Pathology and Laboratory
- Medicine

 NOTE:

- The E/M section is located at the beginning of CPT because these codes are reported by all specialties.
- Medicine section codes classify qualifying circumstances for anesthesia and are reported with Anesthesia section codes.

CPT Category II Codes

CPT category II codes are supplemental tracking codes used for performance measurement. Category II codes are assigned for certain services or tests results, which support nationally established performance measures that have proven to contribute to quality patient care. They are alphanumeric and consist of four digits followed by the alpha character F. Reporting the codes is optional and not a substitute for the assignment of CPT category I codes. When reporting a category II code on the CMS-1500 claim, the submitted charge is zero ($0.00). (When medical practice management software does not allow a $0.00 line-item charge, enter $0.01 instead. The beneficiary is *not* liable for this nominal amount.) CPT category II codes are arranged according to the following categories:

- Modifiers, reported with CPT category II codes only
- Composite codes
- Patient management
- Patient history
- Physical examination
- Diagnostic/screening processes or results
- Therapeutic, preventive, or other interventions
- Follow-up or other outcomes
- Patient safety
- Structural measures
- Nonmeasure code listing

The purpose of reporting category II codes is to facilitate the collection of information about the quality of patient care (e.g., appropriate services provided to patients based on diagnosis). The use of category II is expected to decrease the time required for patient record abstracting and review, thus minimizing the administrative burden on health care providers for tracking patient care quality.

> **Example:** Dr. Ryan is a dermatologist who is participating in a nationwide quality management study about malignant melanoma. CPT category II code 0015F is reported for each patient who receives melanoma follow-up services, which include obtaining a history about new or changing moles (code 1050F), performing a complete physical skin examination (code 2029F), and providing patient counseling to perform a monthly skin self-examination (code 5005F).
>
> Thus, codes 0015F, 1050F, 2029F, and 5005F are reported on the CMS-1500 claim, and the charge for each is zero ($0.00) unless medical practice management software requires entry of a nominal amount, such as $0.01 (for which the patient is *not* responsible). In addition, reason for encounter ICD-10-CM code(s) and CPT category I service/procedure code(s) are reported on the same CMS-1500 claim with appropriate charges entered for each CPT category I code.

NOTE:

Some payers deny claims that contain CPT category II codes. Providers can save category II codes as part of a spreadsheet or database for internal data capture purposes.

CPT Category III Codes

CPT category III codes are temporary codes used to report emerging technology, procedures, and services. The codes facilitate data collection on and assessment of new services and procedures during the FDA approval process or to confirm that a procedure/service is generally provided. According to the CPT coding manual, the "procedure or service is currently or recently performed on humans; and at least one additional criterion (listed in the CPT coding manual) has been met." CPT category III codes are alphanumeric and consist of four digits followed by the alpha character T. CMS designates certain CPT category III codes as covered by Medicare, which means charges are entered when reporting the codes on a CMS-1500 claim.

In the past, researchers were hindered by the length and requirements of the CPT approval process. Thus, CPT category III (temporary) codes were initially released in July 2001 to facilitate the reporting of emerging technology, procedures, and services. They are retired if the emerging technology, procedure, or service is not assigned a CPT category I code within five years. When a category III code is available, it must be reported instead of an unlisted CPT category I code (because reporting an unlisted code does not offer the opportunity for collection of specific data). Category III codes are included as a separate section in CPT (following the category II codes). (HCPCS Level II codes also describe emerging technology, procedures, and services; when an HCPCS Level II code exists, it must be reported for Medicare claims.)

> **Example:** Patient underwent bilateral retinal polarization scan for ocular screening. Results were automated on-site at the provider's office. Report code 0469T. *The code description states, "Sunset January 2028," which means if a permanent code for this procedure is not added as a CPT category I code, it will be deleted.*

CPT Code Format

A five-character code and a narrative description identify each procedure and service listed in CPT. Most procedures and services contain stand-alone descriptions. To save space, some descriptions are not printed in their entirety next to a code number. Instead, the entry is indented and the coder must refer back to the common portion of the code description (or "parent code") that is located before the semicolon. *Indented codes* (or "children codes") are located below the "parent code" description.

Example 1: Locate CPT code 27870 in the coding manual, which has a stand-alone code description.

Example 2: Locate CPT code 27780 in the coding manual, which contains a semicolon in its description. Then, locate code 27781, which has an indented format. The portion of the code description before the semicolon also applies to code 27781, which includes *with manipulation* in its description.

Exercise 9.3 – Organization of CPT

Instructions: Complete each statement.

1. CPT organizes category I procedures and services into six _____.
2. The Evaluation and Management section of CPT is located at the beginning of CPT because these codes are reported by all _____ of physicians.
3. Refer to CPT code 55605. Its code description is _____.
4. The CPT category II code reported for a chronic obstructive pulmonary disease (COPD) patient's status as a *current tobacco smoker* is _____.
5. The CPT category III code reported for a *bilateral optical coherence tomography (OCT), middle ear, with interpretation and report* is _____.

CPT Index

The CPT index is organized by alphabetical main terms and subterms, which contain single codes, ranges of codes, or codes separated by commas.

Example: Locate main term Nasal *Polyp* in the CPT index and its cross-referenced term, which directs the coder to see main term *Nose, Polyp* in the index.

Next, locate main term *Nails* and subterm *Avulsion*, which contains a range of codes to investigate.

Then, locate subterm *Debridement*, which contains multiple codes (separated by a comma) to investigate.

Finally, locate subterm *Evaluation* and its indented subterm *Hematoma, Subungual*, which has one code to verify.

Main Terms and Subterms

The CPT index is organized according to *main terms*, which can stand alone or be followed by modifying terms called *subterms*. Main terms can represent:

- Procedure or service (e.g., arthroscopy)
- Organ or other anatomical site (e.g., ankle)
- Condition (e.g., wound)
- Synonyms (e.g., finger joint or intercarpal joint)
- Eponyms (e.g., Billroth I or II)
- Abbreviations (e.g., EKG)

The Anesthesia main term contains subterms for Anesthesia section codes, and the Surgery, Medicine, category II, and category III sections also index anesthesia services according to anatomical site.

To locate a CPT code, review patient record documentation to locate the service and/or procedure performed and locate the main term in the index (located in the back of the coding manual). Main terms are modified by *subterms* that are *not* indented. (Indented subterms further modify subterms that are not indented.)

Example: For the procedure "surgical temporomandibular joint (TMJ) arthroscopy," refer to the CPT index and locate main term *Temporomandibular Joint (TMJ)* and subterms *Arthroscopy* and *Surgical* 29804. Next, verify code 29804 in the coding manual before reporting it on a claim for submission to a third-party payer. (A diagnosis code must be reported on the claim to justify medical necessity of the procedure.)

 Coding Tip

The descriptions of all codes listed in the index must be carefully investigated before selecting a final code. CPT coding must never be performed solely from the index.

Boldfaced Type

Main terms in the CPT index are printed in boldfaced type. CPT category and subcategory titles and code numbers are also printed in boldfaced type.

Italicized Type

Italicized type is used for the cross-reference terms *See* and *See also* in the CPT index.

Cross-Reference Term

See and *See also* are cross-reference terms that direct coders to an index entry under which codes are listed. No codes are listed under the original entry.

Example: CPT index cross-reference term *See* provides direction to index main term "Arteriovenous Shunt" because no codes are listed for the main term *AV Shunt*.

CPT index cross-reference term *See also* provides direction to index main term "Catheter" where additional codes are listed, which can also be located in the CPT coding manual.

Single Codes and Code Ranges

Index entries for procedures and services may be represented as a **single code**, a **range of codes** separated by a hyphen, a series of codes separated by commas, or a combination of single codes and ranges of codes. All codes listed after a main term and subterms should be reviewed before assigning a code for the procedure or service.

Example: CPT index main term *Acid fast stain* contains just one code.

Subterm *esophagus*, located below main term *Acid perfusion test*, contains two codes separated by commas.

Main term *Acid Reflux* Test contains a range of codes.

Review all codes separated by commas or hyphens in the CPT coding manual to select the most appropriate code.

Inferred Words

To save space in the CPT index when referencing subterms, **inferred words** are used.

Example: The word "of" is inferred and does not actually appear in the CPT index. Locate CPT main term *Abdomen* and subterm *Exploration*, and notice that inferred word "of" does not appear.

Exercise 9.4 – CPT Index

Instructions: Complete each statement.

1. The CPT index is organized by alphabetical main terms printed in _____.

2. The CPT index main term may be followed by indented terms that modify the main term, which are called _____.

3. Italicized type is used for cross-reference terms _____ and *See also* in the CPT index.

4. When a CPT index entry for a procedure contains a _____ of codes separated by a hyphen or a series of codes separated by commas, all codes should be investigated before assigning a code.

5. To save space in the CPT index when referencing subterms, _____ words are used.

CPT Appendices

The **CPT appendices**, located after CPT category III codes, provide additional guidance for proper code assignment. Insurance specialists should carefully review these appendices to become familiar with coding changes that affect the practice annually. (Appendices C, G, H, and I were removed from CPT.)

- *Appendix A* (Modifiers) contains a list of CPT modifiers and detailed descriptions. Place a marker at the beginning of Appendix A because you will refer to it often.

- *Appendix B* (Summary of Additions, Deletions, and Revisions) contains annual CPT coding changes that include added codes and deleted and revised codes and descriptions. Review Appendix B because it is the basis for updating documents and billing tools (e.g., chargemaster, encounter form).

- *Appendix D* (Summary of CPT Add-on Codes) contains a list of add-on codes that are identified throughout CPT with a + symbol. An **add-on code** is reported when another procedure is performed in addition to the primary procedure during the same operative session and must never be reported as a stand-alone code. (Do not report modifier 50 with add-on codes. For bilateral procedures, the add-on code is reported twice. Do not report modifier 51 with add-on codes because payers have already discounted the payment.)

- *Appendix E* (Summary of CPT Codes Exempt from Modifier 51) contains a list of codes that are exempt from modifier 51 reporting rules and that are identified throughout CPT with a forbidden (⊘) symbol.

- *Appendix F* (Summary of CPT Codes Exempt from Modifier 63) contains a list of codes that are exempt from modifier 63.

- *Appendix J* (Electrodiagnostic Medicine Listing of Sensory, Motor, and Mixed Nerves) aligns each sensory, motor, and mixed nerve with its appropriate nerve conduction study code to ensure accurate reporting. There is also a table that indicates the "type of study and maximum number of studies" generally performed for needle electromyogram (EMG), nerve conduction studies, and other EMG studies. The AMA's *CPT Changes 2006: An Insider's View* calls this table a ". . . tool to detect outliers."

- *Appendix K* (Product Pending FDA Approval) contains a list of products that are pending FDA approval but that have been assigned CPT codes. In the CPT manual, these codes are preceded by the flash symbol (✗).

- *Appendix L* (Vascular Families) contains a list of vascular families that is intended to assist in the selection of first-, second-, third-, and beyond third-order branch arteries.

- *Appendix M* (Renumbered CPT Codes–Citations Crosswalk) contains a summary of crosswalked deleted and renumbered codes and citations from 2007 to 2009. (The AMA discontinued the practice of deleting and renumbering codes in 2010.)

- *Appendix N* (Summary of Resequenced CPT Codes) contains a table of CPT codes that do not appear in numeric order. CPT codes are resequenced (instead of deleted and renumbered) so that existing codes can be relocated to a more appropriate location. In the CPT manual, out-of-sequence codes are preceded by the number symbol (**#**).

- *Appendix O* (Multianalyte Assays with Algorithmic Analyses [MAAA] and Proprietary Laboratory Analyses [PLA]) includes administrative codes for procedures that by their nature are typically unique to a single clinical laboratory or manufacturer and CPT category I codes for MAAA and PLA procedures and services.

- *Appendix P* (CPT Codes That May Be Used For Synchronous Real-Time Interactive Audio-Video Telemedicine Services) are reported for encounters that use real-time interactive telecommunications audio-video equipment. In the CPT manual, these codes are preceded by the star (★) symbol. Modifier 95 is reported with Appendix P codes.

- *Appendix Q* appears in CPT 2024; however, it was deleted in September 2023 (after publication of the coding manual) to simplify the reporting of SARS-CoV-2 and COVID-19 product and immunization administration codes. More than 50 were deleted, while vaccine product code 91304 was retained. Deleted codes were replaced with new product codes 91318-91322 and administration code 90480. (Go to **www.ama-assn.org** to locate additional information about Appendix Q and the new vaccine product and immunization administration code.)

- *Appendix R* (Digital Medicine–Services Taxonomy) contains a list of digital medicine services described in CPT according to discrete categories of clinician-to-patient services (e.g., visit), clinician-to-clinician services (e.g., consultation), patient-monitoring services, and digital diagnostic services; they are differentiated by nature of service (e.g., synchronous versus asynchronous communication).

- *Appendix S* (Artificial Intelligence Taxonomy for Medical Services and Procedures) provides guidance about the description and classification of artificial intelligence (AI) applications.

- *Appendix T* (CPT Codes That May Be Used for Synchronous Real-Time Interactive Audio-Only Telemedicine Services) includes codes that may be reported for audio-only services when appended with modifier 93. In the CPT manual, these codes are preceded by the loudspeaker (◄) symbol.

Telemedicine

Telemedicine provides remote medical care using interactive audio and video telecommunications systems that permit real-time communication between the provider, located at a distant site (e.g., physician's office), and the patient, located at the originating site (e.g., patient's home). It is an alternative to in-person face-to-face encounters, which allows patients to receive health care services for minor medical conditions (instead of going to an emergency room) or for chronic conditions that are well managed, from specialists located in other areas of the country, and when patients cannot leave work to see their provider. The availability of *telemedicine* is the result of advancements in clinical decision making and user friendly technology. It is also seen as an affordable option for patients who have high-deductible health insurance plans.

> **Example:** New York State Department of Health (**www.health.ny.gov**) data about *potentially preventable emergency department encounters* identifies common conditions (e.g., ear and sinus infections, sore throats) that represent millions of annual visits to hospital emergency departments. Such encounters could have been avoided or treated elsewhere if patients had been able to schedule an appointment with their primary care providers. Face-to-face encounters with a physician remains the ideal method for having minor conditions addressed; however, if the patient is unable to obtain an appointment for an immediate office visit, the patient can ask whether the issue could be addressed using telemedicine. This results in: (1) cost savings due to avoiding a potentially preventable emergency department encounter, and (2) treatment by the patient's primary care provider. (The patient would schedule an appointment with the provider for follow-up of the condition treated using telemedicine.)

Exercise 9.5 – CPT Appendices

Instructions: Complete each statement.

1. CPT Appendix A contains a list of CPT two-digit _____ and their detailed descriptions.

2. CPT Appendix B contains a summary of code and description additions, deletions, and revisions, which serve as the basis for _____ (or revising) interoffice documents and billing tools.

3. CPT Appendix D contains a summary of add-on codes that are identified throughout CPT with the _____ symbol, and they are never reported as a stand-alone code.

4. CPT Appendix E contains a summary of CPT Codes exempt from modifier 51, and these codes are identified throughout CPT with the _____ symbol.

5. CPT Appendix P contains CPT codes that may be used for synchronous real-time interactive audio-video telemedicine services, which are preceded by the _____ symbol, requiring modifier 95 to be added to each reported code.

CPT Symbols

CPT symbols are located throughout CPT and provide guidance for proper code assignment.

- A *bullet symbol* located to the left of a code number identifies new procedures and services added to CPT.
- A *triangle symbol* located to the left of a code number identifies a code description that has been revised.
- ►◄ *Horizontal triangle symbols* surround new and revised guidelines and notes. These symbols are *not* used for revised code descriptions.

 NOTE:

Review your CPT coding manual to locate codes preceded by the bullet, triangle, and horizontal triangle symbols.

A complete list of code additions, deletions, and revisions is found in Appendix B of CPT. Revisions marked with horizontal triangles (►◄) are *not* included in Appendix B and require review of all CPT guidelines and notes.

; The *semicolon symbol* is used to save space in CPT; thus, some code descriptions are not printed in their entirety next to a code number. Instead, the entry is indented, and the coder must refer back to the common portion of the code description that is located before the semicolon. The common portion begins with a capital letter, and the abbreviated (or subordinate) descriptions are indented and begin with lowercase letters.

Example: Locate code 20910 in the CPT coding manual, which contains a semicolon in its description, and code 20912, which has an indented format. The portion of the code description before the semicolon also applies to code 20912. For a patient who undergoes costochondral and nasal septum cartilage graft procedures during the same operative session, report codes 20910 and 20912 51. Modifier 51 (Multiple procedures) is added so that the payer discounts reimbursement for that reported code.

 Coding Tip ━━━━

CPT is printed using proportional spacing, and careful review of code descriptions to locate the semicolon may be necessary.

+ The *plus symbol* identifies add-on codes (Appendix D of CPT) for procedures that are commonly, but not always, performed at the same time and by the same surgeon as the primary procedure. Parenthetical notes, located below add-on codes, often identify the primary procedure to which add-on codes apply. Add-on codes are exempt from modifier 51. A complete list of codes that are exempt from modifier 51 is found in Appendix E of the CPT manual.

> **Example:** For a patient who undergoes posterior osteotomy of the spine, two cervical vertebral segments, report codes 22210 and 22216. Upon review of the CPT coding manual, notice that code 22216 contains the plus symbol to its left, identifying it as an add-on code.

 Coding Tip

- Do not report codes identified with + (add-on codes) as stand-alone codes; they must be reported with a primary code.
- Do not add modifier 51 (Multiple procedures) to codes identified with the + symbol because payers discount reimbursement for such add-on codes; adding modifier 51 to codes that have the + symbol incorrectly reduces reimbursement even more.
- Do not report modifier 50 (Bilateral procedures) with add-on codes; instead, report the add-on code twice.

⊘ This *forbidden symbol* identifies codes (Appendix E of CPT) that are exempt from modifier 51. These codes are reported in addition to other codes, but they are not classified as add-on codes.

> **Example:** When code 20974 is reported with other procedures performed during the same encounter, do not add modifier 51 (Multiple procedures) because the forbidden symbol appears before the code.

◀ The *loudspeaker symbol* is used to identify codes that may be reported for *audio-only* telemedicine services when appended with modifier 93.

★ The *star symbol* is used to identify codes that may be reported for *audio-video* telemedicine services when appended with modifier 93.

> **Example:** Patient undergoes psychiatric diagnostic evaluation.
> - For a patient who receives synchronous real-time interactive audio-video telemedicine services, report code 90791 95.
> - For a patient who receives synchronous real-time interactive audio-only telemedicine services, report code 90791 93.
> - The star and audio symbols that appear to the left of the code indicate it is reported for real-time interactive audio-video *or* audio-only telemedicine services.

↗ The *flash symbol* indicates codes that classify products pending FDA approval but have already been assigned a CPT code.

> **Example:** Patient was administered an influenza virus vaccine, pandemic formulation, preservative free, which is pending FDA approval. Report code 90671, which contains the flash symbol in front of it.

The *number symbol* indicates out-of-numerical sequence codes.

> **Example:** Patient underwent excision of 4-cm subcutaneous soft tissue tumor of the neck. Report code 21552, which has the number symbol in front of it.

NOTE:

Prior to 2010, when a new code was added and there was no available code in a "code range," a new range of codes was added to accommodate the new code(s). This meant that all codes in a range were deleted (and added as new codes) for certain procedures even though the procedure text and meaning or applicability of the procedure had not changed. Payers typically interpreted a new range of codes as "new codes" to CPT, resulting in payment denials.

The new policy of creating out-of-numerical sequence codes facilitates historical data analysis, reduces the number of codes that providers must revise (e.g., superbill, encounter form), and eliminates the need for payers to modify related reimbursement policies resulting in reduced claims denials.

Resequenced codes appear "out of sequence" in the print version of CPT, but that means the codes are located with procedures to which they are related. CPT code description content determines placement of out-of-sequence codes.

⊃   The *blue reference symbol* located below a code description in some CPT coding manuals indicates that the coder should refer to the *CPT Changes: An Insider's View* annual publication that contains all coding changes for the current year.

⊃   The *green reference symbol* located below a code description in some CPT coding manuals indicates that the coder should refer to the *CPT Assistant* monthly newsletter.

⊃   The *red reference symbol* located below a code description in some CPT coding manuals indicates that the coder should refer to the *Clinical Examples in Radiology* quarterly newsletter.

> **Example:** CPT code 73501 contains reference symbols below its description, which provide direction to coding guidance references.

⋈   The *inverted parens symbol* identifies duplicate proprietary laboratory analyses (PLA) tests. PLA codes are included in Appendix O, and they contain the proprietary name of the procedure. Descriptor language of some PLA codes are identical, and codes are differentiated only by listed proprietary names in Appendix O.

⇅   The *double arrow symbol* is used to identify PLA codes that fulfill CPT Category I criteria (e.g., reportable for third-party payer reimbursement).

Exercise 9.6 – CPT Symbols

Instructions: Complete each statement.

1. The bullet symbol located to the left of a code number identifies _____ procedures and services added to CPT.

2. Horizontal triangle symbols surround _____ guidelines and notes.

3. To save space in CPT, instead of printing code descriptions in their entirety next to a code, the entry is indented and the common portion of the code description is located before the
_____.

4. Codes that classify products pending FDA approval (e.g., vaccines) but that have been assigned a CPT code are indicated by the _____ symbol.

5. Out-of-numerical sequence CPT codes are indicated by the _____ symbol.

CPT Sections, Subsections, Categories, and Subcategories

CPT Category I codes are organized according to six sections that are subdivided into subsections, categories, subcategories headings, and subheadings. Each section contains guidelines, instructional notes, and descriptive qualifiers.

NOTE:

CPT E/M section guidelines refer to categories and subcategories (instead of subsections and categories). Many years ago, the E/M section was a subsection of the Medicine section. When the codes were relocated to the beginning of the CPT coding manual for easy reference, the E/M section was created. The category and subcategory terminology associated with the E/M codes was retained.

CPT Guidelines

Guidelines located at the beginning of each CPT section *should be carefully reviewed before assigning a code* because they define terms and explain the assignment of codes for procedures and services in that section. This means that guidelines in one section do not apply to another section in CPT.

Unlisted Procedures and Services

An **unlisted procedure** or **unlisted service** code is assigned when the provider performs a procedure or provides a service for which there is no CPT code. When an unlisted procedure or service code is reported, a **special report** (e.g., copy of the procedure report) must accompany the claim to describe the nature, extent, and need for the procedure or service along with the time, effort, and equipment necessary to provide the procedure or service.

NOTE:

- Do not add a modifier to CPT unlisted procedure/service codes because they do not include specific descriptions that would justify modifying their meaning.
- Medicare and third-party payers often require providers to report HCPCS Level II national codes instead of unlisted procedure or service CPT codes.

CPT Instructional Notes

CPT instructional notes appear throughout CPT sections to clarify the assignment of codes. They are typeset in two patterns.

- A *blocked unindented note* is located below the title of a subsection, heading (or category), or subheading (or subcategory). It contains instructions that apply to all codes in the subsection, heading/category, or subheading/subcategory.
- An *indented parenthetical* note is located below the
  - Title of a subsection, heading (or category), and subheading (or subcategory)
  - Code description (and the note applies to that code only unless the note indicates otherwise)
- A *parenthetical note* is located in the code description to provide an example. Such notes contain examples in parentheses that are *not* required to appear in the procedural statement documented by the provider.

Coding Tip

Within a code series, parenthetical notes also provide information about deleted codes.

CPT Descriptive Qualifiers

Descriptive qualifiers are terms that clarify the assignment of a CPT code. They can occur in the middle of a main clause or after the semicolon and may or may not be enclosed in parentheses. Make sure you read all code descriptions very carefully to properly assign CPT codes that require descriptive qualifiers.

Example: The descriptive qualifier for code 17000 is *first lesion*, while the descriptive qualifier for code 17003 is *second through 14 lesions, each*.

Exercise 9.7 – CPT Sections, Subsections, Categories, and Subcategories

Instructions: Complete each statement.

1. CPT category I codes are organized according to six _____ that are subdivided into subsections, categories, and subcategories.

2. Defined terms and explanations about code assignment for procedures and services are located in _____, which are located at the beginning of each CPT category I section.

3. When the provider performs a procedure or service for which there is no CPT code, the _____ procedure or service code is reported, and a special report is submitted to the payer.

4. Instructional _____ appear throughout CPT sections to clarify the assignment of codes, and they are located below the title of a subsection, category, or subcategory.

5. Terms that clarify the assignment of a CPT code are called _____ qualifiers.

CPT Modifiers

CPT modifiers clarify services and procedures performed by providers. Although the CPT code and description remain unchanged, modifiers indicate that the description of the service or procedure performed has been altered.

- CPT modifiers are reported as two digits added to the five-character CPT code.
- HCPCS Level II modifiers are reported as two characters added to the five-character CPT code. (HCPCS Level II modifiers were explained in Chapter 8.)
- CPT and HCPCS Level II modifiers reported for Anesthesia services are covered in Chapter 11 of this textbook.

Example: A patient undergoes repair of nasal septal perforations, which was unsuccessful. Report code 30630. Three months later, the patient undergoes repeat repair of nasal septal perforations by a different surgeon. Report code 30630 77. (Modifier 77 indicates a repeat procedure by another physician.)

Functional and Informational Modifiers

When reporting codes with more than one modifier, enter the **functional modifier** (or **pricing modifier** or **payment modifier**) first because it assists in reimbursement decision making (e.g., assistant surgeon). Next, enter the **informational modifier** (or **statistical modifier**), which clarifies aspects of the procedure or service provided for the payer (e.g., procedure performed on right or left side only). (Medicare originally created the terms *functional modifier, payment modifier, pricing modifier, informational modifier*, and *statistical modifier*, which means some payers do not use the terms.) *Functional (payment or pricing) modifiers are reported first*. Then, multiple informational modifiers are reported in any order.

> **Example:** An assistant surgeon participated in the open treatment and internal fixation of left femoral fracture, proximal end, neck. Report code 27236 80 LT.
>
> Modifier 80 (Assistant surgeon), is a functional (payment or pricing) modifier that impacts reimbursement. Modifier LT (Left side) is an informational (statistical) modifier, which indicates that the surgery was performed on the patient's left side, and it does not impact reimbursement.

When multiple modifiers are added to a CPT (or a HCPCS Level II) code and an informational modifier is listed first, third-party payers manually review the claim. (Manual review can slow claims processing and results in reimbursement delays to physicians.)

> Third-party payers, including Medicare administrative contractors (MACs), publish lists of modifiers that impact reimbursement. Because each payer's list is different, a comprehensive list of all possible functional (payment or pricing) modifiers should be developed internally by providers (e.g., clinic, hospital outpatient, physician office). Data abstracting and claims completion software that flags functional (payment or pricing) modifiers will also help remind coding and reimbursement specialists to report them first.
>
> The following is a sample of third-party payers that publish different lists of functional (payment or pricing) modifiers on their websites.
>
> - Novitas Solutions MAC (https://www.novitas-solutions.com) publishes payment modifiers, stating that "informational or statistical modifiers (e.g., any modifier not classified as a payment modifier) should be listed after the payment modifier. If multiple informational/statistical modifiers apply, you may list them in any order (as long as they are listed after payment modifiers)."
>
> - WPS GHA MAC (https://www.wpsgha.com) publishes a pricing modifier fact sheet with a list of modifiers, which are not limited to the first position. "If there is another pricing modifier submitted that is required to be in the first modifier field, these modifiers [from the pricing modifier fact sheet] should be in the second, third, or fourth modifier position."
>
> - Mass General Health Plan (https://resources.allwayshealthpartners.org) publishes a provider payment guidelines document that includes a comprehensive table of modifiers, descriptors, and impact on reimbursement.

Not all CPT or HCPCS Level II modifiers apply to each section of CPT. Coders should contact third-party payers to obtain a list of modifiers and applicable CPT sections because each payer has different reporting requirements.

Reporting Modifiers on Claims

CMS-1500 claims are generated by physicians who perform surgery and provide services to patients who receive treatment on an inpatient or outpatient basis, which is part of *professional billing*. (UB-04 claims are generated by health care facilities that provide inpatient and outpatient services, which is part of *institutional billing*.)

Example: Patient has a history of gallbladder disease. After several hours of acute pain, patient was referred to Dr. S who completed an evaluation of the condition. Dr. S performed a complete history and physical examination in the emergency department and decided to admit the patient to the hospital for an immediate workup for cholecystitis. After evaluating results of laboratory tests and a sonogram, the patient was scheduled for an emergency laparoscopic cholecystectomy. The surgeon was Dr. S, and the assistant surgeon was Dr. A. The surgery was successful, and the patient was discharged the next day and told to return to the office in seven days.

Four days later, the patient returned to Dr. S's office complaining of chest pains. Dr. S performed another examination and ordered the necessary tests for the level 3 E/M service. After reviewing the test results and conferring with the patient's primary care physician, it was determined that the patient was suffering from mild angina.

- The hospital submits a UB-04 claim with ICD-10-PCS procedure codes, and the physicians submit CMS-1500 claims with CPT procedure codes and modifier(s).

- Dr. S submits a CMS-1500 claim (Figure 9-1) for the initial hospital visit with medical decision making of high complexity (99223 57) (Modifier 57 indicates decision for surgery), the laparoscopic cholecystectomy (47562), and established patient office encounter with medical decision making of low level (99213 24). (Modifier 24 indicates an unrelated E/M service was provided by the same physician during a postoperative period.)

- Dr. A submits a CMS-1500 claim (Figure 9-2) for the laparoscopic cholecystectomy 47562 80 (Modifier 80 indicates assistant surgeon).

PROCEDURES, SERVICES, OR SUPPLIES (Explain Unusual Circumstances)	
CPT/HCPCS	MODIFIER
99223	57
47562	
99213	24

Courtesy of the Centers for Medicare & Medicaid Services, www.cms.gov; claim data created by author.

FIGURE 9-1 Completed Block 24D of CMS-1500

PROCEDURES, SERVICES, OR SUPPLIES (Explain Unusual Circumstances)	
CPT/HCPCS	MODIFIER
47562	80

Courtesy of the Centers for Medicare & Medicaid Services, www.cms.gov; claim data created by author.

FIGURE 9-2 Completed Block 24D of CMS-1500

CPT Modifiers According to Reporting Similarities

The AMA and CMS develop new modifiers on a continuous basis, and next available numbers are assigned. This means that there is no relationship among groups of modifier numbers. Reviewing modifiers in strict numeric order does not allow for comparison of those that are related to one another in terms of content; therefore, this chapter organizes modifiers according to reporting similarity. (The inside cover of CPT contains a list of modifiers and titles.)

Evaluation and Management Services

Modifier 24 (unrelated evaluation and management service by the same physician or other qualified health care professional during a postoperative period) is reported with evaluation and management (E/M) service codes to indicate that an E/M service was performed during the standard postoperative period for a condition unrelated to the surgery. The E/M service code to which the modifier is attached must be linked to a diagnosis that is *unrelated* to the surgical diagnosis previously submitted.

Example: One week after surgical treatment to release a frozen shoulder, an established patient received level 3 evaluation and management services for treatment of the flu. Report code 99213 24.

Modifier 25 (significant, separately identifiable evaluation and management service by the same physician or other qualified health care professional on the same day of the procedure or other service) is reported when a documented E/M service was performed on the same day as another procedure because the patient's condition required the assignment of a significant, separately identifiable, additional E/M service that was provided "above and beyond the other service provided or beyond the usual preoperative and postoperative care associated with the procedure performed." The documented medical decision making must "stand on its own" to justify reporting modifier 25 with the E/M code. The separate E/M service provided must be "above and beyond" what is normally performed during a procedure.

> **Example:** During a routine annual examination, it was discovered that the 65-year-old established patient had an enlarged liver expanding the scope of level 4 evaluation and management services. Report codes 99397 and 99214 25.

Modifier 57 (decision for surgery) is reported when the E/M service resulted in the initial decision to perform surgery on the day before or the day of surgery, exempting it from the global surgery package.

> **Example:** The patient received E/M level 4 services for chest pain in the emergency department, and a decision was made to insert a coronary artery stent. Report code 99284 57 in addition to the stent procedure code.

Greater, Reduced, or Discontinued Services

Modifier 22 (increased procedural services) is reported when a procedure requires greater than usual services. Documentation that would support using this modifier includes difficult, complicated, extensive, unusual, or rare procedures.

> **Example:** During surgery, the patient experienced blood loss of 600 cubic centimeters and required intraoperative transfusions. Report the CPT surgery code with modifier 22.

Modifier 52 (reduced services) is reported when a service has been partially reduced or eliminated at the provider's discretion and does not completely match the reported CPT code description.

> **Example:** A surgeon removed a coccygeal pressure ulcer and performed a coccygectomy. However, the surgeon did not use a primary suture or perform a skin flap closure because the wound had to be cleansed for a continued period of time postoperatively. Report code 15920 52. (When the surgeon eventually performs the wound closure procedure, an appropriate code would be reported.)

Modifier 53 (discontinued procedure) is reported when a provider has elected to terminate a procedure because of extenuating circumstances that threaten the well-being of the patient. This modifier applies only to provider office settings and is not reported for elective cancellation (e.g., by the patient) prior to anesthesia induction and/or surgical preparation in the operating suite.

> **Example:** After anesthesia administration, the surgeon inserted the colonoscope and removed it right away because the patient had not been properly prepared for the procedure. Report code 45378 53. The patient received instructions about properly preparing for a colonoscopy procedure, and the procedure was rescheduled.

Modifier 73 (discontinued outpatient procedure prior to anesthesia administration) is reported to describe discontinued procedures *prior to the administration of any anesthesia* because of extenuating circumstances threatening the well-being of the patient. (An ICD-10-CM code to document the reason the procedure was halted is also reported.) This modifier applies only to hospital outpatient and ambulatory surgery center (ASC) settings and is not reported for elective cancellation (e.g., patient changed their mind about undergoing the procedure) prior to anesthesia induction or surgical preparation in the operating suite.

> **Example:** Hospital outpatient developed a heart arrhythmia prior to anesthesia administration, and the laparoscopic cholecystectomy procedure was canceled. Report code 47562 73.

Modifier 74 (discontinued outpatient procedure after anesthesia administration) is reported to describe discontinued procedures after the administration of anesthesia due to extenuating circumstances. (An ICD-10-CM code to document the reason the procedure was halted is also reported.) This modifier applies only to hospital and ASC outpatient settings.

> **Example:** Hospital outpatient was prepped and draped, and general anesthesia was administered. The anesthesiologist noted a sudden increase in blood pressure, and the laparoscopic cholecystectomy procedure was terminated. Report code 47562 74.

Global Surgery

Global surgery modifiers apply to four areas related to the CPT surgical package (Figure 9-3), which includes local infiltration; metacarpal/digital block or topical anesthesia when used; the procedure; and normal, uncomplicated follow-up care. Global surgery modifiers do *not* apply to obstetrical coding, where the CPT description of specific codes clearly describes separate antepartum, postpartum, and delivery services for both vaginal and cesarean deliveries.

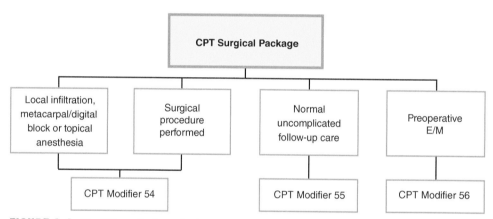

FIGURE 9-3 Modifiers that apply to components of the CPT surgical package

Modifier 54 (surgical care only) is reported when a provider performed only the surgical portion of surgical package and personally administered required local anesthesia. Different provider(s) will have performed preoperative evaluation and/or provided postoperative care.

> **Example:** While on vacation, the patient sustained a tibial shaft fracture and underwent closed treatment by Dr. Ruiz. Upon returning home, the patient received follow-up care in the office from Dr. Cho, a local orthopedist. Dr. Ruiz reports code 27750 54. Dr. Cho reports an appropriate office or other outpatient service E/M code.

Modifier 55 (postoperative management only) is reported when a provider other than the surgeon is responsible for the postoperative management of a surgery that was performed by another provider. Documentation in the medical record should detail the date of transfer of care to calculate the percentage of the fee to be billed for postoperative care. (The modifier is added to the surgical procedure code. Modifier 55 does *not* apply when a second provider occasionally covers for the surgeon and where no transfer of care occurs.)

> **Example:** While on vacation, the patient sustained a tibial shaft fracture and underwent closed treatment by Dr. Charles on May 5. Dr. Charles then arranged for transfer of care to Dr. Smith, an orthopedist in the patient's hometown, on May 6. Upon returning home, the patient received follow-up care on May 8 from Dr. Smith, a local orthopedist. Dr. Smith reports code 27750 55.

Modifier 56 (preoperative management only) is reported when a provider other than the operating surgeon performs preoperative care and evaluation of the patient for surgery (e.g., preoperative clearance).

> **Example:** Dr. Berger preoperatively cleared an established patient during an E/M level 4 service for scheduled surgery by Dr. Jian, and reports code 99214 56.

Special Surgical and Procedural Events

Modifier 58 (staged or related procedure or service by the same physician or other qualified health care professional during the postoperative period) is reported to indicate that additional related surgery is required during the postoperative period of a previously completed surgery and is performed by the same provider. Documentation should include one of the following:

- Original plan for surgery included additional stages to be performed within the postoperative period of first stage of procedure.
- Underlying disease required a second related, but unplanned, procedure to be performed.
- Additional related therapy is required after the performance of a procedure.

Do *not* report modifier 58 when the CPT code description describes multiple sessions of an event.

> **Example:** A surgical wound is not healing properly because of the patient's underlying diabetes. Patient was told prior to the original surgery that if this happened, additional surgery would be required for subcutaneous tissue debridement of the wound. Patient then underwent subcutaneous tissue debridement of the wound. Report code 11042 58 for debridement surgery.

Modifier 59 (distinct procedural service) is reported when same provider performs one or more distinctly independent procedures on the same day as other procedures or services, according to the following criteria:

- Procedures are performed at different sessions or during different patient encounters.
- Procedures are performed on different sites or organs and require a different surgical prep.
- Procedures are performed for multiple or extensive injuries, using separate incisions/excisions; for separate lesions; or for procedures not ordinarily encountered/performed on the same day.

Modifier 59 is *never* added to E/M codes.

> **Example:** Patient has two basal cell carcinomas removed, one from the forehead with a simple closure (11640) and the other from the nose requiring adjacent tissue transfer (14060). Report codes 14060, 11640 51 (forehead), and 11640 59 51 (nose).

CMS created HCPCS Level II modifiers as descriptive subsets of modifier 59, which means the following are reported *instead of modifier 59 on Medicare claims*:

- XE (separate encounter, a service that is distinct because it occurred during a separate encounter)
- XS (separate structure, a service that is distinct because it was performed on a separate organ or structure)
- XP (separate practitioner, a service that is distinct because it was performed by a different practitioner)
- XU (unusual non-overlapping service, the use of a service that is distinct because it does not overlap usual components of the main service)

> **Example:** A patient receives an antibiotic infusion as an outpatient and is discharged. The patient returns later that same day and receives another separate antibiotic infusion. Modifier XE is reported with each CPT medication administration (infusion) code and each HCPCS Level II drug (e.g., clindamycin).

Modifier 63 (procedure performed on infants less than 4 kg) is reported when an infant weighs less than 4 kilograms (kg) because procedures performed for the infant may require increased complexity and provider work. (Appendix A in the CPT coding manual contains a list of codes to which modifier 63 applies.)

> **Example:** Baby Girl Markel's weight was 3.5 kg at the time a diagnostic thoracoscopy was performed. Report 32601 63.

Modifier 78 (unplanned return to the operating/procedure room by the same physician or other qualified health care professional following initial procedure for a related procedure during the postoperative period) is reported for unplanned circumstances that require a return to the operating or procedure room for complications of initial operation. (An ICD-10-CM code to document the surgical complication is also reported.)

> **Example:** The patient's surgical sutures separated, and a 12-cm layer closure of the axillary wound was performed. Report code 12034 78. (An intermediate repair includes the repair and layered closure.)

Modifier 79 (unrelated procedure or service by the same physician or other qualified health care professional during the postoperative period) is reported when a new procedure or service is performed by a provider during the normal postoperative period of a previously performed but unrelated surgery.

> **Example:** Six weeks following cataract surgery performed on the left eye, the patient underwent diathermic repair of retinal detachment, right eye. Report code 67101 79 RT.

Bilateral and Multiple Procedures

Modifier 27 (multiple outpatient hospital E/M encounters on the same date) is reported for patients who receive multiple E/M services performed by different providers on the same day.

> **Example:** A patient was seen in the hospital's emergency department and received level 4 evaluation and management services due to a fractured ankle. The patient was seen later the same day in the urgent care center and provided with level 3 evaluation and management services due to a migraine that did not respond to prescribed medication taken at home. Report codes 99284 27 and 99213 27.

Modifier 50 (bilateral procedure) is a directional modifier that is reported when a procedure is performed bilaterally (on both anatomic structures) during the same operative session and when the code description does not specify that the procedure is bilateral.

> **Example:** Patient underwent bilateral arthrodesis of the knees. Report code 27580 50.

Modifier 50 is *not* reported with add-on codes, which are designated with the plus symbol; instead, report the add-on code(s) *without modifier 50*.

> **Example:** Patient underwent puncture aspiration of three cysts of the right breast and two cysts of the left breast. Report codes 19000 50, 19001, 19001, and 19001. (Code 19000 50 reports two cysts, one from each breast. Add-on code 19001 is reported three times for the three additional cysts. According to Optum's *EncoderPro.com Expert*, directional modifiers are not reported with code 19001. However, some third-party payers may require reporting codes with directional modifiers instead, as 19000 RT, 19001 RT, 19001 RT, 19001 LT, 19001 LT.)

Modifier 50 is *not* reported when code descriptions include anatomic structures that are found bilaterally as well as those *not* found bilaterally.

> **Example:** Patient underwent shaving of a single epidermal 0.2-centimeter lesion, right arm, and a 0.3-centimeter lesion, left arm. Report code 11300 *without modifier 50*. The code description includes "trunk, arms, or legs." Although arms and legs are bilateral structures, the trunk is not; thus, modifier 50 is *not* reported with the code.

Modifier 51 (multiple procedures) is reported when multiple procedures other than E/M services are performed during a single patient encounter by the same provider. The procedures performed are characterized as

- Multiple related surgical procedures performed at the same session

- Surgical procedures performed in combination, whether through the same or another incision, or that involve the same or different anatomy
- Combination medical and surgical procedures performed at the same session

Example: Patient underwent right tibial shaft fracture repair, closed, and left knee arthrodesis. Report codes 27750 and 27580 51.

Repeat Services

Modifier 76 (repeat procedure or service by same physician or other qualified health care professional) is reported when a procedure was repeated because of special circumstances involving the original service and the same physician performed the repeat procedure. Special circumstances include changes in the patient's condition or the need to assess the effect of therapeutic procedures.

Example: The patient underwent initial EKG due to experiencing chest discomfort this morning. A repeat EKG was performed 30 minutes later during the encounter when the patient stated they were starting to experience chest pain. Report codes 93041 and 93041 76.

Modifier 77 (repeat procedure by another physician or other qualified health care professional) is reported when a physician other than the original physician performs a repeat procedure because of special circumstances involving the original study or procedure.

Example: Patient underwent tubal ligation three years ago but became pregnant this year. After C-section delivery for the current pregnancy, patient underwent a second tubal ligation. Report codes 59514 and 58611 77.

Multiple Surgeons

Modifier 62 (two surgeons) is reported when two primary surgeons are required during an operative session, each performing distinct parts of a reportable procedure. Ideally, the surgeons represent different specialties.

Example: A spinal surgeon and a general surgeon work together as primary surgeons to perform an anterior spinal fusion of L5-S1. The spinal surgeon also inserts an intervertebral synthetic cage and performs iliac bone grafting. Each surgeon reports code 22558 62. The spinal surgeon also reports codes 22853 and 20937 (and modifier 51 is *not* added to each code).

Modifier 66 (surgical team) is reported when surgery performed is highly complex and requires the services of a skilled team of three or more surgeons. The procedure reported on the claim for each participating surgeon must include this modifier. The operative reports must document the complexity of the surgery and refer to the actions of each team member.

Example: Reattachment of severed forearm, left. Each surgeon reports code 20802 66 LT.

Modifier 80 (assistant surgeon) is reported when one physician assists another during an operative session. The assistant surgeon reports the same CPT code as the operating physician.

Example: Dr. Luz assisted Dr. Gow during single coronary artery bypass surgery. Dr. Luz reports code 33510 80. (Dr. Gow reports code 33510 without the modifier.)

Modifier 81 (minimum assistant surgeon) is reported when a primary operating physician has planned to perform a surgical procedure alone, but circumstances arise that require the services of an assistant surgeon for a short time. The second surgeon reports the same CPT code as the operating physician.

Example: Dr. Kelly begins an open cholecystectomy procedure and discovers that the gallbladder is the size of a hot dog bun, which necessitates calling Dr. Pietro to assist for a short time. Dr. Kelly reports code 47600. Dr. Pietro reports code 47600 81. (A gallbladder is supposed to be the size of your little finger.)

Modifier 82 (assistant surgeon) (when qualified resident surgeon not available) is reported when a qualified resident surgeon is unavailable to assist with a procedure. In teaching hospitals, the physician acting as the assistant surgeon is usually a qualified resident surgeon. If circumstances arise (e.g., rotational changes) and a qualified resident surgeon is not available, another surgeon may assist with a procedure. The nonresident-assistant surgeon reports the same CPT code as the operating physician.

> **Example:** Resident surgeon Dr. Smith was to assist surgeon Dr. Manlin with a routine laparoscopic appendectomy. Dr. Smith was temporarily reassigned to the emergency department, and Dr. Manlin's partner assisted with the procedure. Dr. Manlin reports code 44970, and Dr. Manlin's partner reports code 44970 82.

Preventive Services

Modifier 33 (preventive service) is reported to alert the third-party payer that a procedure or service was preventive under applicable laws and that patient cost sharing (e.g., coinsurance, copayment, deductible) does not apply when furnished by in-network providers.

> **Example:** The patient's primary care provider provided 20 minutes of smoking and tobacco use cessation counseling in the physician's office setting. Report code 99407 33.

Professional and Technical Components

Modifier 26 (professional component) is reported when the provider either interprets test results or operates equipment for a procedure. Do *not* report this modifier when a specific separately identifiable code describes the professional component of a procedure (e.g., 93010).

> **Example:** Radiologist Dr. Minion interprets a three-view chest x-ray that was performed by a provider at a different facility. Dr. Minion reports code 71047 26.

Mandated Services

Modifier 32 (mandated services) is reported when services (e.g., second or third opinion for a surgical procedure) provided were mandated by a third party (e.g., attorney or payer).

> **Example:** A patient's primary care provider recommends respiratory therapy. The payer arranged for the patient to undergo a level 3 evaluation and management mandated office consultation service by a respiratory specialist. Code 99243 32 is reported.

Unusual Anesthesia

Modifier 23 (unusual anesthesia) is reported when circumstances (e.g., extent of service or patient's physical condition) require anesthesia for procedures that usually require either no anesthesia or local anesthesia.

> **Example:** The 30-year-old patient has an intellectual disability and requires the administration of general anesthesia for ventral hernia repair (instead of regional anesthesia). Code 00832 23 is reported.

Modifier 47 (anesthesia by surgeon) is reported when the surgeon provides regional or general anesthesia in addition to performing the surgical procedure. Modifier 47 is added to the CPT surgery code. It is *not* reported with codes from the Anesthesia section.

> **Example:** The surgeon administers regional anesthesia and performs repair of recurrent inguinal hernia, reducible. Code 49520 47 is reported.

Laboratory Services

Modifier 90 (reference [outside] laboratory) is reported when a laboratory test is performed by an outside or reference laboratory.

> **Example:** The provider orders an automated CBC and automated differential WBC count laboratory test. Arrangements are made with an outside lab to perform the test and bill the physician. The physician reports code 85025 90. (Code 36415 51 is also reported for routine venipuncture.)

Modifier 91 (repeat clinical diagnostic laboratory test) is reported when a clinical diagnostic laboratory test is repeated on the same day to obtain subsequent (multiple) test results. This modifier is not reported when lab tests are repeated to confirm initial results (e.g., due to equipment problems).

> **Example:** The patient underwent serial (repeated) lab tests for cardiac enzyme testing every six hours. Report codes 82657, 82657 91, and 82657 91.

Modifier 92 (alternative laboratory platform testing) is reported when laboratory testing is performed using a kit or transportable instrument that wholly or in part consists of a single-use, disposable analytical chamber. Such testing does not require permanent dedicated space because the testing materials can be carried or transported to the patient care area.

> **Example:** The laboratory technician brought the HIV-1 testing materials to the emergency department and used an HIV-1 single-use testing kit to test the patient. Report code 86701 92.

Multiple Modifiers

Modifier 99 (multiple modifiers) is reported to alert third-party payers that more than one modifier has been added to a procedure or service code. The CMS-1500 claim allows up to four modifiers to be listed after a CPT or HCPCS Level II code, which includes modifier 99 to indicate that "multiple modifiers follow." Thus, when more than four modifiers are reported for the same code, enter modifier 99 on line one. Then, enter all of the additional (multiple) modifiers reported for the same code in CMS-1500 Block 19 (or in the equivalent electronic data field).

> **Example:** An assistant surgeon (80) reports an unusual service (22), bilateral procedure (50), and surgeon-provided general anesthesia services (47) for a lumbar hernia repair procedure (49540). In addition to reporting code 49540 and modifier 99 in Block 24D (line 1), modifiers 22, 47, 50, and 80 are reported in Block 19 of the CMS-1500 claim (Figure 9-4).

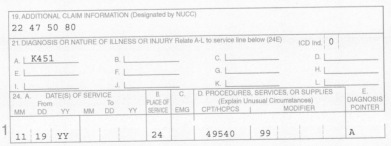

FIGURE 9-4 Block 24D line 1, and Block 19 of CMS-1500 claim, with multiple modifiers entered

The UB-04 claim also allows multiple modifiers associated with the same code to each be reported with the code on separate lines in Form Locator 44. However, modifier 99 is *not* reported on the UB-04 claim.

Example: An assistant surgeon (80) reports an unusual service (22), bilateral procedure (50), and surgeon-provided general anesthesia services (47) for a lumbar hernia repair procedure (49540). Code 49540 is reported on lines 1–4 of the UB-04 claim in Form Locator 44, and one modifier is reported next to the code on each line (Figure 9-5).

42 REV. CD.	43 DESCRIPTION	44 HCPCS / RATE / HIPPS CODE	45 SERV. DATE	46 SERV. UNITS	47 TOTAL CHARGES	48 NON-COVERED CHARGES	49
0490	Repair lumbar hernia	49540 22	1119YY	1	9995 00		
0490	Repair lumbar hernia	49540 47	1119YY	1	0 00		
0490	Repair lumbar hernia	49540 50	1119YY	1	0 00		
0490	Repair lumbar hernia	49540 80	1119YY	1	0 00		

FIGURE 9-5 Form locator 42 (lines 1–4) of UB-04 claim, with multiple modifiers entered

Telemedicine

Modifier 93 (synchronous telemedicine service rendered via telephone or other real-time interactive audio-only telecommunications system) is reported for real-time *telephone* or *audio-only* interactions between a provider and a patient who is located at a distant site from the provider.

Example: Patient underwent psychiatric diagnostic evaluation with medical services via audio-only telemedicine. Report code 90792 93.

Modifier 95 (synchronous telemedicine service rendered via a real-time interactive audio and video telecommunication system) is reported for real-time interactions between a provider and a patient who is located at a distant site from the provider.

Example: Patient underwent psychiatric diagnostic evaluation with medical services via audio-video telemedicine. Report code 90792 95.

Habilitative and Rehabilitative Services

Modifier 96 (habilitative services) is reported for services that

- Help patients learn skills and functioning for daily living that they have not yet developed
- Help patients keep, learn, or improve skills and functioning for daily living

Example: Thirty-month-old child received speech therapy due to a limited expressive vocabulary (speech delay). Report code 92507 96.

Modifier 97 (rehabilitative services) is reported for services that help patients keep, relearn, or improve skills and functioning for daily living that have been lost or impaired because of illness, injury, or disability.

Example: Patient received 15 minutes of direct one-on-one patient contact for therapeutic activities in the physician office setting to improve functional performance as the result of a stroke. Report code 97530 97.

Exercise 9.8 – CPT Modifiers

Instructions: Assign appropriate modifier(s) to each statement. Do *not* assign CPT codes.

_____   1. Assistant surgeon reporting patient's cesarean section, delivery only

_____   2. Cholecystectomy code reported during postoperative period for treatment of leg fracture

(continues)

Exercise 9.8 – continued

_____ 3. Treatment for chronic conditions at same time preventive medicine is provided

_____ 4. Inpatient visit performed by surgeon, with decision to perform surgery tomorrow

_____ 5. Office history and physical examination as preoperative clearance for surgery

_____ 6. Postoperative management of vaginal hysterectomy by a physician other than the surgeon

_____ 7. Repeat gallbladder x-ray series, same physician

_____ 8. Arthroscopy of right elbow and closed fracture reduction of left wrist

_____ 9. Needle core biopsy of right and left breasts

_____ 10. Consultation required by payer

National Correct Coding Initiative (NCCI)

The Centers for Medicare and Medicaid Services (CMS) implemented the **National Correct Coding Initiative (NCCI) program** to promote national correct coding methodologies and to control the improper assignment of codes that result in inappropriate reimbursement of Medicare Part B claims. The NCCI program was also implemented for state Medicaid programs, and separate edit files and manuals are published for it. NCCI program code pairs (or NCCI program edit pairs) cannot be reported on the same claim for the same date of service, and providers use _outpatient code editor (OCE)_ software to detect inappropriate codes and more.

NCCI program _add-on code (AOC) edits_ contain a list of CPT and HCPCS Level II add-on codes with their respective primary codes; a reported add-on code is eligible for payment only when its CPT primary code is also eligible for reimbursement. (A CPT add-on code is preceded by a plus symbol.)

NCCI program _medically unlikely edits (MUEs)_ are used to compare _units of service (UOS)_ with CPT and HCPCS Level II codes reported on claims and indicate the maximum number of UOS allowable by the same provider for the same beneficiary on the same date of service under most circumstances.

> **Example:** A patient undergoes a cataract extraction in the left eye. The claim submitted by the provider contains a 3 in the units column of Block 24, which means the patient underwent cataract extraction surgery on three left eyes. The medically unlikely edit process rejects the claim (because the patient has just one left eye). If a 1 had been entered in the units column of Block 24, the claim would have passed the medically unlikely edit and payment would have been processed.

NCCI program _mutually exclusive edits_ and _procedure-procedure (PTP) code pair edits_ are automated prepayment edits that prevent improper payment when certain codes are submitted together for Part B-covered services. _Mutually exclusive edits_ apply when one procedure or service could not reasonably be performed with the other. When clinical circumstances do justify reporting both codes, add a modifier to either code of the code pair so that payment of both codes might be allowed.

> **Example:** A claim contains CPT codes for initial inpatient E/M services and critical care E/M services (with modifier 59) for the same date of service. Documentation supports initial inpatient E/M services provided at 3 A.M. on the day of admission (when the patient did not require critical care) and critical care services later that same day (when the patient did require critical care).

Procedure-to-procedure (PTP) code pair edits are code pairs (or edit pairs) for which one code is a component of a more comprehensive code, and only the comprehensive code is paid. When clinical circumstances justify reporting both codes, a modifier is added to either code of the code pair for payment consideration. They are used by Medicare administrative contractors to adjudicate provider claims for physician services, outpatient hospital services, and outpatient therapy services; they are _not_ applied to facility claims for inpatient services.

Example of Claims Denial: The patient undergoes a superficial biopsy and a deep biopsy of the same site (during the same operative episode). If CPT codes for both deep and superficial biopsies are reported, NCCI program edits result in claims denial. (When both deep and superficial biopsies are performed on the same site, report only the deep biopsy code.)

Example of Exception: The patient undergoes a superficial biopsy and a deep superficial biopsy of the same site (during the same operative episode). Documentation supports the significant work, effort, and time associated with each biopsy, which means codes for both the superficial biopsy and deep biopsy are reported. A modifier (e.g., 59, Distinct procedural service) is added to the superficial biopsy code so that NCCI program edits do not result in claims denial. (Reduced payment for the superficial biopsy might be processed by the payer after review of documentation.)

When claims are denied based on NCCI program edits, the charges may *not* be billed to Medicare beneficiaries. Since these denials are based on incorrect coding rather than medical necessity, the provider cannot submit a **Notice of Exclusions from Medicare Benefits (NEMB)** to seek payment from the Medicare beneficiary. The NEMB would need to have been signed prior to the procedure or service performed because they are not covered by Medicare.

NCCI program edits are used to process Medicare Part B claims (Table 9-1), and NCCI program coding policies are based on CPT coding conventions, national and local Medicare policies and edits, coding guidelines developed by national societies, standard medical and surgical practice, and current coding practice. NCCI program edits in the outpatient code editor (OCE) are used by MACs to process Medicare Part B claims for outpatient hospital services and by contractors that process state Medicaid claims. Some OCE edits that apply to outpatient hospital services claims differ from comparable edits in the NCCI program used to process physician office services claims.

Example: Code 67911 describes "Correction of lid retraction." A parenthetical note below the code description advises that if autogenous graft materials are obtained during the same operative session, tissue graft code 15769, 20920, or 20922 is reported in addition to code 67911. According to the the NCCI program manual, code 67911 can be reported with a tissue graft code because CPT guidelines and instructional notes provide such coding direction.

TABLE 9-1 Partial Listing of National Correct Coding Initiative (NCCI) Program Edits

NCCI Edit	Description of NCCI Edit	Reason for NCCI Edit
1	Invalid diagnosis code	Invalid diagnosis code entered on claim
2	Diagnosis and age conflict	Diagnosis code includes age range, and age entered is outside of range
3	Diagnosis and sex conflict	Diagnosis code includes sex designation, and sex entered does not match
4	Medicare secondary payer (MSP) alert	Procedure code has MSP alert warning indicator
20	Code2 of a code pair that is not allowed by NCCI even if appropriate modifier is present	Code in column 2 of a code pair is rejected (while column 1 code of the pair is not flagged as an edit)
40	Code2 of a code pair that would be allowed by NCCI if appropriate modifier(s) were present	Code in column 2 of a code pair is rejected (while column 1 code of the pair is not flagged as an edit)

Unbundling CPT Codes

Providers are responsible for reporting the CPT (and HCPCS Level II) code that most comprehensively describes the services provided. NCCI program edits determine the appropriateness of CPT code combinations for claims submitted to MACs. NCCI program edits are designed to detect *unbundling*, which involves reporting multiple codes for a service when a single comprehensive code should be assigned. The practice of unbundling occurs when coders unintentionally report multiple codes when coding guidelines are misinterpreted *or* when multiple codes are intentionally reported to maximize reimbursement.

- Unbundling occurs when one service is divided into its component parts and a code for each component part is reported as if they were separate services.

Example: A 64-year-old female patient undergoes total abdominal hysterectomy with bilateral salpingectomy and oophorectomy. Review CPT Surgery code descriptions for 58150, 58700, and 58720. Reporting codes 58700 and 58720 in addition to 58150 is considered unbundling. If all three codes were submitted on a claim, reimbursement for codes 58700 and 58720 would be disallowed (and the provider might be subject to allegations of fraud and abuse, depending upon intent).

- Unbundling occurs when a code for the separate surgical approach (e.g., laparotomy) is reported in addition to a code for the surgical procedure. Procedures performed to gain access to an area or organ system are not separately reported.

Example: A 54-year-old patient underwent excision of ileoanal reservoir with ileostomy, which required lysis of adhesions to gain access to the site of surgery. Review CPT Surgery code descriptions for 45136 and 44005. Report CPT code 45136 only because code 44005 is a component of the total procedure. Reporting both codes would be considered unbundling.

Exercise 9.9 – National Correct Coding Initiative

Instructions: Complete each statement.

1. To promote national correct coding methodologies and control the improper assignment of codes that result in inappropriate reimbursement of Medicare Part _____ claims, CMS implemented the NCCI program.

2. NCCI program edits are included in the Outpatient Code _____ for use by MACs to process Medicare Part B claims for outpatient hospital procedures and services.

3. NCCI program code pairs that, for clinical reasons, are unlikely to be performed on the same patient on the same day are called mutually _____ edits.

4. When a submitted claim for reimbursement is denied because of incorrect coding rather than medical necessity, the provider cannot submit a Notice of Exclusions from Medicare _____ to seek payment from a Medicare beneficiary.

5. A 34-year-old patient underwent upper gastrointestinal endoscopy, which included visualization of the esophagus, stomach, and duodenum. During endoscopy, brushings collected esophageal specimens and esophageal biopsy was performed. Upon review of CPT Surgery code descriptions for 43235 and 43239, the coder assigned 43239 only (because 43235 is considered a component of the total procedure, 43239). Reporting both codes would be considered _____.

Summary

CPT codes are reported for services and procedures provided by home health care and hospice agencies, outpatient hospital departments, physicians who are employees of a health care facility, and physicians who see patients in their offices or clinics and in patients' homes. To promote national correct coding methodologies and to control the improper assignment of codes that result in inappropriate reimbursement of Medicare Part B claims, the Centers for Medicare & Medicaid Services (CMS) implemented the National Correct Coding Initiative (NCCI) program.

CPT organizes category I procedures and services into six sections: Evaluation and Management (E/M), Anesthesia, Surgery, Radiology (including Nuclear Medicine and Diagnostic Ultrasound), Pathology and Laboratory, and Medicine. Category II codes are optional "evidence-based performance measurements" tracking codes, and category III codes are "emerging technology" temporary codes assigned for data collection purposes. The CPT index is organized by alphabetical main terms printed in boldface, and appendices are located after category III codes.

CPT sections are subdivided into subsections, categories, and subcategories. Guidelines, notes, and descriptive qualifiers are also found in CPT sections, subsections, categories, and subcategories. Two-character modifiers are added to CPT codes to clarify services and procedures performed by providers. Symbols are located throughout the CPT coding book.

Internet Links

JustCoding.com: Go to **www.justcoding.com**, and sign up for the free e-newsletter by clicking on the "eNewsletter Signup" link.

Medicare PFS look-up: Go to **www.cms.gov**, and click on the Medicare link. Scroll down to the Medicare Fee-for-Service Payment heading, and click on the Physician Fee Schedule Look-Up Tool link.

MedlinePlus: www.medlineplus.gov

National Correct Coding Initiative (NCCI) Edits: Go to **www.cms.gov**, and click on the Medicare link. Scroll down to the Coding heading, and click on the National Correct Coding Initiative Edits link.

Review

9.1 – Multiple Choice

Instructions: Select the most appropriate response.

1. Which mandated that CPT codes be reported for outpatient hospital surgical procedures?
   a. Health Insurance, Portability, and Accountability Act of 1996
   b. Healthcare Research and Quality Act of 1989
   c. Medicare Prescription Drug, Improvement, and Modernization Act
   d. Omnibus Budget Reconciliation Act of 1986

2. New, revised, and deleted CPT codes that are provided as an "early release" in July by the CPT Editorial Panel are intended to take effect
   a. after the FDA approves the product.
   b. immediately upon "early release."
   c. six months later.
   d. within a 90-day grace period.

3. The E/M section is located at the beginning of CPT because these codes are
   a. reported by all specialties.
   b. sequenced first on all claims.
   c. the most frequently reported.
   d. used to establish medical necessity.

4. *Arthroscopy, ankle,* and *wound* are examples of _____ in the CPT index.
    a. cross-references
    b. main terms
    c. qualifiers
    d. subterms

5. Which is a CPT index cross-reference term?
    a. Due to   b. *See*   c. *Use*   d. With

6. When a range *or* series of single codes is listed in the CPT index for a procedure or service, the
    a. codes must be reviewed in the CPT manual before a code is assigned.
    b. cross-reference term will direct the coder to another index entry.
    c. range of codes is separated by a comma.
    d. series of single codes is separated by a dash.

7. Codes identified throughout CPT with a forbidden symbol are summarized in Appendix _____.
    a. C   b. D   c. E   d. F

8. Horizontal triangle symbols
    a. identify a revised code description.
    b. mark revisions in Appendix B.
    c. specify new procedures and services.
    d. surround new or revised text.

9. Codes identified with a plus symbol are
    a. add-on codes.
    b. reported with modifier 51.
    c. sequenced first on claims.
    d. stand-alone codes.

10. A code identified by a star symbol indicates that
    a. guidelines and notes are to be reviewed before reporting the code.
    b. it may be reported for synchronous real-time audio-video telemedicine services.
    c. modifier 50 must be added to the reported code.
    d. the code is new to the CPT coding manual.

11. Which are located at the beginning of each CPT section, define terms, and explain the assignment of codes for procedures and services located in a particular section?
    a. Descriptive qualifiers
    b. Guidelines
    c. Notes
    d. Unlisted procedures or services

12. Which are located below the title of a subsection, category/heading, or subcategory/subheading?
    a. Descriptive qualifiers
    b. Guidelines
    c. Notes
    d. Unlisted procedures or services

13. Which requires the submission of a special report that describes the nature, extent, and need for the procedure or service?
    a. Descriptive qualifier
    b. Guideline
    c. Note
    d. Unlisted procedure or service

14. Which code is assigned for physician interpretation of an "unattended sleep study with simultaneous recording of heart rate, oxygen saturation, respiratory airflow, and respiratory effort"?
    a. 95805   b. 95805 90   c. 95806   d. 95806 26

15. A patient was seeking loss-of-wages benefits due to injuries sustained in a motor vehicle accident. The insurance company requested a second opinion regarding injuries and sent the patient for an Independent Medical Exam (IME), where a level 3 outpatient consultation service was provided. The IME physician reviewed medical records from the emergency department, the primary care physician, and pain management center. The IME report was sent to the insurance company. Which code is assigned?

    a. 99243 26   **b.** 99243 32   **c.** 99243 77   **d.** 99243 90

16. A patient presented to the physician's office for removal of 10 skin tags on the torso. During the procedure, the patient became anxious and surgery was discontinued. No skin tags were removed. Which code is reported?

    a. 11200 52   **b.** 11200 53   **c.** 11200 73   **d.** 11200 74

17. The patient underwent osteotomy of cervical spine, anterior approach, single segment, by two surgeons. Which code is reported?

    a. 22220 62   **b.** 22220 66   **c.** 22220 80   **d.** 22220 81

18. The patient underwent a total Thyroxine lab test, which was sent to an outside laboratory but was billed by the physician's office. Which code is reported?

    a. 84436 90   **b.** 84436 91   **c.** 84439 90   **d.** 84437 91

19. If payment of a service or procedure is denied based on National Correct Coding Initiative (NCCI) program edits, the provider

    a. can seek payment from a Medicare beneficiary if an Advance Beneficiary Notice (ABN) was signed by the patient.

    b. expects cash payment from the Medicare beneficiary as a result of having a signed NEMB from the patient on file.

    c. has the office manager initiate the collections process to obtain payment directly from the Medicare beneficiary.

    d. is prohibited from seeking payment from a Medicare beneficiary even when a signed ABN or NEMB was obtained.

20. Patient underwent transcutaneous electrical modulation pain reprocessing for two treatment sessions including placement of electrodes. Which codes are reported?

    a. 0278T, 0278T

    b. 0766T, 0766T

    c. 46999, 46999

    d. 64999, 64999

9.2 – CPT Index

Instructions: Use the CPT index to complete each statement.

1. For abdominohysterectomy, radical, the CPT cross-reference for main term Abdominohysterectomy is _____.

2. For hysterectomy, abdominal, radical, the CPT code is _____.

3. For hysteroscopy with removal of leiomyomata, the CPT code is _____.

4. For total abdominal hysterectomy with partial vaginectomy, the CPT code is _____.

5. For achillotomy, the CPT index cross-reference for main term Achillotomy is _____.

9.3 – CPT Symbols

Instructions: Interpret the use of CPT symbols to respond to each case.

1. A 60-year-old patient presents to the office for a vaccination, and the coder notices a flash symbol before the code to be assigned. The flash symbol means it is pending FDA _____.

2. A 37-year-old patient presents to a local hospital for the birth of a second child. After a difficult labor, the patient undergoes a cesarean section. The patient also undergoes a subtotal hysterectomy due to endometriosis. Codes 59510 and 59525 are reported. The plus symbol that precedes code 59525 means it is a(n) _____ code, and modifier 51 is not added to the code.

3. A patient undergoes genetics counseling for a period of 30 minutes. Code 96040 is reported. The star symbol precedes code 96040, which means that a synchronous _____ service was rendered via a real-time interactive audio and video telecommunications system, and modifier 95 must be added to the code.

4. A patient presents to the emergency department (ED) following an accident in the garage. The patient was working under the car when the jack failed, and the car fell on the patient's chest. Codes 99283 and 44500 are reported for the ED visit. The forbidden symbol precedes code 44500, which means that modifier _____ is not added to the code.

5. Patient underwent radical resection of tumor, scapula. Code 23210 is reported. The semicolon symbol in the code description is used to save space. The description of code 23210 is Radical resection of tumor; _____.

9.4 – CPT Modifiers

Instructions: Assign a CPT modifier to each case.

1. A patient undergoes simple repair of multiple skin lacerations, left foot and toes. The patient also undergoes intermediate repair of left heel laceration. The patient is discharged home after suturing, bandaging, and placing in a soft cast. Codes assigned include 12041 and 12002. Modifier _____ is added to code 12002.

2. An 80-year-old patient undergoes bilateral mastotomy with deep exploration. Code 19020 is assigned. Modifier _____ is added to code 19020.

3. A patient undergoes magnetic resonance imaging (MRI), lower left leg. Dr. Miller interprets the MRI and documents a report. Modifier _____ is added to the CPT code reported for the MRI.

4. Patient underwent incision and drainage (I&D) of a Bartholin's gland abscess done on April 5. The global period is 30 days. The abscess recurred; on April 28, the patient underwent repeat I&D by the same surgeon. Code 56420 was reported for the procedure performed on April 5. Modifier _____ is added to code 56420 for the procedure performed on April 28.

5. A patient underwent biopsy of the prostate gland on October 11, performed by Dr. Smith. The global period is zero days. The pathology results were of uncertain behavior; per the pathologist's recommendations, the patient underwent repeat biopsy on November 15, by Dr. Jones, to obtain a larger sample. Code 55700 was reported for the procedure performed on October 11. Modifier _____ is added to code 55700 for the procedure performed on November 15.

10 CPT Evaluation and Management

Chapter Outline

Overview of Evaluation and Management
Section

Evaluation and Management Section Guidelines

Evaluation and Management Categories and
Subcategories

Chapter Objectives

At the conclusion of this chapter, the student should be able to:

1. Define key terms related to the CPT Evaluation and Management section.
2. Explain the organization of the CPT Evaluation and Management section.
3. Interpret CPT Evaluation and Management section guidelines.
4. Assign CPT Evaluation and Management service codes and modifiers.

Key Terms

advance care planning

care plan oversight
services

case management

concurrent care

consultation

counseling

critical care

delivery/birthing
room attendance
and resuscitation
services

emergency department
service

established patient

face-to-face time

home or residence
services

hospital inpatient and
observation care
service

inpatient neonatal
and pediatric critical
care and intensive
service

medical decision making
(MDM)

newborn care services

new patient

non-face-to-face time

observation care service

office or other outpatient
services

pediatric critical care
patient transport

place of service (POS)

preventive medicine
services

prolonged services

special evaluation
and management
services

standby service

transfer of care

type of service (TOS)

Introduction

The Evaluation and Management (E/M) section is located at the beginning of the CPT coding manual because the codes describe services most frequently provided by physicians and other qualified health care professionals. This makes it easier to locate these frequently reported codes. Accurate assignment of E/M codes is essential to the success of a provider's practice because most revenue generated by the office is based on provision of these services. Before assigning E/M codes, review the guidelines (located at the beginning of the E/M section) and apply any notes (located below category and subcategory titles).

 Coding Tip

Notes located beneath categories and subcategories in the CPT coding manual apply to all codes in the categories or subcategories. Parenthetical notes that are located below a specific code apply to that code only unless the note indicates otherwise.

Most E/M services are cognitive services. This means that the provider must acquire information from the patient, use reasoning skills to process the information, interact with the patient to provide feedback, and respond by creating an appropriate plan of care. E/M services do *not* include significant procedural services (e.g., diagnostic tests or surgical procedures), which are coded separately. However, some services that arise directly from the E/M service provided are included (e.g., cleansing traumatic lesions, closing lacerations with adhesive strips, applying dressings, and providing counseling and educational services), and they are not assigned separate CPT codes.

 NOTE:

The *Medicare National Correct Coding Initiative Policy Manual* provides guidance about assigning procedure codes for the Evaluation and Management section. Go to **www.cms.gov** and enter "Medicare NCCI Policy Manual" in the Search box to navigate to the manual.

Overview of Evaluation and Management Section

The E/M section contains health care categories (e.g., hospital inpatient), which are subdivided into subcategories of services (e.g., initial hospital care, subsequent hospital care). Each subcategory includes E/M services that contain codes and descriptions, which are based on level of medical decision making *or* time. The E/M section is organized according to *place of service (POS)* (e.g., office), *type of service (TOS)* (e.g., preventive medicine service), *content of service* (e.g., medical decision making *or* time), and miscellaneous services (e.g., prolonged services, care plan oversight). The E/M *level of service* reflects the amount of work involved in providing health care to a patient, and correct coding requires the provider to document (1) a medically appropriate history and examination and (2) the level of medical decision making (MDM) for the encounter *or* the total time spent providing services on the date of encounter.

Documentation in the patient record must support the E/M level of service reported. The Centers for Medicare & Medicaid Services (CMS) often refers to E/M codes by level numbers, which often corresponds to the last digit of the CPT code (e.g., 99203 is a level 3 E/M service).

Accurate assignment of E/M codes depends on: (1) identifying the place of service (POS) and type of service (TOS) provided to the patient, (2) determining whether the patient is new or established, (3) reviewing the patient's record for documentation, and (4) using medical decision making *or* time on the date of service to select an appropriate code.

> **Example:** Refer to the Office or Other Outpatient Services category in the E/M section, and notice that it contains two subcategories:
>
> - New patient (contains four codes)
> - Established patient (contains five codes)
>
> Each code represents a level of E/M service, ranked from lowest to highest level. CMS would consider E/M code 99204 a level 4 service.

 NOTE:

- Documentation of a medically appropriate history and examination is required, and E/M code selection will focus on documentation of level of medical decision making *or* time spent on the date of encounter.

Place of Service (POS)

Place of service (POS) refers to the physical location where health care is provided to patients (e.g., office or other outpatient settings, hospitals, nursing facilities, or emergency departments).

> **Example 1:** The provider treated the patient in the office.
> *Place of Service*: Office
> *E/M Category*: Office or Other Outpatient Services

> **Example 2:** The patient received care in the hospital's emergency department.
> *Place of Service*: Hospital Emergency Department
> *E/M Category*: Emergency Department Services

Type of Service (TOS)

Type of service (TOS) refers to the kind of health care services provided to patients (e.g., critical care, hospital inpatient or observation care, nursing facility care, and preventive care).

> **Example 1:** The patient underwent an annual physical examination in the provider's office.
> *Type of Service*: Preventive care
> *E/M Category*: Preventive Medicine Services

> **Example 2:** The hospital inpatient was transferred to the regular medical-surgical unit for recovery from surgery. Patient suddenly stopped breathing and required respirator management by the provider.
> *Type of Service*: Critical care
> *E/M Category*: Critical Care Services

Sometimes *both the TOS and POS* must be identified before the proper code can be assigned.

Example 1: Dr. Smith completed the patient's history and physical examination on the first day of a hospital inpatient admission.

 Place of Service: Hospital

 Type of Service: Initial inpatient care

 E/M Category: Hospital Inpatient or Observation Care Services

 E/M Subcategory: Initial Hospital Inpatient or Observation Care

 E/M Heading: New or Established Patient

Example 2: Dr. Charles saw a new patient (age 38) in the office to perform an annual physical examination.

 Place of Service: Office

 Type of Service: Preventive medicine

 E/M Category: Preventive Medicine Services

 E/M Subcategory: New Patient

 Coding Tip

The CPT Medicine section includes codes describing specialty services (e.g., ophthalmology, psychiatry) that require E/M. When codes for specialty services are reported, a separate E/M service from the CPT E/M section is *not* reported on the same date *unless a significant, separately identifiable E/M service is provided (and modifier 25 is attached).*

Exercise 10.1 – Overview of Evaluation and Management Section

Instructions: Use your CPT coding manual to complete each statement.

1. When a 49-year-old patient is seen in the provider's office for an annual physical examination, the coder should refer to the E/M category entitled _____ Medicine Services.

2. For a 24-year-old patient who received immediate care in the hospital emergency room, the coder should refer to the E/M category entitled _____ Department Services.

3. E/M services codes are based on an appropriate medical history and examination plus time or level of medical decision _____.

4. CMS often refers to E/M codes by level numbers, and the level often corresponds to the last digit of the CPT code. Therefore, code 99215 is a level _____ service.

5. The physical location where health care services are provided to patients is called the _____ of service.

6. The kind of health care services provided to patients is called the _____ of service.

7–10. Elanie Ibraham was seen in the primary care provider's office two months ago and underwent a routine physical examination. The patient returns to the office today with complaints of severe abdominal pain and discomfort. Diagnostic testing revealed Crohn's disease, and a treatment plan was discussed. Identify each of the following for services provided to the patient today.

(continues)

Exercise 10.1 – continued

7. Type of Service: _____ encounter (or visit)

8. Place of Service: physician's _____

9. E/M Category: _____ or Other Outpatient Services

10. E/M Subcategory: _____ patient

Evaluation and Management Section Guidelines

Evaluation and management (E/M) services *guidelines* are general instructions about the assignment of E/M section codes. Reviewing E/M guidelines (and notes) is necessary to the appropriate assignment of E/M codes.

The E/M section guidelines are located at the beginning of the section and include the following:

- E/M guidelines overview
- Classification of Evaluation and Management (E/M) services
- Levels of E/M services
- Unlisted service
- Special report

E/M Guidelines Overview

E/M guidelines apply to most of its categories and subcategories, and separate notes are located below applicable categories and subcategories.

Classification of E/M Services

The E/M section is organized into categories (e.g., office or other outpatient visits) and subcategories (e.g., new patient, established patient). Code descriptions include place and type of service and level of medical decision making *or* time typically required to provide the service. E/M codes often use the last number of each CPT code to represent the level of E/M service provided. Levels within categories and subcategories are not interchangeable. For example, CPT code 99202 is a level 2 office or other outpatient E/M service reported for new patients.

The E/M section contains phrases and definitions for the purpose of selecting an appropriate code.

- New patient and established patient
- Initial and subsequent services
- Split or shared visits
- Multiple evaluation and management services on the same date
- Services reported separately
- History and examination

New and Established Patient

A **new patient** is one who has *not* received any professional services from the physician or qualified health care professional of the exact same specialty and subspecialty who belongs to the same group practice, within the past three years.

An **established patient** is one who *has* received professional services from the physician or other qualified health care professional of the same exact specialty and subspecialty who belongs to the same group practice, within the past three years.

When a physician or other qualified health care professional covers for or is on call for a physician or other qualified health care professional, the encounter is coded as if the responsible physician or other qualified health care professional has provided services. Also, because of the nature of work associated with emergency department care, the E/M Emergency Department Services category does *not* distinguish between new and established patients.

 Coding Tip

- *Professional services* are face-to-face and non-face-to-face services provided by physicians and other qualified health care professionals (e.g., nurse practitioner, physician assistant).

- Definitions of new and established patients include professional services rendered by other physicians and other qualified health care professionals of the exact same specialty and subspecialty in the same group practice.

- CPT Evaluation and Management section guidelines contain a decision tree that can be used to determine new versus established patients.

Example 1: Kerry requested that a prescription be renewed by Dr. Smith's office on January 1, 2023, but did not see the physician. Kerry has been Dr. Smith's patient since an initial office visit on March 15, 2020. On December 1, 2022, Dr. Smith had treated Kerry during an office visit.

New Patient: March 15, 2020

Established Patient: December 1, 2022, and January 1, 2023

Example 2: Dr. Charles and Dr. Black share a practice. Dr. Charles is a general surgeon who treated Alex in the office on July 1, 2022. Alex was first seen by the practice on February 15, 2019, when Dr. Black, also a general surgeon, provided preventive care services. Alex returned to the practice on November 1, 2022, for an annual physical examination conducted by Dr. Black.

New Patient: February 15, 2019, and July 1, 2022.

Established Patient: November 1, 2022

Example 3: Dr. Corey left Southern Tier Physician's Group to join Buffalo Physician Group as a family practitioner. At Buffalo Physician Group, when Dr. Corey provides professional services to patients, are those patients considered new or established?

Answer: Patients who have not received professional services from Dr. Corey or other qualified health care professionals or other physicians of the exact same specialty and subspecialty at Buffalo Physician Group are considered new.

Patients who have been treated by such a provider at Buffalo Physician Group within the past three years are considered established. If any of Dr. Corey's patients from the Southern Tier Physician's Group choose to seek care from Dr. Corey or another physician of the same specialty and subspecialty at the Buffalo Physician Group (and services were provided to them during the past three years), they will be considered established patients.

Initial and Subsequent Services

Some E/M categories (e.g., hospital inpatient services) differentiate services according to whether initial or subsequent services were provided. An initial service is a face-to-face service (e.g., inpatient, observation, nursing facility admission) that is provided to a patient who has not yet received services from a physician or other qualified health care professional in the same specialty or subspecialty. A subsequent service is a face-to-face service (e.g., inpatient, observation, nursing facility stay) that is provided to a patient who has already received services from a physician or other qualified health care professional in the same specialty or subspecialty. For reporting purposes (on CMS-1500 and UB-04 claims), the transition of a patient from the following levels of care is considered a single stay.

- Observation to inpatient care
- Skilled nursing to another nursing facility level of care (e.g., custodial care, intermediate care)

Split or Shared Visits

Physicians and other qualified health care professionals who act as a team during the provision of patient care must apply the *split or shared visits* guideline to determine which provider reports the service for reimbursement. When code selection is based on:

- Medical decision making (MDM), the provider who performed a substantive part of MDM for the number and complexity of problems addressed and who takes responsibility for the care plan that includes risk of complications, morbidity, or mortality of patient management reports the service.
- Time, the provider who spent the majority of face-to-face or non-face-to-face time providing services reports the service.

The amount and complexity of data reviewed and analyzed is used by the provider to select the appropriate E/M code level. In addition, when an independent interpretation of tests and discussion of the management plan or interpretation of tests is performed by the provider, they are used for selection of the appropriate E/M code level.

Multiple Evaluation and Management Services on the Same Date

Patients may receive E/M services in multiple settings (e.g., hospital inpatient care, observation care, nursing facility care) on the same date *or* more than one encounter in the same setting on the same date. When services are provided by the same physician or other qualified health care professional (QHP), including another physician or QHP of the same speciality in a group practice, the following *multiple evaluation and management services on the same date* guidelines apply for reporting purposes. (Refer to the CPT E/M section for details about each guideline.)

- Per day
- Multiple encounters in different settings or facilities
- Emergency department (ED) and services in other settings (same or different facilities)
- Discharge services and services in other facilities
- Discharge services and services in the same facility
- Discharge services and services in a different facility
- Critical care services (including neonatal intensive care services and pediatric and neonatal critical care)
- Transitions between office or other outpatient, home or residence, or emergency department and hospital inpatient or observation or nursing facility

Services Reported Separately

When procedures and services are provided on the same date as a separately identifiable E/M service, the additional procedures and services may be reported.

Example: While being provided with preventive services, the patient asked the provider about symptoms of headache, shortness of breath, and feeling tired. A COVID-19 laboratory test was performed. In addition to an appropriate code for the E/M preventive service, codes for an office or other outpatient E/M service (adding modifier 25 for the significantly, separately identifiable service by same physician on same date) and a COVID-19 laboratory test were reported.

History and Examination

Some E/M services require documentation of a medically appropriate history and examination, the nature and extent of which is determined by the provider. The health care team (e.g., nurse, medical assistant) may collect the information (e.g., chief complaint, history of presenting illness, past history, medication history, vital signs), and the patient can also complete a health care questionnaire or use an electronic health record portal to provide information. The provider is responsible for reviewing all information collected, documenting additional relevant medically appropriate history and examination elements, and authenticating the completed report.

Level of E/M Service

Evaluation and management codes use the last number of each CPT code to represent the level of E/M service. Levels within categories and subcategories are not interchangeable, and each level of E/M service may be reported by physicians or other qualified health care professionals.

> **Example:** CPT code 99202 classifies a level 2 office or other outpatient E/M service reported for new patients, and it requires a medically appropriate history and examination and straightforward medical decision making. Should time be used for code selection, 15 minutes must be met or exceeded on the date of service by the physician or other qualified health care professional is required. CPT code 99211 classifies a level 1 office or other outpatient E/M service reported for established patients, and it is reported when the presence of the physician or other qualified health care professional may *not* be required (e.g., office nurse takes patient's blood pressure and documents it in the record).

Concurrent Care, Transfer of Care, and Counseling

Concurrent care is the provision of similar services, such as hospital inpatient visits, to the same patient by more than one physician or other qualified health care professional on the same day. CMS permits the provision of concurrent care by two or more providers on the same day even if the providers are of the same specialty. To avoid reimbursement denials by third-party payers and Medicare administrative contractors, the attending physician is to add modifier AI (Principal Physician of Record) to the E/M code reported. When possible, each provider should also report different ICD-10-CM diagnosis codes from those reported by other providers who provide E/M services to the patient on the same day.

> **Example:** Laurie was admitted to the hospital on October 5 for an acute myocardial infarction. On October 7, the attending physician (a cardiologist) wrote a physician's order requesting a psychiatrist to consult with the patient regarding anxiety and depression. The cardiologist's insurance specialist should report the ICD-10-CM code for "acute myocardial infarction" to justify inpatient E/M services provided to the patient (and add modifier AI, Principal Physician of Record, to the CPT code reported). The psychiatrist's insurance specialist should report the ICD-10-CM codes for "anxiety and depression" to justify inpatient consultation E/M services provided to the patient. If each provider reported the ICD-10-CM code for "acute myocardial infarction," the provider who submitted the claim first would be reimbursed (and the other provider's claim would be denied).

> **Transfer of care** occurs when a provider who is managing some or all of a patient's problems relinquishes that responsibility to another provider who explicitly agrees to accept this responsibility and who, from the initial encounter, is *not* providing consultative services. The provider transferring care no longer manages these problems but may continue to manage other conditions.

> **Example:** The patient was admitted to the hospital on March 1 by a surgeon for total thyroidectomy that was performed on March 2. During admission, the patient's severe anxiety and depression was initially co-managed with a psychiatrist. Late evening on March 2, the attending physician transferred management of the patient's anxiety and depression to the psychiatrist. At discharge on March 5, the attending physician reported CPT surgery codes for the total thyroidectomy surgery and CPT E/M codes for management of the thyroid condition. The psychiatrist reported CPT E/M codes for management of the patient's anxiety and depression.

(continues)

Concurrent Care, Transfer of Care, and Counseling (*continued*)

CPT has defined **counseling** as a "discussion with a patient and family concerning one or more of the following areas: diagnostic results, impressions, and recommended diagnostic studies; prognosis; risks and benefits of management (treatment) options; instructions for management (treatment) and follow-up; importance of compliance with chosen management (treatment) options; risk factor reduction; and patient and family education."

> **Example:** Weight management counseling services provided to a patient during an E/M encounter visit must be properly documented, along with other required elements, so that the appropriate E/M code can be selected.

Exercise 10.2 – Evaluation and Management Section Guidelines

Instructions: Complete each statement.

1. Tim was seen by Dr. Chambers on February 5 of this year for follow-up of type 2 diabetes mellitus. Tim has been Dr. Chambers' patient since 1984 and was seen for an initial visit that year. Tim returned to the office each year since 1984 for an annual physical examination until last year, when diagnosed with type 2 diabetes mellitus. Since then, Tim has returned for a recheck office visit with Dr. Chambers every three months. Tim is considered a(n) _____ (new or established) patient for Dr. Chambers' practice.

2. Kristin was seen by Dr. Martinez on March 8 six years ago for treatment of influenza. Kristin returned on January 5 one year later for an annual physical examination, which included a prescription for birth control pills. Kristin called the office on April 10 of that same year to request that the local pharmacy be called to refill birth control pills. Dr. Martinez called in the prescription that afternoon. Kristin next returned to the office on April 15 of this year for an annual physical examination. Kristin is considered a(n) _____ (new or established) patient for Dr. Martinez's practice.

3. Dr. Peterson, Dr. Slatterly, and Dr. Vaughan are members of the Medex Pediatric Group Practice. Eric is a 15-year-old boy who was initially seen by Dr. Vaughan on August 5 of last year for a sports physical. Eric returned to the office on September 10 of this year and was seen by Dr. Peterson for treatment of an ear infection. Eric is considered a(n) _____ (new or established) patient for Dr. Peterson's practice.

4–5. The patient was admitted to the hospital on July 4 for treatment of a fractured pelvis, which was sustained while parasailing earlier in the day. On July 5, the attending physician (an orthopedic surgeon) wrote a physician's order requesting a neurologist to consult with the patient regarding numbness of the left foot.

    4. The orthopedic surgeon reports the diagnosis of _____ pelvis to justify inpatient E/M services.

    5. The neurologist reports the diagnosis of _____, left foot, to justify inpatient E/M consultation services.

Levels of E/M Services

The level of E/M service is based on:

- Medical decision making, or
- Time

Medical Decision Making

Medical decision making (MDM) involves assessing the status of a patient's condition, establishing diagnoses, and selecting a management option. (The concept of medical decision making does *not* apply to code 99211.) The four levels of medical decision making include straightforward, low, moderate, and high, and the following elements are considered when selecting an appropriate level of medical decision making:

- Number and complexity of problems addressed during an encounter
- Amount and complexity of data to be reviewed and analyzed
- Risk of complications, morbidity, and mortality of patient management

> **Example:** An Alzheimer's patient who presents for management of diagnosed pneumonia receives evaluation and management services from the physician. The physician documented a medically appropriate history and examination and discussed possible disease management options with the patient's family, including the patient's desire for palliative care. (During the year prior to the Alzheimer's diagnosis, the patient established an advance directive for the health care proxy, which included a do not resuscitate [DNR] order.) The physician would refer to the medical decision making (MDM) table in the CPT E/M guidelines to determine the level of MDM for code selection purposes. If a moderate level of MDM is determined, report code 99214 (Office or other outpatient visit for the evaluation and management of an established patient, which requires a medically appropriate history and examination and moderate level of medical decision making. When using time for code selection, 30 minutes must be met or exceeded on the date of the encounter).

 Coding Tip

The CPT E/M guidelines contain definitions for elements of medical decision making, such as problem, problem addressed, minimal problem, self-limited or minor problem, stable/chronic illness, and many more. Careful review of all definitions is required to determine the level of medical decision making.

The *number and complexity of the problems addressed during an encounter* include:

- When multiple new or established conditions and diagnoses are medically managed or treated during the same encounter, they may affect medical decision making. For example, an older patient with chronic bronchitis who is diagnosed with influenza may require a higher level of medical decision making.
- While signs and symptoms are often associated with a specific condition or diagnosis, each sign or symptom is not necessarily a unique condition. For example, a patient presents with a fever, cough, and body aches, and is diagnosed with influenza; the fever and cough are signs, and the body aches are symptoms, all of which indicate the presence of influenza as the condition.
- Comorbidities (underlying and chronic diseases) are not considered when selecting a level of E/M service *except* when they are medically managed or treated and their presence increases the amount and complexity of data to be reviewed and analyzed or risk of complications and morbidity or mortality of patient management. For example, a patient with comorbidities of diabetes mellitus and hypertension that are well managed is diagnosed with bacterial pneumonia; because the patient's comorbidities are well managed, the amount/complexity of data to be reviewed/analyzed is not increased, and the risk of complications and morbidity or mortality of patient management of the bacterial pneumonia diagnosis is likewise not increased.
- A diagnosis does not, in and of itself, determine complexity or risk because extensive evaluation might be required to conclude that signs or symptoms do not represent a highly morbid condition. For example, the patient presents with a host of signs of symptoms that require extensive testing, with a resultant diagnosis of chronic fatigue syndrome.
- Presenting signs and symptoms that represent a highly morbid condition may "drive" MDM even when the ultimate diagnosis is not highly morbid. For example, a patient presents with severe chest pain and after an electrocardiogram and x-rays, the patient is diagnosed with a diaphragmatic hernia. The severe chest pain is a symptom of a myocardial infarction, which the patient did not experience; however, that symptom represents a highly morbid condition (even though the final diagnosis of diaphragmatic hernia represents a condition that is not highly morbid and can be treated conservatively).

- Evaluation and treatment provided should be consistent with the likely nature of the condition. For example, a patient presents with a swollen ankle and states they have been limping because the ankle hurts. A diagnosis of sprained ankle is consistent with such signs and symptoms (as opposed to possible cancer).

- Multiple problems of a lower severity may, in the aggregate, create higher risk due to interaction. For example, an adult patient presents with a fever of 103 degrees and what they describe as a severe rash of the right lower extremity; the patient is diagnosed with cellulitis. That fever in an adult is extremely high and, therefore, very serious. The patient's description of the rash led to a diagnosis of cellulitis once the physician examined the patient. If the patient had not sought evaluation and management, the cellulitis diagnosis may not have been established and the patient has the potential of developing sepsis (which would require inpatient hospitalization and could result in the patient's death).

The *amount and complexity of data to be reviewed and analyzed* include medical records, ancillary tests, and other information that must be obtained, ordered, reviewed, and analyzed for an encounter. Other information includes that obtained from multiple sources, interprofessional communications not reported separately, and interpretation of tests not reported separately. The ordering of ancillary tests and the review of test results is part of an encounter (and is not considered a subsequent encounter). The ordering of ancillary tests includes those considered but not actually ordered after shared decision making (e.g., physician assistant in discussion with a physician). Data are subdivided into the following categories:

- Tests, documents, orders, and independent historians
- Independent interpretation of tests
- Discussion of management or interpretation of tests with external physician, other qualified health care professional, or another appropriate source

The *risk of complications and morbidity or mortality of patient management decisions* made at the visit and associated with patient problems, diagnostic procedures, and treatments include possible management options selected plus options considered but not selected. This is a process that is determined after shared medical decision making with the patient and family. For example, an older patient who lives alone may be discharged home (instead of to a nursing facility) when home health care is arranged and family and community support are provided. For example, the physician or other qualified health care professional considers prescription drug management, decision for surgery, decision for hospitalization or escalation of hospital inpatient-level care, and decision to not resuscitate or to de-escalate care because of poor prognosis when managing risk.

Remember! The term "risk" relates to risk of complications and morbidity (and even mortality) from the patient's condition or diagnosis, not the risk of medical management provided.

 NOTE:

Refer to CPT coding manual E/M guidelines and *Table 1: Levels of Medical Decision Making (MDM)*, which assists in determining the appropriate level of MDM needed for assigning a code.

The provider is responsible for determining the level of medical decision making, and that decision must be supported by documentation in the patient's chart. CPT includes E/M guidelines that can assist in determining level of medical decision making. The level of medical decision making is selected as follows:

- Straightforward
- Low
- Moderate
- High

Example 1: Determining the level of medical decision making requires complete documentation. Review the progress note to identify:

- Diagnoses documented.
- Whether data were reviewed.
- Management options available to treat the patient.
- Any risk of complications, morbidity, or mortality.

PROGRESS NOTE

SUBJECTIVE: The patient describes an upset stomach for the past five days, and that it just won't go away. The patient denies recent changes in dietary habits or activities. Patient is very upset about recent events in the news.

OBJECTIVE: GI: Normal bowel sounds. No rigidity. Some pain upon deep organ palpation. No organomegaly. Upon review of the record, it is noted that the patient has not complained about this problem in the past.

ASSESSMENT: Dyspepsia due to anxiety.

PLAN: (1) Gaviscon Extra Strength Relief Formula Liquid, 2 to 4 teaspoonfuls 4 times a day after meals and at bedtime. Follow with half a glass of water or other liquid. (2) Referral to Taylor Kaplan, PhD, Clinical Psychologist. (3) Follow-up appointment in one month.

Notice that documentation included a review of data, a diagnosis, and management options. The risk of complications, morbidity, or mortality were not documented.

Example 2: Selecting a level of E/M service is determined by the level of medical decision making for a male patient who was referred by his primary care provider to a specialist; office consultation E/M services were provided to the patient.

SUBJECTIVE: The patient is a 35-year-old new male patient seen today, at the request of his primary care physician, to evaluate his chief complaint of severe snoring. He says that this has gone on for years and that he's finally ready to do something about it because he wakes up frequently during the night from it. He wakes up in the morning feeling very tired and notices that he gets very tired during the day. Review of systems reveals allergies. Denies smoking or alcohol use. He is on no medications.

OBJECTIVE: Blood pressure is 126/86. Pulse is 82. Weight is 185. EYES: Pupils equal, round, and reactive to light and accommodation; extraocular muscles intact. EARS & NOSE: Tympanic membranes normal; oropharynx benign, large uvula. NECK: Supple without jugular venous distention, bruits, or thyromegaly. RESPIRATORY: Breath sounds are clear to percussion and auscultation. EXTREMITIES: Without edema; pulses intact.

ASSESSMENT: Possible sleep apnea. Severe snoring.

PLAN: Patient to undergo sleep study in two weeks. Results to be evaluated to determine whether patient is candidate for laser-assisted uvuloplasty (LAUP) surgery. The written consultation report, including the plan, will be sent to the patient's primary care provider.

To assign the E/M code, the following is determined:

- NEW OR ESTABLISHED PATIENT: The descriptions for all consultation codes include new or established patients. The 35-year old male patient in this example is a *new patient.*
- LEVEL OF MEDICAL DECISION MAKING: CPT's *Table 1: Levels of Medical Decision Making (MDM)*, located in the Evaluation and Management Section Guidelines, contains elements that are used to determine the level of MDM. Two of three elements determine the level of MDM, and for this example the level of MDM is *straightforward*, based on the following:
  - *Number and complexity of problems addressed at the encounter* is *moderate* because "possible sleep apnea" is a previously undiagnosed problem with an uncertain prognosis.

(continued)

- ○ *Amount and/or complexity of data to be reviewed and analyzed* is *minimal or none* because while a sleep study was ordered, its results were not reviewed by the provider during this encounter.

- ○ *Risk of complications and/or morbidity or mortality of patient management* is *low risk of morbidity from additional diagnostic testing or treatment* because while a decision regarding minor surgery will be made after the results of the sleep study are documented, the provider did not document *identified patient or procedure risk factors*.

- • E/M CODE ASSIGNED: 99242

Time

The amount of time a physician or other qualified health care professional spends providing patient care may be used to select an appropriate level of E/M service code. Beginning with CPT 2023, time alone may be used to select an appropriate level of office or other outpatient E/M service code for many E/M categories, such as:

- • Office or other outpatient services
- • Hospital inpatient and observation care services
- • Consultations
- • Nursing facilities services
- • Home or residence services
- • Prolonged services

 NOTE:

Time alone is *not* used to select an emergency department (ED) evaluation and management level of service because of the (1) severity of illness and intensity of services (SI/IS) associated with ED patients, and (2) requirement that ED physicians provide services to multiple patients during an extended period of time.

When time is used to determine an appropriate E/M services codes, the code description provides guidance about the length of time required to select a level of service. Time, for coding purposes, is defined as the total time on the date of the encounter. It includes both face-to-face and non-face-to-face time spent by physicians and other qualified health care professionals who provide services, on the date of the encounter. When a shared or split visit is performed by two or more providers, the distinct time is to be summed. Only the time of one individual should be reported when two or more providers jointly meet with or discuss the patient. Activities performed by clinical staff (e.g., medical assistant, nurse) are not included in the reported time.

- • **Face-to-face time** requires the physician or other qualified health care professional to spend time with the patient, family, or caregiver.

- • **Non-face-to-face time** requires the physician or other qualified health care professional to perform activities that require their participation (e.g., interpreting tests results, writing physician orders for hospital inpatient services). Do *not* count time spent on the performance of other services that are reported separately (using another CPT code), teaching that is general and not limited to that required for the management of a specific patient, or travel.

Example: The attending physician of a hospital inpatient spends *face-to-face time* at the patient's bedside (e.g., examining the patient, performing a review of systems, explaining test results, providing treatment options) and *non-face-to-face time* managing the patient's care at the inpatient unit station (e.g., reviewing tests results, documenting physician orders for diagnostic tests or procedures).

The following activities count toward total time when provided by the physician or other qualified health care professional:

- Care coordination (that is not separately reported using another E/M code)
- Counseling and educating patient, family, or caregiver
- Documenting clinical information in medical record
- Independently interpreting results of ancillary tests (that are not separately reported using another CPT code) and communicating those results to patient, family, or caregiver
- Obtaining and reviewing separately obtained history
- Ordering medications, tests, and procedures
- Performing medically appropriate examination or evaluation
- Preparing to see patient (e.g., reviewing results of ancillary tests)
- Referring patient to and communicating with other health care professionals (when not separately reported with another E/M code)

A *shared or split visit* is defined as an encounter during which the physician and other qualified health care professionals spend face-to-face and non-face-to-face time providing services. The total time spent by the physician and other qualified health care professionals is used to select the appropriate E/M level of service. Activities include patient assessment, management, counseling, and education, and communicating results to patient (or family, caregiver, or guardian) on the date of encounter. When physicians and other qualified health care professionals provide *prolonged services* (e.g., additional time over and above the selected E/M category code), an appropriate E/M prolonged services code may also be reported with the E/M level of service code. Ultimately, it is the provider who is responsible for documenting the total time spent providing services on the date of encounter to justify the level of service code selected.

Unlisted Service

An unlisted service code is assigned when an E/M service is provided for which there is no CPT code (e.g., 99499). When an unlisted procedure or service code is reported, a special report (e.g., copy of documented encounter record) must accompany the claim to describe the nature of, extent of, and need for the procedure or service.

 Coding Tip

Payers often require providers to report HCPCS Level II codes (if available) instead of unlisted procedure or service CPT codes.

Special Report

When an unlisted service code is reported, a special report must be submitted with the insurance claim to demonstrate medical appropriateness. The provider should document the following elements in the special report:

- Complexity of patient's symptoms
- Description of nature of, extent of, and need for service
- Diagnostic and therapeutic procedures performed
- Follow-up care
- Patient's final diagnosis and concurrent problems
- Pertinent physical findings
- Time, effort, and equipment required to provide the service

Exercise 10.3 – Levels of E/M Services and Medical Decision Making

Instructions: Complete each of the following.

1. Which code is reported for a level 3 emergency department service?_____

2. An 89-year-old diabetic patient presented to the hospital emergency room for level 4 evaluation and management of a very painful lower left arm. An x-ray revealed left ulnar fracture. An appropriate medical history and examination was performed, and moderate level of medical decision making was documented. During the encounter, the physician reduced the fracture and applied a short-arm cast (for which a CPT Surgery section code was reported.)

   a. Should an E/M code also be reported for this case? (Yes or No) _____

   b. If so, which code and modifier are reported? (Enter None if no code is reported.)

      _____

3. A 14-year-old patient presented to the primary care provider's office for treatment of a 3 centimeter laceration, which the physician sutured. The physician also administered a tetanus toxoid after confirming that the patient's tetanus immunization status was not up-to-date. Codes for suture repair of the laceration and administration of the tetanus toxoid were assigned from the CPT Surgery and Medicine sections, respectively.

   a. Should an E/M code also be reported for this case? (Yes or No) _____

   b. If so, which code is reported? (Enter None if no code is reported.) _____

4. Dr. Martinez performed a level 3 E/M service to treat an 18-year-old patient in the office for a urinary tract infection. The last time the patient was seen by Dr. Martinez was three months ago during a preventive medicine encounter. Urine culture revealed *Escherichia coli* bacteria. The patient was prescribed antibiotics and instructed to return for recheck in 10 days.

   a. The CPT E/M category is Office or Other Outpatient Services, and the subcategory is _____ Patient.

   b. The appropriate CPT code is _____.

5. Use the case below to assign the E/M consultation code, which requires you to identify the level of medical decision making.

   SUBJECTIVE: A 54-year-old patient is seen in the office by an endocrine specialist for evaluation and management of type 1 diabetes mellitus; the patient also has hypertension. The patient was referred by the primary care provider (PCP) for an opinion about treatment. The patient has no new complaints today and denies chest pain, headache, numbness of the extremities, shortness of breath, or visual changes. The patient has remained on the diet recommended during the last E/M visit with the PCP and regular exercise is part of the daily routine. Home monitoring of blood pressure and glucose levels are within normal limits.

   OBJECTIVE: Blood pressure 130/78. Weight 145. Pulse 78, regular. HEAD, EYES, EARS, NOSE, THROAT: Pupils equal, round, and reactive to light and accommodation. External auditory canals and tympanic membranes negative. Oropharynx benign. NECK: Supple. No bruits, jugular venous distention, or thyromegaly. CHEST: Breath sounds clear to auscultation and percussion. No rubs, rales, rhonchi, or wheezing. HEART: No click, gallop, irregularity, murmur, or rub. EXTREMITIES: Distal pulses intact. No cyanosis, clubbing, or edema. NEUROLOGICAL: Deep tendon reflexes within normal limits and symmetrical. No decreased lower extremity sensation noted. LAB RESULTS: Fasting blood sugar 132. Urinalysis within normal limits.

(continues)

Exercise 10.3 – continued

ASSESSMENT: Type 1 diabetes mellitus, controlled. Hypertension.

PLAN: Glucotrol 5 milligrams daily, every morning. Procardia XL 30 milligrams daily. Relafen 1,000 milligrams daily. Continue home glucose monitoring. SMA-7 and glycosylated hemoglobin today. Return for routine follow-up in three months.

a. What is the level of medical decision making? _____

b. Which E/M code is assigned? _____

Evaluation and Management Categories and Subcategories

The E/M section contains notes unique to each category and subcategory. *Remember to review notes before assigning an E/M code.* (As discussed in Chapter 9, CPT refers to E/M subsections and categories as categories and subcategories, respectively.)

Office or Other Outpatient Services

The *Office or Other Outpatient Services* category of E/M includes the following subcategories:

- New Patient
- Established Patient

Office or other outpatient services are provided in a physician or other provider's office, a hospital outpatient department, or another ambulatory care facility (e.g., stand-alone ambulatory care center). Before assigning an E/M service code from this category, make sure you apply the definition of *new* and *established patient* and consider the following:

- When a patient receives two E/M services from the same provider on the same day and the patient's problem is the same for each encounter, report just one E/M service. (Providers in the same group practice who are in the same exact specialty and same subspecialty submit claims as though they are a single provider.) This means that when E/M office or other outpatient services are provided to the same patient multiple times on the same day for the same problem by the same provider, the highest-level E/M service is reported. *(An exception to this rule is reporting of critical service codes with an E/M service code.)*

- When multiple E/M office or other outpatient services are provided to the same patient on the same day by the same provider and the patient's problems are different for each E/M service, report multiple E/M codes. To justify medical necessity, make sure you link the appropriate diagnosis or condition code to its respective E/M code. Add modifier 25 to the second and subsequent E/M codes.

- When the patient receives office or other outpatient E/M services *on the same day that the patient is admitted to the hospital as an inpatient by the same provider*, report an E/M code for the initial hospital care only. Do not report an office or other outpatient E/M service code.

- When the provider performs a high level of service in the office (e.g., 99205, 99215) and the patient is later admitted to the hospital *on another day as a planned admission*, it may be more appropriate to report a lower-level-of-service initial hospital care E/M code for the hospital admission (because the provider already performed and reported the predominant portion of the E/M during the prior office encounter). (When the patient is admitted on another day but the admission is unplanned, report the appropriate E/M code for the office visit and an appropriate-level-of-service E/M code for the initial hospital care.)

Coding Tip

The provider does not have to redocument the history, review of symptoms, and past/family/social history documented during a previous encounter if the provider documents that the previous information was reviewed and then updates the information. The period of time since the previous encounter should generally be no more than one or two years. In addition, the provider should indicate in the current note where the previous documentation can be found (e.g., Refer to office records dated April 14, YYYY.).

Example 1: Dr. Garcia provides a level 3 E/M service, based on 30 minutes of time, to a new patient in the office for treatment of anxiety. The patient is prescribed medication and referred to a psychologist for therapy. The same patient returns four hours later for anxiety, and Dr. Garcia provides an additional 14 minutes of E/M services. Report code 99203 because the time for both E/M services on the same date of the encounter is totaled (as 30 + 14 = 44 minutes).

Example 2: An 89-year-old established patient receives level 3 E/M services from Dr. James to evaluate prescribed blood pressure medication. The same patient returns five hours later and receives level 4 E/M services from Dr. James to evaluate the patient's hip pain due to falling at home. Report both codes 99213 and 99214 25 because this patient received E/M services for two different problems. (The payer may request copies of the patient record to verify the claim.)

Example 3: An established patient receives level 5 E/M services in the office from Dr. Peterson and is later admitted to the hospital as part of a planned admission, where Dr. Peterson provides level 3 initial hospital care E/M services. The insurance specialist should report code 99223 on the claim for initial hospital inpatient services. (An office or other outpatient services E/M code is not reported when the patient is admitted as a hospital inpatient during the course of an office or other outpatient service.)

Teaching Physicians and Resident Physicians

A *teaching physician* is a physician (other than another resident) who involves and supervises resident physicians in the care of their patients. A *resident physician* (or *resident*) is an individual who participates in an approved graduate medical education (GME) program.

Teaching physicians are no longer required to rewrite in its entirety the key elements of a resident physician's E/M documentation. However, a teaching physician cannot bill for a resident physician's history or physical exam *unless present for a significant portion of the exam*. The teaching physician can select an E/M level of service based on time spent later reviewing the resident's documented history and exam (as part of the medical decision making process), adding it to the history and examination performed by the provider. (These conditions also apply when *any* provider reviews a history and examination performed, for example, six months previously.)

Teaching physicians are also required to substantiate any services reported on a claim by documenting a summary note of services provided personally or directly observed. The summary note can confirm or revise the history of the present illness (HPI), physical examination, and medical decision making activities. (For services such as a single surgical procedure or diagnostic test, the teaching physician can indicate their physical presence during the key portion of the procedure or test.)

Example 1: When all required elements are obtained personally by a teaching physician without a resident present, the teaching physician documents the E/M service as if in a nonteaching setting. The teaching physician's documentation should also include a statement such as, "I performed a history and physical examination of the patient and discussed management with the resident. I reviewed the resident's note and agree with the documented findings and plan of care."

Example 2: When all required elements are obtained by the resident in the presence of or jointly with the teaching physician and documented by the resident, the teaching physician documents their presence during performance of critical or key portion(s) of the service and that they were directly involved in the management of the patient's care. The teaching physician's note should also reference the resident's note. The combination of entries must be adequate to substantiate the level of service billed and the medical necessity of the service. The teaching physician's documentation should also include a statement such as, "I was present with resident during the history and exam. I discussed the case with the resident and agree with the findings and plan of care as documented in the resident's note."

Example 3: When selected required elements of the service (e.g., history and physical examination) are obtained by the resident *in the absence of the teaching physician*, the resident documents the services provided. The teaching physician must independently perform the critical or key portion(s) of the service with or without the resident present and discuss the case with the resident. In this situation, the teaching physician must document that they personally saw the patient, personally performed critical or key portions of the service, and participated in the management of the patient. The teaching physician's note should also reference the resident's note. For payment consideration by the third-party payer, the combined entries of the teaching physician and resident must be adequate to substantiate the level of service billed and the medical necessity of the service. The teaching physician's documentation should also include a statement such as, "I saw and evaluated the patient. Discussed with resident and agree with resident's findings and plan as documented in the resident's note."

Code 99211

Code 99211 is commonly thought of as a "nurse visit" because it is typically reported when ancillary personnel provide E/M services. However, the code can be reported when the E/M service is rendered by any other provider (e.g., nurse practitioner, physician assistant, or physician). CMS "incident to" guidelines apply when the 99211 E/M level of service is provided by ancillary personnel in the office. The guidelines state that the physician and other qualified health care professional must be physically present in the suite of offices when the service is provided. Documentation of a 99211 level of service includes a chief complaint and a description of the service provided. Because the presenting problem is considered of minimal severity, documentation of a history and examination is not required.

Example 1: The office nurse takes and documents the patient's vital signs (blood pressure, height, weight, and body temperature). Report CPT code 99211.

Example 2: The patient comes to the physician's office, and the office nurse administers the monthly intramuscular injection of testosterone enanthate (1 mg) for treatment of male hypogonadism. He had received E/M level 3 services from the physician last week. Report CPT code 96372 (from the Medicine section) and HCPCS Level II national code J3121. Do not report CPT code 99211 because the only service provided was the injection and the patient did not require or receive other E/M services (e.g., taking vital signs). (CPT code 96372 from the Medicine section is reported for the intramuscular injection of the therapeutic, prophylactic, or diagnostic substance.)

Hospital Inpatient and Observation Care Services

Hospital inpatient and observation care services codes are reported by acute care hospitals, inpatient psychiatric facilities, comprehensive inpatient rehabilitation facilities, and partial hospitalization settings. The Hospital Inpatient and Observation Care Services category of E/M includes the following subcategories:

- Initial Hospital Inpatient or Observation Care
- Subsequent Hospital Inpatient or Observation Care
- Hospital Inpatient or Observation Care Services (Including Admissions and Discharge Services)
- Hospital Inpatient or Observation Discharge Services

 NOTE:

When more than one provider (e.g., attending physician and a consultant) delivers inpatient services on the same date of service, the attending physician adds modifier AI (Principal physician of record) to the reported E/M code.

Hospital inpatient and observation care services are provided to hospital inpatients, including partial hospitalization services; they are indicated when the patient's condition requires services or procedures that cannot be performed in any other POS without putting the patient at risk. **Observation care services** include use of a bed and at least periodic monitoring by a hospital's nursing or other staff that is reasonable and necessary to evaluate a patient's condition or determine the need for possible admission to the hospital as an inpatient. It is *not* necessary for the patient be located in an observation area designated by the hospital.

Observation services are reimbursed only when ordered by a physician (or another individual authorized by state licensure law and hospital staff bylaws to admit patients to the hospital or to order outpatient tests). Medicare requires the physician to order an inpatient admission if the duration of observation care is expected to be 48 hours or more. (Other payers require an inpatient admission order if the duration of observation care is expected to be 24 hours or more.) *Partial hospitalization* is a short-term, intensive treatment program where individuals who are experiencing an acute episode of an illness (e.g., geriatric, psychiatric, or rehabilitative) can receive medically supervised treatment during a significant number of daytime or nighttime hours. This type of program is an alternative to 24-hour inpatient hospitalization and allows the patients to maintain their everyday life without the disruption associated with an inpatient hospital stay.

Coding Tip

When using medical decision making *or* time to select a hospital inpatient or observation care code, a continuous service that begins the evening of day one and continues into day two is reported on just one calendar date.

Reporting Codes for Hospitalist Services

The Society of Hospital Medicine defines hospitalists as physicians whose primary focus is the general medical care of hospitalized patients; their activities include patient care, teaching research, and leadership related to hospital medicine. Hospitalists may be employed directly by the hospital, serve as independent contractors, or be part of a group practice of hospitalists.

Example: An orthopedic surgeon admits a 40-year-old patient from the emergency department on May 1 and schedules surgery on May 2 to repair a hip fracture. The surgeon requests that Dr. Jones, an internal medicine hospitalist, evaluate the patient on May 1 for chronic bronchitis and to provide preoperative clearance.

The orthopedic surgeon reports a code for the initial hospital care, and the hospitalist reports a code for the inpatient consultation or a code for the hospital inpatient service, depending on which code the payer accepts. (If the hospitalist had provided E/M services to a Medicare patient, report a code from the Initial Hospital Care subcategory instead of the Inpatient Consultations or Hospital Inpatient Services subcategory.)

Initial Hospital Inpatient or Observation Care

Initial hospital inpatient or observation care services cover the first inpatient encounter the provider has with the patient for each admission. An initial hospital inpatient or observation care code is reported once per hospitalization by the provider. In addition, providers may not bill for both an admission visit and a discharge visit on the same day; for a patient who is admitted and discharged on the same date, report a code from the Hospital Inpatient or Observation Care Services (including Admission and Discharge Services) subcategory. For an observation patient who is admitted as an inpatient by the same provider on the same day as observation care, report an initial hospital inpatient or observation care code only for that day.

A hospital inpatient is someone who is admitted and discharged and has a length of stay (LOS) of one or more days.

- Initial hospital inpatient or observation care codes cover all E/M services provided to a patient by the same provider for a *planned admission*, regardless of where other E/M services were performed (e.g., preoperative history and examination performed in the office just days prior to an elective surgical admission). Report an initial hospital care E/M code only. (An exception is when a surgeon is the primary care provider during an inpatient admission, for which a CPT Surgery code is reported *only*, and inpatient E/M codes are not reported by the surgeon.)

- When a patient receives office or other outpatient E/M services *on the same day as an inpatient admission to the hospital by the same provider*, report an E/M code for the initial hospital inpatient or observation care only. *Do not report an office or other outpatient E/M service code.*

- When a high level of office or other outpatient services is provided in the office and the patient is later admitted to the hospital on another day as a *planned* admission, report a lower-level-of-service initial hospital inpatient and observation care E/M code for the hospital admission (because the provider already performed and reported the predominant portion of the E/M during the office encounter).

- When office or other outpatient services are provided and the patient is later admitted to the hospital on another day as an *unplanned* admission, report the appropriate E/M code for the office visit and an appropriate level-of-service E/M code for the initial hospital inpatient or observation care.

Providers involved in care of the patient but not designated as the attending physician report services from a different category of E/M depending on where services were rendered (e.g., emergency department services).

> **Example:** On the day of inpatient admission, Dr. Thompson provided initial inpatient hospital care E/M level 3 services to a 42-year-old patient who was admitted for antibiotic therapy to treat pneumonia due to *Klebsiella pneumoniae* bacteria. Report code 99223.
>
> If Dr. Thompson had provided level 4 or 5 E/M services to the established patient in the office, resulting in admission the next day, the reported code would be 99214 or 99215 for the office or other outpatient services encounter and code 99221 for the initial hospital inpatient or observation care service.

Subsequent Hospital Inpatient or Observation Care

Subsequent hospital inpatient or observation care includes the review of the patient's record for changes in the patient's condition, the results of diagnostic studies, and the reassessment of the patient's condition since the last assessment performed by the provider.

> **Example:** Dr. Thompson provided subsequent hospital care level 2 services to the 42-year-old patient who was admitted for antibiotic therapy to treat pneumonia due to *Klebsiella pneumoniae* bacteria. Report code 99232.

Hospital Inpatient or Observation Care Services (Including Admission and Discharge Services)

Hospital inpatient or observation care services (including admission and discharge services) are provided to patients who are admitted and discharged on the same date, as follows:

- When a patient is admitted as a hospital inpatient after receiving observation services on the same date, report only an initial hospital inpatient or observation care code. (That code should reflect the services provided by the provider during the patient's observation status.)

- When a patient receives observation services on the same date as the result of services provided at another site of service (e.g., physician's office, hospital ED, or NF), report only an observation or an inpatient care services code. (That code should reflect the services provided by the provider at the other site.)

> **Example 1:** A patient receives 90 minutes of hospital observation care in the emergency department (ED) for an acute asthma attack. The ED physician orders a blood gas analysis laboratory test and an injection of medication to help the patient breathe more easily. The ED physician then orders patient's breathing to continue to be monitored in the hospital observation care unit to ensure that the treatment resolves the patient's problem. Five hours later, the ED physician examines the patient, who has normal vital signs and has resumed normal breathing. The patient is discharged the same day to follow up with the primary care provider. The patient's record reveals documentation of a history and examination, and the level of medical decision making is moderate. Report code 99235 only. (*Do not report ED services code 99283 for this encounter.*)

Example 2: A 38-year-old patient undergoes a scheduled hospital ambulatory surgical procedure and is taken to the recovery room, where they have difficulty awakening from anesthesia and an elevated blood pressure. Both conditions persist during the usual recovery period, and the surgeon orders the ED physician to evaluate the patient. The patient is placed in the hospital's observation care unit, and the ED physician orders the nursing staff to monitor the patient's condition and note any continued abnormalities that could indicate a drug reaction or other postsurgical complications. After four hours in the observation care unit, the patient is no longer lethargic, has a normal blood pressure, and shows no signs of postsurgical complications. The ED physician discharges the patient that same day from the observation care unit to home. The patient record documents a history and examination, and the level of medical decision making is high. Report code 99236. (The coverage of observation services began when the patient was placed in the observation care unit. Services provided to the patient in the hospital's outpatient surgical suite and recovery room are not considered observation care services.)

Example 3: A patient is scheduled to undergo outpatient cataract extraction surgery. The patient expresses a preference for spending the night following the procedure at the hospital despite the fact that the procedure does not require an overnight stay. The hospital registered and treated the patient on an outpatient basis to perform the surgery and then permitted the patient to remain at the hospital overnight (because the patient signed an advance beneficiary notice agreeing to self pay for overnight care). Do not report a code for the overnight stay because it is not covered as medically necessary observation status services. (When a patient is accommodated in this manner, make sure that you notify the patient in advance that the overnight stay is not medically necessary and that the patient will be charged for the additional services. If the patient experiences complications postsurgically that necessitate an inpatient admission, the patient is admitted and a Medicare Part A claim is submitted.)

Hospital Inpatient or Observation Discharge Services

Hospital inpatient or observation discharge services include the final examination of the patient, discussion of the hospital stay with the patient and caregiver, instructions for continuing care provided to the patient and caregiver, and preparation of discharge records, prescriptions, and referral forms. Hospital discharge day management codes are reported for services provided by the provider as part of the final hospital discharge of a patient.

Coding Tip

Do not report a hospital inpatient or observation care service and a hospital inpatient or observation discharge service code for the same date of service.

Example 1: Dr. Taylor provided 30 minutes of hospital discharge services to a 44-year-old patient who was admitted for management of newly diagnosed type 2 diabetes mellitus. The patient responded well to inpatient insulin treatment and, upon examination, is discharged in improved condition. The patient was provided with discharge instructions for diabetes care, including the administration of insulin injections at home. Follow-up appointment in 10 days was scheduled. Report code 99238.

Example 2: Dr. Collins provided 70 minutes of hospital discharge services to a 94-year-old patient who was admitted for surgical treatment of a fractured pelvis. During inpatient hospitalization, the patient developed pneumonia, which was successfully treated. Arrangements were made to transfer the patient to a nursing facility for follow-up care, and orders for pain management were provided. Report code 99239.

Consultations

The *Consultations* category of E/M includes the following subcategories:

- Office or Other Outpatient Consultations
- Inpatient or Observation Consultations

NOTE:

Medicare and some other payers no longer allow providers to report codes from the Consultations category of the E/M section. Providers (e.g., specialists) who deliver consultation services to such patients in a(n)

- Office or hospital outpatient setting are to report codes from the Office or Other Outpatient Services category
- Inpatient setting are to report codes from the Hospital Inpatient or Observation Care Services category
- Nursing facility setting are to report codes from the Nursing Facility Services category

The attending physician reports modifier AI (Principal physician of record) with the initial hospital care code or initial nursing facility care code to distinguish the admitting or attending physician's service from those who provide consultation services.

The OIG reported that most consultation services reported to Medicare in 2001 were inappropriate, and subsequent education efforts to improve reporting failed to produce desired results. Other third-party payers will likely adopt the elimination of CPT's consultation codes. It is unknown whether the AMA will eliminate the "Consultations" category from a future revision of CPT.

> **Example:** On May 1, the patient was seen in the hospital's emergency department (ED) and received level 4 Evaluation and Management services from Dr. Axel (ED physician). This Medicare patient complained of severe shortness of breath, chest pain radiating down the left arm, back pain, and extreme anxiety. The patient was admitted to the hospital on May 1, and Dr. Sanchez (attending physician) provided level 2 initial hospital care. The patient was experiencing severe anxiety during admission, and Dr. Coleman was asked to provide psychiatric consultation; Dr. Coleman provided level 1 inpatient consultation services. Dr. Axel reported code 99284, Dr. Sanchez reported code 99222 AI, and Dr. Coleman reported code 99221.

A **consultation** is an examination of a patient by a health care provider, usually a specialist, for the purpose of advising the attending, primary care, or referring physician in the evaluation and management of a specific problem with a known diagnosis. Consultants may initiate diagnostic and therapeutic services as necessary during the consultative encounter. The following criteria are used to define a consultation:

- The consultation is requested by another provider or source such as a third-party payer. (If the consultation is mandated by a payer or other source, add modifier 32 to the consultation code.)
- The consultant renders an opinion or advice.
- The consultant initiates diagnostic or therapeutic services.
- The requesting provider has documented in the patient's record the request and the need for the consultation.
- The consultant's opinion, advice, and any services rendered are documented in the patient's record and communicated to the requesting provider or source, generally in the form of a written report.

 Coding Tip

- Do not confuse a consultation with a referral. A *referral* is a recommendation to transfer a patient's care from one provider to another. A referring provider does not schedule the appointment or document a request for referral. A referral is not a consultation. To ensure proper coding of the encounter, call the referring provider to inquire whether a consultation was intended instead of a referral.
- No differentiation is made as to patient status (new versus established) when assigning consultation codes.
- When a confirmatory consultation is required by a third-party payer or another party, add modifier 32 to the appropriate code from the Consultations category (non-Medicare patient), Office or Other Outpatient Services category (Medicare office or hospital outpatient), Inpatient Hospital Inpatient and Observation Care category (Medicare inpatient), or Initial Nursing Facility Care subcategory (Medicare nursing facility patient).

Office or Other Outpatient Consultations

The *Office or Other Outpatient Consultation* category includes services provided in the following health care settings:

- Physician's office
- Outpatient or other ambulatory care facility
- Hospital observation services
- Home services
- Domiciliary, rest home, or custodial care
- Emergency department

 Coding Tip

- When a consultant provides follow-up office or other outpatient consultation services, report codes from the Office or Other Outpatient Services, Established Patient category and subcategory.

- When office or other outpatient consultation services are provided to Medicare patients, report codes from the Office or Other Outpatient Services category.

- Guidelines about consultation requests and documentation also apply to consulting providers who report codes from the Office or Other Outpatient Services category.

For a code from the Office or Other Outpatient Consultations subcategory to be reported, the consultation request must be initiated by the attending or primary care physician or another health care provider and the attending or primary care physician must document all consultation requests in the patient's record. The consultant must document a written report that includes the name of the person requesting the consultation, the reason for the consultation, and the way the findings were communicated to the referring health care provider. Any specifically identifiable diagnostic or therapeutic service performed on the same day as the examination may be billed separately. These separate services must be linked to the appropriate diagnosis to ensure that medical necessity criteria are met. (Some Medicare administrative contractors and third-party payers may disallow payment when surgical procedures and E/M services are performed during the encounter.)

Example: On March 15, a 42-year-old patient was seen by Dr. Verde, a general practitioner, due to symptoms of chest pain and heart palpitations. Dr. Verde determined that the patient needed to be evaluated by a specialist and arranged for the patient to be seen in consultation by Dr. Falco, a cardiologist. Dr. Falco provided a level 4 office or other outpatient consultation service to the patient on March 20 and ordered diagnostic testing to establish a definitive diagnosis. (The payer allows CPT consultation codes to be reported.) Code 99244 is reported for the visit to Dr. Falco's office. (If, upon review of diagnostic testing results, Dr. Falco establishes a definitive diagnosis that requires the provision of further E/M services to the patient, report codes from the Office or Other Outpatient Services category of E/M.)

 Coding Tip

- When a consultant provides consultation services in the hospital's emergency department (ED) (at the request of the ED physician), report a code from the Office or Other Outpatient Consultations subcategory of the Consultations subsection.

- When a consultant assumes responsibility for a portion or all management of the case, subsequent care provided by the consultant is reported with the appropriate office or other outpatient services or subsequent hospital inpatient or observation care code.

(continues)

Coding Tip (*continued*)

- A *preoperative clearance* occurs when a surgeon requests that a specialist or another provider (e.g., general practitioner) examine a patient and indicate whether the patient can withstand the expected risks of a specific surgery. This is considered a consultation even if the physician performing the preoperative clearance is the patient's primary care provider. (A written request must be documented in the patient's record.)

 NOTE:

A history and physical examination is often performed by the patient's surgeon (in the office or at the hospital).

Inpatient or Observation Consultations

Inpatient or observation consultation codes are reported when consultation services are provided to non-Medicare inpatients, nursing facility residents, or partial hospitalization patients. Just one consultation code is reported by a consulting provider per non-Medicare admission. When consulting providers participate in the patient's inpatient or observation care, report codes from the Subsequent Hospital Inpatient or Observation Care or Subsequent Nursing Facility subcategory of E/M, depending on health care setting. When follow-up care is provided in the consultant's office, report a code from the Office or Other Outpatient Services category of E/M.

 Coding Tip

- When an inpatient consultation is provided to Medicare patients, consultants report a code from the Initial Hospital Inpatient or Observation Care category or the Initial Nursing Facility Care category.

- Guidelines about consultation requests and documentation also apply to consulting physicians who report codes from the Initial Hospital Inpatient or Observation Care or Initial Nursing Facility Care category.

Example: A 52-year-old patient was admitted to the hospital by the primary care provider (PCP) to control type 2 diabetes mellitus and to evaluate possible gangrene, left foot. The provider ordered inpatient consultation services from an orthopedic surgeon, who provided level 4 E/M initial inpatient consultation services during evaluation of the patient. The orthopedic surgeon told the patient and PCP that immediate surgical debridement was necessary. (Surgical debridement was performed.) (The payer allows CPT consultation codes to be reported.) Report code 99254 57 for the consultation services, along with a code from the CPT Surgery section for surgical debridement. (Modifier 57 is added to code 99254 because the E/M services resulted in a decision to perform surgery. When the orthopedic surgeon provides inpatient and office E/M services to the patient postoperatively, do not report E/M codes. Such follow-up care is part of the global period of surgery; the orthopedic surgeon is paid a fee for having performed the surgery and providing routine follow-up care.)

 Coding Tip

- When consultation services are provided to a nursing facility resident, just one inpatient consultation code (for health plans that allow CPT consultation codes to be reported) or one Medicare patient Initial Nursing Facility Care code may be reported per nursing facility admission, regardless of the length of time the resident remains in the facility (e.g., years). For additional consultation services, report subsequent nursing care visit codes (even when months or years have passed since the initial consultation service).

- For follow-up inpatient and observation consultation services, report codes from the Subsequent Hospital Inpatient and Observation Care subcategory of E/M.

Emergency Department Services

Emergency department services are provided in a hospital, which is open 24 hours for the purpose of providing unscheduled episodic services to patients who require immediate medical attention. A *medical emergency* is the sudden and unexpected onset of a medical condition or the acute exacerbation of a chronic condition that is threatening to life, limb, or sight and that requires immediate medical treatment or that manifests painful symptomatology requiring immediate palliative effort to relieve suffering. A *maternity emergency* is a sudden unexpected medical complication that puts the mother or fetus at risk. A *psychiatric inpatient admission* is an emergency when, based on a psychiatric evaluation performed by a provider (or another qualified mental health care professional with hospital admission authority), the patient is at immediate risk of serious harm to self or others as a result of a mental disorder, and requires immediate continuous skilled observation at the acute level of care.

While emergency department (ED) physicians employed by the facility usually provide ED services, any physician who provides services to a patient registered in the ED may report the ED services codes. This means that the physician does not have to be assigned to the hospital's ED. When services provided in the ED are determined not to be an actual emergency, ED services codes are still reportable if ED services were provided. Typically, the hospital reports a lower-level ED services code for nonemergency conditions.

> **Example:** A 54-year-old patient presented to the hospital ED with the symptoms of abdominal discomfort, severe shortness of breath, and numbness in both hands. The ED physician provided level 5 E/M services, which included diagnostic workup. Report code 99285.

 NOTE:

> When a patient's condition may preclude the completion of a history or an extensive examination, documentation should indicate the constraints imposed by the urgency of the patient's clinical condition and mental status. The ICD-10-CM code should also reflect the urgency of the patient's condition."
>
> **Example:** A comatose patient received emergency department (ED) services during which the physician was unable to perform a history. The patient arrived alone via ambulance to the ED, so family was unable to be interviewed to document a history. The physician completed an examination, and level of medical decision making was high complexity. Report code 99285 because the physician documented the reason a history was unable to be performed.

If a physician provides emergency services to a patient in the office, it is *not* appropriate to assign codes from the Emergency Department Services category of E/M. If the patient's primary care provider (PCP) asks the patient to meet at the hospital's ED as an alternative to the physician's office and the patient is not registered as a patient in the ED, the physician should report a code from the Office or Other Outpatient Services category of E/M. ED services codes are reported only if the patient receives services in the hospital's ED.

When a patient's PCP directs the patient to go to the hospital's ED to receive care and that physician is subsequently asked by the ED physician to evaluate the patient and advise the ED physician as to whether the patient should be admitted to the hospital or be sent home, assign codes as follows:

- If the patient is admitted to the hospital by the patient's PCP, the PCP should report a code for the appropriate level of the initial hospital inpatient or observation care only. All E/M services provided by the PCP in conjunction with an inpatient admission are considered part of initial hospital inpatient or observation care when performed on the same date as the admission. The ED physician who treated the patient in the ED should report the appropriate ED services code.

- If the ED physician, based on the advice of the patient's PCP who came to the ED to evaluate the patient, sends the patient home, the ED physician should report the appropriate ED services code. The patient's PCP should also report an ED services code that describes the services provided in the ED. If the PCP does not come to the hospital to evaluate the patient but provides advice to the ED physician via telephone, the PCP should not report any E/M code.

When an ED physician requests that another provider evaluate an emergency patient, the other provider should report a consultation services code if criteria for providing a consultation have been met (or an appropriate Office or Other Outpatient Services code if the health plan does not allow CPT consultation codes to be reported). If those criteria are not met and the patient is discharged from the ED or admitted to the hospital by another provider, the provider contacted by the ED physician should report an ED services code. If the consulted provider admits the patient to the hospital and the criteria for a consultation have not been met, the provider should report an initial hospital care code.

Other Emergency Services

Other emergency services code 99288 is reported when the provider is in two-way communication contact with ambulance or rescue crew personnel located outside the hospital. The provider directs performance of the following procedures:

- Administration of intramuscular, intratracheal, or subcutaneous drugs
- Administration of intravenous fluids
- Cardiac and pulmonary resuscitation
- Electrical conversion of arrhythmia
- Endotracheal or esophageal obturator airway intubation
- Telemetry of cardiac rhythm

 Coding Tip

- No differentiation is made as to patient status (new versus established) when assigning ED services codes.
- Usually Medicare administrative contractors and third-party payers do not provide a separate payment for services reported as code 99288 because they are considered included in the payment for services (e.g., emergency department services reported with CPT codes or ambulance services reported with HCPCS Level II codes).

Critical Care Services

Critical care is the direct delivery of medical care by a provider to a patient who is critically ill or injured and who requires the full, exclusive attention of the provider. A *critical illness or injury* is one that acutely impairs one or more vital organ systems, jeopardizing the patient's survival. Critical care involves a high level of medical decision making to assess and manage life-threatening conditions (e.g., central nervous system failure, circulatory failure, shock, renal failure, hepatic failure, metabolic failure, respiratory failure, postoperative complications, overwhelming infection, and other vital system functions), to treat single or multiple vital organ system failure, or to prevent further deterioration of vital functions. Critical care is usually, but not always, provided in a critical care area (e.g., coronary care unit, intensive care unit [ICU], pediatric intensive care unit [PICU], respiratory care unit, or emergency care facility). Payers will reimburse critical care services provided in any location as long as the care provided meets the definition of critical care and supporting documentation is in the patient's record.

Critical care services are reported when a provider directly delivers medical care for a critically ill or critically injured patient. Critical care services can be provided on multiple days even if no changes are made to the treatment rendered to the patient, as long as the patient's condition requires the direct delivery of critical care services by the provider. Time spent away from the patient's bedside that is documented in the patient's record qualifies as critical care services (e.g., time spent with family members or surrogate decision makers to obtain the patient's history or to discuss treatment options). The documented progress note must include any family discussion to a specific treatment issue and *explain why the discussion was necessary on that day.*

 NOTE:

Critical care services require personal management by the provider. They are life- and organ-supporting interventions that require personal assessment and manipulation by the provider. Withdrawal of or failure to initiate these interventions on an urgent basis would likely result in sudden and clinically significant or life-threatening deterioration in the patient's condition. The service is of such intensity that the provider must devote their full attention to the patient and, therefore, cannot render services to any other patient during that same period of time.

Critical care time may be continuous or interrupted; the time spent engaged in critical care services is directly related to the patient's care, whether that time was spent at the immediate bedside or elsewhere on the floor or unit. The following services performed elsewhere by the provider represent critical care:

- Spending time at the nursing station reviewing test results
- Discussing the patient's care with other medical staff
- Documenting critical care services in the patient's record
- Obtaining the patient's medical history and discussing treatment options with family members if the discussion is absolutely necessary for the treatment decision under consideration that day

Critical care services include the following procedures, which are not coded or reported separately:

- Blood gases
- Chest x-rays
- Collecting and interpreting physiologic data (e.g., blood pressures, ECG, hematologic data)
- Gastric intubation
- Interpretation of cardiac output measurements
- Pulse oximetry
- Temporary transcutaneous pacing
- Vascular access procedures
- Ventilatory management

Coding Tip

- Just because a patient is located in a critical care unit does not mean that they are receiving critical care; if the patient is stable, report the appropriate subsequent hospital care service code.

- Additional services not included in the list of procedures associated with critical care services, such as Swan-Ganz catheterization (93503) and intubation (31500), are reported separately. Time spent providing such additional services is *not* considered when selecting the critical care services code(s).

When a patient receives critical care services while located in a critical care unit, on a medical or surgical unit, or in the hospital ED, the critical care services codes are reported *in addition to initial hospital care, subsequent hospital care, and initial inpatient consultations service codes.* (Add modifier 25 to the E/M level of service code to report it as a separately identified service provided to the patient.) Documentation of all critical care services provided is crucial, including the length of time the provider spent providing services. Critical care services codes are selected according to the total duration of time the provider spent delivering services to the patient, even if the time spent was not continuous. To calculate duration of time, the provider must devote their full attention to the patient and cannot provide services to any other patient during that same period of time. CPT contains a table that can assist with code assignment according to total duration of critical care provided and applicable code(s).

Coding Tip

- Critical care code 99292 is reported for up to 30 minutes each beyond the first 74 minutes. Throughout CPT, interpret length of time, burn percentage, number of lesions, and so on, as "up to" the number in the code description.

- If critical care services are provided on the same date as a surgical procedure that has a global period and the services are related to the reason for surgery, critical care services are bundled (included) in the reimbursement for the surgical procedure. In this situation, do not report codes for critical care services.

- If critical care services provided are unrelated to the reason for surgery, report codes for services provided (in addition to the surgery code). Attach modifier 24 or 25 to the critical care services code(s). (The surgeon must document that the critical care was unrelated to the surgical procedure performed or was beyond the typical work of pre- or postoperative care associated with the procedure.)

- If the surgeon is also an intensivist, the surgeon should not report codes for critical care services provided to their patient during the pre- or postoperative period. Such critical care services are included in the global surgical fee.

- If a surgeon requires the assistance of another intensivist, the intensivist should report codes for critical care services provided. An *intensivist* is a provider who has received extensive training and experience in critical care and who specializes in the care of critically ill patients, usually in an intensive care unit (ICU). Usually an intensivist has completed a fellowship in critical care following completion of a residency in internal medicine, pulmonary medicine, anesthesia, or surgery. Most intensivists are board-certified or board-eligible in critical care medicine.

- Critical care services are reported for services provided to patients whose age is over 24 months.

- To report critical care services for patients 24 months and younger, refer to codes for critical care pediatric patient transport or codes for inpatient neonatal, infant, and pediatric critical care services.

Example 1: A patient is seen in the hospital ED for trauma as the result of an automobile accident. Level 4 emergency department E/M services are provided, and the ED physician also provides 60 continuous minutes of critical care services. Report the appropriate ED level of service code along with codes 99284 25 and 99291.

Example 2: Dr. Smith delivers critical care services to a patient on June 15 from 8–9 a.m., 10:30–10:45 a.m., and 3:00–3:45 p.m. To assign a critical care services code to this case, total the minutes of critical care services directly delivered by the provider. Codes 99291, 99292, and 99292 are reported.

Nursing Facility Services

Nursing facility services are provided at a nursing facility (NF), skilled nursing facility (SNF), intermediate care facility for individuals with intellectual disability (ICF/IID), long-term care facility (LTCF), or psychiatric residential treatment facility. NFs provide convalescent, rehabilitative, or long-term care for patients, and an assessment must be completed on each patient that meets the resident's medical, nursing, mental, and psychological needs. The patient's functional capacity, identification of potential problems, and nursing plan to enhance (or at least maintain) the patient's physical and psychosocial functions are assessed and documented. The assessments are written when the patient is admitted or readmitted to the facility or when a reassessment is necessary because of a substantial change in the patient's status.

 Coding Tip

No differentiation is made as to patient status (new versus established) when assigning nursing facility services codes.

 NOTE:

Medicare and some other payers do not allow providers to report codes from the Consultations category. Thus, inpatient or observation consultation services for Medicare and other affected nursing facility residents are reported with codes from the Initial Nursing Facility Care subcategories. (Coders should determine whether health plans allow CPT codes from the Consultations category to be reported.)

When more than one provider (e.g., attending physician and a consultant) delivers inpatient services on the same date of service, the attending physician adds modifier AI (Principal Physician of Record) to the reported E/M code.

 Coding Tip

- Report a code for hospital inpatient or observation discharge services, or hospital inpatient or observation care services (including admission and discharge services) and initial nursing facility care *if a patient is discharged and admitted to an NF, SNF, ICF/IID, LTCF, or psychiatric residential treatment facility on the same date.*

- Do not report codes for ED or office or other outpatient services with initial nursing facility care when provided on the same day for the same patient by the same provider. E/M services provided at sites other than

(continues)

> ### Coding Tip (*continued*)
>
> the NF are bundled into initial nursing facility care when performed on the same date as the nursing facility admission by the same provider.
>
> - Do not report codes for initial or subsequent nursing facility care and initial hospital inpatient or observation care on the same date for the same patient by the same provider. Payment for initial hospital care services includes all work performed by the provider in all sites of service on that date.
>
> - Report a code for subsequent nursing facility care when the evaluation of the patient's assessment plan is not required and when the patient has not had a major or permanent change of health status.
>
> - For discharge from a nursing facility, report a code from the nursing facility discharge services subcategory. If the patient has expired, report a code from the nursing facility discharge services if the primary service provided by the provider is pronouncement of death, completion of the death summary, and discussion with the deceased patient's family. The provider must personally visit the patient and document pronouncement of death before midnight on the date the patient expired.

Third-party payers may reimburse E/M services provided in a nursing facility when the purpose of the visit is to fulfill the minimum federal requirement of at least one provider visit every 30 days for the first three months and at least once every 60 days thereafter. The service must also be reasonable and necessary for the diagnosis or treatment of illness or injury or to improve the functioning of a malformed body member. All of the following conditions must be fulfilled:

- The service requires the skill of a physician.
- The service is sufficiently well documented for the level of service and code reported.
- The service is performed by the attending physician, a consulting physician requested by the attending physician, or a named physician requested by the patient or the patient's interested family member or legal guardian.

For an E/M service in an NF to be considered reasonable and necessary, it must be furnished in accordance with accepted standards of medical practice for the diagnosis or treatment of the patient's condition or with the goal of improving the function of a malformed body member, be ordered and furnished by qualified personnel, and meet, but not exceed, the patient's medical need.

> **Example:** On October 14, a 97-year-old patient was transferred from the hospital to the nursing facility in stable condition. The patient's attending physician provided 40 minutes of initial nursing facility care. On November 14, the attending physician provided 10 minutes of subsequent nursing facility care. The patient expired on November 30, and the attending physician was not in attendance. Report codes 99305 (10/14) and 99307 (11/14). (A discharge management code is not reported.)

Home or Residence Services

Home or residence services are provided to individuals in a home or residence to promote, maintain, or restore health and to minimize the effects of disability and illness, including terminal illness. (CPT defines a "home" as a "private residence, temporary lodging, or short-term accommodation, such as a hotel, campground, hostel, or cruise ship." An assisted living facility, domiciliary, group home, or rest home also meets the definition of "home" for CPT coding purposes.) Home or residence services for Medicare patients are provided by nurses, doctors, social workers, therapists, and home health aides. Services are ordered by a provider (instead of treatment in a hospital or SNF) and may result in a shorter acute care hospital or SNF LOS. Home health care programs must be organized, administered, and supervised by a hospital or qualified licensed personnel under the medical direction of a provider. Home services allow patients to recuperate while remaining at home. Since most home health care is temporary and part-time, in addition to providing direct care, the home health staff teaches patients (and their families or others) how to continue needed care (e.g., medication administration, wound care, and therapy).

Coding Tip

Differentiate between new and established patients when reporting codes for home services. Do *not* count travel time when selecting a code based on time.

The home health care provider is responsible for documenting a plan of care and reviewing data. If the written plan of care was not initially prepared by the provider (e.g., prepared by the home health agency), the patient record must include documentation of the provider's contribution to the development of the plan and a review of the specific items entered into the plan. It is not sufficient for a home health agency to maintain documentation in its records for the physician. The provider must maintain their own records, including periodic summary reports provided by the home health agency. Documentation of all face-to-face E/M home services visits and any audiovisual communications with the patient or caretakers must be documented in the patient's record. This documentation must indicate an ongoing knowledge of any changes in the patient's condition, drugs, or other needs and the way they are being addressed.

> **Example:** A primary care physician provides a low level of medical decision making for home services to a 72-year-old established patient to evaluate the status of the patient's wound healing. The patient has been receiving daily skilled wound care. The physician determines that an additional 10 days of daily skilled wound care is needed and documents that order for the home health agency. Report code 99348.

Home Health Agency Face-to-Face Encounters for Medicare Beneficiaries

For Medicare purposes, certifying providers are responsible for documenting all face-to-face encounters with patients in the patient record, and the encounter must occur no more than 90 days prior to the home health start of care date or within 30 days after the start of care. Such face-to-face encounters can be performed using telehealth services at an approved originating site, which is the location of an eligible Medicare beneficiary at the time such services occur. Originating sites must be located in Rural Health Professional Shortage Areas or in counties outside of metropolitan statistical areas, and they can include provider offices, hospitals, critical access hospitals (CAHs), rural health clinics (RHCs), federally qualified health centers (FQHCs), hospital-based or CAH-based renal dialysis centers, skilled nursing facilities (SNFs), and community mental health centers (CMHCs). Nonphysician providers (e.g., certified nurse-midwives, nurse practitioners, physician assistants) can also provide face-to-face E/M home services, but they must inform the certifying physician of any clinical findings exhibited by the patient during the encounter. Then, the provider must document the encounter and countersign the certification. Documentation requirements include:

- Date of face-to-face encounter between the provider and the patient
- Brief narrative describing how the patient's observed clinical condition supports the patient's homebound status and need for skilled services
- Documentation of the encounter (e.g., handwritten, keyboarded, or EHR format) by the certifying provider on the signed/dated certification form or as a signed/dated addendum to the certification

Certifying providers are permitted to verbally communicate the brief narrative describing how the patient's observed clinical condition supports the patient's homebound status and need for skilled services to the home health agency (HHA). The HHA provider documents the encounter on the certification form, and the certifying provider must sign the form.

Prolonged Services

Provider services involving patient contact that are considered beyond the usual service in either an inpatient or outpatient setting may be reported as **prolonged services**. Codes for prolonged services are reported *in addition to* other provider services (e.g., hospital inpatient services). Prolonged services are reported only when the time involved *exceeds* the typical time associated with an E/M service by at least 30 minutes. Prolonged services of less than 30 minutes total duration on a given date are not separately reported because the work involved is included in the total work for the E/M service code. In addition, prolonged services of less than 15 minutes beyond the first hour and less than 15 minutes beyond the final 30 minutes are not reported separately.

Coding Tip

The patient's record must include documentation that supports the E/M level of service code reported, as well as the duration and content of prolonged services that the physician furnished.

- Time the office staff spends with the patient or time the patient remains unaccompanied in the office is not reported using prolonged services codes.

- Time spent waiting for inpatient test results, changes in the patient's condition, end of therapy, or use of facilities is not reported using prolonged services codes.

NOTE:

Codes below the *Prolonged Service with Direct Patient Contact (except with Office or Other Outpatient Services)* subcategory were deleted from CPT 2024. Parenthetical notes provide direction to use codes 99417 and 99418 from the *Prolonged Service With or Without Direct Patient Contact on the Date of an E/M Service* subcategory.

Prolonged Service Without Direct Patient Contact on Date Other Than the Face-to-Face Evaluation and Management Service

Prolonged services without direct patient contact on date other than face-to-face E/M service are reported for non-face-to-face time services that are not provided on the same date as a face-to-face E/M service, such as extensive record review that is related to a face-to-face E/M service provided to a patient on a previous date.

Example: A physician provided level 5 emergency department services with 45 minutes spent face-to-face with an established older adult patient who was seen for senile dementia, hypertension, diabetes mellitus, and arrhythmia. It becomes clear during the encounter that the patient needs to be placed in a skilled nursing facility (SNF) immediately. Upon reflection, the patient's spouse becomes upset about this recommendation, and on the next day the physician spends 50 minutes talking about what the spouse and the patient can expect regarding SNF care. The physician also calls the local SNF to arrange for patient admission and to coordinate the patient's plan of care; 15 minutes are spent during this phone call. The ED encounter was 45 minutes. The total duration of time providing non-face-to-face contact (in addition to the 45 minutes E/M emergency department services) was 65 minutes. Report codes 99285 (ED service) and 99358 (prolonged service on date other than face-to-face E/M service without direct patient contact).

Prolonged Clinical Staff Services with Physician or Other Qualified Health Care Professional Supervision

Prolonged Clinical Staff Services with Physician or Other Qualified Health Care Professional Supervision codes are reported for an office or outpatient setting when clinical staff (e.g., dietician) have prolonged face-to-face time with patients. The physician or qualified health care professional (e.g., nurse practitioner) must provide direct supervision of clinical staff.

> **Example:** An established patient received 20 minutes of office E/M services for a diagnosis of obesity, and code 99213 was reported for the nurse practitioner's provision of services. The patient is participating in a weight loss program, and the dietician also provided 85 minutes of face-to-face time counseling services, under the nurse practitioner's supervision, during the same encounter. Code 99415 was reported for the first 60 minutes of the dietician's time, and code 99416 was also reported for the next 25 minutes of the dietician's time. Thus, the CMS-1500 claim reported codes 99213, 99415, and 99416 for this one encounter.

Prolonged Service With or Without Direct Patient Contact on the Date of an Evaluation and Management Service

Prolonged Service With or Without Direct Patient Contact on the Date of an Evaluation and Management Service codes are reported by physicians or other qualified health care professionals for face-to-face or non-face-to-face patient care. The add-on codes are reported only when the code selected for

- Office or other outpatient service, office consultation, home or residence visit, or cognitive assessment and care plan service.
- Hospital inpatient or observation care services, inpatient consultation, or nursing facility services were based on time alone and when the minimum time required for the highest level of service has been exceeded by at least 15 minutes.

> **Example:** A physician provided level 5 Office or Other Outpatient Services to an acutely ill established patient who was treated for an asthma attack with intermittent bronchial dilation and subcutaneous epinephrine. The physician provided intermittent direct services over a period of 80 minutes. Report codes 99215, 99417, and 99417. CPT's *Total Duration of Established Patient Office or Other Outpatient Services* table in the Prolonged Services category provides guidance about code assignment.

Standby Services

Standby services involve a physician or other qualified health care professional spending a prolonged period of time *without direct (face-to-face) patient contact* waiting for an event to occur that will require the physician's services. Such services must be requested by another provider (e.g., attending physician) and are reported only if the standby time is 30 minutes or longer. However, if a physician who provides standby services performs surgery, the standby services are included in the surgical procedure's global period.

> **Example:** An obstetric surgeon was called in for consultation by the patient's attending physician (a family practitioner) and provided 30 minutes of standby services due to fetal distress, as noted on the fetal monitor. During standby, the fetal distress resolved, the patient went into active labor, and the patient's attending physician (not the obstetric surgeon) delivered the baby vaginally. Report 99360 for the obstetric surgeon (because no cesarean section was required).

Case Management Services

According to CPT, "**case management** is a process in which a physician or another qualified health care professional is responsible for direct care of a patient, and for coordinating and managing access to, initiating, and supervising other health care services needed by the patient." Case management services include medical team conferences with or without direct (face-to-face) contact with the patient or family and require the participation of at least "three qualified health care professionals from different specialties or disciplines, each of whom provide direct care to the patient."

Example: The physician participated in a 30-minute face-to-face medical team conference consisting of three interdisciplinary health care professionals and the patient to discuss a 49-year-old patient's plan of care. Report code 99367.

Care Plan Oversight Services

Care plan oversight services codes are reported by one individual who supervises the home health, hospice, or nursing facility care plan of a patient or resident during a 30-day period. Just one individual may report care plan oversight services for a given period of time, which reflects the sole or predominant supervisory role with a particular patient.

Example: The physician reviewed and revised the hospice agency care plan for a 64-year-old female patient with terminal breast cancer. Care plan oversight services required 25 minutes of the physician's time. Report code 99377.

Preventive Medicine Services

Preventive medicine services include routine examinations or risk management counseling for children and adults who exhibit no overt signs or symptoms of a disorder while presenting to the medical office for a preventive medical physical. Such services are also called *wellness visits*. Discussion of risk factors such as diet and exercise counseling, family problems, substance abuse counseling, and injury prevention are an integral part of preventive medicine. Care must be taken to select the proper code according to the age of the patient and the patient's status (new or established).

 Coding Tip

- Determine the patient's status (new or established) when assigning preventive medicine services codes.
- Preventive medicine services are not reported when a patient who is receiving treatment for a specific disorder returns to the office for a "recheck of a known problem."

When a significant abnormality or preexisting condition is treated during the same encounter as a preventive medicine service (e.g., annual physical exam), it is appropriate to report an office or other outpatient services code in addition to the preventive medicine services code. To report both codes, the preventive medicine services portion of the visit must be documented, and the separate workup for the significant problem must be documented. Add modifier 25 to the appropriate code, and link the appropriate diagnosis code to justify medical necessity.

Example 1: A 24-year-old new patient receives preventive medicine services from a family practitioner. Report code 99385.

Example 2: A 45-year-old established patient receives preventive medicine services as part of an annual physical exam; during examination, the physician notices a breast lump. The physician provides level 3 E/M office or other outpatient services to evaluate the breast lump, which include additional examination and discussion of diagnostic testing plans with the patient. Report codes 99396 and 99213 25.

Counseling Risk Factor Reduction and Behavior Change Intervention

Counseling risk factor reduction and behavior change intervention services are reported by physicians or other qualified health care professionals who provide face-to-face services to promote patients' health and prevent illness or injury.

- Risk factor reduction services are reported for patients who do not have a specific illness, but for whom such counseling might otherwise be used as part of treatment. Patient issues include family problems, substance use, sexual practices, and so on.
- Behavior change interventions are provided to patients who exhibit a behavior that is often considered an illness (e.g., obesity, substance abuse or misuse, tobacco use or addiction).

Example 1: A patient who has been experiencing anxiety and depression receives preventive medicine individual counseling lasting 60 minutes. Report code 99404.

Example 2: A patient with a two-pack per day history of smoking cigarettes receives 10 minutes of individual behavior change intervention counseling and a level 3 E/M service for type 2 diabetes. Report codes 99213 25 and 99406.

Non-Face-to-Face Services

Non-face-to-face services include a variety of modalities. Telephone services are non-face-to-face E/M services that are provided using a telephone to a patient by a physician or other qualified health care professional. Online digital evaluation and medical management are provided using Internet resources to respond to an established patient's online inquiry. Interprofessional telephone/Internet/electronic health record consultations are provided when a treating physician requests the opinion and treatment advice of a consulting physician with specific specialty expertise to assist in the diagnosis and management of a patient's problem without the need for patient's face-to-face contact with the consultant. Digitally stored data services/remote physiologic monitoring services are provided during a 30-day period for an FDA-approved medical device. Remote physiologic monitoring treatment management services are provided to manage a patient's treatment plan for an FDA-approved medical device.

Example 1: A physician called an established patient to discuss the results of laboratory testing and to revise the instructions for taking a prescribed medication. The call was 12 minutes in duration. The patient had previously been seen in the office 10 days ago, and is scheduled to return to the office for follow-up in two months. Report code 99442.

Example 2: A patient emailed Dr. Nguyen to ask whether the prescribed Effexor could be increased from 75 to 150 mg per day, per the recommendation of a marriage counselor. who said the original dosage was not therapeutic for the patient. The physician agreed and instructed the patient to take two 75-mg capsules daily. The patient had been seen by the physician in the office 30 days ago and is scheduled to receive office E/M services in 60 days as part of routine care. The physician spent five minutes providing online digital E/M services. Report code 99421.

Example 3: A patient received an Internet assessment and management service that was provided by an ENT specialist during 60 minutes of medical consultative discussion and review with the patient's treating physician, including a verbal and written report. Report code 99449. (Do not add modifier 95 to code 99449 because the star symbol does not precede the code in the coding manual. The code includes "Internet assessment and management service" in its description.)

Example 4: A physician provided digitally stored data services/remote physiologic monitoring of a patient's blood pressure and respiratory flow rate, including initial set-up and patient education of equipment. Report code 99453.

Example 5: The patient received remote physiologic monitoring treatment management services for 20 minutes on May 1, facilitated by interactive communication between patient and physician during the entire month. Report code 99457.

Special Evaluation and Management Services

According to CPT, **special evaluation and management services** are provided for establishment of baseline information prior to life or disability insurance certificates being issued and for examination of a patient with a work-related or medical disability problem. During special evaluation and management services, the examining provider does *not* assume active management of the patient's health problems.

Example 1: A life insurance company's representative examines a 27-year-old patient at home to determine whether a base life insurance policy will be issued. Report code 99450.

Example 2: A 42-year-old patient who had sustained an on-the-job injury about 10 years ago is evaluated by a court-appointed workers' compensation physician to determine whether the patient's current condition is considered work related. Report code 99456.

Newborn Care Services

Newborn care services are provided to newborns in a variety of health care settings (e.g., hospital, birthing center, and home birth).

Example 1: A 34-year-old patient was admitted to the hospital on May 19 for vaginal delivery, which resulted in a healthy 10-pound newborn. The pediatrician provided newborn care services on May 19 to complete a history and examination of the infant, and on the morning of May 20, the patient and infant were discharged home. Report codes 99460 and 99462 for the newborn case.

Example 2: A 34-year-old patient delivered a healthy 8-pound newborn at home, and the physician in attendance performed a physical examination of the neonate and provided instruction to the parents about initial care. The patient and newborn are scheduled to follow up in the office in three days. Report code 99461 for the newborn case.

Delivery/Birthing Room Attendance and Resuscitation Services

Delivery/birthing room attendance and resuscitation services include attendance at delivery, initial stabilization of the newborn, and delivery/birthing room resuscitation. When delivery room attendance services or delivery room resuscitation services are required, they are reported in addition to newborn care services codes.

> **Example:** Per the request of the patient's delivering physician, a pediatrician was in attendance at the delivery to provide initial stabilization of the newborn. The pediatrician reports code 99464.

Inpatient Neonatal Intensive Care Services and Pediatric and Neonatal Critical Care Services

Inpatient neonatal and pediatric critical care and intensive services are delivered to critically ill neonates and infants by a provider. A *neonate* is a newborn, up to 28 days old. An *infant* is a very young child, up to one year old. The definitions for critical care services codes provided to neonates are the same as those provided to adults. (Refer to the previous section of this chapter for discussion of critical care services definitions and coding guidelines.) Inpatient neonatal and pediatric critical care and intensive services begin on the date of admission, and codes are reported once per day per patient. These codes are reported for each 24-hour period, not according to total duration of critical care; the appropriate code is reported once per day per patient.

Coding Tip

- When a neonate or an infant is no longer considered critically ill (e.g., attains a body weight that exceeds 5,000 grams), report subsequent hospital care codes for inpatient services provided.
- For infants with less than 5,000 grams body weight, who are no longer considered critically ill, report subsequent intensive care services codes.

Pediatric Critical Care Patient Transport

Pediatric critical care patient transport includes the physical attendance and direct face-to-face care delivered by a provider during the interfacility transport of a critically ill or critically injured patient, aged 24 months or younger. *Interfacility transport* is the transfer of a patient from one health care facility to another (e.g., community hospital to children's hospital), and it usually involves use of an ambulance or a helicopter.

> **Example:** A 4-month-old infant requires pediatric critical care patient transport services due to respiratory failure. The infant's pediatrician provided critical care services during a 95-minute interfacility transfer from a rural community hospital, where initial treatment to stabilize the patient was provided, to a specialty children's hospital in a city located 70 miles away. Report codes 99466 (first 74 minutes) and 99467 (16 minutes, which is more than half of the number of minutes specified in the code description).

Inpatient Neonatal and Pediatric Critical Care

Inpatient neonatal critical care services are provided to patients 28 days of age or less. *Inpatient pediatric critical care services* are provided to patients 29 days of age through less than six years of age.

Initial and Continuing Intensive Care Services

Continuing intensive care services codes are reported for services provided subsequent to the day of admission to *very low birth weight* (less than 1,500 grams) or *low birth weight* (1,500–2,500 grams) infants who are no longer considered critically ill.

Example: A 25-day-old infant weighing 1,400 grams received subsequent intensive care services from the pediatrician on days two and three of an inpatient admission. Report codes 99478 and 99478.

Cognitive Assessment and Care Plan Services

Cognitive assessment and care plan services are provided for the comprehensive evaluation of a patient who exhibits signs and symptoms of cognitive impairment to confirm or establish a diagnosis, including its etiology and severity.

Example: Patient underwent cognitive assessment and care planning at an apartment in an assisted living facility. All of the required elements of assessment and care planning were performed and documented. Report code 99483.

Care Management Services

Care management services are provided by providers, other qualified health care professionals, and clinical staff. Services include patient-centered management and support services that are provided to patients who reside at home or in a domiciliary, rest home, or assisted living facility (e.g., coordinating patient care with a home health agency).

Care planning services are provided to patients for the purpose of creating a care plan that contains specific and achievable patient goals that address health problems of a physical, mental, cognitive, social, functional, or environmental origin. According to CPT, elements of a care plan include a "problem list, expected outcome and prognosis, measurable treatment goals, cognitive assessment, functional assessment, symptom management, planned interventions, medical management, environmental evaluation, caregiver assessment, interaction and coordination with outside resources and health care professionals and others, as necessary, and summary of advance directives."

Chronic care management services are provided when the patient's medical and psychological needs require establishment, implementation, revision, or monitoring of the care plan. Such patients receive services for two or more chronic conditions or episodic health conditions, which are expected to be managed for a period of at least 12 months or until the death of the patient and that place the patient at significant risk of acute exacerbation or decompensation, death, or functional decline.

Complex chronic care management services require a minimum of 60 minutes of clinical staff time (under direction of a physician or other qualified health care professional) and for which level of medical decision making is moderate or high.

Principal care management services are provided to patients who require establishment, implementation, revision, or monitoring of a care plan specific to a single, complex chronic medical or psychological condition (e.g., cancer, schizophrenia).

Example: Established patient received level 5 physician office services for treatment of acute bronchitis. During the same encounter, the provider medically managed the patient's brittle type 1 diabetes mellitus and chronic asthma. Patient's care plan was revised to provide education to explain that over-the-counter (OTC) medications cannot be combined with prescribed medications for acute bronchitis because of the risk to stability of the chronic conditions. The patient had numerous questions about not using OTC medications and how they might impact the chronic conditions; the physician provided chronic care management services for 30 minutes to ensure that all of the patient's questions were answered and that the patient understood the treatment plan. Report codes 99215 and 99491.

Psychiatric Collaborative Care Management Services

Psychiatric collaborative care management services are provided when a patient has a diagnosed psychiatric disorder that requires behavioral health care assessment; establishment, implementation, revision, and monitoring of a care plan; and provision of brief interventions. CPT contains a table that can be used to determine code assignment according to: type of service, total duration of collaborative care management over the calendar month, and code(s).

> **Example:** Patient received 1 hour and 45 minutes of initial psychiatric collaborative care management, which included completion and documentation of all required elements was provided for the patient. (One hour and 45 minutes = 105 minutes.) Report codes 99492 and 99494.

Transitional Care Management Services

Transitional care management services are provided to patients in their community setting (e.g., home, assisted living facility). Services are provided for medical and psychosocial problems that require moderate or high level of medical decision making during transitions in care from an inpatient hospital setting, partial hospital, observation status in a hospital, or skilled nursing facility.

> **Example:** A patient was discharged from a nursing facility to home. The provider coordinated home health care services, educated the primary caregiver about follow-up care, and communicated with the patient via telephone on the day after discharge. Level of medical decision making was moderate. Report code 99495 95 (in addition to an appropriate code for nursing facility E/M services).

Advance Care Planning

Advance care planning includes face-to-face services between a physician or other qualified health care professional and a patient, family member, or surrogate for counseling and discussing advance directives, with or without completing relevant legal forms (e.g., health care proxy).

> **Example:** The patient and their daughter met with the patient's primary care physician for 30 minutes of advance care planning, which included an explanation and discussion of the patient's health care proxy. Report code 99497.

General Behavioral Health Integration Care Management

General behavioral health integration care management services are provided by clinical staff for patients with behavioral health and substance abuse conditions, and codes are reported by the supervising physician or other qualified health care professional. Services provided require care management services (face-to-face or non-face-to-face) of 20 or more minutes in a calendar month, a treatment plan, and specified elements of the CPT code description, which include:

- initial assessment or follow-up monitoring, including the use of applicable validated rating scales
- behavioral health care planning in relation to behavioral/psychiatric health problems, including revision for patients who are not progressing or whose status changes

- facilitating and coordinating treatment such as psychotherapy, pharmacotherapy, counseling and psychiatric consultation
- continuity of care with a designated member of the care team

Other Evaluation and Management Services

Other evaluation and management services include pelvic examinations (that are reported in addition to the code for the primary procedure) and unlisted E/M services.

Exercise 10.4 – Evaluation and Management Categories and Subcategories

Instructions: Select the most appropriate response. Be sure to refer to both textbook content *and* CPT Evaluation and Management section guidelines and notes.

1. A 54-year-old patient registers at an urgent care center for COVID-19 testing due to aching, coughing, fatigue, and fever. From which Evaluation and Management category would the code for this encounter be selected?

   a. Consultations

   b. Emergency department services

   c. Office or other outpatient services

   d. Preventive medicine services

2. An established patient receives hospital inpatient discharge day management services from the provider. From which Evaluation and Management subcategory of the hospital inpatient and observation care services category would the code for this encounter be selected?

   a. Hospital inpatient or observation discharge services

   b. Hospital inpatient or observation care services (including admission and discharge services)

   c. Initial hospital inpatient or observation care

   d. Subsequent hospital inpatient or observation care

3. On January 10, a physician provided office E/M services to a 72-year-old patient who is recuperating at home after left hip replacement surgery, and that same physician created an initial home health care plan on the same date. That physician also prepared a subsequent care plan on January 22 to increase the frequency of physical therapy services provided to the patient. Reporting codes from the Care Plan Oversight Services for January 10 and January 22 care plan oversight services is appropriate because

   a. care plan oversight services are reported instead of office or other outpatient services codes.

   b. level of medical decision making for care plan oversight services determines code selection.

   c. the same physician reported care plan oversight services during a 30-day period.

   d. work involved in providing care plan oversight services is not included in office visit codes.

4. A patient was seen in consultation with a hematology specialist for post-COVID recurrent blood clots, and the specialist assumed responsibility for the patient's care after initial consultation. Subsequent office encounters with the specialist should be reported with codes from the _____ category or subcategory.

   a. office or other outpatient consultations

   b. office or other outpatient services

   c. special evaluation and management services

   d. transitional care management services

Exercise 10.4 – continued

5. A patient underwent emergency appendectomy as a hospital inpatient and was discharged home for recuperation. The patient then returned to the hospital, seeking immediate medical attention due to surgical staples separating at the site of incision. From which Evaluation and Management category would the code be selected?

   a. Care management services

   b. Emergency department services

   c. Office or other outpatient services

   d. Prolonged services

6. A 40-year-old patient was admitted to the hospital by the primary care provider (PCP) to control type II diabetes mellitus and to evaluate possible gangrene, left foot. The PCP ordered inpatient consultation services from an orthopedic surgeon, who provided level 4 E/M inpatient consultation services. The orthopedic surgeon told the patient and the PCP that immediate surgical debridement was necessary. Which Evaluation and Management is assigned for the consultation service?

   a. 99244   b. 99244 57   c. 99254   d. 99254 57

7. The physician reviewed and revised the hospice agency care plan for an 84-year-old patient with Alzheimer's disease. For care plan oversight services requiring 25 minutes of the physician's time, CPT code _____ is reported.

   a. 99374   b. 99375   c. 99377   d. 99378

8. The physician provided 70 minutes of hospital inpatient discharge day management services to a 104-year-old patient who was transferred to an assisted living facility. Orders for pain management were provided to the facility. Which Evaluation and Management code(s) is/are assigned?

   a. 99222   b. 99238   c. 99238, 99239   d. 99239

9. A patient with a heart condition is scheduled to undergo a cesarean section. Due to the high-risk nature of the delivery, the attending physician requests standby service from a cardiac surgeon, and 30 minutes later the patient delivers a healthy newborn with no complications. Which Evaluation and Management code is are reported by the cardiac surgeon?

   a. 99026   b. 99027   c. 99360   d. 99464

10. The physician had a 20-minute real-time interactive audio-video telemedicine encounter with an established patient to report results of blood tests, to provide instructions to the patient about lowering the Coumadin dosage, and to answer the patient's questions. A medically appropriate history was documented. Which Evaluation and Management code is reported?

    a. 99213 95   b. 99417 95   c. 99422 95   d. 99499 95

Summary

The E/M section is organized according to place of service (e.g., office, hospital, home, nursing facility, emergency department, or critical care), type of service (e.g., new or initial encounter, follow-up or subsequent encounter), and miscellaneous services (e.g., prolonged service or care plan oversight service). The Evaluation and Management (E/M) section guidelines are located at the beginning of the section and include the following contents: E/M guidelines overview, classification of E/M services, levels of E/M services, unlisted service, and special report.

E/M categories and subcategories contain codes that are classified according to level of services for reporting to third-party payers. Although the last number of some E/M codes represents the level of service (e.g., code 99213 is a level 3 E/M service), the levels within categories and subcategories are not interchangeable. Levels of E/M services include conferences with or about patients, evaluations, examinations, preventive adult and pediatric health supervision, treatments, and other medical services (e.g., determining the need for and location of appropriate care, such as hospice care for a terminally ill patient). The E/M section contains notes unique to each category and subcategory. *Remember to review notes before assigning an E/M code.*

Internet Links

American Academy of Family Physicians (AAFP): https://www.aafp.org

American Academy of Pediatrics (AAP): aap.org

Documentation Guidelines for E/M Services: Go to **cms.gov**; click on the Outreach and Education link, click on the "Get training" link below the Learn heading, click on the Medicare Learning Network® (MLN) link, click on the Publications link, enter Evaluation and Management Services in the Filter On box, click Apply, and click on the 2020-01 link to download the PDF file.

Medicare Learning Network (MLN): Go to **cms.gov**, click on the Outreach & Education link, click on the "Get training" link below the Learn heading, and then click on the Medicare Learning Network® (MLN) link.

Review

10.1 – Multiple Choice

Instructions: Select the most appropriate response.

1. The E/M level of service reflects the
   a. amount of work involved in providing health care to a patient.
   b. kind of health care services provided to a patient.
   c. physical location where health care is provided to a patient.
   d. type of condition for which the patient is being treated.

2. Concurrent care is the provision of similar services to
   a. different patients by the same provider on the same day.
   b. the same patient by more than one provider on the same day.
   c. the same patient by the same provider on different days.
   d. the same patient by the same provider on the same day.

3. Dr. Kim practiced at Hopewell Medical Center until 2020 and then joined the practice with Dr. Evans at the Lakewood Clinic. Which would be considered a new patient at Lakewood Clinic?
   a. Colleen sustained a back injury two years ago and has been under continuous treatment at another facility. Her records were transferred to Lakewood Clinic, and Colleen is going to be seen by Dr. Evans for continuing treatment of the chronic condition.
   b. Henrique, who had last seen Dr. Kim at Hopewell Medical Center in April 2019, is treated by Dr. Kim at the Lakewood Clinic in March 2022.
   c. Raven had a physical performed on June 1, 2020, by Dr. Kim and is seen by Dr. Evans on September 30, 2022, for a sinus condition.
   d. Dorothy was treated last month by Dr. Evans. This week she needs to be seen again, but Lakewood Clinic is closed for the holiday. Dorothy receives synchronous real-time audiovisual telemedicine services from an on-call physician based at Lakewood Clinic who is covering for Dr. Evans.

4. Which involves assessing the status of a patient's condition, establishing diagnoses, and selecting a management option?
    a. Coordination of care
    b. Counseling
    c. Medical decision making
    d. Nature of presenting problem

5. Which is considered when determining the number of diagnoses or management options when selecting the level of medical decision making for the current encounter?
    a. Conditions previously diagnosed and treated, which have now entirely resolved
    b. Evaluation and treatment that is not associated with the likely nature of the condition
    c. Multiple conditions that are medically managed or treated during the current encounter
    d. Time the physician or other qualified health care professional spends providing care

6. Documentation of medical records, ancillary tests, and other information that must be obtained, ordered, reviewed, and interpreted for a patient encounter is associated with which element of medical decision making?
    a. Amount and complexity of data to be reviewed and analyzed
    b. Number and complexity of problems addressed during an encounter
    c. Risk of complications and morbidity or mortality of patient management decisions
    d. Time the physician or other qualified health care professional spends interpreting test results

7. The risk of complications, morbidity, and mortality for patient management decisions made during the encounter includes
    a. analyzing test results.
    b. diagnosing patient conditions.
    c. prescription drug management.
    d. time required to manage care.

8. Two physicians or other qualified health care professionals who provide similar evaluation and management services to the same patient on the same day are providing
    a. concurrent care.
    b. risk management.
    c. standby services.
    d. transfer of care.

9. When a physician documents a discussion about the importance of the patient complying with a weight management program to control their blood glucose, this is considered
    a. concurrent care.
    b. coordination of care.
    c. counseling.
    d. transfer of care.

10. Which is reported using a non-face-to-face service code?
    a. A patient came into the emergency department with severe pain in the lower back. Patient told the physician that recently an MRI was performed at that facility but results were not available yet. The physician looked up the test results and verified that a displaced disc was causing the pain.
    b. A patient involved in a motor vehicle accident came to the emergency department with complaints of a sore neck and blurry vision. The patient was diagnosed with whiplash. The attending physician requested an ophthalmology consultation during the encounter, but no physicians were available so the consultation was scheduled for the following day. The physician instructed the patient to follow up with the primary care physician if symptoms persisted.
    c. A physician called the patient at home to discuss the results of lab tests. After reviewing the reports, the physician believed that further testing was necessary and advised the patient to make an appointment as soon as possible.
    d. During an encounter, a physician recommended physical therapy to a patient with rheumatoid arthritis. The patient expressed concern about which facility to contact and how to get there. Before leaving, the physician provided names and numbers of facilities for treatment, as well as agencies that would assist with transportation needs.

11. A new patient received treatment at a stand-alone urgent care center for flu symptoms with documentation of straightforward level of medical decision making. Which code is assigned?

    a. 99202   **b.** 99203   **c.** 99211   **d.** 99212

12. A six-year-old child undergoes an annual physical examination, and the child's last encounter was one year ago. Which code is reported?

    a. 99211   **b.** 99252   **c.** 99383   **d.** 99393

13. A patient with severe chest pain receives hospital observation services with documentation of a medically appropriate history and examination, moderate level of medical decision making, and discharge the same day. Which code is reported?

    a. 99204   **b.** 99214   **c.** 99222   **d.** 99235

14. A Medicare patient received office consultation services for the first time from a specialist who documented a medically appropriate history and examination during the 45-minute encounter. Which E/M code is reported?

    a. 99204   **b.** 99214   **c.** 99244   **d.** 99253

15. A patient diagnosed with sunburn and blister formation on the tops of the feet was seen in the emergency department with documentation of a medically appropriate history and examination and low level of medical decision making. Which code is reported?

    a. 99213   **b.** 99231   **c.** 99283   **d.** 99288

16. A physician performs a scheduled follow-up visit to a 65-year-old patient in a nursing facility who is recovering from pneumonia. A medically appropriate history and examination and straightforward level of medical decision making were documented. The patient has responded well to the treatment, and no complications are noted. Which code is reported?

    a. 99304   **b.** 99307   **c.** 99341   **d.** 99347

17. A new patient presents to the physician's office with complaints of severe earache, jaw pain, and facial swelling. The physician documented a medically appropriate history and examination. A total time of 50 minutes is documented for the encounter. Which code is reported?

    a. 99204   **b.** 99205   **c.** 99214   **d.** 99215

18. An established patient undergoes a four-month office check-up for medical management of high triglyceride levels, which lasted 20 minutes. A medically appropriate history and examination are documented. Which code is reported?

    a. 99202   **b.** 99213   **c.** 99214   **d.** 99232

19. A subsequent hospital visit was conducted for a 58-year-old patient admitted with an esophageal neoplasm who is spitting up blood. Metastasis is suspected, and the physician documented a medically appropriate examination and high level of medical decision making. Which is reported?

    a. 99233   **b.** 99236   **c.** 99255   **d.** 99285

20. A physician provided initial hospital care for the evaluation and management of a normal newborn infant who was admitted and discharged on March 5. Which code is reported?

    a. 99460   **b.** 99461   **c.** 99462   **d.** 99463

10.2 – Coding Practice

Instructions: Review each case and assign CPT code(s) and appropriate modifier(s).

Office or Other Outpatient Services

1. A 4-year-old established patient received evaluation and management services in the physician's office, which included a low level of medical decision making. The patient is diagnosed with influenza.

2. A 16-year-old outpatient who is a new patient to the office complains of severe facial acne. A medically appropriate history and examination was documented. With a minimal number of diagnoses to consider and a minimal amount of data to review, the level of medical decision making is straightforward.

Hospital Inpatient and Observation Care Services

3. A 50-year-old patient was admitted as a hospital inpatient on October 10 with a diagnosis of pneumonia due to *Staphylococcus aureus*, at which time level 2 E/M services were provided by the attending physician. On October 11 and October 12, the patient received level 2 E/M services. On October 13, the patient was discharged from the hospital in improved condition to follow up with the physician at home; the physician spent 30 minutes performing discharge day management functions.

4. A patient is seen as a hospital inpatient on day two of the hospital stay. The patient had been admitted through the emergency department with status asthmaticus and had been undergoing extensive respiratory therapy over the past 24 to 30 hours. The physician performs a medically appropriate history and examination. The possibility of pneumonia complicating the asthma must be considered. The patient's respiratory condition is still unstable. The level of medical decision making was moderate.

Consultations

5. A 52-year-old patient was sent to a surgeon for an office consultation concerning hemorrhoids, and the health plan allows CPT consultation codes to be reported. A medically appropriate focused history and examination were performed. The consultant recommended treating with medication after straightforward level of medical decision making.

6. A 13-year-old was admitted as a hospital inpatient yesterday for a tympanotomy. Postsurgically, the child developed fever and seizures of unknown origin. A pediatric consultation was requested, and the health plan allows CPT consultation codes to be reported. This was done on the second hospital inpatient day and 24 hours after surgery. A medically appropriate history and examination was documented. The level of medical decision making was high.

Emergency Department Services

7. A patient in the emergency department has a temperature of 103°F and is in acute respiratory distress. Symptoms include severe shortness of breath, chest pain, and gasping. The physician is unable to obtain a history due to the patient's critical condition. The family was interviewed to obtain as much of a history as possible, and the physician performed a medically appropriate examination. The level of medical decision making is high.

8. With two-way communication, the physician provides direction of advanced life support to emergency medical technicians en route to the emergency department with an ambulance patient in apparent cardiac arrest.

Emergency Department Services

9. A patient presents with the complaint of hematemesis. The patient also has a rapid pulse rate and low blood pressure. In the ED, critical care is provided by the ED attending to raise the patient's blood pressure and decrease blood loss. This is done for 70 minutes before the patient is transferred to the surgical suite for an endoscopic procedure to evaluate his esophagus. The ED physician also documents a medically appropriate examination, and the level of medical decision making is high. Due to the patient's serious medical condition, a history cannot be obtained, and family are not in attendance to provide information.

Critical Care Services

10. A physician is called to the intensive care unit to provide care for a patient who received second- and third-degree burns over 50 percent of his body due to a chemical fire. The patient is in respiratory distress and is suffering from severe dehydration. The physician provides support for two hours. Later that day, the physician returns and provides an additional hour of critical care support to the patient.

Nursing Facility Services

11. A 72-year-old patient suffered a cerebral vascular accident. Today the patient is admitted to a skilled nursing facility (SNF) for rehab and medical care. The patient was just discharged from an acute care facility. The SNF medical director documents a medically appropriate history and examination. The physician orders a multidisciplinary rehabilitation care plan and continued treatment of the patient's other conditions, including hypertension and diabetes. The level of medical decision making is high.

12. Subsequent follow-up care is provided for a comatose patient transferred to a long-term care center from the hospital two days ago. The resident shows no signs of consciousness on examination but appears to have developed a minor upper respiratory tract infection with a fever and rales heard on auscultation. The physician performs a medically appropriate history and examination. The physician is concerned that the respiratory infection could progress to pneumonia and orders the appropriate treatment. The level of medical decision making is low.

Home or Residence Services

13. A 64-year-old established patient has diabetes and has been having problems adjusting prescribed insulin doses and has had an onset of dizziness and sensitivity to light. During the home visit, the physician documents a medically appropriate history and examination. The patient's condition is moderately severe, and level of medical decision making is low.

14. A 15-year-old new patient with cystic fibrosis is having problems with the dosage of Pulmozyme, which is a medication used to thin mucus that clogs the lungs. The patient is experiencing moderate throat pain and slight tightness of the chest. The physician makes a home visit, and a medically appropriate history and examination was documented. The level of medical decision making is moderate.

Prolonged Services

15. A patient with asthma presents with acute bronchospasm and moderate respiratory distress and is admitted to hospital observation care at 2 a.m. on August 15. The physician conducts a medically appropriate history and examination, which showed an elevated respiratory rate of 30. The physician provided a total of 100 minutes of face-to-face care. The patient was discharged home at 10 p.m. on August 15. Assign the observation care services code and the prolonged services code.

Standby Services

16. A patient was in the delivery room ready to give birth. When the physician had the patient start pushing, possible complications for the infant were noted and the hospital pediatric neonatal specialist was requested to standby in the delivery room for possible evaluation of this newborn. The pediatric specialist was initially notified at 9:20 a.m. At 10 a.m., the specialist was informed via phone call by the physician that the infant had serial Apgar scores of 9 and 9, which are normal values.

Case Management Services

17. A 72-year-old patient with a history of breast cancer has a suspicious uterine mass. A uterine biopsy was done, which established the diagnosis of carcinoma *in situ* of the uterus. The physician who conducted the surgery participated in a face-to-face meeting with fellow surgeons and discussed the case and the patient's outcome for 30 minutes.

18. A 14-year-old boy twisted his ankle while playing soccer. He received level 3 E/M services from his physician the next morning for which code 99213 was reported on the CMS-1500 claim generated immediately after the visit. The physician ordered an x-ray of the ankle, and the child left the office after the x-ray but did not see the physician. The next day, the patient and his mother came into the office and met with the physician, an orthopedic surgeon, and a rehabilitation therapist. The medical team conference was 45 minutes in duration.

Care Plan Oversight Services

19. A 75-year-old patient was just diagnosed with type 1 diabetes. This means that the patient will be required to self-inject insulin. The physician supervised the coordination of home health care, which required 30 minutes.

20. A 50-year-old patient has brain cancer, and the physician supervised the coordination of hospice services, which required 45 minutes.

Preventive Medicine Services

21. A 13-year-old new patient undergoes initial comprehensive preventive medicine evaluation and management services as part of the school-required sports physical. The patient does not report any medical complaints.

Non-Face-to-Face Services

22. A physician called an established patient to communicate the results of a chest x-ray, which was negative. The call was five minutes in duration. The patient had previously been seen in the office 10 days ago.

23. A patient e-mailed the physician to ask whether taking 500 mg of cinnamon tablets daily would be acceptable, given their prescribed medications. The physician replied via e-mail and approved the 500 mg of cinnamon tablets daily, which required five minutes.

Special Evaluation and Management Services

24. A 58-year-old underwent a medical disability examination due to long-term COPD, severe emphysema, and an inability to work during the past year. The examination was performed by the treating physician. The physician completed a medical history, performed an examination, determined a diagnosis, assessed patient capabilities and stability, calculated impairment, developed a future medical treatment plan, and completed the necessity documentation/certificates and a report.

Newborn Care Services

25. A full-term healthy newborn girl received initial and subsequent hospital care services on July 7 and July 8, respectively.

---

11 CPT Anesthesia

Chapter Outline

Anesthesia Terminology

Overview of Anesthesia Section

Anesthesia Section Guidelines

Anesthesia Subsections

Chapter Objectives

At the conclusion of this chapter, the student should be able to:

1. Define key terms related to the CPT Anesthesia section.
2. Define terminology associated with types of anesthesia.
3. Provide an overview about the Anesthesia section, focusing on organization, services included and excluded, and monitored anesthesia care.
4. Interpret Anesthesia section guidelines.
5. Assign CPT Anesthesia section codes and modifiers.

Key Terms

airway management

analgesia

analgesic

anesthesia

anesthesia conversion factor

anesthesia time unit

anesthesiologist

anesthetic

base unit value

Bier block

capnography

caudal anesthesia

certified anesthesiologist assistant (CAA)

certified registered nurse anesthetist (CRNA)

concurrent medically directed anesthesia procedure

endotracheal tube (ET)

epidural anesthesia

field block

general anesthesia

infiltration anesthesia

intravenous regional anesthesia

local anesthesia

mass spectrometry

moderate (conscious) sedation

modifying unit

monitored anesthesia care (MAC)

peripheral nerve block

physical status modifier

plexus anesthesia

postanesthesia evaluation

postoperative pain management

preanesthesia evaluation

pulse oximetry

qualifying circumstance

regional anesthesia

saddle block anesthesia

sedation

spinal anesthesia

surface anesthesia

Introduction

The Anesthesia section is located after the Evaluation and Management section in the CPT coding manual. Anesthesia codes are reported for services related to the administration of anesthesia (including general and regional), the supplementation of local anesthesia, and other supportive anesthesia services. Anesthesia subsections are organized according to anatomical site, except the last four subsections, which are organized as radiological procedures, burn excisions or debridement procedures, obstetric procedures, and other procedures. Any qualified health care provider who administers analgesic or anesthetic agents is permitted to report codes from the Anesthesia section. Providers include anesthesiologists, certified registered nurse anesthetists (CRNAs), certified anesthesiologist assistants (CAAs), surgeons, and other physicians. However, when the same physician (e.g., surgeon) performs the procedure and administers anesthesia, add modifier 47 to the CPT Surgery section code (and do not report a separate code from the Anesthesia section).

 NOTE:

The *Medicare National Correct Coding Initiative Policy Manual* provides guidance about assigning procedure codes for the Anesthesia section. Go to **www.cms.gov** and enter "Medicare NCCI Policy Manual" in the Search box to navigate to the manual.

Anesthesia Terminology

Anesthesia practitioners are anesthesiologists and *qualified nonphysician anesthetists*, which include certified anesthesiologist assistants and certified registered nurse anesthetists. An **anesthesiologist** is a physician who, after medical school, completes a one-year internship and three-year residency in anesthesia. A **certified anesthesiologist assistant (CAA)** has earned a master's degree from an accredited anesthesia program and has successfully passed the certification exam offered by the National Commission for Certification of Anesthesiologist Assistants (NCCAA). CAAs are part of the anesthesia care team, working under the supervision of a licensed anesthesiologist. A **certified registered nurse anesthetist (CRNA)** is a licensed registered nurse (RN) who has obtained at least one year of acute care nursing experience (e.g., intensive care unit), completed an accredited nurse anesthesia program leading to a doctoral degree, and passed the National Board of Certification and Recertification for Nurse Anesthetists (NBCRNA) national certification exam.

Patients who undergo surgical or other invasive procedures (e.g., radiological procedure) require anesthesia services so the procedure can be performed. **Anesthesia** is the process of inducing a loss of sensitivity to pain in all or part of the body, resulting from the administration of an **anesthetic** (drug or agent that causes a loss of feeling, awareness, and consciousness). An **analgesic** is a drug that reduces pain, such as aspirin, acetaminophen, and ibuprofen; for surgery, other substances (e.g., morphine) are used to cause **analgesia** (loss of pain sensation without loss of consciousness).

Types of Anesthesia

The following types of anesthesia are used in surgical practice:

- General anesthesia
- Local anesthesia
- Regional anesthesia
- Monitored (conscious) sedation

General anesthesia is used for extensive surgeries and involves the administration of anesthetic agents that are inhaled (e.g., sevoflurane combined with nitrous oxide) or administered intravenously (e.g., propofol). They act as hypnotics, muscle relaxants, and painkillers and serve to block any memory of the surgery. General anesthesia renders a patient unconscious, which means the brain doesn't perceive pain signals. To determine the general anesthetic agents to administer, the patient's age and health must be considered, along with the type of surgery to be performed.

Local anesthesia is appropriate for minor surgeries (e.g., dental work, skin biopsy, and suture of a laceration) and involves applying a topical agent (e.g., lidocaine) on the body's surface or injecting a local anesthetic agent (e.g., procaine) for the purpose of numbing a small part of the body. As a result, pain signals are blocked and the patient remains alert. Local anesthesia administration techniques include:

- **Surface anesthesia**: Topical application of local anesthetic cream, solution, or spray to skin or mucous membranes
- **Infiltration anesthesia**: Topical injection of local anesthetic into tissue
- **Field block**: Subcutaneous injection of local anesthetic in area bordering the field to be anesthetized
- **Peripheral nerve blocks**: Injection of local anesthetic in the vicinity of a peripheral nerve to anesthetize that nerve's area of innervation
- **Plexus anesthesia**: Injection of local anesthetic in the vicinity of a *nerve plexus*, which is a network of intersecting nerves (Figure 11-1)

Regional anesthesia is appropriate when there is a need to block pain from a large part of the body (e.g., lower extremity and pelvic surgeries). Regional anesthetic agents are injected into or near the spinal fluid and around a nerve or network of nerves to block the nerve supply to a specific part of the body (Figure 11-2). The patient cannot feel pain in that area when a procedure is performed, and the patient remains awake (or sedated). Intravenous (IV) sedation may be administered prior to regional anesthesia to relax and make the patient drowsy, but the patient remains conscious. Regional anesthesia includes the following:

- **Caudal anesthesia**, or **saddle block anesthesia**: Local anesthetic is injected into the caudal canal, which is the sacral portion of the spinal canal; anesthetized area is the umbilicus, below the navel.
- **Epidural anesthesia**: Local anesthetic is injected into the epidural space where it acts primarily on spinal nerve roots; anesthetized area includes the abdomen, chest, and large regions of the body.

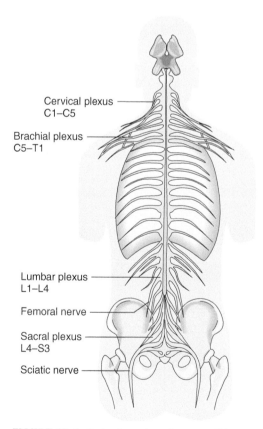

Cervical plexus
C1–C5

Brachial plexus
C5–T1

Lumbar plexus
L1–L4

Femoral nerve

Sacral plexus
L4–S3

Sciatic nerve

FIGURE 11-1 Spinal cord and nerves (Most spinal nerves are named for the corresponding vertebrae.)

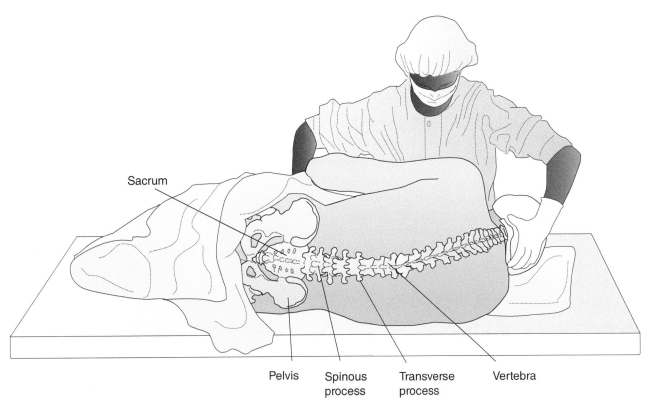

FIGURE 11-2 Correct position for performing a spinal block or inserting an epidural catheter in the lumbar region

- **Spinal anesthesia**: Local anesthetic is injected into cerebrospinal fluid (CSF) at the lumbar spine, where it acts on spinal nerve roots and part of the spinal cord; anesthetized area extends from the legs to the abdomen or chest.
- **Intravenous regional anesthesia**, or **Bier block**: An IV cannula is inserted into the extremity on which the procedure is to be performed and a tourniquet is applied to interrupt blood circulation; then an appropriate volume of local anesthetic is injected into a peripheral vein, anesthetizing the extremity.

Moderate (conscious) sedation is provided by the physician performing the procedure (instead of an anesthesia practitioner), and it uses medication (e.g., benzodiazepine) to help patients feel calm and relaxed during the procedure. While experiencing a drug-induced minimal depression of consciousness, the patient is able to retain control over protective reflexes, such as breathing independently, responding appropriately to verbal commands, and responding appropriately to physical stimulation. Patients also remember little to nothing about the procedure. Moderate (conscious sedation) codes (99151–99157) are located in the Medicine section of CPT.

Example: Patient who underwent partial mastectomy, right breast, with placement of radiotherapy after-loading brachytherapy catheters as an interstitial radioelement, including imaging guidance. The 67-year-old patient received local anesthesia with 30 minutes of moderate (conscious) sedation by the surgeon. An independent trained observer monitored the patient's sedation. Report codes 19301 RT, 19298 RT, 99156, and 99157.

 NOTE:

Sedation is the administration of medication into a vein to relieve pain and anxiety and to make the patient feel calm. Sedation medications are often administered in addition to other forms of anesthesia.

Exercise 11.1 – Anesthesia Terminology

Instructions: Complete each statement.

1. General anesthesia involves the administration of anesthetic agents that are _____ or administered intravenously rendering a patient unconscious, which means the brain does not perceive pain signals.

2. Sedation is the administration of medication to relieve pain and _____, and it makes the patient feel calm.

3. For minor procedures (suture of laceration), it is appropriate to administer _____ anesthesia (e.g., surface or topical anesthesia), applying lidocaine or injecting procaine to block pain signals and allow the patient to remain alert.

4. Regional anesthesia involves injecting anesthetic agents into or near spinal fluid and around a nerve or network of nerves to block the _____ supply to a specific part of the body.

5. Saddle block anesthesia involves locally injecting an anesthetic agent into the _____ canal, which is located at the sacral portion of the spinal canal.

6. Plexus anesthesia involves injecting a local anesthetic in the vicinity of a nerve plexus, which is a _____ of intersecting nerves.

7. Epidural anesthesia involves injecting a local anesthetic into the epidural space where it acts primarily on spinal nerve _____, anesthetizing areas of the abdomen, chest, and large regions of the body.

8. A field block involves the _____ injection of local anesthetic in an area bordering the field to be anesthetized.

9. The topical application of local anesthetic cream, solution, or spray to skin or mucous membranes is called _____ anesthesia.

10. Infiltration anesthesia is the _____ injection of a local anesthetic into tissue.

Overview of Anesthesia Section

The Anesthesia section is organized by anatomic site except for the last four subsections, which are organized as radiological, burn excisions or debridement, obstetrics, and other procedures. Codes are organized according to type of procedure (open, closed, endoscopic), and each anesthesia code relates to corresponding surgical procedures. Because a one-to-one correlation for anesthesia to surgery codes does not exist, one anesthesia code is often reported for many different surgical procedures that share similar anesthesia requirements. One Anesthesia section code is often reported for many different surgical procedures that share similar anesthesia requirements. The Anesthesia section guidelines also include four codes (99100–99140) that are located in the Medicine section, which are used to report qualifying circumstances for anesthesia.

 Coding Tip

Notes located beneath categories, subcategories, headings and subheadings apply to all codes below them. Parenthetical notes located below a specific code apply to that code only unless the note indicates otherwise.

Anesthesia services include preoperative and postoperative evaluations, preparing the patient prior to administration of anesthesia, administration of anesthesia, and anesthesia care and patient monitoring during the procedure. Services also include **airway management** (ensure open airway to patient's lungs) and *fluid management* (administering intravenous fluids to avoid dehydration, maintain an effective circulating volume, and prevent inadequate tissue perfusion). According to the *Medicare National Correct Coding Initiative Policy Manual*, the following services are bundled with the reported anesthesia code.

- Transporting, positioning, prepping, and draping the patient for satisfactory anesthesia induction and surgical procedures
- Placement and monitoring of external monitoring cardiorespiratory and other devices
    - Blood pressure, heart rate, respirations, and temperature
    - **Capnography** (monitoring carbon dioxide levels)
    - *CNS-evoked responses* (monitoring nervous system electrophysiologic responses)
    - Continuous *electrocardiogram* (monitoring heart's electrical activity)
    - Continuous **pulse oximetry** (monitoring arterial oxyhemoglobin saturation)
    - *Doppler flow* (ultrasound to detect blood flow changes)
    - Electroencephalogram (monitoring brain waves)
    - Low oxygen and circuit disconnect alarms
    - **Mass spectrometry** (monitoring proper levels of the anesthetic agent)
- Placement of peripheral IV lines for fluid and medication administration
- Placement of airway tubes (e.g., endotracheal tube, orotracheal tube), including direct or endoscopic laryngoscopy for placement purposes
- Placement of nasogastric or orogastric tube
- Interpretation of laboratory determinations (e.g., arterial blood gases, CBC, blood chemistries, lactate levels)
- Nerve stimulation to determine level of paralysis or localization of nerves
- Insertion of urinary bladder catheter
- Blood sample procurement through existing lines *or* venipuncture or arterial puncture

Monitored Anesthesia Care (MAC)

Monitored anesthesia care (MAC) is the administration of varying amounts of local, regional, and certain mind-altering drugs by an anesthesiologist or a qualified nonphysician anesthetist (e.g., CRNA) during a patient's diagnostic or therapeutic procedure. The Centers for Medicare & Medicaid Services (CMS) defines MAC as "the intraoperative monitoring of the surgical patient's vital physiological signs, in anticipation of the patient's need for general anesthesia or development of adverse physiological patient reaction to the surgery."

During MAC, the anesthesiologist or qualified nonphysician anesthetist administers anesthetic medication through an IV line, monitors the patient's comfort level, and increases or decreases medication as needed (hence the name *monitored anesthesia care*). MAC includes a preoperative visit, intraoperative care, and postoperative anesthesia management. The anesthesiologist or qualified nonphysician anesthetist provides the following services:

- Monitors vital signs and maintains patient's airway and continual evaluation of vital functions
- Diagnoses and treats clinical problems that occur during the procedure
- Administers analgesics, anesthetic agents, hypnotics, sedatives, or other medications as necessary to ensure patient safety and comfort
- Provides other medical services as needed for the safe completion of the procedure

Coding Tip

Because monitored anesthesia care is a physician service provided to an individual patient and is based on medical necessity, reimbursement may be the same amount as for full general anesthesia services if all required services are properly documented. Report the appropriate anesthesia code and add an appropriate anesthesia provider modifier, physical status modifier, and modifier QS (monitored anesthesia care). In addition, report a qualifying circumstances code (from the Medicine section) when indicated. Make sure you report appropriate ICD-10-CM codes that support medical necessity for MAC and identify the reason for the surgical procedure.

NOTE:

When the anesthesiologist provides separate services to surgical patients that are not included as part of the anesthesia service code, such as pain management, modifier 59 or XE (depending on payer requirements) is added to indicate that the service is independent of the anesthesia service.

Exercise 11.2 – Overview of Anesthesia Section

Instructions: Complete each statement.

1. The Anesthesia section is organized by _____ site except for the last four subsections, which are organized as radiological, burn excisions or debridement, obstetrics, and other procedures.

2. When an anesthesiologist provides separate services to surgical patients that are not included as part of the anesthesia service code, such as pain management, modifier _____ or XE (depending on payer requirements) is added to indicate that the service provided is independent of the anesthesia service.

3. The placement of airway tubes (e.g., endotracheal tube), including laryngoscopy, for airway management is included in the reported _____ code.

4. Monitored anesthesia care (MAC) is the administration of varying amounts of local, regional, and certain mind-altering drugs by an anesthesiologist or a qualified nonphysician anesthetist during a patient's diagnostic or therapeutic _____.

5. When reporting a code for monitored anesthesia care, add modifier _____ in addition to appropriate HCPCS Level II provider and physical status modifiers.

Anesthesia Section Guidelines

Anesthesia services are reported by assigning a five-digit procedure code and adding appropriate modifiers. An anesthesiologist or qualified nonphysician anesthetist is responsible for supervising anesthesia services (which include general and regional), supplementation of local anesthesia, and other supportive services so the patient receives appropriate and optimal anesthesia care. The administration of local infiltration, metacarpal/metatarsal/digital block, or topical anesthesia by the operating surgeon or obstetrician is included (bundled) in the surgery code; separate codes are not reported. Such anesthesia is not reported separately because it is included in the surgery code (e.g., surgical procedure fee in physician's office, facility charge at an ambulatory surgical center or hospital outpatient department, and accommodation revenue code for a hospital inpatient).

The anesthesia practitioner is responsible for conducting a **preanesthesia evaluation** (Figure 11-3) of the patient prior to surgery, which includes assessing information from the patient's record, interviewing the patient (e.g., history), conducting a physical examination, evaluating preoperative test results, and ensuring that informed anesthetic consent has been obtained. The preanesthesia evaluation is included (bundled) in the anesthesia services code. If the surgery for which a preanesthesia evaluation was performed is canceled, the anesthesiologist should report an evaluation and management service code (e.g., office or other outpatient consultation or inpatient consultation).

A **postanesthesia evaluation** (Figure 11-4) is also included (bundled) in the anesthesia services code and includes an evaluation of the patient during recovery from anesthesia, as well as evaluation, treatment, and follow-up of possible anesthesia-related complications. When an anesthesiologist or a qualified nonphysician anesthetist provides significant, separately identifiable services (e.g., critical care services, postoperative pain management services, or unrelated ventilator management), the appropriate code(s) are reported for each service.

When an anesthesiologist or qualified nonphysician anesthetist provides anesthesia services, report the code from the CPT Anesthesia section with appropriate modifiers (discussed later in this chapter). (This means that a surgeon performs the surgical procedure while the anesthesiologist or qualified nonphysician

Addressograph

PRE- AND POST-ANESTHESIA EVALUATION RECORD

PRE-ANESTHESIA EVALUATION

HISTORY TAKEN FROM: ❑ Patient ❑ Parent/ Guardian ❑ Significant Other ❑ Chart ❑ Poor Historian ❑ Language Barrier

PROPOSED PROCEDURE:

AGE	GENDER ❑ Male ❑ Female	HEIGHT	WEIGHT	BLOOD PRESSURE	PULSE	RESPIRATIONS	TEMPERATURE	O2 SAT%

PREVIOUS ANESTHESIA:	❑ None
PREVIOUS SURGERY:	❑ None
CURRENT MEDICATIONS:	❑ None
FAMILY HX – ANES. PROBLEMS:	❑ None
ALLERGIES	❑ None
AIRWAY	❑ MP1 ❑ MP2 ❑ MP3 ❑ MP4 ❑ Unrestricted neck ROM ❑ T-M distance = ________
(Enter X in appropriate boxes)	❑ Obesity ❑ ↓ neck ROM ❑ History of difficult airway ❑ Short muscular neck
	❑ Teeth poor repair ❑ Teeth chipped/loose ❑ Edentulous ❑ Facial hair

BODY SYSTEM	COMMENTS
RESPIRATORY	❑ WNL Tobacco Use: ❑ Yes ❑ No ❑ Quit ________ Packs/Day for ____ Years
CARDIOVASCULAR	❑ WNL Pre-procedure Cardiac Assessment:
GASTROINTESTINAL	❑ WNL Ethanol Use: ❑ Yes ❑ No ❑ Quit Frequency ____________ ❑ History of Ethanol abuse
MUSCULOSKELETAL	❑ WNL
GENITOURINARY	❑ WNL
OTHER	❑ WNL
PREGNANCY	❑ WNL ❑ AROM ❑ SROM ❑ Pitocin Drip ❑ Induction ❑ MgDrip Weeks Gestation: ____ G: _____ P: _____ EDC: _______

DIAGNOSTIC STUDIES
ECG
CHEST X-RAY
PULMONARY STUDIES

LABORATORY STUDIES
PT/PTT/INR:
T&S / T&C:
HCG:
LMP:
UA:

OTHER DIAGNOSTIC TESTS

PLANNED ANESTHESIA/MONITORS

PRE-ANESTHESIA MEDICATION

SIGNATURE OF ANESTHESIOLOGIST OR C.R.N.A.

POST-ANESTHESIA EVALUATION

Location	Time	B/P	O_2Sat	Pulse	Respirations	Temperature

❑ Awake ❑ Mask O_2 ❑ Somnolent ❑ Unarousable ❑ Oral/nasal airway
❑ Stable ❑ NC O_2 ❑ Unstable ❑ T-Piece ❑ Intubated ❑ Ventilator
❑ Regional – dermatome level: ❑ Continuous epidural analgesia
❑ Direct admit to hospital room ❑ No anesthesia related complications noted
❑ See notes for anesthesia related concerns ❑ Satisfactory postanesthesia/analgesia recovery

CONTROLLED MEDICATIONS

Medication	Used	Destroyed	Returned

SIGNATURE OF ANESTHESIOLOGIST OR C.R.N.A.

ALFRED STATE MEDICAL CENTER ■ 100 MAIN ST, ALFRED NY 14802 ■ (607) 555-1234

FIGURE 11-3 Sample pre- and postanesthesia evaluation record

anesthetist provides anesthesia services. The surgeon reports code(s) from the Surgery section, and the anesthesiologist or qualified nonphysician anesthetist reports the code from the Anesthesia section.)

Example: An anesthesiologist provides general anesthesia services for a healthy patient who undergoes carpal tunnel surgery. Report code 01810 AA P1.

When the surgeon administers anesthesia *in addition to performing the procedure*, report code(s) from the CPT Surgery section and add modifier 47 (Anesthesia by surgeon) to each code. *Do not add modifier 47 to an anesthesia code.* (This means that the surgeon performs the surgical procedure and provides anesthesia services to the same patient during the same operative session. There is no anesthesiologist or qualified nonphysician anesthetist is in the operating room providing anesthesia services.)

Example: The surgeon provides regional anesthesia services for a 38-year-old patient who undergoes a needle biopsy of the thyroid. Report code 60100 47. Do *not* report code 00322 from the Anesthesia section.

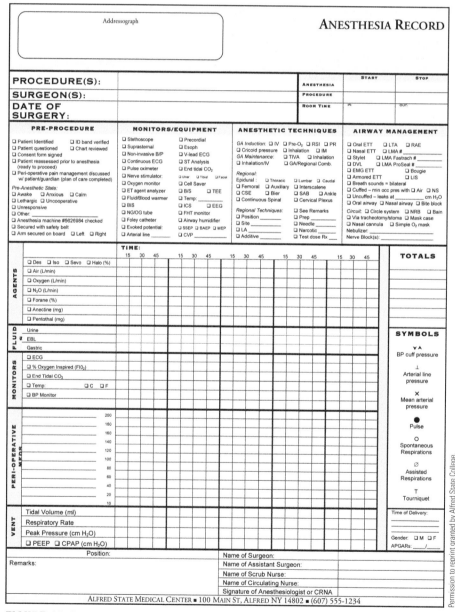

FIGURE 11-4 Sample anesthesia record

Reporting Codes for Unusual Monitoring and Other Services

Standard preparation, monitoring, and procedural services provided during the administration of anesthesia are bundled into the reported CPT Anesthesia code because they are considered integral to provision of the anesthesia service. Although some of these services may never be reported on the same date of service as an anesthesia service, many *could be* provided as part of a separate patient encounter unrelated to the anesthesia service reported on the same date of service. *When a separate procedure or service is provided, modifier 59* (Distinct procedural service) *or XE* (Separate encounter, a service that is distinct because it occurred during a separate encounter) *is added to the reported code so that code bundling edits are bypassed.*

Transporting, positioning, prepping, and draping of the patient for satisfactory anesthesia induction/surgical procedures are included in anesthesia services *along with the following.*

- Placement of external devices including, but not limited to, those for cardiac monitoring, oximetry, capnography, temperature monitoring, EEG, CNS evoked responses (e.g., BSER), and Doppler flow
- Placement of peripheral intravenous lines for fluid and medication administration
- Placement of airway (e.g., endotracheal tube, orotracheal tube)
- Laryngoscopy (direct or endoscopic) for placement of airway (e.g., endotracheal tube)
- Placement of nasogastric or orogastric tube
- Intra-operative interpretation of monitored functions (e.g., blood pressure, heart rate, respirations, oximetry, capnography, temperature, EEG, BSER, Doppler flow, CNS pressure)
- Interpretation of laboratory determinations (e.g., arterial blood gases such as pH, pO2, pCO2, bicarbonate; CBC; blood chemistries; lactate levels) by the anesthesiologist/CRNA
- Nerve stimulation for determination of level of paralysis or localization of nerve(s). Codes for electromyography (EMG) services are for diagnostic purposes for nerve dysfunction. To report these codes, a complete diagnostic report must be present in the medical record.
- Insertion of urinary bladder catheter
- Blood sample procurement through existing lines or requiring venipuncture or arterial puncture

Anesthesia practitioners may report codes for *significant separately identifiable procedures* when:

- Surgery is canceled and the anesthesia practitioner performed a preanesthesia evaluation, for which an E/M code is reported.
- Critical care services are provided by the anesthesia practitioner, for which E/M codes are reported.
- Postoperative management of epidural or subarachnoid drug administration is provided by the anesthesia practitioner, for which Anesthesia code 01996 is reported once daily.
- Postoperative ventilation management is provided by the anesthesia practitioner, for which a Medicine code is reported with modifier 59 or XE.
- Unusual monitoring (e.g., central venous, intra-arterial, pulmonary artery/Swan-Ganz catheterization) is provided during or subsequent to a procedure by the anesthesia practitioner, for which Surgery codes are reported.
- Postoperative pain management is provided after general anesthesia, for which a Surgery code is reported (e.g., epidural injection, peripheral nerve block injection) with modifier 59 *or* XE, depending on payer requirements. (The operating surgeon is *not* permitted to report a code for postoperative pain management.)

Example: An anesthesiologist inserts a percutaneous arterial line (catheter) to monitor the patient while providing the anesthesia services during an intracranial surgical procedure. The moribund patient is not expected to survive without this operation. Later that evening, after the patient had been transferred to the postoperative surgery unit, the anesthesiologist inserted a Swan-Ganz (flow-directed) cardiac catheter. The anesthesiologist reports codes 00210 P5 AA and 93503 59.

(continues)

(continued)

- In the CPT index, locate main term *Anesthesia* and subterm *Intracranial* Procedures to locate code 00210. Modifiers AA (anesthesiologist) and P4 (moribund patient) are added to the code. (Physical status and other modifiers are discussed later in this chapter.)

- Insertion of the percutaneous arterial line (catheter) to monitor the patient is bundled in the 00210 anesthesia code; thus, code 36620 is not separately reported.

- Modifier 59 indicates that the anesthesiologist provided distinct procedures in addition to anesthesia services on the same date.

Emergency Endotracheal Tube Intubation

An **endotracheal tube (ET)** is an artificial airway used for short-term airway management or mechanical ventilation due to potential or actual respiratory system insufficiency. The indications for endotracheal intubation include administration of medications during cardiopulmonary arrest, airway maintenance, oxygenation and ventilation, and secretion control. A CPT code is assigned *only* for a stand-alone emergency endotracheal intubation procedure, such as in a hospital's emergency department (e.g., drug overdose patient). The code is *not* assigned with anesthesia procedure codes because access to the patient's airway is necessary for the administration of general anesthesia.

Example: A patient with sepsis underwent a sternal debridement surgical procedure for which the CRNA provided general anesthesia services. The procedure ended at 2 PM, and anesthesia services were concluded after the patient was transferred from the recovery room to the surgical unit. Late that same night, at the request of the surgeon, the CRNA inserted an endotracheal tube to establish an airway for the patient. Report codes 00550 QZ P3, 31500 59 *or* 31500 XE, depending on payer requirements.

- Modifier QZ (CRNA service without medical direction by physician) is a functional (payment or pricing) modifier that is reported first. Modifier P3 (patient has severe systemic disease) is an informational (statistical) modifier that is reported second. The patient has sepsis, which is a severe systemic disease.

- Modifier 59 (Distinct procedural service) *or* XE (Separate encounter, a service that is distinct because it occurred during a separate encounter) is a functional (payment or pricing) modifier reported with code 31500. That procedure was performed by the CRNA after anesthesia services for surgery had concluded.

Central Venous Access Devices (CVADs)

A *central venous access device (CVAD)* is a thin plastic tube (or catheter) that is inserted (or placed) into a vein and connected to a monitor. After insertion, a chest x-ray is done to verify that the catheter's tip is in the proper location above the heart. It measures a patient's central venous pressure (CVP) as an indicator of circulating blood volume, the heart's effectiveness as a pump, and the patient's vascular tone and response to treatment. CVADs are inserted due to the absence of a suitable peripheral access for fluid administration (e.g., rapid infusion of a high volume of fluid in a patient with *hypovolemia*, which is abnormally decreased blood volume). CVADs are also used for the administration of medications (e.g., potassium chloride and dopamine) that may be harmful to smaller *lumen* (opening) peripheral veins and for the insertion of a pacing wire.

A *central venous pressure (CVP) line* is inserted through a vein in the neck (e.g., external or internal jugular vein) or a vein in the upper chest under the collar bone (e.g., subclavian vein) and then into a large central vein in the chest (e.g., superior vena cava). A *CVP line* is also called a *central venous pressure catheter, central venous catheter (CVC),* or *central venous line (CVL).* A CVP line can also be inserted through a vein in the leg (e.g., femoral) and then into a large central vein below the chest (e.g., inferior vena cava). CVP lines are inserted as external or internal catheters and implanted ports, depending on the patient's condition as well as the frequency and duration of infusions.

- An *external catheter* or *nontunneled catheter* is not implanted under the patient's skin, and it does not require a needle to be inserted into the skin to deliver medications. It is used when the patient requires frequent infusions that last several hours, and it requires a sterile dressing that must be changed once or twice daily. In addition, external catheters may require periodic injections of *heparin* (anticoagulant that prevents blood clots from developing in the catheter). The Cook (cystotomy catheter) is an example of an external catheter. Some nontunneled catheters require just a saline flush, and others require both a saline and a heparin flush. Blood can be drawn from a nontunneled catheter.

- An *internal catheter* (or *tunneled catheter*) is implanted completely under the skin. (The catheter's tip is inserted in the superior vena cava, and the other end is "tunneled" about 6 inches away under the chest's skin and sealed with a Dacron cuff to prevent infection.) An internal catheter requires no special care when it is not being used since it is located completely under the skin. The AshSplit Cath (hemodialysis catheter), Groshong, and Hickman are examples of internal catheters. Some tunneled catheters require just a saline flush, and others require both a saline and heparin flush. Blood can be drawn from a tunneled catheter.

- An *implanted port* is a small reservoir that has a rubber plug attached to the catheter that enters the patient's vein below the collar bone and is threaded into the superior vena cava. The port is implanted underneath the skin (local anesthesia and IV sedation). To access the catheter, the site must be located and cleaned and a special needle is inserted through the skin and into the rubber plug. Blood can be drawn from an implanted port.

Intra-Arterial Lines

An *intra-arterial line* (also called *intra-arterial cannula*, or *intra-arterial catheter*, or *A-line*) is a thin plastic tube, cannula, or catheter that is inserted into an artery and connected to a monitor. Its purpose is to measure immediate changes in intra-arterial blood pressure and concentrations of oxygen and carbon dioxide; it also is used to collect frequent blood samples for lab tests. An A-line is inserted when cardiopulmonary status is unstable or when serial (repeat) blood sampling is necessary.

Swan-Ganz Catheterization

A *Swan-Ganz catheter* is a thin, flexible, flow-directed multilumen plastic tube (or catheter) that is advanced from a peripheral vein into the right atrium and then positioned in a branch of the pulmonary artery. The catheter's balloon tip travels through the pulmonary artery, and pulmonary wedge pressure is measured in front of the temporarily inflated and wedged balloon. *Pulmonary wedge pressure* is the indirect measurement of left atrial pressure that is useful in the diagnosis of left ventricular failure and mitral valve disease. The insertion of a Swan-Ganz catheter serves to obtain diagnostic information about the heart and to provide continuous monitoring of heart function in critically ill patients. The result is that the physician can evaluate circulatory volume due to acute valvular regurgitation, burns, congenital heart disease, heart failure, kidney disease, or shock. It is also used to monitor complications of myocardial infarction and the effects of certain heart medications.

Example: An anesthesiologist inserted a percutaneous arterial line (catheter) to monitor a patient with severe systemic disease while providing anesthesia services during an intracranial surgical procedure. Later that evening, after the patient had been transferred to the postoperative surgery unit and at the request of the surgeon, the anesthesiologist inserted a Swan-Ganz (flow-directed) catheter for cardiac monitoring. The anesthesiologist reports codes 00210 AA P3, 93503 59 *or* 93503 XE, depending on payer requirements.

- Code 00210 is reported for anesthesia services, which includes insertion of a percutaneous arterial line (catheter); thus, code 36620 is not also reported. Modifier AA is a functional (payment or pricing) modifier, which indicates an anesthesiologist provided services, and is reported first. Modifier P3 is an informational (statistical) modifier, which indicates that the patient has a severe systemic disease, and is reported second.

- Modifier 59 (Distinct procedural service) or XE (Separate encounter, a service that is distinct because it occurred during a separate encounter), depending on payer requirements, is reported with the code for insertion of Swan-Ganz catheter for cardiac monitoring purposes. This indicates an unusual monitoring service that is provided in addition to the provision of the anesthesia service during surgery.

Postoperative Pain Management

Postoperative pain management includes the administration of epidural or subarachnoid medications on the date(s) of service after the date of surgery. It is provided by the surgeon as part of the surgical procedure's global package, which means reimbursement is included in the CPT surgery code reported. When postoperative pain management is performed by the anesthesiologist, the surgeon must document the reason such care was transferred to the anesthesiologist. The pain management anesthesia code is reported just once each day that services are provided. Add modifier 59 or XE, depending on payer requirements, on the day of *surgery* to indicate that a distinct procedural service was provided (in addition to administration of anesthesia during surgery that day).

> **Example:** Patient underwent an open reduction internal fixation, left femur, under general anesthesia. The patient had been transferred from the recovery room to the surgical floor. Late that evening, the surgeon requested postoperative pain management by the anesthesiologist who performed a peripheral nerve block injection, left femoral nerve. Report code 64447 59 LT *or* 64447 XE LT, depending on payer requirements.
>
> - Modifier 59 (Distinct procedural service) *or* XE (Separate encounter, a service that is distinct because it occurred during a separate encounter) is a functional (payment or pricing) modifier that is reported first.
> - Modifier LT (Left side) is an informational (statistical) modifier that is reported second.

Anesthesia Modifiers

All anesthesia services require the following types of modifiers to be reviewed for assignment with reported anesthesia codes:

- HCPCS Level II modifiers
- Physical status modifiers
- CPT modifiers

HCPCS Level II Anesthesia Modifiers

When applicable, the following HCPCS Level II modifiers are added (as the first modifier) to reported anesthesia codes:

- AA: Anesthesia services performed personally by anesthesiologist
- AD: Medically supervised by a physician for more than four concurrent procedures
- G8: Monitored anesthesia care for a deep, complex, complicated, or markedly invasive surgical procedure. According to the *CMS National Coverage Policy*, modifier G8 is to be applied to anesthesia codes 00100, 00300, 00400, 00160, 00532, and 00920 only.

> **Example:** Patient undergoes a heart transplant for which general anesthesia was administered by an anesthesiologist. Modifier G8 is reported with the anesthesia service code. (Modifier QS, monitored anesthesia care service, is *not* reported with the anesthesia service code.)

- G9: Monitored anesthesia care for patient who has history of severe cardiopulmonary condition
- QK: Medical direction of 2, 3, or 4 concurrent procedures involving qualified individuals
- QS: Monitored anesthesia care service

> **Example:** An anesthesiologist provided monitored anesthesia care to an otherwise healthy patient who underwent vaginal delivery of a healthy newborn. Report code 01960 AA QS P1.

- QX: Qualified nonphysician anesthetist service with medical direction by physician

Example: A CRNA provided anesthesia services for an otherwise healthy patient who underwent diagnostic arthroscopy, left wrist. The CRNA received medical direction from an anesthesiologist. Report code 01829 QX P1.

- QY: Medical direction of one qualified nonphysician anesthetist by an anesthesiologist

Example: A CAA provided anesthesia services to an otherwise healthy patient who underwent incisional hernia repair. The anesthesiologist provided medical direction in the same operating room. Report code 00832 QY P1.

- QZ: CRNA service without medical direction by physician

Example: A CRNA provided anesthesia services to an otherwise healthy patient who underwent plastic repair of a cleft lip. The anesthesiologist was not in the same operating room and did not provide medical direction. Report code 00102 QZ P1.

Physical Status Modifiers

A **physical status modifier** is added to each reported anesthesia code to indicate the patient's condition at the time anesthesia was administered. The modifier also serves to identify the complexity of services provided. (The physical status modifier is determined by the anesthesiologist or qualified nonphysician anesthetist [e.g., CRNA] and is documented as such in the patient record.) The meaning of physical status modifiers (P1–P6) are located in the CPT coding manual.

Example: An anesthesiologist provided general anesthesia services to a 65-year-old patient with mild systemic disease who underwent total knee replacement. Report code 01402 P2.

CPT Modifiers

CPT modifiers 23, 59, and 74 should be reviewed to determine whether they need to be added to the reported anesthesia codes. Modifier 99 is also reported when multiple modifiers are added to codes. The meanings of each modifier are located in the CPT coding manual.

 Coding Tip

- When a patient's circumstances warrant the administration of general or regional anesthesia (instead of the usual local anesthesia), add modifier 23 to the anesthesia code. The following may require general or regional anesthesia services (when local anesthesia services are usually provided):
  - Extremely apprehensive patients
  - Individuals with an intellectual disability
  - Patients who have a physical condition (e.g., spasticity or tremors)

Example: An anesthesiologist provided general anesthesia services to a 49-year-old patient with chronic obstructive pulmonary disease who underwent extracorporeal shock wave lithotripsy with water bath. The patient was extremely anxious about the procedure, which normally does not require general anesthesia. Report code 00872 AA P3 23.

Coding Tip

- An anesthesiologist or a qualified nonphysician anesthetist reports the anesthesia code with the highest base unit value first. Modifier 59 *or* XE is added to each separately reported anesthesia code or to codes reported for unusual services (e.g., pain management), depending on payer requirements.

Time Reporting

Anesthesia services are reported based on time, which begins when the anesthesiologist or qualified nonphysician anesthetist starts preparing the patient to receive anesthesia and ends when the anesthesiologist or qualified nonphysician anesthetist is no longer in personal attendance. Anesthesia time units are reported for the amount of time the anesthesiologist or qualified nonphysician anesthetist is in personal attendance, providing anesthesia services. Reimbursement for anesthesia services varies according to increments of time. (Nonmonitored time is *not* considered when calculating time units.)

NOTE:

Teaching anesthesiologists must be present with the resident physician during all critical or key portions of the anesthesia service, and they must be immediately available to furnish anesthesia services during the entire procedure. Teaching qualified nonphysician anesthetists who are involved with two concurrent cases must be present with the student nurse anesthetist during pre- and postanesthesia care for each case. They are prohibited from being involved in any other activities (e.g., preanesthesia evaluation of the patient for a third case) when two concurrent cases are ongoing.

Example: A patient undergoes a cataract extraction and requires 90 minutes of MAC by the anesthesiologist, which includes the administration of a sedative along with a retrobulbar injection for regional block anesthesia. Subsequently, an interval of 30 minutes transpires, during which time the patient does not require monitoring by the anesthesiologist. After this period, monitoring commences for 30 additional minutes until the patient is released to the recovery room. The anesthesiologist reports 120 minutes of time on the claim.

Payment for anesthesia services is based on the sum of an anesthesia code-specific base unit value plus anesthesia time units and modifying units multiplied by the locality-specific anesthesia conversion factor. The formula for calculating the anesthesia fee is as follows: [code-specific base unit value + anesthesia time units + modifying units] × locality-specific anesthesia conversion factor. For example, [5 + 3 + 0] × $17.04 = anesthesia fee.

- The code-specific **base unit value** for anesthesia codes represents the degree of difficulty associated with providing anesthesia for a surgical procedure (Table 11-1).
- **Anesthesia time units** are based on the total anesthesia time, and they are reported as one unit for each 15 minutes (or fraction thereof) of anesthesia time. (Anesthesia time begins when the anesthesiologist or qualified nonphysician anesthetist begins to prepare the patient for anesthesia care and ends when the anesthesiologist is no longer in personal attendance.)

NOTE:

Anesthesia time reported includes monitoring during administration of regional block anesthesia and during the procedure. Interval and recovery room times are not included when calculating time, although the anesthesiologist or qualified nonphysician anesthetist is required to document the patient's condition on the recovery room record (Figure 11-5).

TABLE 11-1 Sample Portion of Anesthesia Base Unit Values

CPT Code	Base Unit Value
00100	5
00102	6
00103	5
00104	4
00120	5

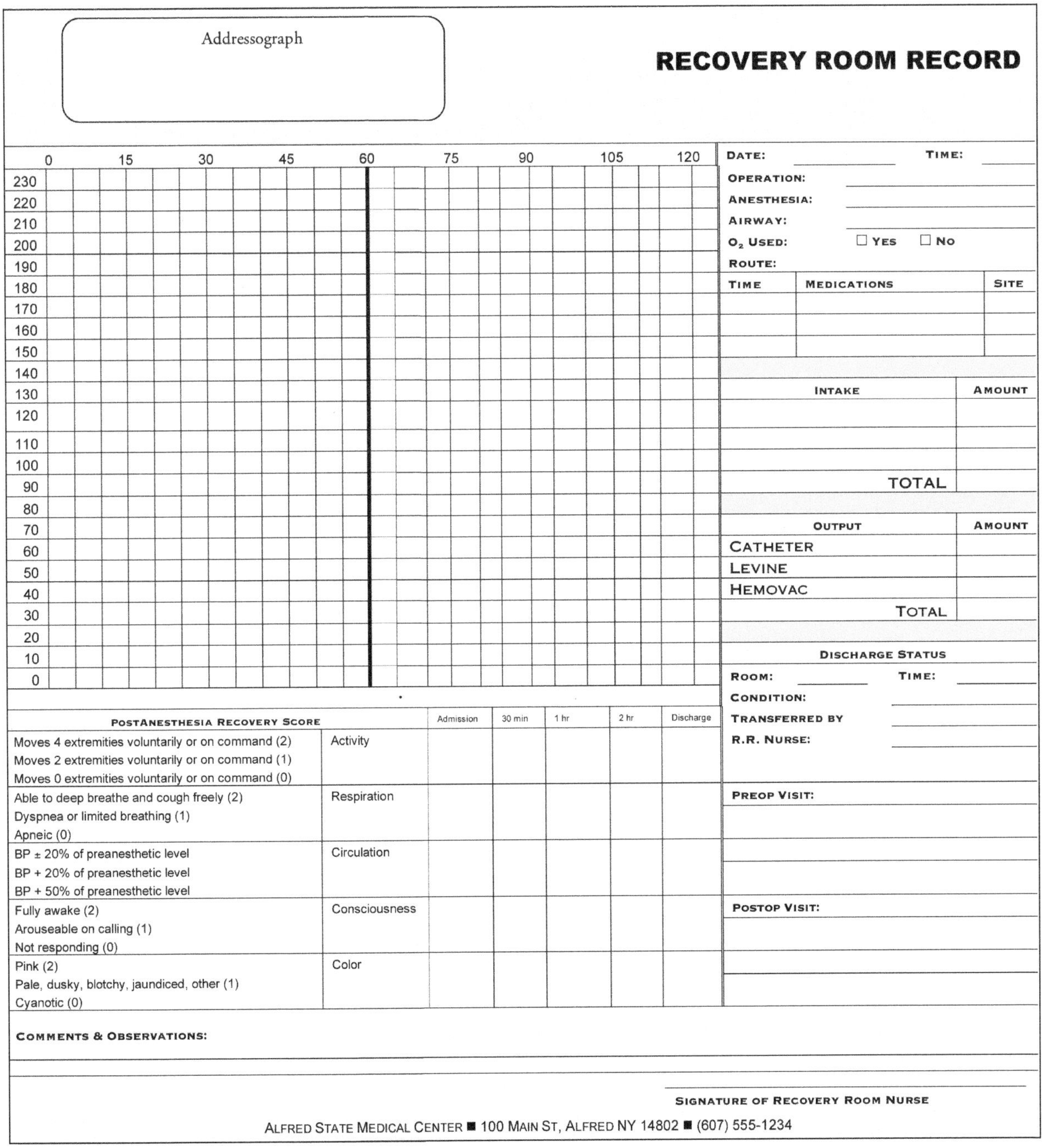

Addressograph

RECOVERY ROOM RECORD

	0	15	30	45	60	75	90	105	120
230									
220									
210									
200									
190									
180									
170									
160									
150									
140									
130									
120									
110									
100									
90									
80									
70									
60									
50									
40									
30									
20									
10									
0									

DATE: TIME:
OPERATION:
ANESTHESIA:
AIRWAY:
O_2 USED: ☐ YES ☐ NO
ROUTE:

TIME	MEDICATIONS	SITE

INTAKE	AMOUNT
TOTAL	

OUTPUT	AMOUNT
CATHETER	
LEVINE	
HEMOVAC	
TOTAL	

DISCHARGE STATUS
ROOM: TIME:
CONDITION:
TRANSFERRED BY
R.R. NURSE:

POSTANESTHESIA RECOVERY SCORE		Admission	30 min	1 hr	2 hr	Discharge
Moves 4 extremities voluntarily or on command (2) Moves 2 extremities voluntarily or on command (1) Moves 0 extremities voluntarily or on command (0)	Activity					
Able to deep breathe and cough freely (2) Dyspnea or limited breathing (1) Apneic (0)	Respiration					
BP ± 20% of preanesthetic level BP + 20% of preanesthetic level BP + 50% of preanesthetic level	Circulation					
Fully awake (2) Arouseable on calling (1) Not responding (0)	Consciousness					
Pink (2) Pale, dusky, blotchy, jaundiced, other (1) Cyanotic (0)	Color					

PREOP VISIT:

POSTOP VISIT:

COMMENTS & OBSERVATIONS:

SIGNATURE OF RECOVERY ROOM NURSE

ALFRED STATE MEDICAL CENTER ■ 100 MAIN ST, ALFRED NY 14802 ■ (607) 555-1234

FIGURE 11-5 Sample recovery room record

- **Modifying units** recognize added complexities associated with the administration of anesthesia, including physical factors and difficult circumstances. Physical factors indicating the patient's condition at the time anesthesia was administered are reported by adding the appropriate physical status modifier (P1–P6) to the anesthesia code. Difficult circumstances are reported with qualifying circumstances codes, located in the CPT Medicine section. The relative values for physical status modifiers and qualifying circumstances codes are located in the current year's American Society of Anesthesiologists (ASA) *Relative Value Guide* publication (Table 11-2).

- The locality-specific **anesthesia conversion factor** is the dollar amount assigned to a geographic location (Table 11-3).

When the patient undergoes more than one procedure during the same operative episode and the anesthesiologist or qualified nonphysician anesthetist provides multiple anesthesia services for the same patient during the same operative session, the anesthesia fee is based on the *highest* code base unit value when multiple stand-alone anesthesia codes are reported (which is added to the total anesthesia time for all services provided). (The anesthesia code with the highest code base unit is reported. The exception is when an anesthesia code has add-on codes, which are also reported, and reimbursement for multiple anesthesia services is based on the sum of the base unit values.)

TABLE 11-2 Sample Portion of Modifying Units and Relative Values

CPT Physical Status Modifier	Relative Value
P1	0
P2	0
P3	1
P4	2
P5	3
P6	0
CPT Qualifying Circumstances Code	**Relative Value**
99100	1
99116	5
99135	5
99140	2

 NOTE:

Base unit values and modifying unit relative values are available as downloadable files at www.cms.gov by entering Anesthesiologists Center in the Search box to locate current anesthesia conversion factors.

TABLE 11-3 Sample Portion of Locality-Specific Anesthesia Conversion Factors

Payer Number	Locality Number	Locality Name	Conversion Factor
00500	00	Alabama	$17.04
00830	01	Alaska	$29.66
00832	00	Arizona	$17.83
00520	13	Arkansas	$16.52

Courtesy of the Centers for Medicare & *Medicaid* Services, www.cms.gov

Example 1: A 22-year-old patient who has chronic asthma underwent a planned vaginal delivery on May 14, during which neuraxial labor anesthesia was administered by an anesthesiologist. Report code 01967 AA P2.

- Anesthesia code 01967 has a base unit value of 5.
- Physical status modifier P2 has a modifying unit relative value of 0.

A review of the patient record indicates 45 minutes of anesthesia time, which is calculated as 3 anesthesia time units (45 ÷ 15 = 3). If a conversion factor of $17.45 is assigned to New York State, payment for anesthesia services is calculated as $139.60. The formula for calculating anesthesia services reimbursement is as follows:

```
STEP 1:  (5 + 3 + 0) × $17.45
STEP 2:  8 × $17.45
AMOUNT:  $139.60
```

Example 2: A 22-year-old patient who has chronic asthma was prepared for a planned vaginal delivery on May 14, during which neuraxial labor anesthesia was administered by an anesthesiologist. Complications required that an emergency cesarean delivery be performed instead of the planned vaginal delivery. Report codes 01967 AA P2, 01968 AA P2, and 99140. (Reimbursement for multiple anesthesia services is based on the sum of each base unit value because code 01968 is an add-on code.)

- Code 01967 has a base unit value of 5.
- Code 01968 has a base unit value of 2.
- Code 99140 has a relative value of 2.
- Physical status modifier P2 has a relative value of 0.

The total length of anesthesia time for both procedures was 75 minutes, which is calculated as 5 anesthesia time units (75 ÷ 15 = 5). If the conversion factor is $17.45, payment for anesthesia services is calculated as $244.30. The formula for calculating anesthesia services reimbursement is as follows:

```
STEP 1:  (5 + 2 + 5 + 2) × $17.45
STEP 2:  14 × $17.45
AMOUNT:  $244.30
```

Example 3: A 39-year-old patient who has otherwise been healthy sustained multiple traumas and was administered general anesthesia by an anesthesiologist during cranial surgery and upper abdominal surgery. Both surgical procedures were performed during the same operative session. (Reimbursement for multiple anesthesia services is based on the highest ASA base unit value when anesthesia for two separate procedures is provided.) Assign codes 00210 AA P5 and 99140. (Do not separately report code 00790 for the administration of anesthesia for the upper abdominal surgery because it was provided during the same operative episode as anesthesia administered for the cranial surgery.)

- Code 00210 has a base unit value of 11.
- Code 99140 has a relative value of 2.
- Physical status modifier P5 has a relative value of 3.

The total length of anesthesia time for both procedures was 120 minutes, which is calculated as 8 anesthesia time units (120 ÷ 15 = 8). If the conversion factor is $17.45, payment for anesthesia services is calculated as $418.80. The formula for calculating anesthesia services reimbursement is as follows:

```
STEP 1:  (11 + 8 + [3 + 2]) × $17.45
STEP 2:  (19 + 5) × $17.45
STEP 3:  24 × $17.45
AMOUNT:  $418.80
```

Medicare defines **concurrent medically directed anesthesia procedures** as "the maximum number of procedures an anesthesiologist or qualified nonphysician anesthetist medically directs within the context of a single procedure and when the procedures overlap each other." The ASA base unit value is reduced for subsequent anesthesia services when the definition of *concurrent medically directed anesthesia procedures* applies to the submission of multiple anesthesia codes. (Base unit value reduction of services is determined by the third-party payer.)

Anesthesia Services

Assign the appropriate CPT code from the Evaluation and Management section when anesthesia services are provided in an office, home, or hospital; this includes consultation services and other medical services. The CPT Medicine section contains codes for reporting *Special Services and Reporting*.

Example: Procedures A through C are concurrent medically directed anesthesia procedures provided by an anesthesiologist on May 20. The start and end times for each procedure represent the periods during which anesthesia time is counted.

Procedure	Start Time	End Time	Number of Concurrent Procedures	Base Unit Value Reduction
A	8:00 AM	8:20 AM	2	10%
B	8:10 AM	8:45 AM	2	10%
C	8:30 AM	9:15 AM	2	10%

- During procedure A, the anesthesiologist medically directed two concurrent procedures A and B from 8:10 AM to 8:20 AM.

- During procedure B, the anesthesiologist medically directed two concurrent procedures A and B from 8:10 AM to 8:20 AM and then procedures B and C from 8:30 AM to 8:45 AM.

- Thus, during each procedure A and B, the anesthesiologist medically directed, at most, two concurrent procedures.

Supplied Materials

When an anesthesiologist or a qualified nonphysician anesthetist provides materials and supplies (e.g., sterile trays and drugs) over and above those usually included with the office visit or other services rendered, report the materials and supplies separately with CPT code 99070 (or an appropriate HCPCS Level II code).

Separate or Multiple Procedures

When multiple surgical procedures are performed during the provision of anesthesia services, report the anesthesia code that represents the most complex procedure performed. However, if the additional anesthesia code for multiple surgical procedures performed is an add-on code, report all codes. The time reported for the provision of anesthesia services is the combined total for all procedures performed.

Unlisted Service or Procedure

When the service or procedure performed is not listed in the CPT coding manual, report an unlisted service or procedure code on the claim and attach a special report to the submitted claim.

Special Report

When a service is provided that is new, variable, rare, or unusual, a *special report* may be submitted with the claim. The special report should include information that defines or describes the nature, event, and need for the procedure as well as the time, effort, and equipment necessary to provide the service. Special reports accompany claims that contain unlisted service or procedure codes.

Qualifying Circumstances

When anesthesia services are provided during situations or circumstances that make anesthesia administration more difficult, report a **qualifying circumstances** code from the CPT Medicine section (in addition to the anesthesia code). Difficult circumstances depend on factors such as extraordinary condition of patient, notable operative conditions, or unusual risk factors. These codes are reported in addition to the anesthesia codes. Qualifying circumstances codes 99100–99140 are located in the CPT Medicine section.

NOTE:

An *emergency condition* results when a delay in treatment of the patient would lead to a significant increase in threat to life or body part.

Example: A 92-year-old patient with controlled hypertension received general anesthesia services from a CRNA and was monitored by an anesthesiologist during total left hip arthroplasty. Report codes 01214 QX P2 and 99100. Modifier QX is a functional (payment or pricing) modifier and is reported first. P2 is an informational (statistical) modifier and is reported second.

Exercise 11.3 – Anesthesia Section Guidelines

Instructions: Complete each statement.

1. Prior to surgery, the provider reviews the patient's record, interviews the patient, conducts a physical examination, evaluates preoperative test results, and ensures that informed anesthetic consent has been obtained as part of the _____ evaluation.

2. Evaluating the patient during recovery from anesthesia and evaluating, treating, and following up possible anesthesia-related complications is part of the _____ evaluation.

3. A patient undergoes a surgical procedure that requires 30 minutes of monitored anesthesia care by the anesthesiologist. Then 15 minutes transpires when the patient does not require monitoring by the anesthesiologist. After this interval, the anesthesiologist commences monitoring for 15 additional minutes until the patient is released to the recovery room. The number of anesthesia time units is _____.

4. A 38-year-old patient who has diabetes mellitus underwent a planned vaginal delivery on November 14, during which neuraxial labor anesthesia was administered by an anesthesiologist. Code 01967 AA P2 is reported (base unit value of 5 and relative value of 0). A review of the patient record indicates 60 minutes of anesthesia time. The conversion factor is $17.45. The payment for anesthesia services is calculated as _____.

5. The physical status modifier for a patient who is on medication for petit mal seizures and who undergoes inguinal herniorrhaphy is _____.

Anesthesia Subsections

The Anesthesia section is organized according to general anatomical areas or services that relate to a number of surgical procedures. For Medicare purposes, just one code from the Anesthesia section is usually reported unless the second and subsequent anesthesia codes are add-on codes. When distinct procedures and services (e.g., Swan-Ganz catheterization) are provided by the anesthesiologist, report separate anesthesia codes and add modifier 59 (distinct procedural service) *or* XE (Separate encounter, a service that is distinct because it occurred during a separate encounter), depending on payer requirements. When more than one code for anesthesia services is reported, the code that describes the anesthesia service for the procedure that has the *highest* base unit value is reported first.

The Anesthesia section includes add-on codes for anesthesia services provided to patients undergoing burn excisions or debridement and obstetrics procedures. The add-on code is reported *in addition to the code for the primary anesthesia service.*

 Coding Tip

Surgical endoscopy/arthroscopy always includes diagnostic endoscopy/arthroscopy. When an anesthesiologist or a qualified nonphysician anesthetist provides anesthesia services for a diagnostic and a surgical endoscopy/arthroscopy performed during the same operative session, report just one anesthesia services code with appropriate modifiers.

Head

Anesthesia services for the Head subsection include procedures on the following anatomical sites: accessory sinuses, ears, eyelids, eyes, facial bones, lips, nose, salivary glands, and skull. Codes for anesthesia services provided for electroconvulsive therapy (ECT) and intraoral and intracranial procedures are also included.

> **Example:** A healthy patient underwent soft tissue biopsy of the accessory sinuses, for which a CRNA provided anesthesia services. The CRNA was supervised by an anesthesiologist. Report code 00164 QX P1.

Neck

Anesthesia services for the Neck subsection include procedures on the following anatomical sites: integumentary system; muscles and nerves of the head, neck, and posterior trunk; esophagus, thyroid, larynx, trachea, and lymphatic system of the neck; and major vessels of the neck.

> **Example:** An anesthesiologist provided anesthesia services to a terminally ill one-year-old patient who underwent laryngoscopy. Report code 00320 AA P4.

Thorax (Chest Wall and Shoulder Girdle)

Anesthesia services for the Thorax (Chest Wall and Shoulder Girdle) subsection include procedures on the following anatomical sites: integumentary system on the extremities, anterior trunk, and perineum; breast; clavicle; scapula; and ribs. Anesthesia services for an electrical conversion of arrhythmias procedure are also included.

Example: A 79-year-old patient underwent bilateral radical mastectomy with internal mammary node dissection (12 lymph nodes). Patient was recently diagnosed with metastatic adenocarcinoma of the breast to the lung. The anesthesiologist provided general anesthesia services. Report codes 00406 AA P5 and 99100.

The surgeon who removes a skin lesion usually provides local anesthesia or monitored anesthesia care (MAC). If general or regional anesthesia services are provided by the surgeon, add modifier 47 to the surgery code. (Do not add modifier 47 to an anesthesia code.) If general anesthesia, regional anesthesia, or MAC is provided by an anesthesiologist or a qualified nonphysician anesthetist, report the appropriate code, physical status modifier, and qualifying circumstances codes. (Add modifier QS to the anesthesia code if MAC is provided.) Also report an appropriate ICD-10-CM diagnosis code to justify medical necessity (e.g., patient with intellectual disability who exhibits severe anxiety about undergoing the procedure).

Example: An anesthesiologist provided monitored anesthesia care (MAC) for a five-year-old patient who underwent a biopsy of the perineum. Report 00400 AA QS P1.

- If the surgeon had provided MAC, report code 56605. (*Do not report modifier QS or modifier 47.*)

- If the surgeon had provided general or regional anesthesia services, report code 56605 47.

Intrathoracic

Anesthesia services for the Intrathoracic subsection include procedures on the following anatomical sites: bronchus, coronary arteries, diaphragm, esophagus, great vessels of chest, heart, lungs, mediastinum, pericardial sac, pleura, sternum, and thorax.

Example: A 39-year-old patient with severe systemic disease underwent sternal debridement for which the anesthesiologist provided general anesthesia services. Report code 00550 AA P3.

Spine and Spinal Cord

Anesthesia services for the Spine and Spinal Cord subsection include procedures on the following anatomical sites: cervical, thoracic, and lumbar spine and spinal cord.

Example: General anesthesia services were provided by an anesthesiologist during an otherwise healthy patient's thoracic spine surgery. Report code 00620 AA P1.

 NOTE:

When a physician performs spinal manipulation under anesthesia, report code 22505. Other manipulation under anesthesia codes (e.g., 23700, manipulation under anesthesia, shoulder joint, including application of fixation apparatus) refers to "reduction" of a fracture. For spinal manipulation without anesthesia, report code 97140 from the CPT Medicine section.

Upper Abdomen

Anesthesia services for the Upper Abdomen subsection include procedures on the upper abdominal wall, liver, major abdominal blood vessels, pancreas, and stomach. This subsection also includes upper gastrointestinal (GI) endoscopy, hernia repairs, and laparoscopy procedures.

Example: An anesthesiologist provides general anesthesia services for a patient who undergoes a liver transplant. Report 00796 AA P5.

Lower Abdomen

Anesthesia services for the Lower Abdomen subsection include procedures on the following anatomical sites: lower abdominal wall, *panniculus adiposus*, or *pannus* (layer of subcutaneous adipose tissue, or fat, below the dermis that contains fat deposits, blood vessels, and nerves). The following anatomical sites are accessed via transabdominal incision: uterus; fallopian tubes; urinary tract, including kidneys and urinary bladder; prostate gland; adrenal glands; lower abdominal vessels; and inferior vena cava. This subsection also includes anesthesia codes for lower intestinal endoscopic procedures and hernia repairs and lower abdomen intraperitoneal procedures including laparoscopy.

Example: An anesthesiologist provided regional anesthesia services to a diabetic patient who underwent total cystectomy. Report code 00864 AA P2.

Perineum

Anesthesia services for the Perineum subsection include procedures on the following anatomical sites: anus, rectum, perineum, vulva, vas deferens, seminal vesicles, testes, penis, vagina, labia, cervix, endometrium, uterus, prostate, urethra, urinary bladder, and ureters.

Example: An anesthesiologist provided general anesthesia services to a hypertensive patient who underwent vulvectomy. Report code 00906 AA P2.

Pelvis (Except Hip)

Anesthesia services for the Pelvis (Except Hip) subsection include procedures on the following anatomical sites: anterior or posterior iliac crest, bony pelvis, interpelviabdominal (hindquarter), pelvis, symphysis pubis, sacroiliac joint, acetabulum, and extrapelvic and intrapelvic obturator nerves.

Example: An anesthesiologist provided general anesthesia services to a chronic asthmatic patient who underwent an open procedure involving the sacroiliac joint. Report code 01170 AA P2.

Upper Leg (Except Knee)

Anesthesia services for the Upper Leg (Except Knee) subsection include procedures on the following anatomical sites: hip joint; upper two-thirds of femur; and arteries, veins, nerves, muscles, tendons, fascia, and bursae of upper leg.

> **Example:** An anesthesiologist provided general anesthesia services to a patient with intellectual disabilities and mild systemic disease who underwent nerve biopsy of the upper leg. Report code 01250 AA P2.

Knee and Popliteal Area

Anesthesia services for the Knee and Popliteal Area subsection include procedures on the following anatomical sites: arteries, veins, nerves, muscles, tendons, fascia, and bursae of knee and popliteal area; lower one-third of femur; knee joint; upper ends of the tibia and fibula; and patella.

> **Example:** An anesthesiologist provided general anesthesia services to a normal healthy patient who underwent diagnostic arthroscopy, left knee. Report code 01382 AA P1.

Lower Leg (Below Knee, Includes Ankle and Foot)

Anesthesia services for the Lower Leg (Below Knee, Includes Ankle and Foot) subsection include procedures on the following anatomical sites: lower leg; ankle; foot; and arteries, veins, bones, nerves, muscles, tendons, and fascia of leg, ankle, and foot.

> **Example:** An anesthesiologist provided general anesthesia services to a normal healthy patient who underwent arthroscopic procedure, right ankle. Report code 01464 AA P1.

Shoulder and Axilla

Anesthesia services for the Shoulder and Axilla subsection include procedures on the following anatomical sites: arteries, veins, nerves, muscles, tendons, fascia, and bursae of shoulder and axillae; humeral head and neck; sternoclavicular joint; acromioclavicular joint; and shoulder joint.

> **Example:** An anesthesiologist provided general anesthesia services to a normal healthy patient who underwent muscle biopsy, left shoulder. Report code 01610 AA P1.

Upper Arm and Elbow

Anesthesia services for the Upper Arm and Elbow subsection include procedures on the following anatomical sites: arteries, veins, nerves, muscle, tendons, fascia, and bursae of upper arm and elbow; humerus; and elbow.

> **Example:** An anesthesiologist provided general anesthesia services to a patient with mild systemic disease who underwent excision of tumor of the right humerus. Report code 01758 AA P2.

Forearm, Wrist, and Hand

Anesthesia services for the Forearm, Wrist, and Hand subsection include procedures on the following anatomical sites: arteries, veins, nerves, muscles, tendons, fascia, and bursae of forearm, wrist, and hand; radius; ulna; wrist; hand bones; distal radius; distal ulna; and hand joints.

Example: An anesthesiologist provided general anesthesia services to a normal healthy but very anxious patient who underwent diagnostic and surgical arthroscopy with bone biopsy, right wrist. Report code 01830 AA P1.

Radiological Procedures

Anesthesia services for the Radiological Procedures subsection include the following: myelography, discography, and vertebroplasty; diagnostic arteriography/venography; cardiac catheterization, including coronary angiography and ventriculography; noninvasive imaging or radiation therapy; and therapeutic interventional radiology involving the arterial/venous/lymphatic systems.

Example: An anesthesiologist provided MAC to a patient with severe systemic disease who underwent cardiac catheterization, including coronary angiography and ventriculography. Report code 01920 AA QS P3.

 NOTE:

- According to National Correct Coding Initiative (NCCI) program guidelines, just one radiological procedure anesthesia code is reported for all anesthesia services provided for radiological procedures performed during the same encounter.
- Radiological supervision and interpretation codes applicable to radiological procedures being performed are reported by the appropriate provider (e.g., radiologist, cardiologist, neurosurgeon, radiation oncologist). These codes are not included (bundled) in anesthesia services codes for radiological procedures, and the appropriate provider must report the radiology procedure or service code.
- Refer to Chapter 17, CPT Radiology, of this textbook for coding rules about radiological procedures and services.

Burn Excisions or Debridement

Anesthesia services for the Burn Excisions or Debridement subsection include the following: second- and third-degree burn excisions or debridement with or without skin grafting according to total body surface area. (Refer to Chapter 12, CPT Surgery I, of this textbook for discussion of total body surface area calculations.)

Example: An anesthesiologist provided general anesthesia services to a two-year-old type 1 diabetic patient who underwent second-degree burn debridement of the chest, 5 percent of total body surface area. Report code 01952 AA P2.

Obstetric

Anesthesia services for the Obstetric subsection include the following: external cephalic version procedure, vaginal delivery, cesarean delivery, urgent hysterectomy following delivery, cesarean hysterectomy without labor analgesia/anesthesia care, abortion procedures, neuraxial labor analgesia/anesthesia for planned vaginal delivery, neuraxial labor analgesia/anesthesia for cesarean delivery following planned vaginal delivery, and cesarean hysterectomy following neuraxial labor analgesia/anesthesia. (Refer to Chapter 16, CPT Surgery V, of this textbook for detailed discussion of obstetric procedures and services.)

Example: An anesthesiologist provided general anesthesia services to a normal healthy patient who suffered a miscarriage and underwent surgery to remove the remaining products of conception. Report code 01965 AA P1.

Other Procedures

Anesthesia services for the Other Procedures subsection include the following: physiologic support for harvesting organ(s) from brain-dead patients, anesthesia for diagnostic/therapeutic nerve blocks and injections, daily hospital management of epidural or subarachnoid continuous drug administration, and unlisted anesthesia procedure(s).

Example: An anesthesiologist managed the continuous drug administration of an epidural for a 50-year-old patient who has chronic obstructive pulmonary disease. Report code 01996 AA P2.

NOTE:

- To report regional intravenous administration of local anesthetic agents or other medication in the upper or lower extremity, assign an Anesthesia code from the appropriate Anesthesia subsection.
- To report a Bier block for pain management, report the "Unlisted procedure, nervous system" code from the Surgery section. A *Bier block* is an intravenous regional block, which involves using a tourniquet to restrict the effects of anesthesia to a region of the body (e.g., leg).
- To report intra-arterial or intravenous injections, including that for pain management, report a code from the Medicine section.

Exercise 11.4 – Anesthesia Subsections

Instructions: Complete each statement below.

1. For Medicare purposes, just one anesthesia code is usually reported unless the second and subsequent anesthesia codes are _____ codes.

2. When procedures on the larynx and trachea are performed on a patient who is younger than one year of age, report code 00326, but do *not* report qualifying circumstances code _____ (anesthesia for patient of extreme age, younger than one year and older than 70) on the same claim.

3. When anesthesia services are provided by an anesthesiologist to a breast cancer patient who undergoes a procedure that involves radical or modified radical breast procedure with internal mammary node dissection, assign code _____ AA P5.

4. When monitored anesthesia care (MAC) is provided by the anesthesiologist or qualified nonphysician anesthetist instead of local anesthesia due to the patient's age or mental status, add HCPCS Level II modifier _____.

5. When anesthesia services are provided for non-invasive imaging or radiation therapy, such as may be required for a patient with an intellectual disability, report code _____ 23.

Summary

The Anesthesia section is located after the Evaluation and Management section in the CPT coding manual, and codes with appropriate modifiers are reported for services related to the administration of anesthesia (including general and regional), supplementation of local anesthesia, and other supportive anesthesia services. The Anesthesia section is organized according to general anatomical areas or services that relate to a number of surgical procedures. For Medicare purposes, just one code from the Anesthesia section is reported unless the second and subsequent anesthesia codes are add-on codes. When separate anesthesia codes are reported, the code that describes the anesthesia service for the procedure that has the *highest* base unit value is reported first.

A physician (e.g., anesthesiologist) is responsible for supervising anesthesia services (which include general and regional), supplementation of local anesthesia, and other supportive services so the patient receives appropriate optimal anesthesia care. The administration of local infiltration, metacarpal/metatarsal/digital block, or topical anesthesia by the operating surgeon or obstetrician is included (bundled) in the surgery code; separate codes are not reported. Anesthesia services include the preparation and monitoring of the patient, as well as the following services: draping, positioning, prepping, and transporting the patient; inserting nasogastric or orogastric tubes; inserting peripheral IV lines for fluid and medication administration; interpreting laboratory results; interpreting monitored functions; placing airway tubes, including laryngoscopy for airway management; positioning external devices for capnography, cardiac monitoring, CNS evoked responses, Doppler flow, pulse oximetry, and temperature; and stimulating nerves to determine level of paralysis or localization of nerve(s).

Internet Links

American Society of Anesthesiologists (ASA): www.asahq.org

Medicare Information for Anesthesiologists: Go to **www.cms.gov**, click on the Medicare link, scroll to the Provider Type heading, and click on the Anesthesiologists link.

Review

11.1 – Multiple Choice

Instructions: Select the most appropriate response.

1. Local anesthesia administration techniques include _____ anesthesia.
   a. caudal, saddle block, and epidural
   b. general, local, and regional
   c. spinal, intravenous regional, and Bier block
   d. surface, infiltration, field block, peripheral nerve block, and plexus

2. CPT Anesthesia subsections are organized by _____ except for the last four subsections, which are organized by type of procedure.
   a. anatomical site
   b. modifying unit
   c. surgical procedure
   d. type of anesthesia

3. Prior to surgery, an anesthesiologist or qualified nonphysician anesthetist reviews the patient record, performs a physical examination, evaluates preoperative test results, and ensures that informed anesthetic consent has been obtained. This service is called
   a. monitored anesthesia care.
   b. postanesthesia evaluation.
   c. postoperative pain management.
   d. preanesthesia evaluation.

4. Which professional evaluates the patient during recovery from anesthesia and evaluates, treats, and follows up possible anesthesia-related complications?
   a. Anesthesiologist or qualified nonphysician anesthetist
   b. Primary care physician who admitted the patient
   c. Recovery room nurse and surgical unit nurse
   d. Surgeon who performed the surgical procedure

5. CPT anesthesia section guidelines include four codes (99100–99140) from the Medicine section, which are used to report
   a. anesthesia services, such as capnography.
   b. distinct procedural services, such as nerve block.
   c. monitored anesthesia care (MAC).
   d. qualifying circumstances for anesthesia.

6. If surgery for which preanesthesia services are performed is canceled, the anesthesiologist should
   a. not report any codes.
   b. report an evaluation and management service code instead of an anesthesia code.
   c. report the anesthesia code for the procedure that was canceled.
   d. report the anesthesia code for the procedure that was canceled and add modifier 53 for discontinued procedure.

7. An anesthesiologist provides anesthesia services for an otherwise healthy five-month-old patient who undergoes a bronchoscopy procedure after a balloon popped near the infant and there was a suspicion that a piece of the balloon could have become lodged in the bronchi. Which code(s) are reported?
   a. 00326 AA P1
   b. 00326 AA P1, 99100
   c. 99100
   d. 99100, 00326 AA P1

8. Code 00218 is reported for anesthesia services provided during an _____ procedure, which is performed on the skull while the patient is in a seated position.
   a. endocranial
   b. innercranial
   c. intercranial
   d. intracranial

9. Which code is used to report anesthesia services for physiological support for harvesting organs from a brain-dead patient?
   a. 01990
   b. 32850
   c. 35600
   d. 38230

10. An anesthesiologist provides anesthesia services for a controlled diabetic patient who undergoes a panniculectomy. Which code is reported?
    a. 00800 AA P2
    b. 00801 AA P2
    c. 00802 AA P2
    d. 00820 AA P2

11. An anesthesiologist provided anesthesia services on an otherwise healthy patient who underwent left corneal transplant. Which CPT code is assigned?
    a. 00144 AA P1
    b. 00580 AA P1
    c. 65410 AA P1
    d. 65710 AA P1

12. An anesthesiologist provided anesthesia services on a 30-year-old patient who underwent thyroidectomy for rare thyroid cancer. Which CPT code is assigned?

  a. 00320 AA P3   **c.** 01442 AA P3
  b. 00322 AA P3   **d.** 60210 AA P3

13. An anesthesiologist provided monitored anesthesia care to a patient with history of severe cardiopulmonary condition who underwent a procedure to access central venous circulation. Which CPT code is assigned?

  a. 00530 AA G9 P3   **c.** 00560 AA G9 P3
  b. 00532 AA G9 P3   **d.** 01916 AA G9 P3

14. An anesthesiologist provided anesthesia services on a patient with mild systemic disease who underwent upper abdomen vascular surgery. Which CPT code is assigned?

  a. 00700 AA P2   **b.** 00770 AA P2   **c.** 00880 AA P2   **d.** 00882 AA P2

15. An anesthesiologist provided anesthesia services on an otherwise healthy patient who underwent open revision of total hip arthroplasty. Which CPT code is assigned?

  a. 01140 AA P1   **b.** 01200 AA P1   **c.** 01215 AA P1   **d.** 27134 AA P1

16. An anesthesiologist provided anesthesia services on a patient with mild systemic disease who underwent popliteal thromboendarterectomy. Which CPT code is assigned?

  a. 01440 AA P2   **b.** 01442 AA P2   **c.** 01400 AA P2   **d.** 35303 AA P2

17. An anesthesiologist provided anesthesia services on an otherwise healthy patient who underwent repair of the Achilles tendon. Which CPT code is assigned?

  a. 01462 AA P1   **b.** 01472 AA P1   **c.** 27650 AA P1   **d.** 28200 AA P1

18. An anesthesiologist provided anesthesia services on a patient with severe systemic disease who underwent an arthroscopic shoulder joint procedure for interthoracoscapular (forequarter) amputation. Which CPT code is assigned?

  a. 01630 AA P3   **b.** 01636 AA P3   **c.** 01710 AA P3   **d.** 23900 AA P3

19. An anesthesiologist provided anesthesia services to a five-year-old otherwise healthy patient who underwent bilateral orchiopexy. Which CPT code is assigned?

  a. 00926 AA P1   **b.** 00928 AA P1   **c.** 00930 AA P1   **d.** 54650 AA P1

20. An anesthesiologist provided anesthesia services on an otherwise healthy patient who underwent phleborrhaphy, right wrist. Which CPT code is assigned?

  a. 01782 AA P1   **b.** 01852 AA P1   **c.** 01916 AA P1   **d.** 37650 AA P1

11.2 – Coding Practice I: Modifiers

Instructions: Review each case and assign CPT anesthesia code(s) and appropriate modifier(s). (Enter the provider-type modifier first, such as 00000 AA P1.) Some cases require assignment of CPT surgery codes and appropriate modifier(s) per chapter content about anesthesia coding guidelines.

1. Regional anesthesia services were provided by an anesthesiologist for a healthy patient who underwent an emergency cesarean section. Later that evening, after the patient had been transferred to the surgical floor, the anesthesiologist inserted a lumbar catheter to provide continuous epidural analgesia pain management (morphine bolus) during the afternoon hours after surgery only.

2. A CRNA (with medical direction by the surgeon) provided general anesthesia services for a controlled diabetic patient who underwent total wrist replacement. Later that evening, after the patient had been transferred to the surgical floor, the CRNA inserted a thoracic epidural catheter to provide continuous postoperative analgesia for pain management. The CRNA monitored the patient's pain management on the day after surgery.

3. A healthy patient underwent total knee replacement surgery; regional anesthesia services were provided by an anesthesiologist.

---

4. An anesthesiologist provided regional pain block for an arthroscopic anterior cruciate ligament repair of the left knee of a healthy 40-year-old patient. The anesthesiologist also performed a femoral nerve block for postoperative pain management later that evening, after the patient had been transferred to the surgical floor.

---

5. A patient with chronic asthma underwent a thoracotomy. The anesthesiologist provided general anesthesia services. Later that evening, after the patient had been transferred to the surgical floor, the CRNA (without medical direction by a physician) inserted an epidural catheter for continuous infusion of morphine for post-operative pain control.

11.3 – Coding Practice II: Anesthesia

Instructions: Review each case and assign the appropriate anesthesia code(s), provider-type modifier(s), and physical status modifier(s). Assign qualifying circumstance code(s) where appropriate. *All anesthesia services were provided by the anesthesiologist, which means that modifier AA is added to each anesthesia code as the provider-type modifier.* Some cases require assignment of CPT surgery codes and appropriate modifier(s) per chapter content about anesthesia coding guidelines. When unusual services are provided by the anesthesiologist, add modifier 59 to those codes.

Head

1. A 77-year-old healthy patient with controlled diabetes mellitus underwent intraocular lens transplant surgery for which general anesthesia was administered.

---

2. A five-year-old healthy child was admitted to the pediatrics floor of an acute care hospital and underwent tympanostomy for which general anesthesia was administered.

Neck

3. A nine-month-old healthy patient underwent emergency tracheostomy under general anesthesia after having sustained injuries in a motor vehicle accident. The child lost consciousness for 60 minutes after the accident and required cardiopulmonary resuscitation.

---

4. A 47-year-old patient with a history of hypertension underwent a partial thyroid lobectomy due to a thyroid tumor. General anesthesia was administered.

Thorax (Chest Wall and Shoulder Girdle)

5. A 33-year-old healthy construction worker fell from a ladder onto a wooden platform and was brought into the emergency room and diagnosed with a concussion; there was no loss of consciousness. The patient went to the operating room for the complicated removal of wood from skin of the left shoulder. The patient received general anesthesia.

---

6. A 14-year-old otherwise healthy child is admitted to the pediatric ward with chest pain, shortness of breath, and possible lordosis. After examination, the diagnosis of pectus excavatum was made. The child had the condition corrected with an open procedure under general anesthesia.

Intrathoracic

7. A 78-year-old smoker with a history of related severe respiratory problems was admitted for shortness of breath, hypertension, and bloody sputum. The patient was diagnosed with severe pneumonia and underwent pneumocentesis performed under general anesthesia.

8. A 45-year-old patient with a history of severe coronary disease and mild hypertension underwent insertion of a permanent pacemaker with epicardial electrodes by thoracotomy. General anesthesia was administered.

Spine and Spinal Cord

9. A 57-year-old patient with a history of osteoporosis underwent posterior arthrodesis in the craniocervical (occipital C2) region. General anesthesia was administered.

10. A 25-year-old patient with heroin dependence and a history of chronic asthma controlled by medication complains today of severe headaches. The patient was admitted to the psychiatric floor of an acute care hospital. After detoxification, the patient still had headaches; increased spinal fluid pressure was noted. The patient underwent diagnostic lumbar spinal puncture performed under regional anesthesia.

Upper Abdomen

11. An obese 56-year-old patient with benign hypertension complained of recurring heartburn. After examination, the patient was admitted for surgery and underwent a transabdominal repair of a diaphragmatic hernia. General anesthesia was administered.

12. An otherwise healthy five-year-old patient underwent percutaneous liver biopsy under general anesthesia.

Lower Abdomen

13. A 54-year-old patient who lost 100 pounds two years ago underwent panniculectomy under general anesthesia. The patient has no significant medical history or chronic conditions.

14. A healthy 36-year-old patient underwent tubal ligation under general anesthesia for voluntary sterilization.

Perineum

15. A 45-year-old healthy patient presented with moderate vaginal bleeding. After being admitted and undergoing lab tests, the patient underwent hysteroscopy with endometrium biopsy under general anesthesia.

16. A healthy 38-year-old patient requested voluntary sterilization and underwent vasectomy. Regional anesthesia was administered.

Pelvis (Except Hip)

17. A healthy volunteer donor offered bone marrow to a needy recipient. The donor underwent bone marrow aspiration of the posterior iliac crest with general anesthesia to provide a sample to test for a match. The donor has no chronic or current medical conditions.

18. An otherwise healthy 14-year-old-male fell while skateboarding and landed on his back. After radiological exam, he was diagnosed with fractured sacroiliac joint. Open treatment of the anterior ring fracture was performed under general anesthesia.

Upper Leg (Except Knee)

19. A 46-year-old female fell while in-line skating and fractured her femur at the proximal end. She underwent open treatment of the femoral fracture with internal fixation under general anesthesia. The patient has type 2 diabetes mellitus, controlled.

20. A 76-year-old female with severe Parkinson's disease fell while getting out of bed. She was unable to walk and was found two days later by her son. She was dehydrated and disoriented. She was seen and evaluated in the emergency department. She was admitted with the diagnosis of a hip fracture. The patient's left hip was repaired with total hip arthroplasty under general anesthesia on the day of admission.

Knee and Popliteal Area

21. A 17-year-old healthy male high school football player's left knee was injured during a game. Examination revealed fractured patella. He underwent open treatment of left fractured patella under general anesthesia.

22. A healthy 15-year-old female high school gymnast's knee was injured during a meet. Radiological examination revealed a torn meniscus. She underwent a surgical arthroscopic procedure of her left knee to repair the meniscus, with general anesthesia.

Lower Leg (Below Knee, Includes Ankle and Foot)

23. A 14-year-old Down syndrome male was stepped on by a horse. Upon radiological exam, it was noted that the child had a trimalleolar fracture. The patient underwent closed treatment of the left trimalleolar fracture without manipulation under general anesthesia.

24. A 23-year-old female who is otherwise healthy was seen in the emergency room with pain, swelling, and disfigurement in her right lower leg. Radiological exam revealed a fractured tibia. She underwent closed reduction and casting under general anesthesia.

Shoulder and Axilla

25. An otherwise healthy 27-year-old male fell while riding his motorcycle. He complained of right shoulder pain and swelling. Upon radiological exam, it was noted that he had a fractured right humerus. He underwent closed treatment of the humeral head under general anesthesia.

26. A healthy 37-year-old female iron worker fell and landed on her left side, dislocating her left shoulder. She underwent closed manipulation, left shoulder joint, which required regional anesthesia.

Upper Arm and Elbow

27. A healthy 21-year-old female college tennis player complained about pain in her left elbow. The joint was swollen and tender. After orthopedic and radiological exam, reconstruction of the lateral collateral ligament was performed under general anesthesia.

28. A 50-year-old healthy bodybuilder felt severe pain in the right upper arm while lifting heavy weights. Radiological exam revealed no rupture of the right biceps tendon. A diagnosis of tendonitis was established. Patient underwent tenodesis the ruptured tendon, right, under general anesthesia.

Forearm, Wrist, and Hand

29. An otherwise healthy 68-year-old male noticed a lump on his left forearm. Examination determined that he needed an incision and drainage of a bursa. The procedure was performed under general anesthesia.

30. A 47-year-old healthy male factory worker caught his lower left arm in a commercial washing machine. The patient sustained a fracture and dislocated distal radius. The patient underwent open reduction of the fracture and dislocation under general anesthesia.

Radiological Procedures

31. A 57-year-old obese patient with hypertension showed possible coronary problems during a stress test. A cardiac catheterization under general anesthesia was performed.

32. A 63-year-old male was diagnosed with a severe glioblastoma multiforme. He underwent radiation therapy under regional anesthesia.

Burn Excisions or Debridement

33. A male firefighter with uncontrolled hypertension sustained severe second-degree burns over 35 percent of his body while on duty. He received general anesthesia during the burn debridement.

34. A 59-year-old healthy female chemical factory worker sustained second-degree burns due to a caustic chemical spill to her left arm. Three percent of her body was burned. She received general anesthesia during burn excision.

Obstetric

35. A healthy 24-year-old female had a normal vaginal delivery under regional anesthesia.

---

36. A controlled non-insulin-dependent diabetic 29-year-old female underwent cesarean delivery with general anesthesia.

Other Procedures

37. A 37-year-old otherwise healthy male has recurring back pain. He underwent spinal disc surgery and continued to need daily epidural continuous drug anesthesia while in the hospital.

---

38. An anesthesiologist provided physiologic support for harvesting organs (for organ donation) from a brain-dead patient.

---

39. A healthy 30-year-old patient underwent insertion of an epidural catheter on the first day of admission. On the second day of admission, the anesthesiologist was responsible for hospital management of continuous epidural drug administration. (Report the Anesthesia code for the second day of admission only.)

---

40. General anesthesia was administered to a six-month-old child with mild systemic disease who underwent anesthesia for a brand new procedure not yet included in CPT. The patient was observed in recovery by the nursing staff and evaluated by the anesthesiologist before being transferred to the pediatric unit of the hospital. The nursing staff placed an IV line for saline and postoperative pain medication.

Chapter Outline

Overview of Surgery Section

Surgery Guidelines

General Subsection

Integumentary System Subsection

Chapter Objectives

At the conclusion of this chapter, the student should be able to:

1. Define key terms related to the General and Integumentary System subsections of CPT Surgery.
2. Provide an overview about the CPT Surgery section, including its organization, format, and content.
3. Interpret CPT Surgery guidelines.
4. Assign codes from the General subsection of CPT Surgery.
5. Assign codes from the Integumentary System subsection of CPT Surgery.

Key Terms

adjacent tissue transfer and rearrangement

biopsy

defect

destruction

diagnostic procedure

donor site

endoscopy

excision

fine-needle aspiration (FNA)

flap

global period

global surgical package

graft

incision

incision and drainage (I&D)

introduction

lumpectomy

mastectomy

Mohs microsurgery

paring and curettement

primary defect

recipient site

reconstruction

removal

repair

revision

rule of nines

secondary defect

separate procedure

shaving

stereotactic localization

stroma

surgical package

suture

therapeutic surgical procedure

tissue approximation

undermining

Introduction

The CPT Surgery section contains codes and code descriptions for surgical procedures performed by physicians. Because procedures can be performed using a variety of methods and in different combinations, the Surgery section contains multiple codes that describe similar procedures. The intention is to allow for coding specificity and to accurately reflect the actual procedure performed. The patient's diagnosis and health status (e.g., normal, healthy patient versus patient with severe systemic disease) guides the physician, who determines whether just one procedure or multiple procedures will be performed during an encounter (e.g., office visit) or operative session (e.g., ambulatory surgery). The documented operative report and other patient record documentation are reviewed to select appropriate codes for reporting to third-party payers. The General subsection includes codes for fine-needle aspiration (FNA) biopsy procedures. The Integumentary System subsection includes codes for procedures performed on the skin, subcutaneous, and accessory structures, nails, and breasts.

Coding Tip

Instructional notes located beneath categories, subcategories, headings, and subheadings apply to all codes under those areas. Parenthetical notes located below a specific code apply to that code only, unless the note indicates otherwise.

NOTE:

The content in Chapters 12 through 16 of this textbook is organized exactly as it appears in the CPT Surgery section. This organization facilitates learning by allowing students to move from one CPT Surgery subsection to the next, in order.

When included in CPT, the Other Procedures code is reported for an unlisted procedure performed on the anatomical site. When reporting an unlisted procedure code, include documentation about the procedure performed with the submitted claim.

The *Medicare National Correct Coding Initiative Policy Manual* provides guidance about assigning procedure codes for the General and Integumentary System subsections. Go to www.cms.gov and enter "Medicare NCCI Policy Manual" in the Search box to navigate to the manual.

Overview of Surgery Section

The CPT Surgery section and its subsections are organized anatomically according to major body area and organ system. Categories and subcategories are organized within subsections according to type of procedure. Selecting the appropriate surgery code requires a careful review of the patient record to determine the procedures and services provided. Before referring to the CPT index to begin the process of locating a surgery code, review the documented operative report (Figure 12-1) to determine the following:

- Major body area (e.g., stomach)
- Organ system (e.g., digestive)
- Surgical approach (e.g., laparotomy)
- Type of procedure performed (e.g., partial gastrectomy)
- Whether multiple procedures were performed during the same operative session (e.g., gastroscopy followed by exploratory laparotomy and removal of a portion of the stomach)

	PREOPERATIVE DIAGNOSIS: Possible uterine polyp.
Name of procedure	**POSTOPERATIVE DIAGNOSIS:** Endometrial polyp.
	PROCEDURE: Hysteroscopy with biopsy.
Surgical approach	The cervix was dilated and hysteroscope was inserted into the
Anatomical site	uterus and the lining of the uterus and openings of the fallopian

tubes were well visualized. One large polyp was noted on the endometrial wall, and a biopsy was taken. The uterus is of normal size and configuration. Biopsy was submitted for pathology examination. Postoperatively the patient is doing well and was taken to the recovery room.

FIGURE 12-1 Sample operative report with name of procedure, surgical approach, and anatomical site highlighted to illustrate how to locate information needed to assign a CPT code

Example 1: When reporting the CPT code for "excision of cervical stump," if an abdominal approach was documented in the operative report, assign code 57540. If a vaginal approach was documented, assign code 57550.

```
57540    Excision of cervical stump, abdominal approach;
57545       with pelvic floor repair
```

Example 2: When reporting the CPT code for "removal of a 0.5-cm malignant lesion of the arm," if a surgical excision was documented in the operative report, assign code 11600.

If a destruction procedure (e.g., laser ablation) was documented, assign code 17260.

Code 11600 includes excision of margins, while code 17260 does not.

CPT code descriptions include the procedure performed, but they do not include the numerous activities integral to the procedure. It would be impractical to list every event common to all procedures of a similar nature in the code's narrative description. Many common activities reflect the principles of medical and surgical care, and while considered acceptable medical/surgical practice, they are not coded separately. In addition, although many activities are common to all procedures, some are integral only to certain groups of procedures.

The services integral to the standard practice of medical/surgical services, for which no separate code is assigned, include

- Cleansing, shaving, and prepping the patient's skin
- Draping and positioning the patient
- Inserting intravenous access for medication
- Administering sedatives (by physician performing procedure)
- Administering local, topical, and regional anesthetic (by physician performing procedure)
- Establishing the surgical approach (identifying anatomical landmarks, making the incision, evaluating the surgical field, and performing simple debridement of traumatized tissue)
- Performing lysis of simple adhesions

- Isolating neurovascular, muscular (including stimulation for identification), bony, or other structures that limit access to surgical field
- Taking surgical cultures
- Irrigating wounds
- Inserting and removing drains, suction devices, dressings, and pumps into the same site
- Closing the surgical incision
- Applying, managing, and removing postoperative dressings, including analgesic devices (e.g., peri-incisional TENS unit, institution of patient-controlled analgesia)
- Documenting preoperative, intraoperative, and postoperative reports, which includes providing photographs, drawings, dictation, and transcription necessary to document services provided
- Identifying surgical supplies (unless third-party payer policy states that they are separately coded and reimbursable)

Example 1: The physician removed cerumen (earwax) impaction prior to performing a myringotomy. The cerumen impaction prevented access to the tympanic membrane, and its removal was necessary for the successful completion of the myringotomy. Report code 69420 (Myringotomy including aspiration and eustachian tube inflation) only. *Do not report a separate code for removal of cerumen impaction.*

Example 2: The physician performed a bronchoscopy to assess the patient's lung anatomy prior to performing a lobectomy (single lobe). Report code 32480, which has a CPT code description of "removal of lung, other than total pneumonectomy; single lobe (lobectomy)." *Do not report a code for the bronchoscopy*, which was performed as a scout endoscopy to assess the surgical field and to establish anatomical landmarks, extent of disease, and so on. When an endoscopic procedure is done as part of an open procedure, such as a lobectomy, it is not separately coded and reported.

If an endoscopy is performed initially to diagnose the patient on the same day as the open procedure, the endoscopy is separately coded and reported. Modifier 58 is added to the endoscopy code to indicate that the procedures are staged or planned services. Also, if endoscopic procedures are performed on distinct, separate areas during the same operative session, separately code and report each procedure (e.g., thoracoscopy and mediastinoscopy). However, if a cursory (brief) evaluation of the upper airway is done as part of a bronchoscopy, do not separately code and report procedures (e.g., laryngoscopy or sinus endoscopy).

Organization of Surgery Section

The guidelines located at the beginning of the Surgery section apply to all codes in the section. The basic organization of the Surgery section is by major body system, which is organized according to anatomical site and type of procedure (Table 12-1). The Surgery section contains the following subsections, which represent major body areas, organ systems, or other designations:

- General
- Integumentary System
- Musculoskeletal System
- Respiratory System
- Cardiovascular System
- Hemic and Lymphatic Systems
- Mediastinum and Diaphragm
- Digestive System
- Urinary System
- Male Genital System
- Reproductive System Procedures
- Intersex Surgery
- Female Genital System
- Maternity Care and Delivery
- Endocrine System
- Nervous System
- Eye and Ocular Adnexa
- Auditory System
- Operating Microscope

TABLE 12-1 Categories Typically Organized Below CPT Surgery Subsections

Category	Description
Incision	Cut made into body tissue during surgery using a knife, electrosurgical unit, or laser
Incision and Drainage (I&D)	Cutting open a lesion (e.g., abscess) and draining its contents
Excision	Removing a portion or all of an organ or another tissue (e.g., skin), using a scalpel or another surgical instrument
Introduction	Injecting, inserting, or puncturing body tissue or scoping an organ
Removal	Eliminating tissue (e.g., amputating a body part) or taking something out (e.g., removing implants, such as buried wire, pins, or screws)
Endoscopy	Visualizing a body cavity using an instrument that can be inserted into the body through a small incision or a natural opening (e.g., nose); endoscopy is also used as a surgical approach for performing other procedures (e.g., laparoscopic cholecystectomy)
Repair	Improving improperly functioning body parts; types of repairs include: • **Grafts:** Any tissue or organ used for implantation or transfer, which involves moving healthy tissue from one site to another to replace diseased or defective tissue • **Suture:** Closing a wound using catgut, glue, silk thread, wire, or other materials (Figure 12-2)
Revision	Modifying a previous procedure (e.g., gastric restrictive procedure) or a device (e.g., shunt)
Reconstruction	Rebuilding a body part, such as the breast
Destruction	*Ablation* (or removal) of benign, premalignant, or malignant tissue by any method, including: • *Chemosurgery:* Using chemicals to destroy diseased tissue, such as for skin cancer • *Cryosurgery:* Applying extreme cold, such as liquid nitrogen, to destroy abnormal tissue cells, such as warts or small skin lesions • *Electrosurgery:* Using an electrical device, such as electrocautery, to destroy abnormal tissue • *LASER (light amplification by stimulated emission of radiation):* Using a device that is filled with a gas, liquid, or solid substance that is stimulated to emit light to a specific wavelength to burn, cut, or dissolve tissue • *Surgical curettement:* Scraping abnormal tissue
Other Procedures	Unrelated procedures, which include arthrodesis, Mohs micrographic surgery, manipulation (of fractures/dislocations), splinting, or casting

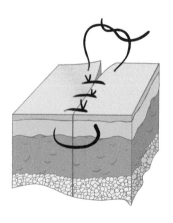

(A)

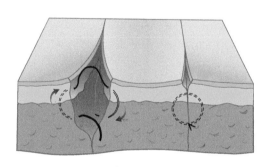

(B)

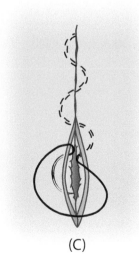

(C)

FIGURE 12-2 (A) Simple interrupted sutures (B) Buried sutures (C) Running subcuticular sutures

Many of the Surgery subsections contain *instructional notes,* which are located just below the title of the subsection, category, or subcategory. Parenthetical notes are located below codes, and they apply to just that code.

> **Example:** The note located above code 11200 in the CPT coding manual provides instruction about methods (e.g., scissoring) for removal, which applies to all codes under "Removal of Skin Tags."
>
> The parenthetical note located below code 11201 in the coding manual indicates that code 11201 is reported with 11200, which means that it is never reported as a stand-alone code. This note applies to code 11201 only.

In the Surgery section, procedures are categorized as diagnostic procedures or therapeutic surgical procedures. **Diagnostic procedures** (e.g., arthroscopy, biopsy, and endoscopy) are performed to evaluate the patient's complaints or symptoms and to establish the diagnosis. **Therapeutic surgical procedures** (e.g., removal, repair) are performed to treat specific conditions or injuries; they include the procedure itself and normal, uncomplicated follow-up care.

Surgery section procedures are typically organized according to the following categories (below the heading of a subsection).

- Incision *or* incision and drainage (I&D)
- Excision
- Introduction or removal
- Endoscopy
- Repair, revision, and reconstruction
- Destruction
- Other procedures

Exercise 12.1 – Overview of Surgery Section

Instructions: Complete each statement.

1. The organization of the CPT Surgery section is according to major body area or _____ system.
2. Endoscopy, arthroscopy, and biopsy are considered _____ procedures.
3. Gastric resection and knee replacement surgeries are considered _____ procedures.
4. The patient underwent cystourethroscopy with brush biopsy of urinary bladder wall. Use your CPT coding manual to identify the following:
   a. Body system: _____
   b. Anatomical site: _____
   c. Surgical approach: _____
   d. Type of procedure performed: _____
   e. Name of the procedure: _____ with _____ of urinary bladder wall
   f. CPT code assigned: _____
5. The physician performed open colectomy with end-to-end anastomosis. Use your CPT coding manual to identify the following:
   a. Body system: _____

(continues)

Exercise 12.1 – continued

b. Anatomical site: _____

c. Surgical approach: _____

d. Type of procedure performed: _____

e. Name of the procedure: _____

f. CPT code assigned: _____

Surgery Guidelines

Guidelines located at the beginning of the CPT Surgery section clarify the assignment of codes and explain terms. Surgery guidelines include the following:

- Services
- CPT surgical package definition
- Follow-up care for diagnostic procedures
- Follow-up care for therapeutic surgical procedures
- Supplied materials
- Reporting more than one procedure/service
- Separate procedure
- Unlisted service or procedure
- Special report
- Imaging guidance
- Surgical destruction
- Foreign body/implant definition

Services

Codes for services that are provided in the office, patient's home, hospital, and other health care facilities are located in the CPT Evaluation and Management (E/M) section. This section also includes codes for consultations and other medical services. Codes for special services and reports are located in the CPT Medicine section.

CPT Surgical Package Definition

Many services performed are integral to the standard of medical/surgical services, such as the cleansing, shaving, and prepping of skin and the insertion of intravenous access for medication. The CPT **surgical package** usually includes the following services, in addition to the surgical procedure performed:

- Local infiltration, metacarpal/metatarsal/digital block, or topical anesthesia
- One related E/M service following the decision for surgery, which includes the history and physical, on the date of the procedure or immediately prior to performance of the procedure
- Immediate postoperative care, which includes documenting the operative report and talking with the family and other physicians or qualified health care professionals
- Documentation of postoperative physician orders
- Evaluation of the patient in the postanesthesia recovery area
- Typical postoperative follow-up care (e.g., removal of sutures)

 NOTE:

The CPT surgical package definition does *not* apply to treatment of patients for surgical complications. Procedures and/or services provided to treat complications are reported in addition to the surgical package CPT code.

CMS Global Surgical Package Definition

The Centers for Medicare & Medicaid Services (CMS) established a national definition for a **global surgical package** (that differs from the definition of the CPT *surgical package*) to ensure that payments are made consistently for the same services across all Medicare administrative contractor jurisdictions. The *global surgical package* definition prevents Medicare payments for services that are more *or* less comprehensive than intended. The CMS global surgical package includes the surgical procedure and a standard package of preoperative, intraoperative, and postoperative services. In addition, CMS categorizes surgeries as major or minor, and it establishes a postoperative **global period** (0, 10, or 90 days) (Figure 12-3) for each surgical procedure, which includes the following policies:

- The global period for major surgery is 0, 10, or 90 days.
- The global period begins the day following surgery.
- The global period includes a one-day preoperative period for major surgery only.

The 90-day global period for major surgery (e.g., open cholecystectomy) includes the day prior to surgery, day of surgery, and 90 days that immediately follow the day of surgery, resulting in a total global period of 92 days.

> **Example:** For a date of surgery on January 1, the
>
> - Preoperative day is December 31
> - Last day of the 90-day postoperative period is April 1
>
> To arrive at April 1, count January 2–31 as 30 days, February 1–28 as 28 days, March 1–31 as 31 days, and April 1 as 1 day, for a total of 90 days *after the day of surgery.* Adding the day prior to surgery (e.g., preoperative day), the day of surgery, and the 90-day postoperative period together results in a total global period of 92 days.
>
> Use the 90-day global period calculator for major surgeries to determine the last date of the postoperative period. Go to https://www.ngsmedicare.com, click on Resources, and click on Tools & Calculators.

CPT Code	Global Period
59050	XXX
59160	010
59200	000
59400	MMM
59525	ZZZ
59812	090
59899	YYY

FIGURE 12-3 Sample of CMS global periods

The global period for minor surgery (e.g., endoscopy) is zero or 10 days, and physician visits on the day of a minor surgical procedure or endoscopy are included in reimbursement for the procedure.

- The zero-day global period includes the day of surgery only.

> **Example:** To determine the zero-day global period for a minor surgical procedure, count the day of surgery only. For a date of surgery on March 5, the last day of the postoperative period is also March 5.

- The 10-day global period includes the day of surgery and the 10 days that immediately follow the day of surgery, resulting in a total global period of 11 days.

> **Example:** To determine the 10-day global period for a minor surgical procedure, count the day of surgery and the 10 days immediately following the date of surgery. For a date of surgery on March 5, the last day of the postoperative period is March 15.
>
> To arrive at March 15, count March 6–15 as 10 days. Adding the day of surgery to the 10-day postoperative period results in a total global period of 11 days.

CMS publishes a list of the global periods for each CPT code in the *Federal Register*, which is used by other payers and also includes alphabetical remark codes that also appear in the global period column:

- 000: Endoscopies and some minor surgical procedures with a 0-day postoperative period
- 010: Minor procedures with a 10-day postoperative period
- 090: Major surgical procedures with a 90-day postoperative period
- MMM: Global period policy does not apply; describes services furnished in uncomplicated maternity cases, including antepartum care, delivery, and postpartum care.
- XXX: Global period policy does not apply.
- YYY: Global period is established by payer and specified as 0, 10, or 90 days (or 000, 010, or 090 days).
- ZZZ: Add-on procedure bundled into primary procedure global period.

 NOTE:

When a patient receives treatment for an unrelated condition during the global period, add modifier 24 to the CPT code for an E/M service or add modifier 79 to the CPT code for a surgical procedure/service.

Instructions for the CMS's global surgical package describe the components of a global surgical package and payment rules for minor surgeries, endoscopies, and global surgical packages that are split between physicians. In addition to the global surgical package policy, other payment policies and claims processing requirements were established for other surgical issues, including bilateral and multiple surgeries. The CMS global surgical package includes the following:

- Preoperative visits after the decision is made to operate, beginning with the day before the day of surgery for major procedures and the day of surgery for minor procedures
- Intraoperative services that are normally a usual and necessary part of a surgical package
- Treatment of complications following surgery (additional services required of the surgeon during the postoperative period because of complications that do not require additional trips to the operating room)
- Postoperative visits (follow-up visits during the postoperative period that are related to recovery from surgery)
- Postsurgical pain management (provided by the surgeon)
- Miscellaneous services (e.g., dressing changes; local incisional care; removal of operative packing; removal of sutures and staples, tubes, drains, and casts; insertion or removal of urinary catheters and nasogastric tubes)

The CMS global surgical package does *not* include the following:

- Initial consultation or evaluation services by the surgeon to determine need for major surgery

NOTE:

For *minor surgery*, the initial consultation or evaluation services by the surgeon *is included* in the global surgical package.

- Services provided by physicians except where the surgeon and the other physician(s) agree on the transfer of care
- Visits unrelated to the diagnosis for which a surgical procedure is performed, except visits due to complications of surgery
- Services provided by other physicians, except when the physicians agree on transfer of care
- Diagnostic tests and procedures, including diagnostic radiological procedures
- Treatment for an underlying condition or an added course of treatment that is not part of normal recovery from surgery
- Clearly distinct surgical procedures during the postoperative period that are *not* for treatment of complications or procedures done in "stages." A new postoperative period begins with each subsequent procedure.
- Treatment for postoperative complications that require a return trip to the operating room (e.g., postoperative wound infection that requires a complex incision and drainage procedure)
- A required, more extensive procedure when a less extensive procedure fails; in this case, the second procedure is payable separately
- For certain services performed in a physician's office, separate payment is no longer made for a surgical tray (HCPCS Level II code A4550)
- Immunosuppressive therapy for organ transplants
- Critical care E/M services unrelated to the surgery

It is important to understand that the procedure being performed determines the global follow-up care; the condition being treated does not. The global surgical packages deal with the procedure(s) performed during the global period by the operating surgeon; only the operating surgeon is associated with that particular global period of follow-up care.

Example: A patient underwent ventral hernia repair performed by a general surgeon and one week later fractured the left ankle. An orthopedic surgeon inserted a pin to repair the fractured ankle. A global follow-up period for the specific surgery performed is associated with the CPT code assigned by each physician. Thus, each physician receives appropriate reimbursement for services provided.

When the patient is seen by the general surgeon for follow-up care related to the ventral hernia repair and such care is provided within the global period, an E/M code for services provided is *not* reported. Payment for such follow-up care is bundled in the CPT code reported for the ventral hernia repair surgery. Likewise, when the patient is seen by the orthopedic surgeon for follow-up care related to the ankle surgery, E/M services are bundled in the CPT code reported for that surgery.

If the patient develops complications subsequent to surgery and receives E/M services within the global period, the respective surgeon should report a CPT code for services provided to receive reimbursement from the third-party payer.

E/M services provided as follow-up to a surgical procedure are included in the reimbursement amount for the surgery, and codes for follow-up E/M services are not reported separately. However, when the patient receives E/M services for an unrelated condition, make sure you report an E/M code to receive reimbursement for services provided.

Example: An excision of a 4.3-cm malignant lesion on the left arm is performed in the office on May 10. The postoperative global period for code 11606 is 10 days. The patient returns to the office on May 15 and is treated for conjunctivitis. The physician should report an appropriate E/M code and add modifier 24 (Unrelated Evaluation and Management Service by the Same Physician During a Postoperative Period) (e.g., 99213 24).

When an E/M service is provided for the purpose of deciding to perform a major surgical procedure, the E/M service is considered a significant, separately identifiable service. Report an appropriate E/M code and add modifier 57 (decision for surgery).

> **Example:** A surgeon provided level 5 consultation services to a patient in the office to determine whether surgery was necessary due to complaints of severe abdominal pain. After evaluation, the ambulance is called and the patient is transported to the hospital, where the surgeon performs an emergency gastrotomy with suture repair of a bleeding ulcer. Report code 43501 (Gastrotomy; with suture repair of bleeding ulcer) and 99245 57 (Office consultation for new or established patient, level 5). Modifier 57 (Decision for surgery) is added to the E/M code.

Local Infiltration, Metacarpal/Metatarsal/Digital Block, or Topical Anesthesia

Local infiltration, metacarpal/metatarsal/digital block, or topical anesthesia, when provided by the physician performing the procedure, is considered part of the procedure. When the surgeon provides general anesthesia, regional anesthesia, or monitored anesthesia care, add modifier 47 to the surgery code.

 NOTE:

> When an anesthesiologist provides general anesthesia, regional anesthesia, or monitored anesthesia care, they report an anesthesia code for services provided. (Refer to Chapter 11, CPT Anesthesia, of this textbook.)

> **Example:** A surgeon injected a local anesthetic in preparation for performing an inguinal hernia repair on a 42-year-old patient. The local anesthetic procedure performed by the surgeon is included in the surgical procedure and is not separately coded and reported.

The management of postoperative pain by the surgeon, including epidural drug administration, is included in the global package with the operative procedure.

Follow-Up Care for Diagnostic Procedures

Diagnostic procedures are performed to evaluate a patient's condition, to determine the nature of a condition, and to distinguish between one disease and another. According to CPT, follow-up care for diagnostic procedures includes only that care related to recovery from the diagnostic procedure itself. Codes for services provided should be reported when a physician treats

- The patient's condition for which the diagnostic procedure was performed
- Other conditions that are not related to the reason for performing the diagnostic procedure

When a patient receives services from the physician who performed the diagnostic procedure and those services are in follow-up to the procedure performed (e.g., suture removal or dressing change), do not report a code for services provided.

Follow-Up Care for Therapeutic Surgical Procedures

Therapeutic surgical procedures are performed for the definitive treatment of a disease or condition rather than for diagnostic or investigative purposes. Follow-up care for therapeutic surgical procedures includes only the care that is typically considered part of the surgical service. The physician generally sees the patient several times as part of normal, uncomplicated follow-up care (e.g., remove sutures, evaluate the results of the surgery, or check for complications). These postoperative visits are included as part of surgery's global period because normal follow-up care services are a necessary component of the surgical process.

Codes for services provided should be reported when a physician treats the following during the postoperative global period:

- Complications (e.g., postoperative wound infection)
- Exacerbations (e.g., macular degeneration that was treated, but worsens, requiring another treatment)
- Recurrence (e.g., return of cancer)
- Presence of other diseases (e.g., appendicitis during global period for gastric resection)
- Injuries (e.g., fracture resulting from car accident)

Supplied Materials

Supplies commonly included in surgical packages (e.g., dressings, tubing, and Steri-Strips) are *not* reported separately. Only those supplies and materials provided by the physician *over and above* supplies usually included with the procedure rendered are reported separately. Assign CPT code 99070 or a specific HCPCS Level II code to report such supplies. (For drugs provided during a procedure, such as the topical administration of Lidocaine, report a HCPCS Level II code.)

The CPT Surgery section procedure codes do not indicate when it is appropriate to report supply items separately. Reimbursement of supplies and materials required to perform the procedure is a specific reimbursement issue, which varies from one third-party payer to another. CMS created specific instructions regarding the separate reporting of "supply" items upon implementation of the practice expense component of the Medicare Physician Fee Schedule, stating that "all supplies, such as surgical trays, are included (e.g., bundled) in the payment for the procedure." Medicare does *not* reimburse the physician for the CPT 99070 supply code. When other payers allow codes for supplies to be reported, the best practice is to report a specific HCPCS Level II supply code (instead of CPT code 99070).

> **Example:** A 42-year-old patient underwent a repair of initial inguinal reducible hernia, right side, with implantation of mesh. Report CPT code 49505 RT and HCPCS Level II code C1781 (supply of mesh). (Do not add modifier 51 to either code.)

Reporting More Than One Procedure/Service

When a physician performs more than one procedure or service on the same date, during the same operative session, or during a postoperative period and the surgical package concept applies, report one or more CPT modifiers to receive reimbursement consideration from third-party payers.

 NOTE:

Refer to Chapter 9, Introduction to CPT Coding, of this textbook for a comprehensive list of modifiers, descriptions, and examples.

Add-on Codes

CPT includes a ✛ (plus) symbol next to add-on codes that describe a service that can be reported only in addition to a primary procedure. Add-on codes can also be identified by specific language in the code descriptor, such as *each additional* or *(List separately in addition to primary procedure)*. Add-on codes are never reported as stand-alone codes because they are considered an integral part of another procedure. They are never reported alone because the procedures they describe would not be performed unless another primary procedure was performed.

Add-on codes allow physicians to separately report procedures and services performed in addition to the primary procedure. The key to identifying add-on codes is determining whether the code always has to be reported with another code. If that is the case, the code is considered an add-on code. Also, add-on codes are exempt from the bilateral procedure and the multiple procedure concept, respectively, which means modifiers 50 and 51 are not added. (Add-on codes are reported twice for bilateral procedures.)

> **Example:** A patient underwent open treatment of three lumbar vertebral fractures. Report codes 22325, 22328, and 22328.
>
> The description for code 22325 includes "one fractured vertebra," and the description for code 22328 states "each additional fractured vertebrae . . . (List separately in addition to code for primary procedure)." This patient underwent treatment for three vertebral fractures, which requires the reporting of three codes. Do not add modifier 51 (Multiple procedures) to the add on codes because they are exempt from that modifier.

Separate Procedure

CPT code descriptions that contain the term **separate procedure** in parentheses are commonly performed as an integral component of a comprehensive service or procedure. When the comprehensive procedure or service is performed, do not report as an additional procedure the code that contains the term *(separate procedure)* in its code description.

> **Example:** The patient underwent sesamoidectomy and excision of a bone cyst of the middle phalanx of the right hand. Report code 26210 F7.
>
> Do not mistakenly report code 26185 in addition to code 26210. Code 26185 contains the term *(separate procedure)* in its code description. The procedure described in code 26185 is a component part of the more comprehensive "excision of bone cyst" procedure.

When a procedure or service that contains *(separate procedure)* in its code description *is performed independently of or is considered unrelated to or distinct from other procedures performed during the same operative session, report the separate procedure code in addition to codes for other procedures (or services).*

Reporting separate procedure codes may be necessary to classify the following:

- Procedure performed during a different session or patient encounter, procedure or surgery, site, or organ system
- Procedure performed through a separate incision or excision
- Separate lesion excised during the same operative session as removal of another lesion
- Treatment of a separate injury (or area of injury for extensive injuries)

Add modifier 59 to the separate procedure code to indicate that the procedure is not considered a component of another procedure, but is a distinct, independent procedure.

> **Example:** A patient underwent a complete salpingo-oophorectomy, bilateral, during the same operative session as a total abdominal hysterectomy. Report code 58150, Total abdominal hysterectomy (corpus and cervix), with or without removal of tube(s), with or without removal of ovary(s). Do not report code 58720, Salpingo-oophorectomy, complete or partial, unilateral or bilateral (separate procedure) because it is considered an integral component of the procedures described for code 58150.

Unlisted Service or Procedure

CPT unlisted service or procedure codes are assigned when no specific code accurately describes the procedure performed. When reporting an unlisted procedure code on an insurance claim, make sure you include a written report (e.g., copy of operative report) that describes the procedure(s) performed. (During the first year that laparoscopic appendectomies and cholecystectomies were performed, no procedure codes were included in CPT. Unlisted procedure codes were reported.)

Example: A physician performs a pressure ulcer excision using a technique that is not described by any existing pressure ulcer codes. Report code 15999, and include a copy of the operative report with the claim.

Special Report

When an unlisted procedure code is reported to a third-party payer, attach a special report to the claim that describes the procedure performed. Special reports may also be required for procedures and services that are rarely provided, unusual, or new (to establish medical necessity). As a minimum, to document a special report, include the following adequate description of the nature, extent, and need for the procedure and time, effort, and equipment necessary to provide the procedure or service. The following additional items may also be documented in a special report: complexity of symptoms, concurrent problems, diagnostic and therapeutic procedures, final diagnosis, follow-up care, and pertinent physical findings.

Example: An ear, nose, and throat specialist performed an experimental procedure on the pharynx of a 14-year-old prodigy opera singer to treat persistent pharyngitis that has not resolved with traditional medical treatment. Conventional procedures to treat the unusual condition are not an option for this patient because they pose too great a risk of damage to the patient's vocal cords. The procedure was approved by the patient's parents, the health care facility at which it was performed, and the third-party payer that will reimburse its costs. Because the procedure is experimental, no CPT code is available. Report 42999, and attach a copy of the transcribed operative report to the claim. The operative report is the "special report" required by the payer to process the claim for reimbursement.

Imaging Guidance

When the description of a surgical procedure code includes *imaging guidance* or *imaging supervision and interpretation* (e.g., CT, fluoroscopy, MRI, nuclear medicine, radiography, ultrasonography), Radiology section guidelines are followed that require documentation of images, anatomic information about the patient, description of imaging guidance, and interpretation of radiologic findings.

Example: Percutaneous breast biopsy, left, with placement of breast clip and imaging of biopsy specimen, including stereotactic guidance. Report code 19081. (Stereotactic guidance pinpoints the exact location of a breast abnormality and is included in the code. A separate Radiology code is *not* reported.)

Surgical Destruction

Surgical destruction is considered part of a surgical procedure, and different methods of destruction are not reported separately unless the techniques substantially differ from the standard management of a problem or condition. (CPT codes are available for exceptions due to special circumstances.) Surgical destruction includes the ablation (or removal) of tissues by any method, including chemical treatment, cryosurgery, electrosurgery, or laser.

Example: A physician performed argon laser treatments on a 6 sq cm congenital port wine stain. Report code 17106.

Foreign Body/Implant Definition

An object that is intentionally placed into the patient is considered an implant while an object that is unintentionally placed (due to ingestion or trauma) is considered a foreign body. However, when an implant shifts from its original position or becomes broken, it is considered a foreign body for coding purposes (especially when it becomes a hazard to a patient). The exception is when CPT coding instructions provide guidance to specific codes that describe the removal of a shifted or broken implant.

Example:

- Patient sustained trauma resulting in a piece of metal being embedded in the left shoulder. Subcutaneous removal of foreign body, left shoulder, was successful. Report code 23330.
- Patient underwent removal of implantable contraceptive capsule, which was inserted two years ago. Report code 11976.

Exercise 12.2 – Surgery Guidelines

Instructions: Complete each statement.

1. The CPT surgical package includes typical _____ follow-up care in addition to the surgical procedure.

2. CMS categorizes surgeries as major or minor and establishes a postoperative _____ period of 0, 10, or 90 days.

3. When the surgeon provides general or regional anesthesia or monitored anesthesia care during a surgical procedure, add modifier _____ to the surgery code.

4. A physician applied sterile dressings after repairing a laceration. The sterile dressings are considered _____, and they are not separately coded and reported.

5. The patient underwent esophageal dilation for esophageal stricture (43450). Then, during the same operative session, the patient was re-prepped and underwent esophagoscopy (43200) to investigate the cause of the esophageal stricture. Upon review of both codes, both are reported, and modifier _____ is added to code 43200 to indicate that a distinct surgical procedure was performed.

6. The global period for a minor surgical procedure performed on March 15 is zero days. The last day of the postoperative period is March _____.

7. The global period for a minor surgical procedure performed on October 4 is 10 days plus the day of surgery. Counting the day of surgery, the last day of the postoperative period is October _____.

8. A surgeon performed an incision and drainage of a facial abscess in the office, which has a 10-day global period. The patient returned to the office three weeks later and was diagnosed with a tonsillar abscess, which was unrelated to the incision and drainage of the facial abscess. Which CPT modifier is added to the most recent E/M code? _____

9. A surgeon provided level 4 E/M services to a patient in the office, which resulted in the decision for surgery. The physician reports the E/M code and adds modifier _____.

10. A physician performed surgery on a patient to destroy 25 lesions. Review the description for CPT code 17004. How many times should code 17004 be reported? _____

General Subsection

The General subsection contains one category *Fine-Needle Aspiration (FNA) Biopsy*. **Fine-needle aspiration (FNA)** involves the removal of fluid from a cyst or cells from a solid mass. Then the cells are examined cytologically. FNA is a percutaneous procedure that is performed with or without imaging guidance. If the cyst or mass is *not* palpable on physical exam, the procedure is typically performed under imaging guidance using fluoroscopy, ultrasound, or computed tomography (CT).

Example 1: A physician aspirates a cyst, without imaging guidance, using FNA technique. Report code 10021.

Example 2: A patient presents with a thyroid nodule. Using CT guidance with radiological supervision and interpretation, an FNA is performed on the thyroid nodule; the material is sent for cytologic review. Report code 10009. Notice the instructional note below code 10010, which states, "Do not report 10009, 10010 in conjunction with 77012." This is an example of a parenthetical note that applies to more than one code. (Directional modifiers, such as LT and RT, are not added to codes in CPT's General subsection.)

Exercise 12.3 – General

Instructions: Assign the CPT code(s) and appropriate modifier(s) to each statement.

1. A patient presents with a palpable left breast mass (non-cystic) for which fine-needle aspiration biopsy is performed.

2. A patient has a nonpalpable thyroid lesion that was identified on a previous thyroid scan. Fine-needle aspiration biopsy of the thyroid lesion is performed under ultrasonic guidance during today's encounter.

Integumentary System Subsection

The Integumentary System subsection includes dermatological procedures, plastic surgery, and components of multiple surgical procedures (e.g., closure, flaps, grafts, and tissue transfer). Integumentary procedures (Table 12-2) are often performed as staged procedures (e.g., flaps and grafts) due to the complexity of services rendered. Integumentary procedures include incision, biopsy, removal, paring/curettement, shaving, destruction, excision, repair, adjacent tissue rearrangement, grafts, flaps, and specialized services (e.g., burn management, Mohs micrographic surgery). (Refer to the definitions of surgical terms earlier in this chapter. Additional terms are defined in Table 12-2.)

The CPT Surgery Integumentary subsection contains the following categories:

- Skin, Subcutaneous and Accessory Structures
- Nails
- Pilonidal Cyst
- Introduction
- Repair (Closure)
- Destruction
- Breast

 Coding Tip

- HCPCS Level II modifiers LT and RT are not added to codes in the Skin, Subcutaneous and Accessory Structures; Nails; Pilonidal Cyst; Introduction; Repair (Closure); or Destruction categories because skin is not a paired organ.
- Add HCPCS Level II modifiers FA through F9 or TA through T9 to codes for procedures performed on the fingernails or toenails.
- Add modifiers 50, LT, or RT to breast procedure codes.

TABLE 12-2 Integumentary Procedures and Definitions

Integumentary Procedure	Definition
Adjacent tissue transfer and rearrangement	Closure of defects by relocating a flap of adjacent normal, healthy tissue from a donor site to a nearby (adjacent) defect, such as a traumatic skin wound or the site of excised lesion; a portion of the flap remains intact to provide a blood supply to the grafted site
Biopsy	Removal and examination of tissue to establish a diagnosis, confirm a diagnosis, or determine the extent of a disease; types of skin biopsies include incisional, punch, and tangential (e.g., shaving)
Flap	Relocation of a mass of tissue (usually skin) that has been partially removed from one part of the body so that it retains its own blood supply
Graft	Any tissue or organ used for implantation or transplant, which involves moving healthy tissue from one site to another to replace diseased or defective tissue
Mohs microsurgery	Technique of excising skin tumors by removing tumor tissue layer by layer, examining the removed portion microscopically for malignant cells, and repeating the procedure until the entire tumor is removed
Paring and curettement	Removal of growths or other material from the wall of a cavity or another surface, as with a curette; paring of lesions (e.g., corns and calluses) seldom, if ever, require local anesthesia
Shaving	Horizontal slicing to remove epidermal and dermal lesions (e.g., without a full-thickness dermal excision); removal includes scissoring or any sharp method

Skin, Subcutaneous and Accessory Structures

The Skin, Subcutaneous and Accessory Structures category includes the following subcategories: Introduction and Removal, Incision and Drainage (I&D), Debridement, Paring or Cutting, Biopsy, Removal of Skin Tags, Shaving of Epidermal or Dermal Lesions, Excision—Benign Lesions, and Excision—Malignant Lesions.

Introduction and Removal

The *Introduction and Removal* category includes a code for percutaneous image-guided fluid collection drainage via catheter of soft tissue abscesses, hematomas, seromas, lymphoceles, and cysts.

Incision and Drainage (I&D)

The I&D category contains procedures that establish a drainage pathway for fluid that forms at sites of infection. CPT I&D procedures include cutaneous and subcutaneous drainage of cysts, fluid collections, infections, hematomas, pustules, and seromas. When a procedure to excise a lesion results in drainage of an area, either as a part of the procedure or as a way to gain access to the lesion, do not report a code for I&D if the excision or another procedure is performed during the same operative session. It is also inappropriate to report a separate code for an I&D of a hematoma if it is performed during the same operative session as excision, repair, destruction, removal, and so on.

> **Example:** A patient undergoes a scheduled procedure to treat a *pilonidal cyst* (entrapped epithelial tissue and hair located in the sacral area at the top of the crease between the buttocks, which can become infected). Treatment options include simple I&D (10080–10081), excision (11770–11772), or a combination of both *if extensive cellulitis is present.*

During simple I&D of a pilonidal cyst, if the provider encounters *extensive cellulitis* (acute inflammation of skin's connective tissue that is caused by infection with bacteria) and the excision of the pilonidal cyst cannot be performed, the provider will prescribe an antibiotic. CPT codes also describe procedures necessary to address complications. Such codes are *not* reported with codes for the original surgery that resulted in the complication. If the original surgery code is reported with the procedure to treat the complication, National Correct Coding Initiative (NCCI) edits will deny reimbursement for the procedure performed to treat the complication.

Example: A patient who underwent a thoracotomy developed a surgical wound infection, which required I&D. Report code 10180 78 for I&D of the (skin) wound infection.

Exercise 12.4 – Incision and Drainage

Instructions: Assign the CPT code(s) and any appropriate modifier(s) to each statement.

1. Complex incision and drainage due to postoperative wound infection following previous open appendectomy.

   _____

2. Incision and drainage of hematoma, skin.

   _____

3. Incision and removal of foreign body, subcutaneous tissue.

   _____

4. Marsupialization acne surgery.

   _____

5. Simple incision and drainage of five infected cysts.

   _____

Lesion Removal

Lesion removal procedures include:

- Excision—Debridement
- Paring or Cutting
- Biopsy
- Removal of Skin Tags
- Shaving of Epidermal or Dermal Lesions
- Excision—Benign Lesions
- Excision—Malignant Lesions

A skin lesion (Figure 12-4) is a pathologic change in tissue (e.g., benign or malignant). To accurately code the removal of lesions, review the patient record to locate the following information:

- Method of removing the lesion (e.g., paring, shaving, or debridement)
- Malignant or benign status of lesion if excision method is performed
- Site or body part where lesion is located
- Size of the lesion in centimeters (Figure 12-5)
- Type of wound closure/repair (e.g., simple, intermediate, or complex)

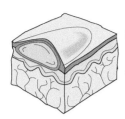

Bulla: (Large blister)
Same as a vesicle only greater than 10 mm
Example:
Contact dermatitis, large second-degree burns, bulbous impetigo, pemphigus

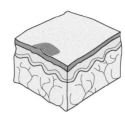

Macule:
Localized changes in skin color of less than 1 cm in diameter
Example:
Freckle

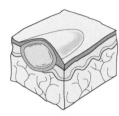

Nodule:
Solid and elevated; however, they extend deeper than papules into the dermis or subcutaneous tissues, greater than 10 mm
Example:
Lipoma, erythema, cyst, wart

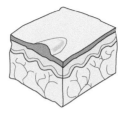

Papule:
Solid, elevated lesion less than 1 cm in diameter
Example:
Elevated nevi

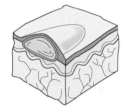

Pustule:
Vesicles or bullae that become filled with pus, usually described as less than 0.5 cm in diameter
Example:
Acne, impetigo, furuncles, carbuncles

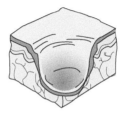

Ulcer:
A depressed lesion of the epidermis and upper papillary layer of the dermis
Example:
Stage 2 pressure ulcer

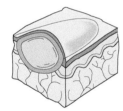

Tumor:
The same as a nodule only greater than 2 cm

Example:
Benign epidermal tumor, basal cell carcinoma

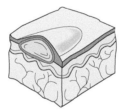

Vesicle: (Small blister)
Accumulation of fluid between the upper layers of the skin; elevated mass containing serous fluid; less than 10 mm
Example:
Herpes simplex, herpes zoster, chickenpox

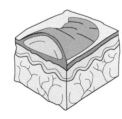

Urticaria, Hives:
Localized edema in the epidermis causing irregular elevation that may be red or pale, may be itchy
Example:
Insect bite, wheal

FIGURE 12-4 Skin lesions

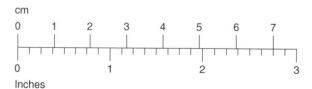

FIGURE 12-5 Lesions are measured in centimeters.
(Note: 2.5 centimeters equals 1 inch.)

NOTE:

- To calculate the size of a lesion, refer to "excised diameter" examples located below the *Measuring and Coding the Removal of a Lesion* subcategory (above the Excision—Benign Lesions category in the Integumentary System subsection). The "excised diameter" includes the size of the lesion plus its margins.
- Documentation of the "excised diameter" should include dimensions for the greatest size (diameter) of the lesion as well as for the margin around the lesion. *When multiple lesions are removed, do not add together the greatest size (or diameter) of each separate lesion even when excised in one ellipse.*
- The margin is the amount of surrounding tissue that must be removed to adequately excise the lesion, and it is calculated as the shortest distance from the lesion to the edge of the skin ellipse.
  - An ellipse is a shape resembling an oval.
  - The narrowest amount of tissue removed from each end of the ellipse is measured and used to calculate the "excised diameter" of the lesion.
  - When multiple lesions are excised using one ellipse, the narrowest margin between lesions is measured and used *in addition to measurements of each end of the ellipse* to calculate the "excised diameter" of each lesion.

> **Example 1:** A 2-cm × 1-cm benign lesion of the cheek was excised in an elliptical fashion with 2-mm margins in all directions. Simple closure was performed. The "excised diameter" is calculated as 2.4 cm because
>
> - The greatest size (or diameter) of the lesion is 2 cm.
> - The narrowest margin of each end of the ellipse is 2 mm (or 0.2 cm), calculated as 0.2 cm × 2 = 0.4 cm.
> - 2 cm + 0.4 cm = 2.4-cm "excised diameter."
>
> Report CPT code 11443. (Do not report a separate code for the simple closure procedure.)

> **Example 2:** One elliptical excision was made to remove two nevi from the patient's left arm. Lesion A was 3 cm in diameter, and lesion B was 2 cm in diameter. Skin margins were 4 mm at each end of the ellipse, and 2 mm between the two lesions. Simple closure was performed. The "excised diameter" of lesion A is 3.5 cm and lesion B is 2.5 cm because
>
> - The greatest size (or diameter) of each lesion is 3 cm and 2 cm, respectively. Do not add together the greatest size (or diameter) of separate lesions even when excised in one ellipse.
> - The narrowest margin of each end of the ellipse is 4 mm (or 0.4 cm). Thus, associate 0.4 cm with each lesion.
> - The narrowest margin between the lesions is 2 mm (or 0.2 cm). Thus, associate 0.1 cm (half of 0.2 cm) with each lesion.
> - 3 cm + 0.4 cm + 0.1 cm = 3.5-cm "excised diameter" of lesion A.
> - 2 cm + 0.4 cm + 0.1 cm = 2.5-cm "excised diameter" of lesion B.
>
> Report CPT code 11404 for lesion A and 11403 51 for lesion B. (Add modifier 51 to the second code because multiple excision procedures were performed during the same session by the same provider on the same site [left arm]. Do not report a separate code for the simple closure procedure. Do not add modifier LT because the codes' descriptions include anatomic structures that are not paired, such as trunk.)

From a coding perspective, benign lesions include neoplasms, fibrous cysts, or other inflammatory cystic lesions. Malignant lesions are typically described as melanoma, basal cell carcinoma, or squamous cell carcinoma. When surgery is performed on a lesion, select the appropriate code according to the lesion's "excised diameter," which includes the lesion plus its margins. (Do not refer to the pathology report for the diameter because placing a lesion in formalin, the formaldehyde solution used to preserve organic specimens, can result in shrinkage.)

> **Example:** A malignant lesion of the nose measuring 1.0 cm in diameter is excised, and the operative report states that excised skin margins are 1.1 cm. The "excised diameter" of the lesion is 2.1 cm (1.0 + 1.1 = 2.1). Therefore, report code 11643 (Excision, malignant lesion including margins, face, ears, eyelids, nose, lips; excised diameter 2.1 to 3.0 cm).

NOTE:

If an operative report describes the diameter of a lesion as having multiple sides, select the largest size as the diameter (e.g., a lesion described as 2 cm × 3 cm × 5 cm is 5 cm in diameter).

Just one type of removal is reported for each lesion, whether it is destruction (e.g., laser or freezing), debridement, paring, curettement, shaving, or excision. CPT notes describe the nature of each of these forms of removal.

When multiple methods are used to remove one lesion, report a code for just one destruction method. *When multiple distinct lesions are removed using different methods*, report a code for each lesion removal and add modifier 59 to each code. Modifier 59 indicates different site, different method, or different type of lesion (e.g., benign versus malignant). Make sure the provider has documented the distinct locations of each lesion in the patient's record.

The biopsy of a lesion involves the partial removal of a lesion, and it is frequently performed at the same time as the removal of the entire lesion to obtain a pathologic specimen. The lesion biopsy is performed first, the tissue is submitted to pathology for evaluation and pathologic diagnosis, and then the lesion is completely removed. When a lesion biopsy is performed as part of a lesion removal, it is considered part of the total procedure and is not assigned a separate code. Types of skin biopsies include incisional, punch, and tangential (e.g., shaving) methods. Report only the CPT code for removal of the lesion.

Lesion removal by any method may require simple, intermediate, or complex closure; it is also possible that a tissue transfer procedure will have to be performed. When the lesion removal requires bandaging, strip closure, or simple closure, the closure is included in the lesion excision and is not coded and reported separately. CPT defines simple, intermediate, and complex repairs, explained later in this chapter.

Simple repair procedures are considered integral to lesion removal. Intermediate and complex repairs (closure), when medically necessary, are coded separately. (For Mohs micrographic surgery, all necessary repairs are coded and reported separately.)

 Coding Tip

- When a benign or malignant lesion is excised and complex closure is performed during the same operative session, two codes are reported.
    - Excision of benign or malignant lesion
    - Complex closure
- However, when a scar is excised followed by complex closure, report the complex repair code only.
- When multiple lesions are excised during the same operative session, report a code for the excision of each lesion.
- When a malignant lesion is excised and the patient returns for further excision to ensure that the malignancy has been completely resected, report a code for excision of a malignant lesion and add modifier 58 (Staged or related procedure...) if surgery was performed within the global surgery period (even when the pathology report documents no residual malignancy).

Refer to the following table when assigning codes for excision of benign or malignant lesions that require wound repair (closure). When using the table to assign codes, it is important to note that

- When multiple lesions are excised during the same operative session, the number of excision codes must be increased accordingly.
- When intermediate or complex repair (closure) is performed to repair defects resulting from excision of multiple lesions, codes are grouped according to the same anatomical sites.

Type of Procedure	# of Codes	Types of Codes
Simple repair	1	Excision
Intermediate repair	2	Excision Intermediate repair
Complex repair	2	Excision Complex repair

Exercise 12.5 – Lesion Removal

Instructions: Assign the CPT code(s) and any appropriate modifier(s) to each statement.

1. A physician excises a 1-cm benign skin lesion, left forearm; the defect is closed with a simple repair.
   _____

2. Punch biopsy of a benign skin lesion on the back and another one on the right arm.
   _____

3. Excision of a 2.1 cm in diameter malignant skin lesion of the nose and two malignant skin lesions of the chest, each 1.5 cm in diameter.
   _____

4. Four warts were removed from the right hand by paring.
   _____

5. A physician excised a 2-cm benign skin lesion from the face.
   _____

Nails

The Nails category includes codes for procedures that are performed to treat a variety of nail conditions, such as infections, trauma, nail dystrophy, and neoplasms. Most nail surgery is performed using local or digital block anesthetic. These procedures are typically performed on toenails but can be done on fingernails as well.

Nondystrophic nails are normal nails with no abnormal development or changes due to aging, injury, or disease. Nail debridement is generally done to treat hypertrophic dystrophic nails and mycotic (fungal) infections. It is performed mechanically by using instruments such as a nail splitter, a nail elevator, and an electrical burr (sander). For lacerations to the nail bed, where the wound extends under the proximal nail fold, a portion or all of the nail plate must be removed in order to visualize the laceration.

 Coding Tip

Report HCPCS Level II modifiers (FA through F9 and TA through T9) with codes for procedures performed on a patient's fingernails and toenails.

Exercise 12.6 – Nails

Instructions: Assign the CPT code(s) and any appropriate modifier(s) to each statement.

1. A diabetic patient was seen by a podiatrist for trimming of nondystrophic nails, which are unaffected by abnormal development or changes in structure or appearance. Following cleansing and drying of all toenails of both feet, clippers are used to cut each nail straight across so that it is in line with the edge of the end of the toe.

   _____

2. Reconstruction of nail bed, second toe on left foot, with graft.

   _____

3. Avulsion of nail plate, simple, 5 nails, right foot.

   _____

4. The physician evacuated blood from a hematoma located beneath a patient's fingernail, second digit, left hand. The physician used an electrocautery needle to pierce the nail plate so the hematoma can drain. Pressure was applied to the nail bed to force the blood from beneath the nail plate. A loose dressing was applied so the area can continue to drain.

   _____

5. Wedge excision of skin of nail fold for ingrown toenail, third digit, right foot.

   _____

Pilonidal Cyst

The Pilonidal Cyst category contains codes for procedures to report excision. A pilonidal cyst contains a tuft of hair that developed as the result of repeated friction, which caused hairs to penetrate the skin; it occurs primarily in the sacrococcygeal area. (For incision of a pilonidal cyst, report the appropriate code from the Incision and Drainage category.)

Exercise 12.7 – Pilonidal Cyst

Instructions: Assign the CPT code(s) and any appropriate modifier(s) to each statement.

1. Excision of complicated pilonidal cyst.

   _____

2. Pilonidal sinus excision, simple.

   _____

3. Excision of extensive pilonidal cyst.

   _____

4. The physician shaved hair adjacent to a simple pilonidal cyst and made an incision to allow drainage of cystic fluid.

   _____

5. The patient presented with an infected pilonidal cyst (complicated). The cyst was incised and drained.

   _____

Introduction

Codes located in the Introduction category include the following procedures: injection of lesion(s); tattooing; subcutaneous injection of filling material (e.g., collagen); insertion, removal, and replacement of tissue expanders; insertion and removal of implantable contraceptive capsules; subcutaneous hormone pellet implantation; and insertion, removal, and removal with insertion of nonbiodegradable drug delivery implants.

CPT codes for intralesional injection(s) into one or more lesions are reported for the treatment of lesions such as keloids, psoriasis, and acne (cystic or nodular). Drugs are injected directly into the lesion, and it is appropriate to report HCPCS Level II national code(s) for medication(s) administered. CPT codes reported are determined by the number of lesions treated (not by the number of injections).

Coding Tip

- Intralesional injection codes are *not* reported for local anesthetic injection in anticipation of chemotherapy or any other definitive service performed on a lesion or group of lesions (e.g., lesion destruction or removal).
- Do not report lesion injection codes with intralesional chemotherapy codes (from the Medicine section) unless separate lesions are injected with different agents. (Add modifier 59 to intralesional chemotherapy code(s) *when performed during the same encounter as lesion injection(s).*)
- The administration (injection) of local anesthesia is included in the surgical procedure performed, and it is not coded separately.

Example: A physician performed intralesional injection of eight lesions. Report code 11901. (Code 11901 is a stand-alone code and requires interpreting the use of a semicolon in the code 11900 description; it does not contain the plus symbol next to the code, which would indicate an add-on code. Do *not* report 11900 and 11901. Report 11901 only based on the injection of eight lesions.)

Exercise 12.8 – Introduction

Instructions: Assign the CPT code(s) and any appropriate modifier(s) to each statement.

1. Patient presented for subcutaneous implantation of estradiol and testosterone compressed crystalline pellets.

   _____

2. A patient presented with acne (cystic), and the physician injected drugs directly into six lesions.

   _____

3. Subcutaneous injection of 15.0 cc of collagen was performed.

   _____

4. Five implantable contraceptive capsules were removed.

   _____

5. Intralesional injection, 12 lesions.

   _____

TABLE 12-3 Medical Terms for Adjacent Tissue Transfer or Rearrangement, Flap, and Graft Procedures

Defect	Wound that is the result of surgical intervention or trauma
Donor site	Anatomical site from which healthy skin is removed
Primary defect	Wound resulting from initial surgical intervention (e.g., excision of lesion) or trauma (e.g., deep abrasions)
Recipient site	Anatomical site to which healthy skin is attached
Secondary defect	Wound resulting from removal of tissue to create flap(s) or graft(s)
Stroma	Supporting tissue (matrix) of an organ
Tissue approximation	Method of replacing sutures with material or substance (e.g., surgical glue), which facilitates enhanced cosmetic results and faster healing of defects
Undermining	Process of using a surgical instrument to separate skin and mucosa from its underlying stroma so that the tissue can be stretched and moved to overlay a defect

Repair (Closure)

The Repair (Closure) category includes the following subcategories, which require knowledge of additional medical terms associated with repair (closure) procedures (Table 12-3):

- Repair—Simple
- Repair—Intermediate
- Repair—Complex
- Adjacent Tissue Transfer or Rearrangement
- Skin Replacement Surgery
- Flaps (Skin and Deep Tissues)
- Other Flaps and Grafts
- Other Procedures
- Pressure Ulcers (Decubitus Ulcers)
- Burns, Local Treatment

Simple, Intermediate, Complex Repairs

Coding wound repairs is sometimes confusing because codes for repairs can be stand-alone procedures and separately reportable services when performed with certain other procedures (e.g., excisions requiring complex repair), or they can be an integral part of a more complex procedure and not separately reportable (e.g., surgical wound closure). Repairs (or closures) are subcategorized as simple, intermediate, and complex.

A *simple repair* is a one-layer closure of superficial wounds that involve the epidermis, dermis, *or* subcutaneous tissue. This type of closure uses a combination of adhesive strips (e.g., Steri-Strips), staples, sutures, and tissue adhesives (e.g., Dermabond surgical glue). Local or topical anesthesia and hemostasis, when provided, are *not* separately coded. For multiple superficial wound repairs, add together the lengths of repairs for *each* group of anatomic sites.

> **Example 1:** Patient underwent 2.0 centimeter single-layer closure of subcutaneous tissue, palm of left hand. Dermis and epidermis layers were then properly aligned, and adhesive strips were applied. Report code 12001. (Do not add informational modifier LT to the code because layers of skin are *not* paired organs.)

> **Example 2:** Patient presented with 1.0 centimeter superficial wound, upper lip, and 3.0 centimeter superficial wound, right upper arm. One-layer closure was performed for each wound, and Steri-Strips were applied. Report codes 12011 and 12002 51.

When performing chemical cauterization, electrocauterization, or wound repair (closure) using adhesive strips only, report an appropriate code from the CPT E/M section.

> **Example:** Physician uses Steri-Strips for superficial wound closure of lacerations, epidermis layer of right forearm, established patient, during a 20-minute office visit. The wound did not require suture closure. Report code 99213. (Do not add informational modifier RT to the code.)

HCPCS Level II code G0168, Wound closure utilizing tissue adhesive(s) only (e.g., Dermabond surgical glue), is a supply code. Therefore, code G0168 is reported in addition to the appropriate wound repair CPT code when an adhesive is used.

Example: Patient sustained a 2.5-centimeter superficial laceration, epidermis of right leg, which was repaired using Dermabond tissue adhesive. Report codes 12001 and G0168.

An *intermediate repair* is a layered closure of wounds that involve epidermis, dermis, subcutaneous, and superficial fascia (e.g., non-muscle fascia). (CPT codes for repair of muscle fascia and muscle are located in the Musculoskeletal System subsection of the Surgery section.) An intermediate repair is considered a deep wound closure, and simple repair of the epidermal, dermal, or subcutaneous layer is *not* coded separately. According to CPT, intermediate repair "includes *limited undermining* (defined as a distance less than the maximum width of the defect, measured perpendicular to the closure line, along at least one entire edge of the defect)" and "single-layer closure of heavily contaminated wounds that have required extensive cleaning or removal of particulate matter."

Example: Patient undergoes layered closure of subcutaneous tissue and superficial fascia wounds, left calf, 5.0 centimeters. Prior to closure, patient underwent extensive removal of glass particles. Report code 12032. Do not report a code for cleaning the wound because, according to CPT, an intermediate repair includes "extensive removal of particulate matter."

A *complex repair* requires the documentation of certain procedures along with simple and intermediate repair (closure) of a wound. (Simple and intermediate repair codes are *not* separately reported with a complex repair code.) According to CPT, complex repair requires one or more of the following procedures: "exposure of bone, cartilage, tendon, or named neurovascular structure; debridement of wound edges; extensive undermining (defined as a distance greater than or equal to the maximum width of the defect, measured perpendicular to the closure line along at least one entire edge of the defect); involvement of free margins of helical rim, vermilion border, or nostril rim; placement of retention sutures. Necessary preparation includes creation of a limited defect for repairs or the debridement of complicated lacerations or avulsions." The excision of benign or malignant lesions, excisional preparation of a wound bed, and debridement of an open fracture or open dislocation are separately coded.

 NOTE:

- Single-layer closure is coded as an intermediate repair if the wound is heavily contaminated and requires extensive cleaning.
- When a physician documents layered closure, do not assume an intermediate repair code is to be reported. Locate documentation of
  - Closure of more than one layer of tissue beneath the dermis. Such closure of tissue layers under the skin uses dissolvable sutures before suturing the dermis and epidermis.

    or
  - Extensive cleaning or removal of foreign matter from a heavily contaminated wound that is closed with a single layer.

Example 1: A complex repair of two scalp lacerations measuring a total of 4 cm is located in the same anatomical site and is the same type of repair. Report code 13121.

Example 2: A complex repair of a 6-cm forehead laceration, 3-cm cheek laceration, and 3-cm chin laceration and an intermediate repair of 3.5-cm lacerations to both hands represent two different sites and types of repairs. Report codes 13132, 13133, and 12042 59. (Report codes 13132 and 13133 for complex repair of the total 12-cm laceration [forehead, cheek, and chin]. Report code 12042 59 for the intermediate repair of the 3.5-cm lacerations of both hands.)

 NOTE:

Modifier 51 (Multiple procedures) is *not* reported with code 13133 because the plus symbol indicates that the code has *modifier 51 exempt* status. However, modifier 59 is reported with code 12042 because notes below Repair (Closure) state, *When more than one classification of wounds is repaired, list the more complicated as the primary procedure and the less complicated as the secondary procedure, using modifier 59* (Distinct procedural service).

Coding Wound Repair (Closure) Procedures

When reporting wound repair (closure) codes, make sure that you do the following:

- Locate documentation about the size of the wound in centimeters, whether angular, curved, or star-shaped.
- Add together the lengths of all wounds for multiple repairs of wounds for each group of anatomical sites, and report just one code for body parts associated with that group of anatomical sites.
- Report the code for the most complicated repair first, followed by less complicated repair codes (with modifier 59, when applicable).
- Report skin debridement codes when
  - Gross contamination requires prolonged cleansing.
  - Large amounts of devitalized or contaminated tissue are removed.
  - Debridement is performed *without* immediate primary wound closure.
- Report codes for extensive debridement of subcutaneous tissue, muscle fascia, muscle, and bone using codes from the Debridement subcategory in the Integumentary System subsection.

Example 1: A diabetic patient is diagnosed with a 2.0-cm $\times$ 2.0-cm posterior left heel ulceration that involves skin, subcutaneous tissues, and the soleus muscle. Debridement at all levels was performed. Report code 11043 for the 4.0-cm treatment area (2.0 cm $\times$ 2.0 cm = 4.0 sq cm).

Example 2: A motorcyclist lost control on a 2-lane country road that was covered with loose stone. Patient suffered an open fracture, right tibia, with extensive abrasions directly over the fracture site, which required debridement down to muscle. The debridement procedure is reported with code 11011. (The open fracture repair code is also reported.)

- For debridement of skin only (e.g., active wound care management), *without* removal of foreign material, report codes from the CPT Medicine section.
- Report codes for the repair of nerves, blood vessels, and tendons (from the specific body system involved, such as nervous, cardiovascular, or musculoskeletal). (However, codes for simple exploration of nerves, blood vessels, and tendons exposed in an open wound are not reported separately.)
- When the physician locates a foreign body and removes it, report a code for its removal only.

In addition, it is important to remember that

- The simple ligation of vessels in an open wound is included in the wound repair code.
- The simple exploration of nerves, blood vessels, or tendons exposed in an open wound is included in the wound repair code *except when dissection is required.*
- The reported wound repair codes are based on length of the wound (in centimeters), wound site, and complexity of repair.
- Wound repairs usually require local anesthesia, and the physician usually performs a neurovascular exam prior to administering the anesthetic. The administration of the local anesthesia is included in the wound repair code.
- When a wound requires one or more of the following, report code(s) from the Wound Exploration—Trauma category of the Musculoskeletal System subsection: debridement; enlargement; extension of dissection (to determine penetration); ligation or coagulation of minor subcutaneous or muscular blood vessels of subcutaneous tissue, muscle fascia, and muscle (not requiring thoracotomy or laparotomy); and removal of foreign bodies.

When the closure of a lesion excision cannot be accomplished by simple, intermediate, or complex closure, the following methods are used:

- Adjacent tissue transfer or rearrangement (Table 12-4)
- Skin replacement surgery

Adjacent Tissue Transfer or Rearrangement

Adjacent tissue transfer or rearrangement involves the closure of defects by relocating a flap of adjacent normal, healthy tissue to a defect. These codes include skin excision and are assigned according to anatomical site.

To determine the correct code, calculate the combined area (as square centimeters) of the defect to be repaired *and the defect created by the tissue transfer*. Do not report a separate code for excision of a lesion or another defect when an adjacent tissue transfer or a rearrangement procedure is performed.

When a procedure is performed to repair a secondary defect (e.g., site of donor advancement flap), report an additional procedure code for the repair (e.g., full-thickness skin graft).

> **Example 1:** Patient previously underwent excision of lesion, chest. Today, the patient undergoes adjacent tissue transfer repair of resulting 1 sq cm skin defect via advancement flap, created from 2 sq cm of adjacent chest tissue. Dressings were applied to both wounds. Report code 14000 (because 1 sq cm + 2 sq cm = 3 sq cm, and the chest is part of the body's trunk).

TABLE 12-4 Adjacent Tissue Transfer and Tissue Rearrangement Methods and Definitions

A Transfer/Rearrangement Method	Definition
Advancement flap	Movement of tissue in a straight line from donor to defect site using a sliding process; once movement is achieved, the flap is sutured in place; advancement flaps are not rotated or moved sideways.
Double pedicle flap	Maintains blood supply from both ends of the flap incision made to create a curvilinear flap contiguous with the defect; flap is pivoted and sutured in place over the defect.
Free flap	Island flap that is detached from donor site and reattached at recipient site via microvascular anastomosis.
Island flap	Flap consisting of skin and subcutaneous tissue with a pedicle comprised only of nutrient vessels; also called *island pedicle flap.*
Myocutaneous flap	Autologous graft consisting of both skin and muscle tissue from the donor site.
Random pattern flap	Myocutaneous flap with a random pattern of arteries.
Rhomboid flap	Random pattern flap that can be raised on any or all corners of a parallelogram configuration, typically 120 and 60 degrees; also called *Limberg flap.*
Rotation flap	Incision made to create a curvilinear flap contiguous with the defect; flap is dissected, freed, pivoted, and sutured in place over the defect.
Tissue rearrangement	Defined by anatomical site and size of defect; includes excision of the defect or lesion; terms used to describe transfer or rearrangement include *Z-plasty, W-plasty, V-Y plasty, rotation flap, advancement flap,* and *double pedicle flap.*
V-Y-plasty	After creation of a V-shaped incision, the edges of the incision are drawn together and sutured, converting the incision to a Y shape.
W-plasty	Both edges of the wound or defect are trimmed into the shape of a W or multiple Ws.
Z-plasty	Involves making an incision along with two additional incisions, one above and another below, creating a Z formation.

> **Example 2:** Patient previously underwent excision of nasal scar, which resulted in a skin defect. Today, the patient undergoes adjacent tissue transfer repair of the 2 sq cm nasal skin defect using an advancement flap (using 4 sq cm of skin from the left cheek). A full-thickness skin graft (using 6 sq cm of skin from right inner thigh) was required to close the 4 sq cm flap left cheek donor site defect. The right inner thigh was repaired using direct closure. Report codes 14060 (because 2 sq cm + 4 sq cm = 6 sq cm) and 15240 51 (which includes direct closure to repair the right inner thigh).

Skin Replacement Surgery Flaps (Skin and Deep Tissues), and Other Flaps and Grafts

CPT graft codes are organized as follows:

- Autograft/tissue cultured autograft
- Acellular dermal replacement
- Allograft/tissue cultured allogeneic skin substitute
- Allograft, skin
- Xenograft, skin

Skin replacement surgery includes surgical preparation and topical placement of an autograft or a skin substitute graft. *Surgical preparation* codes describe initial services performed to prepare a clean and viable wound surface for placement of an autograft, flap, skin substitute graft, or for negative pressure wound therapy. An *autograft* is the transplantation of tissue from the same individual (e.g., harvesting skin from the patient's thigh to graft a defect of the upper arm). *Tissue-cultured autografts* are supplied by laboratories. (Modifier 58 is often added to tissue-cultured autograft codes because labs can only grow a limited amount of tissue and such grafts are often performed as staged procedures.) *Skin substitute grafts* include nonautologous human skin grafts (e.g., acellular dermal), nonhuman skin substitute grafts (e.g., xenograft), and biological products that form a sheet scaffolding for skin growth.

Acellular dermal replacement is a bioengineered artificial skin (e.g., Alloderm). An *allograft* is the transplantation of tissue from someone of the same species (e.g., harvesting skin from another person's thigh to graft a defect on the patient's upper arm). A *xenograft* is the transplantation of tissue from a different species (e.g., harvesting skin from a baboon or a pig to graft a defect on the patient's upper arm).

Types of skin grafts include the following:

- Free skin graft
  - Full-thickness skin graft
  - Split-thickness skin graft
- Pedicle skin graft

Free skin grafts are completely separated from the donor site before being transferred to the recipient site. They are classified as *full-thickness skin grafts* (graft of epidermis and dermis) or *split-thickness skin grafts* (graft of entire epidermis and a portion of the dermis). Full-thickness skin grafts are often harvested from the inguinal folds, supraclavicular region, abdomen, thigh, and postauricular skin (because of the availability of excess skin, which eases primary closure of the donor site). Split-thickness grafts are typically used to repair edematous, infected, or large wounds (e.g., result of burns). *Pinch grafts* (or *patch grafts*) are small full- or split-thickness grafts used to repair chronic lower extremity skin ulcers.

 Coding Tip

- Before reporting codes for free skin grafts, determine whether the graft is full-thickness or split-thickness, what the size of the recipient area is, and where the location of the recipient area is.

- Surgical preparation codes are reported for skin replacement surgery that describe initial services for preparing a clean and viable wound surface for the placement of an autograft, flap or skin substitute graft, or for negative pressure wound therapy.

- Codes for simple debridement of the recipient area do not include repair of the donor site with skin grafts or local flaps. Report additional code(s) when the donor site is repaired in this manner.

Pedicle skin grafts are not immediately completely separated from their donor site. A portion of the graft is transferred to the recipient area, and a remaining portion (the base) is attached to the donor site so that there is a vasculature and nerve supply for the recipient area. Once blood flow to the recipient site is sufficient, the base is grafted to the recipient site.

 Coding Tip

The "delay technique" associated with skin graft procedures is used to improve the blood supply to the base of a flap. This is accomplished by temporarily obstructing the blood supply to the flap to allow a relatively long flap to be transferred onto a narrow pedicle.

When assigning codes for skin grafts, identify the following:

- Type of graft
  - Permanent or temporary
  - Natural or manufactured graft material
  - Use of skin components (e.g., epidermal, dermal, split-thickness, or full-thickness grafts) (Refer to Figure 12-6 to view full-thickness and split-thickness skin grafts.)

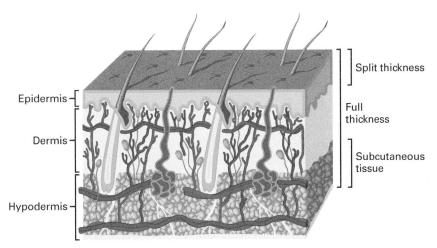

FIGURE 12-6 Depth of full-thickness and split-thickness skin cross sections

- Recipient site (anatomical location)
- Surface area of the recipient site calculated as square centimeters

Just one type of skin graft is usually applied to an anatomical location. Thus, primary free skin graft codes are mutually exclusive of one another. When multiple anatomical locations require different grafts, add modifier 59 to the reported code(s) to indicate that different sites underwent grafting.

When a benign or malignant lesion is excised and surgical preparation and free skin grafting are performed, two codes are reported.

- Excision of lesion code
- Skin graft code

However, when a benign or malignant lesion is excised with flap closure, just the flap closure code is reported.

Generally, debridement of nonintact skin in anticipation of a skin graft is necessary prior to application of the skin graft and is included in the skin graft procedure. When skin is intact, however, and the graft is being performed *after* excisional preparation of intact skin, surgical preparation/creation of recipient site codes are separately reported. The surgical preparation/creation of recipient site codes do not include debridement of nonintact, necrotic, or infected skin, nor is their use indicated with other lesion removal codes, all of which require separate codes to be reported.

> **Example:** Patient underwent repair of a 40 square centimeter full-thickness skin burn of the chest, for which the surgeon had to harvest a full-thickness graft from the abdomen and graft it onto the chest, suturing it onto the wound bed to cover the defect. The donor site surgical wound was closed by suturing the wound edges. Report codes 15200 and 15201.

Refer to Table 12-5 when assigning codes for tissue rearrangement, free skin grafts, flaps (skin and deep tissues), and other flaps and grafts. When multiple tissue rearrangement and free skin graft procedures are required during the same operative session, make sure you report each separately. (The total square centimeters for repair of different defects are not added together.)

Other Procedures

"Other procedures" codes classify the following integumentary system procedures:

- Dermabrasion
- Abrasion
- Chemical peel
- Cervicoplasty
- Blepharoplasty
- Rhytidectomy
- Excision, excessive skin and subcutaneous tissue (including lipectomy)
- Graft for facial nerve paralysis
- Removal of sutures under anesthesia
- Dressing change under anesthesia
- Intravenous injection of agent
- Suction-assisted lipectomy

TABLE 12-5 Assigning Codes for Tissue Transfer or Rearrangement, Free Skin Grafts, Flaps, and Other Flap or Graft

Type of Procedure	# of Codes	Types of Codes
Adjacent tissue transfer or rearrangement	1	• Adjacent tissue transfer or rearrangement
Free skin graft	2 or more	• Free skin graft • Surgical preparation or creation of recipient site *for burn and wound preparation and management procedures only* • Repair of donor site if local flap or skin graft is required
Flap (skin and deep tissue)	1 or more	• Flap (skin and deep tissue) • Repair of donor site if local flap or skin graft is required
Other flap and graft	1 or more	• Flap or graft • Repair of donor site if local flap or skin graft is required

Dermabrasion (Figure 12-7) is performed for conditions such as acne scarring and wrinkles (facial) and rhytids and general keratosis (facial and other than face). The physician uses a rotary device to sand down raised lesions or thickened tissue, regenerating smoother skin.

Example: Patient underwent total face dermabrasion by use of a rotary instrument that penetrates into the dermis layer of skin. Report code 15780.

A *chemical peel* involves the use of chemical agents (e.g., glycolic acid or phenol) to remove wrinkles and abnormal pigmentation. Be sure to determine if treatment is localized to surface layers of the facial skin or the deeper dermal layer.

 N O T E :

Actinic keratosis (AK) is a common sun-induced skin lesion of the epidermis that has the potential to become skin cancer. The most commonly performed treatments for AK includes cryosurgery with liquid nitrogen, topical drug therapy, and curettage. However, AK treatments also include dermabrasion, excision, chemical peels, laser therapy, and photodynamic therapy (PDT).

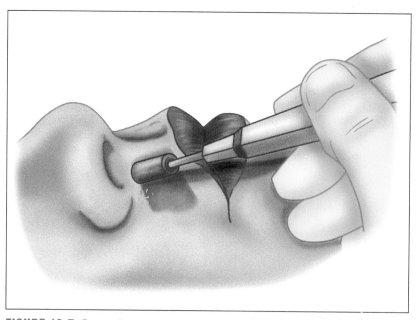

FIGURE 12-7 Dermabrasion

A *blepharoplasty* is any surgical repair of an eyelid. From a coding perspective, blepharoplasty describes the removal of the orbicularis muscle, orbital fat, and excess eyelid skin around the orbit. Make sure you review the operative report to identify the procedure performed and assign appropriate codes. A blepharoptosis repair is performed on the levator muscle of the eyelid. The code selected is based on the surgical approach used to perform the blepharoptosis repair.

Example: Patient underwent blepharoplasty of the left lower eyelid, which required the physician to dissect lower eyelid skin to the subcutaneous and muscle fascial layers and excise excess skin. Report code 15820 E2. (HCPCS Level II modifier E2 is reported to indicate that the procedure was performed on the "lower left, eyelid.")

NOTE:

Medicare reimburses services that are reasonable and necessary to diagnose and treat or to improve the functioning of a malformed body member. When blepharoplasty procedures are performed for cosmetic purposes, they are not covered by Medicare. When the function of the eye is impaired by overlying skin or fatty tissue, the repair is deemed medically necessary and is covered by Medicare.

A *rhytidectomy* involves excising a section of skin to eliminate wrinkles and can be done to reduce *glabellar frown lines*, which are vertical furrows in the forehead area between the eyebrows.

Graft procedures for facial nerve paralysis involve the removal of connective tissue (e.g., fascia) from the body. The graft is transplanted to the face to reanimate previously paralyzed areas.

The removal of sutures by the surgeon is included in the global period associated with that procedure. (The removal of sutures by a physician other than the surgeon who initially placed the sutures is usually reported with an E/M code.)

Abdominal panniculectomy (abdominoplasty) is performed to remove fatty tissue and excess skin from the lower to middle portions of the abdomen. This procedure is typically performed on individuals who have lost considerable weight, resulting in loose-hanging folds of skin in the abdominal area. A lipectomy is the removal of localized subcutaneous fat deposits by suction curettage or blunt cannulization to cosmetically correct obesity and other contour defects.

Example: Patient underwent lipectomy of the submental fat pad. Report code 15838.

When a physician performs a suction-assisted lipectomy, a liposuction cannula is inserted through the fat deposits, removing excess deposits.

Example: Patient underwent suction-assisted lipectomy of the neck. Report code 15876.

Pressure Ulcers (Decubitus Ulcers)

A *pressure ulcer*, or *decubitus ulcer*, or *bedsore*, is an ulceration of the skin and underlying tissue that occurs over a bony prominence (e.g., sacral decubitus). A decubitus ulcer appears in patients confined to bed or immobilized when blood supply is decreased in pressure areas by pressure on the skin, resulting in inflammation and swelling and ultimately necrosis, ulceration, and infection.

The primary excisional procedure of a staged process does not include the flap/graft procedures, which are reported separately. CPT includes notes that provide instruction to report appropriate repair and skin graft codes.

Example: Patient underwent excision of ischial pressure ulcer with ostectomy. Report code 15946.

When a muscle or myocutaneous flap is planned for a subsequent session prospectively (e.g., at the time of the original procedure), report the appropriate flap code and add modifier 58 (Staged procedure).

Burns, Local Treatment

The introduction to the Burns, Local Treatment category states that the application of materials (e.g., Biobrane) is included. To assign appropriate codes for the treatment of burns, review the medical record to identify the following:

- Percentage of body surface
- Severity (depth) of the burn
  - Partial-thickness burns (e.g., first-degree or second-degree)
  - Full-thickness burns (e.g., third-degree)

To determine the extent of body surface involved, the **rule of nines** divides total body surface area (BSA) into nine segments by percentage (Figure 12-8). A better way to estimate the percentage of the body affected by burns is to review the medical record to locate the patient's age. Then, use the *Lund-Browder Diagram and Classification Method Table for Burn Estimations*, which is located in the Destruction, Benign or Premalignant Lesions subcategory in the Destruction category of the Integumentary System subsection in the CPT coding manual. (The surface area for children is estimated differently than that for adults.)

Example: The physician surgically debrided blisters and devitalized tissue that involved less than 5 percent of the total BSA. Report code 16020.

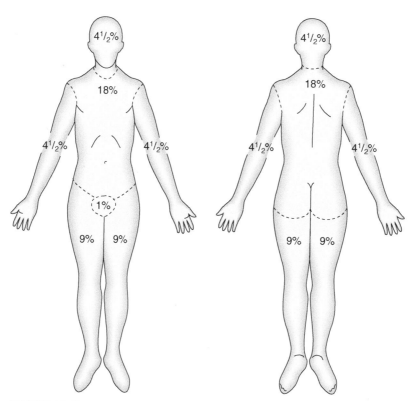

FIGURE 12-8 The rule of nines

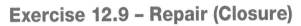

Exercise 12.9 – Repair (Closure)

Instructions: Assign the CPT code(s) and any appropriate modifier(s) to each statement.

1. Simple repair of 3.0-cm scalp laceration.

2. A physician performed a 4-cm wound closure on an established patient using adhesive strips during a level 2 E/M established patient office encounter.

3. Debridement of partial-thickness burn of the right hand involving 1 percent of total body surface.

4. Full-thickness skin graft, free, including direct closure of donor site, trunk (20 sq cm). Surgical preparation of recipient site, trunk (20 sq cm), was also performed during the same operative session.

5. Dermabrasion, total face.

Destruction

Destruction is the ablation of tissue by any method (e.g., electrosurgery, cryosurgery, or laser or chemical treatments). During destruction, excision, incision, removal, repair, or closure procedures, the debridement of nonviable tissue that surrounds a lesion, an injury, or an incision may be necessary to perform the intended procedure. Do not report the debridement codes when the intended procedure (e.g., destruction of lesion) is performed during the same operative session as the debridement procedure; the debridement procedure is considered a necessary part of the total procedure.

Destruction of Benign or Premalignant Lesions and Destruction of Malignant Lesions, Any Method

Each lesion treated is reported as a separate code for the destruction of benign, premalignant, and malignant lesions.

> **Example:** The physician uses a small applicator to apply liquid nitrogen (cryosurgery) directly to the patient's skin to destroy a hypertrophic AK lesion. Report code 17000.

During destruction, excision, incision, removal, repair, or closure procedures, the debridement of nonviable tissue that surrounds a lesion, an injury, or an incision may be necessary to perform the intended procedure. Do *not* report a debridement code when the intended procedure (e.g., destruction of lesion) is performed during the same operative session as the debridement procedure. The debridement procedure is considered a necessary part of the total procedure.

> **Example:** A physician performed laser surgery to destroy a 0.5-cm malignant facial skin lesion. The physician also destroyed a premalignant lesion on skin of the left shoulder using liquid nitrogen. Report codes 17280 and 17000 51.

Mohs Micrographic Surgery

Mohs micrographic surgery is an advanced treatment procedure used to treat basal cell carcinoma and squamous cell carcinoma skin cancers. Dermatologists trained in this technique serve as surgeon, pathologist, and reconstructive surgeon. They use a microscope to trace and ensure the removal of skin cancer to its roots. Mohs micrographic surgery codes are reported instead of excision–malignant lesions codes and surgical pathology codes. Reporting Mohs micrographic surgery and surgical pathology codes on the same claim is inappropriate. A Mohs surgeon who obtains a diagnostic biopsy to make the decision to perform surgery reports the diagnostic biopsy code separately. When Mohs surgery is performed in addition to a skin biopsy on the same day, add modifier 59 to the appropriate biopsy code.

> **Example:** A patient undergoes Mohs micrographic surgery for basal cell carcinoma of the head (behind the left ear). In the first stage, a layer of tissue is removed and the specimen is subdivided into two smaller specimens for pathologic review. In the subsequent stage, the second layer is excised and subdivided into three smaller specimens for pathologic processing. Report codes 17311 and 17312.

Other Procedures

Other Procedures codes classify cryotherapy, chemical exfoliation for acne, electrolysis epilation, and unlisted procedures. When reporting an unlisted procedure code, include documentation about the procedure performed with the submitted claim.

> **Example:** Patient underwent experimental destruction procedure on the skin, which is not currently classified in CPT. Report code 17999.

Exercise 12.10 – Destruction

Instructions: Assign the CPT code(s) and any appropriate modifier(s) to each statement.

1. Destruction of three premalignant facial lesions.

   _____

2. Electrocauterization of 17 skin tags.

   _____

3. Patient underwent removal of five flat warts, using photothermolysis laser (destruction).

   _____

4. Surgical curettement of 1.5 centimeter malignant lesion, trunk.

   _____

5. Laser surgery, 2.3 centimeter malignant lesion, left shoulder.

   _____

Breast

Diagnostic testing used to detect breast cancer may include a mammogram, ultrasonography, magnetic resonance imaging (MRI), FNA, core biopsy, or surgical biopsy. Treatment plans can include a local therapy approach such as breast-conserving surgery or mastectomy, radiation therapy (e.g., internal or implant radiation or external radiation), and breast reconstruction (e.g., implant or tissue transfer).

Because of the unique nature of procedures developed to address breast disease, codes in CPT are established for services (e.g., incision, excision, introduction, repair, and reconstruction). FNA biopsies, core biopsies, open incisional or excisional biopsies, and related procedures performed to procure tissue from a lesion for which an established diagnosis exists are not to be reported separately at the time of a lesion excision unless performed on a different lesion or on the contralateral breast. However, if a diagnosis is not established *and the decision to perform the excision or mastectomy is dependent on the results of the biopsy*, the biopsy is separately reported. Modifier 58 is used to indicate that the biopsy and the excision or mastectomy are staged or planned procedures.

Breast Biopsies

Breast biopsies are performed according to the following methods:

- Fine-needle aspiration (FNA) (Figure 12-9A)
- Needle core biopsy
  - Hand-operated needle
  - Stereotactic localization
- Open biopsy
  - Excisional biopsy
  - Incisional biopsy (Figure 12-9B)

Fine-Needle Aspiration (FNA)

FNA of the breast is reported, depending on whether imaging guidance was used during the procedure. FNA uses a thin needle (e.g., 20- or 22-gauge needle), which is inserted through the mass several times. Suction is applied as the needle is withdrawn to obtain strands of single cells for cytologic diagnosis.

 Coding Tip

Fine-needle aspiration (FNA) of breast tissue procedures are reported with codes from the Introduction subsection of Surgery.

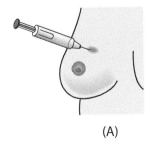
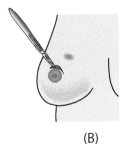

(A)   (B)

FIGURE 12-9 (A) Fine-needle aspiration (B) Incisional biopsy

Needle Core Biopsy

A *needle core biopsy* is obtained using a hand-operated needle (e.g., Trucut or Vim-Silverman) or stereotactic localization. Once the tissue is obtained, it is fixed for routine pathologic section. **Stereotactic localization** is indicated for nonpalpable lesions because it uses specialized three-dimensional imaging to target the lesion. The breast is placed in a fixed position, and a biopsy gun (e.g., 14- or 18-gauge needle) is used to obtain needle core biopsies from the lesion.

Open Biopsy

An *open biopsy* can be excisional or incisional, depending on the amount of lesion removed. An *excisional biopsy* removes the lump or suspicious area in its entirety. An *incisional biopsy* removes a portion of the lesion by slicing into or incising the mass; it is usually performed on large tumors (and the patient undergoes mastectomy later).

 NOTE:

Review the entire operative report to determine whether a breast biopsy is incisional or excisional.

- An *open incisional biopsy* (19101) involves making an incision in the skin of the breast near the site of the suspected mass, identifying the mass, removing a sample of the mass (for pathological evaluation), and performing a layered closure.
- An *excisional biopsy* (19120) involves making an incision in the skin of the breast overlying the site of the mass, dissecting skin and tissue from the mass, removing (excision) the mass (for pathological evaluation), and performing a layered closure. An excisional biopsy is *not* a lumpectomy.
- A **lumpectomy** is a partial mastectomy (19301–19302), also called a *segmental mastectomy* or *quadrantectomy*, that involves making an incision in skin and fascia over the breast mass, excising the breast mass in its entirety, excising a margin (or rim) of healthy tissue, and performing a layered closure. For a lumpectomy *with axillary lymphadenectomy*, the lymph nodes between the pectoralis major and minor muscles along with axillary lymph nodes are removed through a separate incision and performing layered closure.

Example 1: The patient was registered for outpatient surgery on August 1. The surgeon explained that the patient would undergo excisional left breast biopsy in the morning and that if pathology results were positive for cancer, the patient would undergo left breast lumpectomy during the late afternoon. The excisional left breast biopsy was performed at 9 AM, and tissue was positive for adenocarcinoma. The patient returned to the operating room at 2 PM and underwent left breast lumpectomy. Report codes 19120 LT (Excisional breast biopsy) and 19301 58 LT (Breast lumpectomy, staged or related procedure performed by the same physician during the postoperative period). (Modifier 58 is added to just one CPT code. If more than one lumpectomy is performed during the same operative session, modifier 51 is added to each subsequent 19301 code followed by the directional modifier. The pathologist reports an appropriate code from the CPT Pathology and Laboratory section.)

Example 2: During a right breast mass excisional biopsy procedure, breast tissue was sent to the pathologist during the operative procedure for immediate diagnosis. The pathologist examined the specimen and diagnosed a benign lesion. The procedure included layered closure. Report code 19120 RT. (A code for layered closure is *not* separately reported. The pathologist reports an appropriate code from the CPT Pathology and Laboratory section.)

Mastectomy

A **mastectomy** (Figure 12-10) is the surgical removal of all or a portion of the breast. Mastectomies are classified in CPT as follows:

- Partial mastectomy (including lumpectomy)
- Simple or total mastectomy
- Radical mastectomy
- Modified radical mastectomy

Partial mastectomy procedures describe open excisions of breast tissue with specific attention to adequate surgical margins. A *partial mastectomy* involves making an incision through skin and fascia over the breast tumor and clamping lymphatic and blood vessels; the physician then excises the tumor mass along with a section of breast tissue. A partial mastectomy is also called a lumpectomy, quadrantectomy, segmental mastectomy, and tylectomy.

> **Example:** A sentinel node biopsy is performed as part of an axillary lymphadenectomy during a partial right mastectomy procedure. Report code 19302 RT, which includes removal of the sentinel node for biopsy along with other axillary lymph nodes.

Total mastectomy procedures include complete mastectomy, modified radical mastectomy, simple mastectomy, and subcutaneous mastectomy. A *total mastectomy* is the surgical removal of the entire breast, including the pectoral fascia and a sampling of axillary lymph nodes. Radical mastectomy procedures include the removal of pectoral muscles, axillary lymph nodes, and internal mammary lymph nodes. A *radical mastectomy* is a total mastectomy that includes removal of the breast and nipple, pectoralis muscles (major and minor), axillary lymph nodes, and internal mammary lymph nodes. A *modified radical mastectomy* is a total mastectomy that includes removal of the breast and nipple, axillary lymph nodes, and pectoralis minor muscle.

> **Example:** Male patient with advanced, high-grade breast cancer underwent modified radical mastectomy that included removal of pectoral muscles, axillary lymph nodes, and internal mammary lymph nodes. Report code 19306 RT.

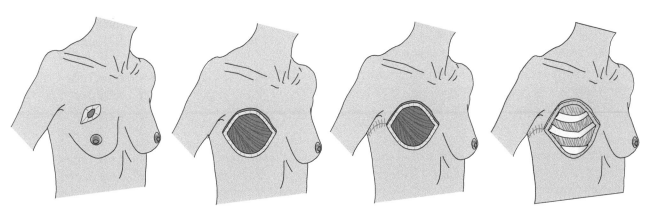

FIGURE 12-10 Types of mastectomies

Breast Repair and Reconstruction

Breast repair procedures include mastopexy (breast lift), breast reduction, breast augmentation with implant, removal of intact breast implant, removal of ruptured breast implant (including implant contents), and insertion or replacement of breast implant. Breast reconstruction procedures include nipple/areola reconstruction, correction of inverted nipples, placement of tissue expander in breast reconstruction, and breast reconstruction using flaps, revision of peri-implant capsule of the breast, peri-implant capsulectomy of the breast, revision of reconstructed breast, and preparation of moulage for custom breast implant (e.g., custom silicone implant for breast deformity).

CPT breast reconstruction codes include the following elements:

- Elevation and transfer of the flap
- Closure of the donor site
- Breast contouring
- Insertion of breast implant or prosthesis, when performed

> **Example:** Patient underwent insertion of a saline-filled breast implant four months post-mastectomy, right breast. Report codes 19342 RT and L8600.
>
> An HCPCS Level II code is reported for the supply of a "silicone or equal" breast implant, which includes a saline implant. Do not report a directional modifier with the code.

Breast reconstruction with transverse rectus abdominis myocutaneous flap (TRAM), single pedicle includes closure of donor site. In addition, TRAM flap codes include the following:

- Creation of the breast pocket
- Elevation of the abdominal flap
- Muscle dissection
- Flap transfer
- Fascial closure (donor site) with or without mesh
- Abdominal closure including umbilicoplasty
- Breast contouring

> **Example:** Patient underwent right breast reconstruction with single-pedicled transverse rectus abdominis myocutaneous (TRAM) flap, which included harvesting the myocutaneous island flap from the abdominal wall, closing the donor site, and shaping the skin flap as a breast. Report code 19367 RT.
>
> A *single-pedicled transverse rectus abdominis myocutaneous (TRAM) flap* is an *island pedicle flap* graft that contains skin, subcutaneous tissue, muscle tissue, and nutrient vessels from the deep muscle layer of the patient's abdominal region.

Because excision of lesions is often done during the same operative session as a mastectomy, breast excisions are not separately reported in addition to the mastectomy code *unless performed to establish the malignant diagnosis before proceeding to the mastectomy.* When a breast excision is performed to obtain tissue to determine pathologic diagnosis of malignancy prior to proceeding to a mastectomy, the excision is separately coded and reported with the mastectomy code and modifier 58 is added to the codes.

Use of other integumentary codes for incision and closure are included in the codes that describe various breast excision or mastectomy codes. Because of the frequent need to biopsy lymph nodes or remove muscle tissue in conjunction with mastectomies, these procedures are included in CPT coding for mastectomy.

It is inappropriate to separately report ipsilateral lymph node dissection with mastectomy codes. When a breast lesion is identified and treated and medical necessity indicates that biopsy of contralateral nodes should be done, report the biopsy or lymph node dissection codes (and add an appropriate directional modifier). Breast reconstruction codes include the insertion of a prosthetic implant, and they are not reported with CPT codes that describe the insertion of breast prosthesis only.

CPT coding for breast procedures generally refers to unilateral procedures, and when performed bilaterally, modifier 50 is added to the code. (A parenthetical note is included as a reminder to report modifier 50 when appropriate.) When breast reconstruction is performed unilaterally, add the applicable HCPCS Level II modifier LT (Left side) or RT (Right side) to the procedure code.

Other Procedures

The Other Procedures code is reported for an unlisted procedure performed on breast. When reporting an unlisted procedure code, include documentation about the procedure performed with the submitted claim.

Example: Patient underwent experimental procedure on the left breast, which is not currently classified in CPT. Report code 19499 LT (and attach a special report to the submitted claim).

Exercise 12.11 – Breast

Instructions: Assign the CPT code(s) and any appropriate modifier(s) to each statement.

1. Excision of two lesions, right breast, identified by the placement of radiological markers for each.

2. Breast reconstruction with single-pedicled transverse rectus abdominis myocutaneous (TRAM) flap, right breast.

3. Lumpectomy, left breast.

4. Physician performed a partial mastectomy of the right breast with right axillary lymphadenectomy and biopsy of the right sentinel node.

5. Patient underwent percutaneous left breast biopsy with placement of a breast localization clip under stereotactic guidance.

Summary

The CPT Surgery section and its subsections are organized anatomically according to major body area or organ system. Guidelines located at the beginning of the CPT Surgery section clarify the assignment of codes and explain terms. The General subsection contains just two codes. The Integumentary System subsection includes dermatological procedures, plastic surgery, and components of multiple surgical procedures (e.g., closure, flaps, grafts, and tissue transfer). Integumentary procedures are often performed as staged procedures (e.g., flaps and grafts) due to the complexity of services rendered.

Internet Links

American Academy of Dermatology (AAD): www.aad.org

Medscape: Go to **www.medscape.com**, and click Register to register for free access to Medscape's clinical information and resources.

National Correct Coding Initiative (NCCI) Edits: Go to **www.cms.gov**, and click on the Medicare link, scroll to the Coding heading, and click on the National Correct Coding Initiative Edits link.

ORlive™ BroadcastMed: Go to **www.orlive.com** to view live webcasts in selected health specialties.

SurgeryTheater: Go to **www.youtube.com**, and enter Surgery Theater in the Search field to locate videos of surgical procedures.

Review

12.1 – Multiple Choice

Instructions: Select the most appropriate response.

1. Which is a therapeutic surgical procedure?
   - **a.** Arthroscopy
   - **b.** Biopsy
   - **c.** Endoscopy
   - **d.** Repair

2. A patient undergoing a surgical procedure was draped and positioned. The surgical area was cleansed and shaved, an IV was started, and a sedative was administered. The surgical approach was identified, and an incision was made. The wound was irrigated, and cultures were taken. The incision was closed, and dressings were applied. The procedure was then dictated and transcribed. A CPT code was assigned to the surgical procedure. Which service is assigned a separate code, in addition to the reported CPT Surgery code?
   - **a.** Administration of a sedative
   - **b.** None of the services are reported separately
   - **c.** Taking cultures and wound irrigation
   - **d.** Transcription of the dictated report

3. Which modifier indicates a staged procedure or service?
   - **a.** 58
   - **b.** 59
   - **c.** 66
   - **d.** 76

4. Which modifier indicates that a patient received treatment for an unrelated condition during the global period?
   - **a.** 51
   - **b.** 57
   - **c.** 59
   - **d.** 79

5. The CMS global surgical package includes
   - **a.** diagnostic tests and procedures, including diagnostic radiological procedures.
   - **b.** initial consultation about the problem by the surgeon to determine the need for surgery.
   - **c.** services provided on the day prior to the day of surgery for major procedures.
   - **d.** treatment for postoperative complications that require a return to the operating room.

6. When an evaluation and management (E/M) service provided is for the purpose of deciding to perform a major surgical procedure, which is reported?
   - **a.** E/M code
   - **b.** E/M code with modifier 57
   - **c.** E/M code with modifier 59
   - **d.** No E/M code is reported because the service is bundled in the surgery code.

7. The code reported for fine-needle aspiration is based on whether
   - **a.** fluid is aspirated from a cyst or cells are aspirated from a solid mass.
   - **b.** imaging guidance is used during the procedure.
   - **c.** masses or cysts are visible or palpable.
   - **d.** the procedure is performed percutaneously.

8. If the operative report describes a lesion as 3.5 cm × 4 cm × 5 cm, which is reported as the diameter?
    a. 3.5 cm   b. 4 cm   c. 5 cm   d. 17.5 cm

9. When Mohs micrographic surgery is performed, Mohs micrographic surgery codes are reported instead of
    a. a diagnostic biopsy code.
    b. debridement codes and a diagnostic biopsy code.
    c. excision–malignant lesion codes and surgical pathology codes.
    d. surgical pathology codes.

10. Wound repair is coded with an appropriate evaluation and management code when the sole repair material used is
    a. adhesive strips.   c. sutures.
    b. staples.   d. tissue adhesives.

11. Evacuation of subungual hematoma. Which CPT code is assigned?
    a. 10140   b. 10160   c. 11740   d. 11750

12. Collagen injection, face, 5.1 cc. Which CPT code is assigned?
    a. 11950   b. 11951   c. 11952   d. 11954

13. Puncture aspiration of abscess on lower left eyelid. Which CPT code is assigned?
    a. 10120 E2   b. 10140 E2   c. 10160 E2   d. 10180 E2

14. Open excision of fibroadenomas, right breast. Which CPT code is assigned?
    a. 19100 RT   b. 19120 RT   c. 19301 RT   d. 21601 RT

15. Suction-assisted abdominal lipectomy. Which CPT code is assigned?
    a. 15876   b. 15877   c. 15878   d. 15879

16. Adjacent tissue transfer of 12 sq cm defect of forehead. Which CPT code is assigned?
    a. 14020   b. 14021   c. 14040   d. 14041

17. Mohs micrographic surgery of upper left arm (first stage) with excision of five specimens. Diagnostic incisional skin biopsy of one scalp skin lesion performed the same day. Which CPT code(s) are assigned?
    a. 11106, 17313   c. 17313
    b. 17313, 11106 59   d. 17313, 11406 51

18. Modified radical mastectomy, left breast, including axillary lymph nodes, excluding pectoral muscles. Which CPT code is assigned?
    a. 19301 LT   b. 19305 LT   c. 19306 LT   d. 19307 LT

19. Epidermal facial chemical peel. Which CPT code is assigned?
    a. 15788   b. 15789   c. 15792   d. 15793

20. Cryosurgery of two plantar warts. Which CPT code(s) are assigned?
    a. 17000, 17000   c. 17000, 17003 51
    b. 17000, 17003   d. 17110

12.2 – Coding Practice

Instructions: Assign the CPT code(s) and appropriate modifier(s) to each case.

General

1. Patient underwent fine-needle aspiration to remove fluid sample from a cyst, anterior neck. Physician palpated the cyst, cleansed the site with Betadine solution, and inserted a 25-gauge needle into the cyst. Approximately 2 cc of fluid were removed. The needle was withdrawn, and a small bandage was placed over the insertion area.

2. Patient underwent fine-needle aspiration to remove a cluster of cells from a solid mass, subcutaneous layer of the left upper quadrant, abdomen. Computed tomography (CT) imaging guidance for needle placement was performed. Physician palpated the mass, cleansed the area with Betadine solution, and inserted a 22-gauge needle into the solid mass. Approximately 1 cc of tissue was removed. The needle was withdrawn, and a small bandage was placed over the insertion area.

Integumentary System

3. A large mass, soft and movable, located on the patient's back between the lower scapular area and midline on the left, was palpated. An elliptical incision was made, a section of the tissue was removed, and the 4.0-cm cyst was resected completely. Bleeding vessels were clamped and coagulated. Penrose drain was left in the wound, and skin edges were closed along with subcutaneous tissue, using interrupted silk sutures.

4. Patient was prepped and draped; after adequate general endotracheal anesthesia, the body was somewhat flexed at the waist to provide adequate exposure after taping in preparation to separate the buttocks at the sacral crease. A probe was inserted into the inferior sinus, and only 3 to 4 cm of fluid were obtained. The area was prepped for excision, and an oval-shaped piece of skin was excised in total, including the simple 5.0-cm subcutaneous pilonidal cyst sinus end. Bleeding was controlled with electrocautery, the area was copiously irrigated with Betadine saline solution and suctioned and sponged off, and vertical mattress sutures of Prolene were placed in layers to obliterate the dead space.

5. Local anesthesia was injected using 1 percent lidocaine with epinephrine 1.5 cc. Incision was made along the postauricular sulcus through the drainage point with retraction applied. A 3.0-cm sebaceous cyst was evident, and it was drained. A small bandage was placed over the incision and drainage site.

6. Split-thickness skin graft of about 7 sq cm was removed from the left thigh, and sterile dressings were applied. A 6-cm malignant lesion was removed from the left calf by a wide excision, including at least 1 cm of normal skin all around, taking it all the way down to include fascia and overlying muscle. Bleeding points were carefully ligated, wound was treated with Hibiclens, and skin graft was applied and sutured in place with 4-0 Mersilene sutures.

7. Patient was using a chain saw, which slipped, and the patient sustained a 5.0-cm laceration to the dorsum of the proximal portion of the left index finger, extending through the extensor tendon and capsule. Debridement of tissue was done to facilitate a better repair of this deep laceration. Tendon and capsule were sutured with five 6-0 silk sutures. Bleeders were ligated with plain catgut. Skin was debrided extensively and approximated with seven sutures of 4-0 Dermal.

8. Patient sustained second-degree burn of the right thigh that was less than 5 percent of the total body surface. The skin was completely necrotic. The right thigh was prepared with pHisoHex, and the wound was debrided using a dermatome. Partial thickness, superficial layer of dead skin tissue was removed. Wound was treated with pHisoHex and cleaned, and a sterile outside dressing was applied.

9. Digital nerve block was applied to numb the top of the right great toe and the left great toe. Blunt dissection of the nail plate from the nail bed, right great toe, was performed and the nail plate was removed. Bleeding was cauterized. Right great toe was bandaged. Next, the left great toenail plate was removed from the nail bed, bleeding was cauterized, and left great toe was bandaged.

10. Patient sustained a 3.0-cm scalp laceration and a 2.0-cm neck laceration after being cut with a knife during a bar fight. Local anesthetic was injected around the scalp and neck laceration sites. Wounds were thoroughly cleansed, explored, and irrigated with a saline solution. One-layer suture repair of scalp and neck wounds was performed.

_____

11. An island pedicle flap was formed on the left thigh with identification and dissection of the femoral artery. The defect was covered by elevating a flap of skin and subcutaneous tissue. The flap was then rotated into the defect, with transfer being accomplished through a tunnel underneath the skin to innervate the artery and vein. The flap was sutured into its new position, and the donor site was closed.

_____

12. Bell's palsy patient underwent harvesting of a graft for residual left facial nerve paralysis. Connective tissue fascia was removed from the fascia lata, right leg. Free fascia graft was transplanted to the face and sutured into place underneath skin to reanimate paralyzed area of the face.

_____

13. Using surgical curettement, 3.0-cm malignant lesion of the neck was destroyed.

_____

14. Procedure: Lumpectomy, left breast. Incision was made through skin and fascia over a left breast mass, and lymphatic and blood vessels were clamped. Tumor mass was excised in its entirety along with normal breast tissue. Drainage tube was placed through a separate stab incision. Layered closure was performed, and a sterile dressing was applied.

_____

15. Right breast cyst was palpated, and needle was inserted into skin of the breast overlying the cyst. Needle was inserted into the cyst, and puncture aspiration facilitated evacuated of fluid into the syringe. Needle was withdrawn, and pressure was applied to the puncture wound.

_____

13

CPT Surgery II

Chapter Outline

Musculoskeletal System Subsection

Respiratory System Subsection

Chapter Objectives

At the conclusion of this chapter, the student should be able to:

1. Define key terms related to the Musculoskeletal System and Respiratory System subsections of CPT Surgery.
2. Assign codes from the Musculoskeletal System subsection of CPT Surgery.
3. Assign codes from the Respiratory System subsection of CPT Surgery.

Key Terms

allogenous

arthrocentesis

arthrodesis

arthroscopy

artificial ankylosis

arytenoidectomy

arytenoidopexy

augmentation

autogenous

backbench work

bronchoscopy

brushing

cadaver donor
    pneumonectomy

cell washing

closed fracture
    treatment

direct laryngoscopy

dislocation

external fixation device

harvesting

immobilize

indirect laryngoscopy

internal fixation device

laryngoscopy

luxation

manipulation

non-segmental
    instrumentation

obturator

open fracture treatment

osteogenesis

osteotomy

percutaneous needle
    biopsy

percutaneous skeletal
    fixation

percutaneous
    vertebroplasty

pneumocentesis

pneumonectomy

recipient lung
    allotransplantation

reduction

replantation

segmental
    instrumentation

skeletal traction

stabilize

subglottic stenosis

subluxation

thoracentesis

thoracoscopy

tracheobronchoscopy

vertebral
    augmentation

Introduction

The Musculoskeletal System subsection includes codes for procedures performed on bones, cartilage, joints, ligaments, muscles, and tendons (including casting and strapping). The Respiratory System subsection includes codes for procedures performed on the nose, accessory sinuses, larynx, trachea and bronchi, lungs, and pleura. CPT guidelines that apply to the subsections are located at the beginning of the Surgery section.

 Coding Tip

> Instructional notes located beneath categories, subcategories, headings, and subheadings apply to all codes in those areas. Parenthetical notes located below a specific code apply to that code only, unless the note indicates otherwise.

 NOTE:

> The content in Chapters 12 through 16 of this textbook is organized exactly as it appears in the CPT Surgery section. This organization facilitates learning by allowing students to move from one CPT Surgery subsection to the next, in order.
>
> When included in CPT, the Other Procedures code is reported for an unlisted procedure performed on the anatomical site. When reporting an unlisted procedure code, include documentation about the procedure performed with the submitted claim.
>
> The *Medicare National Correct Coding Initiative Policy Manual* provides guidance about assigning procedure codes for the Musculoskeletal System and Respiratory System subsections. Go to www.cms.gov and enter "Medicare NCCI Policy Manual" in the Search box to navigate to the manual.

Musculoskeletal System Subsection

The CPT Musculoskeletal System subsection is arranged from head to toe according to body area and includes the following categories:

- General
- Head
- Neck (Soft Tissues) and Thorax
- Back and Flank
- Spine (Vertebral Column)
- Abdomen
- Shoulder
- Humerus (Upper Arm) and Elbow
- Forearm and Wrist
- Hand and Fingers
- Pelvis and Hip Joint
- Femur (Thigh Region) and Knee Joint
- Leg (Tibia and Fibula) and Ankle Joint
- Foot and Toes
- Application of Casts and Strapping
- Endoscopy/Arthroscopy

Each category contains codes for one or more of the following procedures:

- Incision
- Excision
- Introduction or Removal

- Repair, Revision, and/or Reconstruction
- Fracture and/or Dislocation
  - Types of fractures (Table 13-1)
  - Closed and open fracture treatments (Table 13-2)
  - Percutaneous skeletal fixation fracture treatment (Table 13-3)
- Manipulation
- Arthrodesis
- Amputation
- Other Procedures

 Coding Tip

The Other Procedures code is often reported for an unlisted procedure performed on the anatomical site. When reporting an unlisted procedure code, attach documentation (e.g., operative report) that describes the procedure to the submitted claim.

Example: Patient underwent experimental procedure on the spine, which is not currently classified in CPT. Report code 22899.

Musculoskeletal System Instructional Notes

Musculoskeletal System subsection instructional notes include definitions of fractures (e.g., closed and open) and clarify that the type of fracture does not necessarily correspond to the type of treatment (e.g., closed, open, or percutaneous) provided. In addition, types of injury codes include open or closed fractures and joint injuries. Musculoskeletal system instructional notes explain that fracture treatment includes the application and removal of the initial cast, splint, or traction device, with supplies reported separately using a HCPCS Level II code.

Thus, a code for casting, splinting, or applying a traction device is not assigned in addition to the initial fracture treatment code. The exception is Medicare's NCCI coding policy, which states that a significant and separately identifiable evaluation and management service code can be reported with the CPT code for a casting, strapping or traction device when the provider stabilized a fracture or dislocation. In this situation, the patient did not undergo fracture treatment, which will be performed by an orthopedic surgeon. The notes also clarify the excision of subcutaneous soft connective tissue tumors, excision of fascial or subfascial soft tissue tumors, and radical resection of bone tumors.

Example: The 67-year-old patient was taken to the emergency department (ED) by ambulance as the result of an automobile accident. The patient complained of severe abdominal pain and left arm pain. ED services included an MRI for severe abdominal pain, and splenic bruising was diagnosed. The ED physician also diagnosed a left radial and ulnar spinal fracture, which was confirmed upon x-ray. The fracture was stabilized with a strapping device by an orthopedic surgeon. Report codes from the Emergency Department Services category of the Evaluation and Management section, Musculoskeletal System subsection of the Surgery section, and Radiology section. (The ED physician and orthopedic surgeon will also generate a CMS-1500 claim to report the ED service E/M code and fracture treatment code as professional services, respectively.)

 Coding Tip

Open and closed fractures may not receive the same type of treatment. Closed fractures can receive open treatment, and open fractures can receive closed treatment. Either type of fracture can receive **percutaneous skeletal fixation** treatment.

TABLE 13-1 Types of Fractures, Joint Injuries, and Fracture Treatment

Type of Fracture	Definition
Closed fracture (or simple fracture) (Figure 13-1)	• Broken bone(s) do not protrude through skin • No open wounds • Described clinically as "closed"
Dislocation or luxation (Figure 13-1)	• Total displacement of bone from its joint • Subluxation is the partial displacement of a bone from its joint
Open fracture (or compound fracture) (Figure 13-1)	• Broken bone(s) that can be seen through an open wound or that protrudes through skin • Clinically sustained an injury with sufficient force to penetrate skin, subcutaneous tissue, muscle fascia/muscle, and/or bone or joint

TABLE 13-2 Closed and Open Fracture Treatments

Type of Fracture Treatment	Definition

Closed fracture treatment	• Fracture site is not surgically opened or exposed
	• Three methods of treatment
	  ○ With manipulation, or reduction (Figure 13-2), which means that the bones are realigned
	  ○ Without manipulation, which means that the bones are not realigned and a cast or strapping device is placed around the limb to stabilize, or immobilize, it, which secures the bone(s) in fixed position
	  ○ With or without skeletal traction (Figure 13-3), which exerts a pulling force on the affected limb to realign bone or joint

Open fracture treatment	• Fracture site is surgically opened or exposed • With or without *manipulation* (reduction) • With or without *skeletal traction*

TABLE 13-3 Percutaneous Skeletal Fixation Fracture Treatment

Type of Treatment Device	Definition
External fixation device (Figure 13-4)	• Hardware is inserted through bone and skin and held rigid with cross braces outside of the body • Always removed after the fracture has healed • Removal procedure is included in the global service, which means it is *not* separately coded and reported
Internal fixation device (Figure 13-5)	• Pins, screws, and/or plates are inserted through or within the fracture area to stabilize and immobilize the injury • Often called open reduction with internal fixation, or ORIF

Coding Tip

Fracture management codes are found throughout the Musculoskeletal System subsection. The codes include the following:

- Pinning
- Open or closed treatment of the fracture
- Application and removal of the initial cast or splint
- Normal, uncomplicated follow-up care

Do not report separate codes for each of the above services when provided during the same encounter, because they are included in the fracture treatment code. Codes for treatment of fractures and joint injuries (dislocations) are classified according to type of manipulation (reduction) and stabilization (fixation or immobilization).

(continues)

Coding Tip (*continued*)

Physicians perform a *cast windowing* procedure to check for possible infection or a wound's status underneath a cast; code 29730 is reported with modifier 58 (staged procedure) and any applicable directional modifier. *Cast windowing* involves removing a section of the cast, creating a window so that the status of a wound or possible infection can be checked. Then, the section may be reinserted and held in place with casting material.

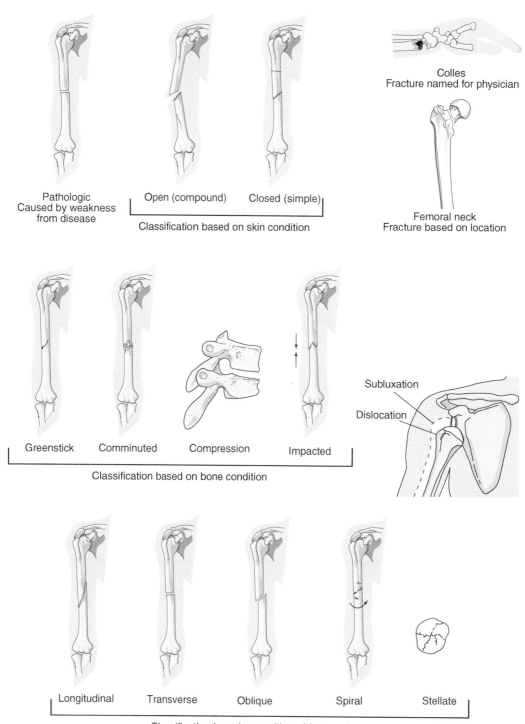

Pathologic
Caused by weakness
from disease

Open (compound)   Closed (simple)

Classification based on skin condition

Colles
Fracture named for physician

Femoral neck
Fracture based on location

Greenstick   Comminuted   Compression   Impacted

Classification based on bone condition

Subluxation

Dislocation

Longitudinal   Transverse   Oblique   Spiral   Stellate

Classification based on position of fracture line

FIGURE 13-1 Fractures and dislocations

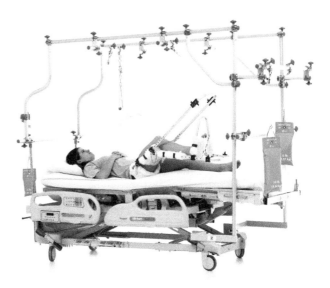

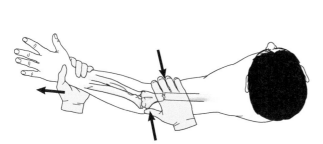

FIGURE 13-2 Closed manipulation (reduction) of fractured left humerus

FIGURE 13-3 Traction

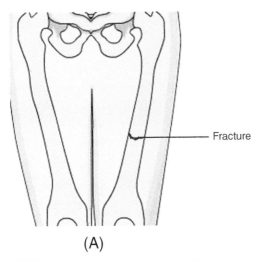

(A)

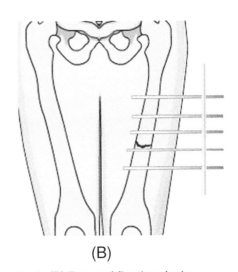

(B)

FIGURE 13-4 External fixation (A) Fracture of femur epiphysis (B) External fixation device stabilizes bone and is removed after bone has healed

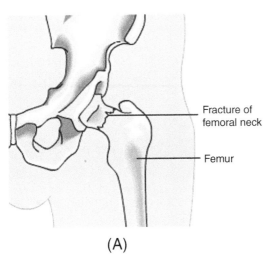

(A)

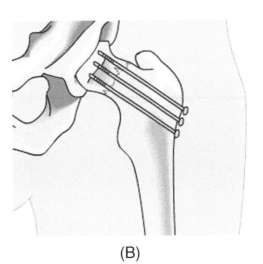

(B)

FIGURE 13-5 Internal fixation (A) Fracture of femoral neck (B) Internal fixation device (e.g., pins) is placed to stabilize the bone and is not removed after the bone has healed

Exercise 13.1 – Musculoskeletal System Instructional Notes

Instructions: Complete each statement.

1. The Musculoskeletal subsection is arranged from head to toe according to _____ _____.
2. Types of injury codes include _____ or _____ and fracture and joint injuries.
3. Open and closed fractures may not receive the same type of _____.
4. Fracture management codes include pinning, open or closed treatment of the fracture, application and removal of the initial cast or splint, and normal _____ uncomplicated care.
5. Codes for treatment of fractures and joint injuries (including dislocations) are classified according to type of _____ or manipulation and stabilization (e.g., fixation, immobilization).

General

The General category contains codes for the following procedures:

- Incision
- Wound Exploration—Trauma (e.g., Penetrating Gunshot, Stab Wound)
- Excision
- Introduction or Removal
- Replantation
- Grafts (or Implants)
- Other Procedures

Incision

An instructional note directs coders to report incision and drainage codes according to specific anatomical sites.

> **Example:** A patient underwent an incision and drainage of a deep abscess, right ankle. Report code 27603 RT, which is located below the Incision subcategory in the Leg (Tibia and Fibula) and Ankle Joint category.

Wound Exploration—Trauma

Wound exploration—trauma codes are reported for the treatment of wound(s) resulting from penetrating trauma (e.g., gunshot or stab wound), and they include the following:

- Surgical exploration and enlargement of the wound
- Extension of dissection (to determine penetration)
- Debridement
- Removal of foreign body(s)
- Ligation or coagulation of minor subcutaneous and/or muscular blood vessel(s) of the subcutaneous tissue, muscle fascia, and/or muscle, not requiring thoracotomy or laparotomy

When major structures or major blood vessels require repair via thoracotomy or laparotomy, do not report the -otomy code. Report the repair code. When a simple, intermediate, or complex repair of wound(s) is performed *alone*, report the appropriate repair code(s) from the Integumentary System section.

> **Example:** A patient was treated for a 2.5-cm stab wound located above the base of the neck. The physician extended the wound to explore and assess damage; it was determined that the injury extended to the muscle. Muscle fascia and subcutaneous tissue were closed in layers, and the skin was closed. Report code 20100.

Excision

Report excision codes for epiphyseal bar procedures (performed on bone) and biopsies performed on muscle or bone.

> **Example:** Patient underwent open bone biopsy of the right femoral shaft. Report code 20245 RT.

Introduction or Removal

Introduction and removal procedure codes are reported for injection procedures, removal of a foreign body, insertion and application of surgical hardware, arthrocentesis, aspirations, and drug delivery. Surgical injections are performed by inserting a needle directly into a joint or tendon sheath, trigger point, or ganglion cyst (Figure 13-6) to aspirate fluid or inject medications. Codes for injections are based on anatomical site. **Arthrocentesis** is a procedure done to puncture a joint for fluid removal or medication injection.

> **Example 1:** A patient underwent aspiration of ganglion cyst, left wrist. Report code 20612 LT.

> **Example 2:** Using ultrasound guidance for needle placement, the physician injected patient's left knee joint with 10 mg of Kenalog (Triamcinolone) for therapeutic relief of knee pain. Report codes 20611 LT and HCPCS Level II code J3301.

> **Example 3:** A patient underwent closed treatment of a left femoral shaft fracture with manipulation and application of an uniplane external fixation system. Report codes 27502 LT and 20690 51 LT. Code 27502 does not specify the use of an external fixation device in its code description; therefore, also report code 20690 with modifier 51. Modifier LT is added to each code to indicate the *left* femoral shaft.

 NOTE:

Code 20690 is reported in addition to the code for treatment of the fracture or joint injury (unless application of an external fixation system is included in the fracture or joint injury code description).

The *insertion of drug-delivery devices*, including manual preparation, is reported as an add-on code with associated procedures, such as arthrotomy, excisional debridement, and so on. Antibiotics or other therapeutic agents are mixed with a carrier substance and shaped into drug-delivery devices (e.g., beads, nails, spacers) and

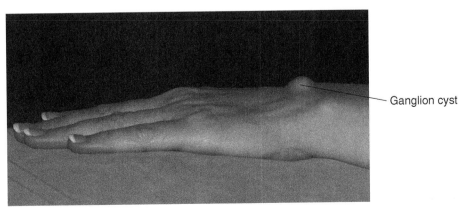

FIGURE 13-6 Ganglion cyst

inserted into subfascial tissue. The *removal of drug-delivery devices* is performed with other procedures such as complex repairs, excisional debridement, tissue transfer, and so on.

> **Example:** Patient underwent osteotomy, right clavicle, with bone graft for malunion with removal of intramedullary drug-delivery device. Report codes 23485 RT and 20703.

When a traumatic injury with an open wound requires surgical debridement but the type of fracture requires manipulation and casting (instead of an external or internal fixation device), report the appropriate code for closed fracture treatment *in addition to the appropriate debridement code.*

> **Example:** A patient underwent closed treatment of tibial fracture with manipulation, application of a cast, and open wound debridement of 15 sq cm of skin using a scalpel around the fracture site. Report codes 27752 and 97597. There is mention of manipulation; therefore, report code 27752. Report code 97597 for the debridement procedure.

Replantation

Replantation is the surgical reattachment of a finger, a hand, a toe, a foot, a leg, or an arm that has been completely severed from a person's body. (A severed body part is also called an amputation.) Replantation codes include arthrodesis, cleansing, debridement, internal fixation, and repair of tendons (as well as the surgical reattachment procedure).

> **Example 1:** A male patient who severed his left arm at the humeral diaphysis in a machine accident underwent replantation of the arm. Wound debridement and shortening were performed on the stump and the amputated part of the arm, along with primary repair of muscles and microsurgical repair of arteries, veins, and nerves and internal fixation. A splint was also applied. Report code 20802 LT.

> **Example 2:** A patient who suffered a partially severed right leg in an automobile accident underwent repair of the cruciate and collateral ligaments of the right knee; suture of tendon, right knee; repair of one arterial blood vessel, right knee; and 7.5-cm complex closure of wound. Report codes 27409 RT, 35226 51 RT, 27380 51 RT, and 13121 51 RT. (Modifier 51 is reported to indicate that multiple procedures were performed *in addition* to the first-listed procedure.)

Grafts (or Implants)

Grafts (or implants) codes are reported when **autogenous** (originating in the patient's body) tissue is obtained through separate skin or fascial incisions, *except when the graft procedure code includes* **harvesting** (removing tissue for transplantation) *the graft (or implant) for which a combination code is reported*. Codes with the ✚ (add-on code) symbol are exempt from modifier. (**Allogenous** grafts involve tissue organ transplanted from one person to another; for example, bone tissue can be obtained from a bone bank. Xenografts are obtained from another species, such as pigs.)

Graft material is harvested (obtained) from bone, cartilage, fascia, or tendon. Harvested bone tissue is transplanted to another site to promote **osteogenesis** (bone growth) or to provide structural stability (e.g., spinal fusion). Harvested cartilage tissue is often used for reconstruction purposes (e.g., facial reconstruction to relieve temporomandibular joint pain). Fascia lata tissue is harvested from gastrocnemius fascia (from the calf) or tensor fascia lata (from the thigh) for soft tissue augmentation (e.g., repair skin defects, such as multiple depressed acne scars or *rhytides*, or wrinkles). (**Augmentation** is the process of enlarging or increasing.) Tendon tissue is harvested for the purpose of repairing another tendon (e.g., reconstruct anterior cruciate ligament).

> **Example:** Costochondral cartilage graft was harvested from the left rib of a four-year-old child for laryngotracheal reconstruction to treat **subglottic stenosis** (narrowing of the airway below the vocal cords, adjacent to the cricoid cartilage). Report codes 31551 and 20910 51.

For bone grafts obtained for spine surgery, just one bone graft code is reported for each operative session (in addition to codes for the definitive procedure, such as spinal fusion) even if graft material is obtained from more than one spinal level (e.g., C1 and C2).

Example: A patient diagnosed with spinal stenosis undergoes laminectomy with cervical spine fusion, which requires harvesting a large structural bone graft from the iliac crest (through a separate incision). Report codes 22800, 20902 51, and 20931 in addition to the spinal fusion procedure code. (Do not add modifier 51 to code 20931 because it is an add-on code.)

Other Procedures

Other Procedures codes classify monitoring of interstitial fluid pressure in detection of muscle compartment syndrome, bone graft with microvascular anastomosis, free osteocutaneous flap with microvascular anastomosis, electrical simulation to aid bone healing, low-intensity ultrasound stimulation to aid bone healing, bone tumor ablation, computer-assisted surgical navigation, and an unlisted procedure. When reporting an unlisted procedure code, include documentation about the procedure performed with the submitted claim.

Example 1: Patient underwent monitoring of interstitial fluid in detection of muscle compartment syndrome. Report code 20950.

Example 2: The patient undergoes bone graft of the left fibula, with microvascular anastomosis. This means that the bone tissue is harvested along with its blood supply (but without overlying skin). (The grafted tissue will be used to reconstruct the patient's right tibial bone, which has a filling defect as the result of trauma; surgery will involve microsurgical anastomosis of blood vessels.) Report code 20955 LT for the "bone graft of left fibula, with microvascular anastomosis."

Exercise 13.2 – General

Instructions: Assign the CPT code(s) and appropriate modifier(s) to each statement.

1. The physician performed an exploration, penetrating wound, neck.

2. Patient underwent exploration of a penetrating wound of the chest, which involved surgical exploration and enlargement of the wound, debridement, removal of a foreign body, and ligation of subcutaneous tissue.

3. Open bone biopsy, superficial, left femur.

4. Patient underwent aspiration of ganglion cyst, right wrist.

5. Patient received a cortisone injection to a single trigger point, which consisted of the trapezius, deltoid, and latissimus dorsi muscles.

6. A patient diagnosed with joint contracture of the right ankle underwent application of a multiplane unilateral external fixation device.

7. A patient severed the right index finger while using a chain saw. The patient underwent successful replantation of the index finger, which included metacarpophalangeal (MCP) joint to insertion of flexor sublimis tendon.

8. Fascia lata graft was harvested using a stripper.

Exercise 13.2 – continued

9. Patient underwent structural bone allograft for spine surgery as part of an arthrodesis, posterior technique, craniocervical (occiput-C2).

_____

10. Electrical stimulation procedure was performed to aid bone healing, invasive type.

_____

Head

Head codes classify procedures performed on the skull, facial bones, and temporomandibular joint (TMJ).

Incision

The Incision code is reported for arthrotomy of the temporomandibular joint.

> **Example:** A patient underwent TMJ arthrotomy to release scar tissue. Report code 21010.

Excision

Excision codes are reported for surgery performed on bone and soft tissue of the face and/or scalp.

> **Example:** Patient underwent TMJ condylectomy. Report code 21050.

Manipulation

Manipulation codes are reported for TMJ manipulation procedures, which requires anesthesia services.

> **Example:** Patient underwent therapeutic TMJ manipulation for which general anesthesia was administered. Report code 21073. (Do not report modifier 50, LT, or RT with code 21073 because the jaw is not a paired organ or body part.)

Head Prosthesis

Head Prosthesis codes describe professional services that involve designing and preparing a prosthesis for a patient. Prostheses are created for rehabilitation patients who have facial, oral, or other anatomical deficiencies that require an artificial ear, eye, or nose or an intraoral **obturator**, which is used to close a gap (e.g., cleft).

> **Example:** A patient was fitted for a mandibular resection prosthesis, which was custom prepared by the physician. Report code 21081.

 Coding Tip

When an outside laboratory prepares the prosthetic device, the physician who fits the device for the patient reports an appropriate evaluation and management code.

Introduction or Removal

Introduction or removal codes are reported for other introduction or removal procedures, such as application of halo-type appliance for maxillofacial fixation (including removal), interdental fixation device (e.g., arch bar) for conditions other than fracture or dislocation (including removal), or injection procedure for TMJ arthrography.

Example: A physician applied a halo-type appliance for maxillofacial fixation, and it was removed 30 days later. Report code 21100. (Do not report a separate code for removal of the halo-type appliance because that procedure is included in the global period for code 21100.)

Repair, Revision, and/or Reconstruction

Reconstruction of the face procedures include LeFort type procedures. *LeFort I* brings the lower midface forward (from the level of the upper teeth) to just above the nostrils. *LeFort II*, or *pyramidal fracture*, is a surgical fracture of the midfacial skeleton at an apex near the superior aspect of the nasal bones. *LeFort III* brings the entire midface forward, from the upper teeth to just above the cheekbones.

Example: A patient underwent a LeFort I reconstruction procedure of the midface, which required reconstruction of two pieces without bone graft. Report code 21142.

 NOTE:

- Colpocleisis, also known as a LeFort procedure, is the surgical repair of a uterine prolapse or a vaginal vault prolapse.
- LeFort I, II, and III fractures are complex bilateral fractures of facial bones that contain large, unstable fragments.
- A Wagstaff-LeFort fracture is an avulsion of the fibula.

Other repair, revision, and/or reconstruction codes are reported for genioplasty, augmentation, and reduction procedures performed on the face, mandible, or forehead. Procedures include reconstruction, osteotomy, arthroplasty, repositioning, augmentation, revision, canthopexy, and reduction.

Example: Patient underwent TMJ arthroplasty with allograft. Report code 21242.

Fracture and/or Dislocation

Fracture and/or dislocation codes are reported for treatment of fractures and/or dislocations of the skull, facial bones, and TMJ.

Example: A physician performs an open reduction and internal fixation of a mandibular fracture. Report code 21470.

Exercise 13.3 – Head

Instructions: Assign CPT code(s) and appropriate modifier(s) to each statement.

1. Arthrotomy of temporomandibular joint, right and left sides.

2. Excision of two facial bones (due to bone abscesses).

3. Maxillofacial impression and custom preparation of speech aid prosthesis.

4. Sliding osteotomy genioplasty, single piece.

5. Reconstruction midface, Lefort II with anterior intrusion.

6. Osteotomy of mandible, segmental.

7. Malar augmentation with prosthetic material.

8. Closed treatment of orbit fracture, with manipulation.

9. Closed treatment of maxillary alveolar ridge fracture.

10. Open treatment of mandibular condylar fracture.

Neck (Soft Tissues) and Thorax

The Neck (Soft Tissues) and Thorax category includes codes for procedures performed on the soft tissues of the neck and thorax (e.g., incision and drainage, excisional biopsies, repairs, revisions, and reconstruction).

Incision

Incision codes are reported for the incision and drainage of abscesses or hematomas, including the deep incision with opening of bone cortex of the thorax.

> **Example:** Patient underwent incision and drainage of deep abscess, soft tissues of thorax, with partial rib ostectomy. Report code 21502.

Excision

Excision codes are reported for excision of soft tissue of the neck or thorax (e.g., biopsy or excision of tumor), radical resection of a tumor, partial and total excision of ribs, costotransversectomy, ostectomy of sternum, sternal debridement, and radical resection of sternum.

> **Example:** Patient underwent costotransversectomy for decompression of paravertebral mass. Report code 21610.

Repair, Revision, and/or Reconstruction

Repair, revision, and/or reconstruction are performed on the soft tissues of the neck (e.g., muscle) and thoracic soft tissues and bones. When procedures are performed to repair superficial wounds, refer to the Integumentary System subsection to assign an appropriate code.

> **Example:** Patient underwent open reconstructive repair of pectus excavatum. Report code 21740.

Fracture and/or Dislocation

Fracture and/or dislocation codes are reported for procedures performed to treat rib and sternum fractures or dislocations.

> **Example:** Patient underwent open treatment of sternum fracture with skeletal fixation. Report code 21825.

Back and Flank

The Back and Flank category contains just one subcategory.

Excision

Back and Flank excision codes are reported for biopsy, tumor excision, and radical resection of tumor procedures performed on the back and flank. When a drain is inserted and/or the incision is repaired with multiple layers of sutures, staples, or Steri-Strips, do not separately report codes for those procedures; they are bundled in Back and Flank codes.

> **Example:** Patient underwent soft tissue biopsy of the back, deep. Report code 21925.

Exercise 13.4 – Neck (Soft Tissues) and Thorax and Back and Flank

Instructions: Assign the CPT code(s) and appropriate modifier(s) to each statement.

1. Deep incision with opening of bone cortex, thorax.

   _____

2. Hyoid myotomy and suspension.

   _____

3. Closed treatment of sternum fracture.

   _____

4. Partial excision of rib.

   _____

5. Sternal debridement.

   _____

6. Needle biopsy, muscle, thorax.

   _____

7. Excision of tumor, subcutaneous soft tissue of back, 2.5 cm.

   _____

(continues)

Exercise 13.4 – continued

8. The physician removed a 4-cm malignant soft tissue tumor, including adjacent tissue, from the patient's flank. Radical resection was performed to remove the tumor and adjacent tissue. The 5-cm surgical wound was repaired with complex closure.

_____

9. Patient underwent biopsy of superficial soft tissues of the back.

_____

10. Biopsy, soft tissue of flank, deep.

_____

Spine (Vertebral Column)

Spine (Vertebral Column) codes classify procedures performed on the cervical, thoracic, and lumbar spine. Vertebral procedures are sometimes followed by arthrodesis, and they may also include bone grafts and instrumentation. When reporting codes for spinal procedures, make sure you differentiate spinal segments (e.g., T1) and interspaces (e.g., T1–T2 interspace) because CPT codes distinguish between them.

- T1–T2 represents two spinal segments of the thoracic vertebrae, at levels 1 and 2.
- L1–L4 represents four spinal segments of the lumbar vertebrae, at levels 1, 2, 3, and 4.
- T1–T2 represents one interspace of the thoracic vertebrae, between levels T1 and T2.
- C1–C2 and C2–C3 represent two interspaces of the cervical vertebrae, between levels C1 and C2 as well as between C2 and C3.

 Coding Tip

- Procedures performed on the bones, connective tissue, and muscles of the spinal column are classified in the Musculoskeletal subsection of CPT Surgery.
- Procedures performed on the spinal cord and spinal nerves are classified in the Nervous System subsection of CPT Surgery.

The notes located just below the Spine (Vertebral Column) category should be reviewed before assigning codes.

- Bone graft procedure codes are reported separately, in addition to arthrodesis procedure codes. For bone grafts in other Musculoskeletal categories, review code descriptions and notes.
- Instrumentation procedure codes are reported in addition to primary procedure codes.
- Vertebral procedures may be followed by arthrodesis and may also include bone grafts and instrumentation.
- When an arthrodesis procedure is performed in addition to another procedure, report the arthrodesis procedure code in addition to codes for other procedures performed. (Add modifier 51 to the arthrodesis procedure code[s].)
- When two surgeons collaborate to perform a spinal procedure during the same operative session on the same patient and each performs a distinct part of the procedure, add modifier 62 to the procedure code reported by each surgeon with the exception of bone graft codes and instrumentation procedures. (Additional procedure codes reported by each surgeon are also reported with modifier 62 if the surgeons continue to work as primary surgeons.)

Example 1: Patient underwent arthrodesis of T1–T3 using local autograft from the ribs. Dual rods were inserted with multiple hooks and sublaminar wires. Report codes 22610, 22614, 22614, 22842, and 20936.

Three thoracic segments were fused; therefore, report codes 22610, 22614, and 22614. (Code 22614 is an add-on code; therefore, do not add modifier 51.) Report code 22842 for insertion of dual rods with multiple hooks and sublaminar wires; it is also exempt from the addition of modifier 51. Code 20936 describes the local autograft from the ribs, and it is exempt from modifier 51.

Example 2: Surgeon A performed a posterior exposure procedure on a patient by making an incision overlying the lumbar vertebrae, separating the fascia and supraspinous ligaments in line with the incision. Surgeon A then lifted ligaments and muscles out of the way. Next, Surgeon B performed a posterior discectomy and fusion at L2, and a partial excision of the vertebral body at L3 was also performed.

- Surgeon A reports code 22612 62.
- Surgeon B reports codes 22612 62 and 22114 51.

Although Surgeon A performed just the posterior exposure part of the procedure, because it is significant to the entire procedure, Surgeon A reports code 22612 with modifier 62 due to having assisted by beginning the surgery. Then, Surgeon B reports code 22612 with modifier 62 due to having assisted by completing the surgery; Surgeon B also reports code 22114 with modifier 51.

Incision

Incision codes are reported for the open incision and drainage of deep abscesses (subfascial) of the following sites:

- Cervical
- Thoracic
- Cervicothoracic
- Lumbar
- Sacral
- Lumbosacral

Example: A patient underwent open incision and drainage of a deep subfascial abscess, sacral region. Report code 22015.

Excision

The Excision subcategory contains a note stating that when two surgeons work together to perform a spinal procedure during the same operative session on the same patient, when each performs a distinct part of the procedure, modifier 62 (Two surgeons) is added to the procedure code reported by each surgeon. (Additional procedure codes are also reported with modifier 62 if the surgeons continue to work as primary surgeons.)

Example: The patient underwent posterior arthrodesis of L1–L2 and L2–L3, which was performed by Dr. Berry. Then, Dr. Thomas performed a minimal discectomy to prepare the L2–L3 interspace for arthrodesis via anterior interbody technique, L3–L4.

Dr. Berry reports codes 22612 62 and 22614 62 for posterior arthrodesis of two levels (L1–L2 and L2–L3). Dr. Thomas reports 22558 62 for anterior interbody technique arthrodesis including minimal discectomy of one level (L3–L4).

Osteotomy

An **osteotomy** is an incision into bone. Spinal osteotomy involves making incisions in vertebral bone to remove pieces or wedges of bone to correct a deformity such as kyphosis, lordosis, or scoliosis (Figure 13-7). Because the osteotomy codes include corpectomy, discectomy, and laminectomy, separate codes are not reported for these procedures when they are documented in the operative report. Osteotomy codes differentiate anterior and posterior approaches.

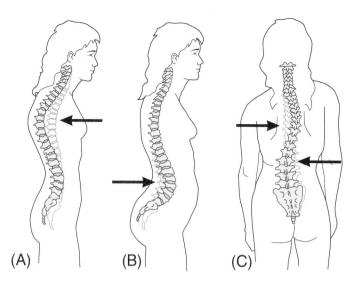

FIGURE 13-7 Spinal deformities (A) Kyphosis (B) Lordosis (C) Scoliosis

Osteotomy procedures include:

- Arthrodesis.

- Instrumentation (report the appropriate code(s) in addition to the primary procedure code).

- Bone graft procedure (report an appropriate code in addition to the primary procedure code).

- Collaboration between two surgeons who perform distinct parts of an anterior spine osteotomy procedure during the same operative session on the same patient (each surgeon adds modifier 62 to reported codes). (Additional procedure codes reported by each surgeon are also reported with modifier 62 if the surgeons continue to work as primary surgeons.) *Read CPT instructional notes carefully because modifier 62 is not reported with certain bone graft or spinal instrumentation procedure codes.*

Spinal osteotomy procedure codes are reported when a portion of the vertebral segment is removed in preparation for realignment of the spine as part of spinal deformity correction.

The three sections of the spinal column are defined as *anterior* (anterior two-thirds of vertebral body), *middle* (posterior third of vertebral body and pedicle), and *posterior* (articular facets, lamina, and spinous process).

The Osteotomy subcategory also includes a note indicating that when two surgeons work together to perform an anterior spine osteotomy procedure during the same operative session on the same patient *and each performs a distinct part of the procedure*, modifier 62 is added to the appropriate procedure codes (reported by each surgeon).

Example 1: Patient underwent spinal osteotomy of spine, posterolateral approach, C1. Report code 22210.

Example 2: Patient underwent anterior osteotomy of the spine with discectomy, T1. Report code 22222. (Do not report a separate code for the discectomy procedure.)

Example 3: Patient underwent anterior spinal osteotomy, L1–L2. Dr. James performed anterior exposure of the spine with mobilization of great vessels. Dr. Smith performed anterior spinal osteotomy of L1–L2 with discectomy. Then Dr. James performed closure procedures. Dr. James reports codes 22224 62 and 22226 62. Dr. Smith also reports codes 22224 62 and 22226 62. (Code 22226 is an add-on code and exempt from modifier 51.)

Fracture and/or Dislocation

Report codes for the following when performed during the same operative session as the treatment of fractures or dislocations.

- Bone graft procedure.
- Arthrodesis.
- Instrumentation procedure.
- Collaboration between two surgeons who perform distinct parts of an open fracture and/or dislocation procedure (each surgeon adds modifier 62 to reported codes). (Additional procedure codes reported by each surgeon are also reported with modifier 62 if the surgeons continue to work as primary surgeons.)

The Fracture and/or Dislocation subcategory also includes a note indicating that when two surgeons work together to treat distinct parts of *open fracture and/or dislocation* procedures during the same operative session and each performs a distinct part of the procedure, modifier 62 is added to the procedure codes. Both surgeons must work together as primary surgeons.

> **Example:** Patient underwent open treatment and reduction of T3–T4 vertebral fracture with grafting. Dr. Lawson performed posterior exposure of the spine with mobilization of great vessels. Dr. Timber performed open treatment and reduction of T3–T4 vertebral fracture with spinal allograft. Then Dr. Lawson performed closure procedures. Dr. Lawson reports codes 22327 62 and 22328 62. Dr. Timber also reports codes 22327 62, 22328 62, and 20931. Codes 22328 and 20931 are exempt from modifier 51.

Manipulation

"Manipulation of spine" under anesthesia is performed to treat back pain and other disorders. The idea is that the patient is more relaxed while under anesthesia, and better spinal manipulation results. The code is reported once for manipulation of any region of the spine, including multiple regions during the same operative session. (For "manipulation of the spine *without* anesthesia," report code 97140 from the Medicine section.)

> **Example:** Patient underwent lumbar spinal manipulation under anesthesia. Report code 22505.

Percutaneous Vertebroplasty and Vertebral Augmentation

Percutaneous vertebroplasty is the process of injecting a material (e.g., cement) into the vertebral body to reinforce that structure using image guidance. **Vertebral augmentation** is the process of creating a cavity followed by injecting material (e.g., cement) under image guidance. Both procedures are typically performed to relieve pain due to (1) vertebral compression fractures (e.g., pathologic fractures due to osteoporosis) and (2) benign and malignant infiltrating vertebral lesions (e.g., aneurysmal bone cysts, giant cell tumor, hemangioma, metastatic cancer, or myeloma). Codes for percutaneous vertebroplasty and vertebral augmentation include bone biopsy when performed, moderate sedation, and imaging guidance necessary to perform the procedure.

Percutaneous vertebroplasty is usually performed with the patient under conscious sedation; a bone cement (that hardens in about 10 minutes) is injected under pressure directly into a fractured vertebra. The cement causes fragments of fractured vertebra to congeal, providing stability. Bone cement is also injected to fill minor spaces in cancellous bone.

> **Example:** Patient underwent percutaneous vertebroplasty under imaging guidance, L1 and L2, to stabilize pathologic fractures due to osteoporosis. Report codes 22511 and 22512. (Code 22512 is exempt from modifier 51 because it is an add-on code.)

Percutaneous Augmentation and Annuloplasty

Percutaneous augmentation and annuloplasty is a minimally invasive technique that is performed under fluoroscopic guidance to treat small tears in the annulus without an associated disc protrusion.

> **Example:** Patient underwent percutaneous intradiscal electrothermal annuloplasty, L5, under fluoroscopic guidance. Report code 22526.

Arthrodesis

Arthrodesis, or **artificial ankylosis**, is the surgical fixation (e.g., fusion) of a joint. Arthrodesis may be performed independently of other procedures; when arthrodesis is performed with another procedure, report the arthrodesis code in addition to the definitive procedure and add modifier 51 to the arthrodesis code if applicable. (Some arthrodesis codes are exempt from modifier 51.)

Arthrodesis performed for reasons other than to correct a spinal deformity is classified according to anatomical approach, such as anterior or anterolateral approach, posterior or posterolateral approach, or anterior or posterior interbody technique. Arthrodesis for spinal deformities (e.g., scoliosis and kyphosis) is also reported according to anatomical approach, such as posterior.

- Spinal instrumentation procedures are reported in addition to the arthrodesis code(s). (Modifier 51 is added to some instrumentation codes.)
- Bone graft procedures are reported in addition to the arthrodesis code(s), and modifier 51 is exempt.

> **Example:** A physician performed posterior arthrodesis of L5–S1 using autogenous iliac bone graft harvested through a separate incision. Report codes 22612 and 20937. (Code 20937 is exempt from modifier 51.)

Exploration

Just one code is reported for exploration of spinal fusion.

- When spinal instrumentation is performed during the same operative session as the exploration of spinal fusion, report an appropriate spinal instrumentation code.
- When instrumentation reinsertion or removal is reported with other procedures (e.g., arthrodesis, decompression, exploration of fusion), add modifier 51 to the spinal instrumentation code(s).
- When exploration of spinal fusion is performed in addition to other definitive procedures (e.g., arthrodesis), add modifier 51 to the "exploration of spinal fusion" code.

Spinal Instrumentation

Spinal instrumentation includes **segmental instrumentation**, which is a fixation at each end of the construct (structure) and includes at least one additional interposed bony attachment. **Non-segmental instrumentation** is a fixation at each end of the construct (structure) that may span several vertebral segments without attachment to the intervening segments. A *vertebral segment* represents a single complete vertebral bone with its associated articular processes and laminae (e.g., C1). A *vertebral interspace* is the non-bony compartment between two adjacent vertebral bodies and it contains the intervertebral disc, which includes the nucleus pulposus, annulus fibrosus, and two cartilaginous endplates.

> **Example:** Patient underwent posterior technique arthrodesis of C1–C2. Autogenous iliac bone graft was used, and it was harvested through a separate incision. Anterior instrumentation of the two vertebral segments was also performed. Report codes 22595, 22845, and 20937. (Code 20937 is exempt from modifier 51.)

Exercise 13.5 – Spine (Vertebral Column)

Instructions: Assign the CPT code(s) and appropriate modifier(s) to each statement.

1. Patient underwent arthrodesis at L4–L5 interspace. Posterior interbody technique laminectomy was performed. Discectomy was also performed to prepare the vertebral interspace for fusion.

   _____

2. Physician performed "spinal manipulation under anesthesia," cervical, thoracic, and lumbar spine.

   _____

3. Patient underwent osteotomy and discectomy of a single cervical spine vertebral segment. Anterior approach was used.

   _____

4. Physician performed arthrodesis using posterior technique of atlas-axis (C1–C2) with internal spinal fixation by wiring the spinous processes.

   _____

5. Patient underwent posterior arthrodesis of L2–L3 for spinal deformity, with casting. Morselized autogenous iliac bone graft was harvested through a separate skin incision.

   _____

Abdomen

The Abdomen subcategory contains codes for:

- Excision
- Other Procedures

   The excision procedure code is reported for excision of abdominal wall tumor. The "other procedures" code is reported for unlisted procedures.

> **Example:** Patient underwent excision of subfascial abdominal wall tumor. Report code 22900.

Shoulder

The Shoulder category contains codes for procedures performed on the clavicle, scapula, humerus head and neck, sternoclavicular joint, acromioclavicular joint, and shoulder joint.

> **Example:** Physician performed removal of a "total shoulder" implant with replacement of a new implant. Report codes 23335 for removal of the implant and 23472 51 for arthroplasty and insertion of a new total shoulder implant.

 NOTE:

To report magnetic resonance imaging (MRI) of the shoulder with intra-articular contrast, report code 23350 (Injection procedure for shoulder arthrography or enhanced CT/MRI shoulder arthrography) in addition to the MRI code (from the Radiology section).

Humerus (Upper Arm) and Elbow

The Humerus (Upper Arm) and Elbow category includes codes for procedures performed on the humerus, elbow, and head and neck of the radius and olecranon process.

> **Example:** Patient underwent closed treatment with manipulation, medial humeral epicondylar fracture. Report code 24565.

Forearm and Wrist

The Forearm and Wrist category includes codes for procedures performed on the radius, ulna, carpal bones, and joints.

> **Example:** A patient was diagnosed with subluxation of extensor carpi ulnaris (ECU) tendon at the wrist. The physician reconstructed the ECU tendon sheath with a retinacular graft harvest from the fourth dorsal compartment. Report code 25275, which includes the procedure for obtaining the graft.

 Coding Tip

- Open carpal tunnel decompression surgery (for carpal tunnel syndrome) is classified in the Nervous System subsection of surgery.
- Surgical endoscopy to release the transverse carpal ligament for treatment of carpal tunnel syndrome is classified below the Endoscopy/Arthroscopy category of the Musculoskeletal System subsection.

Hand and Fingers

The Hand and Fingers category includes codes for procedures performed on the hands and fingers, which include repairs to tendons, nerves, and blood vessels to provide treatment for injuries or to correct deformities. Tendons include two types.

- *Flexor tendons*: Bend the fingers
- *Extensor tendons*: Straighten the fingers

The following procedures are bundled in the tendon repair codes:

- Application of immobilization
- Extension of the excision
- Repair and closure of tendon sheath

Codes for harvesting and inserting tendon grafts from another site, repairing nerves or arteries, and treating fractures are reported in addition to the tendon repair.

> **Example:** A patient underwent percutaneous palmar fasciotomy, right hand for Dupuytren's contracture. Report code 26040 RT.

Exercise 13.6 – Abdomen, Shoulder, Humerus (Upper Arm) and Elbow, Forearm and Wrist, and Hand and Fingers

Instructions: Assign the CPT code(s) and appropriate modifier(s) to each statement.

1. The physician performed an excision of a 4-cm subfascial abdominal wall tumor and the surrounding tissue. Incision was repaired in multiple layers with sutures.

   _____

2. The physician removed subdeltoid calcareous deposits, left shoulder joint, by incising the raised area over the calcium deposits and removing the calcareous deposits.

   _____

3. The physician performed a forequarter interthoracoscapular amputation, right shoulder.

   _____

4. The physician performed removal of a deep foreign body, left shoulder.

   _____

5. Excision of 2-cm malignant tumor from subcutaneous tissue around right elbow.

   _____

6. Percutaneous medial tenotomy for treatment of tennis elbow, right.

   _____

7. Patient who sustained left elbow trauma developed an elbow contracture that required manipulation under anesthesia.

   _____

8. Percutaneous skeletal fixation of left radial fracture.

   _____

9. Injection procedure performed to prep patient for right wrist arthrography.

   _____

10. Left palmar fasciectomy with Z-plasty.

   _____

Pelvis and Hip Joint

The Pelvis and Hip Joint category includes codes for procedures performed on the head and neck of the femur (hip joint).

> **Example:** Patient underwent partial hemiarthroplasty of the left hip with insertion of femoral stem prosthesis. Report code 27125 LT. (Insertion of the femoral stem prosthesis is included in code 27125.)

Femur (Thigh Region) and Knee Joint

The Femur (Thigh Region) and Knee Joint category includes codes for procedures performed on the femur and its tibial plateau and the knee joint.

NOTE:

Arthroscopic knee surgery is a commonly performed procedure, and codes are located under the Endoscopy/Arthroscopy category of the Musculoskeletal System subsection.

The *femur* (Figure 13-8) is the long bone of the thigh, and it articulates with the hip bone, tibia, and patella. The *tibial plateau* is the lower portion of the femur that articulates with the *tibia* (larger of the two lower leg bones). The *knee* is a "hinge" joint comprised of bones, cartilage, ligaments, and tendons. *Ligaments* (e.g., medial collateral ligament) are connective tissue that connects bone to bone (e.g., patella to femur), and they control stability of the knee. Trauma to knee joints can result in ligament tears, which require surgical repair (Figure 13-9).

Example: Patient was diagnosed with an anterior medial left thigh mass, which was 2 × 2 × 1.5 cm in size. With the patient under local anesthesia, biopsy of the mass above the superficial fascia was performed. Report code 27323 LT (because the mass was removed from "above the superficial fascia").

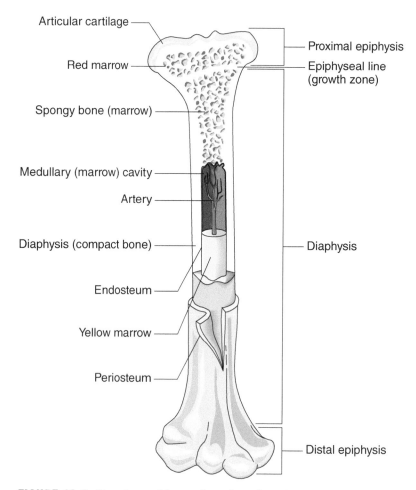

FIGURE 13-8 Structure of femur (long bone), including proximal (near) and distal (far) references to the bone's shaft

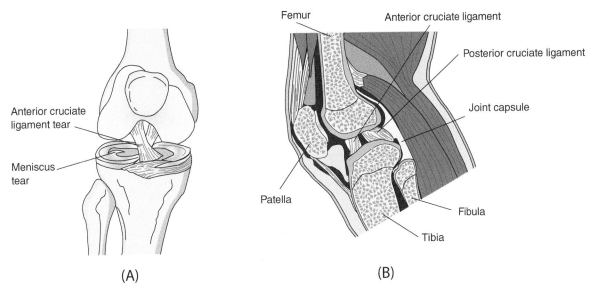

FIGURE 13-9 (A) Meniscus and anterior cruciate ligament tears (B) Knee joint

Leg (Tibia and Fibula) and Ankle Joint

The Leg (Tibia and Fibula) and Ankle Joint category includes codes for procedures performed on the tibia, fibula, and ankle joint.

> **Example:** Patient underwent flexor tenolysis of the right ankle, single tendon. Report code 27680 RT.

Foot and Toes

The Foot and Toes category includes codes for procedures performed on the feet and toes. Hallux valgus repair codes are reported to correct *bunions* (Figure 13-10), which are caused by bone inflammation and swelling and result in medial deviation and axial rotation of the first metatarsophalangeal (MTP) joint. Bunion deformities develop differently, and repair requires different levels of complexity and different techniques, as follows:

- Keller procedure: Simple resection of the base of the proximal phalanx with removal of the medial eminence
- McBride procedure: Distal soft tissue release that corrects soft tissue deformity at the MTP joint
- Mitchell procedure: Complex, double cut osteotomy through the neck of the first metatarsal

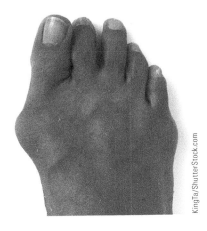

FIGURE 13-10 Bunion

Example: Patient underwent bilateral hallux valgus correction with bunionectomy, sesamoidectomy, and resection of proximal phalanx base. Report code 28292 50.

Exercise 13.7 – Pelvis and Hip Joint, Femur (Thigh Region) and Knee Joint, Leg (Tibia and Fibula) and Ankle Joint, and Foot and Toes

Instructions: Assign the CPT code(s) and appropriate modifier(s) to each statement.

1. Proximal hamstring release, left.

   _____

2. Partial hip replacement with bipolar arthroplasty to treat right hip fracture.

   _____

3. Removal of a foreign body deep in the left thigh.

   _____

4. Complete 1 × 1 × 0.5-cm excision of subcutaneous tumor, posterior left thigh.

   _____

5. Excision of 2-cm bone cyst with autograft of harvested femur graft, left, which was performed during the same operative session.

   _____

6. Decompression fasciotomy of the lateral and posterior compartments, right knee.

   _____

7. Lindholm Operation percutaneous repair of ruptured Achilles tendon, right.

   _____

8. Incision and drainage of infected bursa, left ankle.

   _____

9. Concentric bunion repair procedure, right.

   _____

10. Partial ostectomy to surgically correct bunionette involving the right fifth metatarsal head.

   _____

Application of Casts and Strapping

The Application of Casts and Strapping category includes codes that are reported when the cast (or splint) application or strapping is a(n)

- Replacement procedure performed during or after the period of follow-up care
- Initial service performed *without restorative treatment or procedure* to stabilize or protect a fracture, a dislocation, or another injury and/or to provide comfort to a patient

Example 1: A five-year-old patient was seen in the office to have the left short-arm cast replaced. The patient was playing a game they invented called "bop it," which involved knocking the cast on top of one of the bedposts. The cast cracked and had to be replaced. The patient was instructed to stop playing "bop it." Report code 29075 LT.

Example 2: A seven-year-old male patient injured his left arm while roller skating. A two-view left forearm x-ray at Sylvania Community Hospital's emergency department (ED) revealed fractures of the radial and ulnar shafts. A level III ED evaluation and management service was provided. The patient's arm was placed in a splint to stabilize the fracture, and the parent was informed that treatment would have to be performed the next day because no orthopedic physician was available in the facility or on call. Report codes 99283, 29125 LT, and 73090 LT. (Do not add modifier 57 to the E/M code because surgery was not performed, and do not add modifier 51 to the surgery and radiology codes.)

Upon being informed that treatment would not be performed that day, the parent called the facility from which the family normally receives treatment and asked to speak with the orthopedic surgeon on call. That physician called the parent back within 15 minutes; when the parent explained the circumstances, they were told to bring the x-rays and their child to St. Francis Hospital to meet the surgeon there so an assessment and appropriate treatment could be provided. Upon outpatient evaluation and management (level III) of this new patient by the orthopedic surgeon, the parent was informed that same-day treatment was preferred because waiting until the next day would result in swelling, inflammation, and pain, making it more difficult to treat the fractures. Later that day the patient underwent closed manipulation of radial and ulnar shaft fractures under general anesthesia, and a short-arm cast was applied. The patient remained in the hospital until 10 PM, at which time he was released to return home with his parents. Report codes 25565 and 99203 57.

When one physician applies a cast, splint, or strapping device as initial treatment of a fracture or dislocation and a different physician later performs a restorative treatment or procedure, report "treatment of fracture and/or dislocation" code(s) from the appropriate category in the Musculoskeletal System subsection. (When a cast or strapping is removed by a physician other than the original physician who applied the cast or strapping, report the appropriate cast removal code.)

When a physician performs an initial restorative treatment or procedure and an initial cast, splint, or strap is also applied, the physician is responsible for providing all subsequent fracture, dislocation, and/or injury care. Do not report a code for the application of a cast, splint, or strapping device with the initial restorative treatment or procedure because it is included in the "treatment of fracture and/or dislocation" code.

 Coding Tip

Do not report modifier 58 (staged or related procedure or service by the same physician during the postoperative period) when a temporary cast, splint, or strapping device is applied and the patient later undergoes a restorative treatment or procedure. In addition, do not report evaluation and management service codes unless significant identifiable further services are provided at the time of the cast application or strapping. (Report only the "treatment of fracture and/or dislocation" code.)

Endoscopy/Arthroscopy

The Endoscopy/Arthroscopy category includes codes for procedures performed using an endoscope or arthroscope. Endoscopy is the visual examination of the interior of a body cavity or an organ. **Arthroscopy** (Figure 13-11) is the visual examination of the inside of a joint.

Endoscopic and arthroscopic procedures are diagnostic or surgical, and CPT notes indicate that surgical endoscopy/arthroscopy always includes diagnostic endoscopy/arthroscopy. An endoscopy/arthroscopy is considered diagnostic when it is performed to visualize an abnormality or to determine the extent of disease. When anything in addition to visualization is performed, the endoscopy/arthroscopy procedure is considered surgical.

Example: Patient underwent surgical arthroscopy, left knee, with medical and lateral meniscectomy, which included debridement and shaving of articular cartilage (chondroplasty). Report code 29880 LT.

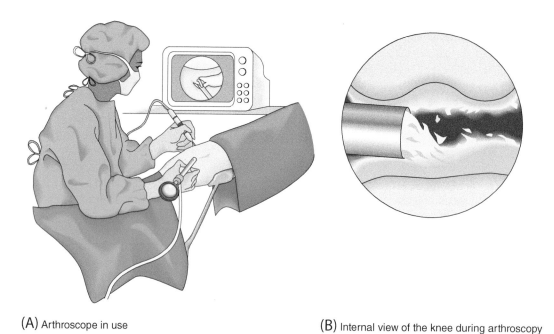

(A) Arthroscope in use   (B) Internal view of the knee during arthroscopy

FIGURE 13-11 Arthroscopic surgery (A) The physician views progress on a monitor
(B) Internal view as diseased tissue is removed during surgery

 Coding Tip

- A surgical endoscopy/arthroscopy always includes a diagnostic endoscopy/arthroscopy. This means that a code for diagnostic endoscopy/arthroscopy is not reported with a code for surgical endoscopy/arthroscopy. A diagnostic endoscopy/arthroscopy code is reported when it is the only endoscopic/arthroscopic procedure performed. (Codes for other procedure codes, other than surgical endoscopy/arthroscopy, can be reported with diagnostic endoscopy/arthroscopy codes.)

- Diagnostic knee arthroscopy is probably the most common type of procedure performed. It is done to examine and diagnose knee joint abnormalities. Diagnostic knee arthroscopy involves inserting an arthroscope through small incisions and using a camera to transmit images onto a monitor so the knee joint's interior can be visualized. During arthroscopic knee surgery, the knee is subdivided into three compartments: medial, lateral, and patellofemoral.

- Surgical knee arthroscopy is often performed to treat diseased or damaged structures of the knee joint (e.g., torn meniscus, meniscal lesions, damaged patella or ligaments, and inflamed or damaged synovium).

Exercise 13.8 – Application of Casts and Strapping and Endoscopy/Arthroscopy

Instructions: Assign the CPT code(s) and appropriate modifier(s) to each statement. (Do not assign CPT E/M codes.)

1. Diagnostic arthroscopy, left elbow, with synovial biopsy.

Exercise 13.8 – continued

2. Patient's left long-arm cast was removed after getting wet, the site was evaluated, and another long-arm fiberglass cast was reapplied. The same physician who applied the first cast removed the wet cast and applied the new cast.

   _____

3. Physician treated flexion contracture of right small finger proximal interphalangeal joint by applying a cast to stabilize the joint.

   _____

4. Patient with diabetic neuropathic ulcers had rigid total contact leg cast applied, left.

   _____

5. Patient sustained nondisplaced fracture of distal left ulna, and emergency department physician applied a molded short-arm static splint for immobilization and protection of the fracture. Patient was referred to orthopedic specialist.

   _____

6. Patient underwent arthroscopic repair of tibial plafond fracture with internal fixation, right.

   _____

7. Surgical arthroscopy of the metacarpophalangeal joint on the right with debridement.

   _____

8. Patient underwent arthroscopic Mumford procedure of distal 1 cm of left clavicle.

   _____

9. Arthroscopic superior labrum anterior/posterior (SLAP) lesion tear repair, right shoulder.

   _____

10. Left knee diagnostic and surgical arthroscopy with medial meniscectomy.

    _____

Respiratory System Subsection

The CPT Respiratory System (Figure 13-12) subsection is arranged according to body area from nose to lungs. It includes the following categories:

- Nose
- Accessory Sinuses
- Larynx
- Trachea and Bronchi
- Lungs and Pleura

Respiratory system categories include one or more of the following procedures:

- Incision
- Excision
- Introduction (and Removal)
- Removal of Foreign Body
- Repair
- Destruction
- Endoscopy
- Other Procedures

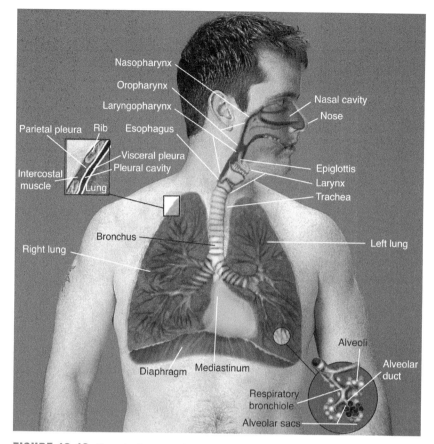

FIGURE 13-12 Respiratory system

The Lungs and Pleura category also contains the following procedures:

- Thoracoscopy (video-assisted thoracic surgery [VATS])
- Stereotactic radiation therapy
- Lung Transplantation
- Surgical Collapse Therapy; Thoracoplasty

Respiratory section guidelines define procedures and provide instruction for the selection of appropriate codes, as follows:

- Approach used for lung procedures
- Amount and type of tissue removed
- Difference between diagnostic and therapeutic procedures
- Ways various removal procedures may be performed

Nose

The Nose category contains codes for procedures that are performed on the nose, nasal septum, intranasal tissue, nasal turbinates, and skin of the nose. (Refer to Figure 13-13 for structure of the upper respiratory system, including nasal anatomy.) Codes for procedures range from simple control of a nosebleed to complex surgery (e.g., rhinoplasty).

 Coding Tip

When the control of bleeding is performed during a procedure on the nose, it is considered an integral part of that procedure and is not separately coded and reported. Thus, codes that classify "control of nasal hemorrhage" are not reported with other procedure codes from the Nose category.

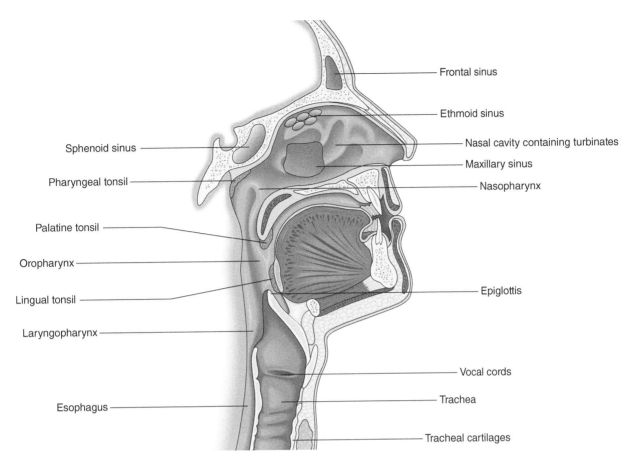

FIGURE 13-13 Structure of the upper respiratory system

Incision

Incision codes are reported for drainage of abscess of hematoma, nasal (internal approach) or nasal septum. A *hematoma* is a localized collection of blood outside of the blood vessels, usually in liquid form within tissue.

Example: Patient underwent drainage of a nasal hematoma via internal approach. Report code 30000.

Excision

Turbinates, or *conchae*, are bony plates covered by spongy mucosa with curved margins. There are three turbinates on each side of the *nasal vestibule* (nose's entrance): inferior, middle, and superior. When surgery is performed on turbinates, it is important to identify the type of turbinate procedure and technique used. Turbinates can be removed by resection or excision with or without endoscopy, cauterization, debridement, laser, cryotherapy, radiofrequency reduction, or ablation. Turbinate excision and submucous resection codes are typically reported for inferior turbinate surgery. These codes can also be reported separately with other surgical procedures performed on the nose (e.g., sphenoid, maxillary, or frontal sinus procedures; septoplasty). Modifier 50 (Bilateral procedure) is added to the reported code when surgery is performed on both sides of the nasal vestibule.

Example: Patient underwent anterior intranasal ethmoidectomy for chronic sinusitis. A partial inferior turbinate excision was performed to gain access to the ethmoid bone. Report code 31200. (Code 30130 is not reported for the partial inferior turbinate excision because it was performed only to gain access to the ethmoid bone.)

Coding Tip

When a turbinate procedure is performed to gain access to the ethmoid bone and a separate diagnosis justifies medical necessity for excision of turbinate or submucous resection of turbinate, report the appropriate code and add modifier 51. (Some third-party payers will not reimburse the turbinate excision or submucous resection because the code descriptions do not specify middle or superior turbinates.)

> **Example:** Patient underwent a total intranasal ethmoidectomy for chronic sinusitis and a complete excision of the inferior turbinate for sleep apnea. Report codes 31201 and 30130 51 because separate diagnoses codes are reported for each procedure.

Introduction

Introduction codes are reported for therapeutic injection into nasal turbinate(s), displacement therapy, and insertion of a nasal septum prosthesis.

> **Example:** Patient underwent Proetz type displacement therapy. Report code 30210.

Removal of Foreign Body

Removal of foreign body codes are reported for removal of a foreign body from the intranasal area (office type procedure) and that requiring general anesthesia or by lateral rhinotomy.

> **Example:** Patient underwent removal of intranasal foreign body via lateral rhinotomy. Report code 30320.

Repair

Nasal repairs include rhinoplasty, repair of nasovestibular stenosis, septoplasty, repair of choanal atresia, lysis of intranasal synechia, fistula repair, septal or intranasal dermatoplasty, and repair of nasal septal perforations.

> **Example:** Patient underwent bilateral nasal septoplasty with cartilage scoring. Report code 30520 50.

Destruction

Destruction codes are reported for ablation of soft tissue of inferior turbinates superficially or intramurally.

> **Example:** Patient underwent submucosal soft tissue ablation of inferior turbinates, bilateral via electrocautery. Report code 30802. Do not add a directional modifier to the code because turbinates are not considered a paired organ or body part.

Other Procedures

Other Procedures codes are reported for the control of nasal hemorrhage, therapeutic fracture of nasal inferior turbinate(s), and unlisted procedures of the nose.

> **Example:** Patient underwent therapeutic fracture of the nasal inferior turbinates. Report code 30930.

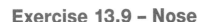

Exercise 13.9 – Nose

Instructions: Assign the CPT code(s) and appropriate modifier(s) to each statement.

1. Physician made therapeutic injections into the mucosa of the right and left turbinates.

   _____

2. Simple excision of polyp from inside of nose, left side, via scalpel. Single-layer closure was also performed.

   _____

3. Removal of nasal mucosa from inside left side of nose for biopsy. Some normal tissue adjacent to diseased mucosa is also removed during biopsy.

   _____

4. Excision of intranasal lesion via lateral rhinotomy, left.

   _____

5. Rhinoplasty for nasal deformity secondary to congenital cleft lip and palate, including columellar lengthening of the tip and septum, with osteotomies.

   _____

Accessory Sinuses

The Accessory Sinuses category contains codes for procedures performed on the maxillary, frontal, ethmoid, and sphenoid sinuses. It also contains unique coding guidelines for endoscopy procedures. (Refer to Figure 13-13 for location of accessory sinuses.)

Incision

Incision codes classify lavage, sinusotomy, and pterygomaxillary fossa surgery. A *lavage* is the washing out of a body cavity, such as the accessory sinuses, with water or a medicated solution. A *sinusotomy* is a surgical incision of the sinus (e.g., treatment of chronic sinus disease). The *pterygomaxillary fossa* is an opening in the skull, through which arteries and nerves pass.

> **Example:** Patient underwent right maxillary sinus lavage by cannulation. Report code 31000 RT.

Excision

Excision codes classify ethmoidectomy and maxillectomy procedures. An *ethmoidectomy* involves removing partitions between the ethmoid sinuses to create larger sinus cavities (e.g., treatment of sinus infections and sinus obstructions). A *maxillectomy* involves removing the upper jaw bone (maxilla) (e.g., treatment of cancer in bones and tissues of roof or hard palate of mouth).

> **Example:** Patient underwent total intranasal ethmoidectomy, left. Report code 31201 LT.

Endoscopy

Endoscopy codes classify unilateral procedures unless the code description indicates otherwise. This means that HCPCS Level II modifier LT or RT is added to the endoscopy code unless the procedure is performed bilaterally and modifier 50 is added to the code.

NOTE:

Modifier 50 is not added to the nasal endoscopy, diagnostic; unilateral or bilateral (separate procedure) because "bilateral" is included in its description. However, modifier LT or RT can be added to the code if the procedure is performed unilaterally.

Diagnostic endoscopy codes include inspection of the interior of the nasal cavity and its meatus, turbinates, and sphenoethmoid recess. When diagnostic endoscopy is performed, the following procedures are bundled in the reported code: administration of local anesthesia, electrocautery, access to different cavities, and some shaving/debridement. (Extensive shaving/debridement is reported with a separate code and modifier 51.) Report just one code when diagnostic endoscopy is performed on all of these areas on one or both sides.

Surgical sinus endoscopy is performed through the nose, using a fiberoptic endoscopy; it includes sinusotomy (when performed) and diagnostic endoscopy. When a physician performs surgical endoscopy of accessory sinuses, evaluation of nasal access regions (diagnostic endoscopy) is also performed as part of the medically necessary service. Do not report a code for diagnostic endoscopy in addition to the surgical endoscopic procedure. This means that when surgical and diagnostic endoscopies are performed during the same operative session, just one code is reported to classify both procedures.

Example: Patient undergoes surgical nasal endoscopy with anterior ethmoidectomy, left; the physician uses the endoscope diagnostically to evaluate other regions of the nasal cavity. Report code 31254 LT. (Do not report code 31231 for the diagnostic nasal endoscopy.)

NOTE:

Recognize the difference between endoscopic and open surgical approaches. An endoscopic nasal surgical approach utilizes a fiberoptic endoscope instrument, which is inserted through the nostril(s). An open nasal surgical approach is performed by making an incision into skin or tissues inside the nasal cavity.

Anatomically, the middle turbinate is part of the ethmoid bone. Therefore, if the middle turbinate is removed during endoscopic polypectomy or endoscopic ethmoidectomy, a code for removal of the middle turbinate is *not* reported.

Example: Patient underwent bilateral nasal surgical endoscopy with total ethmoidectomy and bilateral nasal septoplasty. Report codes 31255 50 and 30520 50 51.

When biopsy of a lesion from the accessory sinuses is obtained as part of an excision, destruction, or other type of removal during the same operative session, do not report a biopsy code in addition to the excision/destruction/removal code. Also, biopsy codes are not separately reported for multiple similar or identical lesions even if the lesions are taken from a different area of the respiratory system.

Example: A patient presents with multiple nasal polyps. Patient undergoes bilateral surgical nasal endoscopy with polypectomy and total ethmoidectomy. Report code 31255 50. (Do not report separate procedure code 31237 for the surgical endoscopy with polypectomy because that procedure is bundled with code 31255.) Even though polypectomy may have been performed prior to total ethmoidectomy, the polypectomy procedure is included in the more invasive ethmoidectomy procedure.

Coding Tip

When a sinusotomy is performed in conjunction with a sinus endoscopy, just one code is reported for both services. If the endoscopy was performed to evaluate the sinus cavity prior to sinusotomy, report just the sinusotomy procedure code. CPT instructions state that a surgical sinus endoscopy always includes sinusotomy and diagnostic endoscopy.

Exercise 13.10 – Accessory Sinuses

Instructions: Assign the CPT code(s) and appropriate modifier(s) to each statement.

1. Bilateral anterior ethmoidectomy via intranasal approach.

   _____

2. Bilateral endoscopic treatment of a nosebleed.

   _____

3. Endoscopic anterior and posterior (total) ethmoidectomy, left, with left maxillary antrostomy.

   _____

4. Nasal endoscopy with biopsy, left.

   _____

5. Endoscopic frontal nasal exploration with removal of tissue from left frontal sinus and diagnostic endoscopy of left turbinates.

   _____

Larynx

The Larynx (Figure 13-14) category contains codes for procedures performed on the epiglottis and larynx and inside the trachea.

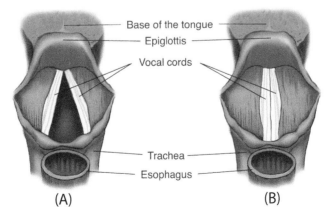

FIGURE 13-14 View of larynx and vocal cords from above. (A) Vocal cords are open during breathing. (B) Vocal cords vibrate together during speech.

Excision

Excision codes classify laryngotomy, laryngectomy, pharyngolaryngectomy, arytenoidectomy or arytenoidopexy, and epiglottidectomy procedures. A *laryngotomy* involves making a surgical incision into the larynx to provide air passage when breathing is obstructed. A *laryngectomy* involves removal of the larynx (voice box). A *pharyngolaryngectomy* is the removal of the hypopharynx (laryngeal part of throat) and larynx. An *epiglottidectomy* is the removal of all or part of the epiglottis (e.g., treatment of sleep apnea).

Example: Patient underwent total intranasal ethmoidectomy, left. Report code 31201 LT.

According to *CPT Assistant* (October 2001), when a total laryngectomy with bilateral radical neck dissection of cervical lymph nodes (31365) is performed, do not add modifier 50 to the code because the larynx is a single midline organ. (A laryngectomy cannot be performed bilaterally.) Instead, report code 31365 for the total laryngectomy and radical neck dissection on one side. Then, report code 38720-59 for the radical neck dissection (total cervical lymphadenectomy) on the other side. The description of code 38720 is "Cervical lymphadenectomy (complete)." Modifier 59 is added to indicate a distinct procedural service.

An **arytenoidectomy** is the excision of arytenoid cartilage, which is located in the bilateral vocal fold. An **arytenoidopexy** is the surgical fixation of arytenoidal cartilage and/or surrounding muscles. Both procedures are done to treat vocal cord paralysis or to improve patient breathing.

Example: Patient underwent endoscopic arytenoidectomy. Report code 31560. (Do *not* report code 31400.)

Introduction

Introduction procedures are performed for emergency endotracheal intubation and to change a tracheotomy tube prior to healing (before an abnormal fistula tract is created by the body).

Example: Patient underwent an emergency endotracheal intubation during provision of critical care services. Report code 31500. (Appropriate code[s] from the E/M critical care services subsection would also be reported.)

Endoscopy

Endoscopy codes include the following types of laryngoscopies, and the documented operative report will indicate the instrumentation used:

- Direct
- Indirect
- Use of operating microscope (for magnification)
- Use of fiberoptic scope (that transmits light)

Laryngoscopy is the visualization of the back of the throat, including the *larynx* (voice box) and vocal cords. **Direct laryngoscopy** is the insertion of a flexible or rigid fiberoptic scope or a rigid laryngoscope to visualize throat structures. **Indirect laryngoscopy** is the insertion of a small hand mirror in the patient's mouth at the back of the throat while the physician wears headgear that contains a mirror and light source; the mirror worn by the physician reflects light into the patient's mouth, allowing the physician to visualize the patient's throat.

Example: Patient underwent indirect diagnostic laryngoscopy. Report code 31505.

Repair

Repair codes classify laryngoplasty and laryngeal reinnervation procedures. A *laryngoplasty* involves reconstruction of the larynx (voice box). A *laryngeal reinnervation* supplies a new, functioning nerve supply to a paralyzed larynx; the purpose is to restore phonation (vocalization).

Example: Patient underwent cricoid split laryngoplasty. Report code 31587.

Exercise 13.11 – Larynx

Instructions: Assign the CPT code(s) and appropriate modifier(s) to each statement. (Do not assign CPT E/M codes.)

1. Emergency department physician places endotracheal tube for a patient in respiratory distress.

   _____

2. Total laryngectomy with unilateral radical neck dissection.

   _____

3. Patient with cricoid split (break in the circular cartilage of the larynx) undergoes laryngoplasty.

   _____

4. Complicated tracheotomy tube change (prior to establishment of fistula tract).

   _____

5. Total laryngectomy with radical neck dissection, right side. Complete cervical lymphadenectomy, left side.

   _____

Trachea and Bronchi

The Trachea and Bronchi (Figure 13-15) category contains codes for procedures performed through the trachea and on tracheal cartilage (carinii) and the bronchi.

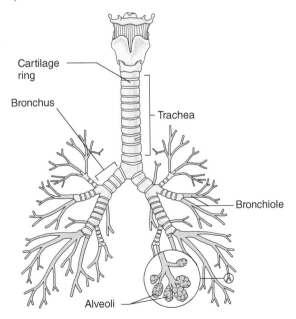

FIGURE 13-15 Trachea, bronchi, bronchial trees, and alveoli (air sacs)

Incision

Incision codes classify tracheostomy, construction of tracheoesophageal fistula and subsequent insertion of an alaryngeal speech prosthesis, tracheal puncture, and tracheostoma revision procedures. A *tracheostomy* involves creating an opening through the neck into the trachea (windpipe); a tracheostomy tube is usually placed into the opening to provide an airway and/or to remove secretions from the lungs. A tracheoesophageal fistula is constructed with insertion of a one-way valve, which is an alaryngeal speech prosthesis, called a *voice button* or a *Blom-Singer prosthesis*, to allow the patient to phonate (vocalize). A *tracheal puncture* involves piercing the trachea with a hollow point needle to aspirate secretions or inject therapeutic agent(s). A *tracheostoma revision* involves incising the stoma area and resecting redundant scar tissue or a poorly healing wound.

Example: Patient underwent emergency transtracheal tracheostomy. Report code 31603.

Endoscopy

A **bronchoscopy** (Figure 13-16) is the visual examination of the interior of the bronchus. A tracheoscopy is the visual examination of the interior of the *trachea* (windpipe). A **tracheobronchoscopy** is the visual examination of the interior of the trachea and bronchus. Endoscopy of the trachea and bronchus is performed with either a flexible fiberoptic scope or a rigid scope, with or without cell washings or brushing. A **brushing** involves combing the mucous lining of the trachea or bronchus with a bronchial brush to collect cells. **Cell washing** involves flushing fluid into an area and removing the fluid, using aspiration technique to collect cells.

Endoscopy procedures also involve use of a bronchoscope, with or without fluoroscopic guidance, to visualize all major lobar and segmental bronchi. These procedures may also include obtaining diagnostic specimens as part of the examination. Fiberoptic bronchoscopy services routinely include inspection of the nasal cavity, pharynx, and larynx. When nasal endoscopy or laryngoscopy is performed, in addition to bronchoscopy, report a code for the bronchoscopy procedure only.

Diagnostic endoscopy of the trachea and bronchi performed during the same operative session as a surgical endoscopy is included in the surgical endoscopy. Do not report a code for diagnostic endoscopy when it is performed with surgical endoscopy.

Diagnostic endoscopy is often performed during an open surgical procedure to evaluate (or scout or investigate) the surgical field. Do not report a code for diagnostic endoscopy when it is performed with an open surgical procedure.

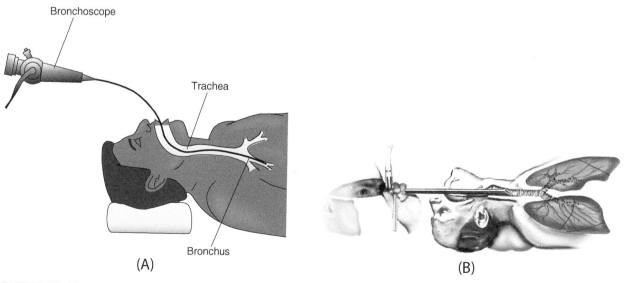

Bronchoscope

Trachea

Bronchus

(A)

(B)

FIGURE 13-16 (A) Flexible bronchoscopy (B) Rigid bronchoscopy

When a surgical endoscopic procedure fails and is converted to an open procedure, do not report a code for the surgical endoscopic procedure. Report only a code for the open procedure.

> **Example:** A patient presents with aspiration of a foreign body. A diagnostic bronchoscopy is performed bilaterally to locate the foreign body, and a surgical bronchoscopy is performed to remove the foreign body from the right bronchus. Report code 31635 RT. (Do not report a code for the diagnostic bronchoscopy.)

Bronchial Thermoplasty

Bronchial thermoplasty codes classify procedures that reduce the amount of smooth muscle in the airway walls in asthmatic patients. *Bronchial thermoplasty* involves introducing a catheter with an electrode array into an area of the lung that is to be treated, and radiofrequency energy is used to heat and reduce the amount of smooth muscle.

> **Example:** Patient underwent flexible bronchoscopy with bronchial thermoplasty, one lobe, right lung. Report code 31660 RT.

Introduction

Introduction codes classify catheterization, catheter aspiration with bronchial brush biopsy, and transtracheal introduction of needle wire dilator/stent or indwelling tube for oxygen therapy procedures.

> **Example:** Patient underwent nasotracheal catheter aspiration to remove sputum from the lungs. Report code 31720. (Do not report a directional modifier because the trachea is not a paired organ.)

Excision, Repair

Excision, Repair codes classify tracheoplasty, carinal reconstruction, bronchoplasty, excision, suture, and revision procedures.

> **Example:** Patient underwent carinal reconstruction. Report code 31766.

Exercise 13.12 – Trachea and Bronchi

Instructions: Assign the CPT code(s) and appropriate modifier(s) to each statement.

1. Emergency transtracheal tracheostomy of 18-month-old child.
   _____

2. Bronchial brush biopsy via transglottic catheterization, right bronchus.
   _____

3. Flexible bronchoscopy to remove a piece of food inhaled into the left bronchus.
   _____

4. Bronchoscopy with bronchial alveolar lavage, right bronchus.
   _____

5. Suture repair of tracheal laceration, cervical region.
   _____

Lungs and Pleura

The Lungs and Pleura (Figure 13-17) category contains codes for procedures performed on the lungs and *pleura* (membrane that envelops the lungs and lines the walls of the pleural cavity).

Incision

Incision codes classify thoracostomy, pneumonostomy, pleural scarification, and decortication procedures. A *thoracostomy* is the construction of an artificial opening through the chest wall, usually for drainage of fluid or release of an abnormal accumulation of air. A *pneumonostomy* is the surgical formation of an artificial opening into a lung (e.g., drainage of abscess). *Pleural scarification* is the injection of a chemical solution into the chest cavity (through a chest tube) to create adhesions between the surface of the lung and inside surface of the chest cavity for the treatment of repeat pneumothorax. *Decortication* is the removal of a constricting membrane or layer of tissue from the surface of the lung to permit the lung to fully expand.

Example: Patient underwent pleural scarification for repeat pneumothorax. Report code 32215.

Excision/Resection

Excision/Resection codes classify pleurectomy, decortication and parietal pleurectomy, and biopsy procedures. *Pleurectomy* is the removal of pleura. *Decortication* is the removal of a constrictive fibrinous covering (to allow the lungs

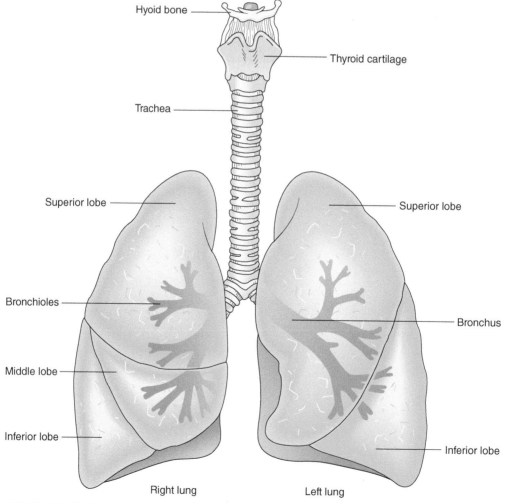

FIGURE 13-17 External view of lungs. Note three lobes in the right lung and two lobes in the left lung

to expand). A *percutaneous pleural biopsy* involves inserting a long needle through skin into the chest wall to obtain pleural tissue (without direct visualization of the pleura). For **percutaneous needle biopsy**, a long needle is inserted through the skin and into other tissue (e.g., chest wall, lung, or mediastinum) to obtain tissue for diagnostic evaluation. *Core needle biopsy* (or *needle core biopsy*) involves using a needle to obtain a core sample of tissue, whereas *fine-needle aspiration (FNA) biopsy* involves using a needle to remove fluid cells for cytological study. However, when a fine-needle aspiration biopsy is documented, report an appropriate code from the General subsection.

> **Example:** Patient underwent parietal pleurectomy. Report code 32310.

Removal

Removal codes classify lung removal, resection and repair of bronchus, resection of apical lung tumor, thoracotomy, and extrapleural enucleation of empyema (empyemectomy) procedures. **Pneumonectomy** is the removal of the entire lung or one or more lobes of the lung. *Thoracotomy* is the surgical incision of the chest wall. *Empyemectomy* is the removal of an *empyema* (abscess in chest cavity between lung and chest wall) in its entirety, including pleural membranes surrounding the abscess.

> **Example:** Patient underwent extrapleural pneumonectomy. Report code 32445.

Introduction and Removal

Introduction and Removal codes classify insertion of indwelling tunneled pleural catheter, tube thoracostomy, placement of interstitial device(s) for radiation therapy guidance, thoracentesis, and pleural drainage procedures. **Thoracentesis** (Figure 13-18A) is the surgical puncture of the chest wall with a needle to obtain fluid from the pleural cavity. It is performed to make a diagnostic evaluation or to drain excess fluid from a patient with severe *pleural effusion* (Figure 13-18B) (fluid in the pleural cavity prevents the lung from fully expanding, making it difficult for the patient to breathe).

Pneumocentesis is the puncture of the pleural space with a transthoracic needle to drain *fluid* or to obtain material for diagnostic study.

> **Example:** Patient underwent thoracentesis via needle for aspiration of fluid from pleural space (pleural effusion). Report code 32554.

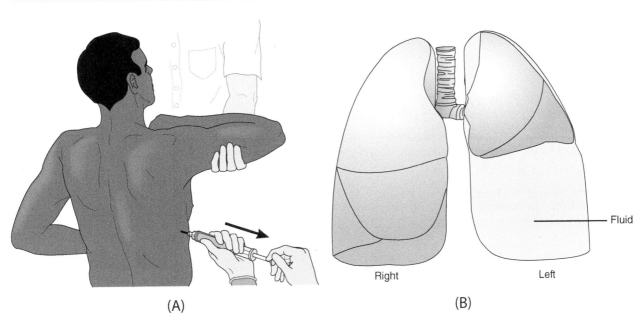

Right   Left   Fluid

(A)   (B)

FIGURE 13-18 (A) Thoracentesis (B) Lung with pleural effusion

Destruction

Destruction codes classify instillation of pleurodesis or fibrinolytic agent procedures. *Pleurodesis agents* (e.g., talc) are instilled to treat recurrent or persistent pneumothorax. *Fibrinolytic agents* (e.g., saline mixture with streptokinase or urokinase) disintegrate or dissolve fibrinous adhesions.

Example: Patient underwent instillation of an agent for pleurodesis via chest tube. Report code 32560.

Thoracoscopy (Video-Assisted Thoracic Surgery [VATS])

A **thoracoscopy** is the visual examination of the pleural cavity, and it provides an alternative to open lung or thoracotomy procedures to treat pleural disorders surgically. Surgical thoracoscopy always includes diagnostic thoracoscopy, which means just the surgical thoracoscopy code is reported when both procedures are performed. However, when an open lung procedure, a thoracotomy, or another open chest procedure immediately follows diagnostic thoracoscopy during the same operative episode, report codes for both procedures (and sequence the open procedure first). When a surgical thoracoscopy is converted to an open procedure, report code(s) for the open lung procedure(s) only; do not report a code for the surgical thoracoscopy procedure.

Example: Patient presents with lower lateral chest wall pain and shortness of breath. Thoracoscopy with diagnostic biopsy of lobulated lung mass is performed. Biopsy reveals mesothelioma. Report code 32608.

Stereotactic Radiation Therapy

The Stereotactic Radiation Therapy code is reported for thoracic target(s) delineation for the purpose of administering stereotactic body radiation therapy. The code is reported just once for an entire course of treatment. *Stereotactic radiation surgery (SRS)* involves identifying and delineating the target(s) for surgery. *Stereotactic body radiation therapy (SBRT)* uses highly potent biological radiation to target a malignant tumor (and codes are reported from the CPT Radiology section). SRS and SBRT procedures usually require the skill of both a surgeon and a radiation oncologist. SRS/SBRT uses a single or up to five fractionated doses of high potent biological radiation, and the high doses of radiation allow a tumor to be precisely localized using four-dimensional imaging. Occasionally, separately reportable *fiducial* (fixed) markers are placed during SRS to ensure proper placement of radiation delivery.

Example: Patient underwent thoracic target delineation for stereotactic body radiation therapy. Report code 32701.

Lung Transplantation

Lung transplants include the following distinct components, and a code is assigned to each by the physician who performs the component procedure:

- **Cadaver donor pneumonectomy**, which involves harvesting the allograft (graft such as lung tissue that is transplanted between genetically nonidentical individuals of the same species) and preserving the allograft with cold preservation solution and cold maintenance

- **Recipient lung allotransplantation**, which includes transplantation of a single or double lung allograft and care of the recipient

- **Backbench work** for lung transplantation, which involves preparing the cadaver donor lung allograft prior to lung transplantation and dissecting allograft from surrounding soft tissues to prepare the pulmonary venous/atrial cuff, pulmonary artery, and bronchus

Example: Patient with severe respiratory system complications due to cystic fibrosis underwent lung transplant procedure to remove diseased lungs and replace them with healthy lungs from a recently deceased donor. Transplant physician performed donor pneumonectomy including cold preservation from cadaver donor, backbench standard preparation of cadaver donor lung allografts, bilateral, and double lung transplant with cardiopulmonary bypass. Report code 32854 for the recipient patient and codes 32850 and 32856 for the cadaver donor lungs.

Surgical Collapse Therapy; Thoracoplasty

Surgical collapse therapy and thoracoplasty codes classify procedures performed to therapeutically collapse a patient's lung(s).

- *Extrapleural resection of ribs* is the removal of rib(s).
- *Thoracoplasty* is the resection of ribs to allow the chest wall to retract, reducing the size of the pleural space.
- *Pneumonolysis* is the division of tissues that attach the lung to the wall of the chest cavity.
- *Therapeutic pneumothorax* is the injection of air into the pleural space.

Example: A patient underwent extraperiosteal pneumonolysis. Report code 32940.

Other Procedures

Other Procedures codes classify total lung lavage, ablation therapy, and unlisted procedures. When a total lung lavage is performed bilaterally, add modifier 50 to the code because its description specifies unilateral. When bronchoscopic bronchial alveolar lavage is performed, go to the Trachea and Bronchi category to locate the appropriate code.

Example: Patient underwent total lung lavage, left. Report code 32997 LT.

Exercise 13.13 – Lungs and Pleura

Instructions: Assign the CPT code(s) and appropriate modifier(s) to each statement.

1. Emergency department physician performed a tube thoracostomy for hemothorax, inserting a tube for drainage.

2. Total lung lavage, right.

3. Percutaneous needle biopsy, pleura.

4. Diagnostic thoracoscopy with lung biopsy (left side) and surgical thoracoscopy with segmental lobectomy (left side) (both procedures performed during same operative session).

5. Patient with severe respiratory system complications due to chronic obstructive pulmonary disease underwent unilateral lung transplant procedure to remove one diseased lung and replace it with a healthy lung from a recently deceased donor. Donor lung also required repair of intrathoracic blood vessel. Transplant physician performed donor pneumonectomy including cold preservation from cadaver donor, backbench standard preparation of cadaver donor lung allografts, and single lung transplant without cardiopulmonary bypass.

Summary

CPT codes in the Musculoskeletal System subsection are reported for procedures on bones, cartilage, joints, ligaments, muscles, and tendons. The subsection is arranged from head to toe according to body area. The Musculoskeletal System subsection also includes codes for fracture management, casting and strapping, and endoscopy/arthroscopy. The CPT Respiratory System subsection is arranged from nose to lungs according to body area.

Internet Links

American Lung Association: www.lung.org

Amilcare Gentili, M.D. (Professor of Clinical Radiology): Go to **www.gentili.net** to locate resources about musculoskeletal radiology.

National Institute of Arthritis and Musculoskeletal and Skin Diseases (NIAMS): www.niams.nih.gov

Northwest ENT Surgery Center: Go to **nwestsurgerycenter.com**, and click on the ENT Surgical Procedures link to locate information about surgical procedures performed on the ears, nose, and throat.

Review

13.1 – Multiple Choice

Instructions: Select the most appropriate response.

1. Which is a type of open fracture treatment?

   a. Closed reduction   **b.** Internal fixation   **c.** Stabilization   **d.** Traction

2. Which is performed to puncture a joint for fluid removal or medication injection?

   a. Arthrocentesis   **c.** Arthroscopy
   b. Arthrodesis   **d.** Artificial ankylosis

3. Musculoskeletal subsection notes state that codes for treatment of fractures and joint injuries (e.g., dislocations) "are categorized by the type of _____ (closed, percutaneous, open) and type of stabilization (fixation, immobilization)."

   a. fixation
   b. fracture
   c. manipulation
   d. resection

4. Open carpal tunnel decompression surgery (for carpal tunnel syndrome) is classified in which CPT Surgery subsection?

   a. Integumentary System
   b. Musculoskeletal System
   c. Nervous System
   d. Operating Microscope

5. The application of casts and strapping are reported when the cast (or splint) or strapping is an initial service performed _____ to stabilize or protect a fracture, a dislocation, or another injury and/or to provide comfort to a patient.

   a. during restorative treatment/procedure
   b. instead of placing a cast (or splint) or strap
   c. when a reduction or manipulation is completed
   d. without restorative treatment/procedure

6. Calcaneus ostectomy for removal of spurs, left foot. Which CPT code is assigned?

   a. 28111 LT   **b.** 28116 LT   **c.** 28118 LT   **d.** 28119 LT

7. Unlisted maxillofacial prosthetic procedure. Which CPT code is assigned?
   - **a.** 21089
   - **b.** 21299
   - **c.** 22899
   - **d.** 23929

8. C3–C4 anterior intervertebral discectomy with decompression of spinal cord and nerve root, including osteophytectomy, performed by two primary surgeons. Which CPT code(s) are reported by Surgeon A?
   - **a.** 63075
   - **b.** 63075 62
   - **c.** 63075, 63075
   - **d.** 63075 62, 63075 62

9. Reconstruction of complete shoulder (rotator) cuff avulsion, chronic, right side. Which CPT code(s) are assigned?
   - **a.** 23130 RT, 23420 RT
   - **b.** 23130 RT, 23420 51 RT
   - **c.** 23410 RT
   - **d.** 23420 RT

10. Incision and drainage of deep abscess, right forearm. Which CPT code is assigned?
    - **a.** 10060
    - **b.** 24310 RT
    - **c.** 25028 RT
    - **d.** 25031 RT

11. When a physician performs surgical nasal/sinus endoscopy with partial ethmoidectomy (anterior) and a septoplasty during the same operative session, report the
    - **a.** septoplasty code (30520).
    - **b.** endoscopy code (31254).
    - **c.** endoscopy code (31254) and the septoplasty code (30520).
    - **d.** endoscopy code (31254) or the septoplasty code (30520).

12. Which is considered part of the ethmoid bone and, if removed during endoscopic polypectomy or endoscopic ethmoidectomy, is not coded and reported separately?
    - **a.** Frontal sinus
    - **b.** Maxillary sinus
    - **c.** Middle turbinate
    - **d.** Nasal vestibule

13. Which is the surgical fixation of arytenoidal cartilage and/or surrounding muscles?
    - **a.** Arytenoidectomy
    - **b.** Arytenoidopexy
    - **c.** Arytenoidostomy
    - **d.** Arytenoidotomy

14. Which procedure is performed to comb the mucous lining of the trachea or bronchus for the purpose of collecting cells?
    - **a.** Brushing
    - **b.** Cell washing
    - **c.** Tracheotomy
    - **d.** Bronchoscopy

15. Which component(s) of a lung transplant are reported as distinct code(s) by the physician who performs the component procedure(s)?
    - **a.** Backbench work for lung transplantation
    - **b.** Cadaver donor pneumonectomy
    - **c.** Recipient lung allotransplantation
    - **d.** Backbench work for lung transplantation, cadaver donor pneumonectomy, and recipient lung allotransplantation

16. Initial cautery to control posterior nasal hemorrhage. Which CPT code is assigned?
    - **a.** 30901
    - **b.** 30903
    - **c.** 30905
    - **d.** 30906

17. Surgical nasal sinus endoscopy with repair of cerebrospinal fluid leak, sphenoid region, right side. Which CPT code is assigned?
    - **a.** 31287 RT
    - **b.** 31290 RT
    - **c.** 31291 RT
    - **d.** 31292 RT

18. A three-year-old child undergoes direct laryngoscopy for fluid aspiration. Which CPT code is assigned?
    - **a.** 31515
    - **b.** 31520
    - **c.** 31520 63
    - **d.** 31525

19. Catheterization with bronchial brush biopsy. Which CPT code is assigned?
    - **a.** 31623
    - **b.** 31717
    - **c.** 31720
    - **d.** 31725

20. Surgical thoracoscopy with excision of a pericardial cyst. Which CPT code is assigned?
    - **a.** 32604
    - **b.** 32658
    - **c.** 32659
    - **d.** 32661

13.2 – Coding Practice: Musculoskeletal System

Instructions: Assign the CPT code(s) and appropriate modifier(s) to each case.

1. Patient sustained a stab wound to the right neck during a domestic dispute and underwent wound exploration. The stab wound was extended, and examination of surrounding bones, connective tissue, muscles, and nerves revealed normal findings. No foreign bodies were found. The area was debrided and irrigated. Coagulation of minor subcutaneous and muscular blood vessels was achieved with electrocautery. The wound was cleaned and closed with 3-0 Vicryl.

    _____

2. Patient underwent reconstruction of the entire forehead and supraorbital rims, requiring grafts, to correct a congenital skeletal deformity. After administration of general anesthesia, scalp and upper eyelid incisions were made to access the surgical site. The forehead bones were reshaped and repositioned, and bone allografts were inserted to augment the forehead and supraorbital rims. Incisions were closed after wires were inserted as fixation devices to maintain the proper shape of the facial bones.

    _____

3. A 13-year-old patient sustained a fractured right femur during a soccer game and underwent open treatment with insertion of two screws and two pins. After administration of general anesthesia, an incision was made over the fracture site and a metal rod was inserted through the bone's shaft to stabilize it. The rod was secured with screws, and the leg was placed in a cast.

    _____

4. Patient underwent incision and drainage of bursa, right knee. Needle was inserted into bursa and fluid was drained from the sac, which was located deep within the knee's soft tissue.

    _____

5. Patient underwent knee replacement surgery four months ago. Today "manipulation of the left knee under general anesthesia" was performed to flex the knee joint and increase its range of motion.

    _____

6. Two-year-old patient underwent reapplication of a long-leg cast to the left femur, which extended from the thigh to the toes. The patient sustained femur fracture four weeks ago when initial reduction was performed and application of long-leg cast was applied. Today that cast was removed and replaced with a long-leg cast due to the patient's age, to ensure optimal bone healing.

    _____

7. Patient underwent open reduction of left tibia fracture four weeks ago, which has a global surgery period of 90 days. Today the orthopedic surgeon cut a hole in the patient's short-leg cast, left, to check for incisional infection due to patient complaints of pain. No infection was noted.

    _____

8. Patient underwent diagnostic arthroscopy of the left elbow due to unexplained pain. Surgeon inserted arthroscope into the left elbow joint to determine presence of disease or injury.

    _____

9. Patient underwent removal of a metal sliver from the index finger, right hand. The surgeon made an incision between the first and second bones of the right index finger. Joint exploration revealed the presence of a metal sliver, which was removed.

    _____

10. Patient underwent closed treatment of fractured tip of the right radius (Colles-type fracture) at distal end, which included application of a short-arm cast.

13.3 – Coding Practice: Respiratory System

Instructions: Assign the CPT code(s) and appropriate modifier(s) to each case.

1. Patient underwent bilateral diagnostic nasal endoscopy. The physician inserted an endoscope into the left nostril to evaluate nasal structures. The right nostril was also examined.

---

2. Patient underwent indirect endoscopy of the larynx with biopsy. The physician used a small, round mirror to examine the vocal cords, tongue, and top of the throat for signs of disease or injury. Biopsy of larynx was performed for evaluation and diagnosis.

---

3. Patient presents with a six-month history of hoarseness. The physician performs a laryngoscopy. The patient is prepped in the usual fashion. A fiberoptic laryngoscope is passed; the vocal cords are examined under direct visualization. Slight swelling is noted. A biopsy sample is taken to be sent to pathology.

---

4. Patient with a history of recurrent spontaneous left pneumothorax was prepped for a thoracoscopy and underwent parietal pleurectomy. An incision was made at the eighth intercostal space, and a thoracoscope was inserted to view patient's lungs. No evidence of disease was found in the lobes. Trocars were then placed, and the pleura was stripped away from the chest wall. A nice surface was accomplished. A chest tube was placed for drainage. The remaining incision was closed with mattress sutures of 4-0 nylon.

---

5. A 45-year-old nonsmoker has had a cough for the last six months. With the patient placed under intravenous sedation, a bronchoscope was passed in the patient's oral cavity. Primary structures of upper area were visualized and found to be normal. The transbronchial area was examined. A biopsy sample was taken of the single lobe of the lung. The patient had minimal blood loss. The bronchoscope was then removed, and the patient returned to the outpatient area in satisfactory condition.

---

6. A patient with bilateral vocal cord paralysis presents for removal of arytenoid cartilage. This is being done to improve the patient's breathing. With the patient placed under general anesthesia, the flexible laryngoscope with operating microscope is inserted into the oral cavity. The pharynx and larynx are examined under the microscope. After adequate visualization is established, the arytenoid cartilage is exposed by excision of the mucosa overlying it and arytenoidectomy performed.

---

7. A 50-year-old patient has difficulty breathing through the left nostril. The patient has a deformity of the septum and presents for a submucous resection of the septum. After making an incision, the lining of the septum is detached. The patient's deviated portion of the septum is removed, and the cartilage portion above is scored. Nasal packing is placed.

---

8. Patient suffers from anosmia. The patient consents to a diagnostic biopsy of intranasal cavities. This procedure is done under local anesthesia delivered to nasal tissue. A small amount of tissue is removed from both intranasal cavities under direct visualization. Minimal bleeding is noted.

---

9. A two-year-old patient presents to the office with a marble in the right side of the nose, per the parent. Using nasal forceps, the marble is removed.

_____

10. A five-year-old patient has a nasal deformity secondary to congenital cleft lip and palate that requires repair. Rhinoplasty is performed by making intranasal incisions and pulling back skin from the nasal bone tip. The bone is shaved and columellar lengthening performed at the tip. The area is irrigated, and nasal packing is placed. The patient has little blood loss.

_____

CPT Surgery III

Chapter Outline

Cardiovascular System Subsection

Hemic and Lymphatic Systems Subsection

Chapter Objectives

At the conclusion of this chapter, the student should be able to:

1. Define key terms related to the Cardiovascular System and the Hemic and Lymphatic Systems subsections of CPT Surgery.
2. Assign codes from the Cardiovascular System subsection of CPT Surgery.
3. Assign codes from the Hemic and Lymphatic Systems subsection of CPT Surgery.

Key Terms

adjuvant techniques

angioscopy

bone marrow aspiration

bone marrow biopsy

cadaver donor cardiectomy with or without pneumonectomy

cardiac ablation

cardiopulmonary bypass

commissurotomy

composite graft

coronary artery bypass graft (CABG)

coronary endarterectomy

cross-over vein graft

cutdown

direct aneurysm repair

embolectomy

en bloc

endovascular aneurysm repair

extracorporeal life support (ECLS)

extracorporeal membrane oxygenation (ECMO)

Maze procedure

modified Maze procedure

nonselective vascular catheterization

nontunneled

pericardiectomy

pericardiocentesis

pericardiotomy

peripherally

recipient heart with or without lung allotransplantation

reconstruction of the vena cava

saphenopopliteal vein anastomosis

selective vascular catheterization

shunting procedure

splenoportography

stab phlebectomy

stented valve

stentless valve

sympathectomy

therapeutic apheresis

thrombectomy

thromboendarterectomy

transmyocardial revascularization (TMR)

tube pericardiostomy

tunneled

valvuloplasty

valvulotomy

vascular family

venous valve transposition

ventricular assist device (VAD)

Introduction

The Cardiovascular System subsection includes codes for procedures performed on the heart and pericardium, arteries and veins, including valves (e.g., mitral and semilunar), and peripheral vascular vessels. The Hemic and Lymphatic Systems subsection includes codes for procedures performed on the spleen, bone marrow and stem cells, (for) transplantation and post-transplantation cellular infusion, lymph nodes, and lymphatic channels. CPT guidelines that apply to the subsections are located at the beginning of the Surgery section.

 Coding Tip

> Instructional notes located beneath categories, subcategories, headings, and subheadings apply to all codes in those areas. Parenthetical notes that are located below a specific code apply to that code only unless the note indicates otherwise.

 NOTE:

> The content in Chapters 12 through 16 of this textbook is organized exactly as it appears in the CPT Surgery section. This organization facilitates learning by allowing students to move from one CPT Surgery subsection to the next, in order.
>
> When included in CPT, the Other Procedures code is reported for an unlisted procedure performed on the anatomical site. When reporting an unlisted procedure code, include documentation about the procedure performed with the submitted claim.
>
> The *Medicare National Correct Coding Initiative Policy Manual* provides guidance about assigning procedure codes for the Cardiovascular System and Hemic and Lymphatic System subsections. Go to www.cms.gov and enter "Medicare NCCI Policy Manual" in the Search box to navigate to the manual.

Cardiovascular System Subsection

Cardiovascular System subsection codes are arranged anatomically and then according to procedure performed. The Cardiovascular System subsection includes the following anatomical sites:

- Heart and pericardium
- Arteries and veins

Cardiovascular System Instructional Notes

Instructional notes located at the beginning of the Cardiovascular System subsection provide instruction on assigning codes for *selective vascular catheterization*. When performed as part of cardiovascular (and radiology) procedures, codes for *selective vascular catheterization* are reported separately.

In addition, parenthetical notes located above the Cardiovascular System subsection title serve as reminders to review other codes and sections in CPT to locate additional codes associated with certain cardiovascular system procedures. (Notes are also located throughout the Cardiovascular System subsection as a reminder to report additional surgery codes with some procedures.)

 Coding Tip

> During cardiovascular procedures, **cardiopulmonary bypass** is often required to divert blood from the heart to the aorta, using a pump oxygenator. Because some procedures can be performed without cardiopulmonary bypass, make sure you review the operative report to determine whether to assign the cardiopulmonary bypass code for the procedure performed.
>
> **Example:** Patient underwent repair of cardiac wound with cardiopulmonary bypass. Report code 33305.

Selective Vascular Catheterization

When reporting codes for selective vascular catheterization, knowledge of the flow of blood (Figure 14-1) throughout the body's circulatory system is crucial. (In fact, it's a good idea to reference an anatomy and physiology textbook such as Cengage's *Body Structures & Functions* when assigning codes to procedures in

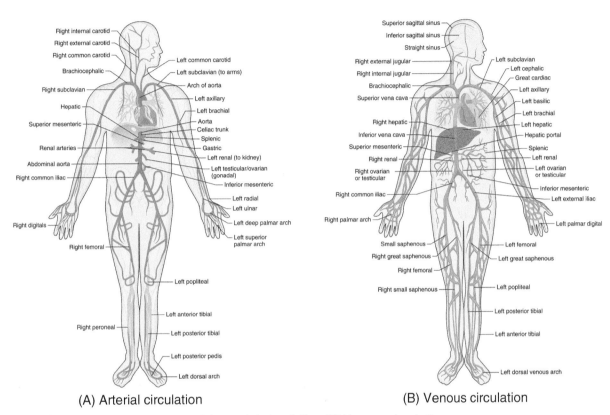

(A) Arterial circulation   (B) Venous circulation

FIGURE 14-1 Circulatory system (A) Arterial circulation (B) Venous circulation

the Cardiovascular System subsection.) Selective vascular catheterization procedures include "vascular injection procedures" and require separate codes to be reported for the following:

- Diagnostic procedure (e.g., carotid angiogram) and/or therapeutic procedure (e.g., balloon dilation via catheter)
- Vascular access (e.g., selective vascular catheterization)

Separate codes are not reported for the administration of local anesthesia, introduction of the needle or catheter, or *injection* of contrast material. (The supply of contrast media *is* assigned an HCPCS Level II code.) In addition, CPT codes are assigned to the point of catheter placement (not guidewire insertion); catheters (or sheaths) are inserted into blood vessels to serve as conduits for the administration of fluids (or gases), access by surgical instruments (e.g., stent), and other tasks (e.g., balloon angioplasty). A guidewire might be inserted beyond placement of the catheter, and no images are taken or procedures are performed at the insertion point of the guidewire; thus, code to the point of catheter placement (not guidewire insertion) (Figure 14-2).

Selective vascular catheterization is the insertion and manipulation or guidance of a catheter (that is attached to a guidewire) into the branches of the arterial system (other than the aorta or the vessel

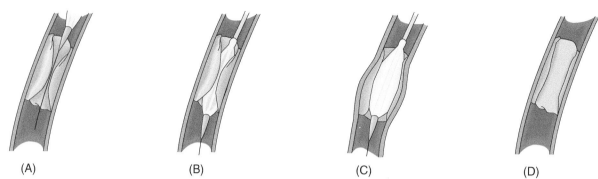

(A)   (B)   (C)   (D)

FIGURE 14-2 (A) Insertion of guidewire into and beyond plaque formation in artery (B) Insertion of catheter with attached balloon through plaque formation in artery (C) Expansion of balloon to compress plaque against arterial walls and open the arterial lumen (D) Compressed plaque, creating wider lumen in artery

punctured) for the purpose of performing diagnostic or therapeutic procedures. Selective vascular catheterization is usually performed under fluoroscopic (moving x-ray) guidance. The code reported for selective vascular catheterization includes introduction of the catheter into the punctured vessel and guidance through all lesser- (or first-) order vessels (to get to the intended vessel that undergoes the diagnostic or therapeutic procedure). Thus, codes are *not* reported for **nonselective vascular catheterization**, which involves introducing the catheter directly into a vessel without further advancement past the punctured vessel or introduction of a catheter into any portion of the aorta or vena cava from any approach (e.g., axillary, brachial, femoral, jugular).

 Coding Tip

When fluoroscopic guidance is provided during selective vascular catheterization, make sure you assign the appropriate supervision and interpretation code from the Radiology Vascular Procedures subsection.

Once the catheter reaches its intended vessel, assign an appropriate code for that selective vascular catheterization. When additional vessels are catheterized for the purpose of performing diagnostic and/or therapeutic procedures, assign codes for selective vascular catheterization of those second- and third- (and beyond) order vessels. First-, second-, and third- (and beyond) order vessel catheterization is discussed next.

A **vascular family** (Figure 14-3) (CPT Appendix L) is a group of vessels that is accessed by the same first-order vessel, and it is supplied by the same primary branch from the aorta. A vascular family can be compared to a tree with branches. The trunk is the aorta, which contains large and small branches. (Think of the aorta as a zero-order vessel because it is a common starting point for catheterization. The femoral artery, as a starting point for catheterization, is an example of another zero-order vessel.) From the starting point, vessels branch outward (similar to a network of streets from a highway) into the following:

- First-order vessels
- Second-order vessels
- Third-order vessels
- Fourth-order vessels

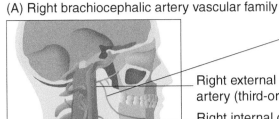

(A) Right brachiocephalic artery vascular family

Right lingual artery
(fourth-order)

Right external carotid
artery (third-order)

Right internal carotid
artery (third-order)

Right common carotid
artery (second-order)

Brachiocephalic
artery (first-order)

✎ NOTE:

The left common carotid artery
is a first-order vessel because it
branches from the aortic arch.
The right common carotid artery
is a second-order vessel because it
branches from the brachiocephalic
artery. The brachiocephalic artery
is a first-order vessel because it
branches from the aortic arch.

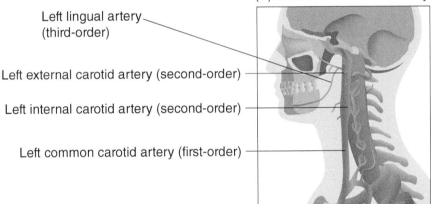

(B) Left common carotid artery vascular family

Left lingual artery
(third-order)

Left external carotid artery (second-order)

Left internal carotid artery (second-order)

Left common carotid artery (first-order)

FIGURE 14-3 Artery vascular families (A) First-, second-, third-, and fourth-order vessels in the right brachiocephalic artery vascular family (B) First-, second-, and third-order vessels in the left common carotid artery vascular family

First-order vessels extend as primary arterial branches from the aorta (e.g., left common carotid artery in the neck and inferior mesenteric artery or common iliac artery in the abdomen). When an *initial* second- or third-order arterial catheterization is performed within a vascular family, report just one code. *Second-order vessels* branch from first-order vessels, and *third-order vessels* branch from second-order vessels. *Fourth-order vessels* branch from third-order vessels. (Refer to Figure 14-3 for an illustration of first-, second-, and third-order vessels of a vascular family.)

Review the operative report to determine which artery (or arteries) underwent diagnostic or therapeutic procedures after having a catheter inserted. Although multiple arteries might be involved in a catheter being threaded from the insertion point to the intended artery, only one code is reported if just one artery undergoes diagnostic or therapeutic procedures.

Example: SELECTIVE VASCULAR CATHETERIZATION INTO FIRST-ORDER VESSELS: After being assaulted, a patient presented to the emergency department, complaining of severe upper left flank pain. Patient underwent left renal angiogram. This required insertion of a catheter into the right femoral artery. The catheter was advanced to the right external iliac and common iliac arteries and aorta and into the left renal artery. Contrast media was injected for visualization of the left renal artery upon x-ray. Report code 36251 LT. The right femoral, right external iliac, and right common iliac arteries underwent nonselective catheterization because they were used to access the left renal artery; no diagnostic or therapeutic procedure was performed on them. (Thus, do not assign catheter placement codes for accessing the right femoral, right external iliac, or right common iliac arteries.)

(continues)

(continued)

> Selective vascular catheterization was achieved by making a small incision in the skin and performing an arterial puncture into the left femoral artery (groin region). A needle containing a stylet (inner wire) was inserted through the skin into the left femoral artery. The stylet was removed and replaced with a guidewire. Under fluoroscopy, the guidewire was advanced through the external iliac artery and common iliac artery and then into the aorta. From the abdominal aorta, the guidewire was advanced into the left renal artery. The needle was removed, and a catheter was inserted over the length of the guidewire until it reached the renal artery. The guidewire was removed, and the catheter was left in place. Under fluoroscopic guidance, contrast media was injected manually with a syringe or with an automatic injector connected to the catheter. (An automatic injector propels a large volume of dye quickly to the angiogram site.) X-rays were taken, and the catheter was slowly and carefully removed. Pressure was applied to the insertion site (to facilitate clotting and to allow the arterial puncture to reseal), and a pressure bandage was applied.

When procedures are performed on multiple arteries along the path of catheterization from first- through to second-, third-, and/or fourth-order vessels, assign an appropriate code for each.

> **Example:** A catheter was introduced into the brachiocephalic artery (first-order) and then inserted into the right common carotid artery (second-order) and the right internal carotid artery (third-order) to the cerebral artery (fourth-order), where contrast media was injected to perform a cerebral angiography. In addition to the cerebral angiography code, report just one selective vascular catheterization code for the cerebral artery. The brachiocephalic, right common carotid, and right internal carotid arteries were used to access the (fourth-order) cerebral artery. No diagnostic or therapeutic procedures were performed on them. Therefore, do not assign selective vascular catheterization codes for catheterization of the brachiocephalic, right common carotid, or right internal carotid arteries.

An add-on code is reported when *additional*

- Selective arterial catheterization of second-order, third-order, and beyond (thoracic or brachiocephalic branch) vessels is achieved using a single first-order artery.
- Second-order, third-order, and beyond (abdominal, pelvic, or lower extremity artery branch) vessels are accessed during selective arterial catheterization.

> **Example:** A catheter was introduced into the left common carotid artery (first-order) and inserted into the left internal carotid artery (second-order). Contrast media was injected and carotid arteriogram performed. The catheter was further advanced into the left cerebral artery (third-order), additional contrast media was injected, and cerebral angiogram was performed. In addition to radiology codes for the carotid arteriogram and cerebral angiogram, report a selective vascular catheterization code for the (second-order) left internal carotid artery and add-on code 36218 for the selective vascular catheterization of the (third-order) cerebral artery. The left common carotid artery was used to access the other two arteries; therefore, a selective vascular catheterization code is *not* assigned.

Coding Tip

When multiple selective arterial catheterization procedures of separate and distinct vascular families are performed during the same operative session, report the appropriate number of units in Form Locator 46 of the UB-04.

> **Example:** Selective arterial catheterization of the thoracic artery and the brachiocephalic artery: Report code 36215 and the number of units on the UB-04 claim (Figure 14-4).

42 REV. CD.	43 DESCRIPTION	44 HCPCS / RATE / HIPPS CODE	45 SERV. DATE	46 SERV. UNITS	47 TOTAL CHARGES	48 NON-COVERED CHARGES	49
		36215		2			

FIGURE 14-4 Reporting selective arterial catheterization code by completing form locators 44 and 46 on the UB-04 claim

Heart and Pericardium

Heart and Pericardium codes describe procedures performed on the heart and pericardium.

Pericardium

The *pericardium*, or *pericardial sac*, is the membrane that surrounds the heart. **Pericardiocentesis** is the insertion of a needle to withdraw fluid from the pericardium. Radiological guidance is often performed with pericardiocentesis, so make sure you report a Radiology code if instructed to do so.

A **tube pericardiostomy** is the insertion of a tube for drainage or specimen collection. A **pericardiotomy** requires thoracotomy as incision for pericardial drainage, fluid collection, or foreign body removal.

Pericardiectomy is the removal of part of the pericardium (to treat chronic pericarditis). Also code the cardiopulmonary bypass if documented in the operative report.

> **Example:** Patient underwent pericardiotomy for removal of blood clot. Report code 33020.

Cardiac Tumor

A *cardiac tumor* is a growth that develops in the heart's *endocardium* (inner lining), *myocardium* (muscle layer), or pericardium. The majority of cardiac tumors are benign, although a percentage are malignant. Methods for diagnosing cardiac tumors include complete history and physical examination and diagnostic procedures such as echocardiogram, electrocardiogram, computed tomography (CT scan), magnetic resonance imaging (MRI), chest x-ray, and coronary arteriogram or angiogram.

Benign cardiac tumors include myxoma, rhabdomyoma, and other rare tumors (e.g., fibroma, hemangioma, lipoma, lymphangioma, neurofibroma, and papillary fibroelastoma). Malignant cardiac tumors include cardiac sarcoma, fibrosarcoma, liposarcoma, and rhabdomyosarcoma. Surgical removal of a cardiac tumor is indicated if it causes an arrhythmia or obstructs blood flow through the heart. When a cardiac tumor cannot be removed, a heart transplant may be required.

> **Example:** Patient underwent resection of intracardiac liposarcoma, resection with cardiopulmonary bypass. Report code 33120.

Transmyocardial Revascularization (TMR)

Transmyocardial revascularization (TMR) uses a high-powered laser to create small channels in the heart muscle to increase blood supply to the myocardium. The procedure also promotes *angiogenesis* (growth of new capillaries) as a blood supply to the heart muscle. TMR is performed to treat severe angina (in patients who are not candidates for coronary artery bypass graft [CABG] or angioplasty surgery), and the procedure may be performed with or without cardiopulmonary bypass. (TMR is usually performed with cardiopulmonary bypass.)

> **Example:** Patient underwent TMR, by thoracotomy. Report code 33140.

Pacemaker or Implantable Defibrillator

A *pacemaker system with lead(s)* (Figure 14-5) regulates the patient's heartbeat to prevent arrhythmias (e.g., atrial fibrillation and bradycardia) and includes a pulse generator (battery and electronic device) and leads

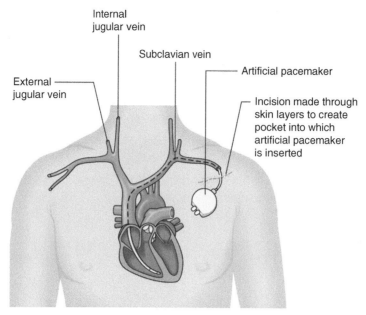

FIGURE 14-5 An artificial pacemaker system is implanted under the skin

(consisting of one or more electrodes). An *implantable cardioverter defibrillator (ICD) system* (Figure 14-6) is similar to a pacemaker in that it includes a pulse generator and leads (containing one or more electrodes), but it uses a combination of antitachycardia pacing and low-energy cardioversion or defibrillating shocks to regulate the patient's heartbeat and prevent arrhythmias (e.g., ventricular fibrillation and ventricular

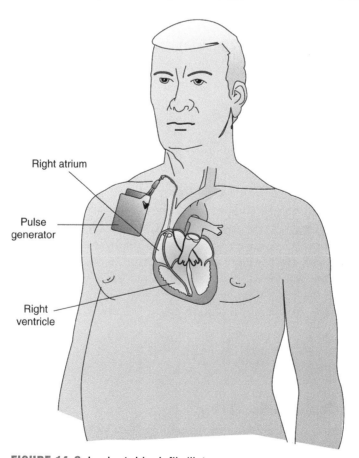

FIGURE 14-6 Implantable defibrillator

tachycardia). *Pulse generators* are implanted internally (permanent) or attached externally (temporary). *Leads that contain electrode(s)* are inserted through a vein using a transvenous approach, or they are inserted on the surface of the heart via thoracotomy. Types of pacemaker and ICD systems with lead(s) include:

- *Single chamber*: Connects a pulse generator to a lead that is inserted in one heart chamber
- *Dual chamber*: Connects a pulse generator to two leads that are inserted in the right atrium and right ventricle
- *Multiple chamber:* Connects a pulse generator to three leads in the right atrium, right ventricle, and left ventricle for biventricular pacing

Example 1: Patient underwent insertion of new permanent pacemaker with transvenous electrode into right atrium. Report code 33206.

Example 2: Patient underwent insertion of permanent pacemaker pulse generator, which was connected to existing dual leads. Report code 33213.

Example 3: Patient underwent insertion of initial permanent implantable defibrillator system pulse generator, dual-chamber transvenous leads, and pacing electrode for left ventricular pacing. Report codes 33249 and 33225. (Do not report modifier 51 with the add-on code.)

Leadless Cardiac Pacemaker

A *leadless cardiac pacemaker system* uses a transcatheter approach to implant a pulse generator with built-in battery in a cardiac chamber (e.g., ventricle).

Example: Transcatheter insertion of permanent leadless pacemaker system, right ventricle, with imaging guidance and device evaluation. Report code 33274.

Replacement of Pulse Generator and Leads

A *replacement pulse generator procedure* is required every 5 to 10 years because of the pulse generator's battery life. Surgery is performed to remove the existing device, disconnect leads, and insert a new pulse generator. Leads are then connected and tested.

Example: Patient underwent permanent pulse generator replacement procedure, single-lead system. Report code 33227.

A more complex *replacement lead procedure* is required when leads fail or the pulse generator becomes infected. Freeing leads from inside each vein for removal is more difficult (than implanting them). Leads follow lengths of veins into heart chambers, and scar tissue forms at multiple sites along that length. Surgeons use a device (e.g., guidewire, sheath) to enclose each lead so that scar tissue is disrupted as the device is advanced toward heart chambers. (Electrocautery is used to heat and vaporize scar tissue. Laser technology is used to vaporize water molecules in scar tissue.) Only after the lead has been freed from its attachments can it be removed from the vein. If devices are not successful in removing each lead, specialized tools are inserted through the femoral vein for lead removal.

Example: Patient underwent replacement of a subcutaneous implantable cardioverter defibrillator (ICD) system with subcutaneous electrode, which required insertion of a new system and electrode, removal of the ICD pulse generator, and removal of the subcutaneous electrode. Report codes 33270, 33241 51, and 33272 51.

Coding Tip

- The CPT *Pacemaker or Implantable Defibrillator* subcategory contains a table of transvenous procedures with codes that are reported for pacemakers and implantable cardioverter-defibrillator systems, which helps clarify code assignment.

- When implantable defibrillator electrodes are removed, a transvenous extraction may be attempted; however, if unsuccessful, a thoracotomy may be required to remove the electrodes.

- When a pacemaker or implantable defibrillator "battery" is changed, it is actually the pulse generator that is changed. Replacement of a pulse generator is reported with two codes: a code for removal of the pulse generator and a code for insertion of a new pulse generator.

- When pacemaker or implantable defibrillator electrodes are replaced, report appropriate code(s) from the *Pacemaker or Implantable Defibrillator* subcategory. Do not report a separate pacemaker removal code, which would be considered overcoding.

NOTE:

When evaluation of a pacemaker system is performed, report a code from the Medicine section. An evaluation is performed after the insertion procedure to determine whether the pacemaker or implantable defibrillator is functioning properly and/or has to be reprogrammed.

Phrenic Nerve Stimulation System

Phrenic Nerve Stimulation System procedures include insertion of the pulse generator, one or more electronic leads, vessel catheterization, imaging guidance, system initiation diagnostic mode, and associated system evaluation. Postsurgical therapeutic activation of the phrenic nerve stimulation system is reported with codes from the CPT Medicine section. *Phrenic nerve stimulation* reanimates the diaphragm of patients with respiratory insufficiency due to central nervous system diagnoses of brain stem injury, congenital central hypoventilation syndrome, spinal cord injury above C4, and idiopathic severe sleep apnea.

> **Example:** Patient underwent insertion of a phrenic nerve stimulation system surgery, which included a pulse generator, two stimulating leads, and one phrenic nerve stimulator transvenous sensing lead. Vessel catheterization, imaging guidance, and initial analysis with diagnostic mode activation were required during the procedure. Report codes 33276 and 33277.

Electrophysiologic Operative Procedures

Electrophysiology is the study of heart arrhythmias; electrophysiologic (EP) procedures analyze heart rhythm abnormalities and include operative ablation or operative incisions and reconstruction of the atria to correct abnormal pathways. The electrophysiology procedure is invasive, similar to a cardiac catheterization, in that electrode catheters are introduced into the right side of the heart from the femoral, brachial, or jugular vein. The catheters positioned in the heart are used to measure and record cardiac rhythm.

- Operative **cardiac ablation (modified Maze procedure)** stops atrial or ventricular fibrillation by using radiofrequency waves (modified electrical energy) to create small scars on the heart's surface. Impulses are redirected and follow a normal electrical pathway through the heart.

- The **Maze procedure** stops atrial fibrillation or atrial flutter by using incisions in heart tissue to stop abnormal heart rhythm.

NOTE:

When the physician performs an "operative" cardiac ablation (also called a Maze procedure), a code is assigned from the CPT Surgery section. Cardiac ablation is sometimes called "cardiac catheter ablation"; however, that procedure is assigned a code from the CPT Medicine section.

Both types of EP procedures require thoracotomy to access the heart, and cardiopulmonary bypass may or may not be used.

Example: Patient underwent operative ablation of ventricular arrhythmogenic focus with cardiopulmonary bypass. Thoracotomy was used to access the heart. Report code 33261.

Subcutaneous Cardiac Rhythm Monitor

A subcutaneous cardiac rhythm monitor is a cardiac event recorder or implantable/insertable loop recorder (ILR), which is placed subcutaneously into a small pre-pectoral pocket. It continuously records the patient's electrocardiographic rhythm, and the device is automatically triggered when rapid, irregular, or slow heart rates are detected.

Example: Patient underwent insertion of subcutaneous cardiac rhythm monitor, which included programming. Report code 33285.

Implantable Hemodynamic Monitors

An implantable hemodynamic monitor is an intravascular device that is implanted via transcatheter approach. It is used for long-term remote (wireless) pulmonary artery pressure monitoring. (A code from the Medicine section is reported for the weekly remote monitoring of pulmonary artery pressures.)

Example: Patient underwent transcatheter implantation of wireless pulmonary artery pressure sensor for long-term hemodynamic monitoring, which included deployment and calibration of the sensor. The physician reviewed recordings of remote monitoring of the wireless pulmonary artery pressure sensor on a weekly basis during the month of July, and the physician prepared a report that included interpretation and trend analysis. Report codes 33289 and 93264.

Heart (Including Valves) and Great Vessels

Repairs to injuries of the heart and/or great vessels (e.g., stab wounds and gunshot wounds) may require cardiopulmonary bypass during the procedure. Many services allow distinct reporting of procedure codes *with or without cardiopulmonary bypass*. When support of cardiac output using devices (e.g., intra-aortic balloon) is documented, report an appropriate code.

 Coding Tip

To report removal of a thrombus in addition to codes for other cardiac procedures performed during the same operative session, a separate incision into the heart is required (to remove the atrial or ventricular thrombus). Add modifier 59 to the appropriate code when it is reported for "removal of a thrombus with coronary bypass" in addition to codes for other cardiac procedures.

Example: Patient underwent repair of cardiac stab wound, with cardiopulmonary bypass. Separate incision was made to remove atrial thrombus. Report codes 33305 and 33315 59.

Cardiac Valves

Cardiac valves are flaps of tissue that keep blood flowing in one direction to allow for the efficient one-way flow of blood through the heart's chambers. *Valvular heart disease* is the abnormality or dysfunction of one or more of the heart's four valves (aortic, mitral, pulmonary, and tricuspid).

- *Valvular atresia*: Valve fails to develop properly and is completely closed at birth
- *Valvular prolapse*: Two valvular flaps do not close properly
- *Valvular regurgitation*: Backflow of blood due to valvular prolapse
- *Valvular stenosis*: Narrowing of one or more cardiac valves

When coding procedures are performed on cardiac valves, first determine the valve involved.

- Aortic
- Mitral
- Tricuspid
- Pulmonary

Then determine the type of procedure performed.

- **Valvuloplasty**: Open-heart surgery during which the surgeon removes the damaged valve and replaces it with a prosthetic, homograft or allograft, stented, or stentless valve (Figure 14-7)

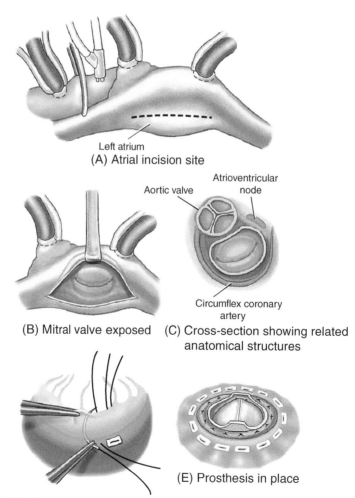

FIGURE 14-7 Mitral valve replacement: (A) Atrial incision site; (B) Mitral valve exposed; (C) Cross-section showing related anatomical structures; (D) Sutures placed in annulus; (E) Prosthesis in place

Coding Tip

When nonsurgical, catheter-based, percutaneous balloon valvuloplasty is performed, report a code from the CPT Medicine section (92986–92990).

- **Valvulotomy**: Open-heart surgery in which an incision is made into a valve to repair valvular damage; includes **commissurotomy**, in which narrowed valve leaflets are widened by carefully opening the fused leaflets with a scalpel

Coding Tip

When multiple valve procedures are performed during the same operative session, add modifier 51 to the second (and subsequent) valve procedure code(s).

NOTE:

A **stented valve** includes framework on which the replacement valve is mounted to provide support for the valve's leaflets. A **stentless valve** is often an actual heart valve obtained from either a human donor (homograft) or a pig, and it does not contain framework. Stentless valves are preferred because they are less obstructive and have improved long-term performance.

Example 1: Patient underwent aortic valvuloplasty with cardiopulmonary bypass. Report code 33390.

Example 2: Patient underwent open replacement of the aortic valve with a stentless tissue valve, including cardiopulmonary bypass. Report code 33410.

Example 3: Patient underwent right ventricular resection for infundibular stenosis, with commissurotomy. Report code 33476.

Other Valvular Procedures

Other Valvular Procedures codes are reported for the repair of non-structural prosthetic valve dysfunction with cardiopulmonary bypass as a separate procedure.

Example: Patient underwent repair of non-structural prosthetic valve dysfunction with cardiopulmonary bypass. Report code 33496.

Coronary Artery Anomalies

An *arteriovenous fistula* is an abnormal passageway between an artery and a vein that allows blood to flow directly into a vein. It can occur as a congenital defect or as the result of trauma. (A fistula can also be surgically created to provide a site for vascular access.) An arteriovenous fistula can occur anywhere in the body, but it most often occurs in the legs or arms. The fistula might eventually develop into an *aneurysm* (bulge in an artery that can weaken the arterial wall and eventually burst, resulting in hemorrhage). For example, a coronary arteriovenous fistula (or coronary artery fistula) is a congenital fistula that is often located between the right coronary artery and the right heart.

> **Example:** Patient underwent a Takeuchi procedure, which involved constructing an intrapulmonary artery tunnel. Report code 33505.

Endoscopy

When an endoscopic approach is used to harvest veins for coronary artery bypass procedures, report code 33508 as an add-on code.

> **Example:** Patient underwent coronary artery bypass graft (CABG) procedure, single coronary venous graft, with endoscopic harvesting of saphenous vein. Report codes 33510 and 33508.

Coronary Artery Bypass Graft (CABG) Procedures

The Cardiovascular System subsection includes coronary artery bypass graft (CABG) procedures, which are organized according to type of graft.

- Venous grafting only for coronary artery bypass
- Combined arterial-venous grafting for coronary bypass (add-on codes)
- Arterial grafting for coronary artery bypass

Coronary artery bypass graft (CABG) (pronounced "cabbage") (Figure 14-8) is a procedure performed to improve the flow of blood to the heart. A blood vessel (called a graft) is removed from the arm, leg, or chest and anastomosed to bypass (detour) the blood flow around a narrowed or blocked coronary artery. (The surgery relieves angina symptoms, improves the patient's ability to exercise, and reduces the patient's risk of a heart attack.) Correctly reporting CABG requires careful review of the operative report to determine the number and type of grafts performed.

 NOTE:

CABG categories include notes about harvesting the saphenous vein graft, an artery, an upper extremity artery or vein, or a femoropopliteal vein segment.

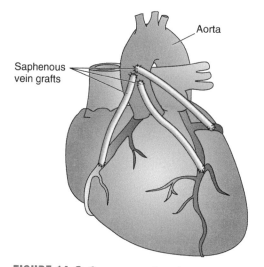

FIGURE 14-8 Coronary artery bypass graft (CABG) using saphenous vein grafts

Venous Grafting Only for Coronary Artery Bypass

CABG procedures that use venous grafts only are *not* reported when CABG procedures use a combination of arterial and venous grafts during the same procedure.

Combined Arterial-Venous Grafting for Coronary Bypass

The add-on codes reported for combined arterial-venous grafts are always reported in addition to codes from the Arterial Grafting for Coronary Artery Bypass subcategory.

Arterial Grafting for Coronary Artery Bypass

Coronary artery bypass procedures that use either arterial grafts only *or* a combination of arterial-venous grafts include the use of the internal mammary artery, gastroepiploic artery, epigastric artery, radial artery, and arterial conduits procured from other sites.

> **Example:** Patient underwent CABG procedure for arteriosclerotic heart disease. A single arterial graft was performed. The sternum was opened, the heart was stopped and cooled, and the patient was connected to cardiopulmonary bypass. A long piece of the saphenous vein was harvested, and one end was attached to the ascending aorta. The other end of the graft was attached to the circumflex coronary artery, just below the blocked area. Report codes 33533 LC and 33517.

 Coding Tip

HCPCS Level II modifiers identify placement of the bypass grafts and are added to the CABG code.

- LC (left circumflex coronary artery)
- LD (left anterior descending coronary artery)
- RC (right coronary artery)

Coronary Endarterectomy

Coronary endarterectomy is performed to remove the inner layer of coronary arteries that contain cholesterol plaques. When a patient's coronary arteries contain extensive cholesterol plaque, a CABG procedure cannot be performed until the plaque is removed via coronary endarterectomy.

> **Example:** Patient underwent coronary endarterectomy of the left anterior descending and left circumflex coronary arteries. During the same operative session, the patient also underwent double CABG. The graft sections were obtained from the internal mammary arteries. Report codes 33534 LC LD, 33572, and 33572.

Single Ventricle and Other Complex Cardiac Anomalies

Procedures performed to correct single ventricle and other complex cardiac anomalies include, for example, the Norwood procedure to repair a single ventricle that has an aortic outflow obstruction and aortic arch hypoplasia. During the procedure, the pulmonary artery is connected to the right ventricle, using a shunt, and the underdeveloped aorta is enlarged and reconstructed.

> **Example:** Patient diagnosed with tricuspid atresia undergoes repair that involves closure of the atrial septal defect and anastomosis of the vena cava to the pulmonary artery. Report code 33615.

Congenital Heart Defects

Congenital heart defects include the following:

- Septal defects
- Sinus of Valsalva defects
- Venous anomalies
- Shunting procedures

- Transposition of great vessels
- Truncus arteriosus
- Aortic anomalies

Septal Defects

The *septum* is tissue that separates the heart's left and right sides. *Septal defects* occur when the tissue doesn't completely close between the heart's chambers (atria or ventricles). This allows oxygen-rich blood from one side of the heart (e.g., left atrium) to mix with oxygen-poor blood on the other side (e.g., right atrium). The extra blood flows through the hole, causing a swishing sound, which is called a *heart murmur* (an extra heart sound).

> **Example:** Patient underwent repair of atrial septal defect, secundum, with cardiopulmonary bypass, without patch. The right atrium was opened, and the size and location of the atrial septal defect was assessed. Due to the small size of the atrial septal tissue, it was closed with a suture. Report code 33641.

The *tetralogy of Fallot* is a congenital heart condition that includes ventral septal defect, stenosis of the infundibulum, hypertrophy of the right ventricle, and an abnormally positioned aorta.

> **Example:** Patient underwent complete repair of tetralogy of Fallot without pulmonary atresia using transannular patch. Report code 33694.

Sinus of Valsalva Defects

The *sinus of Valsalva* (or *aortic sinus*) is an anatomical dilation of the ascending aorta that occurs just above the aortic valve (e.g., left anterior aortic sinus that gives rise to the left coronary artery). Defects include aneurysms and fistulas for which repair and closure procedures are performed.

> **Example:** Patient underwent surgical repair of a sinus of Valsalva aneurysm, with cardiopulmonary bypass. Report code 33720.

Venous Anomalies

Venous anomalies are associated with systemic veins and pulmonary veins and include conditions such as

- *Cor triatriatum* (congenital anomaly in which left atrium or right atrium is divided into two parts by a fold of tissue, membrane, or fibromuscular band; referred to as a heart with three atria)
- *Pulmonary vein stenosis* (abnormal thickening and narrowing of walls of pulmonary veins)
- *Scimitar syndrome* (congenital condition in which an aberrant vessel connects pulmonary vein in right lung to inferior vena cava)
- *Supravalvular mitral ring* (rare congenital defect characterized by an abnormal ridge of connective tissue on the atrial side of the mitral valve)
- *Total anomalous pulmonary venous return (TAPVR)* (rare congenital defect in which all four pulmonary veins do not connect normally to the left atrium but instead drain to the right atrium by way of an abnormal connection)

> **Example:** Patient underwent surgical repair of supravalvular mitral ring via resection of left atrial membrane. Report code 33732.

Shunting Procedures

Shunting procedures are performed to move blood from one area to another, and they are performed for conditions such as

- *Atrial septal defect (ASD)* (opening in atrial septum fails to close after birth)
- *Coarctation of the aorta* (part of the aorta has a very narrow section, similar in appearance to an hourglass timer, reducing blood flow)
- *Patent ductus arteriosus (PDA)* (opening between aorta and pulmonary artery fails to close after birth)
- *Tricuspid atresia* (tricuspid valve is deformed, narrow, or missing)
- *Ventricular septal defect (VSD)* (opening in ventricular septum fails to close after birth)

> **Example:** Patient underwent a shunt procedure of the descending aorta to the pulmonary artery to correct patent ductus arteriosus. Report code 33762.

Transposition of Great Vessels

The *transposition of great vessels* is the congenital reversal of the aorta and pulmonary artery. The pulmonary arteries are supplied by the left ventricle, and the aorta is supplied by the right ventricle—the opposite of the normal arrangement.

> **Example:** Patient underwent repair of transposition of the great arteries with aortic and pulmonary artery reconstruction. Report code 33778.

Truncus Arteriosus

Truncus arteriosus is a congenital malformation in which just one artery arises from the heart to form the aorta and pulmonary artery.

> **Example:** Patient underwent total repair of truncus arteriosus. Report code 33786.

Aortic Anomalies

Aortic Anomalies codes include repair procedures. *Aortic anomalies* result from unusual patterns of aortic development and include conditions such as

- *Tracheal decompression* (or *tracheomalacia*) (softness of cartridge that supports tracheal walls, which can be due to *vascular ring formation* and results in tracheal collapse and decreased airflow)
- *Aberrant vessels* (or *vascular ring formation*) (abnormal growth of vessels, which encircle trachea and esophagus and result in upper airway obstruction)
- *Aortopulmonary septal defect (APSD)* (deficiency in the septum between aorta and pulmonary artery, resulting in abnormal communication between them)
- *Patent ductus arteriosus* (opening between aorta and pulmonary artery fails to close after birth)
- *Coarctation of aorta* (part of the aorta has a very narrow section, similar in appearance to an hourglass timer, reducing blood flow)
- *Hypoplastic aortic arch* (or *interrupted aortic arch*) (absence of a portion of the aortic arch, creating a gap between the ascending and descending aorta)

> **Example:** Patient underwent surgical division of aberrant vessels with aortopexy to correct tracheomalacia. Report codes 33802 and 33800 51.

Thoracic Aortic Aneurysm

An aneurysm (Figure 14-9) is a bulge in an artery that can weaken the arterial wall and eventually burst, resulting in hemorrhage.

> **Example:** Patient underwent transverse aortic arch graft to repair thoracic aortic aneurysm. Cardiopulmonary bypass was provided with profound hypothermia, total circulatory arrest, and isolated cerebral perfusion with reimplantation of arch vessel. Report code 33871.

Endovascular Repair of Descending Thoracic Aorta

Endovascular aneurysm repair procedures involve the placement of grafts to repair defects of the thoracic aorta (e.g., aneurysm, intramural hematoma, penetrating ulcer, traumatic disruption). When fluoroscopic guidance is used during endovascular repair procedures, report a code from the Radiology section (when the Surgery code does not include such guidance).

 NOTE:

Interventional procedures performed with endovascular repair of the descending thoracic aorta are reported separately (e.g., innominate, carotid, subclavian, visceral, or iliac artery transluminal angioplasty or stenting).

> **Example:** Patient underwent placement of proximal extension prosthesis for endovascular repair of descending thoracic aorta dissecting aneurysm, initial extension only. Fluoroscopic guidance confirmed appropriate placement. Report codes 33883 and 75958. (According to Optum's *EncoderPro.com Expert*, modifier 51 is *not* added to the Radiology code.)

Pulmonary Artery

Pulmonary Artery codes describe procedures performed on the pulmonary artery.

> **Example:** Patient underwent repair of pulmonary atresia with ventricular septal defect, by construction or replacement of conduit from right or left ventricle to pulmonary artery. Report code 33920.

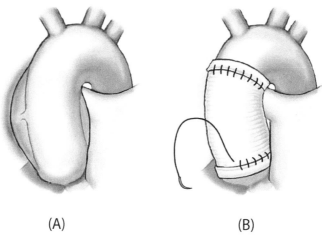

(A)   (B)

FIGURE 14-9 Aortic aneurysm repair (A) Aortic aneurysm
(B) Graft repair of aneurysm

Heart/Lung Transplantation

Guidelines for heart/lung transplantation include three components.

- **Cadaver donor cardiectomy with or without pneumonectomy,** which involves harvesting the allograft (graft such as lung tissue that is transplanted between genetically nonidentical individuals of the same species) and preserving the allograft with cold preservation solution and cold maintenance
- Backbench work, which involves preparing the cadaver donor heart and/or lung allograft prior to lung transplantation and dissecting allograft from surrounding soft tissues to prepare the aorta, superior vena cava, inferior vena cava, pulmonary artery, left atrium, and/or trachea for implantation
- **Recipient heart with or without lung allotransplantation,** which includes transplantation of the allograft and care of the recipient

> **Example:** Patient with severe cardiomyopathy underwent heart transplant procedure to remove a diseased heart and replace it with healthy heart from a recently deceased donor. Transplant physician performed donor cardiectomy including cold preservation from cadaver donor, backbench standard preparation of cadaver donor heart allograft, and heart transplant with cardiopulmonary bypass. Report code 33940 for the donor procedure, and report codes 33944 and 33945 51 for procedures performed on the recipient. Modifier 51 (Multiple procedures) is added to code 33945 only. (Cold preservation is a component of the donor organ harvesting procedure, not the backbench preparation.)
>
> When donor cardiectomy and backbench preparation are performed at a facility other than the transplant facility (and the removed organ is transported to the transplant facility), codes 33940 (donor procedure) and 33944 (recipient procedure) are reported by the first facility. Code 33945 51 (recipient procedure) is reported by the transplant facility.

Extracorporeal Membrane Oxygenation or Extracorporeal Life Support Services

Extracorporeal membrane oxygenation (ECMO) or **extracorporeal life support (ECLS)** provides cardiac and/or respiratory support to the heart and/or lungs, which allow them to rest and recover when patients are sick or injured. The CPT coding manual contains a table of codes for ECMO/ECLS procedures, which helps provide direction to proper codes.

> **Example:** Veno-venous extracorporeal life support was initiated by the patient's physician. Report code 33946.

Cardiac Assist

Cardiac assist procedures include the insertion, implantation, and removal of various devices. A **ventricular assist device (VAD)** provides temporary support for the heart by substituting for left or right heart function (e.g., after myocardial infarction).

> **Example:** Patient underwent percutaneous insertion of intra-aortic balloon assist device into the common femoral artery. Device was then advanced to the distal aortic arch. Report code 33967.

Exercise 14.1 – Heart and Pericardium

Instructions: Assign the CPT code(s) and appropriate modifier(s) to each statement.

1. Patient underwent aortic valve replacement with stentless tissue valve, by division. Cardiopulmonary bypass was provided.

   _____

2. An 18-year-old patient underwent repair of ductus arteriosus by division. Posterolateral thoracotomy was performed to access the heart.

   _____

3. Patient underwent coronary artery bypass surgery using a saphenous vein graft and an internal mammary artery graft.

   _____

4. A seven-year-old child underwent repair of pulmonary atresia with ventricular septal defect by constructing a conduit from the left ventricle to the pulmonary artery.

   _____

5. Patient underwent insertion of permanent pacemaker system with transvenous epicardial electrode (lead), ventricular, via open incision. A pacing electrode was also inserted in the left ventricle to provide a biventricular (dual chamber) pacing system and attached to the inserted pacemaker.

   _____

6. Patient underwent subtotal pericardiectomy, with cardiopulmonary bypass.

   _____

7. Subcutaneous cardiac rhythm monitor was inserted, including programming, in a 54-year-old patient.

   _____

8. Patient underwent sinus of Valsalva fistula repair, with cardiopulmonary bypass.

   _____

9. Operative ablation of ventricular arrhythmogenic focus was performed on a 62-year-old patient, with cardiopulmonary bypass.

   _____

10. Patient underwent transection of pulmonary artery, with cardiopulmonary bypass.

    _____

11. The physician performed pericardiocentesis to drain fluid from the pericardial space, under ultrasonic guidance.

    _____

12. The physician repositioned a previously implanted transvenous pacemaker right ventricular electrode.

    _____

13. Patient underwent banding of pulmonary artery.

    _____

14. The physician opened the right atrium, and a stiff ring was inserted for valvuloplasty of the tricuspid valve.

    _____

Exercise 14.1 – continued

15. Using cardiopulmonary bypass, the physician repaired an artificial prosthetic valve that was malfunctioning due to leakage.

_____

16. The physician performed coronary endarterectomy (open), left anterior descending artery, during the same operative session as coronary artery bypass graft (CABG) procedure (using one arterial graft).

_____

17. The physician performed a Damus-Kaye-Stansel anastomosis procedure.

_____

18. The surgeon repaired transposition of the great arteries via Jatene-type aortic pulmonary artery reconstruction, including closure of ventricular septal defect.

_____

19. The physician repaired an atrial septal defect and ventricular septal defect with patch closure.

_____

20. Using cardiopulmonary bypass, the physician repaired a thoracoabdominal aortic aneurysm using a prosthetic graft.

_____

Arteries and Veins

The Arteries and Veins subsection requires an excellent understanding of the anatomy of vascular structures because it is organized according to artery or vein (and approach). Notes at the beginning of the Arteries and Veins subsection indicate the following:

- Codes for procedures performed on arteries and veins include the establishment of both inflow and outflow by whatever procedures are necessary. This means that separate codes for establishing inflow and outflow are not reported.
- The portion of the operative arteriogram that is performed by the surgeon is included in codes for procedures performed on arteries and veins. (When the radiologist participates by supervising and interpreting an arteriogram, a separate code is reported.)
- When a **sympathectomy** (excision of a segment of the sympathetic nerve) procedure is performed, it is included in the codes for aortic procedures. For example, a lumbar sympathectomy might be performed to improve collateral blood supply to the foot when reconstructive surgery is not possible.

Embolectomy/Thrombectomy

An **embolectomy** is the surgical removal of an _embolus_ (blood clot that circulates throughout the bloodstream), and a **thrombectomy** is the surgical removal of a thrombus (fixed blood clot). Before reporting a code, make sure you identify the type of blood vessel (artery or vein) and the approach used to remove the embolus or thrombus (e.g., catheter and/or incision).

Example 1: Patient underwent carotid embolectomy with catheter, by neck incision. Report code 34001.

Example 2: Patient underwent direct subclavian vein thrombectomy, by neck incision. Report code 34471.

Venous Reconstruction

Venous reconstruction procedures are performed to repair venous valves, the vena cava, and venous transposition. Leg veins contain valves, which contain two leaflets to allow blood to flow in one direction toward the heart. When venous valves become damaged and fail to function properly, the backflow of blood occurs, resulting in varicose veins, pain, leg swelling, hyperpigmentation (skin discoloration), and skin ulcers (breakdown of the skin). Valvuloplasty is performed to repair incompetent valves by opening the vein; exposing the leaflets after dissecting the vein from surrounding tissues; and placing very fine sutures to attach the valve edges to the vein wall, which tightens the valve flaps when the vein is closed.

Reconstruction of the vena cava is performed to correct a congenital defect or to repair the vena cava when the patient sustains trauma or the vena cava is damaged due to long-term drug therapy (e.g., chemotherapy). For example, the obstructed or damaged portion of the vena cava is resected and repaired with an autologous (graft from patient's own body) pericardial patch.

Venous valve transposition is performed to treat chronic deep venous insufficiency. An incision is made to expose the venous valve, and the section of the vein that contains the malfunctioning valve is excised. Then a harvested vein that contains functional valves is anastomosed end-to-end to the remaining vein.

A **cross-over vein graft** procedure involves making an incision to expose the vein's incompetent valve, dividing that section of the vein, and connecting it to a nearby vein that has functioning valves.

A **saphenopopliteal vein anastomosis** involves making an incision to expose the saphenous vein and connecting it to the popliteal vein using end-to-end anastomosis.

> **Example:** Patient developed chronic benign superior vena cava syndrome due to long-term use of central venous catheters for administration of chemotherapy. Reconstruction of vena cava was performed by resecting the obstructed segment and placing an autologous pericardial patch. Report code 34502.

Coding Tip

The list of procedures included with and excluded from endovascular repair of an abdominal aortic aneurysm varies slightly from those associated with endovascular repair of an iliac aneurysm. For example, open femoral or iliac artery exposure is included with endovascular repair of an abdominal aortic aneurysm, but it is reported separately when performed with endovascular repair of an iliac aneurysm.

Repair of Aneurysms

The Arteries and Veins category includes the repair of aneurysms and related procedures.

- Endovascular Repair of Abdominal Aortic Aneurysm and/or Iliac Arteries
- Fenestrated Endovascular Repair of the Visceral and Infrarenal Aorta
- Direct Repair of Aneurysm or Excision (Partial or Total) and Graft Insertion for Aneurysm, Pseudoaneurysm, Ruptured Aneurysm, and Associated Occlusive Disease

An aneurysm is an abnormal "bulging" of a portion of a vessel, usually due to a weakness or thinning of the vessel wall at that location (Figure 14-10). It can be caused by congenital or acquired weakness of the vessel wall. Minimally invasive procedures are performed to implant endovascular devices (e.g., endovascular graft) for treatment of aortic and iliac aneurysms. **Direct aneurysm repair** includes surgical suture of the

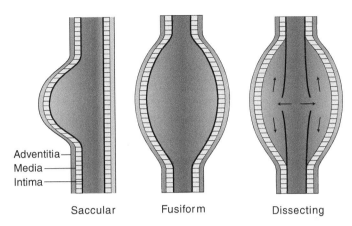

Adventitia
Media
Intima

Saccular   Fusiform   Dissecting

FIGURE 14-10 Three types of aneurysms

sac of an aneurysm and may also include partial or total excision of the arterial segment that contains the aneurysm and insertion of a graft, using end-to-end anastomosis (Figure 14-11).

Because a number of different methods are used to repair abdominal aortic aneurysms, the coder must review the operative report to identify

- Whether an endovascular or direct (open) repair of the abdominal aortic aneurysm was performed
- What the artery and type of exposure were (e.g., open femoral artery exposure for delivery of endovascular prosthesis, by groin incision, unilateral)
- What type of device was used for repair (e.g., modular bifurcated prosthesis)
- What other separately reported procedures or services were provided (e.g., fluoroscopy)

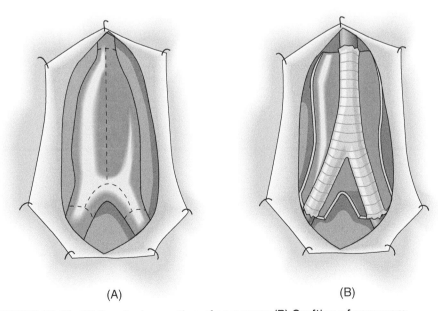

(A)   (B)

FIGURE 14-11 (A) Surgical resection of aneurysm (B) Grafting of aneurysm

Coding Tip

- Codes for endovascular repair of aneurysms include balloon angioplasty with target treatment zone either before or after graft deployment, distal extensions, manipulation, and positioning.
- When assigning codes for aneurysm repair, review the patient record to determine if the type of repair is direct (open) or endovascular. Direct repairs are performed on the thoracic aorta and all other arteries. Endovascular repairs are performed on the thoracic aorta, abdominal aorta, and iliac artery.

Example 1: Patient underwent endovascular repair of descending thoracic aorta (for aneurysm), involving coverage of left subclavian artery origin, initial endoprosthesis plus descending thoracic aortic extension to the level of the celiac artery origin with placement of proximal extension prosthesis for endovascular repair of descending thoracic aorta. Report codes 33880 and 75956. (According to Optum's *EncoderPro.com Expert*, modifier 51 is *not* added to the CPT Radiology code.)

- Notice that the code is located in the *Endovascular Repair of Descending Thoracic Aorta* category of the Cardiovascular System subsection and includes *aneurysm* as an example of a condition for which the procedure is performed.
- Do *not* assign code 33883 for placement of proximal extension prosthesis because the parenthetical note below the code description states, "Do not report 33881, 33883 when extension placement converts repair to cover left subclavian origin. Use only 33880."

Example 2: Patient underwent direct repair with partial excision of aneurysm and graft insertion to treat a left carotid aneurysm. Report code 35001 LT.

Repair of Arteriovenous Fistula

An *arteriovenous fistula* is an abnormal connection or passageway between an artery and a vein, which means blood flows directly from an artery into a vein, bypassing the capillaries. A person may be born with an arteriovenous fistula (congenital fistula), or a fistula may develop after birth (acquired fistula due to trauma or other pathology).

Example 1: Patient underwent repair of a congenital arteriovenous fistula, neck. Report code 35180.

Example 2: Patient sustained a knife wound to the abdomen, and a traumatic arteriovenous fistula developed. Surgical repair of the abdominal arteriovenous fistula was performed. Report code 35189.

Repair of Blood Vessel Other Than for Fistula

Generally, the *repair of blood vessels (other than for fistula)* is due to an injured artery or vein, such as a lacerated or torn blood vessel. Repairs include the following types:

- Direct (e.g., a partly divided vessel or one that has been lacerated longitudinally can be sutured, with the cut ends anastomosed)
- Vein graft (e.g., a piece of saphenous vein is harvested from the patient and sutured over lacerated blood vessel to bypass the abnormal section of the vessel)
- Graft other than vein (e.g., synthetic graft material is sutured end-to-end to the vessel, replacing the excised portion)

> **Example 1:** Patient underwent direct repair of superficial basilic vein, left hand. Report code 35207 LT.

> **Example 2:** Patient underwent repair of peroneal artery with synthetic graft, right lower leg. Report code 35286 RT.

Thromboendarterectomy

A **thromboendarterectomy** is the surgical excision of a thrombus and atherosclerotic inner lining from an obstructed artery. It is typically performed to treat calcified plaque or clot formations that don't respond to balloon angioplasty procedures. Coders must carefully review documentation to distinguish between a thrombectomy (e.g., procedure to remove a thrombus or blood clot) and a thromboendarterectomy (e.g., procedure to remove a thrombus and the lining of the artery, including possible placement of a patch graft).

> **Example 1:** Patient underwent abdominal aortic thromboendarterectomy with patch graft. Report code 35331.

> **Example 2:** Patient underwent carotid thromboendarterectomy with patch graft reoperation 90 days after initial carotid thromboendarterectomy (without patch graft). Report codes 35301 and 35390.

Angioscopy

Angioscopy is the microscopic visualization of substances (e.g., contrast media and radiopaque agents) as they pass through capillaries. The intravenous injection of the substance is performed as part of the procedure.

> **Example:** Patient underwent endovascular repair of infrarenal abdominal aortic aneurysm using aorto-aortic tube prosthesis. Prior to performing the therapeutic portion of the procedure, angioscopy was performed to visualize the interior of the aortic arch. Subsequently, under abdominal aortographic guidance, initial third-order vascular catheterization of left infrarenal artery was performed and atherectomy catheter device was advanced to the aorta. In addition to codes for the endovascular repair (34701, 36247 LT, 75625), report code 35400. (Do not add modifier 51 to code 35400.)

Bypass Graft

Bypass graft procedures are performed on veins and *in situ* veins. Procedures include the use of "other than vein" material (e.g., synthetic graft) as bypass grafts for arteries. Each reported code describes the bypass graft anastomosis location (e.g., carotid-vertebral, carotid-subclavian).

> **Example 1:** Patient underwent bypass graft, with vein, of the left femoral-popliteal artery. Report code 35556 LT.

> **Example 2:** Patient underwent *in situ* vein bypass of the right femoral-popliteal artery. Report code 35583 RT.

> **Example 3:** Patient underwent synthetic bypass graft, common carotid-ipsilateral internal carotid artery, right. Report code 35601 RT.

Composite Grafts

Add-on codes for composite grafts describe harvesting and anastomosis of multiple vein segments as arterial bypass graft conduits. A **composite graft** contains vein and synthetic graft material *or* segments of veins from two or more locations, such as saphenous vein and femoral vein.

Example 1: Patient underwent bypass graft procedure of right femoral-popliteal artery with Gore-Tex synthetic graft and a portion of the right saphenous vein. Report 35556 RT and 35681.

Example 2: Patient underwent bypass graft procedure of right femoral-femoral artery. Vein grafts were obtained from the left brachial and left basilic veins. Report codes 35558 RT and 35682 LT.

 NOTE:

The most common material used for "other than vein" includes synthetic materials such as Gore-Tex.

Adjuvant Techniques

Add-on code(s) for **adjuvant techniques** are additional procedures or techniques that may be required during a *lower extremity* bypass graft procedure. They are performed to improve the *patency* (open and unblocked status of a blood vessel or another tube in the body) of *lower extremity* synthetic or autogenous arterial bypass grafts.

Example 1: Patient underwent right popliteal-tibial bypass grafting with Gore-Tex synthetic graft material. Adjuvant distal vein cuff (DVC) of the popliteal-tibial bypass graft was performed during the same operative session. Report codes 35671 RT and 35685 RT. (Do not add modifier 51 to code 35685.)

Example 2: Patient underwent left femoral-popliteal bypass grafting with polytetrafluoroethylene synthetic material. Adjuvant distal arteriovenous fistula (DAVF) of the femoral-popliteal graft was performed during the same operative session. Report codes 35656 LT and 35686 LT. (Do not add modifier 51 to code 35686.)

Arterial Transposition

Arterial transposition and/or reimplantation procedures are performed to improve arterial blood flow. An add-on code is reported for reimplantation procedures involving *visceral arteries*, which supply blood to the intestines, liver, and spleen.

Example 1: Patient underwent transposition surgery to anastomose the right vertebral artery to the right subclavian artery. Report code 35693 RT.

Example 2: Patient underwent bypass graft surgery of splenorenal artery, during which synthetic graft material was used. Replantation of splenic artery to infrarenal aortic prosthesis was performed during the same operative session to ensure adequate blood supply to the spleen. (The splenorenal artery is a visceral artery because it supplies blood to the spleen and kidneys.) Report codes 35636 and 35697.

Excision, Exploration, Repair, Revision

Excision, exploration, repair, and revision procedures include reoperations, explorations not followed by surgical repair or for postoperative hemorrhage, repair of grant-enteric fistulas, and thrombectomies of arterial or venous grafts, including revision procedures.

Example: Patient underwent exploration for suspected postoperative hemorrhage, chest. Five days ago patient underwent CABG surgery. Report 35820 78.

Vascular Injection Procedures

Vascular injection procedure codes describe common procedures performed to gain venous access for phlebotomy, prophylactic intravenous access, infusion therapy, chemotherapy, and drug administration. They are reported for

- Diagnostic catheterization (e.g., injecting contrast media into vasculature for radiologic imaging)
- Therapeutic (interventional) catheterization (e.g., balloon dilation or stent placement to open narrowed valves and vessels)

 NOTE:

CPT index main term Vascular Injection includes a code for "Unlisted Services and Procedures" as the only entry. (There is no index entry for "Injection, Vascular" in the CPT index. Some codes are listed for the "Catheter" main term in the CPT index.) Thus, coders must become familiar with codes and descriptions in the Vascular Injection Procedures category.

CPT also includes codes for cardiovascular procedures in multiple locations. For example, vascular ultrasound procedures for noncoronary vessels are located in the Cardiovascular Surgery section, but vascular ultrasound procedures for coronary vessels and cardiac catheterizations are located in the Medicine section.

Vascular injection procedures include the following services, *which are not coded and reported separately*:

- Injection of contrast media, with or without automatic power injection

 NOTE:

Although the injection procedure is not reported separately, an HCPCS Level II code for provision of contrast media is reported separately.

- Introduction of needles or catheters

 NOTE:

Although the introduction of a needle or catheter is not reported separately, a CPT code for selective vascular catheterization is reported separately.

- Necessary local anesthesia
- Necessary pre- and postinjection care specifically related to the injection procedure

The following supplies are reported with HCPCS Level II codes if provided during a vascular injection procedure:

- Catheters
- Drugs
- Contrast media

Notes below the Vascular Injection Procedures subcategory provide instruction about coding selective vascular catheterization. (Be sure to review previous content about selective vascular catheterization.)

Codes for vascular injection procedures include the following routes:

- Intravenous
- Intra-arterial–intra-aortic (including placement of shunts for dialysis)
- Venous
- Central venous access procedures

 Coding Tip

- When two separate access procedures (e.g., punctures of two different vessels) are performed, report a separate code for each.
- When a nonselective vascular catheterization is converted to a selective vascular catheterization, report a code for the selective vascular catheterization only.

Vascular injection procedures include the introduction of the catheter or needle into a blood vessel and insertion into lesser- (first-) order vessels. Then when the catheter is inserted as follows for the purpose of performing diagnostic and/or therapeutic procedures, the code(s) for selective vascular catheterization is reported:

- Second-, third- (and beyond) order vessels (e.g., popliteal angiogram)
- Aorta and first-, second-, third- (and beyond) order vessels (e.g., carotid angiogram)

 Coding Tip

Codes for cardiac catheterization are reported from the CPT Medicine section.

 Coding Tip

When a catheter is removed from a vessel, do not report a separate code for that procedure. However, when implantable venous access devices and/or subcutaneous reservoirs are removed, report an appropriate code (e.g., code 36589).

Example: Patient underwent left neck venography with radiological supervision and interpretation. Catheter was introduced into superior vena cava and inserted into left brachiocephalic vein. Catheter was manipulated into left internal jugular vein. Contrast media was injected. Good visualization was obtained. No deformities were noted. Report codes 75860 LT (venography, left internal jugular), 36010 LT (introduction of catheter into superior vena cava), 36011 51 LT (manipulation into left internal jugular vein), and A9698 (contrast media, nonradioactive).

CPT code 36200 is reported just once for "introduction of catheter, aorta" regardless of the number of times the catheter is repositioned in the aorta. When multiple vessels are accessed during catheterization, in different vascular families, report the code for the highest level of selectivity in each vascular family.

Venous procedures are coded according to the type of procedure, patient's age, and the puncture site (e.g., two-year-old patient underwent scalp vein venipuncture, 36405). Make sure you carefully review the patient record and code descriptions to determine whether the procedure was a direct puncture or a cutdown and whether a physician's skill was required.

Therapeutic apheresis is the removal of blood components, cells, or plasma solute and the retransfusion of the remaining components into the patient. Procedure codes are based on blood components.

- White blood cells
- Red blood cells
- Platelets
- Plasmapheresis
- Extracorporeal immunoadsorption and plasma reinfusion
- Extracorporeal selective adsorption or selective filtration and plasma reinfusion

Central Venous Access Procedures

Central venous access procedures include insertion, repair, partial replacement, complete replacement, and/or removal of the catheter or device. The CPT coding manual contains the central venous access procedures table, which provides direction for assignment of proper codes. A venous access device is inserted

- Centrally (e.g., femoral, jugular, or subclavian vein or inferior vena cava)
- Peripherally (e.g., basilic or cephalic vein)

A central venous catheter (CVC) or a central venous access device (CVAD) is used to deliver intravenous fluids and medications and to obtain blood samples. These infusions may be administered for short or prolonged periods, using a single-lumen (allows for infusion of one solution) or multiple-lumen catheter (allows for infusion of several solutions simultaneously).

To be considered a central venous access catheter or device, the tip of the CVC or CVAD must terminate in the subclavian, brachiocephalic, or iliac veins; the superior or inferior vena cava; or the right atrium. (Otherwise, the catheter is considered a midline catheter, MLC.) The device is accessed for use (e.g., administration of medications or hyperalimentation) through a(n)

- Exposed catheter (external to the skin)
- Subcutaneous port
- Subcutaneous pump

CVAD codes are reported according to the patient's age and whether the device is nontunneled (not implanted) or tunneled (implanted).

Peripherally inserted CVADs include peripherally inserted central (venous) catheters (PICCs) and MLCs. The type of catheter inserted depends on the technique used, solutions infused, and duration of the intravenous therapy. Any catheter placed with the tip between the antecubital area and the head of the clavicle is called an MLC. Such placement is typically done for infusion therapy, which is expected to last from one to eight weeks (when the catheter tip doesn't need to terminate in the superior vena cava). The PICC can also be shortened if it is needed for midline placement. It is usually inserted below the antecubital fossa and does not require use of a guidewire.

When reporting codes for central venous access procedures, make sure you determine the following:

- Patient's age
- Whether the catheter was **tunneled** (implanted under the skin and inserted into a vein) or **nontunneled** (not implanted under the skin, such as a short-term intravenous catheter that is inserted directly into a large vein)
- Whether the procedure was done via
  - **Cutdown**: Catheter is inserted directly into a vein through an incision
  - **Peripherally**: Catheter is inserted into peripheral vein using a needle or trocar

NOTE:

Tunneled (implantable) venous access ports are typically used for long-term intravenous therapy, and they contain two parts: catheter and port.

 Coding Tip

Before assigning codes, carefully review CPT coding notes about venous access devices, and refer to the *Central Venous Access Procedures Table* in the coding manual.

Repair of Central Venous Access Device (CVAD) procedures are performed to repair, replace, and/or remove CVADs and central venous catheters (CVCs). These codes do not require selection based on the patient's age or central/peripheral insertion site. However, they do distinguish between nontunneled (with exposed access) and tunneled catheters (require subcutaneous port/pump pocket and connection). They also require knowledge of whether a subcutaneous port or pump was inserted.

Example: Patient underwent mechanical removal of a blood clot from a central venous device using venous access. Report code 36595.

Arterial

Arterial blood gases (e.g., arterial blood oxygen, carbon dioxide, and bicarbonate levels) are commonly performed to diagnose the patient's effectiveness of respiration. To report an arterial puncture for the purpose of obtaining a sample for arterial blood gas analysis, report code 36600. During an arterial puncture, a needle is inserted into the artery to obtain a sample of blood; a catheter is *not* inserted into the artery.

 NOTE:

A heparin flush is performed to maintain patency of the catheter/port and to reduce the risk of blood clotting in the catheter. When a heparin flush is performed as a part of an injection or infusion procedure, it is not separately coded.

Example 1: Patient underwent insertion of a catheter into the artery percutaneously for blood sampling; the catheter was removed after sampling was completed. Report code 36620.

Example 2: Patient underwent a cutdown procedure to access an artery after which a catheter was inserted, the artery was sutured, and the incision was closed in layers. Report code 36625.

Intraosseous

Intraosseous infusion requires insertion of a special needle to puncture the bone marrow cavity (e.g., tibia or femur) to infuse fluids into bone marrow blood vessels.

Example: Patient underwent needle placement for intraosseous infusion. Report code 36680.

Hemodialysis Access, Intervascular Cannulation for Extracorporeal Circulation, or Shunt Insertion

Hemodialysis access procedures include

- Arteriovenous anastomosis, direct
- Insertion of cannulas for prolonged extracorporeal circulation of membrane oxygenation (ECMO)
- Arteriovenous fistula

Arteriovenous hemodialysis access is created by using autogenous venous tissue or inserting a prosthetic graft.

Example 1: Patient underwent forearm vein transposition between the right elbow and the wrist. Report code 36820 RT.

Example 2: Patient underwent open arteriovenous anastomosis of the right cephalic vein. (The cephalic vein is located in the upper arm.) Report code 36818 RT.

Dialysis Circuit

Dialysis circuit procedures and services are performed as part of Hemodialysis treatment, which involves circulating arteriovenous (AV) blood outside of the body through the *dialysis circuit*, which is created using an arterial-venous anastomosis (called an AV fistula) or by placing a prosthetic graft between an artery and vein (called an AV graft). The dialysis circuit is designed for easy and repetitive access, and it contains two segments, the peripheral dialysis segment and the central dialysis segment.

Example: Patient underwent percutaneous mechanical thrombectomy with infusion for thrombolysis. Report code 36904.

Portal Decompression Procedures

Portal decompression procedure codes are reported for the insertion and revision of transvenous intrahepatic portosystemic shunt (TIPS) procedures. A TIPS is inserted to reduce portal pressure associated with portal hypertension. Portal blood flow is diverted into the hepatic vein, which reduces pressure between the portal and systemic circulations.

 Coding Tip

Codes for the insertion or revision of TIPS include radiological supervision and interpretation (e.g., portography and all associated imaging guidance and documentation), which means separate Radiology codes are *not* reported.

Example: Patient underwent insertion of TIPS. Report code 37182.

Transcatheter Procedures

The Transcatheter Procedures subcategory contains instructional notes about reporting codes separately for catheter placement and radiological supervision and interpretation. When transcatheter therapy services are provided, the introduction of the needle and catheter are included in the code for the primary service.

Example 1: Patient underwent open transluminal stent placement of the right femoral artery for revascularization with atherectomy and angioplasty of the same vessel. The catheter was introduced into the right femoral artery (second-order artery), and contrast medium was injected. Femoral magnetic resonance angiogram was performed and revealed blockage of the femoral artery. Repeat femoral magnetic resonance angiogram (Figure 14-12), after stent placement, revealed good arterial circulation in the femoral artery. Report codes 37227 RT, 36246 51 RT, and 73725 51 RT.

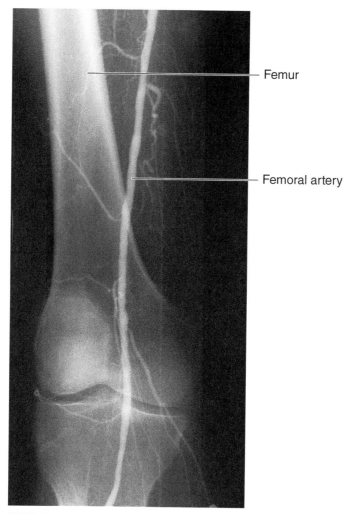

Femur

Femoral artery

FIGURE 14-12 Femoral angiogram. The use of contrast medium makes arteries visible

Example 2: Patient underwent cerebral thrombolysis as therapy for acute ischemic stroke. Report code 37195.

Endovascular Revascularization (Open or Percutaneous, Transcatheter)

Endovascular revascularization procedures are performed for lower extremity occlusive disease, and include open, percutaneous, and transcatheter methods. The CPT codes are inclusive of all services provided for the vessel treated, and codes from one vascular family are reported for the purpose of revascularization.

- *Iliac Vascular Territory*, which is subdivided into the common iliac, internal iliac, and external iliac arteries
- *Femoral/Popliteal Vascular Territory*, which includes the femoral and popliteal arteries in one extremity
- *Tibial/Peroneal Vascular Territory*, which includes the anterior tibial, posterior tibial, and peroneal arteries

Example: Patient underwent percutaneous transluminal angioplasty (Figure 14-13) for endovascular revascularization of the right common iliac, right internal iliac, and right external iliac arteries. Report codes 37220 RT, 37222 RT, and 37222 RT. (Code 37220 is the primary endovascular revascularization code, and code 37222 is reported twice for endovascular revascularization of the two additional arteries.)

Vascular Embolization and Occlusion

Vascular embolization and occlusion codes procedures are performed on arteries, veins, and lymphatics *except* those performed on the central nervous system and the head and neck.

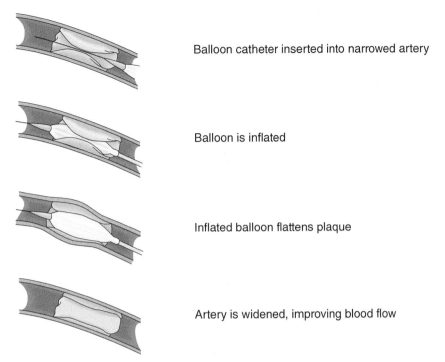

Balloon catheter inserted into narrowed artery

Balloon is inflated

Inflated balloon flattens plaque

Artery is widened, improving blood flow

FIGURE 14-13 Percutaneous transluminal balloon angioplasty

Example: Patient underwent venous vascular embolization, including radiological supervision and interpretation, intraprocedural roadmapping, and imaging guidance necessary to control venous hemorrhage. Report code 37244.

Intravascular Ultrasound Services

Intravascular ultrasound services (IVUS) of noncoronary vessels are performed during diagnostic evaluation and/or therapeutic intervention. These codes are reported in addition to a code for the primary procedure.

Example: Patient undergoes percutaneous transluminal mechanical thrombectomy of dialysis circuit, with diagnostic angiography of dialysis circuit, and intravascular ultrasound service. Report codes 36904 and 37252.

Endoscopy

Endoscopy codes describe vascular endoscopy procedures, and surgical vascular endoscopy always includes diagnostic endoscopy.

Example: Patient underwent surgical vascular endoscopy with ligation of subfascial perforator veins. Report code 37500.

Ligation

Ligation of arteries and veins is performed to control bleeding of a ruptured or dissected (torn) artery/vein. Ligation CPT codes describe

- Ligation, division, and stripping of the saphenous veins. For a **stab phlebectomy**, multiple tiny incisions are made over varicose vein sites. At each stab site, the varicosity is extracted and then the varicose segment is removed. (The stab phlebectomy procedure is not typically performed on saphenous veins.)
- Subfascial ligation of incompetent perforator veins (e.g., connecting superficial veins located below the skin's surface to deep veins in the leg muscle).
- Ligation and division of the short saphenous vein at the saphenopopliteal junction. An incision is made in the skin overlying the short saphenous vein at its junction with the saphenopopliteal vein at the knee. Vessels are dissected and ties are placed around the short saphenous vein, which is divided between the ties.
- Ligation, division, and/or excision of varicose vein "clusters." These are large varicose veins that cannot be effectively treated using the stab phlebectomy technique because they require a larger incision. An open surgical dissection of the vein cluster is made using long incisions rather than short stab incisions.

Example: Patient underwent ligation, division, and stripping of the short saphenous vein, right leg. Report code 37718 RT.

Other Procedures

Other Procedures codes include penile revascularization, penile venous occlusive procedures, and unlisted procedures involving vascular surgery.

Example: Patient underwent penile venous occlusive procedure. Report code 37790.

Exercise 14.2 – Arteries and Veins

Instructions: Assign CPT and HCPCS Level II code(s) and appropriate modifier(s) to each statement. List the Radiology section code first, when applicable, because Arteries and Veins subcategory catheterizations are assigned as additional codes. Assign a HCPCS Level II code for nonradioactive contrast material when applicable.

1. On the initial treatment day, the physician performed transcatheter therapy, which included arterial infusion for thrombolysis of the inferior vena cava. Radiological supervision and interpretation were included.

   _____

2. A physician performed a right upper extremity angiogram, including radiological supervision and interpretation. Catheter was inserted into the right brachial artery, and nonradioactive contrast material was injected to facilitate angiogram imaging.

   _____

3. Physician introduced a catheter into the aorta, injected nonradioactive contrast media, and performed descending thoracic aortography, including radiological supervision and interpretation.

   _____

4. Physician punctured the subclavian vein of a four-year-old, passed a guidewire centrally, and inserted a central venous catheter (nontunneled).

   _____

5. Patient underwent left renal venogram, including radiological supervision and interpretation, which required introduction of a catheter into the inferior vena cava, selective catheter placement into the left renal vein, and selective catheter placement into the left suprarenal vein. Nonradiographic contrast media was injected, and the structures were well visualized.

   _____

Hemic and Lymphatic Systems Subsection

The Hemic and Lymphatic Systems subsection includes the following:

- Spleen
- General
- Transplantation and post-transplantation cellular infusions
- Lymph nodes and lymphatic channels

The Hemic and Lymphatic Systems subsection contains codes that describe procedures on the spleen, bone marrow transplantation services, the lymph nodes and lymph channels, the mediastinum, and the diaphragm. The *hemic system* is a blood-producing system. *Blood* is tissue that consists of plasma, red blood cells, white blood cells, and platelets (or thrombocytes). The *lymphatic system* (Figure 14-14) consists of the spleen, thymus, tonsils, adenoids, vessels that carry lymph, and lymph nodes. The *spleen* (Figure 14-15) produces mature lymphocytes, destroys worn

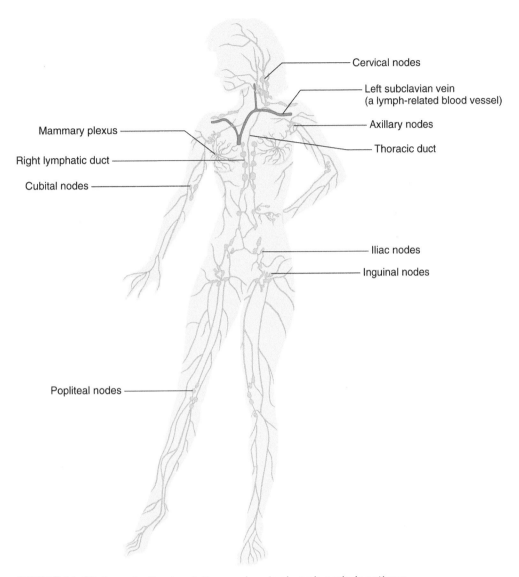

FIGURE 14-14 Lymphatic circulation and major lymph node locations

out red blood cells, and serves as a reservoir for blood. The *thymus* produces T lymphocytes, which are important to the body's immune function. The *tonsils* are located at the back of the throat, and they contain lymphoid tissue that helps fight infections. The *adenoids* are located at the rear of the nose, and they contain lymphoid tissue that helps fight infections. *Lymph* is a clear fluid that contains *chyle* (digestive fluid that contains proteins and fats), some red blood cells, and lymphocytes, which help fight infection and disease. *Lymph nodes* are clusters of bean-shaped nodules that act as the body's filtration system, removing cell waste and excess fluid and helping to fight infection. Lymph nodes are located in the

- Back of the head, just above the hairline (occipital region)
- Neck (cervical region)
- Armpits (axillary region)
- Elbow (cubital region)
- Chest (supraclavicular region)
- Abdomen (retroperitoneal region)
- Groin (inguinal region)
- Knee (popliteal region)

Spleen

Spleen codes are reported for the excision or repair of the spleen, including *en bloc* for extensive disease. (The term **en bloc** means "as a whole.") These codes include laparoscopic procedures performed on the spleen. Instructional notes state that "surgical laparoscopy always includes diagnostic laparoscopy." This means that

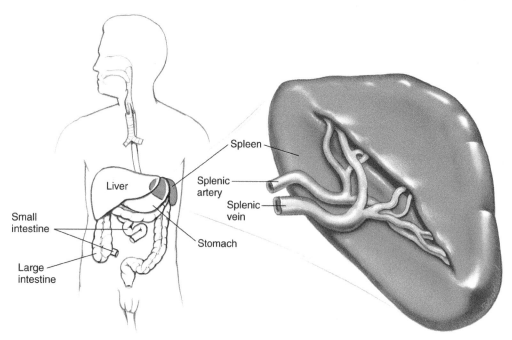

FIGURE 14-15 The spleen performs many important functions related to the immune system

when the physician performs diagnostic and surgical laparoscopies during the same operative session, just the code for surgical laparoscopy is reported.

> **Example:** Patient underwent open repair of ruptured spleen with partial splenectomy. Report code 38115.

When a needle is inserted percutaneously and contrast media is injected into the spleen for direct **splenoportography**, the radiographic visualization of the splenic and portal veins results.

> **Example:** Patient underwent splenoportography, with percutaneous injection of contrast medium into the spleen. Report codes 75810 and 38200 51.

General

The General category includes bone marrow or stem cell procedures and services. *Bone marrow* is spongy material that fills large bones' cavities and consists of two types.

- *Red marrow:* Produces red blood cells, white blood cells, and platelets
- *Yellow marrow:* Replaces red marrow with fatty tissue that does not produce blood cells

Bone marrow contains two types of *stem cells.*

- *Hemopoietic:* Produce red blood cells, white blood cells, and platelets
- *Stromal:* Produce fat, cartilage, and bone and have the ability to differentiate into many kinds of tissue, such as nervous tissue

Codes are reported for the harvesting, aspiration, biopsy, and transplantation of bone marrow and/or stem cells. Codes are also reported for the steps involved in the preservation, preparation, and purification of bone marrow and stem cells prior to transplantation or reinfusion. Stem cells are harvested from a suitable donor (allogeneic) or the patient's bone marrow (autologous).

A **bone marrow aspiration** uses a needle to remove a sample of the liquid bone marrow for examination under a microscope. A **bone marrow biopsy** involves boring a small hole into a long bone (e.g., hip) and using a large, hollow needle to remove bone marrow for examination under a microscope. When bone marrow aspiration and bone marrow biopsy procedures are performed at the same site through the same skin incision (during the same operative session), report just bone marrow biopsy code. When the bone marrow aspiration and bone marrow biopsy procedures are performed at separate sites (e.g., different bones or separate skin incisions in the same bone), report multiple codes.

> **Example:** Progenitor cells (stem cells) were harvested from an umbilical cord after delivery, and they were cryopreserved and kept for transplantation to the neonate later in life or to other recipients. This process required transplantation preparation of hematopoietic progenitor cells and included cryopreservation and storage. Report code 38207.

Transplantation and Post-Transplantation Cellular Infusions

Hematopoietic cell transplantation (HCT) is the autologous or allogeneic infusion of hematopoietic progenitor cells (HPC) obtained from bone marrow, peripheral blood apheresis, or umbilical cord blood. The infusion of HPCs helps restore bone marrow function, while allogeneic lymphocyte infusions are often used to treat chronic myelogenic leukemia. Evaluation and management services provided on the same date of service as infusions are reported with CPT E/M codes and modifier 25.

> **Example:** Hematopoietic cells previously obtained from the patient's bone marrow were implanted because the recipient's immune system had been suppressed using radiation. The autologous harvested cells were injected into the recipient by intravenous drip therapy in a sterile environment. Report code 38241.

Lymph Nodes and Lymphatic Channels

Capillaries surround cells but are not actually connected to cells, which results in the leakage of watery blood plasma (containing oxygen, proteins, glucose, and white blood cells) or lymph (Figure 14-16). This lymph (fluid) is recirculated away from the body's cells in the lymphatic circulatory system, which contains lymphatic channels, called capillaries and lymphatic vessels. The lymph eventually reaches one of about one hundred lymph nodes located throughout the body, which filter the fluid. (Lymph nodes contain white blood cells that filter debris and foreign cells from lymph.) When a patient becomes infected (e.g., bacteria or virus), the number of white blood cells in lymph nodes increases to billions. The lymph nodes work to fight the infection and release the filtered lymph (fluid) back into the bloodstream. Sometimes lymph nodes become infected or abscessed and require surgical treatment.

> **Example:** A patient is diagnosed with cervical lymphadenitis and undergoes incision and drainage. The surgeon makes a skin incision overlying the abscessed cervical lymph node, a needle with a syringe attached is inserted into the lymph node, and the abscess is drained. The wound is closed with Steri-Strips. Report code 38300.

Limited excision of lymph nodes is often performed for *cancer staging*, which is the determination that cancer has or has not spread anatomically from its point of origin. After cancer staging, the complete removal of the lymph nodes, and surgical wound closure is often performed in layers.

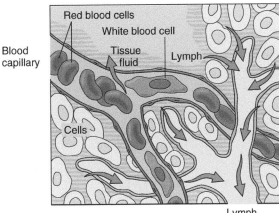

FIGURE 14-16 Lymph circulation showing interaction with blood vessels and cells

Exercise 14.3 – Hemic and Lymphatic

Instructions: Assign the CPT code(s) and appropriate modifier(s) to each statement.

1. Patient underwent bilateral total pelvic lymphadenectomy via laparoscope with multiple periaortic lymph node samplings.

   _____

2. Physician conducted a donor search to locate a suitable match for a transplant patient and arranged acquisition of cells.

   _____

3. Previously frozen stem cells (blood) of a single donor were thawed, without washing.

   _____

4. Bone marrow biopsy, sternum, using trocar.

   _____

5. Allogeneic hematopoietic progenitor (stem) cells were harvested from umbilical and placental blood, cryopreserved, and maintained for transplantation.

   _____

6. Physician sutured lacerations in a ruptured spleen and then resected and removed a damaged segment of the spleen.

   _____

7. Physician performed a total splenectomy.

   _____

8. A patient with idiopathic thrombocytopenic purpura underwent a laparoscopic splenectomy.

   _____

9. Patient underwent suprahyoid lymphadenectomy, left side.

   _____

10. Patient underwent glossectomy with a composite resection, floor of mouth mandibular resection, and radical neck dissection (Commando). Cervical lymphadenectomy (modified radical neck dissection) was performed on the right side.

    _____

Summary

The Cardiovascular System subsection includes codes for procedures performed on the heart and pericardium, valves (e.g., mitral and semilunar), and peripheral vascular vessels (e.g., arteries, veins, and capillaries). Cardiovascular System subsection codes are arranged anatomically and then according to procedure performed.

The Hemic and Lymphatic Systems subsection includes codes for procedures performed on the spleen, lymph nodes, and lymphatic channels.

Internet Links

CTSNet Global I Cardiothoracic Community: www.ctsnet.org

Medcomp vascular access devices: www.medcompnet.com

Vascular & Endovascular Surgery Society: Go to **www.vesurgery.org**, hover over Resources, and click on the FAQs link.

The Gross Physiology of the Cardiovascular System: **www.cardiac-output.info**

The Leukemia & Lymphoma Society: **www.lls.org**

Review

14.1 – Multiple Choice

Instructions: Select the most appropriate response.

1. Codes for selective vascular catheterization procedures are reported separately when performed as part of cardiology and _____ procedures and services.
   a. Evaluation and Management
   b. Medicine
   c. Pathology and Laboratory
   d. Radiology

2. Introducing a vascular catheter directly into a vessel without further advancement past the punctured vessel is called _____ vascular catheterization.
   a. nonselective
   b. selective
   c. superselective
   d. third-order

3. The note located below the Coronary Artery Anomalies subcategory title in the CPT coding manual, which applies to codes 33500–33507, states that basic procedures include _____ when performed during the same operative session.
   a. arterial embolization
   b. coronary artery bypass grafting
   c. endarterectomy or angioplasty
   d. intravascular ultrasound

4. Review code 33286 (Removal, subcutaneous cardiac rhythm monitor). The parenthetical note below code 33286 provides instruction to assign codes 93285, 93291, or 93298 for
   a. Holter monitor and external event recording.
   b. initial implantation, including programming.
   c. removal and reinsertion of a pacing cardioverter.
   d. subsequent electronic analysis and/or reprogramming.

5. When the "battery" of a pacemaker or implantable defibrillator is changed, it is actually the _____ that is changed.
   a. catheter   b. electrode   c. pacemaker   d. pulse generator

6. When reporting codes for selective vascular catheterization, knowledge of the flow of blood throughout the body's circulatory system is crucial. Which is considered a second-order artery of the right brachiocephalic artery vascular family?
   a. brachiocephalic artery
   b. right common carotid artery
   c. right external carotid artery
   d. right internal carotid artery

7. Which is the removal of part of the pericardium?
   a. Pericardiectomy
   b. Pericardiocentesis
   c. Pericardiostomy
   d. Pericardiotomy

8. Which is the removal of a fixed blood clot?
    a. Atherectomy
    b. Embolectomy
    c. Sympathectomy
    d. Thrombectomy

9. The two types of aneurysm repair are
    a. arteriovenous and open.
    b. endocardial and endovascular.
    c. endovascular and direct.
    d. transluminal and direct.

10. *En bloc* means
    a. closed and blocked status of incision.
    b. implanted.
    c. insertion directly into a vein through a blood vessel.
    d. surgical removal as a whole.

11. Injection procedure of radioactive tracer for identification of sentinel node. Which CPT code is assigned?
    a. 36005   b. 38790   c. 38792   d. 38790, 38900

12. Pericardiectomy with cardiopulmonary bypass. Which CPT code(s) are assigned?
    a. 33030, 33935
    b. 33030, 33935 51
    c. 33030, 33935 59
    d. 33031

13. Suture repair of aorta without shunt or cardiopulmonary bypass. Which CPT code is assigned?
    a. 33300   b. 33320   c. 33322   d. 33330

14. A 15-year-old patient is admitted for repair of patent ductus arteriosus by division. Which CPT code is assigned?
    a. 33820   b. 33822   c. 33824   d. 33840

15. Patient with cardiopulmonary insufficiency received 72 hours of daily management of veno-venous extracorporeal life support (ECLS) provided by the physician. Which CPT code(s) are assigned?
    a. 33946
    b. 33946, 33948, 33948
    c. 33948, 33948, 33948
    d. 33949, 33949, 33949

16. Open biopsy of deep cervical nodes. Which CPT code is assigned?
    a. 38500   b. 38510   c. 38520   d. 38525

17. Patient underwent percutaneous transluminal mechanical thrombectomy (extraction of thrombus), arteriovenous fistula. Which CPT code is assigned?
    a. 36825   b. 36831   c. 36832   d. 36904

18. Percutaneous venous transluminal balloon angioplasty, brachiocephalic vein, performed as a distinct procedural service (during the same operative session as the primary CABG procedure). Which CPT code is assigned?
    a. 37236 59   b. 37236 79   c. 37248   d. 37248 59

19. Percutaneous transcatheter retrieval of intravascular foreign body. Which CPT code is assigned?
    a. 37184   b. 37187   c. 37195   d. 37197

20. Direct repair of a ruptured aneurysm of the abdominal aorta. Which CPT code is assigned?
    a. 33877   b. 34701   c. 35082   d. 35092

14.2 – Coding Practice: Cardiovascular System

Instructions: Assign the CPT code(s) and appropriate modifier(s) to each case.

1. A patient presented to the ambulatory surgery center for stripping of the long saphenous veins in the right leg and the long and short saphenous veins in the left leg. The long saphenous veins were stripped from the saphenofemoral junction to the knee.

   _____

2. A patient with a three-year history of mitral regurgitation presented for mitral valve replacement. The procedure began by placing the patient on heart-lung bypass machine. After gaining access to the thoracic cavity, the left atrium was identified. The damaged mitral valve was identified and removed. This was replaced with a biprosthetic valve and sewn in. Total time on bypass machine was 2.5 hours.

   _____

3. A patient presents for pacemaker insertion due to diagnosis of bradycardia. After intravenous sedation was obtained, the entire left chest and neck were prepped. A standard incision was made in the left deltopectoral groove. A small venotomy was made, and permanent pacemaker and transvenous electrodes were inserted with ventricular and atrial leads placed into position. These were tested and found to be functioning properly. The leads were anchored at exit sites from the vein attached to the pacemaker. The pacemaker was tested, was functioning, and was placed in the subcutaneous pocket. All connections are checked. The patient will have another check before discharge from the hospital tomorrow.

   _____

4. A 20-year-old patient presented for surgical treatment of patent ductus arteriosus (PDA). Under general anesthesia, a thoracotomy was done for access to the PDA. After the pericardium was opened to get to the mediastinum, the PDA was identified and closed via ligation.

   _____

5. A two-year-old patient presented to the ED after having fallen in a lake, with a near drowning. The patient was in shock. Regular venous access methods failed, and the emergency department attending physician decided to do a venous cutdown. After a transverse incision over the vein of the patient's ankle was made, a small stab incision was made distal to the first incision for venipuncture cutdown. Two sutures were placed around the vein. A cannula was passed though the incision of the vein. The skin was closed in layers with sutures.

   _____

6. A 45-year-old patient diagnosed with chronic renal failure underwent surgery to facilitate dialysis access. The surgeon created an arteriovenous fistula by other than direct arteriovenous anastomosis with placement of nonautogenous graft access. The patient was prepped and draped in the usual fashion. Dissection was carried down the brachial artery and basilic vein. Prolene sutures were used to expose the vein. A thermoplastic graft was tunneled subcutaneously. The vein graft was sewn end to side. The graft was flushed with saline and then clamped below the anastomosis. The proximal graft at the 4-mm end was beveled and sewn to the small caliber brachial artery. Anastomosis was secured, and the native artery was flushed up through the graft first. All wounds were closed with Vicryl and nylon sutures.

   _____

7. A 57-year-old patient was found to have carotid stenosis after duplex scan and angiogram. The patient presents today for a left carotid thromboendarterectomy with patch angioplasty. The neck area of the patient was prepped. An oblique incision along the sternomastoid muscle was made. Dissection was done through the platysma to the carotid sheath. The hypoglossal and vagus nerves were identified during dissection and preserved with care. The sheath dissection was performed along the anterior border of the left internal jugular vein. The common, external, and internal carotid arteries were dissected. The patient was given heparin, and clamping of the internal carotid did not reveal any changes on EEG monitor. The common and external carotids were clamped. A longitudinal arteriotomy was made. Standard thromboendarterectomy was performed, transecting the proximal end and working distally. The arteriotomy was closed with a patch cut to an ellipse and parachuted into the distal apex. The external and common carotids were opened. There was a good signal in the arteries. No changes were noted on the EEG. The wound was irrigated and closed.

8. The patient had an implantable pacing cardioverter-defibrillator (ICD) placed six months ago. The patient now has a malfunction of this device. After adequate anesthesia, an incision was made and the electrodes were removed from the generator. There was a screw problem with the generator that was producing a noise. The leads were tested and found to be working satisfactorily. The original implantable defibrillator pulse generator was removed, and a replacement implantable defibrillator pulse generator with original dual lead system was inserted. The ICD was placed back in the pocket, and the wound was closed after irrigation with 3-0 and 4-0 Vicryl.

9. A 35-year-old patient has been found to have a pericardial cyst via echocardiogram. After adequate anesthesia, a lateral thoracotomy was performed to gain access to the pericardium. The patient's heart was stopped via cardioplegia infused through a heart-lung bypass machine. The pericardial cyst was seen lying next to the diaphragm. It was removed in total. Drainage tubes were placed. The cardioplegia was reversed. The cyst was sent to pathology for analysis. The wound was closed in layers with Prolene and Vicryl.

10. A patient presented with a history of atherosclerosis. The patient underwent surgery to bypass blocked heart arteries. After anesthesia was administered the surgeon made a thoracic incision. The blockage of the heart was identified. The physician harvested the saphenous vein from the patient's leg to use for coronary artery bypass graft. An opening was made in the aorta, and the grafted vein was sutured to the opening in the aorta at one end and below the blockage at the other end.

14.3 – Coding Practice: Hemic and Lymphatic Systems

Instructions: Assign the CPT code(s) and appropriate modifier(s) to each case.

1. A patient with a history of pancytopenia presented for a bone marrow biopsy. The physician numbed the skin and inserted a needle into the left iliac bone, rotating the needle in an alternating clockwise-counterclockwise motion until the bone cavity was entered. With the needle firmly planted, its core was discharged and the solid bone marrow specimen was collected. The needle was withdrawn, and the specimen was sent for analysis.

2. A 14-year-old patient was in a motor vehicle crash and suffered blunt abdominal trauma. Due to internal bleeding and a ruptured spleen, the patient required a splenectomy. After making the initial abdominal incision, the physician identified the spleen. Splenic blood vessels were tied off. The spleen was removed in total. The remainder of the abdominal cavity was examined for any injuries or bleeding. No injury or additional bleeding was found. The wound was closed in layers.

3. A three-year-old patient with a cystic hygroma of the neck presented for dissection. An incision was made in the neck. The tissue surrounding the hygroma was removed via excision. The hygroma was deep in the neuro-vascular section of the neck. Extensive and deep dissection was required for complete removal. The cystic hygroma was accessed and removed. The skin was closed in multiple layers.

4. A patient underwent pelvic lymphadenectomy, which included removal of all external iliac, hypogastric, and obturator nodes on both sides. The patient has a history of ureteral cancer and now has pelvic pain and swelling. The patient was placed in the supine position. An incision was made over the iliac crest. Blood vessels were identified, and bleeders were cauterized. Enlarged pelvic lymph nodes were identified and removed in total. These were sent to pathology. The wound was closed with sutures.

5. A patient underwent cervical lymph node biopsy, open. The patient's left neck area was prepped and draped in the usual fashion. An incision was made to access the cervical node. A scalene fat pad was identified and excised to access the deeper node. Both the cervical node and the pad were sent to pathology for analysis. The wound was closed in layers.

6. A patient suffered a fall from 20 feet. The patient had internal bleeding and consented to a laparoscopic procedure to identify internal structures that may be causing hemorrhage. The patient was placed in the normal lateral decubitus position. A trocar was placed above the umbilical region through an incision. Gas was introduced into the abdominal cavity. Laparoscopic examination identified damage to the patient's spleen. An additional two incisions were made to insert trocars for the procedure. The spleen was dissected with hemostasis achieved. The spleen was removed via pouch method through the trocar. The three incision sites were closed with sutures.

7. The patient presented for lymphangiography of the right pelvic lymph nodes with radiological supervision and interpretation. The radiologist accessed the patient's vein and injected dye to highlight subcutaneous tissues and lymphatic vessels. A small incision was made to allow for the introduction of a needle and catheter. More dye was injected into the lymphatic vessels. The needle and catheter were secured with a suture. The first set of films was done. The second set of films was done on the next day. After the second set of films, the radiologist removed the catheter and sutured the incision site closed.

8. A patient with a history of chyle in the pleural cavity presented for suturing of the thoracic duct. Via abdominal approach, an incision was made and duct was identified and tied off. The incision was closed in layers with sutures.

9. A patient with leukemia required a bone marrow donor. The physician contacted the national bone marrow donor registry and provided medical information on the patient. A cell donor search for donor hematopoietic progenitor cell acquisition was conducted. The physician received two potential matches.

10. A patient has an enlarged lymph node of the left axillary region. The physician made an incision over the lymph node area after adequate local anesthesia. The lymph node was identified and found to be inflamed; drainage of the axillary lymph node yielded a pustulant material. The area was thoroughly irrigated, and the incision wound was closed with 4-0 Prolene sutures.

Chapter 45

CPT Surgery IV

Chapter Outline

Mediastinum and Diaphragm Subsection

Digestive System Subsection

Urinary System Subsection

Chapter Objectives

At the conclusion of this chapter, the student should be able to:

1. Define key terms related to the Mediastinum and Diaphragm, Digestive System, and Urinary System subsections of CPT Surgery.
2. Assign codes from the Mediastinum and Diaphragm subsection of CPT Surgery.
3. Assign codes from the Digestive System subsection of CPT Surgery.
4. Assign codes from the Urinary System subsection of CPT Surgery.

Key Terms

anoscopy

cholecystectomy

colectomy

colonoscopy

colostomy

complex fistulectomy

cystoscopy

cystourethroscopy

diagnostic endoscopy

endoscopic retrograde cholangiopancreatography (ERCP)

enterectomy

enterolysis

esophagogastroduodenoscopy (EGD)

esophagogastroscopy

esophagoscopy

gastrectomy

hepatotomy

ileostomy

laparoscopy

laser-assisted uvulopalatoplasty

lithotripsy

nephrectomy

Nissen fundoplasty

ostomy

palatopharyngoplasty

percutaneous lithotomy

peritoneoscopy

proctectomy

proctosigmoidoscopy

rhinoplasty

second-stage fistulectomy/ fistulotomy

seton

sigmoidoscopy

stoma

subcutaneous fistulectomy

submuscular fistulectomy

surgical endoscopy

transurethral resection of the prostate (TURP)

transurethral ureteroscopic lithotripsy

upper GI endoscopy

ureterolithotomy

urethroplasty

Whipple procedure

Introduction

The Mediastinum and Diaphragm subsection includes codes for procedures performed on the mediastinum and diaphragm. The Digestive System subsection includes codes for procedures performed on gastrointestinal (GI) tract organs as well as the teeth, palate and uvula, adenoids and tonsils, Meckel's diverticulum and mesentery, appendix, biliary tract, pancreas, abdomen, peritoneum, and omentum. The Urinary System subsection includes codes for procedures performed on the kidneys, ureters, bladder, and urethra.

 Coding Tip

Instructional notes located beneath categories, subcategories, headings, and subheadings apply to all codes in those areas. Parenthetical notes that are located below a specific code apply to that code only, unless the note indicates otherwise.

 NOTE:

The content in Chapters 12 through 16 of this textbook is organized exactly as it appears in the CPT Surgery section. This organization facilitates learning by allowing students to move from one CPT Surgery subsection to the next, in order.

When included in CPT, the Other Procedures code below is reported for an unlisted procedure performed on the anatomical site. When reporting an unlisted procedure code, include documentation (e.g., special report) about the procedure performed with the submitted claim.

The *Medicare National Correct Coding Initiative Policy Manual* provides guidance about assigning procedure codes for the Mediastinum and Diaphragm subsection and the Digestive System and Urinary System subsections. Go to **www.cms.gov** and enter "Medicare NCCI Policy Manual" in the Search box to navigate to the manual.

Mediastinum and Diaphragm Subsection

Mediastinum and Diaphragm subsection categories include the following:

- Mediastinum
- Diaphragm

The *mediastinum* is the space in the thoracic cavity between the lungs that contains the aorta, the esophagus, the heart, and other structures.

The *diaphragm* is the thin muscle below the heart and lungs that separates the chest from the abdomen. It functions in respiration by contracting during inspiration, which means that the size of the chest cavity expands when a person is breathing in. Procedures to repair two types of hernias are included in the Diaphragm category.

- Hiatal hernia (Figure 15-1)
- Diaphragmatic hernia

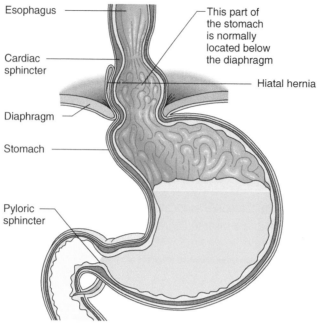

FIGURE 15-1 In a hiatal hernia (or hiatal hernia), part of the stomach protrudes through the esophageal opening in the diaphragm

Example 1: Patient underwent resection of mediastinal cyst. Report code 39200.

Example 2: Patient underwent resection of the diaphragm, with simple repair. Report code 39560.

Exercise 15.1 – Mediastinum and Diaphragm

Instructions: Assign the CPT code(s) and appropriate modifier(s) to each statement.

1. The physician performed a complex repair during resection of the diaphragm, closing the residual defect with synthetic graft material.

   _____

2. Mediastinotomy to remove foreign body using transthoracic approach, including median sternotomy.

   _____

3. Patient underwent repair, laceration of diaphragm.

   _____

4. Physician inserted a mediastinoscope through an incision in the sternal notch and performed a mediastinal lymph node biopsy.

   _____

5. Physician repaired an acute traumatic diaphragmatic hernia.

   _____

Digestive System Subsection

The *digestive system* (Figure 15-2) begins at the mouth and extends to the anus. The upper digestive tract consists of the mouth, pharynx, esophagus, and stomach. The esophagus passes through the diaphragm and enters the stomach between its body and fundus. The stomach lies below the diaphragm and is composed of the fundus (upper portion under the diaphragm), body (middle), and antrum (lower).

The liver, gallbladder, and pancreas are digestive accessory organs that produce enzymes and substances that assist with digestion in the small intestine. The absorption of nutrients into the bloodstream occurs in the small intestine (Figure 15-3). The pyloric sphincter controls the passage of digested food from the stomach into the duodenum (first part of the small intestine). The small intestine also contains the jejunum and the ileum, where the ileocecal valve allows for the controlled passage of digested material into the large intestine. The last section of the digestive tract is called the large intestine (Figure 15-4). It includes the cecum, colon, rectum, and anus. The appendix, located off the large intestine, has no known function.

NOTE:

When a lesion of the *mucocutaneous margin* (mucous membrane and skin) borders the digestive tract, it may appear that treatment (e.g., biopsy, destruction, or excision) requires the reporting of codes from multiple subsections of CPT Surgery. In fact, codes from just *one* of the following CPT subsections are reported:

- Integumentary system
- Digestive system

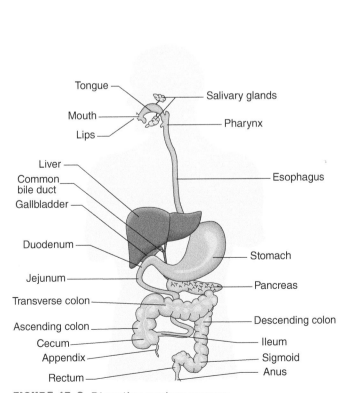

FIGURE 15-2 Digestive system organs

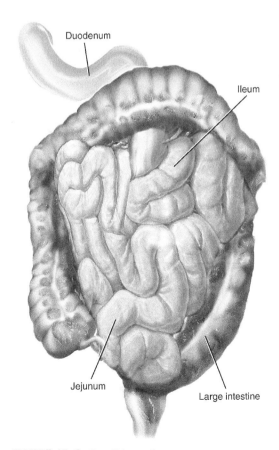

FIGURE 15-3 Small intestine

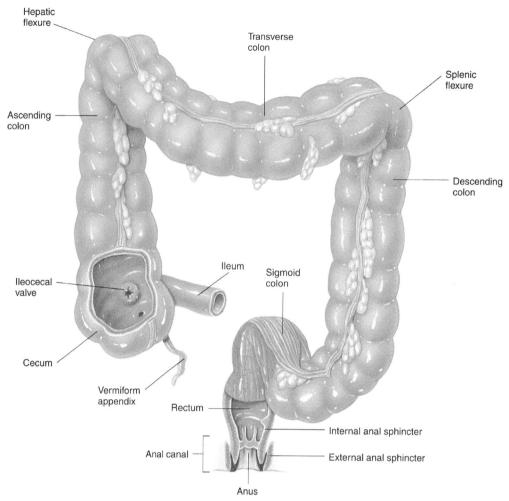

FIGURE 15-4 Large intestine

Digestive system procedures diagnose and treat disorders of the digestive system (e.g., gastrointestinal endoscopy, laparoscopy, and gastric analysis). Similar to other Surgery subsections, procedures are organized first by anatomical area and then by type.

Example: Patient underwent upper gastrointestinal endoscopy of the esophagus, stomach, and duodenum, with specimen collection via brushing technique. Report code 43235.

Digestive System subsection codes are reported for open, endoscopic, and laparoscopic procedures. The operative report must be carefully reviewed to correctly identify the surgical approach. For gastrostomy (Figure 15-5) procedures, carefully review code descriptions because codes reported are based on surgical approach.

Example: Patient underwent flexible transoral esophagogastroduodenoscopy with directed placement of percutaneous gastrostomy tube. Report code 43246.

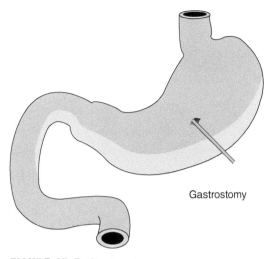

FIGURE 15-5 Gastrostomy

 NOTE:

The CPT Medicine section also contains codes for digestive system procedures in its Gastroenterology subsection, including codes for diagnostic tests such as electrogastrography. Such tests are generally included in endoscopic procedures, which means that they are not separately coded and reported.

Codes for procedures performed on the oral cavity (Figure 15-6) are organized according to the following anatomical sites:

- Lips
- Vestibule of mouth
- Tongue and floor of mouth
- Dentoalveolar structures

- Palate and uvula
- Salivary glands and ducts
- Pharynx, adenoids, and tonsils

Lips

Procedures performed on the lips (e.g., biopsy of lip) include:

- Excision
- Repair (cheiloplasty)
- Other procedures

When a procedure is performed on the *skin* of the lip, report an appropriate code from the Integumentary System subsection. Do *not* report codes from both subsections for the same lip procedure.

Example 1: Patient underwent a lip biopsy. Report code 40490.

Example 2: Patient underwent incisional biopsy of the skin of the lip. The surgeon removed a skin lesion from the lateral side of the bottom lip. Report code 11106 (from the Integumentary System subsection).

Cheiloplasty is the plastic surgery of the lips. To properly assign codes, review the operative report to determine the vertical height associated with the repair (e.g., up to one-half vertical height or over one-half vertical height).

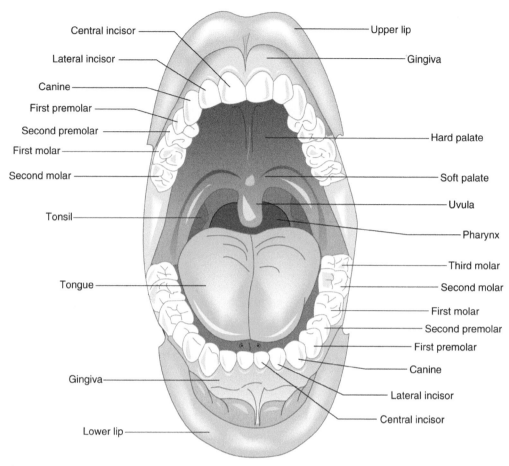

FIGURE 15-6 Oral cavity

The *full-thickness* repair of a lip laceration is reported with a code from the Repair (Cheiloplasty) category. Do *not* report a code from the Integumentary System subsection instead of *or* in addition to full-thickness repairs of lip lacerations. (Simple and intermediate repairs of *skin* on the lip are reported with codes from the Integumentary System subsection.)

For procedures performed to repair cleft lip and nasal deformities, review the operative report to identify whether the procedure is

- Primary or secondary
- One-stage or two-stage

A primary procedure repairs the cleft lip/nasal deformity without recreating the defect. A secondary procedure recreates the defect and includes reclosure to repair the cleft lip/nasal deformity. For a **rhinoplasty** (repair of skin defect of the nose using harvested tissue or plastic surgery to change the nose's shape or size), report a code from the Respiratory subsection.

Example 1: Patient underwent full-thickness repair of the vermilion border of the upper lip. Patient sustained a laceration while replacing spark plugs in a classic 1967 Pontiac Bonneville. Report code 40650.

Example 2: Patient underwent up to half vertical height full-thickness repair of the lower lip due to laceration acquired during a bar fight. The wound extended through the full thickness of the lip, including the vermilion border. Wound size was up to one-half the vertical height of the lip. Report code 40652.

Vestibule of Mouth

Procedures performed on the vestibule of the mouth, which includes mucosal and submucosal tissue (inner lining) of the lips and cheeks, include:

- Incision
- Excision, destruction
- Repair
- Other procedures

Example: The patient has a habit of sucking on toothpicks; during a recent automobile accident, a toothpick became embedded in submucosal tissue in the mouth. Patient underwent simple removal of embedded foreign body (toothpick). Report code 40804.

Tongue and Floor of Mouth

Procedures performed on the tongue and floor of the mouth include:

- Incision
- Excision
- Repair
- Other procedures

When reporting codes for excision of a tongue lesion, review the operative report to identify the

- Location of the lesion (e.g., posterior one-third or anterior two-thirds of the tongue)
- Type of excision (partial or complete/total)

 NOTE:

When a partial glossectomy with bilateral radical neck dissection is performed, report code 41135 for the glossectomy and radical neck dissection on one side. (There is just one tongue, which means modifier 50 cannot be added to code 41135.) Report code 38720 59 for the radical neck dissection on the other side. (Modifier 59 is added to indicate a distinct procedural service.)

Example: Patient underwent partial glossectomy with unilateral radical neck dissection. Report code 41135.

Dentoalveolar Structures

Procedures performed on dentoalveolar structures (e.g., teeth or gums) include:

- Incision
- Excision, destruction
- Other procedures

(Commonly performed dental procedures are included in the *Current Dental Terminology* [CDT].)

Example: Patient underwent drainage of gum abscess. Report code 41800.

Palate and Uvula

Procedures performed on the hard and soft palates and the uvula include:

- Incision
- Excision, destruction
- Repair
- Other procedures

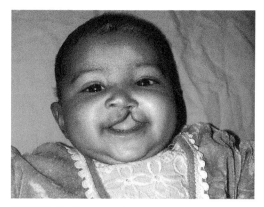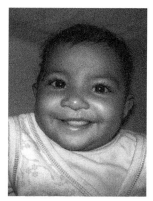

FIGURE 15-7 A child with a cleft palate before and after treatment

A **palatopharyngoplasty** is performed to treat oropharyngeal obstructions; it involves surgically resecting excess tissue from the uvula, soft palate, and pharynx to open the airway (e.g., cure extreme cases of snoring with or without sleep apnea).

 NOTE:

A **laser-assisted uvulopalatoplasty** procedure uses a laser technique to remove tissue from the uvula, soft palate, and pharynx. CPT does not list a specific code for laser-assisted uvulopalatoplasty. Therefore, report HCPCS Level II code S2080. Because more than one treatment session may be required to achieve optimal results, subsequent visits to repeat the laser-assisted uvulopalatoplasty are included in the global period for the code reported. Therefore, a code for each repeat session is *not* reported separately during the global period.

For codes that describe cleft palate repairs (Figure 15-7), the size and location of the cleft determine the type of repair performed (and reported code).

Example: The patient underwent primary plastic repair of cleft lip/nasal deformity, complete, unilateral. During the same operative session, the patient also underwent palatoplasty for cleft palate, with closure of alveolar ridge, soft tissue only. Report codes 40700 and 42205 51.

Salivary Gland and Ducts

Procedures performed to treat conditions involving the salivary gland and salivary ducts (e.g., abscess, cyst, and tumor) include:

- Incision
- Excision
- Repair
- Other procedures

The selection of a code for the excision of a parotid tumor or the parotid gland is based on the following:

- What amount of tissue was excised
- Where the location was (e.g., lateral lobe)
- Whether the procedure included nerve dissection
- Whether the procedure included radical neck dissection

Example: Patient underwent excision of a parotid tumor with radical neck dissection on the right and complete cervical lymphadenectomy on the left. Report code 42426 RT for excision of the parotid tumor and radical neck dissection on the right side. Also, report code 38720 59 LT for the complete cervical lymphadenectomy on the contralateral (left) side. Add functional modifier 59 (Distinct procedural service) to indicate that a distinct procedural service was provided, followed by informational modifier LT (Left side). (*Note*: When surgeons document "excision... with bilateral radical neck dissection, two codes are required as described in this example. Modifier 50 cannot be added to indicate "bilateral radical neck dissection" because separate prep and draping is required to performed dissection of lymph nodes on the contralateral side.)

Pharynx, Adenoids, and Tonsils

Procedures performed on the pharynx, adenoids, and tonsils include:

- Incision
- Excision, destruction
- Repair
- Other procedures

The pharynx contains three segments.

- *Nasopharynx*: Located above the soft palate
- *Oropharynx*: Area between the soft palate and the upper portion of the epiglottis, including the tonsils
- *Hypopharynx*: Extends from the upper edge of the epiglottis to the larynx/esophagus juncture

A variety of techniques and approaches are used when treating conditions of the pharynx (e.g., oral, cervical, thoracic, and horizontal or lateral neck incisions).

Example: Patient underwent removal of a lesion of the pharynx via oral approach using curettage. Report code 42808.

Tonsillectomy and Adenoidectomy

Procedures performed to remove diseased tonsils or adenoids include the following techniques:

- Cryogenic
- Electrocautery
- Laser

The selection of a tonsillectomy or adenoidectomy code is based on the following:

- Type of procedure performed (e.g., primary or secondary)
- Age of the patient

A primary procedure code is reported the first time the tonsils or adenoids are removed. A secondary procedure code is reported when there is tissue regrowth requiring subsequent removal. The age of the patient is a factor because age increases the complexity (level of difficulty) of the procedure and lengthens the recovery time.

Separate codes are included to report hemorrhage control following tonsillectomy and adenoidectomy procedures. Make sure you report these procedure codes with modifier 78 to indicate the return to the operating room for a related procedure performed during the postoperative (global) period.

Codes reported for the radical resection of tonsils include the removal of the tonsils, tonsillar pillars, retromolar trigone, and any infected portions of the maxilla and mandible. Radical resection may also include a hemi- or total glossectomy and/or a full neck dissection.

Coding Tip

Tonsillectomy and adenoidectomy are routinely performed bilaterally, and modifier 50 is not added to the codes.

A limited pharyngectomy is performed to remove a small portion of the pharyngeal wall (e.g., pyriform sinus).

Example: A six-year-old patient underwent tonsillectomy and adenoidectomy. Report code 42820.

Exercise 15.2 – Oral Cavity

Instructions: Assign the CPT code(s) and appropriate modifier(s) to each statement.

1. Patient underwent alveoloplasty to remove sharp areas or undercuts of alveolar bone, one quadrant.

2. Surgeon used a scalpel to slice off a cancerous portion of the vermilion border of the patient's lip; mucosal advancement was performed after excision.

3. Surgeon made an incision through submucosal tissue and removed a lesion in the vestibule of the mouth. Wound repair was not required.

4. Patient underwent simple incision of the lingual frenum to free the tongue.

5. Patient underwent intraoral left parotid gland sialolithotomy.

6. Surgeon repaired a tear at the pharyngoesophageal junction.

7. Physician performed an incision and drainage of a tonsillar abscess.

8. Surgeon removed an eight-year-old patient's tonsils and adenoids.

9. Physician controlled secondary oropharyngeal hemorrhaging, status post-tonsillectomy, by using cellulose sponges that expanded when placed in the tonsillar cavity.

10. Physician performed a tonsillectomy on a 12-year-old patient.

Esophagus

Procedures performed on the esophagus include:

- Incision
- Excision
- Endoscopy
- Laparoscopy

- Repair
- Manipulation
- Other procedures

When assigning codes to procedures performed on the esophagus, review documentation carefully to identify the approach (e.g., incision or endoscopy).

Example: Patient underwent esophagotomy via cervical approach, with removal of foreign body. Report code 43020.

Endoscopy

Endoscopic procedures performed to visualize digestive system organs generally use a flexible fiberoptic tube. (Rigid instruments are also used to perform endoscopy.) GI endoscopy is performed to diagnose and treat disorders of the GI tract. Codes are assigned according to the type of instrument used and the anatomical area visualized.

- **Esophagoscopy** is the direct visualization of the esophagus from the cricopharyngeus muscle (upper esophageal sphincter) to and including the gastroesophageal junction (and may include examination of the proximal region of the stomach via retroflexion when performed), using an endoscope.
- **Upper GI endoscopy** (**esophagogastroscopy**) is the direct visualization of the esophagus and the stomach.
- **Esophagogastroduodenoscopy (EGD)** (Figure 15-8) uses a fiberoptic endoscope to visualize the esophagus, stomach, and proximal duodenum.
- **Endoscopic retrograde cholangiopancreatography (ERCP)** involves passing an endoscope through the esophagus, stomach, and duodenum to the ducts of the biliary tree and pancreas. A small plastic tube is passed through the endoscope, through which dye is injected (to allow for visualization of the ducts on x-rays). A radiologist then takes x-rays to diagnose liver, gallbladder, bile duct, and pancreas problems.

Endoscopic procedures are considered diagnostic or surgical, and surgical endoscopy always includes diagnostic endoscopy. This means that when both procedures are performed during the same operative session, report the code for surgical endoscopy only.

- **Diagnostic endoscopy** is performed to visualize an abnormality or determine the extent of disease.
- **Surgical endoscopy** is performed when anything in addition to visualization is performed (e.g., removal of foreign body).

Example: Patient underwent diagnostic flexible sigmoidoscopy and biopsy of a lesion during the same operative session. Report code 45331. Do *not* report the code for the diagnostic endoscopy.

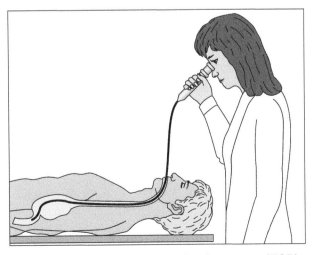

FIGURE 15-8 Esophagogastroduodenoscopy (EGD)

Endoscopic biopsy codes are reported just once regardless of the number of biopsies performed. Likewise, endoscopic polyp or lesion removal codes are reported just once regardless of the number of polyps or lesions treated.

Example 1: Patient underwent flexible esophagoscopy with multiple biopsies. Report code 43202.

Example 2: Patient underwent flexible esophagoscopy with removal of five polyps by hot biopsy forceps. Report code 43216 (just once even though five polyps were removed).

The endoscopic treatment of *esophageal varices* (uneven, enlarged, tortuous veins) (Figure 15-9) includes the following:

- Ligation (similar to the technique used to band hemorrhoids)
- Endoscopic injection of a sclerosing agent (e.g., concentrated saltwater) after passing sclerotherapy needle through scope

Example 1: Patient underwent flexible esophagoscopy with band ligation of esophageal varices. Report code 43205.

Example 2: Patient underwent direct ligation of esophageal varices. Physician accessed the esophagus through a thoracic incision and ligated the varices with sutures. Report code 43400.

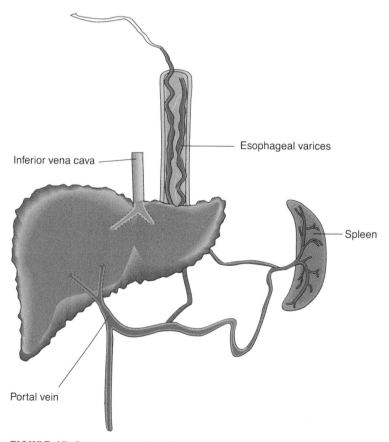

FIGURE 15-9 Esophageal varices

Example 3: Patient underwent ligation at the gastroesophageal junction for preexisting esophageal perforation. The physician ligated the junction of the stomach and esophagus, and a gastrostomy was created for feeding. Report code 43405. Do not report a code for the gastrostomy because it is considered as a separate procedure in CPT, which means it is included as part of the procedure performed in code 43405.

Procedures performed to treat gastroesophageal reflux disease (GERD) typically use moderate (conscious) sedation and radiofrequency energy delivered via endoscopy. The physician performs an EGD with ultrasound examination, and radiofrequency energy is subsequently applied through the endoscope to the muscle of the lower esophageal sphincter and/or the gastric cardia to treat GERD.

Example: Patient underwent upper GI endoscopy of the esophagus, stomach, and duodenum with delivery of thermal energy to the lower esophageal sphincter muscle for treatment of GERD. Report code 43257.

Endoscopic retrograde cholangiopancreatography (ERCP) combines upper gastrointestinal (GI) endoscopy and x-rays to detect and treat bile and pancreatic duct problems, such as blockages due to tumors, gallstones that become stuck in ducts, inflammation and infection due to trauma or illness, sclerosis (scarring) of ducts, and pseudocysts (accumulation of fluid and tissue debris). For example, if gallstones are present in the gallbladder (or bile duct), the doctor can remove them through the endoscope. Biopsies may also be taken for evaluation by the pathologist.

Example: Patient underwent diagnostic ERCP with single biopsy. Report code 43261.

When a sphincterotomy of the bile duct or pancreatic duct is performed, it includes a diagnostic ERCP. A guidewire is advanced into the biliary tree, and an electrocautery current is applied to make the incision. However, when the patient undergoes gallstone and pancreatic duct stone removal and a sphincterotomy is performed during the same operative session, two codes are reported.

Example: A patient undergoes ERCP basket removal of gallstones following a sphincterotomy. Report codes 43262 and 43264 51.

Laparoscopy

A **laparoscopy**, or **peritoneoscopy**, is the examination of the peritoneal contents using a laparoscope that is inserted through the abdominal wall.

- *Closed laparoscopy* is the insufflation of the abdominal cavity and is performed using a percutaneously placed needle.
- *Open laparoscopy* is the insufflation of the abdomen and is performed using a trocar, which is placed under direct vision after making a small celiotomy incision.

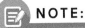 **NOTE:**

Surgical laparoscopy always includes diagnostic laparoscopy, which means a separate code is *not* reported for the diagnostic laparosopy.

Example: Patient underwent surgical laparoscopy with Nissen esophagogastric fundoplasty. Report code 43280. (**Nissen fundoplasty** involves mobilizing the lower end of the esophagus by suturing the fundus of the stomach around the circumference of the lower esophagus at the esophagogastric junction.)

Manipulation

When endoscopic esophageal procedures are performed, the advancement of the endoscope through the esophagus expands any stricture. The dilation is considered an integral part of the esophagoscopy procedure. This means that a code for dilation of the esophagus without the use of an endoscope is *not* reported with a code for endoscopy of the esophagus (even if the operative report documents esophageal dilation during endoscopy).

 NOTE:

Esophageal dilation (without endoscopy) is usually performed under fluoroscopic guidance. Report the appropriate fluoroscopic guidance (x-ray) code in addition to the dilation code, when performed.

Example: The physician uses fluoroscopy to insert a guidewire and to dilate the esophagus by passing dilators over the guidewire. Report codes 43453 and 74360. (Fluoroscopy is for radiological guidance during the procedure.)

Other Procedures

The free transfer of a short segment of jejunum is usually performed after portions of the pharynx or esophagus have been resected (e.g., cervical esophageal and hypopharyngeal carcinoma).

Example: Patient underwent free jejunum transfer with microvascular anastomosis. Report code 43496.

Stomach

Procedures performed on the stomach include:

- Incision
- Excision
- Laparoscopy
- Introduction
- Bariatric surgery
- Other procedures

Stomach procedures include the following:

- **Gastrectomy** (removal of all or a portion of the stomach), which is typically performed to treat ulcers (Figure 15-10) or malignancy.
- Roux-en-Y gastric bypass and small bowel reconstruction procedures that use a Y-shaped anastomosis, which includes the intestines.
- Surgical laparoscopic procedures performed on the stomach. Codes reported for procedures involving the field of bariatric surgery use laparoscopic techniques to perform gastric restrictive procedures for morbid obesity.
- Naso- or orogastric tube placement that requires a physician's skill and fluoroscopic guidance (reported when the nursing staff is unable to successfully insert the tube). Do not report a code when the nursing staff inserts the tube.
- Gastric restrictive procedures involving placement of an adjustable gastric band.

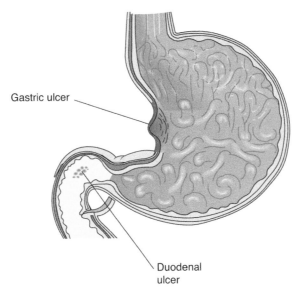

Gastric ulcer

Duodenal
ulcer

FIGURE 15-10 Gastric and duodenal ulcers

- Gastric restrictive procedure, which includes two reconstructive anastomoses (biliopancreatic diversion with duodenal switch).
- Gastric bypass procedure, which includes Roux-en-Y gastroenterostomy.

Example: Patient underwent surgical laparoscopic gastric restrictive procedure, which included gastric bypass and Roux-en-Y gastroenterostomy, roux limb 150 cm. Report code 43644.

Exercise 15.3 – Esophagus and Stomach

Instructions: Assign the CPT code(s) and appropriate modifier(s) to each statement.

1. Physician inserted a flexible esophagoscope into the esophagus and removed a lesion using snare technique.

2. Surgeon made an incision in the left posterior chest wall into the esophagus to remove a foreign body from the esophagus.

3. Physician inserted a balloon endoscopically for tamponade of bleeding esophageal varices.

4. Dr. Smith performed a partial cervical esophagectomy, and then Dr. Jones performed a jejunum transfer with microvascular anastomosis.

5. The physician passed an endoscope through the patient's mouth and visualized the entire esophagus, stomach, duodenum, and jejunum. One lesion was removed from the small intestine using biopsy forceps. Another small intestinal lesion was removed using a snare.

6. Patient underwent incision of the pyloric muscle.

(continues)

Exercise 15.3 – continued

7. The physician performed an open revision of a previously performed gastric restrictive procedure and reversed the previously partitioned stomach to restore normal gastrointestinal continuity.

   _____

8. Using fluoroscopic guidance (lasting 15 minutes), the physician repositioned a gastric feeding tube through the duodenum.

   _____

9. The physician performed a laparoscopic surgical gastric restrictive procedure with gastric bypass and Roux-en-Y gastroenterostomy (roux limb length 75 centimeters).

   _____

10. The physician performed laparoscopic gastric restrictive procedure by revising the adjustable gastric restrictive device component.

   _____

Intestines (Except Rectum)

Procedures performed on the intestines (except rectum) include:

- Incision
- Excision
- Laparoscopy
- Enterostomy—external fistulization of intestines
- Endoscopy, small intestine
- Endoscopy, stomal
- Introduction
- Repair
- Other procedures

Because codes located in the Intestines (Except Rectum) subsection describe similar-sounding procedures (e.g., enterolysis, enterectomy, and enteroenterostomy), coders must carefully review operative report documentation to ensure correct code assignment.

Incision

Enterolysis (freeing of intestinal adhesions) is described as a separate procedure code, and it is considered an integral component of hernia repair codes. Therefore, do not report the enterolysis code when other surgical procedures include the lysis of intestinal adhesions. However, if documentation indicates that enterolysis was extensive and added significantly to the procedure, add modifier 22 (Increased procedural services) to the enterolysis code. A condition that can result from the development of intestinal adhesions is *volvulus* (Figure 15-11) (twisting or displacement of intestines, causing obstruction), which requires enterolysis surgery.

Example: Patient underwent reduction of volvulus via laparotomy. Report code 44050.

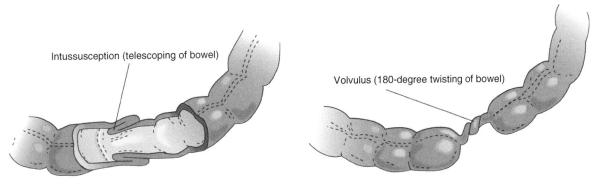

Intussusception (telescoping of bowel)

Volvulus (180-degree twisting of bowel)

FIGURE 15-11 Bowel obstructions can be caused by an intussusception or a volvulus

Excision

Enterectomy (resection of small bowel segments) procedure codes describe resection of a segment of the intestine, and they require the coder to determine the

- Amount of tissue removed
- Type of repair performed

An *enteroenterostomy* is the creation of an artificial external opening or fistula in the intestines.

> **Example:** Patient underwent enterectomy, which involved resection of two segments of the small intestine with anastomosis. Report codes 44120 and 44121. (Do not add modifier 51 to code 44121.)

Colectomy is the removal of part or all of the large intestine (e.g., colon); however, a partial colectomy is more common. Four types of partial colectomies include removal of

- All/part of the right colon (e.g., right colectomy)
- All/part of the left colon (e.g., left colectomy)
- All/part of the rectosigmoid colon (e.g., anterior resection)
- The lower rectosigmoid colon, rectum, and anus (e.g., abdominal perineal resection)

> **Example:** Patient underwent total colectomy with proctectomy and ileostomy. Report code 44155.

Laparoscopy

Surgical laparoscopy includes diagnostic laparoscopy, which means if both procedures are documented a code for the surgical laparoscopy only is reported. However, when a diagnostic laparoscopy (e.g., peritoneoscopy) *only* is performed, report the (separate procedure) code.

> **Example:** Patient underwent laparoscopic jejunostomy for feeding. Report code 44186.

Enterostomy—External Fistulization of Intestines

An **ostomy** refers to surgically creating an opening in the body for the discharge of body wastes. (A **stoma** is a surgically created opening between the ureter, small intestine, or large intestine through to the abdominal wall.) Ostomy procedures are organized according to the portion of the digestive tract that is brought to the surface. (They may be permanent or temporary.) Types of ostomies are the following:

- **Colostomy**: A portion of the colon or rectum is removed, and the remaining colon is brought to the abdominal wall (Figure 15-12).
- **Ileostomy**: The colon and rectum are removed, and the small intestine is brought to the abdominal wall.

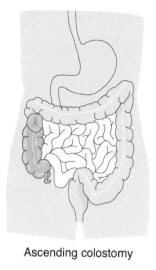

Ascending colostomy

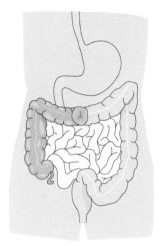

Transverse colostomy

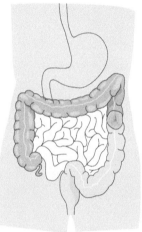

Descending colostomy

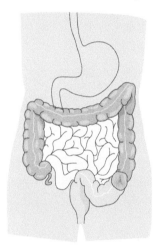

Sigmoid colostomy

FIGURE 15-12 Colostomy locations (Blue section may be surgically removed if colostomy is permanent)

A *continent ileostomy*, or *Kock pouch*, is a surgical variation of an ileostomy. A reservoir pouch is created inside the abdomen using a portion of the terminal ileum, a valve is constructed in the pouch, and a stoma is brought through the abdominal wall. A catheter is inserted into the pouch several times each day to empty feces from the reservoir.

Example: Patient underwent continent ileostomy. Report code 44316.

Endoscopy, Small Intestine and Endoscopy, Stomal

Jejunal feedings are performed via small intestinal endoscopy. This type of endoscopy is an enteroscopy that is performed beyond the second portion of the duodenum. During this procedure, a thin tube is passed through the gastrostomy tube into the stomach and advanced; a direct puncture is *not* made into the jejunum.

Example: Patient underwent small intestinal endoscopy with enteroscopy beyond the second portion of the duodenum and single biopsy. Report code 44361.

Introduction

The introduction of a long gastrointestinal (GI) tube with an inflatable balloon at the end (e.g., Miller-Abbott) is performed to clear GI strictures.

> **Example:** Patient underwent introduction of a Miller-Abbott GI tube to clear GI strictures. Report code 44500.

Repair

Repair codes are reported for procedures performed to repair the small intestine.

> **Example:** Patient underwent the suturing of a single perforation of the small intestine. Report code 44602.

Other Procedures

Other procedures codes are reported for procedures performed to exclude the small intestine from the pelvis by implanting mesh or other prosthesis or by using native tissue. When the small intestine is elevated to prevent damage from radiation therapy, mesh, other prosthesis, or native tissue is used. An instructional note below the code provides instruction to report therapeutic radiation treatment codes from the Radiology Oncology subsection of the Radiology section.

> **Example:** Patient underwent exclusion of the small intestine from the pelvis with placement of mesh. Report code 44700.

Meckel's Diverticulum and the Mesentery

Diverticula (Figure 15-13) are small pouches (herniations) in the colon that bulge outward through weak spots. *Diverticulosis* is the presence of diverticula in the mucosa and submucosa, through or between fibers of the colon's major muscle layer. Diverticulosis is almost always located in the descending or sigmoid colon.

Meckel's diverticulum is a common congenital abnormality of the GI tract that results in a pouch in the wall of the small bowel that contains remnants of fetal GI tissue. The diverticulum may contain gastric, stomach, ectopic, or pancreatic tissue. Treatment includes excision of Meckel's diverticulum.

> **Example:** Patient underwent excision of Meckel's diverticulum. Report code 44800.

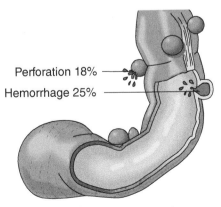

Perforation 18%
Hemorrhage 25%

FIGURE 15-13 Diverticula in the sigmoid colon

Appendix

Appendectomies are performed laparoscopically or through an open abdominal incision. An instructional note below states that when an incidental appendectomy is performed during intra-abdominal surgery, it is not reported separately. When an appendectomy is performed for an indicated purpose (e.g., inflamed) during the same operative session as another major procedure, report the appropriate appendectomy add-on code.

Example 1: Patient underwent laparoscopic appendectomy for acute appendicitis. Report code 44970.

Example 2: Patient underwent excision of Meckel's diverticulum. During surgery, the physician noted that the appendix was inflamed and enlarged; an appendectomy was also performed. Report codes 44800 and 44955. (Do not add modifier 51 to code 44955, and do not add modifier 59 to that code because an incidental appendectomy does not require a separate surgical prep or incision.)

Colon and Rectum

Procedures performed on the colon and rectum include:

- Incision
- Excision
- Destruction
- Endoscopy

- Laparoscopy
- Repair
- Manipulation
- Other procedures

Endoscopic procedure codes specify the type of instrument used, the purpose of the endoscopy, and the site involved. When reporting codes for colonoscopies (e.g., colostomy or rectum), the coder must also determine the approach and the extent of colonoscopy. GI endoscopic procedures involve the small bowel, colon, and rectum and include the following:

- **Proctosigmoidoscopy:** Visual examination of the rectum and sigmoid colon
- **Sigmoidoscopy:** Visual examination of the entire rectum and sigmoid colon and may include a portion of the descending colon (Figure 15-14)
- **Colonoscopy:** Visual examination of the entire colon, from the rectum to the cecum, and may include the terminal ileum (Figure 15-15)

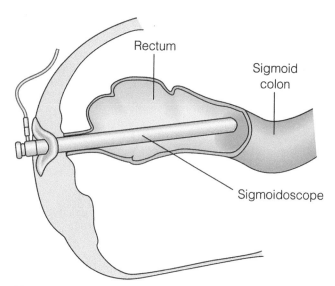

FIGURE 15-14 Sigmoidoscopy

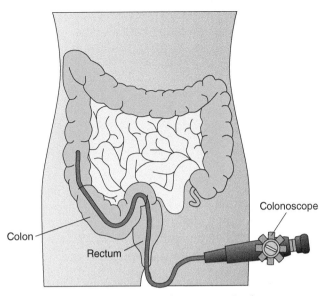

FIGURE 15-15 Colonoscopy (posterior view)

Proctosigmoidoscopy and sigmoidoscopy procedures are typically performed without anesthesia. Colonoscopies usually require sedation to avoid severe patient discomfort. Only the code for the most extensive endoscopic procedure involving the colon is reported when multiple endoscopies are performed during the same encounter.

> **Example:** Patient underwent sigmoidoscopy and colonoscopy during the same operative session. Report code 45378 for the colonoscopy only. (Do not report a code for the sigmoidoscopy because the endoscope was passed through the sigmoid colon to perform the colonoscopy. Visual examination of the sigmoid colon was performed on the way to visual examination of the rest of the colon.)

For a *colonoscopy through stoma*, the scope is inserted through the large intestine's stoma, called a colostomy that includes the following sites: sigmoid colostomy, transverse colostomy, descending colostomy, and ascending colostomy. For an *ileoscopy through stoma*, the scope is inserted through the ileostomy in the small intestine.

> **Example 1:** Patient underwent colonoscopy through stoma with endoscopic stent placement. Report code 44402.

> **Example 2:** Patient underwent diagnostic ileoscopy through stoma, which included multiple biopsies. Report code 44382.

When multiple services are provided during an endoscopic procedure, report a code for each. Multiple services are reimbursed according to multiple endoscopic payment rules (e.g., discounted reimbursement for second and subsequent procedures). An exception to this rule is follow-up treatment of bleeding due to the endoscopic procedure.

Different techniques are used to remove lesions or polyps (Figure 15-16) through an endoscope. A *hot biopsy forceps* uses tweezer-like forceps connected to a monopolar electrocautery unit and a grounding pad. *Bipolar cautery* uses an electric current that flows from one tip of the forceps to the other and does not require a

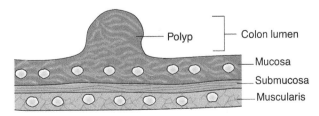

FIGURE 15-16 Colon polyp

grounding pad. An *electrocautery snare* uses a wire loop to encircle, not grasp, the polyp. *Cold biopsy forceps* does not use electrocoagulation; the polyp is simply pulled from the colon wall. *Laser technique* is most suitable for treatment of rectal lesions and uses a waveguide to deliver the laser beam through the endoscope to the lesion (e.g., YAG laser).

> **Example:** Patient underwent removal of a polyp by snare technique during a colonoscopy. During the same operative session, another area of the colon was also biopsied. Report code 45385 for the colonoscopy with polypectomy and code 45380 59 for colonoscopy with biopsy. Add modifier 59 to code 45380 because the colon biopsy was performed as a distinct and separate procedure, using different instruments.

A **proctectomy** is the surgical removal of the rectum. (Do not confuse this procedure with a *prostatectomy*, which is the excision of the prostate gland.) An *ileoanal anastomosis* (or *J-pouch*, *pull-through*, or *endorectal pull-through*) is a common alternative to conventional ileostomy, and it is not considered an ostomy because there is no stoma. The colon and most of the rectum are surgically removed, and an internal pouch is created from the terminal portion of the ileum. An opening at the bottom of the pouch is attached (anastomosed) to the anus so that existing anal sphincter muscles can be used for continence.

> **Example:** Patient underwent proctopexy via abdominal approach. Report code 45540.

Anus

Procedures performed on the anus include:

- Incision
- Excision
- Introduction
- Endoscopy

- Repair
- Destruction
- Other procedures

Anoscopy is a diagnostic procedure during which anal mucosa and the lower rectum are visualized using an anoscope. Anoscopy is typically performed to detect hemorrhoids (Figure 15-17), polyps, anal fissures, and anal bleeding.

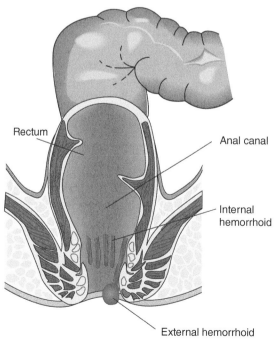

Rectum

Anal canal

Internal hemorrhoid

External hemorrhoid

FIGURE 15-17 Hemorrhoids: internal and external

For hemorrhoidectomy procedures, identify what approach was used, where the hemorrhoid(s) were located (e.g., internal or external), and whether a fissurectomy was also performed. The most commonly performed procedure is a hemorrhoidectomy by simple ligature (e.g., rubber band). (Report the appropriate code once regardless of the number of hemorrhoids removed.) Simple hemorrhoidectomy procedures do not include plastic repair; complex and extensive hemorrhoidectomy procedures do require plastic repair. When multiple methods are used to remove multiple hemorrhoids, report a code for each method.

Example: Patient underwent hemorrhoidopexy for prolapsing internal hemorrhoids via stapling. Report code 46947.

When reporting codes for the surgical treatment of anal fistulas, apply the following definitions:

- **Subcutaneous fistulectomy**: Removal of an anal fistula, without division of the sphincter muscle
- **Submuscular fistulectomy**: Removal of an anal fistula, including division of the sphincter muscle
- **Complex fistulectomy**: Excision of multiple fistulas
- **Second-stage fistulectomy/fistulotomy**: Use of a **seton**, such as a large silk suture or rubber bands, to cut through the fistula; the seton is left in place until later removal

Example: Patient underwent subcutaneous fistulectomy. Report code 46270.

Exercise 15.4 – Intestines (Except Rectum), Meckel's Diverticulum, Mesentery, Appendix, Rectum, and Anus

Instructions: Assign the CPT code(s) and appropriate modifier(s) to each statement.

1. After performing an emergency cesarean section (C-section), the physician noticed that the appendix was distended, resulting in medical necessity for an appendectomy performed during the same operative session. Code 51514 was reported for the emergency C-section as the primary procedure. Which add-on code is assigned for the appendectomy performed during the same operative session?

2. The physician performed intestinal adhesions enterolysis.

3. The physician resected two segments of small intestine and performed an anastomosis between the remaining intestinal ends. An open approach was used for this surgery.

4. The physician repaired a defect in the mesentery with sutures.

5. The physician performed a laparoscopic partial colectomy with end colostomy and closure of the distal segment.

6. The physician drained a pelvic abscess through the rectum.

7. The physician removed a portion of the rectum through combined open abdominal and transsacral approaches, with anastomosis.

8. The physician performed rigid proctosigmoidoscopy and obtained brushings.

(continues)

Exercise 15.4 – continued

9. The physician performed a flexible sigmoidoscopy and removed a polyp. The physician inserted the sigmoidoscope through the anus and advanced the scope into the sigmoid colon. The lumen of the sigmoid colon and rectum were well visualized, and the polyp was identified and removed with hot biopsy forceps. The sigmoidoscope was withdrawn upon completion of the procedure.

10. The physician inserted a colonoscope through the anus and advanced the scope past the splenic flexure. Two polyps were identified and removed by hot biopsy forceps.

Liver

Procedures performed to treat liver injuries and diseases include:

- Incision
- Excision
- Liver transplantation
- Repair
- Laparoscopy
- Other procedures

Liver injuries include gunshot wounds, stab wounds, and blunt trauma; treatment includes various methods of hemorrhage control. The management of liver hemorrhage may require a simple suture of the liver wound, or it may require complex suturing of the liver wound or injury, with or without hepatic artery ligation.

Other procedures codes are reported for the exploration of a hepatic wound, extensive debridement, coagulation, and/or packing of the liver.

A **hepatotomy** (open drainage of abscess or cyst) is performed in one or two stages, but when it is performed as a two-stage procedure, the code is not reported a second time.

Example 1: Patient underwent wedge biopsy of the liver. Report code 47100.

Example 2: Patient underwent surgical laparoscopy with ablation of one liver tumor, using cryosurgery under ultrasound guidance. Report codes 47371 and 76940.

Example 3: Patient underwent reexploration of a hepatic wound to remove packing material. Report code 47362.

Biliary Tract

Procedures performed on the organs and duct system, which creates, transports, stores, and releases bile into the duodenum (as part of the digestive process), include:

- Incision
- Introduction
- Endoscopy
- Laparoscopy
- Excision
- Repair
- Other procedures

The *biliary system* includes the following digestive accessory organs and structures (Figure 15-18):

- Gallbladder
- Bile ducts inside the liver
- Bile ducts outside the liver
- Hepatic ducts
- Common bile duct
- Cystic duct

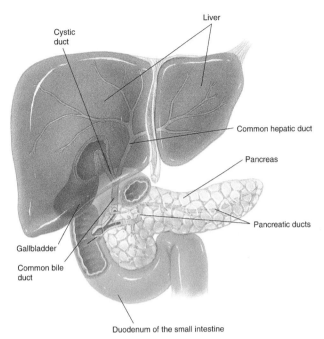

Cystic duct
Liver
Common hepatic duct
Pancreas
Pancreatic ducts
Gallbladder
Common bile duct
Duodenum of the small intestine

FIGURE 15-18 Digestive accessory organs (liver, gallbladder, and pancreas)

A **cholecystectomy** (surgical removal of the gallbladder) (Figure 15-19) can be performed laparoscopically or as an open procedure. During a cholecystectomy, common duct exploration and dilation procedures are often performed through the same incision. An operative cholangiography may also be performed during the same operative session.

Coding Tip

When a cholecystectomy is attempted laparoscopically and converted to an open procedure, report a code for the open cholecystectomy procedure only.

Example: Patient underwent open cholecystostomy with removal of gallbladder calculus. Report code 47480.

Pancreas

Procedures performed on the pancreas, including pancreas transplantation, include:

- Incision
- Excision
- Introduction
- Repair
- Pancreas transplantation
- Other procedures

The **Whipple procedure** is the excision of the pancreas, duodenum, bile duct, and stomach with reconstruction; code assignment is based on the extent of the excision. The code reported for an internal anastomosis of the pancreatic duct is based on the approach.

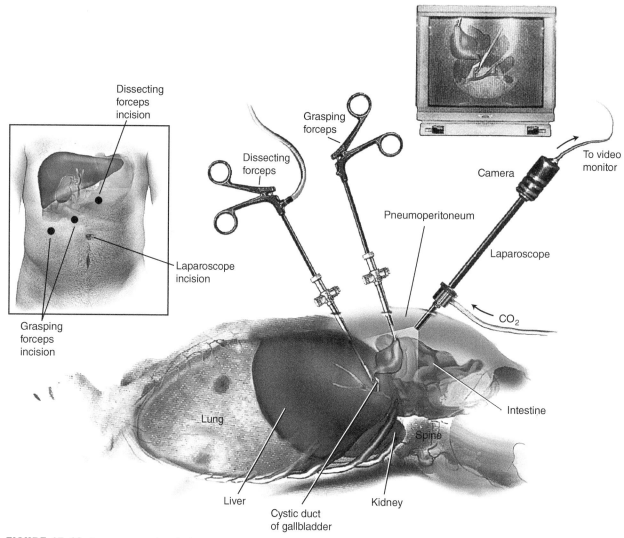

FIGURE 15-19 Laparoscopic cholecystectomy (lateral view)

Example: Patient underwent placement of a peripancreatic drain for pancreatitis. Report code 48000.

Abdomen, Peritoneum, and Omentum

Procedures performed on the abdomen, peritoneum, and omentum include:

- Incision
- Excision, destruction
- Laparoscopy
- Introduction, revision, removal
- Repair
- Suture
- Other procedures

When reporting codes, make sure you review the operative report to determine whether the procedure was performed via laparotomy or laparoscopy.

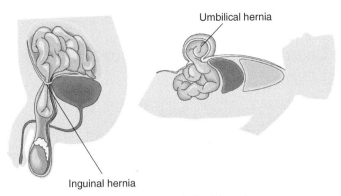

FIGURE 15-20 Inguinal and umbilical hernias

A *hernia* is the protrusion of internal organs (e.g., intestines) through a weakening in the musculature. To report codes for hernia repair procedures, determine the

- Hernia site (e.g., inguinal, lumbar, or femoral) (Figure 15-20)
- Patient's age
- Type of hernia (initial or recurrent)
- Clinical presentation of the hernia (e.g., reducible, incarcerated, strangulated, or recurrent)
- Use of mesh

Hernia repairs (herniorrhaphies) include

- Traditional/conventional (physician pushes bulging tissue back into the abdominal cavity and sutures surrounding muscle in place)
- Mesh repairs (uses mesh, such as Marlex or Prolene, instead of sutures to repair incisional or ventral hernias)
- Laparoscopic (typically performed to repair bilateral and recurrent hernias)

 Coding Tip

- Neonatal diaphragmatic hiatal hernia repairs are not included in the Digestive System subsection. To report codes for these repairs, refer to the Mediastinum and Diaphragm subsection.
- Implantation of mesh or other prosthesis is reported for incisional or ventral hernia repairs. When mesh or other prosthesis is used to repair other types of hernias, do *not* separately report a code. (The mesh code is also reported with Integumentary System codes for closure after debridement of necrotizing soft tissue infection.)
- When strangulated organs are repaired in addition to a strangulated hernia, report a code for each procedure performed.
- When a hernia repair is performed during another open abdominal procedure, a code for the hernia repair is reported only if it was performed through a different incisional site. Add modifier 59 (Distinct procedural service) to the hernia repair code. An incidental hernia repair during the course of an abdominal procedure is not coded and reported.

Exercise 15.5 – Liver, Biliary Tract, Pancreas, Abdomen, Peritoneum, and Omentum

Instructions: Assign the CPT code(s) and appropriate modifier(s) to each statement.

1. Hepatotomy for open drainage of abscess or cyst, 1 stage.

   _____

2. Surgeon removed segments II, III, and IV (the whole left lobe) of the liver from a living donor.

   _____

3. The physician performed radiofrequency ablation of a liver tumor via an open laparotomy.

   _____

4. The physician performed laparoscopic cholecystectomy with common bile duct exploration.

   _____

5. The physician performed a cholecystostomy with removal of calculus.

   _____

6. Subsequent to a previous peritoneocentesis (performed at a different operative session), the physician withdrew fluid and performed infusion and drainage of fluid from the abdominal cavity (peritoneal lavage).

   _____

7. The physician reopened a recent laparotomy incision, before the incision had fully healed, to drain a postoperative infection.

   _____

8. The physician performed laparoscopic repair of an initial inguinal hernia.

   _____

9. The physician performed a two-centimeter reducible epigastric hernia repair.

   _____

10. The physician repaired an initial, reducible, inguinal hernia with hydrocelectomy in a five-month-old infant.

   _____

Urinary System Subsection

The *urinary system* consists of the kidneys, ureters, urinary bladder, and urethra (Figure 15-21). Blood flows through the renal arteries to the kidneys, where waste materials are filtered and urine is formed. Urine is transported from the kidneys to the bladder by the ureters, and the urine ultimately passes out of the body through the urethra.

 NOTE:

The *ureter* is the tube that conveys urine from each kidney to the urinary bladder; there are two ureters. The *urethra* is the tube that conveys urine from the urinary bladder to the outside of the body.

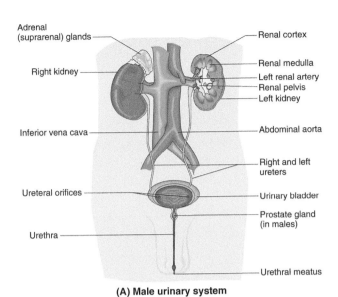
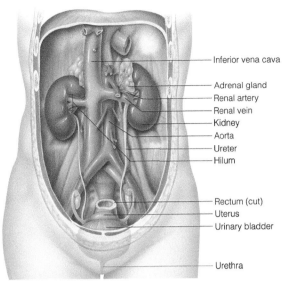

(A) Male urinary system   **(B) Female urinary system**

FIGURE 15-21 Urinary system (A) Male (B) Female

A urinary tract infection is a common disorder of the urinary system and may involve different areas of the urinary tract (e.g., urethritis, prostatitis, cystitis, and pyelonephritis). Other urinary system disorders affect the pressure within the urinary system, affect stagnation of flow (stasis), and cause the formation of stones (calculi).

Urinary system function can also be affected by disorders such as obstruction (e.g., benign prostatic hypertrophy or strictures), which typically form in three places within the ureter.

- Ureteropelvic junction (between ureter and renal pelvis)
- Ureterovesical junction (between ureter and bladder)
- Ureter/iliac arteries

Various methods are used to treat urinary disorders, including open procedures and endoscopy or laparoscopy. Diagnostic urodynamic procedures (study of urine storage and voiding functions) include tests such as the following:

- Cystometrogram
- Uroflowmetry
- Urethral pressure profile (UPP)
- Neuromuscular studies
- Voiding pressure (VP) studies

Urinary system procedures are organized according to anatomical site and surgical approach (e.g., open, incision, percutaneous, endoscopic, or laparoscopic), including endoscopic and open procedures.

Many procedures include the phrase *exclusive of radiologic service*, which means that an additional code from the Radiology section is assigned to report the radiologic service performed.

> **Example:** Patient underwent renal endoscopy through established nephrostomy, with biopsy. Report code 50555.

Urinary system procedures are organized according to anatomical site.

- Kidney
- Ureter

- Bladder
- Urethra

Kidney

Procedures performed on the kidney include:

- Incision
- Excision
- Renal transplantation
- Introduction

- Repair
- Laparoscopy
- Endoscopy
- Other procedures

The *kidneys* filter and clean the blood, producing urine that carries waste. In renal (kidney) failure, filtration of blood is slowed or stopped (due to obstruction, bacterial infection, or injury). This causes waste products and other toxic substances to build up in the blood. These problems can lead to renal failure, resulting in the need for treatment such as surgery or dialysis.

The removal of urinary calculi (stones) (Figure 15-22) is coded according to the anatomical site (e.g., renal pelvis, bladder, or urethra) and approach (e.g., open incision, percutaneous, or endoscopic).

Example: Patient underwent left nephrolithotomy to remove urinary stones. Report code 50060 LT.

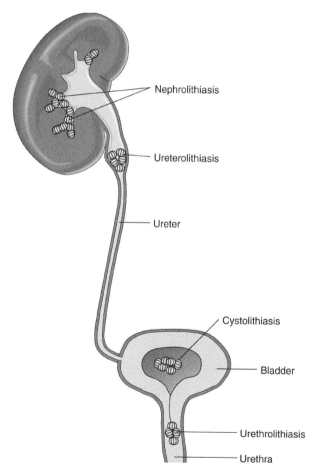

FIGURE 15-22 Common locations of urinary calculi (stone) formation: nephrolithiasis (kidney stone), ureterolithiasis (ureter stone), cystolithiasis (urinary bladder stone), and urethrolithiasis (urethral stone)

Nephrectomy (surgical removal of a kidney) requires review of the operative report to identify the

- Type of procedure (e.g., partial or total)
- Surgical approach (e.g., laparoscopic or open)
- Other structures removed

Example: Patient underwent laparoscopic partial nephrectomy, left. Report code 50543 LT.

When a surgeon performs a retrograde pyelography (or retrograde ureteropyelography), one or both of the ureters are catheterized and contrast is injected slowly through the catheter.

Example: Patient underwent injection procedure for left ureterogram, existing access. Report code 50431 LT. The number (#) sign that precedes the code indicates a resequenced code, which means it is out of numerical order in CPT.

Extracorporeal shock wave lithotripsy (ESWL) is a nonoperative procedure that uses ultrasonic shock waves to break up stones in the renal pelvis or ureter (Figure 15-23). The patient then passes the stones in urine, with minimal discomfort. **Percutaneous lithotomy** and **lithotripsy** is a two-stage procedure that requires a percutaneous nephrostomy and dilation of the nephrostomy tract. Instruments (e.g., a basket or lithotripter) are inserted via nephrostomy, and the stones are removed.

Example: Patient underwent extracorporeal shock wave lithotripsy on the left side to pulverize kidney stones. Report code 50590 LT.

Renal transplantation procedures include three distinct components.

- Harvest of the kidney from a cadaver or living donor
- Physician backbench work, which includes standard preparation of a cadaver or living donor allograft prior to transplantation
- Allotransplantation (e.g., organ removal, if required, and transplantation of the allograft)

The procurement of kidneys involves harvesting organs from a cadaver or living donor. Once the kidney is received by the hospital, backbench standard preparation is performed to prepare the kidneys for transplantation. The actual transplantation of the kidney (Figure 15-24) into the recipient is also reported. During kidney transplants, a patient's nonfunctioning kidney(s) might not be removed. A code is reported when the nonfunctioning kidney(s) are removed. Add modifier LT (Left side) or RT (Right side) for unilateral kidney transplant and nonfunctioning resection procedures. Add modifier 50 (Bilateral procedure) when both kidneys are transplanted or both nonfunctioning kidneys are resected.

Example: Patient underwent left kidney transplant, including backbench standard preparation of living donor renal allograft. Left kidney was obtained from a living donor. Report codes 50365 LT, 50325 51 LT (recipient), and 50320 LT (donor).

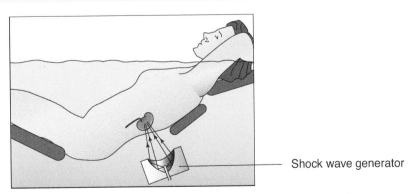

FIGURE 15-23 **Extracorporeal shock wave lithotripsy (ESWL)**

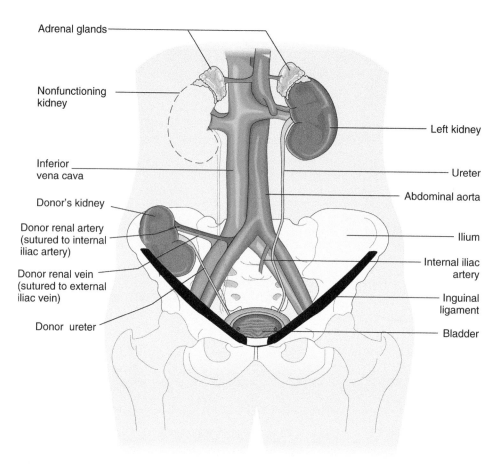

FIGURE 15-24 Renal (kidney) transplantation

Ureter

Procedures performed on the ureter include:

- Incision and biopsy
- Excision
- Introduction

- Repair
- Laparoscopy
- Endoscopy

The *ureters* convey urine from the kidneys to the urinary bladder. The walls of the ureters contain muscle that propels urine using wavelike motions called *peristalsis*. Procedures performed on the ureters are based on two approaches.

- Open endoscopic
- Laparoscopic

To facilitate the passage of urine through the ureter(s), a physician may insert a ureteral stent. Stents used to relieve or prevent ureteral obstruction can be placed during the course of another diagnostic or therapeutic intervention. Stents may be temporary, and the physician may remove a temporary stent and insert another type of stent (e.g., indwelling).

A **ureterolithotomy** is the surgical removal of stones from the ureter. The procedure should identify the ureteral location from which the stone was removed.

- Upper one-third of ureter
- Middle one-third of ureter
- Lower one-third of ureter

Ureteral anastomosis procedures are mutually exclusive procedures, and codes for these procedures are not usually reported for the same operative session. However, if during the same operative session, an anastomosis is performed on one ureter and a different anastomosis is performed on the other ureter, add modifiers LT (Left side) and RT (Right side) to each code (to describe the service performed on each respective ureter).

"Ureterostomy, transplantation of ureter to skin," is mutually exclusive of "ureterostomy, ureterocolon conduit, and urinary undiversion" procedures unless performed on different locations. When reporting a ureterostomy code for the transplantation of the ureter to skin with another ureter procedure code, add modifier 59 (Distinct procedural service) and modifier LT or RT to both procedure codes.

Ureteral endoscopy is the visualization of the ureter(s) using an endoscope. Review the operative report to locate the procedure performed through the endoscope (e.g., biopsy).

Example: Patient underwent ureterolysis, with repositioning of left ureter for retroperitoneal fibrosis. Report code 50715 LT.

Bladder

Procedures performed on the bladder include:

- Incision
- Removal
- Excision
- Introduction
- Urodynamics
- Repair
- Laparoscopy
- Endoscopy (e.g., cystoscopy, urethroscopy, cystourethroscopy)
- Transurethral surgery
- Vesical neck and prostate

The *urinary bladder* is a hollow organ that serves as a reservoir for urine until it passes from the body (via urination). Urine enters the urinary bladder from the ureters and exits through the urethra.

Coding Tip

Urethral catheterization codes (Figure 15-25) are reported only when performed independently.

- When urethral catheterization is performed preceding surgery, a code is not separately reported. Urethral catheterization is considered integral to preoperative services provided and represents the standard of medical practice.
- When urethral catheterization or urethral dilation is necessary to accomplish a more extensive procedure, a code for the urethral catheterization or urethral dilation is not separately reported.

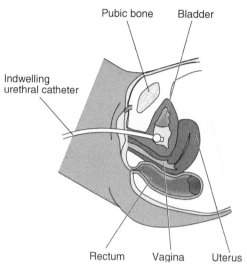

FIGURE 15-25 Indwelling urethral catheter in a female patient

Open excisional procedures of the bladder include the excision of urachal cysts and sinuses, cystostomy (Figure 15-26), cystectomy, and pelvic exenteration. Diagnostic urodynamic procedures are performed to study urine storage and voiding functions, and the codes may be reported separately or in combination when more than one procedure is performed. (Report as many codes as necessary to completely describe procedures performed.) Urodynamics includes cystometrogram (CMG), uroflowmetry (UFR), urethral pressure profile studies, neuromuscular studies, and voiding pressure studies.

A *cystometrogram* records urinary bladder pressure at various volumes, which is useful in diagnosing bladder outlet obstruction and other voiding dysfunctions.

- A simple cystometrogram measures the bladder's capacity, sensation, and intravesical pressure.
- A complex cystometrogram is a procedure in which the physician uses a rectal probe to differentiate abdominal pressure from bladder pressure. Components of complex cystometry include the placement of the transurethral catheter and anal probe, measurement of voiding cystometry and intra-abdominal pressure, and other provocative maneuvers (e.g., patient position changes and trials of anticholinergics or muscle depressants).

Uroflowmetry measures the amount of urine that flows from the urinary bladder per second.

- Simple uroflowmetry measures voiding time and peak flow using nonautomated equipment.
- Complex uroflowmetry measures/records mean, peak flow, and time to reach peak flow during continuous urination, and it is performed using automated equipment.

UPP studies (urethral closure pressure profile) describe tests for measuring urethral pressure. A UPP records pressures along the urethra using a special catheter. Electromyography studies measure anal or urethral sphincter muscle activity during voiding and urine flow rate. This study is usually performed on patients with voiding dysfunctions.

Voiding pressure (VP) studies involve placing a transducer into the urinary bladder to measure the patient's urine flow rate and pressure during emptying of the urinary bladder. Intra-abdominal VP (e.g., rectal, gastric, and intraperitoneal) can also be measured.

Example 1: Patient underwent simple uroflowmetry. Report code 51736.

Example 2: Patient underwent complex uroflowmetry, which required the use of calibrated electronic equipment. Report code 51741.

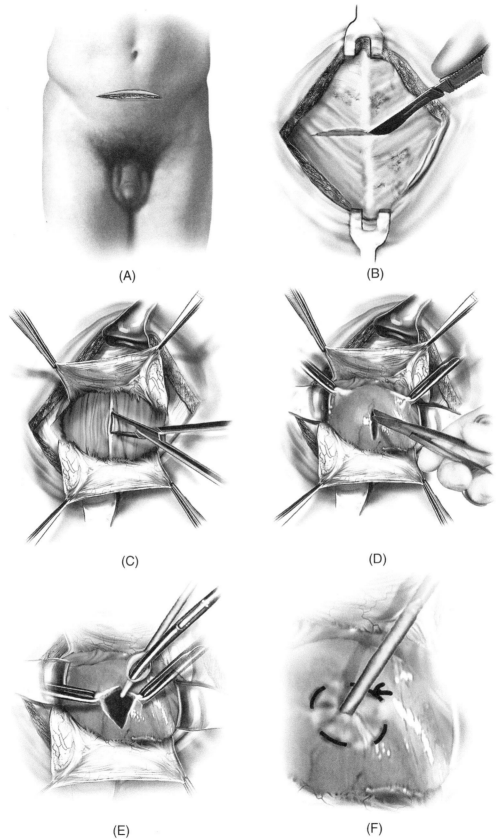

(A)

(B)

(C)

(D)

(E)

(F)

FIGURE 15-26 Open cystostomy (A) Incision site (B) Fascia incised (C) Muscle split (D) Bladder incised (E) Cystostomy tube inserted (F) Cystostomy tube secured with purse-string suture

Urinary endoscopy procedures are organized according to

- Anatomical area (e.g., urethra, prostate, or ureter)
- Procedure performed (e.g., cystourethroscopy with insertion of indwelling ureteral stent)

Cystoscopy, or **cystourethroscopy** (Figure 15-27), allows for the direct visual examination of the urinary bladder and urethra.

> **Example:** A cystourethroscope was passed through the urethra and urinary bladder to examine the urethra, bladder, and ureteral openings. No other procedure was performed. Report code 52000.

Transurethral surgery is performed on the

- Urethra and bladder
- Ureter and pelvis

It is important to review the operative report to identify the anatomical site for the surgery performed. Diagnostic procedures (e.g., bladder biopsy) and therapeutic procedures (e.g., steroid injection into a urethral stricture) are accomplished using a transurethral approach. Transurethral surgeries include diagnostic cystoscopy, which is not reported separately.

When a physician performs a urethral dilation to determine the size of the cystoscope to be inserted, do not code and report the dilation procedure separately. However, when the physician performs a cystourethroscopy with transurethral dilation for a urethral stricture, assign an appropriate code.

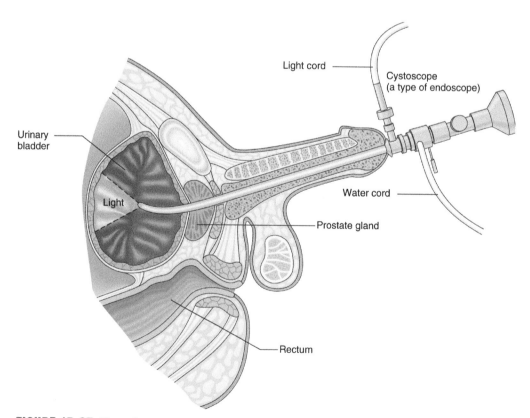

FIGURE 15-27 Use of a cystoscope to examine the interior of the bladder in a male

Cystourethroscopy with removal of foreign body, calculus, or ureteral stent from urethra or bladder is described as simple or complicated.

Before a transurethral therapeutic or diagnostic intervention procedure is performed, a direct visual examination is performed using a cystourethroscope. The cystoscope is passed through the male urethra to visualize the urethra, prostate, and bladder.

Instructional notes clarify the reporting of temporary stents and self-retaining indwelling stents. Indwelling ureteral catheters are inserted into the renal pelvis via the ureter to allow drainage (e.g., when a tumor is impinging on the ureters). Gibbons and double-J stents are the most common ureteral stents.

When a surgeon performs a **transurethral ureteroscopic lithotripsy** (instead of an ESWL), a cystoscope is inserted through the urethra into the bladder and a ureteroscope is passed into the ureters. Instruments passed through the ureteroscope into the ureters are used to manipulate and disintegrate stones (utilizing transcystoscopic electrohydraulic shock waves, ultrasound, or laser).

Transurethral resection of the prostate (TURP) is an initial resection of the prostate gland via transurethral approach using an electrosurgical device. Specific codes are included for laser treatment of the prostate gland. TURP codes include vasectomy, meatotomy, cystourethroscopy, urethral calibration, dilation, and/or internal urethrotomy. Codes for these procedures, when performed during the same operative session as a TURP, are not reported separately.

The physician may perform a prostatectomy using different methods, such as transurethral two-stage prostatectomy *or* transurethral destruction of the prostate using *either* microwave thermotherapy *or* radiofrequency.

Urethra

Procedures performed on the urethra include:

- Incision
- Excision
- Repair
- Manipulation
- Other procedures

The *urethra* is a muscular tube that discharges urine from the urinary bladder. In males, the urethra also serves as a passageway for semen. Codes assigned for urethral procedures will vary depending on the gender of the patient.

Example 1: Female patient underwent total urethrectomy, including cystostomy. Report code 53210.

Example 2: Male patient underwent total urethrectomy, including cystostomy. Report code 53215.

To report codes properly for urethral excision procedures, locate the diagnosis in the patient's record.

Example 1: Patient underwent excision of urethral polyp, distal urethra. Report code 53260.

Example 2: Patient underwent excision of urethral caruncle. Report code 53265.

For **urethroplasty** (repair of the urethra), identify whether the procedure was staged *and* which stage was performed.

> **Example 1:** Patient underwent urethroplasty, first stage, to repair stricture. Report code 53400.

> **Example 2:** Patient underwent urethroplasty, second stage, to form a urethra. Procedure included urinary diversion. Report code 53405.

> **Example 3:** Patient underwent one-stage urethroplasty to reconstruct a male anterior urethra. Report code 53410.

For dilation of urethral stricture, identify the surgical approach, patient's sex, and whether dilation was initial or subsequent.

> **Example 1:** Male patient underwent initial dilation of urethral stricture by passage of sound or urethral dilator. Report code 53600.

> **Example 2:** Male patient underwent subsequent dilation of urethral stricture by passage of sound or urethral dilator. Report code 53601.

> **Example 3:** Male patient underwent initial dilation of urethral stricture by passage of filiform and follower. Report code 53620.

> **Example 4:** Female patient underwent initial dilation of urethra including suppository and instillation. Report code 53660.

 Coding Tip

Urethral repair codes are performed to treat urethral wounds or injuries (urethrorrhaphy). When urethroplasty is performed, do not report a separate code for urethrorrhaphy because suture to repair wound or injury is included in the urethroplasty procedure.

Exercise 15.6 – Urinary System

Instructions: Assign the CPT code(s) and appropriate modifier(s) to each statement.

1. Physician made an open incision and inserted multiple drain tubes to drain an infection (abscess) from the right kidney.

   _____

2. The physician pulverized a renal calculus by directing extracorporeal shock wave therapy through a water cushion placed against the left side of the patient at the location of the kidney stone.

   _____

(continues)

Exercise 15.6 – continued

3. The physician removed a kidney stone (calculus) by making an incision in the right kidney.

_____

4. The interventional radiologist inserted a percutaneous nephrostomy catheter into the right renal pelvis for drainage. Fluoroscopic guidance was provided.

_____

5. The physician performed laparoscopic ablation of a solid mass from the posterior hilum of the left kidney.

_____

6. The physician made an incision in the left ureter through the abdominal wall for examination of the ureter and insertion of a catheter for drainage.

_____

7. The physician examined the patient's right and left renal and ureteral structures with an endoscope, which passed through an established opening between the skin and the ureter (ureterostomy). The physician also inserted a catheter into the ureter.

_____

8. The physician revised a surgical opening between the skin and the right ureter.

_____

9. Patient underwent left antegrade urography, including radiological supervision and interpretation. The physician performed an injection procedure through an indwelling ureteral catheter for the ureterography.

_____

10. The physician performed a transurethral resection of a postoperative bladder neck contracture using a resectoscope.

_____

11. The physician inserted a special instrument through the cystourethroscope to fragment a calculus in the ureter using electrohydraulics.

_____

12. The physician inserted a suprapubic catheter in the bladder to aspirate urine.

_____

13. The physician performed a sling procedure using synthetic material to treat a male patient's urinary incontinence.

_____

14. The physician made an initial attempt to treat a male patient's urethral stricture using a dilator.

_____

15. The physician performed a transurethral destruction of the prostate using microwave therapy.

_____

Summary

The Mediastinum and Diaphragm subsection includes codes for procedures performed on the mediastinum and diaphragm. The Digestive System subsection includes procedures to diagnose and treat disorders of the digestive system (e.g., gastrointestinal endoscopy, laparoscopy, and gastric analysis). Similar to other Surgery subsections, procedures are organized first by anatomical area and then by type. Digestive System subsection codes are also reported for open, endoscopic, and laparoscopic procedures. The operative report must be carefully reviewed to correctly identify the surgical approach. Urinary System subsection procedures are organized according to anatomical site and surgical approach (e.g., open, incision, percutaneous, endoscopic, or laparoscopic). The subsection also separates endoscopy procedures from open procedures. Many procedures include the phrase "exclusive of radiologic service," which means that an additional code from the Radiology section is assigned to report the radiological service performed.

Internet Links

American College of Gastroenterology (ACG): Go to **www.gi.org**, and click on the Patients link to access information about diseases and treatments.

Society of American Gastrointestinal and Endoscopic Surgeons (SAGES): www.sages.org

Urology Care Foundation: **www.urologyhealth.org**

WebSurg's Online university of IRCAD: **www.websurg.com**

Review

15.1 – Multiple Choice

Instructions: Select the most appropriate response.

1. Which types of hernias are assigned codes from the Mediastinum and Diaphragm subsection of Surgery?
    a. Abdominal and epigastric
    b. Hiatus and diaphragmatic
    c. Incisional and inguinal
    d. Umbilicus and femoral

2. Procedures performed on the gallbladder, bile ducts, hepatic ducts, and cystic ducts are assigned codes from which anatomical category of the Digestive System subsection of Surgery?
    a. Abdomen, Peritoneum, and Omentum
    b. Biliary Tract
    c. Liver
    d. Ureter

3. Hernia repair codes are located in which category of the Digestive System subsection of Surgery?
    a. Abdomen, Peritoneum, and Omentum
    b. Anus
    c. Appendix
    d. Rectum

4. Which procedure(s) has/have age as a factor in determining the correct code?
    a. Colonoscopy
    b. Esophagotomy and esophagoscopy
    c. Palatopharyngoplasty
    d. Tonsillectomy and adenoidectomy

5. When assigning codes for a ureterolithotomy procedure (50610–50630), which correctly describes the location in the ureter from which the stone was removed?
    a. Right or left side of ureter
    b. Upper-left, lower-left, upper-right, or lower-right quadrant of ureter
    c. Upper, middle, or lower one-third of ureter
    d. Upper or lower half of ureter

6. Diagnostic procedures (e.g., uroflowmetry) that are performed to study urine storage and voiding functions are assigned a code from which subcategory of the Bladder category in the Urinary System subsection of Surgery?
    a. Bladder
    b. Endoscopy
    c. Laparoscopy
    d. Urodynamics

7. Codes for urethral catheterization are reported when performed _____ another urinary bladder procedure.
    a. in combination with
    b. independently of
    c. preceding surgery for
    d. as a more extensive procedure than

8. Which gastrointestinal (GI) endoscopy procedure involves injecting dye through a tube in the endoscope to allow for visualization of the ducts on x-rays?
    a. Endoscopic retrograde cholangiopancreatography (ERCP)
    b. Esophagogastroduodenoscopy (EGD)
    c. Esophagoscopy
    d. Upper GI endoscopy (esophagogastroscopy)

9. When the patient is scheduled to undergo sigmoidoscopy, and the procedure is halted after proctoscopy, the CPT code for _____ is reported.
    a. colonoscopy
    b. proctoscopy
    c. sigmoidoscopy
    d. transverse colonoscopy

10. When a hernia repair is performed through a different incisional site during another open abdominal procedure, which modifier is added to the hernia repair code?
    a. 51   b. 58   c. 59   d. 79

11. Excision of mediastinal tumor. Which CPT code is assigned?
    a. 39200   b. 39220   c. 39401   d. 39402

12. Destruction of dentoalveolar lesion. Which CPT code is assigned?
    a. 41825   b. 41826   c. 41827   d. 41850

13. Simple revision of colostomy. Which CPT code is assigned?
    a. 44320   b. 44322   c. 44340   d. 44345

14. Incision and drainage of ischiorectal abscess. Which CPT code is assigned?
    a. 45020   b. 46040   c. 46045   d. 46060

15. Proximal subtotal pancreatectomy with total duodenectomy, partial gastrectomy, choledochoenterostomy, and gastrojejunostomy with pancreatojejunostomy. Which CPT code is assigned?
    a. 48150   b. 48152   c. 48153   d. 48154

16. Peritoneoscopy with partial laparoscopic colectomy and anastomosis. Which CPT code(s) are assigned?
    a. 44140
    b. 44204
    c. 49320, 44140
    d. 49320, 44204

17. Open drainage of retroperitoneal abscess. Which CPT code is assigned?
    a. 49020   b. 49060   c. 49405   d. 49406

18. Intraoral incision and drainage of hematoma of tongue, submandibular space. Which CPT code is assigned?
    a. 41008   b. 41009   c. 41015   d. 41017

19. Cystourethroscopy with resection of 1.1-cm bladder tumor. Which CPT code is assigned?
    a. 52224   b. 52234   c. 52235   d. 52240

20. Female patient underwent reconstructive urethroplasty. Which CPT code is assigned?
    a. 53410   b. 53420   c. 53430   d. 53431

15.2 – Coding Practice: Mediastinum and Diaphragm

Instructions: Assign the CPT code(s) and appropriate modifier(s) to each case.

1. A patient is found to have a cyst-like lesion per magnetic resonance imaging (MRI) of the mediastinum. This is to be removed. An incision is made by the physician from the shoulder blade to the spinal column of the thoracic area. Muscles are retracted, and the rib cage is exposed. After gaining access to the thoracic cavity, the physician identifies the cyst and resects it. The specimen is sent to pathology. The wound is closed in layers.

_____

2. A 45-year-old patient has an acute traumatic diaphragmatic hernia. After adequate general anesthesia, an abdominal incision is made in the epigastric region. A moderate amount of abdominal tissue is protruding through the hernia into the diaphragm. These contents are moved back into proper placement. The opening of the diaphragm is closed with sutures.

_____

3. Via transabdominal approach, the physician performs imbrication by overlapping diaphragm tissue to ensure that the diaphragm is in the correct position and the eventration is corrected.

_____

4. A lacerated diaphragm tear measuring 2.5 cm is repaired with sutures.

_____

5. A patient is being seen to confirm the diagnosis of sarcoidosis. An endoscopic examination of the mediastinum is done under general anesthesia. After making an incision in the area of the sternum, the scope is inserted. The trachea, bronchi, and lymph nodes are examined. A lymph node biopsy is taken. The scope is withdrawn, and the incision is closed with sutures.

_____

15.3 – Coding Practice: Digestive System

Instructions: Assign the CPT code(s) and appropriate modifier(s) to each case.

1. A patient had the signs and symptoms consistent with a perforated viscus. After discussion, the patient consented to suture repair of the gastric ulcer. The patient was placed in a supine position. After adequate anesthesia, attention was turned to the anterior abdominal wall. A midline incision was made. Gross contamination was visualized. This was suctioned out. The perforated gastric ulcer was visualized, and copious irrigation with 3 liters of warm saline was performed. All gross evidence of contamination was gone. Checking was done, hemostasis was throughout, and the skin incision was closed.

_____

2. A patient presented with a lesion of the lip; due to the patient's history of smoking, it was determined to remove the lesion and send it to analysis to rule out carcinoma. After adequate anesthesia, a wedge excision was done of the lower lip to remove the lesion. The defect was closed with a small flap and sutures.

_____

3. A patient with the diagnosis of carcinoma of the stomach presented for a hemigastrectomy. With the patient in the supine position and after adequate level of general anesthesia, the abdomen was prepped and draped in usual sterile fashion. An upper midline incision was made to access the abdominal cavity. The abdominal ligament was retracted to the right side of the incision. The stoma was mobilized. The duodenum was divided away from the stomach. The tumor was identified. The stomach tumor was transected with cautery, and a specimen was sent for evaluation by pathology. The distal margin of the remaining stomach was cleaned. Staples were used to close the curvature area of the stomach. The abdomen was closed with running Prolene for the fascia. The skin was closed with staples.

_____

4. An 18-year-old patient has a history of chronic tonsillitis. Under general anesthesia, the physician separated the tonsils from the tonsil bed by blunt and sharp dissection followed by the snare. No gross bleeding was found. The adenoids were extracted by the adenotome followed by the sharp curette. Again, no gross bleeding was found. The patient had minimal blood loss.

---

5. A 72-year-old patient presented to the emergency department with a 14-hour history of acute right inguinal pain and obstructive symptoms. Examination found a tender nonreducible mass in the right groin. Patient consented to surgical intervention via exploration and correction of possible hernia. After adequate anesthesia, the patient had an oblique preperitoneal incision through the fascia. The peritoneal cavity was entered. A strangulated loop was found along with the femoral hernia. The lower edge of the inguinal ligament was grasped with clamps, and interrupted Prolenes were used to close the femoral defect using Coopers ligament repair. The defect was closed up to the edge of the external iliac vein. Once the repair was completed, the wound was irrigated with saline. The bowel was inspected and appeared to be totally revascularized, with no evidence of necrosis and no need for resection. The femoral hernia sac was reduced and resected using electrocautery. The abdominal wall was closed with interrupted polypropylene sutures for the anterior wall fascia. A Jackson-Pratt drain was brought out through a separate stab wound. The subcutaneous tissue was closed with interrupted 3-0 Vicryl, and the skin was closed with staples.

---

6. A patient with chronic cholelithiasis presented for a cholecystectomy. An infraumbilical incision was made, and a trocar was inserted into the abdominal cavity. After insufflation of the cavity, the laparoscope was inserted through the trocar. Two additional incisions were made to place trocars—one on the right side and one on the left. The gallbladder was identified. It was noted to be slightly enlarged and grayish in color. Multiple stones were palpable inside the gallbladder. Tissue surrounding the gallbladder was dissected. The cystic duct and artery were clipped and then cut. The gallbladder was dissected from the liver bed and removed through the umbilical trocar site. Careful irrigation of the cavity was done. The patient had minimal blood loss.

---

7. A 19-year-old patient presented to the hospital with a history of bloody stools of three weeks' duration. The patient was prepped for a sigmoidoscopy. The sigmoidoscope was passed without difficulty to about 40 cm. The entire mucosal lining was erythematous. There was no friability of the overlying mucosa and no bleeding noted anywhere. No pseudopolyps were noted. Biopsies were taken at about 30 cm; these were thought to be representative of the mucosa in general. The scope was retracted; no other abnormalities were seen.

---

8. A patient with a history of breast cancer presented for a biopsy of the liver to confirm metastatic disease. The abdomen was exposed by an incision through the skin, fascia, and muscle. A wedge-shaped section of the liver was resected. This specimen was sent to pathology.

---

9. A patient was found to have a sublingual abscess of the mouth. After consent and normal prep, an incision up through the supramylohyoid muscle was made. The superficial abscess was identified, an extraoral incision made, and clear liquid fluid was drained from the abscess.

---

10. A 45-year-old patient has been diagnosed with a right parotid gland mass via examination and radiograph films. The patient presented for excision of this mass. After adequate anesthesia, the initial incision was made near the midpoint of the mandible. Skin flaps were retracted to expose the right parotid gland. The facial nerve was visualized. A mass was identified on the lateral lobe of the right parotid gland, and it was carefully dissected free from the space with attention not to damage the facial nerve. The mass was sent in total to pathology for analysis.

15.4 – Coding Practice: Urinary System

Instructions: Assign the CPT code(s) and appropriate modifier(s) to each case.

1. A patient with the complaint of hematuria presented for an endoscopic examination under conscious sedation. A cystourethroscope was passed through the structures of the urinary system. A lesion was identified on the trigone; this was fulgurated. The cystourethroscope was removed.

   _____

2. A patient was diagnosed with a urethral calculus as confirmed by x-ray. Endoscopic treatment was warranted to remove this stone. A cystourethroscope was passed through the urethra, and the stone was extracted through the endoscope. The remaining structures of the system were examined and found to be normal. The cystourethroscope was removed.

   _____

3. The patient consented to cystourethroscopy with possible bladder tumor removal. After the endoscope was inserted through the urethra, the bladder was entered. A lesion approximately 3.0 cm in size was identified in the bladder. This was resected and taken out through the scope. Minimal bleeders were cauterized. The remainder of the bladder was normal in appearance. The cystoscope was removed.

   _____

4. Imaging was used to assist in the percutaneous insertion of a guidewire, and a catheter was inserted to drain and collect fluid from the right kidney for analysis. The catheter was removed, and a bandage was applied.

   _____

5. The patient was placed on a table. Water-filled bellows using coupling gel to make contact with the skin of the patient's right back were positioned at the area of the kidney stone. Extracorporeal shock wave therapy was administered and directed in short bursts toward the bellows for a total of 35 minutes. The process was overseen by the attending physician, who monitored the fragmentation of the stone. The patient was discharged with instructions to drain urine and collect stone fragments.

   _____

6. An endoscope was passed through the urethra. The urethra was normal in appearance, as was the bladder upon examination. The cystourethroscope was then directed to the right ureter. Slight narrowing was seen in the distal third of this ureter. A double-J stent was placed in the right ureter. The left ureter was then examined and found to be normal. The stent will be removed at a later date.

   _____

7. With the patient under general anesthesia, a midline incision was made over the abdominal cavity wall. After the bladder was accessed, a right ureterocele was identified. This was repaired via an incision made in the bladder. All bleeders were cauterized. Minimal blood loss was noted. The bladder was closed with absorbable sutures. A urethral Foley catheter was placed. The fascia and muscle were closed with staples. The skin was closed with sutures.

   _____

8. The patient consented to a renal biopsy. The skin of the back was punctured with the biopsy needle after administration of anesthesia. The needle was advanced to the right kidney. The core of the needle was used to collect the tissue specimen. The needle core was removed to preserve the specimen for pathology. Another core was inserted in the needle, and the same method was used to collect two more specimens. The skin puncture wound was closed with two sutures.

   _____

9. The patient underwent nephrolithotomy to remove a kidney stone. After incision to the back and access to the left kidney was achieved, the stone was identified and removed. Examination of the remainder of the kidney was found to be normal in appearance. The kidney was closed with sutures. A drainage tube was inserted. The tube was allowed to drain outside the body via access through another small incision. The main incision was closed in layers.

_____

10. A patient presented for the first stage of urethroplasty. After an abdominal incision was made, the urethra was identified. The strictures were seen. An incision was made over the first stricture area. The area was opened wide and sutured to the edge of the mucosa. The second stricture area was handled in the same method. The patient will return in eight weeks for stage two of this repair.

_____

16 | CPT Surgery V

Chapter Outline

Male Genital System Subsection

Reproductive System Procedures Subsection

Intersex Surgery Subsection

Female Genital System Subsection

Maternity Care and Delivery Subsection

Endocrine System Subsection

Nervous System Subsection

Eye and Ocular Adnexa Subsection

Auditory System Subsection

Operating Microscope Subsection

Chapter Objectives

At the conclusion of this chapter, the student should be able to:

1. Define key terms related to the Male Genital System, Reproductive System Procedures, Intersex Surgery, Female Genital System, Maternity Care and Delivery, Endocrine System, Nervous System, Eye and Ocular Adnexa, Auditory System, and Operating Microscope subsections of CPT Surgery.
2. Assign codes from the Male Genital System subsection of CPT Surgery.
3. Assign codes from the Reproductive System Procedures subsection of CPT Surgery.
4. Assign codes from the Intersex Surgery subsection of CPT Surgery.
5. Assign codes from the Female Genital System subsection of CPT Surgery.
6. Assign codes from the Maternity Care and Delivery subsection of CPT Surgery.
7. Assign codes from the Endocrine System subsection of CPT Surgery.
8. Assign codes from the Nervous System subsection of CPT Surgery.
9. Assign codes from the Eye and Ocular Adnexa subsection of CPT Surgery.
10. Assign codes from the Auditory System subsection of CPT Surgery.
11. Assign codes from the Operating Microscope subsection of CPT Surgery.

Key Terms

antepartum care	anterolateral approach	cochlear implant	corpectomy
anterior approach	burr hole	conization	costovertebral approach

delivery services

discectomy

enucleation of the eye

evisceration of ocular contents

exenteration of the orbit

extracapsular cataract extraction (ECCE)

hysteroscopy

intersex surgery

intracapsular cataract extraction (ICCE)

laminectomy

laminotomy

lateral extracavitary approach (LECA)

LEEP electrodissection conization

loop electrodissection conization

myringotomy

neuroplasty

neurorrhaphy

neurostimulator

ocular implant

omentectomy

oophorectomy

operating microscope

orbital implant

osteophytectomy

postpartum care

salpingo-oophorectomy

stereotaxis

tenosynovitis

transpedicular approach

tympanoplasty

tympanostomy

vaginal birth after cesarean (VBAC)

Introduction

The Male Genital System subsection includes codes for procedures performed on the male genitalia and accessory organs. The Reproductive System Procedures subsection includes codes for the placement of needles into pelvic organs and/or genitalia for subsequent interstitial radioelement application. The Intersex Surgery subsection contains just two codes for male-to-female as well as female-to-male sex change procedures. The Female Genital System subsection includes codes for procedures performed on female genitalia and accessory organs. The Maternity Care and Delivery subsection includes codes for procedures performed and services provided for obstetrics, including antepartum, delivery, and postpartum care.

 Coding Tip

Instructional notes located beneath categories, subcategories, headings, and subheadings apply to all codes in those areas. Parenthetical notes that are located below a specific code apply to that code only unless the note indicates otherwise.

The Endocrine System subsection includes codes for procedures performed on endocrine glands. The Nervous System subsection includes codes for procedures performed on the central and peripheral nervous systems. The Eye and Ocular Adnexa subsection includes codes for procedures performed on the eyeball, anterior segment, posterior segment, ocular adnexa, and conjunctiva. The Auditory System subsection includes codes for procedures performed on the external ear, middle ear, internal ear, and temporal bone (middle fossa approach). The Operating Microscope subsection contains a code that is reported in addition to the primary procedure code when an operating microscope is used during a surgical procedure to perform microsurgery techniques.

CPT guidelines that apply to the subsections are located at the beginning of the Surgery section.

 NOTE:

The content in Chapters 12 through 16 of this textbook is organized exactly as it appears in the CPT Surgery section. This organization facilitates learning by allowing students to move from one CPT Surgery subsection to the next, in order.

When included in CPT, the Other Procedures code below is reported for an unlisted procedure performed on the anatomical site. When reporting an unlisted procedure code, include documentation about the procedure (e.g., special report) performed with the submitted claim.

The *Medicare National Correct Coding Initiative Policy Manual* provides guidance about assigning procedure codes for the Male Genital System, Reproductive System Procedures, Intersex Surgery, Female Genital System, Maternity Care and Delivery, Endocrine System, Nervous System, Eye and Ocular Adnexa, Auditory System, and Operating Microscope subsections. Go to www.cms.gov and enter "Medicare NCCI Policy Manual" in the Search box to navigate to the manual.

Male Genital System Subsection

The *male genital system* (Figure 16-1) includes the prostate, seminal vesicles, penis, testicles (testes) (Figure 16-2), epididymis, tunica vaginalis, vas deferens, scrotum, and spermatic cord. Codes are reported for procedures performed on the male genital system. Code assignment is determined according to

- Approach (e.g., incision, destruction, excision, or introduction)
- Reason for surgery

  When an orchiectomy (removal of testis) procedure is performed, identify the following:

- Type of procedure (simple or radical)
- Surgical approach
- Additional procedures performed

Example 1: Patient underwent radical orchiectomy (removal of testis on the right) due to testicular tumor, inguinal approach. Report code 54530 RT.

Example 2: Patient underwent simple orchiectomy on the left, inguinal approach, which was performed prophylactically to prevent the release of hormones that may promote tumor metastasis. Report code 54520 LT.

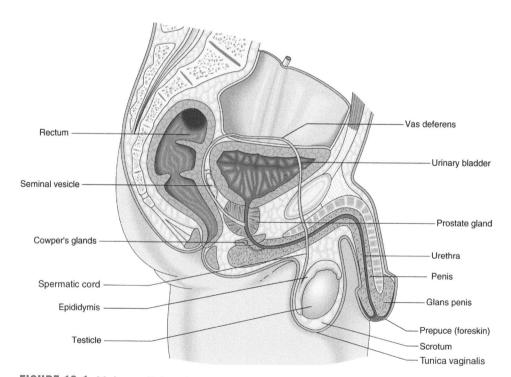

FIGURE 16-1 Male genital system

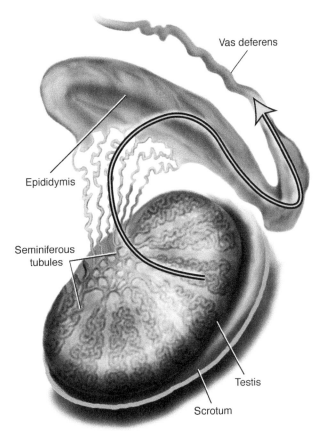

FIGURE 16-2 Male testicle

Example 3: Patient underwent right orchiopexy via abdominal approach for intra-abdominal testis. Report code 54650 RT.

Example 4: Patient underwent laparoscopic orchiopexy, left, for intra-abdominal testis. Report code 54692 LT.

The *vas deferens* is the tube that carries spermatozoa from the testis, and it is the structure upon which a vasectomy procedure is performed (Figure 16-3). A *varicocele* (Figure 16-4) is an abnormal dilation of the veins of the spermatic cord in the scrotum. Treatment typically involves ligation of spermatic veins or excision of the varicocele. For excision or ligation of a varicocele, review the operative report to locate the approach.

- Laparoscopic
- Abdominal

Example 1: Patient underwent vasectomy procedure. Report code 55250. Do not add modifiers 50, LT, or RT to the code because its description includes the phrase *unilateral or bilateral*. The code also includes postoperative semen examination to determine whether the semen contains sperm.

Example 2: The patient underwent ligation of spermatic veins for varicocele. Report code 55530.

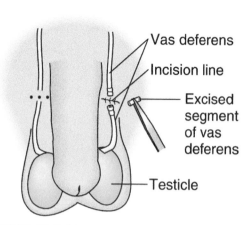

FIGURE 16-3 Vasectomy procedure

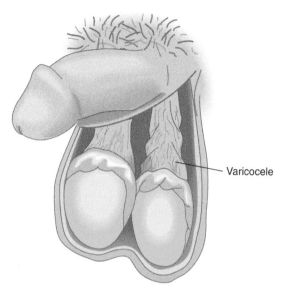

FIGURE 16-4 Varicocele affecting the left testicle

Benign conditions of the prostate gland include infection, inflammation, and benign prostatic hyperplasia (BPH) (also called benign prostatic hypertrophy, BPH). Men with benign prostate disease experience difficulty urinating (voiding). The degree of prostate involvement determines the therapeutic approach. For severe BPH, surgical procedures performed to restore urine flow include the following:

- Transurethral resection of the prostate (TURP) (Figure 16-5)
- Subtotal open prostatectomy (subtotal perineal prostatectomy)
- Subtotal prepubic prostatectomy
- Subtotal retropubic prostatectomy

Example: Patient underwent complete transurethral electrosurgical resection of the prostate using an electrocautery knife, including control of postoperative bleeding. During the same operative session, complete vasectomy was performed as well as meatotomy, cystourethroscopy, urethral calibration and dilation, and internal urethrotomy. Report code 52601.

Prostate cancer treatment may involve surgery, chemical destruction, electrocautery, or radiation. Surgical procedures that are performed to treat localized prostate cancer include radical prostatectomy, laparoscopic radical prostatectomy, and cryoablation.

A prostate biopsy includes the following types:

- Needle
- Punch
- Incisional

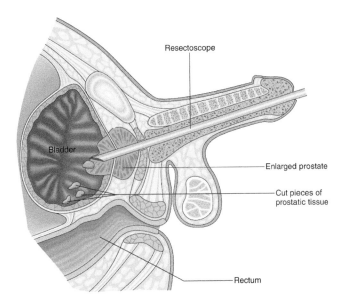

FIGURE 16-5 A transurethral resection of the prostate (TURP) is performed to treat benign prostatic hypertrophy

The "transperineal placement of needles or catheters into prostate for interstitial radioelement application, with or without cystoscopy" describes a procedure performed for interstitial radioelement application. The code is reported for the transperineal placement of needles or catheters only. A parenthetical note directs the coder to the Radiology section to separately report the radioelement application codes.

> **Example:** Patient underwent transperineal placement of needles into prostate for interstitial radioelement application and remote afterloading high dose rate radionuclide interstitial brachytherapy, 1 channel. Report codes 55875 and 77770. The parenthetical note located below code 55875 directs the coder to report the code for interstitial radioelement application.

Exercise 16.1 – Male Genital System

Instructions: Assign the CPT code(s) and appropriate modifier(s) to each statement.

1. The physician excised diseased scrotal tissue.

2. The physician removed a lesion from the left spermatic cord by dissection and excision.

3. The physician made an incision into the scrotum to search for the right testis, which failed to descend into the scrotum.

4. The physician performed a peroneal radical prostatectomy to remove the entire gland along with the seminal vesicles and the vas deferens.

5. The physician destroyed extensive condyloma of the penis using a chemosurgery technique.

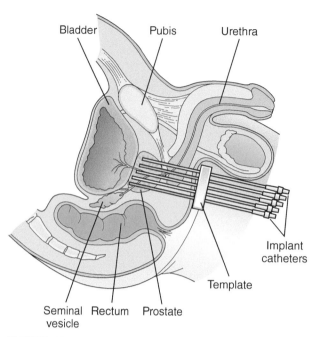

FIGURE 16-6 Insertion of implant catheters through perineum into prostate and seminal vesicles

Reproductive System Procedures Subsection

The reproductive system procedures subsection contains a code to report the placement of needles or catheters into pelvic organs and/or genitalia (Figure 16-6) for subsequent interstitial radioelement application. The code is *not* reported when needles or catheters are inserted into the prostate gland.

Example: Patient underwent insertion of catheters into the uterus to facilitate radiation therapy. Report code 55920.

 NOTE:

Radioelement application includes radioactive isotopes (e.g., iodine-125) contained within tiny seeds that remain inside the pelvic organs or genitalia to deliver radiation during an extended period of time (e.g., months). This method targets the prescribed body area, minimizing radiation exposure to normal tissue.

Intersex Surgery Subsection

Intersex surgery (Figure 16-7) is performed as a series of staged procedures to transform the normal adult genitalia of one sex to that of the other sex (genital reconstructive surgery or sex reassignment surgery).

- For male-to-female intersex surgery, portions of the male genitalia are removed and female external genitals are formed.
- For female-to-male intersex surgery, a penis and scrotum are formed using pedicle flap grafts and free skin grafts and a prosthesis is inserted.

Example: Patient underwent female to male intersex surgery. Report code 55980.

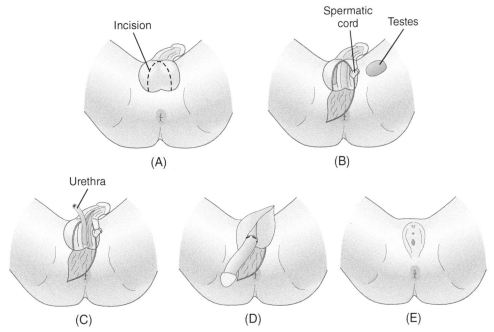

FIGURE 16-7 Sex reassignment surgery: (A) To change male genitalia to female genitalia, an incision is made into the scrotum. (B) The flap of scrotal skin is retracted, and the testes are removed. (C) Skin is then excised from the penis but remains attached, and a shorter urethra is created. (D) All but a stump of the penis is then removed. (E) Excess skin is used to create labia (external genitalia) and the vagina

Exercise 16.2 – Reproductive System Procedures and Intersex Surgery

Instructions: Assign the CPT code(s) and appropriate modifier(s) to each statement.

1. Patient underwent placement of a needle into the bladder for the purpose of subsequent interstitial radioelement application.

   _____

2. Intersex surgery was performed to dissect the penis and remove portions of it to fashion a clitoris-like structure. The urethral opening was moved, and a vagina was created by dissecting and opening the perineum. Labia were created using scrotal skin and adjacent tissue.

   _____

3. In the fourth of a series of staged intersex surgeries, the physician formed a penis and scrotum using pedicle flap grafts and free skin grafts. Prostheses were placed in the penis and testicles, and the vagina was closed.

   _____

Female Genital System Subsection

Female Genital System subsection codes are reported for procedures performed on the *female genital system* (Figure 16-8), including vulva, perineum, introitus, vagina, cervix uteri, corpus uteri, oviduct/ovary (fallopian tube), ovary. *In vitro* fertilization (IVF) procedures are also reported from this subsection.

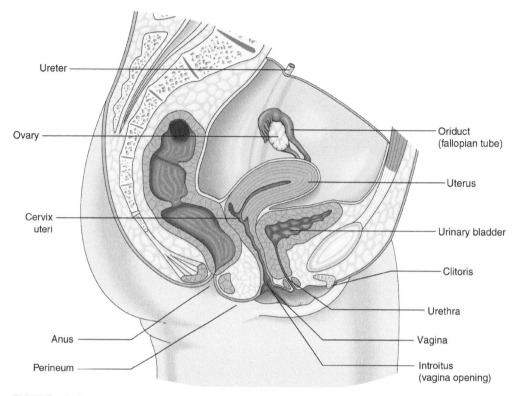

FIGURE 16-8 Female genital system

When reporting codes for procedures performed on the female genital system, review the operative report to identify the following:

- Anatomy on which the procedure was performed (e.g., vulva)
- Surgical approach

 NOTE:

Codes in the Female Genital System subsection are reported for procedures performed on patients who are *not* pregnant. To report codes for patients who are pregnant, refer to the Maternity Care and Delivery subsection.

 Coding Tip

- All laparoscopic procedures and nonobstetrical dilation and curettage procedure codes are located in the Female Genital System subsection.
- Some female genital procedures are located in other subsection categories of the CPT coding manual, such as the open destruction of endometriomas, which is located in the Digestive System subsection, Abdomen/Peritoneum/Omentum category, Excision/Destruction subcategory.

For vulvectomy procedure codes, refer to the following definitions when reviewing the operative report (to select the type of procedure performed):

- *Simple procedure*: Removal of skin and superficial subcutaneous tissues
- *Radical procedure*: Removal of skin and deep subcutaneous tissue

- *Partial procedure*: Removal of less than 80 percent of the vulvar area
- *Complete procedure*: Removal of greater than 80 percent of the vulvar area

When an open sling operation is performed for stress incontinence, report a code from the Female Genital System subsection. When a laparoscopic sling operation is performed, report a code from the Urinary System subsection.

Coding Tip

Make sure you read CPT code descriptions carefully. When the code description states "with or without" another procedure, that other procedure is *not* reported separately.

> **Example:** Patient underwent anterior colporrhaphy, repair of cystocele, and cystourethroscopy. Report code 57240. Do not report a separate code for the cystourethroscopy.

A pelvic exam under anesthesia is a routine evaluation of the surgical field, and it is reported with a code *only if performed separately*. This procedure is included in all major and most minor gynecological procedures, and it is *not* reported separately when performed during the same operative session as another female genital system surgical procedure.

Endoscopy codes are reported for examination and magnification, and codes distinguish among anatomical sites (e.g., vulva, vagina, cervix uteri, and oviduct/ovary). Abnormalities of the female genital system (e.g., cancer, tumors, human papilloma virus [HPV], and pruritus) are commonly diagnosed and treated with examination and magnification. For example, laparoscopy/hysteroscopy is performed to visualize the corpus uteri (Figure 16-9).

When dilation of the vagina or cervix is performed during the same operative session as another vaginal approach procedure, do not report the dilation procedure separately. When a pelvic examination under anesthesia is performed during the same operative session as a dilation and curettage (Figure 16-10), report the code for the dilation and curettage only.

Conization of the cervix (removal of a cone-shaped piece of tissue) is reported for fulguration, dilation and curettage, and repair procedures. Conization procedures can also be performed through use of a cold knife or laser or through loop electrode excision. Make sure you review the operative report carefully to assign the appropriate code.

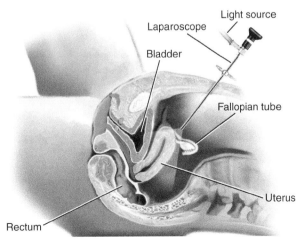

FIGURE 16-9 Laparoscopy/hysteroscopy

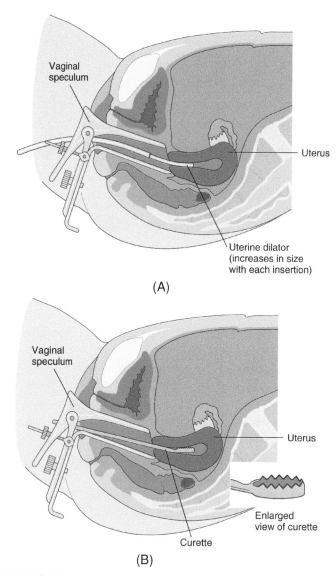

(A)

(B)

FIGURE 16-10 Dilation and curettage: (A) Dilation is the expansion of the cervical opening. (B) Curettage is the removal of material from the endometrial lining of the uterus

 Coding Tip

Physicians use the terms *loop conization* and *LEEP (loop electrosurgical excision procedure) conization* interchangeably in operative reports. **Loop electrodissection conization** is a deep dissection of the cervix using a loop wire (instead of the traditional surgical scalpel). **LEEP electrodissection conization** is a more superficial dissection of the cervix using a loop wire.

For abdominal hysterectomy procedures, make sure you review the operative report to identify whether the fallopian tubes and/or ovaries were removed during the same operative session as the hysterectomy. Then read the code descriptions carefully to select the appropriate code.

When reporting a code for vaginal hysterectomy (Figure 16-11), determine whether the surgical approach is open or laparoscopic.

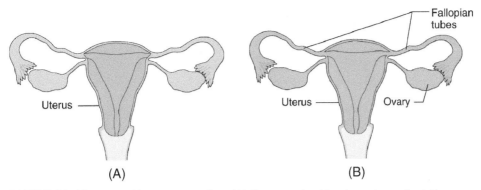

FIGURE 16-11 Vaginal hysterectomies: (A) For a vaginal hysterectomy, just the uterus and cervix are removed. (B) For a vaginal hysterectomy with bilateral salpingo-oophorectomy, the cervix, uterus, fallopian tubes, and ovaries are removed

Coding Tip

The code description "with or without removal of tube(s), with or without removal of ovary(s)" indicates that these procedures are bilateral. Therefore, do not report modifier 50 with codes containing such descriptions.

Hysteroscopy is the direct visualization of the cervical canal and uterine cavity using a hysteroscope. It is performed to examine the endometrium and to carry out surgical procedures (e.g., removal of cervical polyp). When a dilation and curettage is performed during the same operative session as a hysteroscopic biopsy or polypectomy, do not report a separate code for the dilation and curettage.

Oviduct/Ovary procedures are performed on the fallopian tubes and endoscopic procedures performed on the ovaries. Make sure you review the operative report to differentiate therapeutic procedures performed using surgical laparoscopy or hysteroscopy from those performed for diagnostic laparoscopy.

Review the operative report to determine the surgical approach before coding a tubal ligation procedure (e.g., ligation, transaction, or other occlusion of the fallopian tubes) (Figure 16-12).

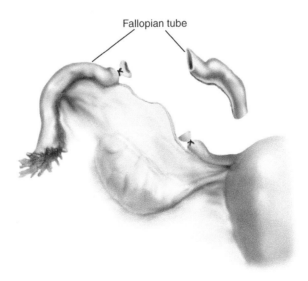

FIGURE 16-12 Tubal ligation

- Abdominal or vaginal approach
- Vaginal or suprapubic approach
- Laparoscopic

Example: Patient underwent a total abdominal hysterectomy during which routine lysis of adhesions was performed to access the abdomen. Report code 58150. (Do *not* report code 58660.)

Procedures performed on the ovaries are based on surgical approach.

- Open (e.g., oophorectomy performed via open surgery)
- Laparoscopic (e.g., laparoscopic oophorectomy)

An **oophorectomy** (removal of the ovaries) is often performed due to ovarian cancer. An ovarian malignancy is also resected by performing a bilateral **salpingo-oophorectomy** (removal of both fallopian tubes and ovaries) and an **omentectomy** (removal of the omentum).

In vitro fertilization (IVF) procedures are performed during a one- to seven-day period from the time the *oocyte* (immature female reproductive cell, or egg) was aspirated from the ovary until the embryo is transferred to the uterus or is cryopreserved. IVF procedures include both male and female gametes in addition to the subsequent embryos that develop. The physician who performs the oocyte retrieval reports a code for follicle puncture for oocyte retrieval, any method, to describe these services.

 Coding Tip

Any associated laboratory procedures performed during *in vitro* fertilization are reported separately with codes from the CPT Pathology and Laboratory section.

Exercise 16.3 – Female Genital System

Instructions: Assign the CPT code(s) and appropriate modifier(s) to each statement.

1. The physician performed a tubal ligation (vaginal approach), postpartum, bilateral, during same hospitalization (as delivery). (Do not code the delivery.)

   _____

2. The physician performed colpocentesis to aspirate fluid from the peritoneum through the vaginal wall.

   _____

3. The physician harvested a mature egg from its follicle for *in vitro* fertilization.

   _____

4. The physician inserted an intrauterine device (IUD).

   _____

5. The physician performed laparoscopic electrical cautery destruction of an ovarian lesion with the assistance of a fiberoptic laparoscope.

   _____

Maternity Care and Delivery Subsection

In clinical terms, pregnancy is subdivided into trimesters.

- First trimester (fetal organ development)
- Second trimester (well-baby visits at the physician's office)
- Third trimester (baby maturity and delivery at 38–40 weeks)

In coding terms, the three stages of uncomplicated pregnancy care include services provided as part of total obstetrical care, and pregnancy confirmation is reported with an appropriate E/M code (not as part of antepartum care).

- Antepartum care
- Delivery of the baby
- Postpartum care

Total obstetrical care does not include diagnostic procedures (e.g., ultrasound, amniocentesis, or special screening tests), physician office visits for unrelated conditions incidental to pregnancy, and additional visits due to high-risk conditions or medical complications of pregnancy (e.g., cardiac conditions, diabetes mellitus, hyperemesis, hypertension, neurological conditions, premature rupture of membranes, preterm labor, or toxemia). Codes for these services are separately reported from the CPT Evaluation and Management and Medicine sections. For treatment of surgical complications associated with pregnancy (e.g., appendectomy, cholecystectomy, hernia repair, or removal of ovarian cyst or Bartholin cyst), codes from the Surgery section are reported separately.

Most maternity care and delivery procedures include just what is described in the code description. Additional procedures performed on the same day as a maternity care and delivery service are reported separately, except for the following services, which are included in the code for maternity care and delivery:

- Fetal monitoring during labor
- Episiotomy
- Delivery of the placenta

Services that are reported separately when performed during maternity care and delivery include the following:

- Amniocentesis (Figure 16-13)
- Chorionic villus sampling
- Cordocentesis
- Fetal contraction stress test
- Fetal nonstress test
- Insertion of cervical dilator
  (e.g., laminaria and prostaglandin)
- External cephalic version with or without tocolysis
- Limited or complete obstetric ultrasound
- Fetal biophysical profile
- Fetal echocardiography
- Administration of Rh immune globulin

Antepartum Services

Antepartum care begins with conception and ends with delivery, and it includes the following:

- Initial prenatal history and examination
- Subsequent prenatal history and examinations
- Documentation of weight, blood pressures, and fetal heart tones
- Routine chemical urinalysis (e.g., glucose)
- Monthly visits up to 28 weeks' gestation
- Biweekly visits to 36 weeks' gestation
- Weekly visits until delivery

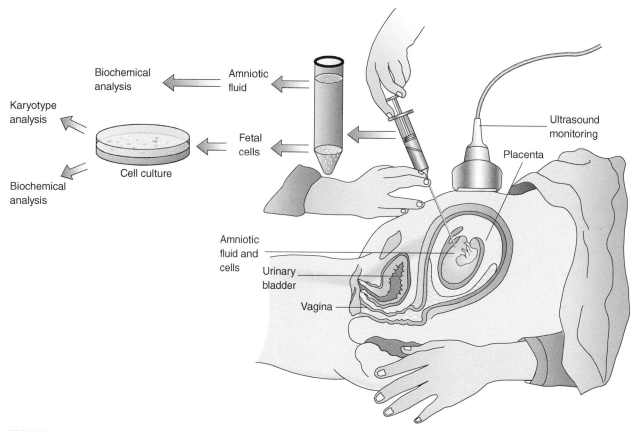

FIGURE 16-13 Amniocentesis and preparation of specimen for amniotic fluid analysis

The previously listed services are included with total obstetrical care, and they are not reported separately. Services that are reported separately with a code from the Evaluation and Management or Surgery section of CPT (in addition to a code for delivery services) include the management of the following:

- Medical problems *unrelated* to pregnancy
- Complications related to pregnancy

> **Example:** Patient develops gestational diabetes, which complicates the pregnancy. Patient requires additional office visits to monitor blood sugar and weight. Report an appropriate evaluation and management service code for each office visit during which the patient's gestational diabetes is managed.

When a physician provides *antepartum care only* (e.g., patient's care is transferred to another physician or patient relocates out of the area), report an appropriate evaluation and management code for the first through third antepartum care visit. For the fourth and subsequent visits, report the code for antepartum care, depending on the number of visits.

Delivery Services

Delivery services (e.g., vaginal delivery, cesarean delivery, and delivery after previous cesarean delivery) begin with the admission of the patient to the hospital and end with delivery of the placenta (Figure 16-14). Services include the following:

- Admission of the patient to the hospital
- Admission history and physical examination

- Management of uncomplicated labor
- Vaginal delivery (with or without episiotomy and/or with or without forceps) or cesarean delivery

The induction of labor (e.g., Pitocin [oxytocin]) during delivery is included in the code for delivery services. The artificial rupture of membranes (AROM) prior to delivery is also included in the delivery services code.

Services provided during delivery that are reported separately include the following:

- Fetal scalp blood sampling
- External cephalic version
- Administration of regional anesthesia (e.g., epidural)

The delivery of the placenta is included in the delivery service, and it is *not* reported in addition to the delivery service. When the patient delivers vaginally prior to admission to the hospital and subsequent delivery of the placenta is performed by a physician in the hospital, a separate code is reported.

Services that are reported separately with a code from the Evaluation and Management or Surgery section of CPT (in addition to a code for delivery services) include the following:

- Management of surgical problems that develop during the postpartum period
- Admission to the hospital for observation prior to delivery
- Medical complications of pregnancy, labor, and/or delivery that require additional resources (e.g., diabetes, hypertension, toxemia, preterm labor, or premature rupture of membranes)
- Tubal ligation performed after delivery

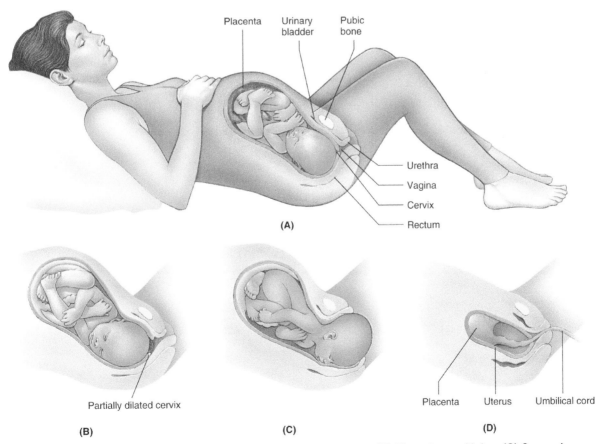

FIGURE 16-14 Stages of labor (A) Position of the fetus before labor (B) First stage of labor (C) Second stage of labor, fetal delivery (D) Third stage of labor, delivery of the placenta

Coding Tip

- Multiple births create the potential for complications during pregnancy, and they present coding challenges. (Report the ICD-10-CM diagnosis code for multiple gestation.)
- When performing diagnostic tests on multiple fetuses (e.g., amniocentesis or biophysical profile), more work is usually required because the procedure must be performed and documented for each fetus. To indicate additional work, report the appropriate code with modifier 22 or report the code for each fetus. (Report an ICD-10-CM diagnosis code for multiple gestation.)

Example: Patient received routine obstetric care, which included antepartum care, vaginal delivery of twins, and postpartum care. Report codes 59400 and 59409 51.

Postpartum Care

Postpartum care begins after vaginal or cesarean section delivery and includes the recovery room visit; any uncomplicated inpatient hospital and outpatient postpartum visits; follow-up care for episiotomy; and repair of cervical, vaginal, or perineal lacerations, including follow-up care. During delivery, if a vaginal laceration occurs and the repair is minimal, it is included in the delivery services. The repair of the vaginal laceration is not coded separately.

Coding Tip

- When a physician provides all or part of the antepartum and/or postpartum care but does not perform the delivery due to termination of pregnancy by abortion or referral to another physician for delivery, report antepartum and postpartum codes.
- When a physician performs only the delivery, report a "delivery only" code.

Example: The on-call obstetrician performs an emergency cesarean section on a colleague's patient. The on-call obstetrician reports code 59514. The patient's obstetrician reports codes for antepartum and postpartum care.

Delivery After Previous Cesarean Delivery

Codes for delivery after previous cesarean section are reported whether an attempted vaginal birth (after previous cesarean delivery) is successful or a repeat cesarean is performed. A **vaginal birth after cesarean (VBAC)** is a planned vaginal birth after previous cesarean section. Different codes are reported for planned versus unplanned VBAC procedures.

Example: Patient who had undergone previous cesarean delivery received routine obstetric care including antepartum care, vaginal delivery for the current pregnancy, and postpartum care. Report code 59610.

Abortion

Abortion treatment codes are based on the method used and type of abortion, and medical treatment of a spontaneous complete abortion during any trimester (e.g., miscarriage) is reported with an appropriate E/M code.

- *Incomplete abortion*: Miscarriage in which part, but not all, of the uterine contents are expelled

- *Induced abortion*: Deliberate termination of pregnancy

- *Missed abortion*: Miscarriage in which a dead fetus and other products of conception remain in the uterus for four or more weeks

- *Septic abortion*: Abortion-related pelvic and uterine infection

Example: Patient underwent treatment for a septic abortion, which was completed surgically. Report code 59830.

Exercise 16.4 – Maternity Care and Delivery

Instructions: Assign the CPT code(s) and appropriate modifier(s) to each statement.

1. The physician treated an ectopic pregnancy by removing the fallopian tube and ovary through an incision in the lower abdomen.

   _____

2. Using ultrasonic guidance, the physician inserted an amniocentesis needle through the abdominal wall into the interior of the pregnant uterus and directly into the amniotic sac to collect amniotic fluid for diagnostic analysis.

   _____

3. Using ultrasonic guidance, the physician inserted an amniocentesis needle through the abdominal wall into the cavity of the pregnant uterus and into the umbilical vessels to obtain fetal blood for cordocentesis procedure.

   _____

4. The physician used an external monitor to record fetal heart rate changes during a fetal nonstress test.

   _____

5. A physician provided all antepartum (7 visits) and postpartum obstetrical care but did not perform the delivery.

   _____

Endocrine System Subsection

The *endocrine system* (Figure 16-15) includes the following glands:

- Adrenal (2)
- Gonads (ovaries in females, testes in males) (2)
- Pancreas (islets of Langerhans) (1)
- Parathyroid (divided into four lobes) (1)
- Pituitary (divided into two lobes) (1)
- Thymus (1)
- Thyroid (divided into two lobes) (1)

The Endocrine System subsection includes procedures performed on the endocrine glands and the carotid body.

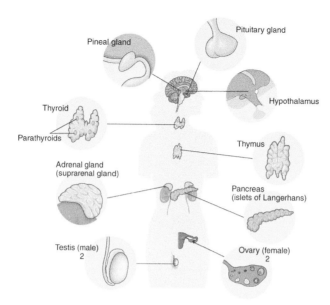

FIGURE 16-15 Endocrine glands

Coding Tip

Codes for procedures performed on pituitary and pineal glands are located in the Nervous System subsection.

Thyroid Gland

Thyroid Gland procedures are increasingly complex involving excision of the thyroid gland.

A "total or subtotal resection" is the removal of both the left and right lobes of the thyroid gland. A "limited neck dissection" is the removal of a limited number of lymph nodes. A "radical neck dissection" is the total removal of lymph nodes from one side (or both sides) of the neck.

NOTE:

When a radical neck dissection is performed during the same operative session as the resection of a unilateral organ (e.g., larynx), modifier 50 is not added to the procedure codes. The thyroid gland is a unilateral organ that contains two lobes. Thus, modifiers 50, LT, and RT are *never* added to thyroid gland procedure codes.

Example: A physician suspects lymphoma in a patient who has signs of diffuse neck swelling. A large-core needle biopsy of the right lobe of the thyroid gland is performed. The tissue is sent for histopathology. Report code 60100.

Parathyroid, Thymus, Adrenal Glands, Pancreas, and Carotid Body

The types of procedures performed on the parathyroid, thymus, adrenal glands, and carotid body include excision, laparoscopy, and other procedures. The *carotid body* is tissue that contains many capillaries, and it is located at the point where the carotid artery branches in the neck. It contains cells that sense oxygen and carbon dioxide blood levels so that information is sent to the brain's medulla to regulate heart rate.

Surgery performed on the adrenal glands can be performed as open or laparoscopic procedures. Make sure you review the operative report to identify the surgical approach to report the appropriate code.

The exploration of parathyroid glands is often performed using a cervical approach. In cases where further exploration is needed, the physician uses a transthoracic approach.

Example: Patient underwent laparoscopic exploration with partial removal of the left adrenal gland, performed from a transabdominal approach. Report code 60650 LT.

Exercise 16.5 – Endocrine System

Instructions: Assign the CPT code(s) and appropriate modifier(s) to each statement.

1. The physician determines the location of a thyroid cyst, using palpation, and aspirates it.

_____

2. The physician performed a total thyroid lobectomy on the right and a contralateral subtotal lobectomy on the left, including isthmusectomy.

_____

3. The physician removed remaining thyroid tissue on one side, following an earlier partial thyroidectomy.

_____

4. Patient underwent percutaneous core needle biopsy of the thyroid gland.

_____

5. Patient underwent incision and drainage of an infected thyroglossal duct cyst of the neck, which was the result of incomplete closure of the embryonic thyroglossal duct between the thyroid gland and the back of the tongue.

_____

6. The physician performed a laparoscopic exploration of the left adrenal gland through the abdomen with partial adrenalectomy, left.

_____

7. The physician explored the parathyroid glands. During the same operative session, a parathyroid autotransplantation was also performed.

_____

8. Patient underwent partial adrenalectomy, left, with biopsy, dorsal approach.

_____

9. The physician surgically removed the parathyroid glands.

_____

10. The physician removed a carotid body tumor, which was located just above the bifurcation of the left carotid artery.

_____

Nervous System Subsection

The *nervous system* (Figure 16-16) includes the following:

- Central nervous system (brain and spinal cord)
- Peripheral nervous system (12 pairs of cranial nerves extending from the brain and 31 pairs of spinal nerves extending from the spinal cord)

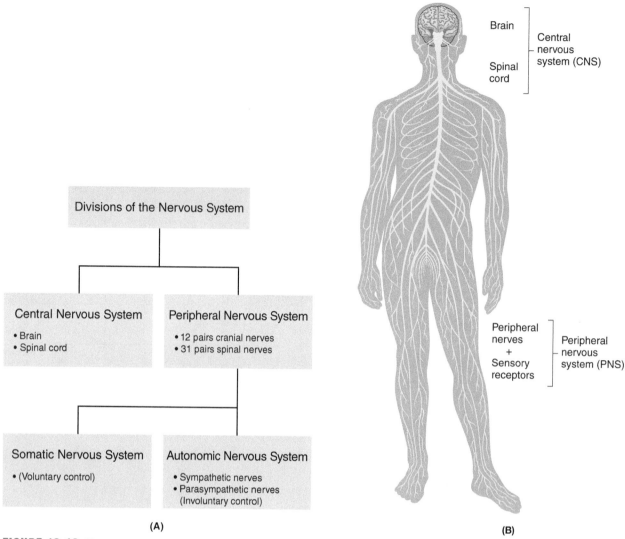

FIGURE 16-16 Nervous system (A) Divisions of the nervous system (B) Structure of the central nervous system and peripheral nervous system

Codes for Nervous System subsection procedures are arranged anatomically.

- Skull, meninges, and brain
- Spine and spinal cord
- Extracranial nerves, peripheral nerves, and autonomic nervous system

Nervous system procedures are performed using a variety of approaches (e.g., craniectomy, craniotomy, and laminectomy) and for specific purposes (e.g., decompression and drainage of hematomas).

> **Example:** Patient underwent a bilateral surgery to create burr holes with drainage of hematoma, extradural. Report code 61154 50. Add modifier 50 (Bilateral procedure) to the code because the parenthetical note below the code description states, "For bilateral procedure, report 61154 with modifier 50."

Skull, Meninges, and Brain

Skull, Meninges, and Brain (Figure 16-17) procedures are organized according to the following:

- Injection, drainage, or aspiration
- Twist drill, burr hole(s), or trephine
- Craniectomy or craniotomy
- Surgery of skull base

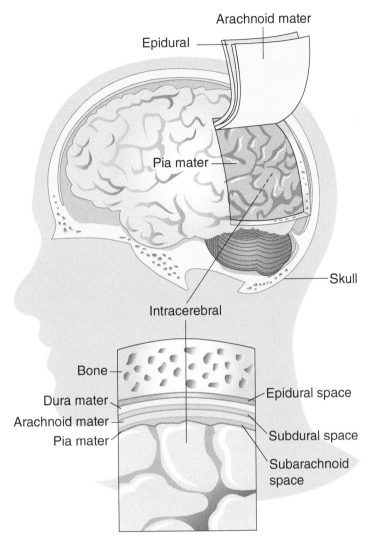

FIGURE 16-17 Skull, meninges, and brain

- Endovascular therapy
- Surgery for aneurysm, arteriovenous malformation, or vascular disease
- Stereotaxis
- Stereotactic radiosurgery (cranial)
- Neurostimulators (intracranial)
- Repair
- Neuroendoscopy
- Cerebrospinal fluid (CSF) shunt

A **burr hole** is a small opening in the skull made with a surgical drill. This procedure is often necessary when intracranial surgery (e.g., craniotomy or craniectomy) is planned. The burr hole provides access to intracranial contents, it alleviates pressure in preparation of further surgery, and it allows the placement of an intracranial pressure monitoring device. (These services are integral to the performance of subsequent services, and they are not to be separately coded or reported.)

When burr holes, punctures, and/or taps are created for the purpose of performing drainage procedures (e.g., hematoma, abscess, or cyst) and additional procedures are performed, the burr hole and drainage procedure is not separately coded and reported (unless it is performed as a staged procedure). In addition, many intracranial procedures include bone grafting; such grafts are not separately coded and reported.

Example 1: Patient underwent ventricular puncture through previous burr hole with injection of medication. Report code 61026. (The ventricular puncture through a previous burr hole describes the approach to access a specific area of the brain.)

Example 2: A patient with an open head injury and a contrecoup subdural hematoma underwent a craniectomy on the right side for the open head injury and creation of a burr hole on the left side of the skull to drain the subdural hematoma. Report codes 61304 and 61154 51 LT. Do not add a directional modifier to the code 61304. Add modifiers 51 (Multiple procedures) and LT (Left side) to the second code because creation of the burr hole on the left side and drainage of the subdural hematoma are separate services not integral to the craniectomy, and a parenthetical note located below the description of code 61154 states, "For bilateral procedure, report 61154 with modifier 50."

Surgery of Skull Base

Surgery of skull base codes contain instructional notes that define anatomical areas included (e.g., skull base includes the base of the anterior, middle, and posterior cranial fossae). Notes further indicate that skull base surgery often requires the skills of several different surgical specialties that work together. Skull base surgery requires review of the operative report to identify the following variables:

- What the size of the lesion or tumor is
- What the anatomy of the individual patient is
- Whether this is an initial procedure to treat the condition or a reoperation

Surgery of skull base codes are arranged anatomically (anterior, middle, and posterior cranial fossae), and they are further subdivided according to the following:

- Approach procedures (provide adequate exposure to the intracranial field so the definitive procedure, such as excision of lesion, can be performed)
- Definitive procedures (e.g., resection, excision, transection, ligation, and obliteration), which include primary closure of dura, mucous membranes, and skin
- Repair and/or reconstruction of skull defects of skull base procedures (reported separately when cranioplasty, extensive dural grafting, extensive skin grafts, or local or regional myocutaneous pedicle flaps are required)

When skull base surgery is performed, a code for each procedure is reported by the surgeon who performed that aspect of the procedure: approach procedure, definitive procedure, and repair and/or reconstructive procedure. Generally, one surgeon performs the approach procedure, which exposes the area (e.g., lesion) to be treated. Another surgeon then performs the treatment (e.g., excision of lesion). A third surgeon repairs the defect created by the treatment (e.g., free tissue graft of dural defect created by excision of lesion). When one surgeon performs both the approach procedure and the definitive procedure, that surgeon reports both codes on the same claim; modifier 51 is added to the secondary procedure.

 NOTE:

Skull base surgery procedures are not typically considered "staged" because definitive closure of the surgical field (e.g., dura, subcutaneous tissues, or skin) must be performed to avoid serious infections (e.g., osteomyelitis or meningitis).

Example: The patient underwent resection of neoplastic vascular lesion, base of anterior cranial fossa, extradural, which required an extradural craniofacial approach to the anterior cranial fossa along with lateral rhinotomy, ethmoidectomy, and sphenoidectomy. Report codes 61600 and 61580 51. (The code for the definitive procedure, in this case a resection, is reported first.)

Codes distinguish between procedures performed extradurally (outside the dura) or intradurally (within the dura). The dura mater is the outermost, fibrous, and toughest of the three meninges (Figure 16-18) that surround the brain and spinal cord.

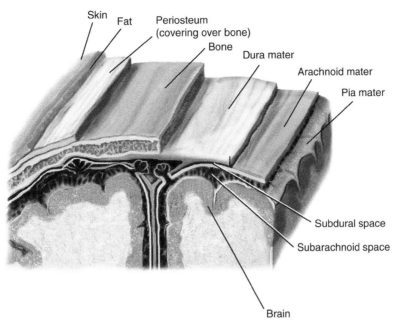

FIGURE 16-18 Meninges (dura mater, arachnoid mater, and pia mater) and other anatomical structures that protect the brain

Some Surgery of Skull Base codes are add-on procedures. They are not reported alone; they must be reported with another procedure code.

> **Example:** A surgeon performed a resection of an infectious lesion of the parasellar area and a transection of the carotid artery in a petrous canal, without repair. (No repair and/or reconstruction of surgical defects of the skull base was required.) Report codes 61607 and 61611. (The approach procedure was performed by a different surgeon; therefore, do not report a code for an approach procedure.) (Code 61611 is exempt from modifier 51.)

Neurostimulators (Intracranial)

Craniotomy procedure codes are usually bundled with craniectomy codes. Thus, when a craniotomy is performed during the same operative session as a craniectomy, report only the craniectomy code. Do not report the craniotomy code in addition to the craniectomy code.

> **Example:** When a patient undergoes "craniectomy or craniotomy for implantation of neurostimulator electrodes" during the same operative session as the creation of "twist drill or burr hole(s) for implantation of neurostimulator electrodes," only code 61860 is reported. Code 61850 is not reported in addition to code 61860.

Cerebrospinal Fluid (CSF) Shunt

A CSF shunt (Figure 16-19) is used to eliminate excess CSF in cases of hydrocephalus.

> **Example:** A child underwent creation of a ventriculo peritoneal shunt. Report code 62223.

Spine and Spinal Cord

The Spine and Spinal Cord percutaneous procedures are performed on the spine and include spinal injections and extracranial and peripheral nerve injections. To report procedure codes properly, review the operative report to identify the following:

- What the anatomical site is (e.g., epidural or facet joint nerves)
- Whether the procedure is diagnostic or therapeutic

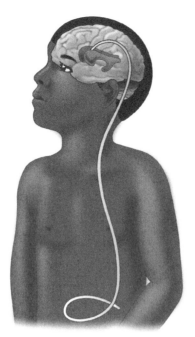

FIGURE 16-19 A cerebrospinal shunt allows drainage of cerebrospinal fluid (CSF) from the brain into the peritoneal cavity

- What type of substance is injected (e.g., contrast media or neurolytic substance)
- Whether the injections are continuous

Example: Patient underwent percutaneous lysis of epidural adhesions procedure under fluoroscopic guidance on June 14. Hypertonic saline solution was administered during the procedure. Report code 62264. (Do not report a separate code for fluoroscopic guidance.)

 Coding Tip

- A code from the Anesthesia section is reported for the daily hospital management of continuous epidural or subarachnoid drug administration performed with services assigned for the injection of diagnostic or therapeutic substances.

- For a spinal puncture procedure, the administration of local anesthesia is included. Reporting a separate code for the administration of local anesthesia (e.g., nerve block or facet block) is inappropriate.

- When an anesthetic block procedure is performed and cerebrospinal fluid is withdrawn during the same operative session (to make room for the anesthetic), do not report a code for diagnostic lumbar puncture. Report a code for the nerve (or other) block only because the removal of CSF is not done for diagnostic purposes.

- A partial vertebral corpectomy is the "removal of a substantial portion of the body of the vertebra. In the cervical spine, the amount of bone removed is defined as at least one-half of the vertebral body. In the thoracic and lumbar spine, the amount of bone removed is defined as at least one-third of the vertebral body."

Catheter Implantation

The *implantation* of an epidural or intrathecal catheter placement involves penetration of the dura.

> **Example:** Patient underwent implantation of tunneled epidural catheter for long-term medication administration via external pump. Report code 62350.

Reservoir/Pump Implantation

Programmable and nonprogrammable infusion pumps provide long-term access to the vascular or nervous system for the administration of medications. When electronic analysis and reprogramming of a programmable implanted pump is performed at the same time as refilling and maintenance, report a separate code.

> **Example:** Patient underwent implantation of a subcutaneous reservoir for intrathecal drug infusion. Report code 62360.

Endoscopic Decompression of Neural Elements and/or Excision of Herniated Intervertebral Discs

Endoscopic decompression of neural elements and excision of herniated intervertebral discs include percutaneous, endoscopic, and open surgical approaches. Visualization includes direct and indirect.

> **Example:** Patient underwent endoscopic decompression of lumbar spinal cord, which included laminotomy and excision of herniated intervertebral disk. Report code 62380.

Posterior Extradural Laminotomy or Laminectomy for Exploration/Decompression of Neural Elements or Excision of Herniated Intervertebral Discs

A **laminotomy** involves the removal of part of the lamina from one side of the vertebra. A **laminectomy** is the excision of the entire posterior arch or lamina of a vertebra. When reporting codes for a laminectomy or laminotomy (hemilaminectomy) procedure, determine the following:

- Anatomical site
- Surgical approach
- Type of procedure performed

Coding Tip

- A laminotomy is also known as a hemilaminectomy. Therefore, review of the operative report to differentiate between laminectomy and laminotomy (or hemilaminectomy) is required.
- When a laminotomy is performed during the same operative session as a laminectomy, the laminotomy code is not reported separately.

When codes are reported for laminotomy procedures, just one vertebral interspace in a specific area of the spine is accessed. When additional interspace(s) are accessed for laminotomy during the same operative session, report appropriate add-on code(s) in addition to the primary procedure code.

> **Example:** Patient underwent hemilaminectomy, decompression of nerve root(s), partial facetectomy, C1-C2 and C2-C3 interspaces. Report codes 63040 50, 63043, and 63043. According to the parenthetical notes below each code, modifier 50 (Bilateral procedure) is added to the code 63040, while code 63043 is reported twice.

Transpedicular or Costovertebral Approach for Posterolateral Extradural Exploration/Decompression

Extradural exploration/decompression procedures are performed using a transpedicular or costovertebral approach.

- A **transpedicular approach** is performed through and inside the pedicle (segment between transverse process and vertebral body) of a thoracic vertebra to access a thoracic disc. This approach does not require retraction of the spinal cord, but it may involve removal of the lamina and facet joint.

- A **costovertebral approach** is performed where the ribs articulate (connect) with thoracic vertebrae. (*Costovertebral* refers to that area of the thoracic spine where the rib meets the vertebra.) The physician makes an incision laterally to the spine, cutting through epidermis, dermis, subcutaneous tissue, fascia, muscle tissue, and a section of rib.

> **Example:** Patient underwent decompression of spinal cord at T1 via costovertebral approach. Report code 63064.

Anterior or Anterolateral Approach for Extradural Exploration/Decompression

A **discectomy** is the removal of an intervertebral disc. Make sure you review the operative report to identify the *number of interspaces removed* (e.g., C1-C2 describes one interspace, and C1-C2 and C2-C3 describe two interspaces) (Figure 16-20).

A **corpectomy** is the removal of a portion of the vertebra and adjacent intervertebral discs. Its purpose is for the decompression of the spinal cord and spinal nerves. A bone graft is placed to reconstruct the spine and provide stability. Make sure you review the operative report to identify the *number of segments removed* (e.g., C1 describes one segment, and C1-C2 describes two segments) (Figure 16-20).

 Coding Tip

- **Osteophytectomy** is the removal of bone spurs to relieve compression of the spinal cord or nerve roots.

- The placement of graft material (obtained from the ilium or the removed rib) into the disc space is reported with a code, when performed. Grafting is performed to allow for proper spacing between vertebrae and to promote spinal fusion.

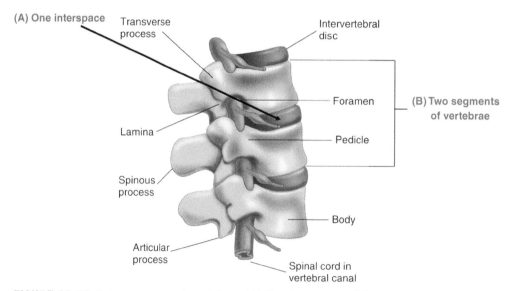

FIGURE 16-20 Interspaces and vertebrae (A) One interspace (B) Two segments of vertebrae

Exploration/decompression procedures are performed using an anterior or anterolateral approach.

- An **anterior approach** involves making an incision overlying the intervertebral disc by cutting through epidermis, dermis, subcutaneous tissue, fascia, and muscle tissue.
- An **anterolateral approach** involves making an incision along (and removing) the rib that corresponds to the vertebra that is located above the compressed intervertebral disc.

> **Example:** Patient underwent anterior discectomy with decompression of spinal cord, including osteophytectomy, C2-C3. Report code 63075.

Lateral Extracavitary Approach (LECA) for Extradural Exploration/ Decompression

For the **lateral extracavitary approach (LECA)**, a midline incision is made in the area of the affected vertebral segment (e.g., fractured vertebra or vertebral tumor), and the incision is inferiorly curved out to the lateral plane. Paraspinous muscles are mobilized medially (denervating and devascularizing these structures). The muscles are lifted from the spinous process, and they are divided and lifted from the ribs, exposing the vertebral segment.

> **Example:** Patient underwent complete vertebral corpectomy with decompression of spinal cord, T1. Report code 63101.

Incision

Laminectomy procedures are also called decompression surgery and involve creating space to enlarge the spinal canal by removing lamina, which is the posterior portion of a vertebra. The purpose of the procedure is to relieve pressure on the spinal cord and nerves.

> **Example:** Patient underwent one-stage cervical laminectomy procedure with cordotomy and section of both spinothalamic tracts. Report code 63197.

Excision by Laminectomy of Lesion Other Than Herniated Disc

When reporting codes for excision by laminectomy of lesion other than herniated disc, review the operative report to identify the following:

- Anatomical site
  - Cervical
  - Thoracic
  - Lumbar
  - Sacral
- Type of procedure performed
  - Excision or occlusion of arteriovenous malformation of spinal cord
  - Excision or evacuation of intraspinal lesion other than neoplasm, extradural
  - Excision of intraspinal lesion other than neoplasm, intradural
  - Biopsy/excision of intraspinal neoplasm, extradural or intradural

An add-on code is reported for osteoplastic reconstruction of dorsal spinal elements following a primary intraspinal procedure, such as laminectomy with drainage of intramedullary cyst/syrinx to subarachnoid space. (Do *not* add modifier 51 to the add-on code.)

> **Example:** Patient underwent laminectomy for excision of intraspinal neoplasm, extradural, thoracic. Report code 63276.

Excision, Anterior or Anterolateral Approach, Intraspinal Lesion

An excision code is reported for "vertebral corpectomy (vertebral body resection), partial or complete, for excision of intraspinal lesion, single segment; each additional segment." An add-on code is reported for each additional segment in addition to the code for the single segment. (Do *not* add modifier 51 to the add-on code.)

> **Example:** Patient underwent partial vertebral corpectomy for excision of an intraspinal lesion, extradural, C1 and C2. Report codes 63300 and 63308.

Stereotaxis

Stereotaxis uses a stereotactic guidance system to allow the physician to determine three-dimensional coordinates to

- Create a lesion on the spinal cord (to alleviate chronic pain in a particular part of the body).
- Stimulate the spinal cord percutaneously (to create a lesion that will block pain).
- Facilitate the biopsy, aspiration, or excision of a spinal cord lesion.

> **Example:** Patient underwent stereotactic percutaneous electrical stimulation of the spinal cord to create a lesion to block severe pain. Report code 63600.

Stereotactic Radiosurgery (Spinal)

Spinal stereotactic radiosurgery uses externally generated ionizing radiation to inactivate or eradicate spinal targets without the need to make an incision.

> **Example:** Patient underwent particle beam stereotactic radiosurgery, one spinal lesion. Report code 63620.

Neurostimulators (Spinal)

A spinal **neurostimulator** system includes an electrode and a pulse generator that are implanted along the spine to alleviate pain or control spasms. Neurostimulator codes describe procedures performed to implant, revise, and place neurostimulators along the spine. Codes for the implantation or placement and removal or revision of the neurostimulators are reported separately.

> **Example:** Patient underwent percutaneous implantation of neurostimulator electrode array, epidural. Report code 63650.

 Coding Tip

Initial and subsequent electronic analysis and programming of neurostimulator pulse generators are reported with Medicine section codes.

Repair

When reporting repair codes, do *not* add modifier 63 (Procedure performed on infants less than 4 kg). (Modifier 63 is added to indicate significantly increased complexity and physician work associated with procedures performed on infants who weigh less than 4 kg.) It is not appropriate to add modifier 63 to these repair codes because the additional complexity and work is already included in the procedure codes.

> **Example:** Patient underwent repair of meningocele, 10 cm in diameter. Report code 63702.

Shunt, Spinal CSF

Shunt, Spinal CSF procedures are performed on the lumbar spine (not the brain).

> **Example:** Patient underwent creation of percutaneous shunt, lumbar, subarachnoid-peritoneal. Report code 63741.

 Coding Tip

For CSF shunt procedures performed on the brain, report codes located under the Skull, Meninges, and Brain category.

Extracranial Nerves, Peripheral Nerves, and Autonomic Nervous System

Extracranial Nerves, Peripheral Nerves, and Autonomic Nervous System procedures are performed on these types of nerves. To report procedure codes properly, review the operative report to identify the following:

- Anatomical site (e.g., somatic nerve or sympathetic nerve)
- Type of procedure performed (e.g., injection or neurostimulator implantation)

Introduction/Injection of Anesthetic Agent (Nerve Block), Diagnostic or Therapeutic

The introduction or injection of an anesthetic agent (e.g., nerve block) is performed on somatic and sympathetic nerves for diagnostic and therapeutic reasons (e.g., pain management).

- *Somatic nerves* control voluntary movements (performed by skeletal muscles) and conscious sensation (e.g., hearing, sight, and touch), and they include voluntary motor and sensory nerves.
- *Sympathetic nerves* are part of the involuntary autonomic nervous system and originate in the thoracic and lumbar regions of the spinal cord; they inhibit (or oppose) the physiological effects of the parasympathetic nervous system (e.g., contract blood vessels, increase heart rate, and reduce digestive secretions).

To properly report codes (e.g., nerve blocks), review the operative report to identify the following:

- Type of substance injected (e.g., anesthetic or neurolytic)
- Nerves involved (e.g., somatic or sympathetic)
- Type of block (e.g., single, multiple, or regional)
- Duration of the infusion

> **Example:** Patient underwent injection of anesthetic agent, vagus nerve, which required fluoroscopic imaging guidance. Report codes 64408 and 77002.

 Coding Tip

When injections into an area *surrounding the spinal cord* are performed, report pain management codes from the Medicine section (instead of injection into nerve codes).

Neurostimulators (Peripheral Nerve)

A peripheral nerve neurostimulator system includes an electrode and a pulse generator that are implanted along peripheral nerves to alleviate pain or control spasms. Codes for the implantation or placement and removal or revision of the neurostimulators are reported separately.

> **Example:** Patient underwent percutaneous implantation of neurostimulator electrode array, cranial nerve. Report code 64553.

 Coding Tip

Initial and subsequent electronic analysis and programming of neurostimulator pulse generators are reported with Medicine section codes.

Destruction by Neurolytic Agent (e.g., Chemical, Thermal, Electrical, or Radiofrequency), Chemodenervation

Procedures that include destruction by neurolytic agent (e.g., chemical, thermal, electrical, or radiofrequency), somatic or sympathetic nerves also include the injection of other therapeutic agents, such as corticosteroids.

> **Example:** Patient underwent destruction by neurolytic agent, intercostal nerve. Report code 64620.

Neuroplasty (Exploration, Neurolysis, or Nerve Decompression)

Neuroplasty is the freeing or decompression of an intact nerve from scar tissue. Neuroplasty also includes decompression, exploration, external neurolysis, and/or nerve transposition, which are not coded and reported separately. A code for the use of an operating microscope during internal neurolysis (included in neuroplasty) procedures is reported from the Neuroplasty heading in addition to the neuroplasty code.

Carpal Tunnel Release

The *carpal tunnel* receives its name from the eight bones in the wrist (carpals) that form a tunnel-like structure. The tunnel is filled with flexor tendons that control finger movement and provide a pathway for the median nerve to reach sensory cells in the hand.

Repetitive flexing and extension of the wrist (e.g., repetitive motion injuries due to a job such as keyboarding or assembly line work) may cause a thickening of the protective sheaths that surround each of the tendons. When the tendon sheaths become swollen (*tenosynovitis*), increased pressure is applied to the median nerve, producing carpal tunnel syndrome.

Carpal tunnel syndrome (Figure 16-21) is a painful progressive condition caused by compression of the median nerve at the wrist. Symptoms usually begin with numbness, pain, and weakness in the hand and wrist. Then pain radiates up the arm. As symptoms worsen, a tingling sensation may result along with decreased grip strength.

Surgical treatment of carpal tunnel syndrome includes surgery to release compression of the median nerve. (Anti-inflammatory drugs and hand/wrist splinting are also used to reduce tendon swelling.) However, when the

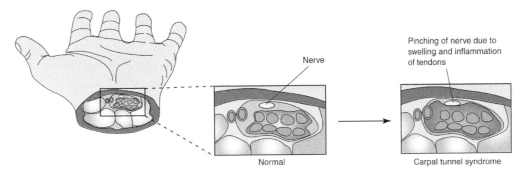

FIGURE 16-21 Carpal tunnel syndrome

release of the transverse carpal ligament is performed endoscopically, report a code from the Musculoskeletal System subsection.

> **Example 1:** Patient underwent an open procedure that included neuroplasty and transposition of the median nerve at the carpal tunnel, left wrist, which required use of the operating microscope for internal neurolysis. Report codes 64721 LT and 64727.

> **Example 2:** Patient underwent surgical endoscopy for release of transverse carpal ligament, right wrist. Report code 29848 RT.

Transection or Avulsion

Transection or avulsion procedures involve surgically removing a nerve (e.g., eliminate pain).

> **Example:** Patient underwent lingual nerve transection due to continuous pain and burning sensation of the tongue. Report codes 64721 LT and 64727.

Excision

Excision procedures are performed on somatic and sympathetic nerves.

> **Example:** Patient underwent excision of neuroma, digital nerves, left thumb, and left second digit. Report codes 64776 FA and 64778 F1.

Neurorrhaphy and Neurorrhaphy with Nerve Graft, Vein Graft, or Conduit

Neurorrhaphy (repair of nerves) procedures include the suture and anastomosis of proximal nerves (e.g., facial-spinal and facial-hypoglossal). For neurorrhaphy with nerve graft procedures, the operative report should be reviewed to identify the following:

- Anatomical site (e.g., head and neck, hand or foot, or arm or leg)
- Length of the nerve graft (e.g., up to 4 cm in length or more than 4 cm in length)

> **Example:** Patient underwent suture of brachial plexus nerve. Report code 64861.

Exercise 16.6 – Nervous System

Instructions: Assign the CPT code(s) and appropriate modifier(s) to each statement.

1. Burr holes were drilled into the infratentorial area for exploratory craniotomy.

(continues)

Exercise 16.6 – continued

2. Burr holes were created, and a ventricular reservoir was implanted.

3. The physician inserted a subcutaneous (infusion) pump for connection to a ventricular (brain) catheter.

4. The physician reprogrammed a cerebrospinal fluid shunt on a patient with an implanted programmable cerebrospinal fluid valve and shunt system to decrease the shunt pressure.

5. The physician punctured cerebrovascular fluid shunt tubing with a needle to drain fluid to determine functioning.

6. Gill laminectomy with decompression of lumbar nerve roots.

7. Diagnostic lumbar spine puncture.

8. Laminectomy with creation of lumbar shunt for drainage of excess cerebrospinal fluid.

9. Replacement (insertion) of a nonprogrammable epidural drug infusion pump.

10. Decompression of spinal cord with removal of herniated disc via costovertebral approach, T1.

11. Nerve block, left axillary nerve.

12. Lumbar paravertebral facet joint injections, two levels, left side.

13. Single-level intercostal nerve block injection, left.

14. Excision of neuroma, left sciatic nerve.

15. Percutaneous implantation of neurostimulator electrode array, cranial nerve.

Eye and Ocular Adnexa Subsection

Eye and Ocular Adnexa procedures are performed on the eyeball, anterior and posterior segment, ocular adnexa, and conjunctivae (Figure 16-22). When reporting codes, review the operative report to identify the following:

- Anatomical site (e.g., eyeball)
- Type of procedure (e.g., retinal repair)

Eye and Ocular Adnexa codes also include surgery to remove eyelid lesions and the repair or reconstruction of orbits, eyeballs, and eyelids.

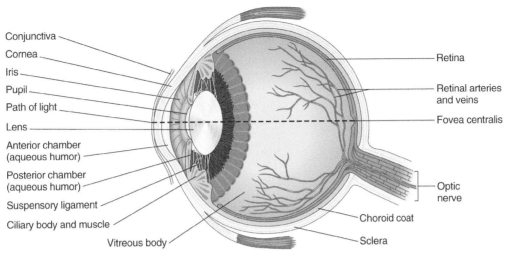

Conjunctiva
Cornea
Iris
Pupil
Path of light
Lens
Anterior chamber (aqueous humor)
Posterior chamber (aqueous humor)
Suspensory ligament
Ciliary body and muscle
Vitreous body

Retina
Retinal arteries and veins
Fovea centralis
Optic nerve
Choroid coat
Sclera

FIGURE 16-22 Eye and ocular adnexa

Coding Tip

Ophthalmologic procedures are also located in the

- Integumentary System subsection (CPT Surgery) (e.g., shaving of epidermal lesions from the eyelid)
- Musculoskeletal System subsection (CPT Surgery) (e.g., orbital wall decompression with nasal/sinus endoscopy)
- Medicine section (e.g., diagnostic/therapeutic ophthalmologic services)

NOTE:

The following HCPCS Level II modifiers are added to Eyelid heading codes when appropriate:

- E1 (upper left eyelid)
- E2 (lower left eyelid)
- E3 (upper right eyelid)
- E4 (lower right eyelid)

Eyeball

The *eyeball*, or *globe*, contains the choroid, retina, and sclera. The *sclera* is the white of the eye that comprises the eye's outer layer; it contains fibrous tissue that maintains the eye's shape and protects the eye's inner layers. The *cornea* is the transparent layer on the eye's surface; it covers the iris and pupil and provides focusing power. The *uvea* is the eye's vascular layer, which includes the choroid, ciliary body (ciliary muscle), and iris. The *choroid* is the opaque layer behind the retina that contains blood vessels. The *iris* is colored tissue that surrounds the pupil. The *pupil* is the black opening in the center of the iris that permits light to enter the eye. The *lens* is a clear, flexible, curved structure that focuses images on the retina. The *ciliary body*, or *ciliary muscle*, adjusts the shape of the lens and focuses light rays onto the retina. The *retina* contains nerve tissue.

An **evisceration of ocular contents** includes removal of the contents of the eyeball (choroid, ciliary muscles, iris, lens, retina, and vitreous); the sclera remains intact. (An implant may or may not be placed into the scleral shell.)

An **enucleation of the eye** includes severing the eyeball from extraorbital muscles and the optic nerve and removing it. (An implant may or may not be placed and attached to extraocular muscles.)

An **exenteration of the orbit** includes the removal of orbital contents and may also include removal of bone, muscle, and/or the myocutaneous flap. When a skin graft is placed, report a code from the Integumentary subsection (in addition to the exenteration of the orbit code). When the eyelid is repaired, report a code from the Reconstruction Area of the Eyelids subheading (in addition to the exenteration of the orbit code).

Procedures performed to modify an ocular implant alter the shape of a prosthesis to create a better fit. An **orbital implant** is inserted outside the muscular cone into the eye socket, and an intraocular lens (IOL) is placed. An **ocular implant** is inserted inside the muscular cone.

> **Example:** Patient underwent secondary insertion of ocular implant (after having undergone previous evisceration) into the scleral shell, left eye. Report code 65130 LT.

CPT differentiates between the removal of a foreign body located in the eye and removal of implanted material (e.g., ocular implant). When coding the removal of a foreign body from the external eyeball, review the operative report to identify the following:

- Where the location is (e.g., intraocular)
- Whether a foreign body is embedded
- Whether a slit lamp was used

Most foreign bodies of the eye are located in the cornea and conjunctiva. Fluorescein staining with slit lamp inspection is used to visualize a corneal foreign body or abrasion.

For laceration repairs of ocular structures, an extensive conjunctival laceration may also include a graft or flap. The repair of a laceration includes use of a conjunctival flap and restoration of anterior chamber by air or saline injection. Do *not* separately code and report these procedures.

> **Example:** Patient underwent the removal of foreign body, left external eye, superficial conjunctiva. Report code 65205 LT.

Anterior Segment

Anterior Segment codes are reported for procedures performed on the anterior segment of the eye, which includes the cornea, anterior chamber, anterior sclera, iris, ciliary body (ciliary muscle), and lens.

- Corneal transplant (e.g., keratoplasty) is a common procedure that includes use of fresh or preserved grafts and preparation of donor material.

- Radial keratotomy (Figure 16-23) corrects myopia; the surgeon makes numerous radial incisions (like the pattern of spokes of a wheel) extending from the pupil to the periphery of the cornea. (The procedure was accidentally discovered by Dr. Svyatoslav Fyodorov, who removed pieces of glass from a patient's eye and noted that the patient's eyesight improved after removal of the glass. The lacerations to the cornea resulted in the improved eyesight.)

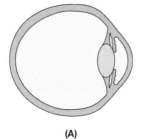
(A)

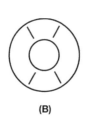
(B)

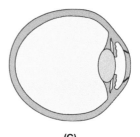
(C)

FIGURE 16-23 Radial keratotomy (A) Cross-section of eye prior to surgery (B) Small incisions are made in the cornea from the middle outward. (C) Radial keratotomy causes the cornea to become flatter, improving vision

- Cataract removal codes include the following procedures, which are not separately coded and reported:

  - Anterior and posterior capsulotomy
  - Iridectomy
  - Iridotomy
  - Lateral canthotomy
  - Subconjunctival or subtenon injections

  - Use of viscoelastic agents, enzymatic zonulysis, and other pharmacologic agents
  - Implantation of an IOL prosthesis *when performed during the same operative session*

The following two surgical methods are typically used to remove the lens and cataracts:

- **Intracapsular cataract extraction (ICCE)**: Removal of lens and surrounding capsule

- **Extracapsular cataract extraction (ECCE)**: Removal of lens and anterior portion of capsule

The extracapsular cataract removal with insertion of an IOL (Figure 16-24) is a common procedure. An iridectomy, trabeculectomy, and anterior vitrectomy may also be performed during the same operative session as the cataract removal. Codes for these procedures are *not* reported separately.

 Coding Tip

When an iridectomy is performed to accomplish the cataract extraction, it is considered an integral part of the procedure and is not reported separately.

Example: A patient presents with a cataract and evidence of glaucoma, left eye. Trabeculectomy is performed on August 15 as treatment for the glaucoma. Extracapsular cataract extraction with insertion of IOL prosthesis is performed on August 30 as treatment for the cataract. Report codes 66170 LT (August 15) and 66984 LT (August 30). (Code 99070 or C1780 is also reported.)

Posterior Segment

Posterior segment procedures are performed on the vitreous, retina or choroid, and sclera. Vitreous procedures include the removal and aspiration of vitreous and other fluids. Retina or Choroid procedures include repair, prophylaxis, and destruction. Some retinal detachment repair procedures are also performed on the vitreous.

Example: Code 67108 is reported for the repair of a retinal detachment. The code includes the following procedures: vitrectomy, air or gas tamponade, focal endolaser photocoagulation, cryotherapy, drainage of subretinal fluid, scleral buckling, and/or removal of lens by same technique. This means that separate codes are not reported for the included procedures.

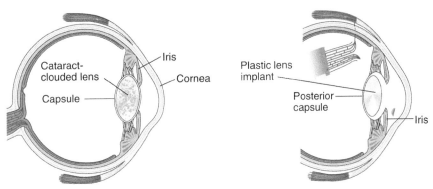

FIGURE 16-24 Cataract extraction with placement of intraocular lens

Ocular Adnexa

The *ocular adnexa* includes the orbit, eye muscles, eyelids, eyelashes, conjunctiva, and lacrimal apparatus. The *orbit*, or *eye socket*, is the bony cavity in the skull that contains and protects the eyeball (and its associated blood vessels, muscles, and nerves). The eye muscles work together to enable binocular vision. The eyelids protect the eyeball and keep its surface moist. The eyebrows and eyelashes prevent debris from getting into the eyes. The *conjunctiva* is a mucous membrane that lines the underside of each eyelid and forms a protective covering over the exposed surface of the eyeball. The *lacrimal apparatus*, or *tear apparatus*, contains structures that produce, store, and remove tears.

These codes are reported for procedures performed on the eyelid that involve more than skin. Many of these codes also include surgery to correct *strabismus*, which is improperly aligned eyes, such as cross-eyes (one eye points inward) and walleye (one eye points outward). Such codes are reported for exploration, excision, and decompression procedures performed on the orbit, in addition to injections and orbital implants.

Strabismus surgery is performed on extraocular muscles to realign the eyes. Each strabismus surgery code reflects a procedure performed on one eye (unilateral), which means that modifier 50 is added to the appropriate code when the procedure is performed on both eyes. Two methods are used to correct the alignment of eye muscles.

- Recession: Lengthening the muscle
- Resection: Shortening the muscle

For a recession procedure, the muscle is detached from the attachment site on the surface of the eyeball and reattached along the surface of the eye. For a resection procedure, a small portion of the muscle is removed and the eye muscle is reattached to the original insertion site.

 Coding Tip

> Codes for the treatment of orbital bone fractures (e.g., frontal, sphenoid, zygomatic, maxilla, ethmoid, and lacrimal) are located in the Musculoskeletal System section.

When it is medically necessary to inject sclerosing agents during the same operative session as surgery to correct glaucoma, that service is included in the glaucoma surgery.

Example: Patient underwent removal of an embedded foreign body, left lower eyelid. Report code 67938 E2.

Conjunctiva

Conjunctiva procedures include the following:

- Incision and drainage
- Excision and/or destruction
- Injection
- Conjunctivoplasty
- Other procedures
- Lacrimal system

Example: Patient underwent incision and drainage of a conjunctival cyst of the right upper eyelid. Report code 68020 E3.

A *trachoma* is a chronic inflammation of the conjunctiva in which granulations form. The physician uses biomicroscopic guidance to remove the conjunctival follicles with a cotton tipped swab or a curette without making an incision. Physicians often use biomicroscopic guidance (e.g., an optical instrument that looks like a microscope with two eyepieces) to treat trachoma. A slit lamp (e.g., a specialized magnifying microscope used to examine the structures of the eye) is also used with the biomicroscope.

NOTE:

Per the CPT note below the "Eye and Ocular Adnexa" subsection, do not report code 69990 (microsurgical techniques requiring use of operating microscope) in addition to codes 65091–68850. Use of the operating microscope is not reported separately because it is considered an essential part of eye and ocular adnexa procedures.

When a subconjunctival injection with a local anesthetic is performed as part of a more extensive anesthetic procedure (e.g., peribulbar or retrobulbar block), do not separately code and report the injection procedure. The injection procedure is considered a routine part of the anesthetic procedure and does not represent a separate service.

Conjunctivoplasty codes describe plastic surgery procedures performed on the conjunctiva. The following procedures are included in conjunctivoplasty codes, which means that they are *not* coded and reported separately: incision and drainage, excision and/or destruction, and injection of conjunctiva.

The lacrimal system keeps the cornea and conjunctiva moist through tear production. Codes reported for procedures performed on the lacrimal system include incision, excision, repair, and probing and/or related procedures.

A common procedure is the repair of the *lacrimal puncta*, which are small openings in the inner canthus of the eyelids that channel tears. There are two puncta in each eye, an upper and lower punctum. Thus, when both puncta in one eye are treated, report the appropriate code twice. According to *CPT Assistant* (June 1996), when all puncta in both eyes are treated (four puncta), codes 68705 and 68760–68761 are reported four times.

Example: Patient underwent closure of all four lacrimal puncta via laser surgery, both eyes. Report codes 68760 E1, 68760 E2, 68760 E3, and 68760 E4.

Exercise 16.7 – Eye and Ocular Adnexa

Instructions: Assign the CPT code(s) and appropriate modifier(s) to each statement.

1. Removal of foreign body from cornea of right eye, using a slit lamp.

2. Modification of ocular implant with replacement of pegs, right eye.

3. Cryotherapy destruction of corneal lesion, left eye.

4. Endoscopic goniotomy, right eye, for congenital glaucoma.

5. Insertion of iris-supported intraocular lens four weeks after right cataract removal.

6. Extracapsular cataract removal with insertion of intraocular lens prosthesis, left eye.

7. Aspiration of vitreous fluid, pars plana approach, right eye.

8. Diathermy of a retinal lesion for a patient with progressive diabetic retinopathy, both eyes.

(continues)

Exercise 16.7 – continued

9. Scleral reinforcement with graft, left eye.

___

10. Prophylactic treatment of retinal detachment, left eye, using cryotherapy.

___

11. Fine-needle aspiration of orbital contents, right eye.

___

12. Strabismus surgery that included a recession procedure of two horizontal muscles, both eyes.

___

13. Removal of chalazions from right upper eyelid and left upper eyelid.

___

14. Injection of corticosteroid into subconjunctival space, left eye.

___

15. Closure of a total of four lacrimal puncta using collagen plugs, both eyes.

___

Auditory System Subsection

The Auditory System (Figure 16-25) subsection is organized anatomically according to the following:

- External ear
- Middle ear
- Inner ear
- Temporal bone, middle fossa approach

Instructional notes direct the coder to otorhinolaryngologic service codes in the Medicine section for diagnostic services performed on the auditory system.

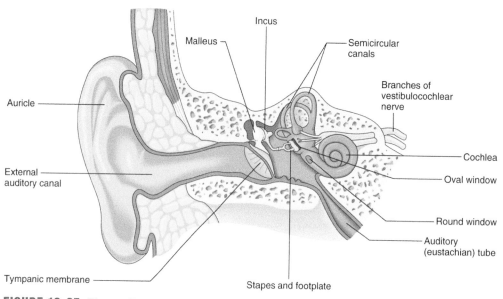

FIGURE 16-25 The auditory system

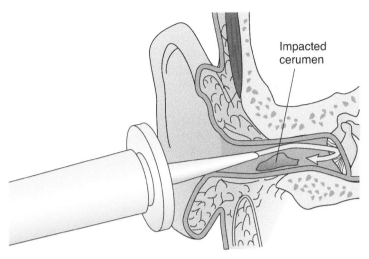

FIGURE 16-26 Removal of impacted cerumen

 Coding Tip

Most procedures in the Auditory System subsection are unilateral. Report modifier LT (Left side), RT (Right side), or 50 (Bilateral Procedure) as appropriate.

External Ear

The *external ear* includes the auricle (or pinna) and the external auditory meatus (or ear canal). The incision, excision, removal of foreign body, repair, and other procedures are performed on the external ear.

A frequently performed procedure is the "removal of impacted cerumen using irrigation/lavage, one or both ears" (Figure 16-26), which is reported with modifier 50 when the procedure is performed bilaterally or modifiers LT or RT when performed on one side. (For removal of cerumen that is *not* impacted, report an appropriate E/M code.)

> **Example:** Patient underwent biopsy, external ear, left. Report code 69100 LT.

Middle Ear

The *middle ear* includes the tympanic membrane, auditory ossicles, muscles, and conduction pathways. A commonly performed procedure is "tympanostomy (requiring insertion of ventilation tube), local or topical anesthesia." This procedure is typically performed on children who have chronic ear infections. *Auditory osseointegrated implant* surgery embeds a titanium prosthesis into the skull, attaching a small *external speech (or sound) processor* to the prosthetic *abutment* to allow sound vibrations to be transmitted to the inner ear for improved hearing.

A **myringotomy**, or **tympanostomy**, is the surgical incision of the tympanic membrane, and it is usually performed to release pressure or fluid. A **tympanoplasty** is the repair or reconstruction of the eardrum (Figure 16-27).

> **Example:** Patient underwent complete mastoidectomy, left ear. Report code 69502 LT.

Inner Ear

The *inner ear* includes the cochlea, saccule, acoustic nerve (e.g., auditory portion), semicircular canals, utricle, and superior and inferior vestibular nerves (e.g., vestibular portion). A labyrinthotomy procedure is performed using a transcanal approach, and all required infusions performed on initial and subsequent days of treatment are included in the reported code.

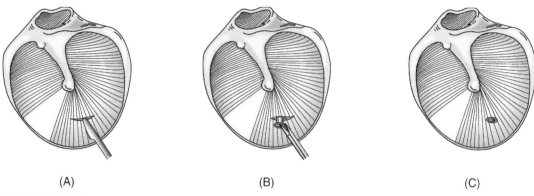

FIGURE 16-27 Tympanoplasty (A) Tympanic membrane incision (B) Tube placement
(C) Tympanoplasty completed

A **cochlear implant** is an implanted electronic device for treatment of sensory deafness. A vestibular nerve section using a transcranial approach includes the removal of the semicircular canals as well as bone over the internal auditory canal.

Example: Patient underwent cochlear device implantation with mastoidectomy, right and left ears. Report code 69930 50.

Temporal Bone, Middle Fossa Approach

Temporal bone, middle fossa approach codes are reported for nerve decompression or repair procedures. A common procedure performed to repair facial nerve damage is total nerve decompression, which is used to treat symptoms of *Bell's palsy* (unilateral paralysis of facial muscles resulting from dysfunction of the 7th cranial nerve, probably due to a viral infection).

Example: Patient underwent decompression of the internal auditory canal, left ear. Report code 69960 LT.

Exercise 16.8 – Auditory System

Instructions: Assign the CPT code(s) and appropriate modifier(s) to each statement.

1. Simple incision and drainage, abscess, left external ear.

_____

2. Removal of a button from the left ear canal of a 2-year-old child.

_____

3. Plastic surgeon reduced the size of a protruding right ear.

_____

4. With the patient under general anesthesia, the physician removed ventilating tubes from both ears.

_____

5. Replacement of electromagnetic bone conduction hearing device and removal of old device, left ear.

_____

6. Mobilization of stapes on the left.

_____

7. Physician implanted cochlear devices bilaterally.

_____

Exercise 16.8 – continued

8. Removal of temporal bone tumor, left side.

   _____

9. A physician treated a patient who was diagnosed with a tumor of the left facial nerve by performing total decompression for left facial nerve repair, which included grafting the nerve.

   _____

10. Decompression of internal auditory canal, right side.

    _____

Operating Microscope Subsection

When an **operating microscope** is used during a surgical procedure to perform microsurgery techniques, report add-on code 69990 in addition to the primary procedure code.

 Coding Tip

Do *not* report code 69990 for

- Visualization with a magnifying loupe or corrected vision.

- Procedures for which use of an operating microscope is an inclusive component. (Refer to Operating Microscope heading notes for a list of excluded codes.)

Example: Patient underwent vestibular nerve section, transcranial approach, with use of an operating microscope. Report codes 69950 and 69990.

Exercise 16.9 – Operating Microscope

Instructions: Assign the CPT code(s) and appropriate modifier(s) to each statement.

1. An otolaryngologist used a magnifying loupe to perform a left tympanic membrane repair.

   _____

2. Diagnostic direct laryngoscopy with use of an operating microscope.

   _____

3. The physician uses an operating microscope while performing a partial mastectomy via tylectomy, right breast.

   _____

4. Microsurgical epididymovasostomy, bilateral.

   _____

5. The physician used an operating microscope to perform a hypophysectomy.

   _____

Summary

For procedures performed on the male genital system, code assignment is determined according to approach (e.g., incision, destruction, excision, or introduction) and reason for surgery. Reproductive System Procedures include the placement of needles into pelvic organs and/or genitalia for subsequent interstitial radioelement application. Intersex surgery is performed as a series of staged procedures to transform the normal adult genitalia of one sex to that of the other sex (genital reconstructive surgery or sex reassignment surgery).

Codes in the Female Genital System heading are reported for procedures performed on patients who are *not* pregnant. (Codes for patients who are pregnant are reported from the Maternity Care and Delivery heading.) When reporting codes for procedures performed on the female genital system, review the operative report to identify the anatomy on which the procedure was performed (e.g., vulva, perineum, introitus, or vagina) and the surgical approach.

The three stages of pregnancy care include services provided as part of total obstetrical care: antepartum care, delivery of the baby, and postpartum care. Total obstetrical care does *not* include diagnostic procedures, physician office visits for unrelated conditions incidental to pregnancy, and additional visits due to high-risk conditions or medical complications of pregnancy. Codes for these services are separately reported from the Evaluation and Management and Medicine sections of CPT. The treatment of surgical complications associated with pregnancy are separately reported with codes from the Surgery section.

The Endocrine System subsection includes procedures performed on the endocrine glands and the carotid body. Codes for Nervous System subsection procedures are arranged anatomically (skull, meninges, and brain; spine and spinal cord; and extracranial nerves, peripheral nerves, and autonomic nervous system). Nervous system procedures are performed using a variety of approaches for specific purposes.

The Eye and Ocular Adnexa subsection describes procedures performed on the eyeball, anterior and posterior segment, ocular adnexa, and conjunctivae. When reporting codes, review the operative report to identify the anatomical site and type of procedure. The Auditory System subsection is organized anatomically according to the external ear; middle ear; inner ear; and temporal bone, middle fossa approach. When an operating microscope is used during a surgical procedure to perform microsurgery techniques, report add-on code 69990 in addition to the primary procedure code when appropriate.

Internet Links

American Academy of Family Physicians: Go to **www.aafp.org**, click on the FPM Journal link, scroll down and click on the Topic Collections link, go to the Coding & Practice Management heading, and click on the Coding link.

American Academy of Otolaryngology—Head and Neck Surgery: www.entnet.org

American Association of Neurological Surgeons: www.aans.org

American College of Obstetricians and Gynecologists: Go to **www.acog.org**, hover over the Practice Management link, and then click on the Coding link.

Center for Male Reproductive Medicine (CMRM) and Vasectomy Reversal: www.malereproduction.com

Center for Male Reproductive Medicine and Microsurgery: www.maleinfertility.org

The Eye Digest: www.scribd.com/eyeMD

FamilyDoctor.org: Go to **www.familydoctor.org**, hover over the Family Health link, and click on the Pregnancy and Childbirth link to locate articles.

Lacrimedics, Inc.: Go to **www.lacrimedics.com**, and click on the Patients link.

Office on Women's Health: www.womenshealth.gov

Society for Endocrinology: www.endocrinology.org

Review

16.1 – Multiple Choice

Instructions: Select the most appropriate response.

1. The tube that carries spermatozoa from the testis is the
   a. prostate gland.
   b. urethra.
   c. varicocele.
   d. vas deferens.

2. Which procedure involves the direct visualization of the cervical canal and the uterine cavity and is performed to examine the endometrium?
   a. Colposcopy
   b. Hysteroscopy
   c. LEEP electrodissection conization
   d. Loop electrodissection conization

3. According to the notes below the Maternity Care and Delivery subsection of Surgery, which is included in codes reported for maternity care and delivery?
   a. Cordocentesis
   b. Episiotomy
   c. Fetal nonstress test
   d. Insertion of cervical dilator

4. How many glands are included in the endocrine system?
   a. 7
   b. 9
   c. 13
   d. 15

5. When more than one interspace is accessed for laminotomy during the same operative session, report the
   a. appropriate add-on code(s) in addition to the primary procedure code.
   b. primary code once for each interspace accessed.
   c. primary code only.
   d. primary code with modifier 51.

6. Which surgical approach used in extradural exploration/decompression involves making an incision overlying the intervertebral disc and cutting through epidermis, dermis, subcutaneous, fascia, and muscle tissue?
   a. Anterior approach
   b. Anterolateral approach
   c. Costovertebral approach
   d. Transpedicular approach

7. Which nerves are part of the involuntary autonomic nervous system, originate in the thoracic and lumbar regions of the spinal cord, and inhibit the physiological effects of the parasympathetic nervous system?
   a. Cranial
   b. Median
   c. Somatic
   d. Sympathetic

8. Which is the freeing or decompression of an intact nerve from scar tissue?
   a. Neuroma
   b. Neuroplasty
   c. Neurorrhaphy
   d. Neurostimulator

9. When all puncta in both eyes are treated during the same encounter, the appropriate code is reported
   a. once.
   b. twice.
   c. three times.
   d. four times.

10. Which includes the tympanic membrane, auditory ossicles, muscles, and conduction pathways?
    a. Cochlea
    b. Inner ear
    c. Middle ear
    d. Outer ear

11. Plastic repair of the penis due to epispadias distal to external sphincter. Patient was diagnosed with incontinence. Which CPT code is assigned?
    a. 54360
    b. 54380
    c. 54385
    d. 54390

12. Patient placed under anesthesia and an impacted foreign body removed from vagina. Which CPT code is assigned?
    a. 57110
    b. 57111
    c. 57135
    d. 57415

13. Surgical treatment of ovarian ectopic pregnancy with vaginal salpingectomy, left side. Which CPT code is assigned?
    - **a.** 59120 LT
    - **b.** 59130 LT
    - **c.** 59140 LT
    - **d.** 59150 LT

14. Excision of thyroglossal duct cyst. Which CPT code is assigned?
    - **a.** 60200
    - **b.** 60280
    - **c.** 60281
    - **d.** 60600

15. Intersex surgery, female to male. Which CPT code(s) are assigned?
    - **a.** 55970
    - **b.** 55980
    - **c.** 54125, 55970
    - **d.** 54125, 55980

16. Replacement of cerebrospinal fluid shunt using operating microscope. Which CPT code(s) are assigned?
    - **a.** 62220, 69990
    - **b.** 62223
    - **c.** 62225
    - **d.** 62230, 69990

17. Insertion of catheters into uterus to facilitate radiation therapy. Which CPT code is assigned?
    - **a.** 49320
    - **b.** 51045
    - **c.** 52005
    - **d.** 55920

18. Laceration repair of right conjunctiva by mobilization and rearrangement, with hospitalization. Which CPT code is assigned?
    - **a.** 65270 RT
    - **b.** 65272 RT
    - **c.** 65273 RT
    - **d.** 65285 RT

19. Patient diagnosed as having dislocated lens in left eye. Physician performed intracapsular removal of lens. Which CPT code is assigned?
    - **a.** 66920 LT
    - **b.** 66930 LT
    - **c.** 66940 LT
    - **d.** 66982 LT

20. Transcanal labyrinthectomy, right ear. Which CPT code is assigned?
    - **a.** 69801 RT
    - **b.** 69905 RT
    - **c.** 69910 RT
    - **d.** 69915 RT

16.2 – Coding Practice: Male Genital System and Intersex Surgery

Instructions: Assign the CPT code(s) and appropriate modifier(s) to each case.

1. A biopsy needle was passed up the urethra. Using manual guidance, the surgeon identified the prostate gland and performed a punch biopsy. The needle was withdrawn.

2. The patient had been diagnosed with hydroceles, which are scheduled to be removed via excision. First, an incision was made into the patient's scrotum. The hydrocele on the right was identified and dissected free. The left side of the patient's body was treated in the same manner for the hydrocele there.

3. The patient has a papilloma of the penis, which is destroyed via laser surgery.

4. After being informed of all of the risks, the parents of a newborn male patient consented to a circumcision. Regional dorsal penile block (anesthesia) was administered by the physician performing the circumcision. The foreskin of the penis was clamped, and excess skin was trimmed. The clamp was left in place, and antibiotic ointment was applied.

5. After adequate general anesthesia, the patient's scrotum was incised. The spermatic cord was identified, dissected, and cross-clamped. The right testis was carefully pushed up from the scrotum and excised. All vessels were clamped, and all bleeders were cauterized. The left testis was removed using a similar method. The spermatic cord was cross-clamped and cut.

6. Patient underwent bilateral vasectomy including postoperative semen examination. The skin over the spermatic cord was injected with a local anesthetic. The scrotum was exposed via an incision, and the tubular structures of this organ were identified. The vas deferens was identified and cut with a small section of the tube removed. The same method was performed on the opposite side.

7. A subtotal perineal prostatectomy was being performed for prostate cancer. An incision was made at the scrotum. A urethrotomy was used to enlarge the penile urethra. The prostate was dissected via the use of an instrument. The prostate as well as supporting anatomical structures were removed. All bleeding was controlled with cauterization.

8. Patient underwent reduction of torsion of the left testis. An incision was made in the patient's scrotum. The twisted left testis was identified. The testis was carefully detangled. Excellent blood flow was seen. Four sutures were used to anchor the testis to the wall of the scrotum to prevent further twisting.

9. Second-stage operation was done with the goal of constructing a penis and scrotum. This was done using multiple grafts from the patient's skin and clitoris. A penile prosthesis was implanted into the constructed organ.

10. The new construction of a vagina was the goal in this staged procedure. Using tissue from the patient's penis, a clitoris structure was fashioned. The perineum of the patient was opened to form a vagina. The sides of the vagina were lined with skin grafts to add stability.

16.3 – Coding Practice: Reproductive System Procedures and Female Genital System

Instructions: Assign the CPT code(s) and appropriate modifier(s) to each case.

1. The patient has a diagnosis of recurrent cervical carcinoma with metastatic disease to the uterus, ovaries, fallopian tubes, and urinary bladder. After discussing surgical risks, the patient consented to pelvic exenteration, which included an abdominal hysterectomy. An incision was made at the pubic area. The fascia and muscle were retracted. The cervix, uterus, ovaries, and fallopian tubes were identified and excised. The bladder was found to have numerous lesions; it was also removed. The ureters were transplanted to the skin to allow for urine flow. An ileal urinary conduit, in which the ureters are implanted into a segment of small bowel, was done. Patient also underwent placement of needles into pelvic organs in preparation for subsequent interstitial radioelement application, which will be scheduled postoperatively.

2. An endoscope was inserted into the vulva and passed into the uterus. After gaining access to the cavity, a biopsy of the endometrium was done. The scope was withdrawn.

3. An incision was made in the umbilical region for the insertion of laparoscope; a second incision was made on the right side of the abdomen to pass additional trocars. A Falope ring was inserted and advanced through the trocar to the area of the fallopian tubes. This ring was clamped around both fallopian tubes to provide occlusion.

4. A colposcope was inserted into the patient. This allowed for visualization of the female genital organs. The vagina was found to be normal. The cervix had an area of fibrous tissue, which was biopsied. The endocervical area had an area of inflammation, and curettage was performed.

5. After inserting a speculum into the vagina, the physician was able to visualize a vaginal cyst directly. Forceps were used to clamp the cyst. The cyst was excised and sent to pathology for analysis. The speculum was removed.

6. After inserting a speculum into the vagina, the physician identified a Bartholin gland; the cyst was directly visualized. An incision was made, and the cyst was dissected free of the surrounding tissue and mucosa. The wound was closed in layers with absorbable sutures.

7. After insertion of a speculum into the vagina, laser ablation was performed to cauterize the outer cells of the cervix.

8. The physician performed a salpingostomy and identified a damaged right fallopian tube.

9. After insertion of a speculum into the vagina, a catheter was passed that contained several small embryos. With the use of the catheter, the embryos were transferred and implanted in the uterus.

10. After an abdominal incision was made, the left ovary was identified. The ovarian cysts were located and removed in total. The incision was closed with sutures.

16.4 – Coding Practice: Maternity Care and Delivery

Instructions: Assign the CPT code(s) and appropriate modifier(s) to each case.

1. A neonatologist attached a fetal monitoring electrode to the scalp of the fetus in utero as part of prenatal testing during labor. The physician read, interpreted, and made notations on the tracing coming from the electrode data.

2. A patient at 39 weeks' gestation presented in labor. The patient has requested a VBAC (vaginal birth after cesarean). After 20 hours in labor, fetal distress was noted. The patient required a cesarean delivery. All antepartum and postpartum routine care was provided by the delivering physician.

3. A patient with five fetuses presents for fetal reduction due to severe preeclampsia. Using the potassium chloride method, two fetal sacs are injected. At the conclusion of the procedure, the patient has three fetal sacs intact.

4. At 11 weeks' gestation, the patient had an incomplete abortion. Due to profuse vaginal bleeding, evacuating the uterus was necessary. Dilation and curettage was done with suction of any remaining products of conception.

5. A patient presents after having delivered the baby vaginally en route to the hospital in a private motor vehicle. The patient's spouse saw a large "Delivery" notice and arrived at the facility's shipping and receiving entrance. Staff brought a bed to that entrance and transported the patient to the emergency department. The newborn was taken directly to the neonatal intensive care unit (NICU) for evaluation. The placenta had not been delivered on route to the hospital. Using abdominal massage, the placenta was delivered.

_____

6. An ectopic pregnancy was confirmed by ultrasound. Via a vaginal approach, the pelvic cavity was visualized and examined. All products of conception were removed using curettage. The pelvic cavity was lavaged with saline solution. The patient's right fallopian tube was affected. This tube was excised.

_____

7. After normal prenatal care, this patient presented in labor at 38 weeks. An episiotomy was done to facilitate delivery. A normal healthy newborn was born via vaginal delivery. The episiotomy was repaired. The patient was discharged with the baby and received postpartum follow-up care in the office.

_____

8. The patient presents for a level 4 E/M encounter in the office. Her estimated gestational age was 26 weeks. The patient reports heavy vaginal bleeding overnight. After insertion of the speculum, the uterus was examined. Slight bleeding was noted. The patient has had a complete spontaneous abortion. No products of conception are seen. There is no need for surgical intervention.

_____

9. Routine prenatal care was rendered to this patient, who presented at 41 weeks in labor. The patient was examined, and the fetus was found to be in a breech position. The fetus was turned via external cephalic version using an abdominal approach. After turning of fetus, an episiotomy was performed. A normal healthy 10-pound infant was born via vaginal delivery. The episiotomy was repaired. Postpartum care was delivered.

_____

10. Uterine evacuation and curettage to remove a hydatidiform mole.

_____

16.5 – Coding Practice: Endocrine System

Instructions: Assign the CPT code(s) and appropriate modifier(s) to each case.

1. The patient's neck was palpated, and a mass was identified on the left. Local anesthesia was administered, and the position of the mass was confirmed again by palpation. A percutaneous core needle was inserted through the skin and underlying tissue into the thyroid mass. The needle was withdrawn with the sample inside the core. The sample will be sent for analysis.

_____

2. After adequate general anesthesia, a cervical incision was made. Skin, fascia, and muscle were retracted to expose the thyroid gland. A severely enlarged left lobe of the thyroid was found. The left lobe of the thyroid gland was removed in total and sent to pathology for analysis. Parathyroid glands were carefully inspected and found to be normal. These were not removed but were left intact. All bleeders were cauterized. The skin and muscle were closed in layers.

_____

3. After adequate general anesthesia, a midline abdominal incision was made. The retroperitoneal area was identified and found to be normal. The adrenal glands were directly visualized. The left adrenal gland was removed in total. A biopsy sample was taken from the right adrenal gland.

_____

4. After adequate general anesthesia, an incision was made along the thyroglossal duct cyst. A portion of the hyoid bone was removed, and recurrent thyroglossal duct cyst was excised. Wound was packed for secondary closure.

5. After adequate general anesthesia, a cervical incision was made to expose the thyroid and parathyroid glands. The parathyroid glands were directly visualized. The right parathyroid gland was removed.

6. After several small incisions were made in the patient's back, the laparoscope was introduced. The adrenal gland on the right was identified and examined. It was normal in appearance. The left adrenal gland was found to be enlarged at the tip. This section was removed and passed through the trocar. The scope was removed and the skin incision closed with sutures.

7. After a cervical incision was made, the muscles of the neck were separated to expose the thyroid and parathyroid glands. The right lobe was normal in appearance and size. The left upper thyroid gland had a goiter measuring approximately 3.0 cm. This lobe with the goiter was removed.

8. Based on thyroid biopsy, this patient presented for a total thyroidectomy due to thyroid carcinoma. The neck area was cleaned and draped in the usual fashion. Under general anesthesia, the patient had a cervical incision. A radical neck dissection was performed. After the muscles of the neck were separated, the gland was exposed. Direct visualization showed the gland to be cystic and nodular in nature. The right lobe of the gland was removed first, followed by the left lobe. The parathyroid glands were inspected and appeared to be normal. The thyroid gland in total was removed and sent to pathology for analysis along with cervical lymph nodes. All bleeders were cauterized. The incision was closed in layers with staples and sutures.

9. Under general anesthesia, a cervical incision at the previous incision site was done. The neck muscles were divided and retracted. The thyroid area was exposed. The absent left lobe of the thyroid was noted. The right lobe of the thyroid was examined. It was found to be very nodular in appearance. This lobe was removed as part of a secondary thyroidectomy, which involved removing all remaining thyroid tissue following previous removal of the left lobe. The parathyroid glands were examined and appeared normal. The specimen of the right lobe was sent to pathology. The muscles were retracted back and closed with staples. The incision was closed in layers.

10. After the patient's adrenal area was accessed through a midline abdominal incision, the retroperitoneal space was explored. A mass was identified adjacent to the left adrenal gland. This was removed along with the left adrenal gland *in toto*, which also appeared abnormal. The incision was closed.

16.6 – Coding Practice: Nervous System

Instructions: Assign the CPT code(s) and appropriate modifier(s) to each case.

1. After the patient was placed in a prone position, an incision was made over the upper spinal area. Epidural drug infusion device was implanted as a subcutaneous reservoir. The incision was closed with sutures.

2. The greater occipital nerve, left, was identified, and a nerve block (anesthetic agent) injection was performed.

3. The patient presented with a laceration of the digital nerve of the left hand. This was repaired with sutures.

_____

4. Percutaneous neurostimulator electrode array device implantation through skin to cranial nerve.

_____

5. The patient presents with a meningocele approximately 4.0 cm in diameter. This was repaired after placing the patient in a prone position and making an incision. Access was gained to the dura of the thoracic spinal region. The bulging tissue was carefully placed into normal position. The incision was closed.

_____

6. The patient was placed on their left side. After local anesthesia, the needle was inserted at the lumbar region. The sheath of the needle was pulled back; cloudy fluid was seen. This fluid was collected in the hollow portion of the needle.

_____

7. This patient presented for drainage of a brain abscess. After a burr hole was drilled, the cranium was accessed to reveal the site of the abscess. The abscess was drained.

_____

8. The patient presented with an arteriovenous (AV) malformation. A craniotomy was performed to gain access to the brain and the site of the malformation. This was done without difficulty. Blood vessels leading to the malformation were identified and ligated. The malformation measured approximately 2.0 cm in size. It was carefully repaired via supratentorial resection. The bone portion from the craniotomy was replaced and secured.

_____

9. The patient presented with a nerve compression, left leg. An incision was made overlying the compressed sciatic nerve midpoint. Neuroplasty involved identifying scar tissue and dissecting it to release the sciatic nerve.

_____

10. The patient presented for a replacement of a lumbosubarachnoid cerebrospinal fluid shunt, which was performed by first incising at the original incision site. A moderate number of adhesions were seen, which were removed. The old shunt was also removed. A new shunt was placed in the same position.

_____

16.7 – Coding Practice: Eye and Ocular Adnexa

Instructions: Assign the CPT code(s) and appropriate modifier(s) to each case.

1. The patient presented with a foreign body sensation of the left eye. Under slit lamp examination, a small metallic foreign body was identified. This object was slightly embedded in the lower corneal area. It was removed via a small incision, using the slit lamp for guidance.

_____

2. The patient presented for correction of strabismus (crossed eyes). The left eye was immobilized with a speculum. Incisions were made in the conjunctiva. The horizontal lateral muscle was identified and incised. The horizontal lateral muscle was sutured distally to the sclera. The horizontal medial rectus muscle was surgically incised and sutured in the same manner.

_____

3. After injection of a local anesthetic agent, the left upper eyelid was examined closely. A large chalazion was seen. The chalazion was resected in total. A moderate area of infection was noted, and this was drained. The infectious area was flushed with saline solution.

_____

4. After the injection of a local anesthetic agent, an incision was made on the patient's right side at the site of the medial canthal tendon. Dacryocystectomy was performed via careful dissection, with the lacrimal sac identified and removed.

_____

5. The patient presented with a corneal lamellar on the right side. This was excised using scleral scissors. Antibiotic ointment was applied.

_____

6. Using a laser, short bursts were administered to the patient's left eye. This iridotomy was performed to allow for the movement of fluid in the anterior chamber and to treat the patient's glaucoma.

_____

7. Using a xenon arc for photocoagulation and prophylaxis of a retinal tear, right eye, spots were made on the patient's retina. This provided a good seal of the tear.

_____

8. With the patient under local anesthesia, the right lower eyelid is palpated and a foreign body is found in the upper-right quadrant near the posterior surface. The lid was everted and an incision made under the site. The foreign body was removed.

_____

9. The patient presented with a tumor of the lacrimal gland. An incision was made in the lid crease of the left upper eyelid. This had to be extended down into the lacrimal fossa. An osteotomy was necessary to gain access to the entire mass. The mass was removed in total. The incisional wound was closed.

_____

10. After making an incision in the patient's left eye at the junction of the cornea and sclera, the eye was entered. Extracapsular cataract removal was accomplished, and the soft portion of the lens was removed. This removed the entire cataract, leaving the capsule of the eye intact. An intraocular lens (IOL) was inserted. The incision was closed, and antibiotic injection was done.

_____

16.8 – Coding Practice: Auditory System

Instructions: Assign the CPT code(s) and appropriate modifier(s) to each case.

1. Impacted cerumen was removed from the left and right ears, using lavage and suction instrumentation. After removal, the ear canals were inspected. No evidence of infection was seen.

_____

2. Decompression of the left internal auditory canal was performed for hearing maintenance in a neurofibromatosis patient. No postoperative complications were documented, and radiological and audiological follow-up will be scheduled.

_____

3. The patient reported a buzzing sound from the left ear. Direct examination identified an insect-like foreign object in the canal. Using a cerumen spoon, the object was removed.

_____

4. Using the punch biopsy method, a specimen was taken from the right external auditory canal.

_____

5. With the patient under general anesthesia, an incision was made at the left auricular region and tympano-plasty with mastoidectomy was performed. The outer bone of the mastoid was removed, and the mastoid antrum was entered. The tympanic membrane was identified and perforated. The eardrum was brought forward. The middle ear was examined. A cholesteatoma was found and removed. The ossicular chain was identified and examined and found to be normal.

_____

6. Through the ear canal of the patient's left ear, the aural polyp was identified under direct examination. With an ear snare, the polyp was removed from the middle ear. Antibiotic drops were placed in the canal. Minimal bleeding was noted.

_____

7. After the patient's right auditory canal was examined, an abscess was noted. This required drainage. An incision was made over the location of this external abscess. The abscess was drained, with a thick yellowish material seen. Antibiotic ointment and dressing were applied.

_____

8. The patient underwent bilateral myringotomy, including aspiration and eustachian tube inflation, under local anesthesia.

_____

9. Patient underwent removal of tumor, left temporal bone, which required vertical incision anterior to left auricle, extending it superiorly to expose temporalis muscle. The muscle was divided and craniotomy performed to expose the dura over temporal lobe of brain. After elevating the dura, the tumor was isolated and excised. Bone plug was returned to skull, incision was sutured, and dressing was applied.

_____

10. The patient presented seven months postmastoidectomy for simple debridement of the left cavity. This was done under direct visualization using suction. Skin and debris were removed from the left side of the mastoid. No infection was observed. The skin and debris removed appeared normal in appearance.

_____

16.9 – Coding Practice: Operating Microscope

Instructions: Assign the CPT code(s) and appropriate modifier(s) to each case.

1. The patient underwent transcanal labyrinthotomy with cryosurgery and multiple perfusion of vestibuloactive drugs. After anesthesia, an incision was made posterior to the ear canal on the right and the external ear was exposed. The operating microscope was brought into the field to facilitate the placement of a temporary stapes plate. The cryolaser was used to debride tissue present in the area.

_____

2. A patient presented with a fistula of the left salivary gland. This area was incised to expose the fistula, and the operating microscope was used to get a better view of the fistula for the purpose of closure.

_____

3. A neonatal patient presented with a diaphragmatic hernia. Under adequate anesthesia, an abdominal incision was made. The operating microscope was used to identify all vessels and small arteries. This was in part due to the size of the infant. The hernia sac was exposed and dissected free, sutures were placed to close the diaphragmatic hernia defect, and the external incision was closed in layers.

_____

4. Patient underwent arthrodesis, anterior interbody, with C3 nerve root decompression, disc space preparation, discectomy, and osteophytectomy. Operating microscope was used to facilitate surgery.

_____

5. The patient had an injury to the left pinky finger. The volar plate required repair. The digit was incised at the interphalangeal joint space. The operating microscope was used to identify the area of instability. The plate was sutured to the distal bone. The wound was closed with sutures.

_____

6. An incision was made over the skin at the site of the injured blood vessel, left hand, third finger. The operating microscope was brought into the field to help identify the vessel and used to assist in the dissection. Direct repair of the vessel with sutures was performed. The surgical incision was closed with sutures.

_____

7. Patient underwent microvascular anastomosis with free omental flap pedicled on to the left gastroepiploic vessel to reconstruct a defect.

_____

8. The patient presented with a lesion of the pharynx. The patient's oral cavity was assessed using the operating microscope, and the lesion was identified. After identification, the laser was brought into the field to perform the excision. Minimal bleeding was noted.

_____

9. The patient presented with several small lesions of the epiglottis. Epiglottidectomy was performed using the operating microscope.

_____

10. Patient underwent nerve repair for a peripheral nerve injury, left hand, to restore innervation. Operating microscope was used for nerve allograft, three nerves, using nonvascularized cable nerves. Incision was made, tissues were dissected to locate damaged nerves, which were resected and removed. Nerve allografts were attached to each end of resected nerves, suturing proximal and distal ends into place. Region was infused with heparin solution and saline to prevent clot formation. Operative wound was repaired in layers.

_____

CPT Radiology

Chapter Outline

Radiology Terminology

Overview of Radiology Section

Radiology Section Guidelines

Radiology Subsections

Chapter Objectives

At the conclusion of this chapter, the student should be able to:

1. Define key terms related to the CPT Radiology Section.
2. Define radiology terminology related to planes of view, positioning and radiographic projection, and radiology procedures.
3. Summarize the organization, format, and content of the CPT Radiology section.
4. Interpret CPT Radiology Section guidelines.
5. Assign codes from the CPT Radiology section.

Key Terms

angiography

anteroposterior projection

aortography

arthrography

bone density study

cardiac blood pool imaging

component coding

computed axial tomography (CT) (CAT)

computed tomography angiography (CTA)

contrast agent

contrast material

coronal plane

cystography

diagnostic mammography

Doppler ultrasonography

dosimetry

dual energy x-ray absorptiometry (DEXA) (DXA)

fluoroscopy

global service

interventional radiologic procedure

lateral projection

magnetic resonance angiography (MRA)

magnetic resonance imaging (MRI)

mammography

midsagittal plane

nuclear imaging

nuclear medicine

oblique projection

parenterally

plane of view

positron emission tomography (PET)

posteroanterior (PA) projection

professional component

radiation oncology

radiographic projection

radiologic guidance

radiological supervision and interpretation

radiologist

radiology

radionuclide

radiopharmaceutical therapy

sagittal plane

screening mammography

single photon emission computerized tomography (SPECT)

systemic radiation therapy

technical component	transverse plane	ultrasound	view
therapeutic port film	ultrasonography	venography	x-ray

Introduction

The CPT Radiology section includes subsections for diagnostic radiology (diagnostic imaging); diagnostic ultrasound; radiologic guidance; breast, mammography; bone/joint studies; radiation oncology; and nuclear medicine. These subsections are further subdivided into anatomical categories. The Diagnostic Radiology (Diagnostic Imaging) subsection includes noninvasive and invasive diagnostic and therapeutic (interventional) procedures, as well as computed (or computerized) tomography and magnetic resonance imaging.

 NOTE:

Procedures frequently performed by radiologists that are located in other CPT sections include

- Noninvasive vascular diagnostic studies (Medicine section)
- Invasive (or interventional) radiology services (Surgery section), such as
  - Injection procedures
  - Transcatheter procedures

When included in CPT, the Other Procedures code is reported for an unlisted procedure performed on the anatomical site. When reporting an unlisted procedure code, include documentation about the procedure performed (e.g., special report) with the submitted claim.

The *Medicare National Correct Coding Initiative Policy Manual* provides guidance about assigning procedure and service codes for the Radiology section. Go to **www.cms.gov** and enter "Medicare NCCI Policy Manual" in the Search box to navigate to the manual.

Radiology Terminology

Radiology is a branch of medicine that uses imaging techniques to diagnose and treat disease. A **radiologist** is a physician who has undergone specialized training to interpret diagnostic x-rays, perform specialized x-ray procedures, and administer radiation for the treatment of disease (e.g., cancer). Terms unique to the radiographic procedures include the following:

- Planes of view
- Positioning and radiographic projection

> **Example:** Axial is a standard plane of reference for most radiology codes. For example, axial images depict the long axis of the body, from the head to foot.

Planes of View

Terminology that describes **planes of view** (Figure 17-1) used when performing radiology procedures includes the following:

- **Coronal plane** (or *frontal plane*): Divides the body into anterior or ventral and posterior or dorsal portions at a right angle to the sagittal plane, separating the body into front and back; also called ventral or dorsal plane
- **Midsagittal plane**: Vertically divides the body through the midline into two equal left and right halves

- **Sagittal plane**: Vertically divides the body into unequal left and right portions
- **Transverse plane** (or *horizontal plane* or *axial plane*): Horizontally divides the body into superior and inferior portions

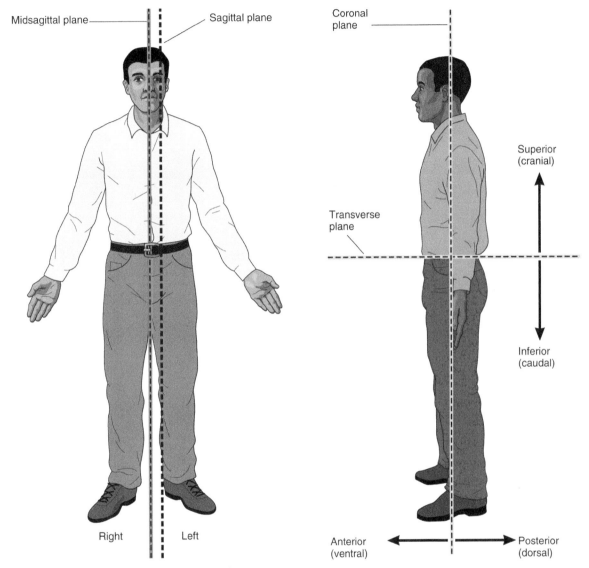

FIGURE 17-1 Planes that separate body structures

Positioning and Radiographic Projection

Patients are positioned for radiographic procedures so that a certain part of the body is placed closest to the x-ray film. The patient's position in relation to the x-ray camera is the **view** (e.g., code 71045 specifies a single view of the chest). **Radiographic projection** (Figure 17-2) describes the path that the x-ray beam travels through the body, from entrance to exit. An *x-ray beam* is made up of invisible electromagnetic energy waves called *photons*, which are emitted from a radiation machine and are used to produce images (x-rays) and treat disease (e.g., cancer). Radiographic projections include the following:

- **Anteroposterior projection**: Patient is positioned with their back parallel to the film; the x-ray beam travels from front to back, or anterior to posterior
- **Lateral projection**, or *side view*: Patient is positioned at a right angle to the film; the x-ray beam travels through the side of the body

- **Oblique projection**: Patient is positioned with the body slanted sideways toward the film, halfway between a parallel and right-angle position; the x-ray beam travels through this angle of the body
- **Posteroanterior (PA) projection**: Patient is positioned facing the film and parallel to it; the x-ray beam travels from back to front, or posterior to anterior

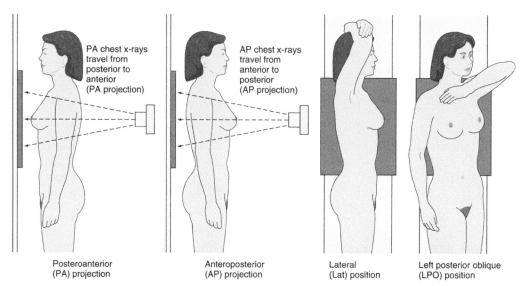

FIGURE 17-2 Radiographic projections

Radiology Procedures

Radiology procedures include the following:

- **Angiography**: x-ray of a blood vessel after injection of contrast material (Figure 17-3)
- **Aortography**: x-ray of the aorta after injection of contrast material
- **Arthrography**: x-ray of a joint after injection of contrast material
- **Computed axial tomography (CT) (CAT)**: x-ray of horizontal and vertical cross-sectional views or "slices" of the body that are computer-processed to create three-dimensional, or 3D, images
- **Computed tomography angiography (CTA)**: x-rays of different angles create cross-sectional images of organs, bones, and tissues to visualize blood flow in arterial and venous vessels throughout the body
- **Cystography**: x-ray of the urinary bladder after injection of contrast material
- **Fluoroscopy**: Continuous x-ray beam generates a movie-like image that is viewed on a monitor; used for invasive procedures such as intravenous/intra-arterial catheterization and extracorporeal shock wave lithotripsy
- **Magnetic resonance imaging (MRI)**: Noninvasive x-ray procedure uses an external magnetic field to produce a two-dimensional view of an internal organ or structure such as the brain or spinal cord
- **Nuclear imaging**: Noninvasive x-ray procedure creates an image by measuring radiation emission, or radiation "uptake," of body areas after the administration of a **radionuclide**, which is a radioactive material, such as an isotope of iodine
- **Positron emission tomography (PET)**: x-ray images of the body are produced after the administration of radioisotopes, which track metabolism or blood flow, not anatomy

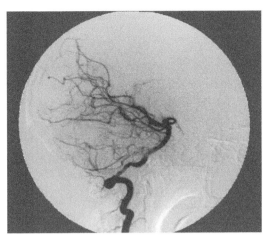

FIGURE 17-3 Angiography

- **Single photon emission computerized tomography (SPECT)**: 3D x-ray images of internal organs are produced after administration of a radioactive material, which visualize anatomy *and* function
- **Ultrasound**, or **ultrasonography**: High-frequency sound waves bounce off internal organs and create echoes; the echo pattern is displayed on the ultrasound machine monitor; an *echo* is the effect of a sound that reflects off a distant surface and returns to its source, just like the sound produced when you yell into a well and your voice "bounces back"
- **Venography**: x-ray of a vein is taken after injection of contrast material
- **x-ray**: Radiographic visualization or imaging of internal body structures that uses low-dose high-energy radiation (High-dose high-energy radiation is used to treat diseases such as cancer.)

When a radiology procedure is performed, a device called a *block* (e.g., lead apron) made of lead or another heavy metal is placed between the radiation beam and that portion of the patient's body that requires protection from radiation.

The international unit of exposure dose for x-rays or gamma rays is called a *roentgen*, abbreviated as R or r. (Roentgen is named after Professor Wilhelm Konrad Roentgen, who discovered x-rays in 1895.) A unit of *radiation absorbed dose (rad)* is the amount of radiant energy absorbed in a tissue. Newer radiation terminology includes the term *gray*, abbreviated as *gy*, named for British physician L. Harold Gray (1905–1965) (an authority on the use of radiation for cancer treatment). (One gray equals 100 rads.) A *roentgen-equivalent-man (rem)* is the unit of measurement that includes different biological responses to different kinds of radiation. The radiation quantity measured by rem is called an *equivalent dose*. (A millirem is one-thousandth of a rem, the unit for measuring equivalent dose.)

Exercise 17.1 – Radiology Terminology

Instructions: Complete each statement.

1. The branch of medicine that uses imaging techniques to diagnose and treat disease is called _____.

2. A physician who has undergone specialized training to interpret diagnostic x-rays, perform specialized x-ray procedures, and administer radiation for the treatment of disease is called a _____.

(continues)

Exercise 17.1 – continued

3. The transverse plane horizontally divides the body into superior and _____ portions.

4. The coronal plane divides the body into anterior or ventral and posterior or _____ portions at a right angle to the sagittal plane, separating the body into front and back.

5. The sagittal plane vertically divides the body into _____ left and right portions.

6. The midsagittal plane vertically divides the body through the midline into two _____ left and right halves.

7. The path that the x-ray beam travels through the body, from entrance to exit, is called the radiographic _____.

8. The patient's position in relation to the x-ray camera is called the _____.

9. For an anteroposterior projection, the patient is positioned with their back _____ to the film.

10. For a lateral projection, the patient is positioned at a right angle to the film and the x-ray beam travels through the _____ of the body.

11. For an oblique projection, the patient is positioned with the body _____ the film and slanted sideways.

12. For a posteroanterior (PA) projection, the patient is positioned _____ to the film and facing it.

13. An x-ray of a blood vessel after injection of contrast material is called _____.

14. Ultrasound (or ultrasonography) uses high-frequency sound waves that bounce off internal organs and create _____, which are displayed on an ultrasound machine monitor as a pattern.

15. Nuclear imaging is a noninvasive x-ray procedure that creates an image by measuring radiation emission, or radiation "uptake," of body areas after the administration of a _____, which is a radioactive material such as an isotope of iodine.

Overview of Radiology Section

The Radiology section includes subsections for diagnostic radiology (diagnostic imaging); diagnostic ultrasound; radiologic guidance; breast, mammography; bone/joint studies; radiation oncology; and nuclear medicine. Procedure descriptions include the

- Type of service (e.g., modality)
- Anatomical site
- Use of contrast material

Professional Versus Technical Components

For radiology coding, the physician responsible for the professional and technical components of an examination must be determined. (Professional and technical components are reimbursement issues, which means that there are no CPT guidelines or notes explaining the three options.) Radiology procedures include the following three components:

- **Technical component:** Use of equipment and supplies and the employment of radiologic technologists to perform diagnostic imaging examinations and administer radiation therapy treatments
- **Professional component:** Services provided by the physician, which include supervising the performance of a diagnostic imaging procedure, interpreting imaging films, and documenting the imaging report
- **Global service:** Combined technical and professional components, as reported with a CPT Radiology code

Most radiology procedures require both professional and technical components, and the following modifiers are added to radiology codes as appropriate:

- 26 (Professional component)
- TC (Technical component)

NOTE:

Some radiology codes include only a professional component, and modifier 26 is *not* added to these codes (e.g., therapeutic radiology treatment planning codes and weekly radiation therapy management codes).

Modifier 26 is added to the radiology code when a radiologist supervises the radiologic procedure, interprets the radiographic image, and documents a report (but does not perform the radiologic procedure). This indicates that only the professional component was provided.

Modifier TC is added to the radiology code when the provider or facility performs the radiologic procedure. (A radiologist employed by another facility interprets the radiographic image and documents the report. That radiologist adds modifier 26 to the radiology code.)

When a provider owns the equipment and performs both the technical and the professional components, a global service CPT code is reported. A modifier is *not* added to the radiology code. (Hospitals own radiology equipment, and they employ radiologic technicians who perform x-rays and employ or contract with radiologists who interpret radiographic images and document reports.)

NOTE:

Depending on the contract negotiated between radiologists and the health care facility

- Radiologists are considered employees of the health care facility (e.g., hospital) or contractors.
- The facility submits claims to obtain reimbursement for all services provided to patients (including professional services), or the radiologists use a medical billing service to submit claims for professional services.

Example 1: Patient undergoes a complete chest x-ray, minimum of four views, which is performed on an outpatient basis at the hospital. Report code 71048. The patient's primary care provider had completed a requisition for the chest x-ray after having evaluated the patient in the office for shortness of breath. The radiologic technician takes the x-ray, and the radiologist interprets the image and documents an x-ray report. A copy of the x-ray report is mailed to the patient's primary care provider. The hospital reports the x-ray code as a global service.

Example 2: Patient undergoes a complete wrist x-ray, minimum of three views, which is performed at a freestanding radiology clinic. Report code 73110. The patient's primary care provider had completed a requisition for the wrist x-ray after evaluating the patient in the office for severe wrist pain earlier that day. The clinic's radiologic technician takes the x-ray, and the clinic's radiologist interprets the image and documents an x-ray report. A copy of the x-ray report is mailed to the patient's primary care provider. The clinic reports the x-ray code as a global service.

Example 3: The patient is seen by the primary care provider, who evaluates a lump on the right pinky finger. The office has x-ray equipment and takes a two-view x-ray of the hand. The x-ray is interpreted by a hand specialist who is located in another office. The primary care provider reports code 73120 TC. The hand specialist reports code 73120 26.

Use of Modifiers with Radiology Codes

Modifiers commonly added to Radiology codes include

- 52 (Reduced services), to indicate that a service is partially reduced at the physician's discretion.

Example: Patient underwent ultrasound exam of swollen tonsils. Code 76536 is reported for "Ultrasound, soft tissues of head and neck (e.g., thyroid, parathyroid, parotid) real time with image documentation." Because just tonsillar tissue was evaluated, code 76536 52 is reported.

- 76 (Repeat procedure by same physician or other qualified health care professional), to describe a repeat procedure by the same physician on the same date of service. ("Same physician" refers to either the same physician or a physician in the same specialty or group.)

Example: A patient presents to the emergency department (ED) with blunt abdominal trauma. Complete acute abdomen series with supine, erect, and decubitus views and single-view chest x-ray was performed. The patient became unstable several hours later in the ED, and the x-ray was repeated. Code 74022 76 is reported for the repeat x-ray.

Coding Tip

- Modifier 50 (Bilateral procedure) is not added when code descriptions specify "bilateral." Radiology code descriptions must be carefully reviewed to determine whether modifier 50 should be added (when code descriptions do not specify "bilateral" and the procedure performed was bilateral).
- HCPCS Level II anatomical modifiers LT (Left side) and RT (Right side) are added to radiology codes when appropriate. These modifiers are reported to identify a specific side of the body.

Complete Procedure

The term *complete* as included in radiology code descriptions refers to the number of views required for the study of a designated body part. Code descriptions include language that indicates what constitutes a *complete study* for a specific type of radiologic procedure.

Example 1: Patient underwent complete mastoid x-ray. Report code 70130.

Example 2: Patient underwent temporomandibular joint (TMJ) arthrography, which included radiological supervision and interpretation. The radiologist also performed an injection procedure for the TMJ arthrography during the same encounter. Report codes 70332 and 21116.

Both components comprise a complete procedure when performed by the same physician (e.g., radiologist), and two codes are reported by that physician. However, when two physicians are involved in performing each component of the procedure, each physician submits the code for their respective portion of the procedure performed.

Evaluation and Management (E/M) Services

When the radiologist provides E/M services as part of the radiographic procedure (e.g., invasive or interventional radiology), a CPT E/M code is *not* reported. The services provided by the radiologist include a minimal history and examination to determine the following:

- Reason for the examination
- Presence of allergies
- Acquisition of informed consent
- Discussion of follow-up
- Review of the patient record

The level of medical decision making is usually characterized by:

- Whether the invasive or interventional procedure should be performed
- Whether any comorbidities (coexisting conditions) may impact the procedure
- What discussion and education took place with the patient

However, when a significant, separately identifiable E/M service is provided by the radiologist *distinct from the radiographic procedure*, an appropriate E/M code is reported (e.g., initial radiation oncology consultation to determine whether to proceed with treatment).

Example: The patient's primary care provider requests that a radiologist provide consultation services to render an opinion about the patient's candidacy for a uterine embolization procedure. The radiologist performs a comprehensive history and examination and reviews the patient's record. A pelvic MRI is performed to assist in medical decision making. The radiologist reports a code from the Office or Other Outpatient Consultations category of the CPT E/M section.

Exercise 17.2 – Overview of Radiology Section

Instructions: Complete each statement.

1. Procedure descriptions for codes in the Radiology section include type of _____, anatomical site, and use of contrast material.

2. Services provided by the radiologic technologist include performing diagnostic imaging examinations and administering radiation therapy treatments, and they are considered the _____ component.

3. Services provided by the physician include supervising the performance of a diagnostic imaging procedure, interpreting imaging films, and documenting the imaging report, and they are considered the _____ component.

4. Combined technical and professional components reported with a CPT radiology code are considered a _____ service.

5. When a significant, separately identifiable evaluation and management (E/M) service is provided by the radiologist _____ *from the radiographic procedure*, an appropriate E/M code is reported.

Radiology Section Guidelines

Guidelines located at the beginning of the Radiology section provide instruction about the following:

- Subject listings
- Separate procedures
- Unlisted service or procedure
- Special report

- Supervision and interpretation, imaging guidance
- Administration of contrast material(s)
- Written report(s)
- Foreign body/implant definition

Instructional notes appear throughout the Radiology section to provide coding clarification and direction.

Subject Listings

When radiologic services are performed by or under the responsible supervision of a physician (e.g., radiologist) or other qualified health care professional, radiology codes are reported.

Separate Procedures

Some procedures are considered an integral component of a total service or procedure and are identified by the descriptor *separate procedure*. These codes are *not* reported in addition to the code for the primary or total x-ray procedure unless unrelated to or distinct from other procedures provided.

> **Example:** Patient undergoes laparoscopic cholecystectomy with intraoperative cholangiogram and fluoroscopy. Report codes 47563 (surgeon) and 74300 (radiologist).

Unlisted Service or Procedure

As in other CPT sections, unlisted procedure codes are reported for a service or procedure that is not adequately described or listed in CPT.

Special Report

When a service is new, unusual, or rarely provided, a special report is attached to the submitted claim to validate the medical necessity and appropriateness of the service.

Supervision and Interpretation, Imaging Guidance

Imaging procedures may require a surgical procedure to access the imaged area (e.g., injection of contrast material), or a surgical procedure may require image guidance (e.g., lung biopsy with fluoroscopic guidance). When a surgical procedure requires imaging guidance and the code description includes imaging guidance and associated radiological supervision and interpretation, do not report a separate code for the imaging service.

> **Example:** Patient undergoes injection procedure and antegrade pyelography through a previously placed nephrostomy. The physician provided supervision and interpretation of the pyelography. Report code 50431. Do *not* report a separate code from the CPT Radiology section because the code description includes "all associated radiological supervision and interpretation."

When a surgical procedure or a service (e.g., Medicine section) requires imaging guidance and the code description does *not* include imaging guidance and associated radiological supervision and interpretation, report a separate code for the imaging service *in addition to* the surgical procedure or service code.

> **Example:** Patient undergoes venous catheterization for selective organ blood sampling with image guidance. Report codes 36500 and 75893. The Radiology code is also reported because the Surgery code description does not include "imaging guidance and associated radiological supervision and interpretation."

(The radiological supervision and interpretation, imaging guidance, concept does not apply to Radiation Oncology procedures.)

Interventional Radiology Procedures

Interventional radiology procedures (e.g., catheterization, injection of contrast media) are used to diagnose and treat conditions using percutaneous or minimally invasive techniques under imaging guidance. Due to the complexity of interventional radiology procedures, **component coding** allows for reporting a CPT Radiology code *and* a CPT Surgery code to completely describe the service provided (when a combination code does not exist). Component coding provides a mechanism for reporting interventional procedures whether performed by a single physician or by different physicians (e.g., one physician performs the procedure and the other performs the imaging supervision and interpretation).

- When two different physicians (e.g., surgeon and radiologist) perform the surgical and radiological components, each physician reports the code(s) for their component of the procedure performed. The radiological portion of the procedure is designated as **radiological supervision and interpretation**.
- When one physician performs the procedure and provides radiological supervision and interpretation, that physician reports code(s) for both components.

Example 1: Patient underwent hospital outpatient injection procedure and antegrade nephrostogram through a previously placed nephrostomy. The hospital and physician each report CPT Surgery section code 50431 for institutional and professional coding, respectively. A separate CPT Radiology section code is *not* reported because the code description includes the injection, antegrade nephrostogram, and "all associated radiological supervision and interpretation."

Example 2: Patient underwent hospital outpatient needle biopsy of the liver under fluoroscopic guidance. The hospital and physician each report CPT Surgery section code 47000 for institutional and professional coding, respectively, and the hospital reports CPT Radiology section code 77002.

Administration of Contrast Material(s)

A **contrast agent**, or **contrast material** (or contrast medium), is a radiopaque substance (solid or liquid) that is administered to provide better radiographic visualization of organs studied. The contrast agent is administered orally, rectally, intravenously, percutaneously, or through inhalation or urinary catheterization. A *contrast medium injection device* (Figure 17-4) is used to deliver a predetermined amount of contrast, typically for vascular imaging procedures.

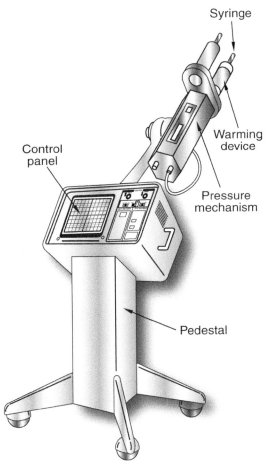

FIGURE 17-4 Contrast medium injection device

NOTE:

Radiologic procedures are performed with contrast, without contrast, or with and without contrast. Separate codes are available in the Radiology section to describe all of these combinations.

Contrast agents are radiopaque (impenetrable by x-rays or other forms of radiation), and they block x-ray beams and provide excellent contrast for body structures. Common contrast agents include barium sulfate (gastrointestinal studies), organic iodine (vascular and renal studies), and iodized oils (myelography). Contrast materials make body structures appear white on x-rays.

Coding Tip

Radiology codes that contain the description "with contrast" include intravascular, intra-articular, or intrathecal administration of contrast material. When contrast material is administered orally or rectally, the administration of the contrast material is not reported separately. It is included in the radiologic procedure performed.

NOTE:

The supply of contrast material is not included in radiology procedure codes. HCPCS Level II codes are reported for the supply of contrast material (e.g., A4641).

Written Report(s)

The written report, documented and authenticated by the interpreting individual (e.g., radiologist), is considered an integral part of a radiologic procedure or interpretation. Therefore, before reporting the radiology procedure code on an insurance claim, the documented report must be available in the patient's record.

NOTE:

Code of Federal Regulations, 42 CFR (Conditions of Participation for Hospitals) requires the radiologist or other practitioner who performs radiology services to sign reports of their interpretations. Authentication may include signatures, written initials or computer entry. (Electronic signatures require verification methods to ensure accuracy of the entry, such as encryption.)

Radiology guidelines state that the interpreting individual must sign a written report as an integral part of a radiologic procedure. However, the guidelines do *not* specify content or format.

When a teaching physician reviews a radiographic image interpreted by a resident, the teaching physician is responsible for documenting a note indicating that the image was reviewed with the resident, and the teaching physician agreed with the resident's interpretation. (If the teaching physician disagreed with the resident's interpretation, the teaching physician is responsible for documenting a corrected report.) Before a claim is submitted to Medicare for payment, the radiologic report must be authenticated by the teaching physician (and a statement of agreement with the resident's interpretation must be documented by the teaching physician).

Foreign Body/Implant Definition

An object that is intentionally placed into the patient is considered an implant while an object that is unintentionally placed (due to ingestion or trauma) is considered a foreign body. However, when an implant shifts from its original position or becomes broken, it is considered a foreign body for coding purposes (especially when it becomes a hazard to a patient). The exception is when CPT coding instructions provide guidance to specific codes that describes the removal of a shifted or broken implant.

Exercise 17.3 – Radiology Section Guidelines

Instructions: Complete each statement.

1. Radiological procedures that are completed as an integral component of a total service or procedure are called _____ procedures.
2. A radiological procedure that is provided to patients but that is not included in the current edition of the CPT coding manual is called a(n) _____ procedure.
3. Due to the complexity of interventional radiology services, _____ coding allows for reporting a radiology procedure code and a surgical procedure code to completely describe the service provided.
4. A radiopaque substance administered to provide better radiographic visualization of organs studied is called _____ agents, material, or medium.
5. CPT Radiology guidelines state that the interpreting individual must sign a documented _____ report as an integral part of a radiologic procedure.

Radiology Subsections

The CPT Radiology section includes seven subsections.

- Diagnostic radiology (diagnostic imaging)
- Diagnostic ultrasound
- Radiologic guidance
- Breast, mammography
- Bone/joint studies
- Radiation oncology
- Nuclear medicine

Radiology is the medical specialty that uses x-rays (e.g., radiant energy) to diagnose and treat injuries and disease. Radiology imaging includes radiography (x-rays, including fluoroscopy), computed tomography (CT), computed tomographic angiography, magnetic resonance imaging (MRI), magnetic resonance angiography (MRA), and specialized radiography (e.g., myelography, hysterosalpingography, aortography, angiography).

Diagnostic Radiology (Diagnostic Imaging)

The Diagnostic Radiology (Diagnostic Imaging) subsection includes codes for the:

- Head and neck
- Chest (Figure 17-5)
- Spine and pelvis
- Upper extremities
- Lower extremities
- Abdomen
- Gastrointestinal tract
- Urinary tract
- Gynecological and obstetrical
- Heart
- Vascular procedures
- Other procedures

The Diagnostic Radiology (Diagnostic Imaging) subsection includes diagnostic and therapeutic procedures, computed tomography (CT) (Figure 17-6), magnetic resonance imaging (MRI), and magnetic resonance

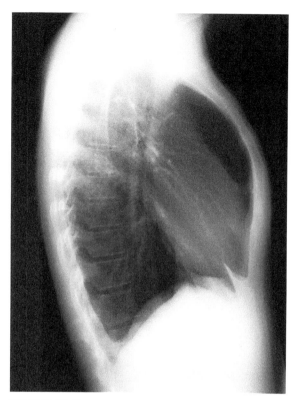

FIGURE 17-5 Lateral chest x-ray. Bones of the spine are white, and soft tissues are shades of gray

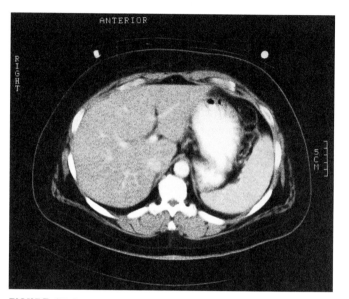

FIGURE 17-6 Abdominal CT scan in which the liver is predominant in the upper left and the stomach is visible in the upper right

angiography (MRA). These diagnostic procedures can be as simple as a routine chest x-ray or as complex as a carotid angiography, which requires selective vascular catheterization.

To code diagnostic radiology procedures accurately, identify the following:

- Anatomical site
- Type of procedure
- Number of views
- Laterality of the procedure (e.g., unilateral or bilateral)
- Use of contrast media

CPT allows for various combinations of codes to address the number and type of radiographic views. For a given radiographic series, the procedure code that most accurately describes what was performed is appropriate.

A variety of combinations of views necessary to obtain medically useful information are included in the Diagnostic Radiology subsection. A complete review of available codes for radiographic procedures ensures accurate coding so that the most comprehensive code is reported (to describe services performed). Do not report multiple codes to describe a service when a combination code is available.

 NOTE:

A careful review of the radiology code description is required so that the most comprehensive code is reported. The radiologic report will indicate the number of views.

When radiographic procedures are repeated during the same encounter due to substandard quality, just one code is reported. However, if after reviewing initial films the radiologist elects to obtain additional views to render further interpretation, determine the third-party payer's policy regarding multiple procedures. Generally, the CPT code that describes the total service provided is reported even if the patient was released from the radiology suite and had to return for additional services.

Descriptions of many radiology codes refer to a "minimum" number of views. When more than the minimum number specified in the code description is performed and a more specific code is not available, report one code for the highest level of service. (When additional x-rays are necessary due to a change in the patient's condition, report separate radiology codes as appropriate.)

Example 1: A three-view x-ray of the shoulder was obtained. Report code 73030.

Example 2: The patient presented to the ED with the complaint of severe shortness of breath. A single-view chest x-ray was obtained. A repeat chest x-ray, four views, was obtained several hours later after it was noted that the patient was experiencing labored breathing unrelieved by medication. Report codes 71045 and 71048 59. (Modifier 59 indicates that the second x-ray was a separate procedure.)

Radiographic procedures are performed without contrast, with contrast, or with and without contrast. (Invasive diagnostic imaging that involves the use of contrast material is discussed later.) Separate codes are available to describe all of these combinations of contrast usage.

Preliminary scout radiographs obtained prior to contrast administration or delayed imaging radiographs are often performed. When a CPT code is available to report scout radiographs, it is reported. If there is no CPT code, the scout radiograph procedures are included in the reported code for the primary procedure.

Fluoroscopy

According to *CPT Assistant*, when radiologic supervision and interpretation are performed during surgical procedures, fluoroscopy (Figure 17-7) is included in the radiologic procedure. This means that codes for physician or other qualified health care professional time during fluoroscopy (76000) are *not* reported in addition to the radiologic procedure code.

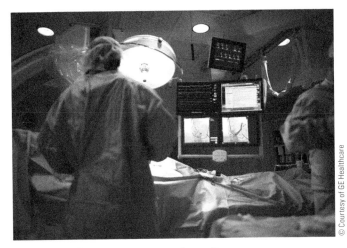

© Courtesy of GE Healthcare

FIGURE 17-7 Fluoroscopy and monitors ensure proper positioning of implantable cardioverter defibrillator/pacemaker

Example: Patient underwent a laparoscopic cholecystectomy and an intraoperative cholangiogram with fluoroscopy. Report codes 47563 (surgical component) and 74300. Do *not* report code 76000 (fluoroscopy) because it is included in code 74300.

Interventional Radiologic Procedures

Interventional radiologic procedures involve the administration of contrast material orally (by mouth, such as for an upper GI), rectally (by rectum, such as a barium enema), or **parenterally** (other than by mouth or rectum, such as implantation, infusion, or injection).

 Coding Tip

The administration of oral or rectal contrast material is included as part of the radiologic procedure code. (Do *not* report a separate code for the administration of oral or rectal contrast material.) However, it is acceptable to report an HCPCS Level II code for the supply of the contrast material.

When spinal radiologic procedures are performed using CT, MRI, or magnetic resonance angiography (MRA) and the code description includes the phrase *with contrast*, do not report a code for intravenous (IV) injection. The IV injection procedure is included in the radiologic procedure code. However, when an intrathecal injection is performed, report a separate code. (*Intrathecal* refers to the fluid-filled space between layers of tissue that cover the brain and spinal cord.)

Example 1: Patient underwent CT of the cervical spine, with IV injection of contrast material. Report code 72126.

Example 2: Patient underwent CT of the thoracic spine, with intrathecal injection of contrast material. Report codes 72129 and 62284.

For intra-articular injection of contrast material, report the appropriate joint injection code. When an IV line is placed for administration of contrast material, it is not coded or reported. Placement of the IV line is included in the radiologic procedure code.

Example: Patient underwent left femoral venography, which required placement of an IV line and injection of contrast material. Report codes 75820 and 36005. (Do *not* report code 36000 for placement of the IV line.)

 NOTE:

For urogenital radiography, the insertion of a urethral catheter is included in the radiographic procedure code and not separately reported. However, a code from the CPT Surgery section for the injection procedure to administer dye or radionuclide material is reported.

Example: Patient underwent cystography (three views), which involved insertion of a catheter through the patient's urethra into the bladder and injection of contrast material. x-rays were taken from various angles at various stages of filling to visualize the bladder. Report codes 74430 and 51600. (Do *not* report a code for catheter insertion.) (The supply of dye is reported with a code from HCPCS Level II.)

Computed Tomography (CT) and Computed Tomographic Angiography (CTA)

CT (or CAT) is an x-ray of horizontal and vertical cross-sectional views or "slices" of the body (Figure 17-8), which are computer-processed to create 3D images.

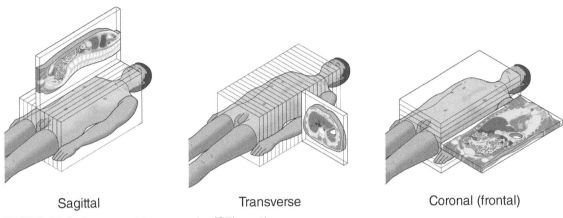

Sagittal   Transverse   Coronal (frontal)

FIGURE 17-8 Computed tomography (CT) sections

CTA (Figure 17-9) is a less invasive technique that uses x-ray beams to image blood vessels. (Until the introduction of CTA, vascular evaluation was performed primarily using invasive angiography procedures, which required catheterization.)

> **Example 1:** Patient underwent CT of the abdomen, with contrast material. Report code 74160.

> **Example 2:** Patient underwent CTA of the abdomen, first without contrast material and then followed by the injection of contrast material, and image post processing. Report code 74175.

Do not report a code for the injection of contrast material for a "with contrast" CTA procedure. However, the supply of the contrast material is reported separately with an appropriate HCPCS Level II code. (The administration of oral or rectal contrast materials does not qualify as "with contrast." Such contrast materials are not typically used in CTA because they obscure the vasculature.)

> **Example:** The patient underwent a CTA of the abdominal aorta with contrast material, including bilateral iliofemoral lower extremity runoff. Post processing of the image was performed. Report code 75635.

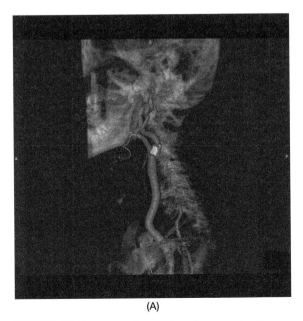
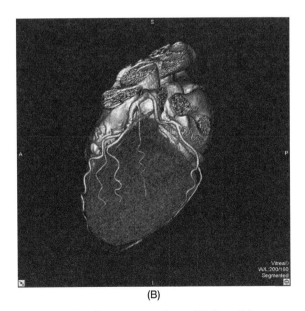

(A)   (B)

FIGURE 17-9 Three-dimensional computed tomography angiography (CTA) reconstructions (A) Carotid arteries (B) Coronary arteries

Magnetic Resonance Imaging (MRI)

Magnetic resonance imaging (MRI) (Figure 17-10) produces high-quality anatomical images. Code descriptions include studies performed without contrast materials, with contrast materials, and without contrast material followed by injection of contrast materials.

Example: A diagnostic MRI of the brain (Figure 17-11) was performed without contrast material. Report code 70551.

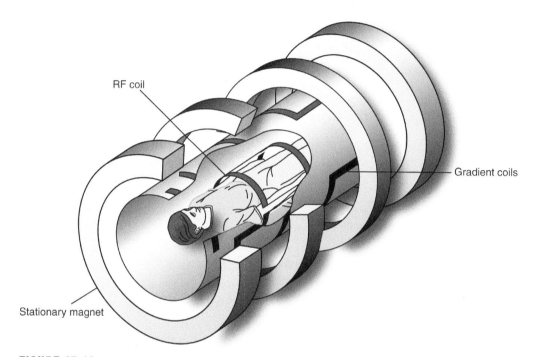

FIGURE 17-10 Magnetic resonance imaging (MRI) unit, which includes stationary magnet, radio frequency coil, and gradient coils

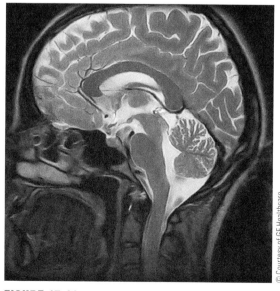

© Courtesy of GE Healthcare

FIGURE 17-11 Magnetic resonance imaging (MRI) of the brain

Magnetic Resonance Angiography (MRA)

Magnetic resonance angiography (MRA) is a noninvasive diagnostic study that is used to evaluate disorders of arterial and venous structures. MRA is performed to visualize the arteries and vessels without invasive procedures, and it is performed on MRI machines that contain hardware and software enhancements. Post processing procedures to create the images are included in MRA codes.

> **Example:** Patient underwent MRA of the abdomen with contrast material. Report code 74185.

Vascular Procedures

Some vascular radiographic procedures performed on the aorta and arteries are designated as selective or nonselective. The radiographic procedure codes are reported in addition to appropriate catheterization codes from the Surgery section. (Chapter 14 of this textbook contains content about coding of arterial catheterization procedures.)

- *Selective vascular catheterization* is the insertion and manipulation or guidance of a catheter into the branches of the arterial system (other than the aorta or the vessel punctured) for the purpose of performing diagnostic (e.g., angiography) or therapeutic (e.g., endarterectomy) procedures. Selective vascular catheterization includes introduction of the catheter and all lesser-order selective catheterizations used in the approach.

> **Example:** The insertion of the catheter from the aorta into the right common and internal carotid arteries is a selective vascular catheterization procedure. (The catheter was inserted into the aorta from the brachial artery, which is a nonselective vascular catheterization procedure.)

- *Nonselective vascular catheterization* is the introduction of a catheter into a vessel and guidance of the catheter into lesser- (or first-) order vessels. (A nonselective catheterization code from the Surgery section is *not* reported with a selective radiological supervision and interpretation code.)

> **Example:** The introduction of a catheter into the femoral artery and threading of the catheter into the aorta is a nonselective vascular catheterization procedure. (If the catheter is further threaded from the aorta into another vessel, such as the brachiocephalic artery, a selective vascular catheterization procedure is performed.)

For diagnostic angiography or venography (radiological supervision and interpretation) (Figure 17-12), the following interventional procedures are included in the procedure code:

- Contrast injections, angiography, roadmapping, and/or fluoroscopic guidance for the intervention
- Vessel measurement
- Post angioplasty/stent angiography

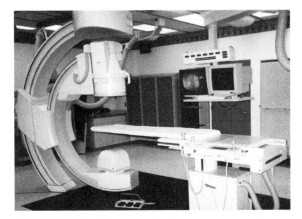

FIGURE 17-12 Vascular imaging equipment

Codes for the above procedures are not coded separately when performed during the same session as an angiography or a venography.

For diagnostic angiography or venography performed during the same session as an interventional procedure, the angiography or venography is separately coded and reported if

- No prior catheter-based angiographic study is available during a full diagnostic study *and the decision to intervene is based on the diagnostic study*
- A prior angiographic study is available, but documentation indicates the following:
  - The patient's clinical condition has changed since the prior study.
  - There was inadequate visualization of anatomy and/or pathology.
  - There was a clinical change during the procedure that requires new evaluation.

> **Example:** Patient underwent selective catheter placement into the left common carotid artery with angiography of ipsilateral (same side) intracranial carotid circulation, extracranial carotid, and cervicocerebral arch. Procedure included associated radiological supervision and interpretation for angiography. Report code 36223 LT. (Do *not* report a separate angiography code.)

Vascular Procedures—Transcatheter Procedures

Therapeutic transcatheter radiological supervision and interpretation code(s) include the following services:

- Contrast injections, angiography/venography, roadmapping, and fluoroscopic guidance for the intervention
- Vessel measurement
- Completion angiography/venography

Codes for the above procedures are *not* coded separately when performed during the same session as a therapeutic transcatheter procedure.

> **Example:** Patient underwent angiography through existing catheter for follow-up study for transcatheter therapy, via infusion. Report code 75898.

Other Procedures

Other procedure codes are reported for professional time associated with fluoroscopy, radiological examinations not included previously in CPT, cineradiography and videoradiography, consultation on x-ray examination, 3D rendering, computed tomography follow-up study, magnetic resonance spectroscopy and elastography, and unlisted fluoroscopic procedures.

> **Example:** A 5-year-old child swallowed a coin and underwent single-view nose-to-rectum radiologic examination to detect the foreign object. Report code 76010.

Exercise 17.4 – Diagnostic Radiology (Diagnostic Imaging)

Instructions: Assign the CPT code(s) and appropriate modifier(s) to each statement. When a radiopharmaceutical agent is provided, assign the appropriate HCPCS Level II code(s).

1. Cardiac magnetic resonance imaging for morphology and function revealed no abnormalities of the heart, cardiac structures, heart valves, and cardiac function.

   _____

Exercise 17.4 – continued

2. Orthodontic cephalogram.

_____

3. Retrograde angiography, left brachial artery, images were taken to visualize the vessel. The procedure was facilitated by injection of contrast material into a catheter that was inserted into the left brachial artery. The radiologist provided supervision and interpretation.

_____

4. Radiological examination, sacrum and coccyx, two views.

_____

5. Magnetic resonance spectroscopy (MRS).

_____

Diagnostic Ultrasound

Diagnostic ultrasound uses high-frequency sound waves (e.g., mechanical oscillations) to produce an image. Radiologic ultrasound codes are organized according to anatomical site. Radiologic ultrasound procedures are often performed as follow-up studies for inconclusive diagnostic radiology procedures. They are also performed intraoperatively (e.g., during endoscopic procedures). Ultrasound is also used as guidance for biopsies, cyst localization, invasive procedures (e.g., ablation of renal cysts), paracentesis, pericardiocentesis, placement of radiation therapy fields, and thoracentesis.

Ultrasound display modes include

- _A-mode_, or _amplitude modulation_: One-dimensional display that reflects the length of time a sound reaches a structure and is reflected back
- _B-scan_, or _brightness mode_, or _gray-scale ultrasound_: Two-dimensional display that reflects sound waves bouncing off tissues or organs; the diagnostic ultrasound produces a two-dimensional cross-sectional view of tissues that cannot be seen directly (e.g., used to locate a lesion and determine its shape)
- _M-mode_, or _motion mode_: One-dimensional display that reflects the _movement_ of structures
- _Real-time scan_: Two-dimensional display of structures and movement that indicates the movement, shape, and size of the tissue or organ

Ophthalmic ultrasound includes the following:

- _Biometric A-scan_: Diagnostic ultrasound that produces a one-dimensional view of normal and abnormal eye tissue and precise measurements of the eye's length (e.g., dimensions of an orbital lesion and exact depth of a foreign body)
- _Biomicroscopy_: Optical instrument that looks like a microscope, with two eyepieces; uses a _slit lamp exam_ (high-intensity light source that is focused to shine as a slit to view anterior structures of the eye) (e.g., conjunctiva, cornea, eyelid, iris, natural crystalline lens, sclera)
- _Corneal pachymetry_: Noninvasive ultrasound procedure that determines thickness of the cornea (e.g., prior to performing LASIK surgery)
- _Quantitative A-scan_: Diagnostic ultrasound that produces quantitative data about the posterior eye segment and evaluates tissue consistency, mobility, and vascularity (e.g., size of an orbital lesion)

Complete and Limited Ultrasound Procedures

To report a code for a "complete" ultrasound, the documented report must contain a description of all elements or the reason that an element could not be visualized (e.g., organ is surgically absent). A complete study includes visualization and diagnostic evaluation of all major structures within the anatomical location.

If fewer/less than the required elements for a complete exam are documented (e.g., limited number of organs or limited portion of region evaluated), report the "limited" code for that anatomical region. A limited study could include a follow-up examination, or it might address just a single quadrant or single diagnostic problem. (A "limited" exam of an anatomical region is not reported during the same session as a "complete" exam of the same region.)

 Coding Tip

Abdomen and retroperitoneum ultrasound codes are described as:

- Complete (e.g., entire abdomen)
- Limited (e.g., single organ or single quadrant)

A limited ultrasound of a single organ or a single quadrant is also performed as follow-up to a complete ultrasound procedure. For example, a complete abdominal ultrasound revealed an abnormality of a single organ. Patient was placed on a therapeutic regimen (e.g., medications). A limited abdominal ultrasound of that organ was performed as follow-up to determine whether abnormality still existed.

 NOTE:

ED physicians perform limited ultrasound procedures to evaluate a specific problem, and diagnostic ultrasound results are used to determine subsequent treatment.

Example 1: Patient underwent complete ultrasound of the abdominal region, B-scan and real time with image documentation. Report code 76700. (A complete ultrasound of the abdomen describes all major abdominal structures, and organ-specific findings are reported, such as the liver and spleen.)

Example 2: Patient underwent limited ultrasound of the abdomen, B-scan and real time with image documentation. Report code 76705. (A limited ultrasound of the abdomen describes a problem-specific study, such as the presence or absence of intraperitoneal fluid.)

 Coding Tip

When there is no corresponding limited ultrasound procedure code for a complete procedure and a limited ultrasound was performed, add modifier 52 (Reduced Services) to the complete code.

Example: Patient underwent a fetal Doppler echocardiography, continuous wave; spectral display was unable to be performed. Report code 76827 52. The CPT code description is "Doppler echocardiography, fetal, pulsed wave and/or continuous wave with spectral display; complete." Because the "spectral display" was not performed, modifier 52 (Reduced services) is added to the code because a complete procedure was not performed.

Doppler Ultrasound

Doppler ultrasound is effective in the evaluation of major arteries and veins, of the heart, and in obstetrics for fetal monitoring. **Doppler ultrasonography** evaluates movement by measuring changes in the frequency of echoes reflected from moving structures. It uses diagnostic ultrasound to detect moving structures (e.g., blood cells) and measures their direction and speed. Doppler ultrasound allows for real-time viewing of blood flow, which cannot be obtained by other methods.

 Coding Tip

Austrian mathematician and physicist (Johann) Christian Doppler is known for a principle called the Doppler effect (frequency of a sound wave appears to change as the source moves toward or away from you).

Example: Patient underwent ultrasound of transplanted kidney, real time with image documentation, with duplex Doppler studies. Report code 76776.

 Coding Tip

Review Non-Invasive Vascular Diagnostic Studies subsection codes located in the Medicine section to report venous Doppler studies and duplex scans.

Obstetrical Ultrasound Procedures

An ultrasound of the pregnant uterus includes fetal and maternal evaluation for single and multiple gestations, with limited and follow-up exams.

Example: Patient underwent fetal biophysical profile with nonstress testing to assess amniotic fluid and fetal breathing, tone, and movement. Report code 76818.

Fetal echocardiography is performed ultrasonically according to specific criteria.

Example: Patient underwent fetal echocardiography, cardiovascular system, real time with image documentation (2D), with M-mode recording. Report code 76825.

For patients known to be pregnant (e.g., established diagnosis of pregnancy), it is appropriate to report an obstetrical ultrasound code. However, when a patient does not have an established diagnosis of pregnancy and undergoes an ultrasound evaluation (e.g., dysmenorrhea or pelvic pain), report a nonobstetrical ultrasound code.

Example: A patient with an established diagnosis of pregnancy presents with symptoms that necessitate an ultrasound evaluation of the pelvis. Report an obstetrical ultrasound code even if the outcome of the procedure is that the patient is not pregnant (e.g., ultrasound confirms that miscarriage occurred).

Ultrasonic Guidance Procedures

Ultrasonic guidance procedures include the use of ultrasound when certain procedures (e.g., ultrasonic guidance for endomyocardial biopsy) are performed.

Report *either* a diagnostic ultrasound *or* a guidance ultrasound code (but not both) for the same patient during the same encounter.

Example: Patient underwent ultrasound guidance for endomyocardial biopsy performed during the same encounter. Report codes 93505 and 76932.

Other Procedures

The code for "ultrasound study, follow-up" is *not* reported in addition to other echocardiograph procedures or ultrasound guidance procedures because it is reported for a follow-up procedure performed on the same day. Other procedures include ultrasound bone density measurement and interpretation, targeted ultrasound to detect lesions, elastographic ultrasound, intraoperative ultrasonic guidance, and unlisted ultrasound procedures.

Example: Patient underwent elastographic ultrasound to detect three target lesions. Report codes 76982, 76983, and 76983.

Exercise 17.5 – Diagnostic Ultrasound

Instructions: Assign the CPT code(s) and appropriate modifier(s) to each statement.

1. Radiologist performed a complete abdominal ultrasound, real time, with image documentation.

2. The patient, known to have an intrauterine pregnancy based on previous physician evaluation, underwent single-gestation transabdominal real-time ultrasound of pregnant uterus with image documentation, first trimester.

3. Patient underwent fetal biophysical profile, with nonstress testing, due to suspicion that fetus was in distress.

4. Abdominal ultrasound with real time and image documentation, stomach.

5. Ophthalmic diagnostic ultrasound for left corneal pachymetry.

Radiologic Guidance

Radiologic guidance is performed during a procedure to visualize access to an anatomical site. The Radiologic Guidance subsection includes codes for fluoroscopic guidance, computed tomography guidance, and magnetic resonance imaging (MRI) guidance (Table 17-1).

TABLE 17-1 Radiologic Guidance and the Purpose of Each

Category	Purpose

Fluoroscopic Guidance	• Guidance for placement, replacement, or removal of:
	  ○ Catheter
	  ○ Central venous access device (CVAD)
	  ○ Needle

Computed Tomography Guidance	• Guidance for stereotactic localization • Guidance for needle placement • Guidance and monitoring of parenchymal tissue ablation • Guidance for placement of radiation therapy fields
Magnetic Resonance Imaging (MRI) Guidance	• Guidance for needle placement • Guidance and monitoring of parenchymal tissue ablation

Example: A 75-year-old patient underwent fluoroscopic guidance for visualization of the subclavian vein during placement of a nontunneled central venous catheter. Report codes 36556 and 77001. (Do not report modifier 51 with add-on code 77001.)

Radiologic Guidance Notes

Notes located below the Radiologic Guidance subsection provide guidance for code assignment. For example, when Surgery section code descriptions state, "fluoroscopic guidance is included," a separate code from the Fluoroscopic Guidance category is *not* assigned. However, when a note below a Surgery code indicates that when a radiologist provides supervision and interpretation of the image, a separate code from the Radiologic Guidance category may be assigned. Other notes include parenthetical lists of codes that are not reported with Radiologic Guidance subsection codes.

Example: Add-on code 77003 (fluoroscopic guidance) is *not* reported with code 62270 (lumbar puncture) because parenthetical notes below the codes specify that the codes are not reported together.

Exercise 17.6 – Radiologic Guidance

Instructions: Assign the CPT code(s) and appropriate modifier(s) to each statement.

1. Fluoroscopic guidance for percutaneous needle placement during liver (needle) biopsy.

2. Stereotactic biopsy (including burr hole) of intracranial lesion with mapping using computed tomography (CT), brain. CT required radiologist supervision and interpretation to identify brain coordinates for stereotactic biopsy.

3. Magnetic resonance imaging guidance for radiofrequency ablation of osteoid, left tibia.

4. Three-year-old patient underwent insertion of non-tunneled central venous catheter, which used fluoroscopic imaging guidance.

5. Radiofrequency percutaneous ablation, liver tumor with magnetic imaging guidance and monitoring.

Breast, Mammography

Mammography (Figure 17-13) is a radiological examination of the soft tissue and internal structures of the breast.

- **Screening mammography** (Figure 17-14A) is performed when a patient presents without signs and symptoms of breast disease (e.g., routine annual screening for early detection of unsuspected breast cancer).
- **Diagnostic mammography** (Figure 17-14B) includes an assessment of suspected disease (e.g., suspicious mass is palpated on physical examination) and diagnostic mammography codes are reported when an abnormality is found or suspected.

 NOTE:

Mammography code descriptions do not specify male or female, which means that the codes can be reported for either female or male patients.

Example: Patient underwent bilateral screening mammography with computer-aided detection, which was reviewed and interpreted by the radiologist. Report code 77067. Do not add modifier 50 because "bilateral" is included in the code description.

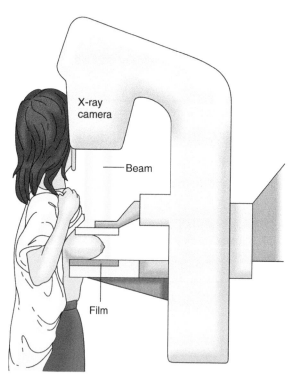

FIGURE 17-13 In mammography, the breast is flattened and then radiographed from above

Exercise 17.7 – Breast, Mammography

Instructions: Assign the CPT code(s) and appropriate modifier(s) to each statement.

1. Magnetic resonance imaging, right and left breasts.

   _____

2. Bilateral screening mammography.

   _____

3. Diagnostic digital breast tomosynthesis, left.

   _____

4. Mammary ductogram, multiple ducts of the right breast, including supervision and interpretation.

   _____

5. Magnetic resonance imaging mammography, left breast, without contrast material, including computer-aided detection.

   _____

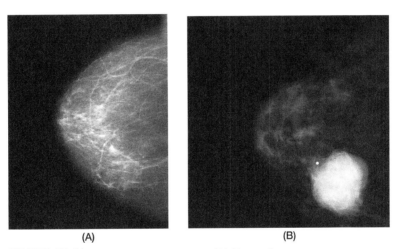

(A)   (B)

FIGURE 17-14 **Mammogram images (A) Normal mammogram
(B) Large breast mass is visible, lower right**

Bone/Joint Studies

Bone and joint studies are radiological procedures performed to detect bone density, bone age, bone length, and bone marrow supply, and to assess vertebral fractures. A **bone density study** evaluates diseases of the bone and are used to assess the response of bone disease to treatment. The studies assess bone mass (e.g., density) of the wrist, radius, hip, pelvis, spine, or heel.

Dual energy x-ray absorptiometry (DEXA or **DXA)** is a bone density study that uses two x-ray beams with different levels of energy pulsing alternately (e.g., two-dimensional projection) to create the image. Results are scores that are reported as standard deviations of the bone density of a person at the age of peak bone mass (e.g., 30 years of age). (Both men and women undergo DEXA imaging.) To code DEXA studies properly, determine the type of skeletal bone mass being measured.

- Axial skeleton (e.g., hips, pelvis, or spine)
- Appendicular skeleton (e.g., peripheral bones such as wrist or heel, vertebra)

Example 1: Patient underwent DXA bone density study of the hips and pelvis. Report code 77080.

Example 2: Nine-day-old infant underwent osseous survey. Report code 77076.

Exercise 17.8 – Bone/Joint Studies

Instructions: Assign the CPT code(s) and appropriate modifier(s) to each statement.

1. Bone age study.

2. Joint survey, single view, left knee and ankle joints.

3. Limited osseous survey radiological examination to detect osteoporosis.

4. Vertebral fracture assessment via dual-energy x-ray absorptiometry.

5. Bone length scanogram study.

Radiation Oncology

Radiation oncology is the specialty of medicine that utilizes high-energy ionizing radiation in the treatment of malignant neoplasms and certain nonmalignant conditions. Distinct therapeutic modalities (methods) are directed at malignant and benign lesions. Modalities include brachytherapy, hyperthermia, stereotactic radiation, and teletherapy.

Radiation oncology codes include professional services and technical procedures that are organized according to the following types of treatment provided:

- Consultation (clinical management)
- Clinical treatment planning (external and internal sources)
- Medical radiation physics, dosimetry, treatment devices, and special services
- Stereotactic radiation treatment delivery
- Other procedures
- Radiation treatment delivery
- Neutron beam treatment delivery
- Radiation treatment management
- Proton beam treatment delivery
- Hyperthermia
- Clinical intracavitary hyperthermia
- Clinical brachytherapy

Consultation (Clinical Management)

Codes from the CPT E/M, Surgery, and/or Medicine sections are reported by the radiation oncologist who does the following:

- Provides preliminary consultation services

- Evaluates a patient prior to the decision to treat
- Delivers full medical care (in addition to treatment management)

Consultation (clinical management) services provided by the radiation oncologist include evaluation of the patient, determination of the need for radiation therapy, identification of site(s) of treatment, assessment of therapy goal(s), and the coordination and sequencing of combined modality therapy with other oncology specialists. The radiation oncologist subsequently orders and coordinates the technical planning and execution of the treatment with ancillary staff, including radiation therapists, dosimetrists, and physicists. (The treatment is supervised by the radiation oncologist.)

Consultation services provided by radiation oncologists are the same as those provided by other physicians (e.g., a referral is required for initial consultation). The initial consultation is reported with an appropriate CPT Evaluation and Management (E/M) code for outpatient consultation services or inpatient consultation services. (The code is reported just once per course of radiation therapy.) (Refer to Chapter 10 of this textbook for clarification about assignment of consultation codes.)

Once the radiation oncologist has determined the appropriate radiation therapy, the best course of treatment is established. During radiation treatment, patients are monitored closely for adverse reactions that require immediate care. Thus, ongoing patient evaluation is provided as necessary. These services are reported with radiation oncology treatment management codes, *not* E/M service codes.

When a patient completes the course of radiation therapy, the patient continues to see the radiation oncologist during regular follow-up visits. The radiation oncologist monitors the patient's progress and reaction to treatment. This follow-up care is reported with codes from the CPT E/M section (the same as any other established patient follow-up care).

Clinical Treatment Planning (External and Internal Sources)

Clinical treatment planning is performed for each radiation therapy patient, and it includes interpretation of special testing, tumor localization, *treatment volume determination* (region within the body to which radiation therapy is directed), treatment time/dosage determination, choice of treatment modality, determination of number and size of treatment *ports* (sites on the skin where radiation beams enter the body), selection of appropriate treatment devices, and other procedures.

Radiation is administered by a machine outside the body (*external radiation*), is placed inside the body (*internal radiation*) (Figure 17-15), or uses unsealed radioactive materials that travel throughout the body (**systemic radiation therapy**). The internal radiation source is usually sealed in a small container called an *implant* (e.g., thin wire, catheter, ribbon, capsule, or seed) and inserted directly into the body. The type of radiation administered depends on what type of cancer it is, where it is located, how far into the body the radiation has to go, what the patient's general health and medical history are, whether the patient will have other types of cancer treatment, and other factors. Most patients receive external radiation, and some receive both external and internal or systemic radiation therapy.

Clinical treatment planning and tumor mapping are critical to identifying the location, extent, and volume of tumor(s) to be treated and all critical and sensitive structures surrounding them. The radiation oncologist plans the appropriate course of therapy that will allow for maximum benefit while protecting surrounding tissues and structures. Clinical treatment planning may involve ordering and interpreting special tests such as CT scans, lymphangiography, MRI scans, and radionuclide scans and/or surgical exploration with biopsy. Markers may also be placed for the purpose of treatment planning and tumor localization.

 Coding Tip

Debulking (surgical removal of part of a malignant tumor; also called *cytoreduction surgery*) may be performed to enhance the effectiveness of radiation oncology treatment.

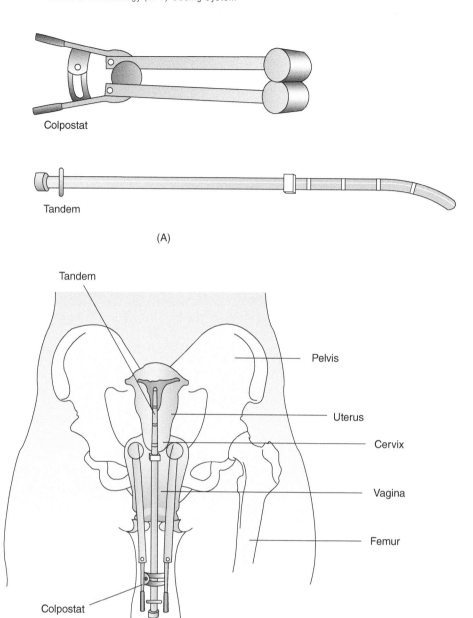

FIGURE 17-15 Radium implant devices (A) Colpostat and tandem (B) Placement of colpostat and tandem within vagina and uterus

Therapeutic radiology treatment planning codes are described according to type of planning, as follows:

- Simple
  - Single treatment area of interest
  - Single port or simple parallel opposed ports
  - Minimal (simple or no) *blocking* (device, such as lead, that shields or protects critical or sensitive organs)
  - No interpretation of special tests for localization of tumor volume
- Intermediate
  - Two separate treatment areas
  - Three or more converging ports

- ○ Multiple blocks to protect critical or sensitive organs
- ○ Special time/dose constraints
- ○ Interpretation of special tests for localization of tumor volume

- Complex
  - ○ Three or more separate treatment areas
  - ○ Highly complex blocking to protect critical or sensitive organs
  - ○ Custom shielding blocks
  - ○ Tangential ports
  - ○ Special *wedges* (treatment beam-modifying devices that act to change the beam intensity profile)
  - ○ Special *compensators* (irregularly shaped beam-modifying devices used to reconfigure beam intensity so it matches irregular tissue contour)
  - ○ Rotational or special beam considerations
  - ○ Combination of therapeutic modalities
  - ○ Interpretation of complex testing procedures (e.g., CT and MRI localization)
  - ○ Possible special laboratory testing

Simulation clinical treatment planning uses a simulator to determine various treatment ports to be used during radiation therapy. The simulator can orient a radiation beam toward a patient according to parameters that imitate the treatment proposed for actual therapy (but it does not deliver radiation therapy). Simulation may be carried out on a dedicated conventional simulator or by use of a CT scanner, radiation therapy treatment unit (e.g., linear accelerator), or other diagnostic imaging equipment (e.g., fluoroscopy, CT, or MRI). Simulation is complex because custom shielding blocks are designed, and the simulation must be coordinated with information from treatment planning CT scans and isodose plan data. Therapeutic radiology simulation-aided field setting codes are described according to type of setting.

- Simple
  - ○ Simulation of single treatment area
  - ○ Single port or parallel opposed ports
  - ○ Minimal (simple or no) blocking of critical or sensitive organs

- Intermediate
  - ○ Simulation of three or more converging ports
  - ○ Two separate treatment areas
  - ○ Multiple blocking of critical or sensitive organs

- Complex
  - ○ Simulation of tangential (peripheral) portals (or ports)
  - ○ Three or more treatment areas
  - ○ Rotation or arc therapy
  - ○ Three-dimensional (3D)
  - ○ Computer-generated 3D reconstruction of tumor volume and surrounding critical or sensitive normal tissue structures (using CT scans or MRI data in preparation for noncoplanar or coplanar therapy)
  - ○ Simulation uses documented 3D beam's eye view volume-dose displays of multiple or moving beams
  - ○ Documentation with 3D volume reconstruction and dose distribution is required

Example: Radiation oncologist provided simple therapeutic radiology treatment planning services, which consisted of a single area of malignancy with a single port or opposing ports parallel to each other and basic or no blocking. Report code 77261.

Medical Radiation Physics, Dosimetry, Treatment Devices, and Special Services

"Medical radiation physics, **dosimetry** (measurement and calculation of radiation treatment doses), treatment devices, and special services" codes are reported by the health care facility (e.g., hospital). There is no professional component for most of these services. (Reimbursement for the radiation oncologist's professional component is included in reimbursement for clinical treatment planning and radiation treatment management codes.)

A basic radiation dosimetry calculation is a photon calculation that includes central axis depth dose, time dose factor (TDF), nominal standard dose (NSD), gap calculation, off-axis and tissue inhomogeneity factors, as well as calculation of nonionizing radiation surface and depth dose. Dosimetry may be repeated during the course of treatment as required. That CPT code is reported as many times as necessary during a course of radiation therapy. However, codes for teletherapy isodose planning services are reimbursed just once per course of treatment.

Intensity modulated radiation therapy (IMRT) uses high-precision radiotherapy to precisely target cancerous tumors with higher radiation doses by using strategically positioned beams to minimize collateral damage to healthy cells. IMRT varies the intensity of radiation exposure depending on whether tumor is present in the beam pathway. The radiation therapy consists of multiple pencil thin beams (or beamlets) calculated to hit tumors with high-dose radiation beams and sensitive normal tissues with modulated lower-intensity beams, leaving them mostly unaffected. Planning for IMRT involves the use of computer programs that calculate the beam angle configurations and dosage intensities. The CPT code reported for an IMRT plan includes dose-volume histograms for target and critical structure partial tolerance specifications. A CPT code is reported for IMRT delivery, and includes guidance and tracking, when performed.

Brachytherapy isodose calculation is also reimbursed just once per course of treatment. The number of units billed for brachytherapy isodose calculation (simple, intermediate, or complex) should equal the number of brachytherapy treatments provided within the billing period. When billing is done for multiple treatment devices, there must be documentation in the clinical record to support the medical necessity of each device or set of devices.

The use of a treatment device is based on the clinical judgment of the radiation oncologist and is influenced by the patient's anatomy and disease state. The selection and use of any treatment device requires medical necessity, radiation oncologist involvement, and a written and signed order for each device. The radiation oncologist must be directly involved in the design, selection, and placement of any device and must document their involvement with each device.

Treatment devices include the following:

- Beam-shaping devices are called blocks, and they are placed in an external radiation beam to modify its shape to either contour the beam around target structures or to shield normal tissues.
- Immobilization devices (e.g., thermoplastic face and body masks, bite-block head holders, Styrofoam body casts, and breast boards) are used to restrict patient movement during treatment.
- Beam-modifying devices include wedges, compensators, and boluses.
- Shielding devices include bite blocks, eye shields, and testicular shields.

Codes for treatment devices are reported at the onset of the treatment. They may be reported again later during the course of treatment if additional or new devices are required.

Codes for medical physics and medical radiation physics consultations are reported for patients undergoing radiation therapy. Although the radiation oncologist orders these procedures, they generally have little involvement in the actual procedure. The medical radiation physics measurements are used to evaluate a treatment plan. After these procedures are completed, treatment management and delivery is established. Continuing medical physics consultation is reported "per week of therapy," which means that it may be reported after multiple radiation treatments *if those treatments occurred during one week of treatment. If, however, the multiple radiation treatments occurred over a period of multiple different weeks, the continuing medical physics consultation code would be reported once for each week of treatment.*

Example: Radiation oncologist designed and constructed a simple block treatment device. Report code 77332.

Stereotactic Radiation Treatment Delivery

Stereotactic radiation treatment delivery includes the following types:

- *Stereotactic radiosurgery (SRS)*: Radiation therapy that focuses high-powered x-rays onto a small area, such as a brain, liver, lung, or other lesion; it is a single-session treatment that has such a dramatic effect on its target that the result is considered "surgical"; however, it is not actually considered a surgical procedure; also referred to as *gamma knife* or *cyberknife*.
- *Stereotactic body radiation therapy (SBRT)*: Radiation therapy that uses special equipment to position a patient and precisely deliver smaller doses of radiation over several days to bone, liver, and lung tumors in the body; SBRT is not administered to brain tumors; exposure to normal tissue is minimized; also called extracranial *radiotherapy*.

Example: Patient underwent radiation treatment delivery, which used stereotactic radiosurgery to deliver one large radiation dose to the brain tumor. Report code 77371.

Radiation Treatment Delivery

Radiation treatment delivery codes are reported for the administration of radiation therapy *per treatment*. A nonphysician may deliver radiation treatment; however, the radiation oncologist is responsible for checking and documenting the accuracy of the treatment. The radiation oncologist must also treat any adverse reactions to treatment and monitor the effects of radiation therapy on the tumor and surrounding tissues. (Radiation treatment delivery includes ongoing patient evaluation, and codes for such evaluation are not reported separately.)

- Radiation treatment delivery is measured in units of *MeV* (*megaelectron volts* or *megavolts*), which is 1 million electron volts.
- **Therapeutic port films** are x-rays taken during delivery of radiation treatment that utilize the treatment beam of the machine. Portal films demonstrate the exact shape, size, and area covered by the treatment beam during an actual treatment.

Example: Complex radiation therapy delivery was directed to three distinct treatment areas, and 11 MeV was administered. Report code 77412.

Neutron Beam Treatment Delivery

Neutron beam radiation therapy is an external radiation treatment that uses higher linear energy transfer to treat certain tumors (e.g., salivary gland tumors) due to increased susceptibility, as compared with conventional radiation therapy. An interventional radiologist provides this treatment at a facility equipped with a superconducting accelerator (cyclotron). Pretreatment planning usually involves CT to locate and determine the tumor volume prior to radiation therapy.

Example: Patient underwent high-energy neutron radiation treatment delivery 1 isocenter with coplanar geometry and blocking. Report code 77423.

Radiation Treatment Management

Radiation treatment management is reported in units of five fractions or treatment sessions even though the service need not be performed on consecutive days. For radiation treatment management purposes, a *fraction* is a single session of radiation treatment delivered to a specific area of interest. The number of calendar days between treatment fractions is not relevant as long as the treatment is directed to the same area and is part of a single course of therapy. Thus, a claim is submitted with the treatment code for every five treatments. *Multiple fractions* that represent two or more treatment sessions furnished on the same day are counted separately *if there has been a distinct break in therapy sessions*. (Refer to the *Radiation Management and Treatment Table* in the CPT coding manual for guidance about assignment of codes.)

> **Example:** Radiation treatment management of 20 daily treatments during a 4-week period. Report codes 77427, 77427, 77427, and 77427.

 NOTE:

- When a patient who has completed a course of radiation therapy returns with a recurrent tumor and treatment is provided to the same area, report codes for a separate course of radiation therapy.
- HCPCS Level II codes for radioactive materials, when supplied by the radiation oncologist, are reported in addition to codes for radiation therapy.

Reimbursement for weekly radiation therapy management includes payment for normal follow-up care during therapy and for three months following its completion.

> **Example:** Radiation oncologist provided radiation therapy management for a course of treatment that consisted of two single sessions (fractions). Report code 77431.

Proton Beam Treatment Delivery

Compared to photon beams, proton beams deliver higher radiation doses to tumors, and proton beams do not exceed the radiation tolerance of normal tissue. Proton beam treatment delivery is a modality that consists of delivering smaller doses to intervening normal tissues and organs. Codes are reported according to the following types of treatment:

- *Simple*: Single treatment area utilizing a single nontangential/oblique port, custom block with or without compensation
- *Intermediate*: One or more treatment areas utilizing two or more ports or one or more tangential/oblique ports, with custom blocks and compensators
- *Complex*: One or more treatment areas using two or more ports per treatment area with matching or patching fields and/or multiple isocenters, with custom blocks and compensators

> **Example:** Patient underwent intermediate proton treatment delivery to two treatment areas using two ports per treatment area and custom blocks. Report code 77523.

Hyperthermia and Clinical Intracavitary Hyperthermia

Hyperthermia involves the use of an external heat-generating source (e.g., ultrasound or microwave) to produce localized heating. Hyperthermia is usually performed immediately before or after a session of external beam radiation therapy. Typically, three to six applications of hyperthermia per course of radiation therapy are required. When hyperthermia is generated by intracavitary probe(s), report code 77620.

> **Example:** Patient underwent hyperthermia treatment, which was generated by an interstitial probe that used 10 interstitial applicators. Report code 77615.

Clinical Brachytherapy

Brachytherapy (Figure 17-16) involves the use of radioactive isotopes for internal radiation, and codes are reported according to the following applications:

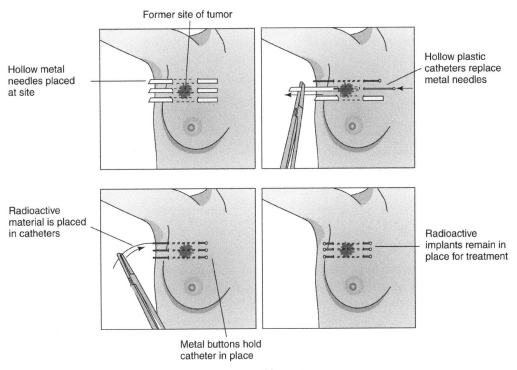

Former site of tumor

Hollow metal needles placed at site

Hollow plastic catheters replace metal needles

Radioactive material is placed in catheters

Radioactive implants remain in place for treatment

Metal buttons hold catheter in place

FIGURE 17-16 Brachytherapy for treatment of breast cancer

- *Simple*: Application has 1 to 4 sources/ribbons
- *Intermediate*: Application has 5 to 10 sources/ribbons
- *Complex*: Application has greater than 10 sources/ribbons

A *source* is an intracavitary placement or permanent interstitial placement. A *ribbon* is a temporary interstitial placement. Intracavitary brachytherapy is performed by placing applicators containing radioactive materials directly into or around a tumor area. A common use of intracavitary brachytherapy is the treatment of carcinoma of the endometrium (uterus) or cervix.

Intracavitary and interstitial applications are seldom used as the sole modality of radiation treatment. Interstitial brachytherapy is performed with needles, ribbons, or wires containing radioactive materials that are inserted directly into and around a cancerous area. The devices remain in place over a period of many days while delivering their relatively low-intensity radiation directly into the tumor. These applications are often used in conjunction with external beam radiation therapy to bring the total dose up to the desired level.

Example: Radiation oncologist supervised the handling and loading of a radiation source. Report code 77790.

Exercise 17.9 – Radiation Oncology

Instructions: Assign the CPT code to each statement.

1. A special teletherapy port plan for the total body.

   _____

2. The patient underwent a hyperthermia treatment that was generated by an intracavitary probe.

   _____

(continues)

Exercise 17.9 – continued

3. A therapeutic radiology simulation-aided field setting of a single treatment area with a single port was performed.

   _____

4. Patient underwent superficial voltage radiation treatment delivery, external, on May 5.

   _____

5. The surface application of low-dose-rate radionuclide source for clinical brachytherapy was provided.

   _____

Nuclear Medicine

Nuclear medicine involves the use of radioactive elements (e.g., radionuclides and radioisotopes) for diagnostic imaging (e.g., scan) and **radiopharmaceutical therapy** (destroys diseased tissue, such as a malignant neoplasm). The isotope emits gamma rays as it deteriorates, which enables the radiologist to visualize internal abnormalities (e.g., tumors). The images created by the contrast media (radioactive element) are detected by a gamma camera.

Nuclear medicine codes do not include the provision of radium, which means that the nuclear medicine report must be reviewed to identify the diagnostic or therapeutic radiopharmaceutical provided. Then an appropriate HCPCS Level II code is reported for the radiopharmaceutical administered. (The injection of the radionuclide is included as part of the procedure, and a separate injection code is *not* reported.)

The Nuclear Medicine subsection contains codes for diagnostic and therapeutic procedures with diagnostic procedures organized by body system (e.g., endocrine system). Common diagnostic nuclear medicine procedures include bone scans, cardiac scans (e.g., thallium scan and MUGA), renal scans, thyroid scans, and hepatobiliary scans (e.g., HIDA scans). Therapeutic nuclear medicine procedures are used to treat diseases such as chronic leukemia, hyperthyroidism, and thyroid cancer.

Endocrine System

Nuclear medicine is commonly used to evaluate thyroid function (e.g., thyroid update). *Uptake* is the absorption by a tissue of a substance, material, or mineral and its permanent or temporary retention.

A thyroid uptake test measures thyroid function to determine how much iodine the thyroid absorbs (expressed as a percentage of the administered radioiodine present in the thyroid gland at a specific time after administration). Thyroid imaging (scan) is performed to assess anatomical size and physiologic function. A radioactive tracer (e.g., iodide-123 capsule or technetium-99m injection) is administered, which allows blood flow and vascularity of the thyroid to be monitored by imaging at different intervals.

> **Example:** Patient underwent thyroid imaging with vascular flow and radioactive tracer. Report code 78013 (and an HCPCS Level II code for the radioactive material administered).

Hematopoietic, Reticuloendothelial, and Lymphatic System

Bone marrow imaging evaluates bone marrow functioning and irregular marrow tissue expansion (e.g., malignancy or infection). A radiopharmaceutical radiotracer (e.g., radiolabeled sulfur colloid) is injected, and images are obtained after a two- to three-hour delay using a special camera (e.g., scintillation or gamma camera). The camera takes images by detecting gamma radiation from the radionuclide in bone marrow as it "scintillates" (e.g., emits energy in a flash of light) when coming in contact with the camera's detector.

For whole blood volume determination, the radiopharmaceutical volume-dilution technique evaluates plasma and red cell volume by using radiolabeled protein tracers (e.g., iodinated serum albumin) and autologous radiolabeled red blood cells. The procedure involves collecting blood and recording blood counts to calculate volumes using formulas that compare the dilution factor from a standard sample of each radiotracer.

A lymphatics and lymph nodes imaging code is reported for lymphoscintigraphy. The injection of a radioactive tracer is included in the lymphoscintigraphy procedure. Modifier 26 (Professional Component) is added to the lymphoscintigraphy code only if the professional component was performed by the physician.

Example: Patient underwent a platelet survival study. Report code 78191.

Gastrointestinal System

Tomographic single-photon emission computed tomography (SPECT) is used for evaluation of the anatomy and functionality of the liver. A radiolabeled sulfur colloid is injected, and imaging of the distribution of gamma radiation emitted from the radiopharmaceutical is performed. SPECT imaging is performed by rotating a single- or multiple-head camera around the patient to provide 3D computer-reconstructed views of cross-sectional slices of the liver. For imaging done with a vascular flow test, red blood cells are labeled to enable imaging of the blood flow through the liver.

Example: Patient underwent acute gastrointestinal blood loss imaging. Report code 78278.

Musculoskeletal System

Single and dual photon absorptiometry are noninvasive techniques used to measure the absorption of the photon beam (e.g., mono- or dichromatic) by bone material. The device is placed directly on the patient and uses a small amount of radionuclide to measure the bone mass absorption. This provides a measurement of the bone mineral density of cortical bone and can be used to assess an individual's response to treatment at different intervals.

Example: Patient underwent a bone density study with single photon absorptiometry, vertebral column and rib cage. Report code 78350.

Cardiovascular System

Myocardial perfusion and cardiac blood pool imaging may be performed at rest or during stress. When performed during exercise and/or pharmacologic stress, report an appropriate stress test code from the Medicine section. **Cardiac blood pool imaging** uses a gamma camera for sampling, which is performed repetitively over several hundred heartbeats during the transition of the radionuclide (e.g., technetium-99m) through the central circulation.

Nuclear imaging for noncardiac vascular flow studies is performed to evaluate arterial or venous peripheral vascular diseases or injuries. In radionuclide angiography, red blood cells are tagged with radioactivity and injected intravenously. A scintillation camera takes a series of dynamic images every two to three seconds immediately after injection, followed by static images.

For myocardial perfusion study, PET myocardial imaging is typically performed on patients with coronary artery disease and left ventricular dysfunction. PET scanning is also used in diagnostic and therapeutic procedures for malignant tumors. PET is a noninvasive nuclear medicine technique that produces 3D images of the distribution of radioactivity (e.g., emission of positrons) similar to a CT scan. However, PET uses radiopharmaceuticals instead of dye and x-rays. When the radiopharmaceutical agent is injected into the blood, a positron scanner detects, measures, and displays metabolism of tissues (e.g., heart and brain) and many types of tumors. PET scans are also used to diagnose dementia. (Report appropriate HCPCS Level II codes for radiopharmaceutical diagnostic imaging agents or "tracers," in addition to CPT codes for PET scan procedures.)

Example: Patient underwent single-study myocardial imaging, PET, and metabolic evaluation. Report code 78459.

Respiratory System

Pulmonary ventilation imaging illustrates the regional distribution of inspired air throughout the lungs, including clearance dynamics and uptake. A pulmonary perfusion imaging procedure is used to diagnose pulmonary emboli (Figure 17-17) and pulmonary trauma. The procedure consists of imaging a patient twice.

- Once after inhalation of a radioactive aerosol to determine pulmonary ventilation
- Once again after injection of a radioactive particulate to determine lung perfusion

Example: Patient underwent pulmonary ventilation and perfusion imaging. Report code 78582.

Nervous System

Radiology Nervous System codes are reported for brain imaging, cerebral vascular flow, cerebrospinal fluid flow/leakage, and radiopharmaceutical dacryocystography radiographic procedures.

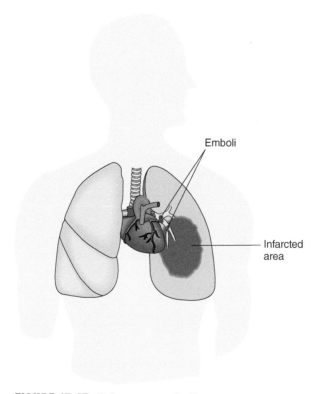

FIGURE 17-17 Pulmonary emboli

Example: Patient underwent radiopharmaceutical dacryocystography. Report code 78660.

Genitourinary System

Radiology Genitourinary System codes are reported for kidney imaging, kidney function study, urinary bladder residual study, ureteral reflux study, and testicular imaging radiographic procedures.

Example: Patient underwent multiple kidney imaging studies with vascular flow and function, with and without pharmacological angiotensin intervention as a converting enzyme inhibitor. Report code 78709.

Other Procedures

Radiology Other Procedures codes include tomographic SPECT imaging, which allows for evaluation of complex anatomy. A radionuclide is introduced, and the distribution of gamma radiation emitted is detected with a camera that rotates around the patient. A 3D computer reconstructs views of cross-sectional slices of the body. When scanning for an inflammatory process, gallium is the radiopharmaceutical used.

Example: Patient underwent single-area, single-day imaging, tomographic single-photon emission computed tomography (SPECT) for radiopharmaceutical localization of a stomach tumor. Report code 78803 (and an HCPCS Level II code for the radiopharmaceutical agent).

Therapeutic (Nuclear Medicine)

When radiopharmaceutical therapy is administered orally or intravenously, the reported code includes the mode of administration (e.g., injection or infusion). When intra-arterial, intracavitary, or intra-articular administration is the method used for radiopharmaceutical therapy, an appropriate injection and/or procedure code is reported in addition to the therapy code. When imaging guidance and radiological supervision and interpretation are provided for intra-arterial, intracavitary, or intra-articular administration, appropriate code(s) are reported in addition to the therapy and administration codes.

Example: Patient underwent radiopharmaceutical therapy for chronic leukemia, by oral administration. Report code 79005.

Exercise 17.10 – Nuclear Medicine

Instructions: Assign the CPT code to each statement.

1. Therapeutic nuclear medicine radiopharmaceutical is injected directly into a vein.

2. The physician determines the location of the sentinel node(s) using scintigraphy nuclear medicine imaging.

3. The physician administered a radiolabeled monoclonal antibody by intravenous infusion for radiopharmaceutical nuclear medicine therapy.

4. Patient underwent aerosol pulmonary ventilation and perfusion nuclear medicine imaging.

5. Patient underwent cardiac shunt detection nuclear medicine procedure.

Summary

Radiology is a branch of medicine that uses imaging techniques to diagnose and treat disease. A radiologist is a physician who has undergone specialized training to interpret diagnostic x-rays, perform specialized x-ray procedures, and administer radiation for the treatment of disease (e.g., cancer). The Radiology section includes subsections for diagnostic radiology (diagnostic imaging); diagnostic ultrasound; radiologic guidance; breast, mammography; bone/joint studies; radiation oncology; and nuclear medicine. Procedure descriptions include the type of service, anatomical site, and use of contrast material. Radiology guidelines are located at the beginning of the section, and they should be carefully reviewed prior to the assigning of codes.

Internet Links

Hospital for Special Surgery: Go to **www.hss.edu**, click on Conditions, and click on a letter that corresponds with the first letter of condition or treatment to be researched.

LearningRadiology: www.learningradiology.com

RadiologyInfo.org: www.radiologyinfo.org

Review

17.1 — Multiple Choice

Instructions: Select the most appropriate response.

1. Which are the types of radiographic projection?
    a. Anteroposterior, lateral, oblique, and posteroanterior
    b. Anteroposterior, posteroanterior, midsagittal, and sagittal
    c. Coronal, midsagittal, sagittal, and transverse
    d. Coronal, transverse, lateral, and oblique

2. Which are the three components of a radiologic procedure?
    a. Coronal, transverse, and lateral
    b. Posteroanterior, midsagittal, and sagittal
    c. Simple, intermediate, and complex
    d. Technical, professional, and global

3. Which is a common contrast agent administered to provide better radiographic visualization of organs studied?
    a. Barium sulfate
    b. Betadine
    c. Iodized sodium
    d. Sulfuric acid

4. Which is used for the rectal administration of contrast material?
    a. Barium enema
    b. Implantation
    c. Infusion
    d. Injection

5. The *component coding* concept applies to _____ radiology procedures, which are used to diagnose and treat conditions using percutaneous or minimally invasive techniques under imaging guidance.
    a. foreign body removal
    b. implant replacement
    c. interventional
    d. unlisted

6. Biometric A-scan, quantitative A-scan, and corneal pachymetry are considered
    a. types of ophthalmic ultrasound.
    b. types of x-rays.
    c. radiographic projections.
    d. ultrasound display modes.

7. Brachytherapy, hyperthermia, stereotactic radiation, and teletherapy are considered
   a. dosimetry techniques.
   b. external heat-generating sources.
   c. therapeutic modalities for radiation oncology.
   d. treatment devices.

8. Which includes the use of equipment and supplies and the employment of radiologic technologists to perform diagnostic imaging examinations and administer radiation therapy treatments?
   a. Complete procedure
   b. Global service
   c. Professional element
   d. Technical component

9. In CPT, many radiological services include image guidance in their code descriptions, which means _____ radiological supervision and interpretation codes for image guidance are not reported.
   a. contrast material
   b. separate
   c. therapeutic
   d. unlisted

10. A patient underwent a nuclear medicine procedure in which radionuclides were administered to destroy a malignant neoplasm. For nuclear medicine purposes, radionuclides are an example of _____ elements and destruction of the malignant neoplasm is considered the _____ procedure.
    a. radioactive, diagnostic
    b. radioactive, radiopharmaceutical
    c. radiopharmaceutical, gamma ray
    d. therapeutic, gamma ray

11. Complete radiological exam of paranasal sinuses. Which CPT code is assigned?
    a. 70140   b. 70160   c. 70210   d. 70220

12. Chest x-ray, four views. Which CPT code is assigned?
    a. 71045   b. 71046   c. 71047   d. 71048

13. Computed tomography of the cervical spine without contrast on a patient, repeated the same day. Which CPT code(s) are assigned?
    a. 70450, 70450 76   b. 72125, 72125 76   c. 72126 76   d. 72127 76

14. Hip x-ray, two views, performed on the right side of the patient. Which CPT code is assigned?
    a. 73501 RT   b. 73502 RT   c. 73521 RT   d. 73525 RT

15. Selective adrenal angiography, left side, with radiological supervision and interpretation. Which CPT code is assigned?
    a. 75726 LT   b. 75731 LT   c. 75733 LT   d. 75736 LT

16. Screening mammography, bilateral breasts. Which CPT code is assigned?
    a. 77065 50   b. 77066   c. 77067   d. 77067 50

17. Red cell survival study. Which CPT code is assigned?
    a. 78110   b. 78120   c. 78130   d. 78140

18. Radiopharmaceutical localization of tumor using tomographic SPECT of uterus, single day imaging, performed twice by the same physician during the same encounter. Which CPT code(s) are assigned?
    a. 78803
    b. 78803 51
    c. 78803 77
    d. 78803, 78803 76

19. Radiopharmaceutical therapy by intracavitary administration. Which CPT code is assigned?
    a. 79200   b. 79403   c. 79440   d. 79445

20. Therapeutic radiology treatment planning, simple. Which CPT code is assigned?
    a. 77261   b. 77262   c. 77263   d. 77280

17.2 — Coding Practice: Diagnostic Radiology (Diagnostic Imaging)

Instructions: Assign the CPT code(s) and appropriate modifier(s) to each case. When a radiopharmaceutical agent is provided, assign the appropriate HCPCS Level II code(s).

1. One-view x-ray of abdomen reveals no abnormal soft tissue masses, gas shadows, or calcifications. Liver and spleen not enlarged. Visualized bones appear normal.

2. Following administration of oral contrast medium, gallbladder x-ray indicates satisfactory concentration, the outline is normal, and no calculi are detected. Impression: Normal gallbladder series. (In addition to the CPT code, assign the HCPCS Level II for supply of contrast medium.)

3. Serial small bowel x-ray series shows normal progression of barium from the rectum through the small intestine. The jejunum and ileum show a normal caliber and position. There is no evidence of filling defect or obstruction. The mucosal pattern is normal. Impression: Normal small bowel series. (In addition to the CPT code, assign the HCPCS Level II for supply of barium, which is a contrast medium.)

4. AP and oblique x-rays of the right portion of the rib cage show no evidence of fracture or other abnormality of the visualized ribs.

5. x-ray of the skull in three views shows calvarium to be intact. There is no evidence of any abnormal calcification or increased intracranial pressure. Sella turcica is normal in size and shape. There are a few teeth in the mandible, and there is poor visualization of the lamina dura.

6. Left hand x-ray in two views shows some osteoporosis of the visualized bones. There is no evidence of fracture or dislocation. Calcification is seen in the arteries around the wrist.

7. Radiologic examination of chest, one view, at 72 inches shows the heart to be transverse in position. Significant enlargement is not apparent on this study. At both bases, there is noted air-bronchogram effect associated with pulmonary infiltration. The thoracic aorta shows atheromatous calcification, and the right acromioclavicular joint shows degenerative arthrosis, as does the thoracic spine, which also shows a scoliosis with convexity toward the right.

8. Drip technique infusion urography reveals that the right renal length is approximately 11.3 cm, and the left is approximately 10.8 cm. Right kidney is higher than the left. Following Renografin, there was minimal delay in excretion from the kidneys and rather poor concentration bilaterally throughout the study, particularly on the right. As far as can be seen, the renal collecting structures are grossly normal. Drip infusion urography shows poorly functioning kidneys. For this reason, one cannot fully assess the kidneys or ureters. As far as can be seen, significant pathology is not apparent. (In addition to the CPT code, assign the HCPCS Level II for supply of Renografin, which is contrast material.)

9. x-ray of sella turcica reveals that the cranial vault is intact. Sella turcica was normal in size and shape. There are no intracranial calcifications.

10. x-ray of cervical spine, two views, was performed; there is no fracture or dislocation identified. Alignment is normal. There is no disc space narrowing. Neural foramina are patent bilaterally. There are no cervical ribs and no soft tissue calcifications in either side of the neck.

11. x-ray, right and left knees, in frontal, oblique, and lateral projections reveals no fracture or dislocation and no joint effusion. Impression: Negative examination of both knees.

12. Left wrist x-ray in frontal and lateral projections reveals an anatomical reduction of the distal radial epiphysis.

13. After administration of intravenous contrast dye, soft tissue structures of the neck are identified via computed tomography (CT) scan. The thyroid and parathyroid glands are seen. The right parathyroid gland shows a cyst-like structure. (In addition the CPT code, assign the HCPCS Level II for supply of contrast medium.)

14. CT scan of lumbar spine reveals a right curvature of 3 mm. The vertebra at L4 has a moderate amount of bone spur. Conclusion: Scoliosis.

15. A complete view of the heart and cardiac structures via magnetic resonance imaging (MRI) revealed no abnormalities. Heart valves were normal in appearance. Cardiac function was normal. Conclusion: Normal imaging of the heart.

17.3 — Coding Practice: Diagnostic Ultrasound

Instructions: Assign the CPT code to each case.

1. The pregnant uterus is examined via a transabdominal view. Estimated gestation is 16 weeks. A single fetus is observed. No abnormalities of the fetus or placenta are seen. Maternal anatomy was also imaged and determined to be normal. Real-time imaging is provided during this ultrasound.

2. The scrotum is normal in size. All tissue within appears normal. The testes are normal in appearance. The epididymis appears normal in structure.

3. An aortic aneurysm screening ultrasound with real time image documentation was performed to visualize blood flow through the abdominal aorta and to identify any defects. The abdominal aorta appears normal in structure and without defects.

4. Ultrasound of soft tissue of the neck with real time image documentation allowed visualization of normal soft tissue, including the thyroid, parathyroid, and parotid glands.

5. Patient with unexplained vaginal bleeding underwent transvaginal ultrasonography, which was performed after inserting the ultrasound probe two inches into the vagina canal. The transducer was slowly turned, and images were transmitted to the monitor. Impression: Lesion, anterior wall of vagina.

17.4 — Coding Practice: Radiologic Guidance

Instructions: Assign the CPT code(s) and appropriate modifier(s) to each case.

1. Computed tomography guidance for needle placement, radiological supervision, and interpretation.

   _____

2. The radiologist performed magnetic resonance imaging guidance for needle placement with radiological supervision and interpretation.

   _____

3. Patient underwent percutaneous needle biopsy, right biceps muscle, with fluoroscopic guidance for needle placement.

   _____

4. Radiologist provided computed tomography guidance services during placement of radiation therapy fields.

   _____

5. Radiologist provided computed tomography guidance during a procedure for stereotactic localization.

   _____

17.5 — Coding Practice: Breast, Mammography

Instructions: Assign the CPT code(s) and appropriate modifier(s) to each case.

1. Patient underwent magnetic resonance imaging, left breast, with computer-aided detection for real-time lesion detection.

   _____

2. Patient underwent magnetic resonance imaging, left breast, to detect a suspected lesion.

   _____

3. A diagnostic digital breast tomosynthesis, bilateral, was performed to produce three-dimensional (3D) mammography to detect abnormalities and perform morphological analysis.

   _____

4. Patient underwent mammary galactogram, multiple ducts, right breast, with radiological supervision and interpretation.

   _____

5. Patient underwent bilateral screening mammography and bilateral screening digital breast tomosynthesis.

   _____

17.6 — Coding Practice: Bone/Joint Studies

Instructions: Assign the CPT code to each case.

1. Patient underwent limited osseous survey radiologic examination for possible metastases.

   _____

2. Patient underwent joint radiography with manual application of stress performed by radiologist, right and left knees, to visualize joint characteristics in other than routine positioning.

   _____

3. Patient underwent magnetic resonance imaging to determine bone marrow blood supply.

   _____

4. Patient underwent dual-energy x-ray absorptiometry (DXA), bone density study, axial skeleton, including vertebral fracture assessment.

_____

5. Patient underwent orthoroentgenogram for bone length studies.

_____

17.7 — Coding Practice: Radiation Oncology and Clinical Brachytherapy

Instructions: Assign the CPT code to each case.

1. Patient underwent radiation treatment during which 4 MeV (megavoltages) were delivered to the thyroid area.

_____

2. Therapeutic radiology port images were completed to verify accurate positioning of treatment portals for a patient undergoing external beam radiation therapy.

_____

3. Patient underwent high energy neutron radiation treatment delivery, 1 isocenter with coplanar geometry with wedge.

_____

4. Patient underwent 2-channel remote afterloading high dose rate radionuclide interstitial brachytherapy, including basic dosimetry, for treatment of stomach cancer.

_____

5. Patient underwent hyperthermia generated by intracavitary probes for the purposes of increasing cell metabolism and the potential for cell destruction as treatment of a malignancy.

_____

17.8 — Coding Practice: Nuclear Medicine

Instructions: Assign the CPT code to each case. Do *not* assign HCPCS Level II codes for supply of radioactive contrast material.

1. Positron emission tomography (PET) scan of the chest region reveals no soft tissue masses or bony abnormalities. Ribs, mediastinum, and heart are normal.

_____

2. Nuclear medicine imaging of the liver and spleen reveals the liver to be of normal size with homogeneous uptake. The spleen is enlarged and is almost the same size as the liver. There is also increased activity in the spleen. I do not see any focal areas of diminished activity, and there is no significant bone marrow uptake. Conclusion: Splenomegaly.

_____

3. Nuclear medicine whole body bone and joint scan reveals uptake was noted in the nasal area of the sphenoid sinuses. The remainder of the scan is normal. No masses, bony abnormalities, or metastatic disease is seen.

_____

4. Patient underwent nuclear medicine imaging including vascular flow, thyroid gland.

_____

5. Patient underwent oral administration of radiopharmaceutical therapy.

_____

CPT Pathology and Laboratory

Chapter Outline

Overview of Pathology and Laboratory Section

Pathology and Laboratory Section Guidelines

Pathology and Laboratory Subsections

Chapter Objectives

At the conclusion of this chapter, the student should be able to:

1. Define key terms related to the CPT Pathology and Laboratory Section.
2. Summarize the organization, format, and content of the CPT Pathology and Laboratory section.
3. Interpret CPT Pathology and Laboratory Section guidelines.
4. Assign codes from the subsections of CPT Pathology and Laboratory.

Key Terms

adjuvant
aliquot
analyte
antibody
antigen
arterial puncture
assay
Bethesda System
Chemstrip automated urine analyzer

Clinical Laboratory Improvement Act of 1988 (CLIA)
cytogenetics
cytopathology
definitive identification
dipstick
evocative
fluorescence *in situ* hybridization (FISH)

Gram stain
gross examination
hematology
immunoglobulin
immunology
microbiology
microtechnique
necropsy
phlebotomy

presumptive identification
qualitative assay
quantitative assay
reagent strip automated urine analyzer
specimen
venipuncture

Introduction

The CPT Pathology and Laboratory section includes subsections for organ or disease-oriented panels, drug assays, therapeutic drug assays, evocative/suppression testing, consultations (clinical pathology), urinalysis, molecular pathology, genomic sequencing procedures and other molecular multianalyte assays, multianalyte assays with algorithmic analyses, chemistry, hematology and coagulation, immunology, transfusion medicine, microbiology, anatomical pathology, cytopathology, cytogenetic studies, surgical pathology, *in vivo* (e.g., transcutaneous) laboratory procedures, other procedures, reproductive medicine procedures, and proprietary laboratory analyses.

 NOTE:

The *Medicare National Correct Coding Initiative Policy Manual* provides guidance about assigning procedure and service codes for the Pathology and Laboratory section. Go to **www.cms.gov** and enter "Medicare NCCI Policy Manual" in the Search box to navigate to the manual.

Overview of Pathology and Laboratory Section

CPT pathology and laboratory codes describe services performed on specimens (e.g., body fluids, tissue, or cytological specimens) to evaluate, prevent, diagnose, or treat a disease. A **specimen** (e.g., blood, urine, tissue from an organ) is tissue submitted for laboratory or pathological evaluation. Types of examinations include the following:

- Biophysical
- Chemical
- Cytological
- Hematological
- Immunohematological
- Microbiological
- Pathological
- Serological

Example: A wound culture is obtained from the smear of an infected area. The infective organism is identified as the result of growing the organism on a culture plate and microscopically reviewing the specimen or serologically testing the organism (e.g., antistreptolysin O titer).

Most clinical laboratory service codes include a technical component; however, some include both a technical and a professional component. In addition, because many pathology and laboratory procedures can be performed using different methods, patient record documentation must be reviewed along with code descriptions and instructional notes.

New *proprietary laboratory analyses (PLA)* codes were added to CPT effective January 2016 and are available to any clinical laboratory or manufacturer that wants to specifically identify their commercially available tests that are used on human specimens. PLA test codes are published quarterly at the **https://www.ama-assn.org** website, with new codes effective in the quarter following their publication. The CPT coding manual now includes PLA codes, and new codes will continue to be published quarterly at the AMA's website.

 NOTE:

Hospitals include CPT pathology and laboratory codes on a chargemaster, which is used to report services (and supplies) for inpatients, outpatients, and emergency department patients. ICD-10-PCS codes are not assigned to pathology and laboratory procedures that are performed on an inpatient hospital basis because such services do not impact diagnosis-related group (DRG) assignment and facility reimbursement.

 NOTE:

Depending on the contract negotiated between pathologists and the health care facility

- Pathologists are considered employees of the health care facility (e.g., a hospital) or they are considered contractors.
- The facility submits claims to obtain reimbursement for all services provided to patients (including professional services) *or* the pathologists use a medical billing service to submit claims for professional services.

Specimens and Specimen Collection

Laboratory codes describe the *performance* of lab tests. These codes do not include *collection of the specimen* (e.g., venipuncture, fingerstick, or lumbar puncture) used to perform the test.

For laboratory-testing purposes, a specimen includes tissue (e.g., blood, sputum, and urine) that is submitted for individual and separate examinations and/or pathological diagnosis. Specimen collection is reported separately, in addition to the laboratory test performed. Collection methods vary from those requiring no patient preparation to invasive-type procedures, and the reason for the test typically determines the appropriate collection method. Special collection methods (e.g., urethral catheterization or suprapubic aspiration) are indicated when a specimen cannot be obtained by more common techniques.

> **Example:** With an indwelling urinary catheter in place, a specimen is obtained by inserting the needle into the catheter. The urine is aspirated and placed in a sterile urine container for laboratory testing.

Venipuncture, or **phlebotomy**, is the puncture of a vein using a needle for the purpose of drawing blood, and it is the most common method of collecting blood specimens. **Arterial puncture** is the puncture of an artery using a needle for the purpose of drawing blood. For safety purposes, after venipuncture, the used needle is placed in an approved *sharps container* made of hard, damage-resistant plastic (Figure 18-1).

 Coding Tip

A venipuncture code is reported just once per encounter for each type of specimen, regardless of the number of specimens drawn.

Professional and Technical Components

Certain laboratory procedures contain both a professional (e.g., physician) component and a technical component. The *professional component* includes ordering, reviewing, and interpreting a pathology or laboratory procedure and service by a physician (e.g., pathologist, primary care physician) or other qualified health care professional (e.g., physician assistant). The *technical component* includes, but is not limited to, the cost of equipment, supplies, and technician salaries for pathology or laboratory procedures and services. The technical component is typically billed on the date the patient underwent the pathology or laboratory procedure and service.

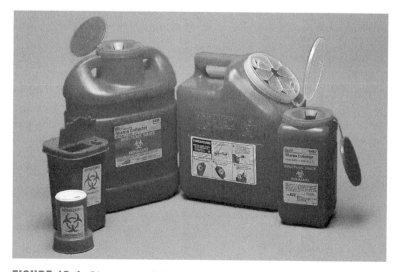

FIGURE 18-1 Sharps containers

Coding Tip

When a pathology and laboratory procedure or service code description includes both the technical and professional components, and one of the components was not performed, report the appropriate code with modifier

- 26, to indicate that only the professional component was performed
- TC, to indicate that only the technical component was performed

Pathologists often oversee the clinical pathology laboratory department and assume overall responsibility for test results. When reporting codes for professional and technical components of clinical pathology and laboratory services, standard practice is for the pathologist to report the *professional component* of services. Clinical pathology professional services include the following:

- Directing and evaluating quality assurance and control procedures (e.g., ensuring that tests and procedures are properly performed, recorded, and reported; validating test methodologies)
- Supervising laboratory technicians
- Recommending follow-up diagnostic tests, when appropriate

The hospital or CLIA-approved independent facility reports the *technical component*, which represents costs associated with laboratory equipment, supplies, and nonphysician personnel. The hospital's technical component does *not* include the pathologist's professional services.

NOTE:

Most laboratory services reported with CPT codes are paid by Medicare according to the laboratory fee schedule, which is discussed in Chapter 20, Insurance and Reimbursement Overview, of this textbook.

Coding Tip

Modifier 90, Reference (Outside) Laboratory, is reported with pathology and laboratory codes to indicate that an outside laboratory performed the service. Specimen handling is assigned a code from the Special Services, Procedures and Reports subsection of the Medicine section.

Pathology and laboratory services can be provided by a physician or by technologists under the supervision of a physician. Although most codes describe clinical laboratory tests, physician laboratory and pathology services are also included. Physician laboratory and pathology services include the following:

- Surgical pathology services
- Cytopathology, hematology, and blood-banking services that require a physician
- Clinical consultation services
- Clinical laboratory interpretation services

Typically, pathology and laboratory specimens are prepared by laboratory personnel with a pathologist assuming responsibility for the integrity of the results. Certain tests are personally reviewed by the pathologist. Very few CPT pathology and laboratory codes require patient contact; however, occasionally a pathologist provides evaluation and management services. Such services are reported with appropriate CPT evaluation and management codes.

Clinical Laboratory Improvement Act of 1988 (CLIA)

To perform certain pathology and laboratory tests (and to submit claims to Medicare and Medicaid), physician office labs must obtain certification under the **Clinical Laboratory Improvement Act of 1988 (CLIA)**. A waiver is available for small office labs that perform only basic testing (e.g., urine dipsticks and fingerstick glucose testing), and a special CLIA waiver number is assigned to these labs. The list of approved tests is updated periodically, which means that physician office labs must determine if they still qualify for a waiver.

 Coding Tip

When reporting CLIA waived services to Medicare or Medicaid, add HCPCS Level II modifier QW to pathology and laboratory codes.

National Coverage Determinations (NCDs)

The Centers for Medicare & Medicaid Services (CMS) developed National Coverage Determinations (NCDs), which define coverage for services and procedures. Medicare administrative contractors (MACs) apply national coverage determinations nationwide, and local coverage decisions (LCDs) supplement the NCDs. Pathology and laboratory NCDs were developed to

- Simplify administrative requirements for clinical diagnostic services.
- Promote national uniformity in processing Medicare claims.

Pathology and Laboratory Section Tables

The following tables are located in the Pathology and Laboratory section of CPT.

- Definitions and Acronym Conversion Listing (in the Drug Assay subsection)
- Definitive Drug Classes Listing (in the Definitive Drug Classes category of the Drug Assay subsection)
- Medical Decision Making (in the Instructions for Selecting a Level of Pathology Clinical Consultation Services category of the Pathology Clinical Consultations subsection)
- Molecular Pathology Gene Table (prior to Pathology and Laboratory Guidelines)
- Table (in the Genomic Sequencing Procedures and Other Molecular Multianalyte Assays subsection)

Exercise 18.1 – Overview of Pathology and Laboratory Section

Instructions: Complete each statement.

1. Although most clinical laboratory service codes include a technical component, some include both a technical and a(n) _____ component.

2. Review of patient record documentation is necessary before assigning pathology and laboratory codes because many procedures can be performed using different _____.

3. Hospital coders usually do not assign pathology and laboratory codes because they are included on a(n) _____, which is used by providers to report services provided to patients.

4. CPT laboratory codes describe the performance of lab tests, and they do not include collection of the _____, which is performed using different methods and is reported separately.

5. The puncture of a vein using a needle for the purpose of drawing blood as a common method of collecting blood specimens is called venipuncture, or _____.

Exercise 18.1 – continued

6. A routine venipuncture is assigned CPT code _____, and it is reported in addition to the laboratory procedure code.

7. For a cutdown venipuncture procedure, age 1 or over, CPT code _____ is assigned.

8. When a pathology and laboratory procedure code description includes technical and professional components, and both components were not performed, modifier _____ is added to the code to indicate that only the professional component was performed.

9. When an outside laboratory performs pathology and laboratory services, add modifier _____ to the reported code.

10. To perform certain pathology and laboratory tests (and to submit claims to Medicare and Medicaid), physician office labs must obtain _____ under the Clinical Laboratory Improvement Act (CLIA) of 1988.

Pathology and Laboratory Section Guidelines

Guidelines located at the beginning of the Pathology and Laboratory section provide instruction about the following:

- Services in pathology and laboratory
- Separate or multiple procedures
- Unlisted services or procedures
- Special reports

Services in Pathology and Laboratory

Pathology and laboratory services are provided by a physician (e.g., a pathologist) or by technologists under responsible supervision of a physician. The unit of pathology service is a *specimen*, which is tissue that is submitted for individual and separate examination and pathological diagnosis. When multiple specimens are received for pathological examination, each specimen is considered a single unit of service and each is reported with a separate code.

Example 1: Two separately identified skin lesions are submitted for individual examination and diagnosis. Report codes 88305 and 88305 59. (Modifier 59 is added to indicate that the second lesion was evaluated as a "distinct procedural service.")

Example 2: The uterus (with or without tubes and ovaries) is considered one specimen and is reported with code 88305 (when the uterus is removed for prolapse and shows no other abnormalities), 88309 (for neoplasia), or 88307 (for other conditions).

Example 3: A cell block prepared from cytology fluids, bone marrow aspirates, or fine-needle aspirates is coded as 88305. (A *block* is a portion of tissue obtained from a specimen that is placed in a support medium, such as paraffin. A *section* is a thin slice of tissue prepared from a block that is examined.)

Separate or Multiple Procedures

It is appropriate to separately code and report multiple pathology and laboratory procedures that are provided on the same date of service. However, it is *not* appropriate to report tests that are repeated simply to confirm initial results (because of an equipment malfunction or technician error) or when a series of tests is performed (e.g., glucose tolerance tests). These services are considered part of the originally ordered test, and codes for repeated tests are not separately coded and reported.

> **Example:** The physician ordered an automated hemogram with automated platelet count. The laboratory also conducted a manual platelet count as a confirmatory test for quality control purposes. Report code 85027. (Do not report code 85032, manual platelet count, because it was conducted by the laboratory for quality control purposes.)

Unlisted Service or Procedure

A service or procedure that is provided for which there is no CPT code is reported with an "unlisted service or procedure" code.

> **Example:** An unlisted immunology procedure is reported with code 86849 (and a special report is attached to the submitted insurance claim).

Special Report

When an unlisted procedure or service code is reported on a claim, a "special report" is attached to the submitted claim to clarify the service or procedure performed. A service or procedure that is rarely performed, unusual, variable, or new may require a special report to be submitted so the third-party payer can determine the medical appropriateness of the service or procedure. The special report should include a description of the nature, extent, and need for the procedure. In addition, the following items may be included:

- Complexity of symptoms
- Final diagnosis
- Pertinent physical findings
- Diagnostic and therapeutic procedures
- Concurrent problems
- Follow-up care

Modifier 51, Modifier 90, and Modifier 91

- Modifier 51 (Multiple procedures) is *not* added to pathology and laboratory codes.
- Modifier 90 (Reference [outside] laboratory) is added to a laboratory procedure code when the procedure is performed by an organization other than the physician or other qualified health care professional. Reporting the modifier alerts the third-party payer that an outside laboratory will submit a claim for reimbursement. (Outside lab personnel or courier services use special equipment to facilitate the transportation of specimens to the laboratory facility. For such specimen handling, report codes from the Special Services, Procedures and Reports subsection in the Medicine section.)
- Modifier 91 (Repeat clinical diagnostic laboratory test) is added to pathology and laboratory codes when procedures or services are repeated on the same date of service to obtain multiple results.

> **Example 1:** A patient undergoes a comprehensive metabolic panel laboratory test. Because of abnormal blood urea nitrogen (BUN) test results, the patient undergoes a repeat BUN test as an individual test. Report codes 80053 and 84520 91.

> **Example 2:** The physician's office collects a urine specimen from a patient, and an outside laboratory picks up the specimen for which an automated urinalysis with microscopy has been ordered. Report code 81001 90 for the urinalysis. The outside laboratory may also report code 99000 for specimen handling, which is located in the Special Services, Procedures and Reports subsection of the Medicine section.

Exercise 18.2 – Pathology and Laboratory Section Guidelines

Instructions: Complete each statement.

1. The unit of pathology service is a(n) _____, which is tissue submitted for individual and separate examination and pathological diagnosis.

2. During the same operative session, the surgeon submitted "incidental appendix" tissue and a section of fallopian tube (as the result of a sterilization procedure) for pathological evaluation. Refer to the notes located below the Surgical Pathology subsection (codes 88300–88399) to determine whether one or two codes are reported. Code 88302 is reported _____ (once/twice).

3. It is appropriate to separately code and report multiple pathology and laboratory procedures that are provided on the _____ date of service.

4. A service or procedure that is provided for which there is no CPT code available is reported with an unlisted code, and a(n) _____ report is attached to the submitted claim.

5. When procedures or services are repeated on the same date of service to obtain multiple results, add modifier 91 to the reported pathology and laboratory code(s). It is *not* appropriate to add modifier _____ to pathology and laboratory codes.

Pathology and Laboratory Subsections

The Pathology and Laboratory section is organized according to type of procedure performed or service provided. Pathology and laboratory procedures are listed alphabetically within each subsection, which include the following:

- Organ or disease-oriented panels
- Drug assay
- Therapeutic drug assays
- Evocative/suppression testing
- Pathology clinical consultations
- Urinalysis
- Molecular pathology
- Genomic sequencing procedures and other molecular multianalyte assays
- Multianalyte assays with algorithmic analyses
- Chemistry
- Hematology and coagulation

- Immunology
- Transfusion medicine
- Microbiology
- Anatomic pathology
- Cytopathology
- Cytogenetic studies
- Surgical pathology
- *In vivo* laboratory procedures
- Other procedures
- Reproductive medicine procedures
- Proprietary laboratory analyses

Organ or Disease-Oriented Panels

Organ or disease-oriented panels are a defined group of tests that are administered for a certain purpose. The panels were developed for coding purposes only and are not considered clinical parameters. The tests listed below each panel identify the components of that panel.

To report an organ or disease-oriented panel code, all tests listed below the panel must be performed. No substitutions can be made.

Example: Patient underwent a general health panel. Report code 80050, which must include all of the following procedures:

- Comprehensive metabolic panel
- Blood count, complete (CBC); automated and automated differential WBC count *or* Blood count, complete (CBC), automated (85027) and appropriate manual differential WBC count
- Thyroid-stimulating hormone (TSH)

Individual laboratory codes are *not* reported in addition to the general health panel code.

When only one or several of the tests associated with a panel are performed, do not report the panel code. Instead, report codes for each individual test performed.

Example: Patient underwent a glucose test and a sodium test. Report codes 82947 and 84295. (Do *not* report basic metabolic panel code 80048.)

When laboratory tests are performed in addition to those required for an organ or disease-oriented panel, separate codes are reported for the additional tests (in addition to the panel code).

Example: Patient underwent a basic metabolic panel test and an albumin test. Report codes 80048 and 82040.

Drug Assay and Therapeutic Drug Assays

Drug testing procedures are located in three subsections of pathology and laboratory, and code selection is dependent on the purpose and type of patient results obtained.

- Therapeutic drug assays
- Drug assay
- Chemistry

An **assay** (e.g., lab test) is the measurement of the amount of a constituent in a specimen. Therapeutic drug assay procedures are performed using blood, cerebrospinal fluid, plasma, or serum to monitor the patient's clinical response to a known, prescribed, or over-the-counter medication. The two major categories include the following:

(1) *Presumptive drug class procedures* identify possible use or non-use of a drug or drug class. They may be followed by a definitive test in order to specifically identify drugs or metabolites.

(2) *Definitive drug class procedures* are qualitative or quantitative tests that identify possible use or non-use of a drug. These tests identify specific drugs and associated metabolites, if performed. (A presumptive test is not required prior to a definitive drug test.)

Qualitative assays detect whether a particular substance is present. **Quantitative assays** detect the amount of a substance in a specimen.

The material for drug class procedures may be any specimen type unless otherwise specified in the code descriptor (e.g., urine, blood, oral fluid, meconium, hair). Procedures can be qualitative, semiquantitative, or quantitative depending on the purpose of the testing. Therapeutic drug assay procedures are typically quantitative tests and the specimen type is whole blood, serum, plasma, or cerebrospinal fluid. When the same procedure(s) is performed on more than one specimen type (e.g., hair and urine), the appropriate code is reported separately for each specimen type using modifier 59 (Distinct procedural service).

Drugs or classes of drugs may be commonly assayed first by a presumptive screening method followed by a definitive drug identification method. Presumptive methods include immunoassays, enzymatic methods, chromatographic methods without mass spectrometry, or mass spectrometry without adequate drug resolution by chromatography.

Drugs or classes of drugs may be assayed first using a presumptive screening method followed by a definitive drug identification method. The drug class and methodology must be determined when reporting codes for presumptive procedures.

Example 1: Patient underwent alcohol drug screen (Drug Class List A) using an instrumented test system. Report code 80305.

Example 2: Patient underwent definitive drug testing for three or more types of anabolic steroids on the same encounter date. Report code 80328.

Example 3: Patient underwent a total digoxin therapeutic drug assay procedure to monitor the clinical response to treatment. (The patient's blood was drawn for this laboratory procedure.) Report code 80162.

Example 4: Patient underwent Breathalyzer testing for presence of alcohol (ethanol). Report code 82075.

Evocative/Suppression Testing

Evocative/suppression test panels include the administration of evocative or suppressive agents and the baseline and subsequent measurement of their effect on chemical constituents. They are reported for the laboratory component of the testing protocol. (**Evocative** means to cause a specific response; this term is used to describe various tests intended to cause production of hormones or other secretions.)

Coding Tip

Report a code from the CPT Medicine section for administration (e.g., infusion) of the evocative or suppressive agents. To locate the administration of agent code, refer to the Hydration, Therapeutic, Prophylactic, Diagnostic Injections and Infusions, and Chemotherapy and Other Highly Complex Drug or Highly Complex Biologic Agent Administration subsection of CPT Medicine.

Physician attendance and monitoring during evocative/suppression testing is reported with codes from the CPT Evaluation and Management section.

Pathology Clinical Consultations

The physician (e.g., pathologist) review of laboratory test results is *not* a separately reportable service. However, when a pathologist is requested to provide pathology clinical consultation services regarding pathology and/or laboratory test results, pathology clinical consultation codes are reported. (Other pathology consultative codes are assigned for consultative review of tissue specimen slides and pathologic consultation during surgery.) The pathology clinical consultation requires

- Clinical assessment, evaluation of pathology and laboratory findings, or other clinical/diagnostic information that requires additional medical interpretative judgment
- Preparation of a written report

Example: A surgeon orders a pathology clinical consultation to determine a patient's suitability for surgery based on the results of pathology and laboratory findings. The pathologist documents a written consultation report for a highly complex clinical problem that includes a 60-minute comprehensive review of the patient's medical records, including the patient's history and current pathology laboratory results, and a high level of medical decision making about the patient's candidacy for surgery. Report code 80505.

NOTE:

A pathologist who provides a pathology clinical consultation service *that includes examination of the patient* reports an appropriate evaluation and management code (e.g., outpatient, inpatient, or consultation). The pathologist is responsible for ensuring that criteria for reporting the evaluation and management code (e.g., time or medical decision making) have been met and a report has been appropriately documented in the medical record.

When reporting a pathology clinical consultation code, the appropriate level of services provided is determined by (1) total time documented for the provision of pathology clinical consultation services on the date of consultation, or (2) level of medical decision making.

Urinalysis

Most urine tests are performed to diagnose or monitor renal or urinary tract disease. Urine testing is easily performed and does not require an invasive skin puncture. Urine collection containers (Figure 18-2) used for routine urinalysis are made of material that is clear (translucent), and they have lids that can be secured to prevent spills during transport. For example, protein in the urine may indicate glomerulonephritis, and urine cultures monitor the effectiveness of antibiotic treatment for urinary tract infections.

Urinalysis codes are reported for the analysis of one or more components of the urine. The reported code is based on method (e.g., dipstick), purpose (e.g., a pregnancy test), or element evaluated (e.g., bilirubin, bacteriuria screen).

Quantitative urine tests often require a timed collection. Timed urine collection is often performed because substances (e.g., hormones, proteins, and electrolytes) are excreted over a 24-hour period. Because exercise, hydration, and body metabolism affect excretion rates, these time periods may range anywhere from 2 to 24 hours.

A **reagent strip automated urine analyzer** (or **Chemstrip automated urine analyzer**) (Figure 18-3) is used to determine various components in the urine (including glucose, albumin, hemoglobin, and bile concentrations, as well as urinary pH, specific gravity, protein, ketone bodies, nitrites, and leukocyte esterase). A **dipstick** (Figure 18-4) is a small strip of plastic that is infused with a chemical that reacts to products in urine by changing color. It is considered preliminary and may be performed for screening purposes.

 Coding Tip

Analysis of urine is also included in other Pathology and Laboratory subsections. For example, a urine chloride test is reported with a code from the Chemistry subsection.

The appropriate handling and storage of urine is necessary to prevent changes that adversely impact accurate results. Many **analytes** (substance or chemical compound undergoing analysis) require the use of preservatives so that they remain viable during the collection period. The choice of preservative depends on the type of collection. For example, sodium fluoride is used to preserve glucose in a 24-hour urine collection.

Example: Nonautomated urinalysis by dipstick, without microscopy. Report code 81002.

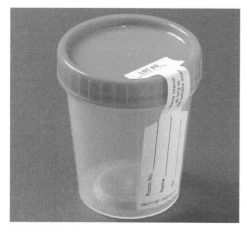

FIGURE 18-2 Urine collection container

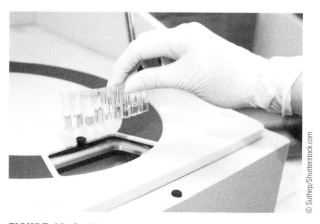

FIGURE 18-3 Chemstrip automated urine analyzer

© Suthep/Shutterstock.com

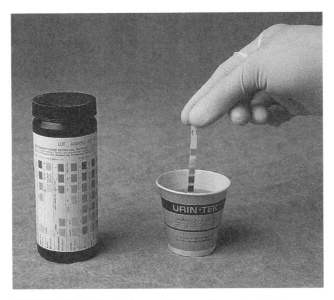

FIGURE 18-4 Dipstick used for routine urinalysis

Molecular Pathology

Molecular pathology laboratory procedures involve the analysis of nucleic acid to detect gene variants, which may be indicative of certain conditions (e.g., constitutional disorders, neoplasia, histocompatibility enzymes). They are organized as Tier 1 and Tier 2 molecular pathology laboratory procedures. CPT incorporates the Human Genome Organization–approved gene names in code descriptions along with proteins or diseases associated with the genes. Molecular pathology notes indicate that any procedures performed prior to cell lysis, such as microdissection, are to be reported separately, and an extensive list of definitions is also included.

- Tier 1 molecular pathology laboratory procedures include gene-specific and genomic procedures according to the *analyte* (substance or chemical compound undergoing analysis) or the *allele* (genetic variants).

- Tier 2 procedures are not listed in Tier 1, and they are reported according to level of technical resources and interpretive professional work required. (Tier 2 procedures are performed less frequently than Tier 1 procedures.)

- If a tested analyte is not represented by a Tier 1 or a Tier 2 code, report the unlisted molecular pathology procedure code.

Example: Patient underwent the *BRCA1* and *BRCA2* gene analysis laboratory procedure to determine the risk for hereditary breast and ovarian cancer. Report code 81162.

Coding Tip

When tests require that a physician or other qualified health care professional interpret the results, and the provider performs the interpretation only, add modifier 26 (Professional component) to the code.

Genomic Sequencing Procedures and Other Molecular Multianalyte Assays

Genomic sequencing procedures (GSPs) and other molecular multianalyte assays are DNA or RNA sequence analysis methods that simultaneously assay multiple genes or genetic regions relevant to a clinical situation.

> **Example:** Patient underwent genome sequence analysis for Huntington's disease. Report code 81425.

Multianalyte Assays with Algorithmic Analyses

Multianalyte Assays with Algorithmic Analyses (MAAAs) are performed to determine discrete genetic values, properties, or characteristics, and the results are potentially of independent medical significance or useful in the medical management of a patient (e.g., determine patient's risk for certain diseases).

> **Example:** Patient underwent oncology (ovarian) biochemical assays of two proteins (CA-125 and HE4), utilizing serum, with menopausal status, with the algorithm reported as a risk score. Report code 81500.

Chemistry

Chemistry codes are reported for quantitative tests unless the code description indicates otherwise. (Presumptive and/or definitive drug testing procedures are reported with drug assay codes.) Chemical tests performed on body materials are obtained from any source (e.g., blood or urine) unless the code description specifies otherwise. Codes in the Chemistry subsection are listed in an alphabetical order.

To properly assign codes from the Chemistry subsection, locate the code that describes the analyte to be tested (the specific substance to be analyzed).

When a chemistry test is performed on multiple specimens from different sources, or on specimens that are obtained at different times, the analyte is reported separately for each source and for *each* specimen.

> **Example:** Patient underwent two lab tests to determine total bilirubin levels. A specimen was obtained during the morning and afternoon on April 5. Report codes 82247 and 82247 91.

Stool includes waste products of digested food bile, mucus, epithelial cells, and bacteria. Stool studies are performed to evaluate bowel function (e.g., for intestinal bleeding, infections, infestations, inflammation, malabsorption, and diarrhea).

> **Example:** Patient underwent occult blood testing by peroxidase activity, qualitative, feces, one determination. Report code 82272.

Body fluids can be tested for blood urea nitrogen (BUN) and creatinine to determine whether the fluid is urine. For example, code 84560 is reported for uric acid testing, other source, which is helpful in obstetrics to differentiate amniotic fluid from urine.

Hematology and Coagulation

Hematology is the study of the function and disorders of blood (Figure 18-5). *Coagulation* is the process of blood clotting. Hematology and coagulation laboratory tests are performed to evaluate blood and blood clotting, such as CBC, clotting factor tests, clotting inhibitor tests, and prothrombin and thrombin time. Bone marrow, smear interpretation, is also included in the Hematology and Coagulation subsection. (Bone marrow biopsy and cell block interpretations are reported with a code from the Surgical Pathology subsection.)

Platelet count codes are integrated into the blood count series of codes. Codes for the current manual microscopic review of blood describe the microscopic examination of a blood smear with a manual differential leukocyte (WBC) count.

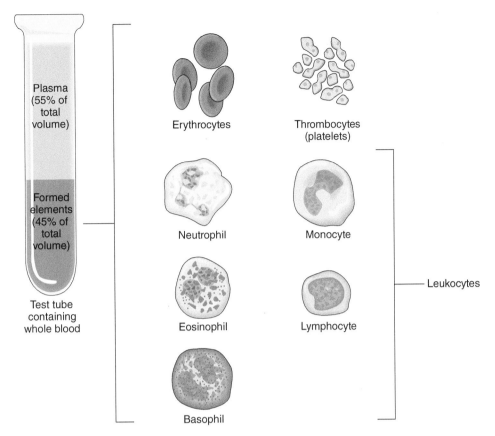

FIGURE 18-5 Blood components

Automated CBC and automated differential WBC count tests are performed when blood is tested to determine the following levels:

- Hemoglobin (Hgb)
- Hematocrit (Hct)
- Red blood cell (RBC)

- White blood cell (WBC)
- Platelet

The automated differential WBC count determines the number of basophils, eosinophils, monocytes, lymphocytes, and neutrophils. (When a manual cell count of erythrocytes, leukocytes, or platelets is performed, the appropriate code is reported for *each* type.)

Example 1: Patient underwent manual CBC to determine Hct, Hgb, erythrocyte, and leukocyte levels. Report codes 85014, 85018, 85032, and 85032 59. (Code 85032 is reported twice to reflect testing of each erythrocyte and leukocyte level.)

Example 2: Patient underwent an automated CBC and an automated differential WBC count. Report code 85025 *or* codes 85027 and 85004, depending on the laboratory's processing of the WBC differential.

Specific methodologies for measuring D-dimer fibrin degradation products, based on the sensitivity of the analysis, are differentiated as

- Qualitative or semiquantitative
- Quantitative
- Ultrasensitive, qualitative or semiquantitative

Example: Patient underwent qualitative fibrin degradation products D-dimer test. Report code 85378.

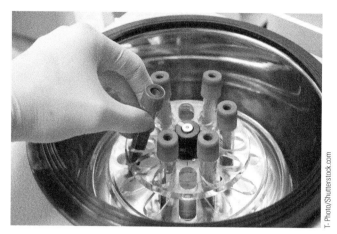

FIGURE 18-6 Serological centrifuge

Immunology

Immunology is the study of the immune system. Immunology procedures include antigen and antibody laboratory studies and tissue typing. Antigen and antibody studies measure the reaction of

- **Antigens** (Ag): Foreign substances that elicit the formation of antibodies
- **Antibodies** (Ab): Proteins in the body made by the immune system that fight infection and disease

(An **adjuvant** is a substance administered with an antigen that enhances the response to the antigen.) Figure 18-6 contains a serological centrifuge, which is used to spin test tubes of blood to test for agglutination reactions (clumping of blood cells). Hemagglutination (agglutination of red blood cells) is a method used to visualize antigen–antibody reactions.

> **Example:** Patient underwent HIV-1 antibody test to determine exposure to human immunodeficiency virus and subsequent antibody development. Report code 86701.

Immunoglobulins are proteins produced by plasma cells that help fight infection. Some immunoglobulins (e.g., gamma globulins) are involved in immune responses to bacteria or foreign substances (e.g., allergens or transplanted tissue). Immunoglobulins include IgA, IgD, IgE, IgG, and IgM. Codes are also reported for the quantitative and qualitative measurement of IgE.

> **Example:** Patient underwent quantitative allergen-specific IgE testing, five allergens. Report code 86003 five times.

Tumor antigen procedures indicate the presence of a tumor marker in the patient's blood.

> **Example:** Patient with previously treated stage II and stage III breast cancer underwent immunoassay for tumor antigen CA 125 to test for recurrence of breast cancer. Report code 86304.

Laboratory tests performed to identify specific antibodies are performed using a multistep method. Tissue typing procedures are performed to determine compatibility between a recipient and donors for organ or bone marrow transplants.

> **Example:** Patient underwent human leukocyte antigen (HLA) typing of single antigen A10. Report code 86812. (HLA determines graft acceptance.)

Transfusion Medicine

Transfusion medicine codes are often reported by blood banks, and they describe blood preparation services for transfusion. For transfusion services, report the appropriate CPT code as well as an HCPCS Level II code for the blood product transfused. (The service code is reported with the date of service for the transfusion, not the date the blood was collected.) When autologous blood is collected but not transfused, report the appropriate code with the number of units collected but not transfused.

The collection, modification, treatment, and processing of autologous blood specimens for transplantation are described as (1) predeposited or (2) intra- or postoperative salvage. When processing and storage costs are incurred for unused blood or blood products, the provider may submit charges when patient-specific preparation was done (e.g., blood typing and cross-matching).

> **Example:** Patient underwent transfusion of one unit of frozen blood, which included freezing (and preparation) as well as thawing. Report code 86932. (If the type of blood product had been stated in the example, such as plasma, report the more specific HCPCS Level II code P9017 instead.)

 NOTE:

A transfusion ambulatory payment classification (APC) payment is paid once per day regardless of the number of units or different types of products transfused when reporting codes for a health care facility (e.g., hospital outpatient department).

Microbiology

Microbiology is the study of microbes (e.g., bacteria, parasites, and viruses). Microbiology codes include bacteriology, mycology, parasitology, and virology, and the codes are intended to describe primary definitive (or final) bacterial cultures. To properly assign microbiology codes, determine the following:

- Source
- Handling method
- Stains performed
- Identification technique used

It is appropriate to separately report multiple procedures when various microbiology testing procedures are performed.

Microscopic examinations evaluate cytologic specimens to identify bacteria and other infecting organisms (e.g., determining hormone receptor assay results, chromatin identification, culture and sensitivity testing). Microbiology subsection notes provide instruction about the presumptive identification of microorganisms and definitive identification.

- **Presumptive identification** is the identification by colony morphology, growth on selective media, Gram stains, or up to three tests (e.g., catalase, oxidase, indole, or urease).
- **Definitive identification** of microorganisms is the identification to the genus or species level that requires additional tests (e.g., biochemical panels or slide cultures). The word "definitive" refers to the final culture that identifies the organism. Reporting these codes indicates that a specific organism genus or group (e.g., *Staphylococcus, Salmonella*, or *Streptococcus*) has been identified.

When additional studies involve molecular probes, chromatography, or immunologic techniques, report the codes separately in addition to definitive identification codes. For multiple specimens/sites, add modifier 59 to the microbiology code. For repeat laboratory tests performed on the same day, add modifier 91 to the microbiology code.

A **Gram stain** is a method of classifying all bacteria as gram positive or gram negative. The shape of the organism (e.g., spherical or rod-shaped) may also be helpful in the identification of the infecting organism. When the Gram stain indicates Gram negative rods, the infection may be caused by *Escherichia coli*. With knowledge of Gram stain results, the physician can initiate antibiotic treatment based on the organism's identity.

> **Example:** A fluorescent stain for bacteria, primary source smear with interpretation, was performed. Report code 87206.

Anatomic Pathology

Anatomical pathology codes are reported for physician (pathologist) services only. Physician services involved in performing **necropsy** (autopsy) are specific to the following:

- Portions of the body
- Gross examination
- Regional examination
- Forensic examination
- Infant/stillborn

> **Example:** The pathologist performed a gross and microscopic autopsy that included the brain of a stillborn infant. Report code 88029. (**Gross examination** involves visually evaluating a specimen with the naked eye.)

Cytopathology

Cytopathology is the study of diseased cells. Specimen cells are typically obtained using brushing, washing, needle biopsy, or fine-needle aspiration. Thus, the patient record must be reviewed to determine the collection method to correctly report cytopathology codes. Cytopathology subsection codes are reported for various cytopathology procedures, as follows:

- Cytopathology collection methods (e.g., brushings, fluids, smears, washings)
- Cervical or vaginal cytopathology physician interpretation
- Cytopathological smears and cytopathology of fluids, washings or brushings from sources other than cervical or vaginal
- Cytohistologic studies of fine-needle aspirate
- Cervical and vaginal screening for cells collected in preservative fluid using an automated thin manual layer preparation.
- Flow cytometry tests

Pap smear (Figure 18-7) screening and physician interpretation using different methods for preparation, screening, and reporting are reported with cytopathology codes.

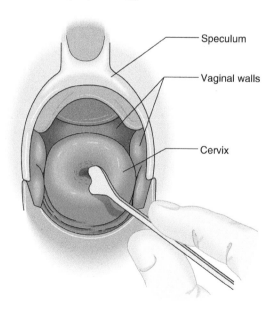

FIGURE 18-7 Performing a Pap smear

- Bethesda System of reporting
- Non-Bethesda reporting
- Thin-layer preparations
- Automated screening with any system of reporting

The **Bethesda System** is a format for reporting cervical/vaginal cytology that includes a state of specimen adequacy, the general category (e.g., if the specimen is within normal limits), and a descriptive diagnosis (e.g., benign cellular changes). (HCPCS Level II codes P3000 and P3001 for screening Papanicolaou smears also describe cytopathology services.)

 Coding Tip

Cytopathology notes provide instruction to report its codes in addition to the screening code when these additional services are provided.

- Cytopathology, cervical or vaginal (any reporting system), requiring interpretation by physician
- Cytopathology, slides, cervical or vaginal, definitive hormonal evaluation (e.g., maturation index, karyopyknotic index, estrogenic index) (List separately in addition to code[s] for other technical and interpretation services.)

Example: Cytopathology evaluation of fine-needle aspirate, interpretation, and report. Report code 88173.

Cytogenetic Studies

Cytogenetics is the study of the cell and its heredity-related components, including chromosomes. Cytogenetic studies are performed to study cellular ("cyto") structure and function related to heredity ("genetics"). They are performed based on the nature of the disorder for which the patient is being tested because the cell culture and analytical standards are disease dependent, not tissue dependent.

Example 1: Tissue culture for non-neoplastic disorders, lymphocyte. Report code 88230.

Example 2: Tissue culture for neoplastic disorders, solid tumor. Report code 88239.

Cryopreservation services are provided for the freezing, storage, and subsequent thawing of cells, as well as the expansion of established cell lines for subsequent laboratory testing. For some testing procedures (e.g., tests for genetic disorders), the cell line is frozen to preserve the culture, and subsequent thawing must be done before an analysis can be completed. (An **aliquot** is a portion of a specimen used for testing.)

Example 1: Cryopreservation, freezing and storage of cells, each cell line. Report code 88240.

Example 2: Thawing and expansion of frozen cells, each aliquot. Report code 88241.

White blood cells (e.g., T lymphocytes) are typically used as the specimen for chromosome analysis. *Chromosomal breakage syndromes* include genetic disorders that are usually transmitted in a genetic autosomal recessive mode. The syndromes are characterized by a defect in DNA repair mechanisms and a predisposition to cancer. Codes for chromosome analysis for breakage syndromes are described according to the

- Name of the specific syndrome being investigated (e.g., Fanconi anemia)
- Specific technique for analysis

Codes for cytogenetic studies describe the

- Type of tissue cultured
- Special culture techniques or treatments of the culture

- Numbers of cells studied and analyzed
- Special analysis techniques used

Thus, submitting a claim for a single cytogenetic study typically requires reporting three or more codes.

Example: Cytogenetic study of a standard karyotype on peripheral blood lymphocytes is reported with a code for lymphocyte culture (88230), a code for chromosome analysis counting 15 to 20 cells, two karyotypes with banding (88262), and a code to describe the physician work of interpretation and report of the cytogenetic testing performed (88291).

Molecular cytogenetics includes the **fluorescence *in situ* hybridization (FISH)** method, which is performed to detect submicroscopic changes in chromosomes (e.g., genetic disorders, such as Williams syndrome) or for identification of unknown chromosomal material. Chromosomal aberrations can also be identified using FISH analyses in patients with other constitutional or acquired (e.g., neoplastic) disorders.

Example: Molecular cytogenetics test, DNA probe fluorescent *in situ* hybridization (FISH) test. Report code 88271.

Surgical Pathology

Surgical pathology includes the gross and microscopic examination of specimens submitted for pathologic evaluation (Figure 18-8). (A *specimen* is tissue submitted to the pathology department for evaluation; it is also the unit of service used to report surgical pathology codes.) Surgical pathology levels of service are determined by the following:

- Type of exam

- Type of tissue

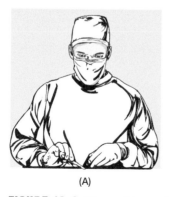
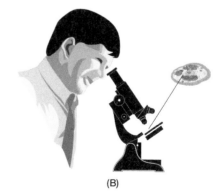

(A)   (B)

FIGURE 18-8 Tissue biopsy (A) A small piece of tissue is surgically removed (B) Pathologist views tissue under microscope, looking for presence of disease

When multiple individual tissue specimens are submitted from the same patient, a separate code is reported for each specimen.

> **Example:** Two separate frozen sections of breast tissue were evaluated by the pathologist during surgery. Report codes 88331 and 88332.

Surgical pathology instructional notes provide instruction that surgical pathology services include accession, examination, and reporting. *Accession* is the assignment of a number to record the order of tissue acquisition; an *accession number* is assigned to each pathology case (e.g., 05-00101 for the facility's 101st case in 2005).

Notes also identify and define the *specimen* as the unit of service for reporting surgical pathology codes. These codes are reported according to the extent and complexity of the evaluation.

- Level I surgical pathology code is reported for any specimen the examining pathologist believes can be accurately diagnosed *without* microscopic examination.
- Level II surgical pathology code is reported when gross *and* microscopic examination is performed to confirm identification of a specimen or the absence of disease.
- Level III through level VI codes are reported when gross and microscopic examinations are performed, and these codes describe levels of service for specimens that require increasingly complex levels of physician (pathologist) work, from lowest to highest, due to a presumed presence of disease. Code descriptions include specimen sites and specific types of disease.
  - Uncomplicated specimen (e.g., hemorrhoids)
  - Single complicated specimen (e.g., kidney resection)
  - Multiple complicated specimens (e.g., breast with regional lymph nodes)

> **Example:** Cervical carcinoma was diagnosed upon endocervical biopsy. Patient subsequently underwent a hysterectomy. Pathologist examined the endocervix and uterus. Codes 88305 and 88309 are reported whether or not residual cancer is found.

Pathology consultation services describe the opinion or advice about the presence or absence of diseased or abnormal tissue, as requested by another physician. The consulting pathologist prepares consultation reports and written interpretations about slides or other material received from another facility.

Pathology consultations performed during surgery are also interoperative pathology examinations that assist in determining an immediate surgical course (e.g., breast biopsy resulting in total mastectomy during same operative episode). Pathological consultations during surgery include macroscopic (gross) tissue reviews only, frozen sections, or cytological examinations.

> **Example:** A sigmoid colon biopsy is sent to the pathologist during surgery for immediate diagnosis. The pathologist examines the specimen and provides a pathological diagnosis of diverticulosis without microscopic examination of the tissue. Report code 88329.

In Vivo (e.g., Transcutaneous) Laboratory Procedures

The *in vivo* (e.g., transcutaneous) procedures describe bilirubin and hemoglobin tests.

 NOTE:

A total transcutaneous bilirubin test is usually performed on newborns to diagnose jaundice, and testing is done four times a day or more to monitor the condition and determine the efficiency of therapy.

> **Example:** Patient underwent total transcutaneous bilirubin test. Report code 88720.

Other Procedures

Other procedures include laboratory and pathology procedures that are not included in previous or subsequent Pathology and Laboratory categories.

> **Example:** Patient underwent sweat collection via iontophoresis. Report code 89230.

Reproductive Medicine Procedures

Reproductive medicine procedures include new technology and evolving reproductive medical practices such as the following:

- Oocyte/embryo culture and fertilization techniques
- Oocyte/embryo biopsy techniques
- Freezing, thawing, and storage techniques

(These procedures are performed in highly specialized clinical laboratories.)

When reporting the culture and fertilization of oocytes, report the appropriate code one time for the culture and fertilization, regardless of the number of eggs fertilized.

> **Example:** Patient underwent culture and fertilization of six embryos in less than four days. Report code 89250 just once.

Co-culture techniques performed on tissue cultures of human embryo, oviductal, uterine, granulosa, or other cells involve the isolation of the cells, culture, plating, and the co-culture of these cells with human embryos. This procedure may involve microscopic and cytochemical examination of culture cells to determine their viability or functionality.

The preparation of embryo for transfer, using any method, includes removing the embryo(s) from culture, preparing the embryo(s) for transfer, loading the embryo(s) into a catheter, transporting the embryo(s) to the transfer room for transfer to the patient, and examining the catheter after transfer to ensure that no embryo(s) are retained.

Coding Tip

Microtechnique is a micromanipulation technique used for preparing an embryo for transfer.

The preparation and examination of the oocyte prior to fertilization (e.g., stripping of the granulosa, cumulus oophorous, and corona radiation and verifying extrusion of the first polar body) are included in assisted oocyte fertilization procedures. Preparation and examination procedures are *not* separately coded and reported during oocyte fertilization.

Sperm identification and preparation prior to injection into the cytoplasm of the oocyte are coded and reported separately with sperm isolation and preparation codes, as appropriate.

NOTE:

Methods of assisted oocyte fertilization include the following:

- Intracytoplasmic sperm injection (ICSI)
- Subzonal insertion (SZI)
- Partial zona dissection (PZD)

Sperm identification from aspiration other than seminal fluid (e.g., from the vas deferens or epididymis) excludes identification of sperm from seminal fluid.

The work of identifying sperm does *not* include the work of assisted oocyte fertilization by any method (e.g., microtechnique), which is reported with a separate code.

> **Example 1:** Simple preparation sperm isolation procedure with semen analysis, in preparation for insemination. Report code 89260.

> **Example 2:** Assisted oocyte fertilization, microtechnique, nine oocytes. Report code 89280.

Proprietary Laboratory Analyses

Proprietary Laboratory Analysis (PLA) procedures include proprietary clinical laboratory analyses conducted by a single (sole-source) laboratory *or* licensed/marketed to multiple providing laboratories that are cleared/approved by the Food and Drug Administration (FDA). These advanced diagnostic laboratory tests (ADLTs) and clinical diagnostic laboratory tests (CDLTs) are defined under the Protecting Access to Medicare Act (PAMA) of 2014. The range of medical laboratory tests include multianalyte assays with algorithmic analyses (MAAA) and genomic sequencing procedures (GSPs). Codes in the Proprietary Laboratory Analyses subsection are released on a quarterly basis to expedite reporting, and they are published electronically at the AMA website (**www.ama-assn.org**).

> **Example:** Patient underwent proprietary laboratory analysis which included red blood cell antigen typing, DNA, human erythrocyte antigen gene analysis of 35 antigens from 11 blood groups, utilizing whole blood, and common RBC alleles. Report code 0001U.

Exercise 18.3 – Pathology and Laboratory Subsections

Instructions: Assign CPT code(s) and appropriate modifier(s) to each statement.

1. Physician orders a routine urinalysis to be completed by an outside lab.

   _____

2. Quantitative therapeutic drugs assay to determine lithium level. Routine venipuncture.

   _____

3. Organ or disease-oriented panel for electrolytes.

   _____

4. Patient underwent surgery to remove a basal cell carcinoma, which was submitted to the pathologist intraoperatively for diagnosis and evaluation of adequacy of the surgical margins. Intraoperative surgical pathology consultation included one basal cell carcinoma tissue block specimen, which required frozen section to confirm the adequacy of excision.

   _____

5. The physician's office staff performed a urine pregnancy test using dipstick reagents that chemically react with urine. A change in color indicated positive findings and the presence of hormones found in the urine of women in early pregnancy.

   _____

6. Specimen collection via arterial puncture and blood gas determination (pH only).

   _____

7. Organ or disease-oriented lipid panel and blood sodium test.

   _____

(continues)

Exercise 18.3 – continued

8. A sigmoid colon biopsy specimen was sent for surgical pathology, gross and microscopic examination.

_____

9. Reptilase test.

_____

10. C-reactive protein test.

_____

11. T-cell count test using flow cytometry.

_____

12. Serologic blood typing, Rh (D) factor.

_____

13. Bacteria culture, urine, for quantitative colony count.

_____

14. Autopsy, gross and microscopic examination, including brain and spinal cord.

_____

15. Antibody identification test for leukocyte antibodies.

_____

16. Transcutaneous quantitative hemoglobin (Hgb) in vivo lab test.

_____

17. Caffeine halothane contracture test (CHCT) for malignant hyperthermia susceptibility, including interpretation and report.

_____

18. Agar antibiotic sensitivity study to assess whether methicillin would be effective for a patient diagnosed with a staphylococcal B infection.

_____

19. Collection of sweat from a patient via iontophoresis to rule out cystic fibrosis.

_____

20. Cryopreservation of an embryo.

_____

Summary

CPT pathology and laboratory codes describe services performed on specimens (e.g., body fluids, tissue, or cytological specimens) to evaluate, prevent, diagnose, or treat a disease. Most clinical laboratory service codes include a technical component, and some include both a technical and a professional component. The Pathology and Laboratory section is organized according to type of procedure performed, and procedures are listed alphabetically within each subsection. Because many laboratory and pathology tests can be performed using different methods, patient record documentation must be reviewed along with code descriptions and instructional notes. Guidelines located at the beginning of the Pathology and Laboratory section provide instruction about services in pathology and laboratory, separate or multiple procedures, subsection information, unlisted services or procedures, and special reports.

Internet Links

Clinical Laboratory Improvement Amendments (CLIA): Go to **www.cdc.gov/clia**

National Coverage Determinations for Laboratory Services: Go to **www.cms.gov**, click on the Medicare link, then scroll down to the Coverage heading, click on the Medicare Coverage - General Information link, click on the Medicare Coverage Center link located below the Related Links heading, click on the Lab NCDs – ICD-10 link, and scroll down and click on the Index of Lab NCDs link to view them.

Review

18.1 – Multiple Choice

Instructions: Select the most appropriate response.

1. Coders usually do not assign codes to pathology and laboratory procedures that are performed on an _____ basis because such services do not impact _____ assignment and facility reimbursement.
   a. inpatient, diagnosis-related group (DRG)
   b. inpatient, prospective payment system (PPS)
   c. outpatient, diagnosis-related group (DRG)
   d. outpatient, prospective payment system (PPS)

2. CPT Pathology and Laboratory section codes describe the _____ of laboratory and pathology services.
   a. conveyance of blood and other fluid samples
   b. performance, collection, and clinical consultation
   c. specimen handling by an outside laboratory
   d. transportation to a local hospital laboratory

3. Which modifier is added to pathology and laboratory codes when procedures or services are repeated on the same date of service to obtain multiple results?
   a. 59   c. 91
   b. 90   d. QW

4. When an unlisted procedure or service code is reported, what is attached to the submitted claim to clarify the service or procedure performed?
   a. Authentication number   c. Special report
   b. Copy of entire patient record   d. Verification code

5. Which subsection of Pathology and Laboratory contains codes that are often reported by blood banks?
   a. Drug Testing and Therapeutic Drug Assays
   b. Hematology and Coagulation
   c. Other Procedures
   d. Transfusion Medicine

6. Which is a substance administered with an antigen to enhance the response to the antigen?
   a. Adjuvant   c. Assay
   b. Aliquot   d. Specimen

7. IgA, IgD, IgE, IgG, and IgM are considered
   a. analytes.   c. immunoglobulins.
   b. antigens.   d. specimens.

8. Physician attendance and monitoring during evocative or suppressive agent testing is reported with codes from the _____ section.
   a. Clinical Pathology Consultation
   b. Evaluation and Management
   c. Medicine
   d. Surgery

9. Which is the study of diseased cells?
   a. Cytology
   b. Cytopathology
   c. Immunology
   d. Pathology

10. Codes from the _____ subsection of Pathology and Laboratory are reported for tests performed to study cellular structure and function related to heredity.
    a. Anatomical Pathology
    b. Cytogenetic Studies
    c. Cytopathology
    d. Organ or Disease-Oriented Panels

11. A patient presents with symptoms of dehydration. The physician ordered an electrolyte panel, which included carbon dioxide (bicarbonate), chloride, potassium, and sodium. Which CPT code(s) are assigned?
    a. 80047
    b. 80048
    c. 80051
    d. 80053

12. Routine urinalysis. Which CPT code is assigned?
    a. 81000
    b. 81001
    c. 81002
    d. 81003

13. Qualitative fetal hemoglobin. Which CPT code is assigned?
    a. 83030
    b. 83033
    c. 83036
    d. 83045

14. Qualitative analysis of organic acids, three specimens. Which CPT code(s) are assigned?
    a. 83919
    b. 83919, 83919, 83919
    c. 83919, 83919 51, 83919 51
    d. 83919, 83919 91, 83919 91

15. Alkaline phosphatase isoenzymes. Which CPT code is assigned?
    a. 84060
    b. 84075
    c. 84078
    d. 84080

16. CBC, automated, including Hgb, Hct, RBC, WBC, and platelet count. Which CPT code(s) are assigned?
    a. 85004, 85014
    b. 85025
    c. 85027
    d. 85032

17. ABO, Rh, and MN blood typing for paternity testing. Which CPT code is assigned?
    a. 86900
    b. 86901
    c. 86905
    d. 86910

18. Thromboplastin time, partial (PTT) in plasma. Which CPT code is assigned?
    a. 85347
    b. 85670
    c. 85730
    d. 85732

19. RBC antibody screen, two different serum techniques. Which CPT code(s) are assigned?
    a. 86850
    b. 86850, 86850
    c. 86850, 86850 51
    d. 86850, 86850 91

20. *Chlamydia* culture. Which CPT code is assigned?
    a. 87110
    b. 87270
    c. 87487
    d. 87810

18.2 – Coding Practice: Pathology and Laboratory Section

Instructions: Assign CPT code(s) and appropriate modifier(s) to each case.

1. ORGAN OR DISEASE-ORIENTED PANELS: A patient's blood is sent for obstetric panel testing, and the following tests were performed as a result: automated CBC, automated differential WBC, HBsAg, rubella antibody, qualitative syphilis test, RBC antibody screen, ABO blood typing, and Rh (D) blood typing.

   _____

2. ORGAN OR DISEASE-ORIENTED PANELS: A patient's blood is sent for the following tests: albumin, total calcium, carbon dioxide (bicarbonate), chloride, creatinine, glucose, phosphorus inorganic (phosphate), potassium, sodium, and urea nitrogen (BUN). Automated CBC was also performed.

   _____

3. URINALYSIS: Urinalysis, automated with identification of sediments via microscope.

   _____

4. OTHER PROCEDURES: Sperm isolation procedure including sperm wash and complete semen analysis.

   _____

5. EVOCATIVE/SUPPRESSION TESTING: Patient underwent combined rapid anterior pituitary evaluation panel, which included ACTH, LH, FSH, prolactin, HGH, cortisol, and TSH testing. Intramuscular injection of protirelin (Thyrel thyrotropin-releasing hormone, TRH) 250 mg as the suppressive agent. (In addition to the Pathology and Laboratory code, assign a code from the Medicine section for intramuscular injection and a code from the HCPCS Level II J Codes Drugs section for supply of protirelin.)

   _____

6. MICROBIOLOGY: Microorganism antigen detection by immunofluorescent technique of primary source for _Bordetella pertussis_.

   _____

7. CHEMISTRY: _Helicobacter pylori_ blood test.

   _____

8. HEMATOLOGY AND COAGULATION: Blood cell count for hematocrit level.

   _____

9. CHEMISTRY: Direct measurement of blood gases, O_2 saturation level.

   _____

10. SURGICAL PATHOLOGY: Intraoperative surgical pathology consultation of breast tissue, single specimen, with frozen section. Pathological diagnosis was adenocarcinoma. After partial mastectomy, breast tissue was submitted for surgical pathology gross and microscopic examination, level V. (Do not code the mastectomy.)

    _____

11. MICROBIOLOGY: Tissue examination by KOH slide to detect fungi, nails.

    _____

12. CHEMISTRY: Testing of blood for level of TSH and thyroid hormone (T3) uptake.

    _____

13. DRUG ASSAY: Urine sample used to perform drug screening using a chromatographic method.

    _____

14. IMMUNOLOGY: Blood test for antinuclear antibodies (ANA) to rule out SLE.

_____

15. IMMUNOLOGY: Lymphocytotoxicity assay, visual crossmatch, with titration.

_____

16. IMMUNOLOGY: *Shigella* antibody titer testing of blood sample.

_____

17. MICROBIOLOGY: Infectious agent genotype analysis by nucleic acid (DNA) for cytomegalovirus.

_____

18. TRANSFUSION MEDICINE: Coombs test for RBC antibody screen using the microtiter plates serum technique.

_____

19. SURGICAL PATHOLOGY: Gross and microscopic pathology examination of nasal mucosa tissue (submitted by surgeon after nasal mucosa biopsy).

_____

20. *IN VIVO* LABORATORY PROCEDURES: Total bilirubin, transcutaneous, *in vivo* lab test.

_____

21. REPRODUCTIVE MEDICINE PROCEDURES: Preparation of embryo for transfer via catheter.

_____

22. CHEMISTRY: Radioimmunoassay of blood for total prostate specific antigen (PSA).

_____

23. CONSULTATIONS (CLINICAL PATHOLOGY): Clinical pathology consultation, limited review of patient records, straightforward decision making, requiring 15 minutes.

_____

24. SURGICAL PATHOLOGY: Gross and microscopic examination of tissue resulting from Dupuytren's contracture surgery.

_____

25. MOLECULAR PATHOLOGY: Gene analysis to detect abnormal atrophin 1 (ATN1) alleles for confirmation of dentatorubral-pallidoluysian atrophy (DRPLA) condition.

_____

26. CYTOPATHOLOGY: Cervical Pap smear using Bethesda System with manual screening and computer-assisted rescreening under physician supervision.

_____

27. CYTOGENIC STUDIES: Bone marrow tissue culture for neoplastic disorder.

_____

28. OTHER PROCEDURES: Specimen of knee joint synovial fluid for cell count.

_____

29. GENOMIC SEQUENCING PROCEDURES AND OTHER MOLECULAR MULTIANALYTE ASSAYS: Genomic sequencing analysis panel of all required genes completed to detect aortic dysfunction or dilation condition.

_____

30. PROPRIETARY LABORATORY ANALYSES: Proprietary laboratory analysis syphilis test, non-treponemal antibody, immunoassay, qualitative rapid plasma reagin (RPR).

_____

Chapter Outline

Overview of Medicine Section

Medicine Section Guidelines

Medicine Subsections

Chapter Objectives

At the conclusion of this chapter, the student should be able to:

1. Define key terms related to the CPT Medicine Section.
2. Summarize the organization, format, and content of the CPT Medicine section.
3. Interpret the CPT Medicine Section guidelines.
4. Assign codes from the subsections of CPT Medicine.

Key Terms

adjuvant chemotherapy

allergen

allergen immunotherapy

allergy sensitivity test

autonomic function test

biofeedback

cardiac catheterization

cardiography

chemotherapy

chiropractic manipulative
    treatment (CMT)

duplex scan

echocardiography

electrocardiography

electromyography

gamma globulin

hemodialysis

immune globulin (Ig)

immune serum globulin

intradermal test
    (intracutaneous)

intravenous push

manometry

minimally invasive
    procedure

multiple sleep latency

narcosynthesis

needle
    electromyography

noninvasive procedure

oscilloscope

osteopathic manipulative
    treatment (OMT)

patch test
    (epicutaneous)

peritoneal dialysis

pharmacologic
    management

physiatrist

physical medicine and
    rehabilitation

polysomnography

psychotherapy

puncture, prick,
    or scratch test
    (percutaneous)

renal dialysis

sleep laboratory

sleep staging

sleep study

Introduction

The Medicine section is the last section of CPT, and its codes for noninvasive or minimally invasive diagnostic and therapeutic procedures and services can be reported along with those from all other sections.

 NOTE:

The *Medicare National Correct Coding Initiative Policy Manual* provides guidance about assigning procedure and service codes for the Medicine section. Go to **www.cms.gov** and enter "Medicare NCCI Policy Manual" in the Search box to navigate to the manual.

Overview of Medicine Section

The Medicine section includes codes for procedures and services that apply to various medical specialties (e.g., gastroenterology, ophthalmology, otorhinolaryngology, and psychiatry) and different types of health care providers (e.g., physical therapists, occupational therapists). Medicine section procedures are *noninvasive* or *minimally invasive* diagnostic and therapeutic procedures and services. **Noninvasive procedures** require no surgical incision or excision, and they are not open procedures. **Minimally invasive procedures** include percutaneous access. Medicine is the last section of CPT, and its codes can be reported along with those from all other sections.

 NOTE:

When included in CPT, the Other Procedures code is reported for an unlisted procedure performed on the anatomical site. When reporting an unlisted procedure code, include documentation about the procedure performed with the submitted claim.

Exercise 19.1 – Overview of Medicine Section

Instructions: Complete each statement.

1. When no surgical incision or excision is required to perform a procedure, it is considered _____, as opposed to invasive.

2. Percutaneous access procedures are considered minimally _____, as opposed to noninvasive.

3. Codes from the Medicine section _____ (can/cannot) be reported with codes from other CPT sections.

4. The CPT Medicine section contains codes for diagnostic and _____ procedures and services.

5. The CPT Medicine section includes procedures and services that apply to various medical _____ and different types of health care providers.

Medicine Section Guidelines

Guidelines located at the beginning of the Medicine section provide instruction about the following:

- Add-on codes
- Separate procedures
- Unlisted service or procedure
- Special report
- Imaging guidance
- Supplied materials
- Foreign Body/Implant Definition

Instructional notes appear throughout the Medicine section to provide coding clarification and direction. Almost every Medicine subsection contains notes unique to that subsection.

Add-On Codes

Add-on codes are reported for procedures and services performed in *addition* to a *primary procedure*. Modifiers 50 (bilateral procedure) and 51 (multiple procedures) are not reported with add-on codes; instead, report the add-on code twice for a bilateral procedure. They are identified in the CPT with a plus symbol (✚). A parenthetical note located below an add-on code identifies the primary procedure to which an add-on code applies.

> **Example:** A six-year-old patient received the DTaP (diphtheria, tetanus toxoids, acellular pertussis) vaccine with physician counseling, for which codes 90460, 90461, 90461, and 90700 are reported. (Do not add modifier 51 to code 90461 or 90700.)

Separate Procedures

Some procedures and services located in the Medicine section are considered an integral component of a complete procedure or service, and they are identified by the description "separate procedure." Do not report a "separate procedure" code in addition to a code for the comprehensive (or complete) procedure *unless the "separate procedure" is performed independently or is distinct from other services provided at the same time.*

When a "separate procedure" is performed independently or is distinct from other services provided at the same time, add modifier 59 (Distinct Procedural Service) to the "separate procedure" code. Modifier 59 indicates that the procedure was performed as a distinct, independent procedure.

> **Example:** Patient underwent orthoptic training and gonioscopy, performed by a physician. Report codes 92065 and 92020 59.

Bundled CPT Medicine Section Codes

When reporting codes for outpatient hospital services and physician office services, use outpatient code editor (OCE) software or national correct coding initiative (NCCI) software to identify bundled codes for procedures and services considered necessary to accomplish the major procedure. Bundled procedure and services codes are *not* separately coded and reported with the major procedure code. Reporting the component codes in addition to the major procedure code is considered *unbundling*, which is fraud.

> **Example:** Patient underwent a stress test. Report code 93015. (Do *not* report codes 93016, 93017, and/or 93018 with code 93015. Doing so is considered unbundling.)

Multiple CPT Medicine Section Codes

When multiple procedures and/or services are performed on the same date, report a separate code for each procedure and/or service.

> **Example:** An established patient received 60 minutes of outpatient individual psychotherapy, and after psychotherapy the psychologist prepared a mandatory progress report and submitted it to the third-party payer. Report codes 90837 and 90889.

Unlisted Service or Procedure

CPT unlisted procedure and service codes are assigned when there is no specific code that accurately describes the procedure or service performed. When reporting an unlisted procedure code to a third-party payer, submit a written report (e.g., a copy of an operative report) that describes the procedure or service performed.

Special Report

When an unlisted procedure or service code is reported to a third-party payer, a special report is submitted that describes the procedure or service performed. Special reports may also be required for procedures and services that are rarely provided or are new in order to establish that the procedure is necessary. As a minimum, documentation in a special report includes an adequate definition or description of the nature, extent, and need for the procedure or service; and the time, effort, and equipment necessary to provide the procedure or service.

Additional items may also be documented in a special report including complexity of symptoms, concurrent problems, diagnostic and therapeutic procedures, final diagnosis, follow-up care, and pertinent physical findings.

Imaging Guidance

When imaging guidance or imaging supervision and interpretation is performed as part of a Medicine procedure, the Radiology guidelines apply.

Supplied Materials

Supplies and materials provided by the physician (e.g., drugs or sterile trays) other than those typically included with a procedure or service are reported separately. Report CPT code 99070 or a specific HCPCS Level II code for materials and supplies provided.

> **Example:** Patient underwent chemotherapy administration (intramuscular) of vincristine sulfate, 1 mg. Report CPT code 96401 and HCPCS Level II code J9370. (HCPCS Level II code J9370 is more specific than CPT code 99070, which is a nonspecific supplies and materials code.)

Foreign Body/Implant Definition

An object that is intentionally placed into the patient is considered an implant while an object that is unintentionally placed (due to ingestion or trauma) is considered a foreign body. However, when an implant shifts from its original position or becomes broken, it is considered a foreign body for coding purposes (especially when it becomes a hazard to a patient). The exception is when CPT coding instructions provide guidance to specific codes that describe the removal of a shifted or broken implant.

Exercise 19.2 – Medicine Section Guidelines

Instructions: Complete each statement.

1. Instructional _____ appear throughout the Medicine section to provide coding clarification and direction.
2. When multiple procedures and/or services are performed on the same date, report a(n) _____ code for each procedure and/or service documented.
3. Add-on codes are reported for procedures and services performed in addition to a primary procedure, and they are identified in CPT with a(n) _____ symbol.
4. Some procedures and services located in the Medicine section are considered an integral component of a complete procedure or service, and they are identified by the description "_____ procedure."
5. Supplies and materials provided by the physician, other than those typically included with a procedure or service, are reported with CPT code 99070 or a specific HCPCS Level _____ code for materials and supplies provided.

Medicine Subsections

Medicine subsections include the following:

- Immune globulins, serum or recombinant products
- Immunization administration for vaccines/toxoids
- Vaccines, toxoids
- Psychiatry
- Biofeedback
- Dialysis
- Gastroenterology
- Ophthalmology
- Special otorhinolaryngological services

- Cardiovascular
- Noninvasive vascular diagnostic studies
- Pulmonary
- Allergy and clinical immunology
- Endocrinology
- Neurology and neuromuscular procedures
- Medical genetics and genetic counseling services
- Adaptive behavior services
- Central nervous system assessments/tests (e.g., neurocognitive, mental status, speech testing)
- Health behavior assessment and intervention
- Behavior management services
- Hydration, therapeutic, prophylactic, diagnostic injections and infusions, and chemotherapy and other highly complex drug or highly complex biologic agent administration

- Photodynamic therapy
- Special dermatological procedures
- Physical medicine and rehabilitation
- Medical nutrition therapy
- Acupuncture
- Osteopathic manipulative treatment
- Chiropractic manipulative treatment
- Education and training for patient self-management
- Non-face-to-face nonphysician services
- Special services, procedures, and reports
- Qualifying circumstances for anesthesia
- Moderate (conscious) sedation
- Other services and procedures
- Home health procedures/services
- Medication therapy management services

Immune Globulins, Serum or Recombinant Products

An **immune globulin (Ig)** (**gamma globulin** or **immune serum globulin**) is a sterilized solution obtained from pooled human blood plasma, which contains immunoglobulins (or antibodies) that protect against infectious agents that cause various diseases. (Antibodies are substances in blood plasma that fight infection.) Immune globulins are administered to patients who need to use someone else's antibodies to help fight off or prevent illnesses from occurring. Ig formulations produced from donors include high levels of antibodies against hepatitis B (hepatitis B immune globulin-HBIG), rabies (rabies immune globulin-RIG), tetanus (tetanus immune globulin-TIG), and varicella (chicken pox; varicella zoster immune globulin-VZIG).

 NOTE:

The administration of an Ig provides temporary protection and is *not* considered an immunization, which provides longer-term protection.

Immune globulin codes are reported for the *supply of the immune globulin product*, which includes broad-spectrum and anti-infective immune globulins, antitoxins, and other isoantibodies. The *administration* of an immune globulin is reported separately with a code from the Therapeutic, Prophylactic, and Diagnostic Injections and Infusions subsection of the Medicine section.

 Coding Tip

Modifier 51 (Multiple procedures) is *not* reported with Immune Globulins, Serum, or Recombinant Products codes when performed with another procedure.

- Intravenous infusion
- Subcutaneous infusion
- Intramuscular or subcutaneous injection
- Intravenous push

Example: Intramuscular injection of 250 units of human tetanus immune globulin (TIg) was administered to a patient. Report codes 96372 and 90389.

Immunization Administration for Vaccines/Toxoids

Immunization administration for vaccines/toxoids codes are reported in addition to codes from the Medicine subsection entitled *Vaccines, Toxoids*. (When a significant separately identifiable E/M service is also provided, report an appropriate code from the CPT E/M section in addition to the immunization administration for vaccines/toxoids codes.) The immunization administration for vaccines/toxoids include the following:

- Administrative staff services (e.g., appointment scheduling, preparing a patient's record, and submitting an insurance claim to a payer)
- Clinical staff services (e.g., taking vital signs, assessing past reactions and contraindications, preparing and administering the vaccine/toxoid, monitoring reactions, and documenting in the record)

The following types of immunization administration for vaccines/toxoids are reported:

- Intradermal, intramuscular, percutaneous, and subcutaneous injections
- Intranasal and oral administration

The immunization administration of *pediatric* vaccines/toxoids with counseling by a physician or other qualified health care professional is reported to accurately describe the work involved, which includes patient/family counseling provided by the physician during the administration of a vaccine/toxoid. The codes are reported for each component of the vaccine(s) administered.

Example: A six-year-old patient received immunization administration (intramuscular injection) of the MMR (measles, mumps, rubella) vaccine. Physician discussed the vaccine composition with the patient's mother, including risks and benefits. Report codes 90460, 90461, 90461, and 90707.

Coding Tip

- Report immunization administration for vaccines/toxoids codes in addition to vaccine/toxoid codes.
- Do not report immunization administration codes for the administration of allergy injections or testing, chemotherapy, placement of catheters, transfusions, or venipuncture. Refer to the appropriate Surgery or Medicine subsection for reporting such codes.

Vaccines, Toxoids

Vaccines/toxoids codes identify the vaccine/toxoid product only. They are reported with immunization administration for vaccines/toxoids codes.

Example: An 18-year-old patient received immunization administration (subcutaneous injection) of an MMR booster. Report codes 90471 and 90707.

Coding Tip

- Do not add modifier 51 (Multiple Procedures) to vaccines/toxoids or immunization administration for vaccines/toxoids codes.
- When vaccines/toxoids codes are reported during an E/M preventive medicine encounter, add modifier 25 to the evaluation and management code.
- New vaccines have been approved for use by the Food and Drug Administration (FDA) over recent years. CPT created a new symbol (✔) to indicate that FDA approval is pending, which means it is anticipated that the vaccines will receive FDA approval, but that approval was pending at the time of publication. Once the vaccine is approved by the FDA, the symbol will be removed.

Reporting Evaluation and Management Service Codes with Immunization Administration and Vaccines/Toxoids Codes

There is considerable confusion regarding whether a provider should report an evaluation and management (E/M) service for an encounter for immunization administration of vaccines/toxoids. Correct coding depends on whether the provider performed a medically necessary E/M service *in addition to the immunization administration*. To assign an E/M code in addition to the immunization administration code, the E/M service must exceed services included with immunization administration codes.

 NOTE:

Reporting E/M service code 99211 does not require the presence of the physician or the documentation of key components.

Example: Physician provided a level 3 E/M service to a 48-year-old established patient to medically manage hypertension. During the same encounter, the physician administered a flu shot (influenza vaccine, inactivated [IIV], subunit, adjuvanted, intramuscular injection). Report codes 99213 25, 90471, and 90653.

Psychiatry

Psychiatrists, psychologists, and licensed clinical social workers report psychiatry codes for psychotherapy services, which include the following:

- Interactive complexity
- Psychiatric diagnostic procedures
  - Psychotherapy
  - Other psychotherapy
  - Other psychiatric services or procedures

 Coding Tip

- Psychiatric evaluation and management (E/M) services are reported by physicians, nurse practitioners, and physician assistants. Psychologists and licensed clinical social workers do not report codes from the CPT E/M section.

- Psychiatric consultation includes examination of the patient, exchange of information with the primary care physician or other pertinent individuals (e.g., family members and caretakers), and preparation of reports. Because no psychiatric treatment is provided during a psychiatric consultation, report the appropriate evaluation and management consultation code.

Interactive Complexity

Interactive complexity refers to specific communication factors that complicate the delivery of a psychiatric procedure, such as difficult communication with verbally undeveloped patients. The interactive complexity code is reported as an add-on code in addition to codes for diagnostic psychiatric evaluation, psychotherapy, psychotherapy performed with evaluation and management, and group psychology.

Psychiatric Diagnostic Procedures

Psychiatric diagnostic evaluation services include documentation of the patient's history, mental status, and recommendations. Evaluation may also include communication with the patient's family and others, along with review and ordering of diagnostic studies.

> **Example:** Patient received interactive psychiatric diagnostic interview examination services as the result of the parents finding out that patient was being routinely bullied at elementary school. Report code 90791.

Psychotherapy

Psychotherapy is the treatment of mental illness and behavioral disturbances in which the provider uses definitive therapeutic communication in an attempt to alleviate emotional disturbances, reverse or change maladaptive patterns of behavior, and encourage personality growth and development.

> **Example:** Patient underwent 30 minutes of psychotherapy. Report code 90832.

Other Psychotherapy

Psychotherapy for crisis involves an urgent assessment and history of a patient's crisis state, which is typically life threatening or complex, requiring immediate attention to a patient in high distress. A mental status exam and disposition is included, and treatment consists of psychotherapy, mobilization of resources to defuse the crisis and restore safety, and implementation of psychotherapeutic interventions to minimize the potential for psychological trauma.

Psychoanalysis attempts to gain insight into a patient's motivations and conflicts to change maladaptive behavior (e.g., an inability to cope with the challenges of everyday living). The psychoanalysis code is reported on a per-day basis. Do not confuse psychoanalysis and psychotherapy codes. The psychoanalysis code refers to the practice of psychoanalysis (e.g., patient is treated by a physician who is credentialed to practice analytic therapy, and psychoanalysis is the treatment being used).

Family psychotherapy involves the patient's family in the treatment process, and the dynamics within the family are the focus of the psychotherapeutic sessions. Family psychotherapy may be performed with or without the patient present. Codes reported are based on whether the patient is present or not and whether multiple family groups are being treated.

> **Example:** Psychotherapy was provided on May 5 to the families of three different patients who reside in a drug treatment center. Report code 90849 on the insurance claim for *each* patient.

Other Psychiatric Services or Procedures

Other psychiatric services or procedures include the following:

- Pharmacologic management
- Narcosynthesis for psychiatric diagnostic and therapeutic purposes
- Therapeutic repetitive transcranial magnetic stimulation (TMS) treatment
- Electroconvulsive therapy
- Individual psychophysiological therapy incorporating biofeedback training
- Hypnotherapy
- Environmental intervention for medical management
- Psychiatric evaluation of hospital records
- Interpretation or explanation of psychiatric examination/procedure results
- Preparation of report of patient's psychiatric status, history, treatment, or progress for the benefit of other physicians, agencies, or third-party payers

Pharmacologic management is the evaluation of a patient's medications for effect (such as a patient's reaction to medication), proper dosage (e.g., a therapeutic dose), and renewal of prescribed medications. Pharmacologic management is provided by a physician (such as a psychiatrist) to a patient who undergoes psychotherapy from a nonphysician colleague (e.g., a psychologist or a licensed clinical social worker) or when a patient's condition is being effectively treated by psychotropic drugs alone. Generally, the patient does not receive other services from the physician during the encounter. When an evaluation and management (E/M) service is provided by the physician or other qualified health care professional, the pharmacologic management is included in the E/M service. It is not coded and reported separately. (The psychotherapy provided during pharmacologic management is minimal and is also not coded or reported separately.)

Narcosynthesis is a form of psychotherapy that is provided when the patient is under the influence of a drug, such as a sedative or narcotic (e.g., a barbiturate, benzodiazepine-type drug that is administered intravenously). The administration of a medication to release inhibitions allows a patient to discuss issues that are too difficult to verbalize otherwise.

Electroconvulsive therapy is used to treat depression or life-threatening psychosis (e.g., severe affective disorders or schizophrenia) and involves the application of electric current to the brain through scalp electrodes. The term *electroconvulsive* refers to a convulsive response to an electrical stimulus. In electroconvulsive therapy, it is necessary to monitor the patient (e.g., management of the seizure, observation, and decisions regarding further treatment). If the psychiatrist also administers anesthesia for the electroconvulsive therapy, report the appropriate anesthesia code (00104), which includes cardiac and oxygen saturation monitoring.

> **Example:** Patient underwent narcosynthesis for psychiatric diagnostic and therapeutic purposes. Amytal (amobarbital), 125 milligrams was injected prior to therapy. Report codes 90865, 96372, and J0300.

Biofeedback

Biofeedback is a technique that trains the patient to gain some control over autonomic body functions. Biofeedback services include the following:

- Reviewing the patient's history
- Preparing the biofeedback equipment
- Placing electrodes on the patient

- Reading and interpreting responses
- Monitoring the patient
- Controlling muscle responses

 Coding Tip

During individual psychophysiological therapy that incorporates biofeedback training, a separate biofeedback training code is *not* reported.

The code for biofeedback services may include different types of administration (e.g., electromyogram application), and it is intended to identify all methods of biofeedback provided, even when more than one modality is performed during the same session. Electromyogram is a nerve conduction study that plots the electrical activity produced by muscle contractions. **Manometry** is a diagnostic test that measures muscle function using a pressure-sensitive tube.

> **Example 1:** Patient underwent 15 minutes biofeedback of perineal muscles for bladder training to prevent urinary incontinence. Treatment included use of manometry. Report code 90912.

> **Example 2:** Patient underwent 30 minutes of individual psychophysiological therapy that included biofeedback training and behavior-modifying psychotherapy. Report code 90875. (Do *not* report a code for biofeedback training.)

Dialysis

The Dialysis subsection includes the following:

- Hemodialysis
- Miscellaneous dialysis procedures

- End-stage renal disease services
- Other dialysis procedures

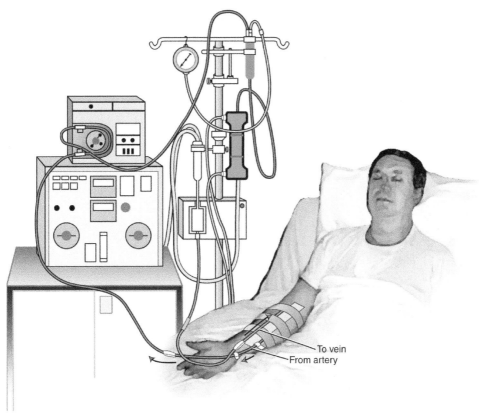

FIGURE 19-1 Hemodialysis filters waste from the patient's blood. Blood leaves the body via an artery, is filtered, and then is returned into a vein

Renal dialysis artificially removes toxic waste products from the body when the patient's kidneys are unable to perform this function because of disease or deterioration. Dialysis is used for acute, temporary kidney failure (e.g., acute renal failure) or chronic renal failure (e.g., end-stage renal disease). The following types of dialysis are used, depending on the patient's condition and whether the patient is experiencing acute or chronic renal failure:

- **Hemodialysis**: Process of removing waste products, toxins, and excess fluids from the blood; patient's blood is diverted into a dialyzer, where it is treated and returned into the patient's circulation by another tube inserted into a different blood vessel (Figure 19-1)

- **Peritoneal dialysis**: Soft catheter is inserted into abdominal cavity and dialysate fluid is infused at intermittent times

 Coding Tip

All evaluation and management (E/M) services related to end-stage renal disease (ESRD) and rendered during dialysis are included in the dialysis procedure code. An E/M service related to ESRD performed on the day of dialysis is not separately coded and reported. When the patient receives E/M services for a completely different condition that is not related to ESRD, report an appropriate E/M service code and add modifier 25 (significant, separately identifiable E/M service by the same physician on the same day as the procedure or other service).

Hemodialysis

Hemodialysis service codes include all E/M services related to the patient's renal disease *on the day of the hemodialysis procedure.* These codes are reported when hemodialysis services are provided to ESRD and non-ESRD patients in an inpatient setting and to non-ESRD patients in an outpatient setting.

Example: A 54-year-old patient was admitted as a hospital inpatient for treatment of ESRD. Admission date was August 5, and discharge date was August 10. The patient underwent hemodialysis procedures on August 5, 7, and 9, which included evaluation by the attending physician. Report codes 90935, 90935, and 90935. (Attending physician should report appropriate inpatient evaluation and management service codes with modifier 25 for provision of services unrelated to ESRD and the hemodialysis procedure on those dates. For other dates, such as August 6, 8, and 10, the attending physician should report appropriate inpatient E/M service codes for daily care and discharge services.)

Miscellaneous Dialysis Procedures

Miscellaneous dialysis procedures codes include peritoneal dialysis, hemofiltration, and other continuous renal replacement therapies (for single physician evaluation or repeated physician evaluations).

Example: Patient underwent peritoneal dialysis, which required repeated physician evaluations on the same date of treatment. Report code 90947.

End-Stage Renal Disease (ESRD) Services

ESRD services are typically performed as outpatient procedures, they are age-related, and reimbursement is usually made according to a monthly capitated payment method.

NOTE:

A *capitated payment method* is the result of an agreement between a third-party payer and a health care provider in which the provider agrees to provide services to a patient in return for a fixed monthly payment.

- ESRD services codes are reported *once per month per patient* (every 30 days). The appropriate code is reported just once, at the conclusion of a full month of ESRD services.

  Example: A 48-year-old patient received ESRD-related services two times each week during the entire month of June. Report code 90960.

- ESRD service codes can also be reported when less than a *full month of services* are provided to a patient. The appropriate code is reported for each day of service (e.g., when a patient requires less than a month's ESRD services after inpatient hospitalization).

  Example: A 54-year-old patient was hospitalized for ESRD from July 5 to July 20, and upon discharge received outpatient ESRD services on July 22, 24, 26, 28, and 30. Report codes 90970, 90970, 90970, 90970, and 90970 for outpatient ESRD services.

Coding Tip

- For patients under 20 years of age, ESRD codes include monitoring of nutrition, assessment of growth and development, and parental counseling.
- ESRD codes include physician services related to establishing a dialyzing cycle, evaluation and management of the dialysis visits, and patient management during the dialysis, provided during a full month.

Other Dialysis Procedures

Other dialysis procedures include dialysis training (e.g., completed course of training, an individual training session), hemoperfusion (e.g., using activated charcoal or resin), and unlisted dialysis procedures (inpatient or outpatient).

> **Example:** Patient completed an entire course of outpatient dialysis training during the month of June. Report code 90989.

Exercise 19.3 – Immune Globulin Products, Immunizations, Psychiatry, Biofeedback, and Dialysis

Instructions: Assign CPT code(s) and appropriate modifier(s) to each statement.

1. IMMUNE GLOBULINS, SERUM, OR RECOMBINANT PRODUCTS: Intramuscular injection, rabies immune globulin (RIg), human.

2. IMMUNIZATION ADMINISTRATION FOR VACCINES/TOXOIDS: Oral immunization administration, 2-dose rotavirus vaccine. Patient is 18 months old.

3. PSYCHIATRY: A 60-minute individual psychotherapy session provided via synchronous real-time telemedicine using audio video teleconference software.

4. BIOFEEDBACK: Biofeedback training for anxiety using EMG and EEG modalities.

5. DIALYSIS: A 10-year-old patient received ESRD dialysis-related services daily from July 1 through July 3.

Gastroenterology

The Gastroenterology subsection includes codes for gastroenterology tests (e.g., motility, acid perfusion) and also includes the following:

- Gastric physiology
- Other procedures

 Coding Tip

Gastroenterology tests are frequently performed in conjunction with gastrointestinal (GI) endoscopic procedures. Do *not* report codes separately from the Gastroenterology subsection of the Medicine section with Surgery section GI endoscopic procedures.

Gastroenterology procedures (Table 19-1) are found in the Surgery section. Related diagnostic services are found in the Pathology and Laboratory and Radiology sections.

> **Example:** Patient underwent gastric motility (manometric) studies. Report code 91020.

TABLE 19-1 Gastroenterology Procedures and Services

Procedure	Description
Esophageal or gastric intubation and collection of washings	• Tube is inserted through nose or mouth into esophagus or stomach. • One or more washings are obtained for *cytology* (study of cells).
Esophageal, gastric, or duodenal motility	• Tube is inserted through patient's nose or mouth into the esophagus, stomach, or duodenum. • Tube is slowly withdrawn to test muscles for weakness or abnormality (manometry).
Acid perfusion test of esophagus (or Bernstein test)	• Nasogastric tube is inserted into the esophagus. • Mild hydrochloric acid is poured through the tube in an attempt to recreate and evaluate gastric reflux symptoms. • Test is done to determine whether chest pain is due to acid reflux and not a cardiac condition.
Gastroesophageal reflux test	• Electrode is inserted through nasal catheter into esophagus to determine pH levels. • Electrode remains in esophagus over a period of time to obtain multiple levels (to determine acid reflux or non-acid reflux).
Esophageal balloon distention provocation study	• Local anesthetic is administered to numb the throat. • Balloon is inserted into esophagus and is expanded in multiple sites to increasing degrees to provoke chest pain. • This is done to rule out a cardiac source of existing chest pain.
Gastric analysis test (or Hollander test)	• Nasogastric tube is inserted through patient's nose or mouth into the stomach. • Stimulant is injected into the stomach (e.g., histamine, insulin, pentagastrin, calcium, or secretin). • Gastric contents are suctioned through the tube and are analyzed.
Gastric saline load test	• Nasogastric tube is inserted through patient's nose or mouth into the stomach. • Gastric contents are suctioned, and stomach is filled with saline. • After 30 minutes, gastric contents are resuctioned and measured to determine presence of impaired gastric emptying.
Breath hydrogen test	• Patient's exhalations are tested for hydrogen to determine whether undigested food is entering the duodenum. • Test is administered over a period of 3 to 5 hours, after patient has fasted for 12 hours and has swallowed test sugars (e.g., fructose, lactose, or lactulose).
Placement of intestinal bleeding tube	• Intestinal bleeding tube is inserted through mouth into duodenum. • Tube is monitored and used to suppress bleeding, if present.
Gastric intubation for aspiration or lavage	• Nasogastric tube is inserted through patient's nose or mouth into the stomach. • Gastric contents are suctioned to remove ingested poisons or to decompress intestinal blockage.
Gastrointestinal (GI) tract imaging	• Patient swallows a capsule that provides color imaging as it passes through the GI system. • Data are transmitted from the capsule to a data recorder.
Rectal sensation, tone, and compliance test	• Balloon is inserted into the patient's rectum and gradually inflated. • Reactions to various levels of inflation are studied.
Anorectal manometry	• This measures pressure of anal sphincter to diagnose constipation or incontinence.
Pulsed irrigation of fecal impaction (or pulsed irrigation evaluation, PCE)	• Automated enema is inserted for cases of chronic constipation when the patient has no voluntary bowel control (e.g., a paraplegic patient).
Electrogastrography (EGG)	• Electrodes are attached to the patient's abdomen. • Myoelectrical activity is detected and recorded.

Ophthalmology

Ophthalmology services include the following:

- General ophthalmological services
- Special ophthalmological services
- Contact lens services
- Spectacle services (including prosthesis for aphakia)

General Ophthalmological Services

General ophthalmological services codes are reported for new or established patient examinations. A physician (such as an ophthalmologist) can report an appropriate evaluation and management (E/M) service code instead of a general ophthalmological service code. *Do not report a general ophthalmological services code in addition to an E/M service code.*

Ophthalmologists have a choice when assigning codes for E/M services because they provide unique and specialized services that do not match criteria associated with E/M codes. Instead of reporting codes from the E/M section, an ophthalmologist may report codes from the Medicine section. These codes describe intermediate and comprehensive levels of service, which are defined by CPT.

When services provided are less than those described by general ophthalmological services codes, the ophthalmologist should report the appropriate E/M codes.

- Intermediate ophthalmological services include history, general medical observation, external ocular and adnexal examination, and other diagnostic procedures as indicated. This may include the use of mydriasis for ophthalmoscopy.

> **Example:** Established patient was seen in the office by the ophthalmologist for evaluation of glaucoma. Interval history, external examination, ophthalmoscopy, biomicroscopy, and tonometry were performed to evaluate the patient's response to glaucoma treatment. Report code 92012.

- Comprehensive ophthalmological services include a general evaluation of the complete visual system (e.g., history, general medical observation, external and ophthalmoscopic examinations, gross visual fields and basic sensorimotor examination, biomicroscopy, examination with cycloplegia or mydriasis, and tonometry). In addition, diagnostic and treatment procedures are included. Comprehensive services may be performed during multiple sessions or visits.

> **Example:** An established patient previously diagnosed with glaucoma was seen in the ophthalmologist's office. The ophthalmic technician tested the patient's visual acuity, gross visual field by confrontation, ocular motility including primary gaze alignment, and intraocular pressures. The ophthalmologist examined the patient's ocular adnexae, including lids, lacrimal glands, lacrimal drainage, orbits, and preauricular lymph nodes. The pupils and irises were also examined. The ophthalmologist performed a slit lamp examination of the corneas, anterior chambers, and lenses. The patient's bulbar and palpebral conjunctivae were also inspected. The ophthalmologist prescribed medication and ordered lab work. Report code 92014.

Special Ophthalmological Services

Special ophthalmological services codes are significant, separately identifiable services, which means they are reported in addition to general ophthalmological examination services, when performed.

 Coding Tip

Routine ophthalmoscopy is included in general ophthalmological services. However, other special ophthalmological services are not included, and they should be coded and reported separately when performed (e.g., a determination of refractive state).

Determination of refractive state establishes whether a prescription is required for vision correction. It is performed using an eye chart and refractor (a device that contains a wide range of lens strengths that can be easily and quickly changed). The fitting of glasses or contact lenses is *not* included with determination of refractive state services.

Example: Patient underwent determination of refractive state. Report code 92015.

Contact Lens Services and Spectacle Services (Including Prosthesis for Aphakia)

When contact lens or spectacle services are provided, supply of the contact lenses or spectacles (glasses) is not included. Report an appropriate HCPCS Level II code for the supply of materials.

Example: Patient underwent fitting of bifocal spectacles. Ophthalmologist provided "sphere, bifocal, plano to plus or minus 4.00d, per lens" glasses to the patient. Report codes 92341 and V2200.

Special Otorhinolaryngologic Services

Special Otorhinolaryngologic services include the following:

- Vestibular function tests, without electrical recording
- Vestibular function tests, with recording (e.g., ENG)
- Audiologic function tests

- Evaluative and therapeutic services
- Special diagnostic procedures
- Other procedures

When otorhinolaryngologic services are performed during an evaluation and management (E/M) service, do not code and report the component procedures separately (e.g., otoscopy, tuning fork test, whispered voice test). Special otorhinolaryngologic services that are *not* typically included in a comprehensive otorhinolaryngologic evaluation are reported separately.

Example: An otorhinolaryngologist performed a level 4 E/M service in the office, which included documenting the established patient's history, an external inspection of the ears, and a rhinoscopic examination of the nose. Otoscopic examination of the external auditory canals and tympanic membranes revealed negative findings. Hearing assessment was performed with tuning forks, whispered voice, and finger-rub techniques. Report code 99214 from the E/M section. Do *not* report separate codes for the hearing assessments performed.

 NOTE:

During an E/M service, when the physician also performs nasal function studies, code 92512 is also reported.

Audiologic function tests with medical diagnostic evaluation codes include testing of both ears. Do *not* add modifier 50 (Bilateral procedure) to these codes.

Example: Patient underwent a pure-tone screening test, air only, both ears. Report code 92551.

Codes for audiometric tests are reported separately only when calibrated electronic equipment is used. For pure-tone audiometry, earphones are used. The patient responds to different tone pitches (frequencies). Air and bone thresholds are similar to pure-tone audiometry procedures, except a bone oscillator is used instead of earphones.

Example: Patient underwent pure-tone audiometry, air and bone, one ear. Report code 92553 52. Modifier 52 (Reduced services) is added because audiometry was performed for one ear (instead of both ears). A directional modifier is *not* added to the code.

Cardiovascular

Cardiovascular services include the following:

- Therapeutic services and procedures
- Cardiography
- Cardiovascular monitoring services
- Implantable, insertable, and wearable cardiac device evaluations
- Phrenic nerve stimulation system
- Echocardiography
- Cardiac catheterization
- Intracardiac electrophysiological procedures/studies
- Peripheral arterial disease rehabilitation
- Noninvasive physiologic studies and procedures
- Home and outpatient international normalized ratio (INR) monitoring services
- Other procedures

Coding Tip

- Many therapeutic and diagnostic cardiovascular procedure codes include intravenous or intra-arterial access, electrocardiographic monitoring, and agents administered by injection or infusion. Therefore, do not separately report these codes for routine access, monitoring, injection, or infusion services.
- Cardiovascular code descriptions often state "with interpretation," or "tracing only," whereas others describe the total (global, technical, and professional) service. Be sure to carefully review code descriptions before reporting a code.

Therapeutic Services and Procedures

Therapeutic services performed during a heart catheterization, after the diagnostic images are obtained, are reported in addition to the heart catheterization codes (e.g., balloon angioplasty). Therapeutic procedures include the following:

- Cardiopulmonary resuscitation
- Transcutaneous pacing
- Cardioversion
- Circulatory assist procedures
- Thrombolysis
- Transcatheter placement of stents
- Percutaneous transluminal coronary balloon angioplasty
- Atherectomy

Percutaneous coronary artery interventions include stent placement (Figure 19-2), atherectomy, and balloon angioplasty (Figure 19-3). For a given coronary artery and its branches, report only the most complex intervention, regardless of the number of stent placements, atherectomies, or balloon angioplasties performed in that coronary artery and its branches. (Stent placement is considered more complex than an atherectomy. An atherectomy is considered more complex than a balloon angioplasty.) Do not add modifier 59 to codes reported for percutaneous coronary artery stent placement, atherectomy, or balloon angioplasty. These interventions are reported with an appropriate modifier to indicate in which coronary artery the procedure was performed. These modifiers are the following:

- LC (left circumflex coronary artery)
- RC (right coronary artery)
- LD (left anterior descending coronary artery)

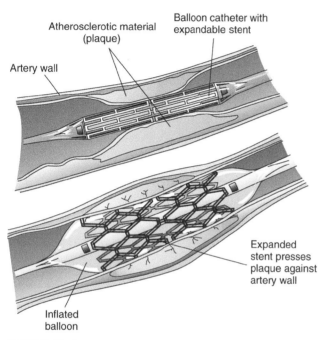

FIGURE 19-2 A stent is inserted after balloon angioplasty to prevent restenosis of the treated artery

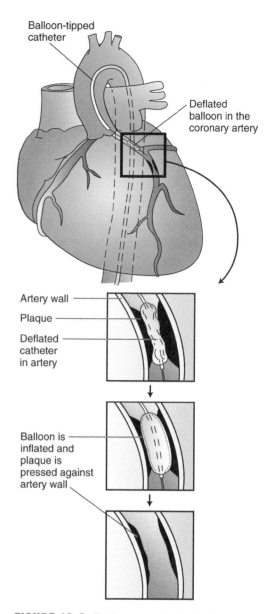

FIGURE 19-3 Balloon angioplasty is performed to open a blocked coronary artery

 Coding Tip

Medicare recognizes the following three coronary arteries for reimbursement purposes when considering first and additional vessel interventions:

- Left anterior descending
- Left circumflex
- Right coronary

Therefore, it is possible to report up to three percutaneous interventions if an intervention is performed in each of the three coronary arteries or their branches.

- The first procedure is reported with a primary code that describes the most complex procedure performed.
- Procedures performed in other coronary arteries are reported with the add-on codes.

When cardiopulmonary resuscitation (CPR) is performed *without* other evaluation and management services, the time required to perform CPR is not included in determining the critical care or other time-based evaluation and management services. Codes from the E/M section are reported for time-based critical care services and prolonged management services.

> **Example:** A "code blue" is called on a hospital inpatient. The responding physician directs cardiopulmonary resuscitation. After the patient is resuscitated, the patient's attending physician resumes patient care. Report code 92950 for CPR.

Cardiography

Cardiography, or **electrocardiography**, is a diagnostic procedure that records the heart's electronic activity with a cardiograph and produces a cardiogram (or electrocardiogram, ECG, or EKG) (Figure 19-4). Cardiography codes are reported for routine electrocardiograms and other procedures (e.g., vector cardiogram, 24-hour monitoring, and patient demand recordings when ordered by the provider). Be sure to identify the total, professional, and technical components (and appropriate modifiers) before reporting cardiography codes.

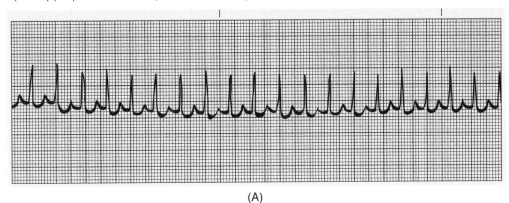

(A)

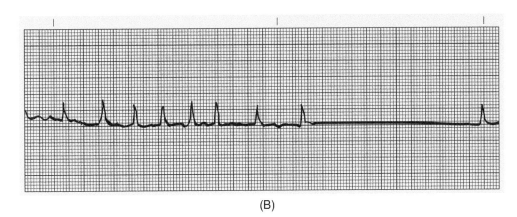

(B)

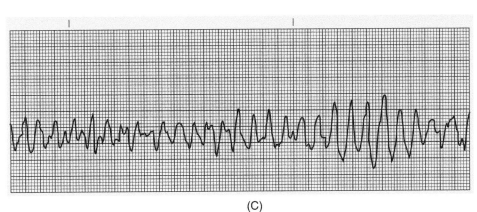

(C)

FIGURE 19-4 Electrocardiogram showing disruptions of heart rhythms (A) Paroxysmal atrial tachycardia (PAT) (B) Atrial fibrillation (C) Ventricular fibrillation

The routine monitoring of EKG rhythm and hemodynamics, including cardiac outputs, is included as part of critical care evaluation and management services. Therefore, do not separately report EKG rhythm strip and cardiac output measurement review codes with critical care services.

> **Example:** Patient underwent routine ECG (tracing only) in the physician's office. Report code 93005.

Cardiovascular Monitoring Services

Cardiovascular monitoring services (e.g., pacemaker programming) use in-person and remote technology to assess cardiovascular rhythm (electrocardiogram) data. Holter monitors, mobile cardiac telemetry monitors, event monitors, and long-term continuous recorders are used for cardiovascular monitoring services.

> **Example:** Patient underwent transtelephonic rhythm strip pacemaker evaluation of the multiple lead pacemaker system for a period of 60 days, which included physician analysis, review, and documented report. Report code 93293 just once.

Implantable, Insertable, and Wearable Cardiac Device Evaluations

Cardiac device evaluation services are diagnostic medical procedures using in-person and remote technology to assess cardiac device therapy and cardiovascular physiologic data.

> **Example:** Patient underwent a 30-day remote interrogation device evaluation that required a subcutaneous cardiac rhythm monitor system. Analysis of recorded heart rhythm data, and physician analysis, review and report were included. Report code 93298.

Phrenic Nerve Stimulation System

Phrenic nerve stimulation involves using a technique to reanimate the diaphragm of patients who have respiratory insufficiency due to central nervous system conditions, such as brain stem injuries, congenital central hypoventilation syndrome, idiopathic severe sleep apnea, and spinal cord injury above C4. Diaphragm pacing leads are placed around phrenic nerves bilaterally and attached to electrodes implanted in a subcutaneous pocket. The electrodes are connected outside the body to a stimulator device worn on the skin. The stimulator device sends electrical impulses to electrodes, causing the diaphragm to contract (helping the patient to breathe).

The phrenic nerve stimulation system subcategory includes codes for therapy activation, subsequent interrogation, interrogation and programming, and programming during a polysomnogram.

> **Example:** Patient underwent therapy activation of implanted phrenic nerve stimulation system, including interrogation and programming. Report code 93150.

Echocardiography

Echocardiography (Figure 19-5) is a diagnostic procedure that uses ultrasound to obtain two-dimensional images of the heart and great arteries (aorta, vena cavae). Echocardiography codes include the total procedure. When just the professional component is performed, add modifier 26 to the code.

> **Example:** Patient underwent transesophageal echocardiography for congenital cardiac anomalies, which included placement of the probe, image acquisition, and interpretation and report. Report code 93315.

Cardiac Catheterization

Cardiac catheterization (Figure 19-6) is an invasive diagnostic medical procedure that includes several components. The procedure begins when the physician introduces one or more catheters into peripheral arteries and/or veins. Cardiac catheterizations include introduction, positioning (and repositioning) of catheter(s), recording

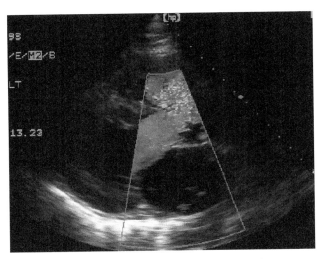

FIGURE 19-5 Echocardiography: The large area of red shows the flow of blood through an abnormal opening between the aorta and right atrium

of intracardiac and/or intravascular pressure(s), and final evaluation and preparation of a report. (A table of *Cardiac Catheterization Codes* in the CPT coding manual provides coding guidance.)

Cardiac output measurement is routinely performed during cardiac catheterization procedures. These codes are not reported in addition to cardiac catheterization codes.

Fluoroscopic guidance procedures are integral to invasive intravascular procedures, and codes for such procedures are not reported separately.

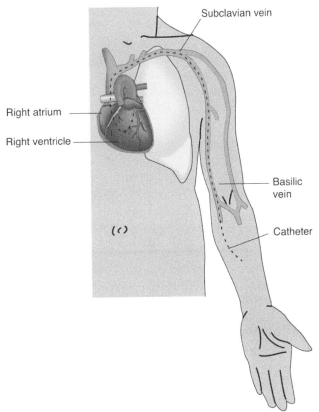

Subclavian vein

Right atrium

Right ventricle

Basilic vein

Catheter

(c)

FIGURE 19-6 Cardiac catheterization: Once the catheter is inserted in the heart, a contrast medium is injected and an angiogram is performed to detect coronary vessel patency (openness)

When reporting codes for cardiac catheterization procedures, review patient-record documentation to determine the following:

- Catheter placement
- Injection procedure
- Supervision and interpretation of fluoroscopic guidance

The femoral artery is the most common access point for cardiac catheterization (such as left heart catheterization, aortography, coronary angiography, internal mammary artery injection, vein bypass graft injection, and for other left heart procedures and coronary artery interventions). Right heart catheterization and pulmonary arteriography are most often performed via the right femoral vein. Each catheter is then positioned in a branch vessel or a cardiac chamber. During the catheterization procedure, recordings are made for measurement of intracardiac and intravascular pressure, oxygen saturation or blood gases, and cardiac output.

Angiography, frequently performed during a diagnostic catheterization, may require the assignment of a separate code. Angiography involves injecting a contrast medium and imaging the vessel (e.g., in order to determine the location or severity of obstructive lesions or abnormalities). Repositioning the catheter may be necessary during the procedure to perform injection of contrast for angiography. A final evaluation of all data and a report are required.

> **Example:** Patient underwent combined right and left heart catheterization, which included intraprocedural injection for left ventriculography with imaging supervision and interpretation. Report code 93453.

Endomyocardial biopsy provides tissue for direct pathologic evaluation of cardiac muscle using a special biopsy catheter with a bioptome tip (an open tip that closes to obtain tissue sample) to obtain myocardial tissue samples. To monitor a cardiac transplant patient for signs of rejection, the physician inserts a bioptome-tip catheter and, under fluoroscopy, advances it to the right ventricle. The instrument obtains myocardial tissue that is submitted for pathologic examination.

Insertion of a Swan-Ganz catheter is included in the cardiac catheterization codes. It is not separately reported *except when performed as a separate and distinct procedure from the heart catheterization*. A Swan-Ganz catheter is a flexible, multiple-lumen, balloon-tipped flotation catheter that is introduced through a major peripheral vein (e.g., the jugular or subclavian). It is passed under pressure waveform guidance, with or without fluoroscopy, through the right atrium, right ventricle, and pulmonary artery. The balloon is inflated and the tip measures the retrograde transmission of pressure from the left side of the heart (left ventricular end-diastolic pressure), as well as central venous pressure. With the balloon deflated, the catheter measures pulmonary artery systolic, diastolic, and mean pressures; it then allows infusion (and some patients are fitted with pacing electrodes).

> **Example:** During postoperative recovery after a heart catheterization, the patient's condition became unstable, and the physician inserted a Swan-Ganz flow-directed catheter for evaluation and monitoring. Report code 93503.

Intracardiac Electrophysiological Procedures/Studies

Intracardiac electrophysiological procedures and studies describe services that record, map, or change heart conduction (e.g., recording bundle of His, mapping tachycardia during repair surgery). Many of these codes contain instructional notes that indicate their use with other codes. Intracardiac electrophysiological procedures (EP) may be diagnostic or therapeutic, and these procedures include the insertion and repositioning of catheters.

Peripheral Arterial Disease Rehabilitation

Peripheral arterial disease (PAD) is a disease in which plaque builds up in arteries that carry blood to the head, organs, and limbs; plaque consists of cholesterol, calcium, fat, fibrous tissue, and other substances in the blood. PAD rehabilitation includes physical exercise that consists of a series of sessions, each session lasting 45–60 minutes, and involves use of either a motorized treadmill or a track.

> **Example:** During a series of three sessions, as part of PAD rehabilitation with supervision by an exercise physiologist, the patient exercised on a motorized treadmill for 45 minutes. Report codes 93668, 93668, and 93668.

Noninvasive Physiologic Studies and Procedures

Noninvasive physiologic studies and procedures include bioimpedance-derived physiologic cardiovascular analysis, electronic analysis of antitachycardia pacemaker system, temperature gradient studies, and so on.

> **Example:** Patient underwent a procedure for determination of venous pressure. Report code 93770.

Home and Outpatient International Normalized Ratio (INR) Monitoring Services

Home and Outpatient International Normalized Ratio (INR) Monitoring Services describe warfarin therapy management, which involves ordering, reviewing, and interpreting new INR test result(s), patient instructions, and dosage adjustments. Modifier 25 is added to the reported E/M code when a significantly, separately identifiable evaluation and management (E/M) service is provided on the same day as INR monitoring services. Codes for INR monitoring services are also *not* reported with E/M non-face-to-face services for telephone or online digital E/M services for home when the E/M services address home and outpatient INR monitoring.

> **Example 1:** Anticoagulant management was provided to a patient taking warfarin, which included the review and interpretation of a new home international normalized ratio (INR) test result, and patient instructions. The patient's dosage is unchanged. No additional tests are required. Report code 93793.

> **Example 2:** Patient received level 3 emergency department services for management of uncontrolled type 1 diabetes mellitus and face-to-face patient training for initiation of home international normalized ratio (INR) monitoring, which included use and care of the INR monitor, obtaining a blood sample, instructions for reporting home INR test results, and documentation of the patient's ability to perform testing and report results. Report codes 99283 25 and 93792.

> **Example 3:** Patient received level 3 established patient office encounter evaluation and management services that included anticoagulant management of warfarin. Report code 99213 only. (Do not report code 93793.)

Other Procedures

Cardiac rehabilitation is a customized program of exercise and education. Cardiac rehabilitation programs typically last about three to six months, during which the patient works with cardiologists, nurse educators, dietitians, exercise rehabilitation specialists, occupational therapists, physical therapists, psychologists, and psychiatrists. Because the cardiac rehabilitation codes describe comprehensive services provided by a physician for cardiac rehabilitation, all services related to cardiac rehabilitation are included. Thus, it would *not* be appropriate to report a separate evaluation and management service code unless it is an unrelated, separately identifiable service.

 Coding Tip

All intracardiac electrophysiological procedures/studies codes are exempt from modifier 51.

> **Example:** On November 15, 20, and 25, a patient received physician services for outpatient cardiac rehabilitation without continuous ECG monitoring. Report codes 93797, 93797, and 93797 for each date of service.

Noninvasive Vascular Diagnostic Studies

Noninvasive vascular diagnostic studies (e.g., a duplex scan) include ultrasound scanning to display two-dimensional structure and motion and arterial and venous studies. They identify the following anatomical structures or areas to be studied. (A **duplex scan** is a noninvasive test that is performed to evaluate a vessel's blood flow.)

- Cerebrovascular arterial studies
- Extremity arterial studies (including digits)
- Extremity venous studies (including digits)

- Visceral and penile vascular studies
- Extremity arterial-venous studies
- Other noninvasive vascular diagnostic studies

Example: Patient underwent a duplex scan of lower extremity arteries, bilaterally. Report code 93925.

Exercise 19.4 – Gastroenterology, Ophthalmology, Otorhinolaryngology, Cardiovascular, Noninvasive Vascular Diagnostic Studies

Instructions: Assign CPT code(s) and appropriate modifier(s) to each statement.

1. GASTROENTEROLOGY: Gastric motility manometric studies.

   _____

2. OPHTHALMOLOGY: Comprehensive ophthalmological therapeutic evaluation services, new patient, one visit.

   _____

3. SPECIAL OTORHINOLARYNGOLOGIC SERVICES: Diagnostic otolaryngologic examination under general anesthesia.

   _____

4. CARDIOVASCULAR: Percutaneous transcatheter placement of intracoronary stents in left anterior descending coronary artery and right inferior coronary artery with coronary angioplasty.

   _____

5. NONINVASIVE VASCULAR DIAGNOSTIC STUDIES: Duplex scan of extracranial arteries, complete bilateral study.

   _____

Pulmonary

Pulmonary codes are reported for ventilation management and pulmonary diagnostic testing, rehabilitation, and therapies. When pulmonary services are provided during an evaluation and management (E/M) encounter (e.g., hospital inpatient visit, emergency department service, office visit), report a code from the Pulmonary subsection of the Medicine section in addition to the appropriate E/M code.

- _Ventilator management_ is provided to patients in hospital inpatient and observation care settings, nursing facilities, and for whom home care is provided

Example: A hospital inpatient was treated with a mechanical ventilator that was applied with a mask over the nose and mouth to assist with breathing due to emphysema. Initial ventilator management services were provided on April 5, and subsequent ventilator management services were provided on April 6 and 7. Report codes 94002, 94003, and 94003. (Do not report modifier 51 with code 94003.)

- _Pulmonary diagnostic testing, rehabilitation, and therapies_ includes laboratory procedures and interpretation of test results (e.g., spirometry, vital capacity, and thoracic gas volume)

Example: During a level 3 outpatient E/M service to evaluate cystic fibrosis, the established patient underwent outpatient pulmonary function testing to assess maximum breathing capacity and maximal voluntary ventilation. The physician interpreted the results of testing and adjusted the patient's medications. Report codes 99213 25 and 94200. (Modifier 25 is reported with the E/M code to indicate that a significant, separately identifiable E/M service was provided by the same physician on the same day of the pulmonary function testing procedure.)

Allergy and Clinical Immunology

The Allergy and Clinical Immunology subsection includes the following:

- Allergy testing
- Ingestion challenge testing
- Allergen immunotherapy

Allergy Testing

Allergy sensitivity tests are performed on skin (cutaneous) and mucous membranes to identify the source of a patient's allergies (e.g., pollen as a source). Allergy skin tests include

- **Puncture, prick, or scratch test (percutaneous):** Tiny drops of purified allergen extracts are pricked or scratched into the skin's surface. The test is performed to identify allergies to pollen, mold, pet dander, dust mites, foods, insect venom, and penicillin (Figure 19-7).
- **Intradermal test (intracutaneous):** Purified allergen extracts are injected into the skin of patient's arm (Figure 19-8). The test is performed when an allergy to insect venom or penicillin is suspected.
- **Patch test (epicutaneous):** An allergen is applied to a patch, which is placed on skin. The test is performed to identify substances that cause contact dermatitis, such as latex, medications, fragrances, preservatives, hair dyes, metals, and resins.

Example: Patient underwent two patch tests. Report codes 95044 and 95044.

Ingestion Challenge Testing

Ingestion challenge testing includes the sequential and incremental ingestion of test items. Examples of test items include drugs, foods, and other substances. Patient assessment and monitoring activities (e.g., blood pressure) that are performed during ingestion challenge testing are *not* separately reported. However, intervention therapy (e.g., injection of epinephrine), when performed, is reported separately along with appropriate evaluation and management service code(s).

Example: Patient underwent 120 minutes of ingestion challenge testing (strawberries). Report code 95076.

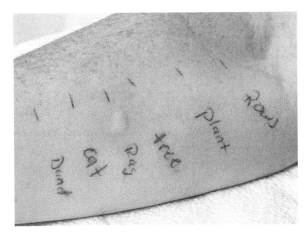

FIGURE 19-7 In scratch (percutaneous) tests, allergens are placed on the skin, the skin is scratched, and the allergen is labeled. Reactions usually occur within 20 minutes. Pictured is a reaction to ragweed

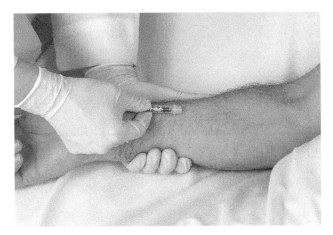

FIGURE 19-8 Intradermal skin test

Allergen Immunotherapy

Allergen immunotherapy (also known as allergy shots, allergy vaccines, desensitization shots, or hypo-sensitization shots) contains small amounts of **allergens** (allergy-causing substances to which a patient reacts) to increase the patient's tolerance to allergens. Code descriptions indicate whether the allergenic extract is provided or not.

 NOTE:

An allergen immunotherapy dose is the amount of antigen administered in a single injection from a multiple-dose vial.

Example: A primary care provider administers a single allergy injection using allergenic extract that was previously prepared by an allergist and brought to the office by the patient. Report code 95115.

Allergen immunotherapy is administered on a schedule; patients typically receive treatment once or twice a week for about three to six months, and then once a month for three to five years. There are usually two phases of treatment.

- The buildup phase, during which patients receive shots one or two times per week for about three to six months

- The maintenance phase, during which patients receive shots every two to four weeks for five months or longer

Endocrinology

Continual glucose (blood sugar) monitoring for up to 72 hours involves the subcutaneous placement of a sensor from which data are sent to a monitor. The patient calibrates the monitor on a daily basis.

Example: Dr. Jones was provided with a printout of recorded data from a subcutaneous sensor inserted into a patient. The sensor facilitated ambulatory continuous glucose monitoring of interstitial tissue fluid for 72 hours. Dr. Jones analyzed and interpreted the data and prepared a report. Report code 95251.

Neurology and Neuromuscular Procedures

Neurology and neuromuscular diagnostic and therapeutic services include:

- Sleep medicine testing
- Routine electroencephalography (EEG)
- Electrocorticography
- Range-of-motion testing
- Electromyography
- Ischemic muscle testing and guidance for chemodenervation
- Nerve conduction tests

- Intraoperative neurophysiology
- Autonomic function tests
- Evoked potentials and reflex tests
- Special EEG tests
- Neurostimulators, analysis-programming
- Other procedures
- Motion analysis
- Functional brain mapping

Sleep Medicine Testing

Sleep testing includes sleep studies and polysomnography, which are performed for the continuous monitoring and recording of various physiological parameters of sleep for six or more hours. Sleep testing is usually done in a health care facility's **sleep laboratory**, which is managed by a sleep technologist who explains and performs the sleep studies. (Sleep studies and polysomnographies are ordered, reviewed, and interpreted by physicians.) Sleeping rooms typically contain regular (not hospital) beds, an attached bathroom, and a television.

Sleep medicine testing codes include physician review and interpretation of data, and the preparation of a report.

- **Multiple sleep latency** is the observation of a patient during at least a six-hour period of sleep and includes assessment of sleep latency (dormancy) and/or wakefulness after the sleep period.

- **Sleep studies** evaluate adult and pediatric patients during sleep by monitoring brainwaves, heart rate, and eye movements. They are performed to diagnose sleep disorders, which include breathing, movement, and neurologic disorders that occur at night. Electrodes are applied to the patient's scalp, sides of the head, below the chin, chest, and legs. A sensor is placed next to the nose and mouth to measure airflow. A pulse oximetry clip is placed on the patient's finger to measure blood oxygen levels. Patients are also videotaped while asleep.

- **Polysomnography** is a sleep study that includes sleep staging with additional parameters of sleep (e.g., belts can be placed around the rib cage and abdomen to measure breathing movements). **Sleep staging** includes a 1-4 lead EEG, electro-oculogram (EOG), and submental electromyogram (EMG). Parameters that determine the polysomnography code to report include the following:

○ Airflow	○ Gas exchange by oximetry
○ Body positions	○ Gastroesophageal reflux
○ Continuous blood pressure monitoring	○ Motor activity movement
○ Electrocardiogram	○ Penile tumescence
○ End tidal gas analysis	○ Snoring
○ Extended EEG monitoring	○ Transcutaneous monitoring
○ Extremity muscle activity	○ Ventilation and respiratory effort

Example: A patient with a history of sleep apnea undergoes a sleep study, during which the patient is monitored for six hours. Polysomnography includes the measurement of respiration, airflow, muscle activity, continuous monitoring of blood pressure, and sleep staging with EEG, electro-oculogram, and submental electromyogram. Report code 95808.

Routine Electroencephalography (EEG)

EEG procedures include the use of the following, when appropriate:

- *Hyperventilation*: Deep or rapid breathing
- *Photic stimulation*: Reaction to light

Extended EEG codes are reported to test various stages of activity and sleep. (A *Long-Term EEG Monitoring Table* in the CPT coding manual provides guidance for code assignment.)

Example: Patient underwent a 60-minute EEG test, which included photic (pertaining to light) stimulation. Report code 95812.

Electrocorticography

Electrocorticography (ECoG) procedures include the recording of an EEG from electrodes directly on or in the brain. An ECG code is reported when an electrocorticogram is performed during surgery or after the physician has inserted electrodes into the brain for EEG recording.

Example: Patient underwent electrocorticography during brain surgery. Report code 95829 (in additional to appropriate brain surgery codes from the Surgery section).

Range-of-Motion Testing

Range-of-motion testing codes are reported for muscle testing, range-of-motion measurements and reports, and Tensilon testing for myasthenia gravis. The *Tensilon test* involves injecting the drug Tensilon (or its generic, edrophonium chloride) into a vein to block the action of the enzyme that breaks down the neurotransmitter acetylcholinesterase. The patient is then observed for rapid improvement in strength (e.g., use of eye muscles).

Example: Patient underwent range-of-motion measurements (including physician report) of each extremity. Report code 95851.

Electromyography

Electromyography (EMG) is a test that is used to detect nerve function by measuring the electrical activity generated by muscles. **Needle electromyography** testing involves inserting needle electrodes into skeletal muscles and observing the electrical activity of those muscles using an **oscilloscope** (a device that displays electrical waveforms on a monitor) and a loudspeaker.

Example: Patient underwent limited needle EMG study of the left bicep muscle. Report code 95870.

Ischemic Muscle Testing and Guidance for Chemodenervation

Ischemic muscle testing and guidance for chemodenervation services are performed to treat various neurological conditions.

Example: Patient underwent ischemic limb exercise test with collection of several specimens to determine the presence of muscle metabolites. Report code 95875.

Nerve Conduction Tests

Nerve conduction tests are performed for sensory conduction, motor conduction, or Hoffman's reflex (H-reflex) (knee jerk reflex). For sensory conduction and H-reflex testing, electrodes are placed directly over the nerve; for motor conduction testing, electrodes are placed over the motor point of a specific muscle; then, electrical stimulation is applied. Amplitude, conduction velocity, and latency of the stimulation are measured.

Example: Patient underwent three nerve conduction studies due to left leg numbness. Report code 95908.

Intraoperative Neurophysiology

Intraoperative neurophysiology testing codes are reported when performed during a surgical procedure. (The primary procedure code is reported as the first-listed procedure.)

Example: Patient underwent EEG needle electromyography of one extremity, during which 15 minutes of intraoperative neurophysiology testing was also performed. Report codes 95860 and 95940.

Autonomic Function Tests

Autonomic function tests evaluate autonomic nervous system functioning (e.g., heart or lungs).

Example: Patient underwent autonomic function testing, during which patient was instructed to perform the Valsalva maneuver and then lie on a tilt table. The patient's blood pressure was monitored both during the maneuver and while on the tilt table. Report code 95922.

Evoked Potentials and Reflex Tests

A *short-latency somatosensory evoked potential study* involves electrically stimulating nerves to evaluate their responsiveness to the body's superficial surface and internal structures (e.g., the organs). (The appropriate code is reported according to testing site.) A *central motor evoked potential study* uses low-voltage electrodes, which are placed on the scalp and target sites to test the nervous system's pathway. A *visual evoked potential (VEP) test* of the central nervous system (CNS) involves stimulating the eye using the checkerboard or flash technique to monitor the patient's response. An *orbicularis oculi* (blink) test is monitored with sensors.

> **Example 1:** Patient underwent a short-latency somatosensory evoked potential study, stimulation of any/all peripheral nerves or skin sites, recording from the central nervous system; in upper limbs. Report code 95925.

> **Example 2:** Patient underwent VEP testing of the CNS using the flash technique. Report code 95930.

Special EEG Tests

Continuous electroencephalographic monitoring services codes are reported when a separately identifiable long-term or monitoring service is performed.

> **Example:** Patient underwent EEG during carotid artery (nonintracranial) surgery. Report code 95955.

Neurostimulators, Analysis-Programming

Neurostimulators and analysis-programming codes are reported when a previously implanted neurostimulator pulse generator system is electronically analyzed to determine battery status, pulse amplitude and duration, rate, and so on.

> **Example:** Patient underwent electronic analysis of implanted neurostimulator pulse generator system without reprogramming. Report code 95970.

Other Procedures

Other procedures codes are reported for the refill and maintenance of implantable infusion pumps or reservoirs for drug delivery, for canalith repositioning, per day, and for an unlisted neurological or neuromuscular diagnostic procedure.

> **Example:** Patient with terminal cancer undergoes a procedure to have implantable pump located in the spine refilled and maintained to ensure delivery of 500 mg of morphine sulfate, which is the loading dose prescribed for palliative care. Report codes 95990 and S0093.

Motion Analysis

Motion analysis codes are reported for services performed during major diagnostic or therapeutic decision making. During human motion analysis, patient movements are recorded, digitized, copied onto a computer, and processed. When a physician reviews and interprets the results of motion analysis and documents a written report, the appropriate code is reported just once in addition to the motion analysis tests performed. Modifier 51 is added to that review and interpretation code when the service is provided during the same encounter as motion analysis testing.

> **Example:** In the motion analysis lab, a patient is instructed to walk along a special walkway that includes a pressure sensor platform, which is positioned on the walkway. As the patient walks, pressure data are recorded and later analyzed for areas of the foot (e.g., hallux, heel, and metatarsal heads). The peak pressure is calculated for all areas, and the highest pressure is measured. Report code 96001. (Do not report bilateral 50 or directional modifiers LT or RT.)
>
> Next, the patient undergoes testing for dynamic plantar pressure measurements during walking, dynamic surface electromyography during walking or other functional activities, and dynamic fine wire electromyography during walking or other functional activities. Codes 96001, 96002, and 96003 are reported. The provider then reviews and interprets all test results and prepares a written report. Code 96004 is reported.

Functional Brain Mapping

Functional brain mapping is a process by which a series of tests is administered by a physician or a psychologist to assess cognition, language, memory, movement, and sensation. The results of testing are documented in a report to identify expected versus observed locations of brain activity documented as the patient performs assigned tasks.

During functional brain mapping, the patient undergoes functional neuroimaging of the brain, which is also called functional magnetic resonance imaging (fMRI) of the brain. Report a Radiology code (e.g., Magnetic resonance imaging, brain, functional MRI) in addition to the functional brain mapping code when a physician or psychologist entirely administers the functional brain mapping.

> **Example:** Dr. Sanders performs a functional brain mapping with fMRI on a 49-year-old patient who has been experiencing memory losses and motor problems to assess cognition, language, memory, movement, and sensation. Report codes 96020 and 70555.

Medical Genetics and Genetic Counseling Services

Medical genetics and genetic counseling services are reported when a trained genetic counselor meets with an individual, couple, or family to investigate the family's genetic history and to assess risks associated with genetic defects in offspring.

> **Example:** A married couple, who was referred to a trained genetic counselor by their fertility doctor, received 60 minutes of medical genetic counseling. Report codes 96040, 96040. (Code 96040 is reported for *each* 30-minute session of counseling.)

Adaptive Behavior Services

Adaptive behavior services include adaptive behavior assessments and adaptive behavior treatment for deficient adaptive behaviors (e.g., impaired communication), maladaptive behaviors (e.g., repetitive behaviors), and other impaired functioning (e.g., difficulty following instructions).

> **Example:** Patient underwent 30 minutes of behavior identification–supporting assessment. Report codes 97152, 97152.

Exercise 19.5 – Pulmonary, Allergy/Clinical Immunology, Endocrinology, Neurology, Medical Genetics

Instructions: Assign CPT code(s) to each statement.

1. PULMONARY: Total vital capacity measurement.

   _____

2. ALLERGY AND CLINICAL IMMUNOLOGY: Intracutaneous tests using allergenic extracts (cat hair, pollens, mixed vespid venom protein) for delayed skin reaction.

   _____

3. ENDOCRINOLOGY: Physician provided analysis and interpretation of ambulatory continuous glucose monitoring of interstitial tissue fluid via subcutaneous sensor for a 72-hour period, and a report was generated.

   _____

4. NEUROLOGY AND NEUROMUSCULAR PROCEDURES: Electroencephalogram (EEG), including recording for comatose patient.

   _____

5. MEDICAL GENETICS AND GENETIC COUNSELING SERVICES: Medical genetics and genetic counseling services, 60 minutes, face-to-face with patient and family.

   _____

Central Nervous System Assessments/Tests (e.g., Neuro-Cognitive, Mental Status, Speech Testing)

Central nervous system assessments/tests codes are reported when tests are performed to measure cognitive function of the central nervous system (e.g., cognitive processes, visual motor responses, and abstractive abilities). Several testing procedures are included, such as psychological testing which includes psychodiagnostic assessment of personality, psychopathology, emotionality, and intellectual abilities (e.g., WAIS-R, Rorschach, and MMPI tests). (*Central Nervous System Assessments/Tests Tables* in the CPT coding manual provide guidance for code assignment.)

> **Example:** Patient underwent developmental speech and language delay screening, using a standardized instrument, with scoring and documentation. Report code 96110.

Health Behavior Assessment and Intervention

Health behavior assessment and intervention codes are reported for tests that identify the psychological, behavioral, emotional, cognitive, and social elements involved in the prevention, treatment, or management of physical health problems. The focus of the assessment is not on mental health, but on biopsychosocial factors that are considered important to physical health problems and treatments. Health and behavior intervention procedures are used to modify factors affecting the patient. The focus of the intervention is to improve the patient's health and well-being by using cognitive, behavioral, social, and/or psychophysiological procedures.

Health and behavior assessment/intervention codes describe services associated with an acute or chronic illness that does not meet the criteria for psychiatric diagnosis, prevention of a physical disability, and maintenance of health. If the patient requires psychotherapy or other psychiatric services/procedures and/or health and behavior assessment/intervention, report the primary service performed for each date of service.

> **Example:** A psychiatrist performed a health behavior assessment of a child who was diagnosed with leukemia and who was suffering from severe distress and combativeness to chemotherapy administration. Report codes 96156.

Behavior Management Services

Behavior management services are reported for behavior management and modification services that are provided to multiple-family groups (without the patient present) and administered by a physician or other qualified health care professional. The goal is to teach participants interventions that can be used to effectively manage the patient's mental or physical health diagnosis.

> **Example:** One-hour face-to-face multiple-family group behavior management and modification training included the parents of patients with a mental health diagnosis (without the patient present), with administration by a physician. Report code 96202.

Hydration, Therapeutic, Prophylactic, Diagnostic Injections and Infusions, and Chemotherapy and Other Highly Complex Drug or Highly Complex Biologic Agent Administration

The hydration, therapeutic, prophylactic, diagnostic injections and infusions, and chemotherapy and other highly complex drug or highly complex biologic agent administration codes include:

- Hydration
- Therapeutic, prophylactic, and diagnostic injections and infusions (excludes chemotherapy and other highly complex drug or highly complex biologic agent administration)
- Chemotherapy and other highly complex drug or highly complex biologic agent administration

 NOTE:

Patient record documentation should include physician verification of the patient's treatment plan and direction of staff who provide injection and infusion services.

The following services are included, which means they are not separately coded and reported:

- Administration of local anesthesia
- Intravenous (IV) insertion
- Access to indwelling IV, subcutaneous catheter, or port
- Flushing performed upon completion of infusion
- Routine syringes, tubing, and other supplies

When multiple injections or infusions or combination services are provided, report the initial code only once except *when two separate intravenous (IV) sites are required*. When the length of infusion time is included in the code description, report the code based on actual infusion time.

Hydration

Hydration codes are reported for the intravenous infusion of prepackaged fluids and electrolytes (e.g., normal saline and normal saline with potassium chloride, up to 30 mEq). When reporting these codes, review the patient record for documentation that the physician supervised

- Patient assessment (e.g., history and examination)
- Patient consent (e.g., discussion of risks and benefits)
- Patient safety (e.g., proper dose was administered; patient's response to infusion, including adverse reaction)
- Staff members who provided infusion services (e.g., the nursing staff)

Example: Patient received initial intravenous infusion hydration of 1,000 cubic centimeters lactated Ringer's (pH–balanced electrolyte solution) for 60 minutes. Report codes 96360 and J7120.

Therapeutic, Prophylactic, and Diagnostic Injections and Infusions

Therapeutic, prophylactic, and diagnostic injections and infusions codes are reported for the administration of substances (other than hydration) and drugs. When reporting these codes, review the patient record for documentation that the physician supervised

- Patient assessment
- Patient safety
- Patient consent
- Staff members who provided injection and/or infusion services

Example 1: Patient underwent therapeutic injection (intramuscular) of kanamycin sulfate, 500 mg. Report codes 96372 and J1840.

Example 2: Patient underwent routine insertion of an IV catheter for one-hour IV infusion of 1,000 milliliters of potassium chloride and magnesium sulfate. Report codes 96365 and S5013.

Example 3: Patient, age 54, underwent nontunneled central venous access catheter (CVAC) procedure prior to one-hour intravenous infusion of 1,000 milliliters of potassium chloride and magnesium sulfate drug therapy. Report codes 36556, 96365, and S5013.

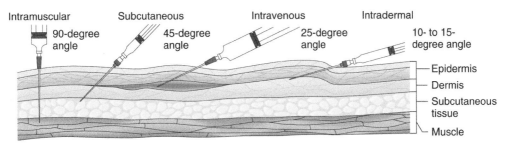

FIGURE 19-9 Angles of injection for administration of therapeutic, prophylactic, and diagnostic medications

Staff members who administer therapeutic, prophylactic, and diagnostic injections (Figure 19-9) and infusions undergo special training to learn how to assess patients, provide informed consent, monitor patient safety, and administer injections and infusions. **Intravenous push** is an

- Injection administered by a health care professional who is in constant attendance to administer the injection and observe the patient
- Infusion of 15 minutes or less

 Coding Tip

- Any fluid used to administer a drug (e.g., flushing of IV with saline solution between drug therapies) is considered incidental hydration, and a separate hydration code is not reported.
- Report HCPCS Level II codes for the supply of drugs (e.g., J0280, aminophylline).
- The administration of IV fluids to maintain line patency (unblocked condition) is not separately coded and reported.

Chemotherapy and Other Highly Complex Drug or Highly Complex Biologic Agent Administration

Chemotherapy is the treatment of cancer with drugs that serve to destroy cancer cells or slow the growth of cancer cells, keep cancer from spreading to other parts of the body, and prevent recurrence of the cancer. Chemotherapy administered in addition to other cancer treatments, such as surgery and/or radiation therapy, is called **adjuvant chemotherapy**.

Codes are reported for the parenteral administration of chemotherapeutic agents, which means that the chemotherapy is administered by a route *other than by mouth*, such as implantation (of a catheter or port), infusion, or injection.

 Coding Tip

To report chemotherapy infusion, select the appropriate code(s) from the chemotherapy administration series of codes. These codes can be separately billed when an E/M service is rendered on the same day as the chemotherapy administration.

- The flushing of a vascular access port (e.g., saline solution) prior to the administration of chemotherapeutic agents is integral to the chemotherapy administration. It is not coded and reported separately.
- When infusion of hydrating solutions (e.g., saline solution) or drugs (e.g., heparin) other than antineoplastic drugs is a necessary and integral part of a procedure, a code for that infusion is *not* reported separately.

Example: The infusion of a hydrating solution is started prior to the administration of chemotherapy. The infusion of the hydrating solution is included in the reported chemotherapy code, and it is not reported separately.

There are many chemotherapy drugs currently available to treat cancer, and chemotherapy is administered in a variety of ways, depending on the drugs used and the type of cancer.

Oral chemotherapy is administered by mouth in the form of a pill, capsule, or liquid, while parenteral methods of chemotherapy administration include the following:

- Implantation of a catheter or port into a central vein or body cavity
- Infusion or injection of intravenous (IV) chemotherapy into a vein
- Injection of intramuscular (IM) chemotherapy into the muscle
- Injection of subcutaneous (SQ) chemotherapy under the skin

When different techniques are used to parenterally administer chemotherapy (e.g., injection, infusion, implantation) *during the same encounter*, report a separate code for each parenteral method.

Example 1: A patient diagnosed with malignant melanoma, skin of scalp, undergoes one hour of intravenous infusion of chemotherapy and intralesional chemotherapy administration to the scalp lesion. Report codes 96405 and 96413.

Example 2: A patient was administered three injections of antineoplastic drugs and an infusion of antineoplastic drugs for two hours during one encounter. Report codes 96401, 96401, 96401, 96413, and 96415.

When an intravenous infusion of saline (an antiemetic) or other nonchemotherapy drug is administered at the same time as the chemotherapeutic agent(s), *these infusions are not coded and reported separately*. However, the supply of the drugs *is* reported separately with HCPCS Level II codes. If hydration or intravenous infusion is administered on the same day, but sequentially rather than at the same time as the chemotherapeutic agents, codes for the infusions are reported. Modifier 59 (Distinct Procedural Service) is added to these codes to indicate that the infusions were administered at different times.

 Coding Tip

Report code 96365 (IV infusion, for therapy, prophylaxis, or diagnosis, initial; up to one hour) to indicate an infusion of drugs (e.g., antihypertensive medication) *other than antineoplastic drugs*. Code 96366 is reported for each additional hour of infusion, up to eight hours.

Example: Patient receives nonchemotherapy infusions for 60 minutes. Report code 96365 along with the HCPCS Level II code[s] for the drugs administered.

Chemotherapy and other highly complex drug or highly complex biologic agent administration services are independent of the patient's evaluation and management (E/M) services and may occur sequentially on the same day. If performed, the appropriate E/M code should be reported as an additional code. Preparation of chemotherapy agent(s) is included in the service for administration of the agent, and it is not coded and reported separately.

Medications (e.g., antibiotics, steroidal agents, antiemetics, narcotics, analgesics, and biological agents) administered independently or sequentially as supportive management of chemotherapy administration are separately coded and reported, as appropriate. It is appropriate to report separately the appropriate HCPCS Level II code(s) for the supply of chemotherapy drugs in addition to the code(s) for chemotherapy administration.

Exercise 19.6 – Adaptive Behavior Services, CNS Assessments/Tests, Health Behavior Assessment/Intervention, Injections/Infusions/Chemotherapy Administration

Instructions: Assign CPT code(s) to each statement.

1. ADAPTIVE BEHAVIOR SERVICES: Family adaptive behavior treatment guidance administered by physician with patient, face-to-face, including guardians and caregivers, 60 minutes.

   _____

2. CENTRAL NERVOUS SYSTEM ASSESSMENT/TESTS: Assessment of aphasia to determine speech and language functions, including interpretation and report, 1 hour.

   _____

3. HEALTH BEHAVIOR ASSESSMENT AND INTERVENTION: Health behavior invention with patient, face-to-face, 30 minutes, to modify emotional and cognitive factors that impact patient's physical health.

   _____

4. INJECTIONS/INFUSION/CHEMOTHERAPY ADMINISTRATION: A patient received intravenous (IV) push of ceftriaxone sodium antibiotic 250 mg through an existing IV line. The IV was flushed with normal saline before and after administration of the antibiotic to check for patency and to clear the IV line. (Also assign an HCPCS Level II code for supply of drug.)

   _____

5. INJECTIONS/INFUSION/CHEMOTHERAPY ADMINISTRATION: Intravenous infusion of methotrexate, 50 mg, 2 hours, as chemotherapy treatment for osteosarcoma. (Also assign an HCPCS Level II code for the medication.)

   _____

Photodynamic Therapy

Photodynamic therapy is administered by

- External application of light to destroy premalignancies
- Endoscopic application of light that activates photosensitive drugs to ablate abnormal tissue

 Coding Tip

A photodynamic therapy code is reported for each exposure session, *not* for each lesion treated.

Photodynamic therapy (PDT) is the application of a photosensitizing agent (e.g., 20 percent topical aminolevulinic acid HCl) directly onto a patient's lesions to treat premalignant cells (e.g., nonhyperkeratotic actinic keratosis) or abnormal cells. The patient returns for a scheduled encounter during which a photodynamic therapy illuminator (light) is directed on the treated lesions. A cytotoxic reaction results when the topical agent applied to the lesions is irradiated, killing premalignant or abnormal cells, preventing their spread.

> **Example:** On May 1, single unit dosage of 20 percent topical aminolevulinic acid HCl was applied and illuminated/activated as the photosensitive drug. The patient underwent photodynamic therapy via external application of light to destroy premalignant lesions of the skin and adjacent mucosa. Report codes 96567 and J7308.

Special Dermatological Procedures

Special dermatological procedures codes describe dermatology procedures that are usually (but not always) performed in addition to an appropriate evaluation and management (E/M) service code.

> **Example:** During a level 3 outpatient consultation encounter, the dermatologist performed a history and examination, and level of medical decision making was low. The dermatologist used ultraviolet light (actinotherapy) to treat the two areas of acne frontalis. Report codes 99243 and 96900.

Physical Medicine and Rehabilitation

Physical medicine and rehabilitation is a branch of medicine that focuses on the prevention, diagnosis, and treatment of disorders of the musculoskeletal, cardiovascular, and pulmonary systems that may produce temporary or permanent impairment. A **physiatrist** is a physician who specializes in physical medicine and rehabilitation and treats acute/chronic pain and musculoskeletal disorders. Physiatrists also treat disorders of the musculoskeletal system that result in severe functional limitations (e.g., a baby with a birth defect, the victim of a bad car accident, an older adult person with a broken hip). Physiatrists coordinate the long-term rehabilitation process for patients with spinal-cord injuries, cancer, stroke, brain injuries, amputations, and multiple sclerosis or other neurological disorders. The specialty focuses on the restoration of function to people with problems ranging from simple physical mobility issues to those with complex cognitive involvement.

Physiatrists offer a broad spectrum of medical services (e.g., the prescription of drugs or assistive devices such as a brace or artificial limb). However, they do not perform surgery. Physiatrists use diverse modalities (any physical agent applied to produce therapeutic changes) that include therapies such as heat and cold, electrotherapies, massage, biofeedback, traction, and therapeutic exercise. (The CPT coding manual provides definitions of documentation components required for physical therapy evaluations, such as body regions.)

> **Example 1:** Patient underwent diathermy. Report code 97024.

> **Example 2:** A diabetic patient presents for treatment of a chronic open wound on the left foot. The wound measures 4 cm $\times$ 3 cm (or 12 sq cm), and the physician treats it by using surgical scissors to perform sharp selective debridement. Report code 97597.

Medical Nutrition Therapy

Medical nutrition therapy includes

- Type of assessment
- Individual or group therapy
- Length of time

> **Example:** Patient underwent medical nutrition therapy reevaluation and assessment. The provider spent 30 minutes face-to-face with the patient. Report codes 97803 and 97803.

Acupuncture

Acupuncture treatment includes face-to-face patient contact for 15-minute increments of time and according to whether electrical stimulation was provided.

Example: Patient underwent acupuncture, which included five needles. The provider spent 30 minutes of one-on-one contact with the patient. Report codes 97810 and 97811.

Exercise 19.7 – Photodynamic Therapy, Dermatology, Medical Nutrition Therapy, Acupuncture

Instructions: Assign CPT code(s) to each statement.

1. PHOTODYNAMIC THERAPY: External application of light for photodynamic therapy of premalignant lesion, forehead, after application of aminolevulinic acid HCl photosensitive drug 10% gel, 10 mg, August 14. (Also assign an HCPCS Level II code for supply of drug.)

   _____

2. SPECIAL DERMATOLOGICAL PROCEDURES: Actinotherapy ultraviolet light for treatment of severe psoriasis.

   _____

3. PHYSICAL MEDICINE AND REHABILITATION: Patient was immersed in Hubbard tank for burn tissue cleansing, 15 minutes.

   _____

4. MEDICAL NUTRITION THERAPY: Patient underwent initial assessment and intervention for medical nutrition therapy, face-to-face, 15 minutes.

   _____

5. ACUPUNCTURE: Patient received acupuncture, 10 needles, 30 minutes.

   _____

Osteopathic Manipulative Treatment

Manipulative and body-based practices focus primarily on the structures and systems of the body, including the bones and joints, the soft tissues, and the circulatory and lymphatic systems. **Osteopathic manipulative treatment (OMT)** is a manual treatment performed by a physician, during which emphasis is placed on normal body mechanics and manipulative methods to detect and correct structure. Osteopathic practice includes diagnostic and therapeutic techniques (e.g., musculoskeletal manipulations as well as prescriptions and other therapies) and preventive measures. Combining available medical procedures with OMT provides patients with the most comprehensive care. The osteopathic codes are reported according to the number of body regions treated. It is also appropriate to report codes for other restorative modalities and procedures performed on the same day when medically necessary.

Coding Tip

- A provider who performs OMT cannot report anesthesia services separately (e.g., nerve blocks and epidural injections) for OMT.
- According to Medicare, postoperative pain management after OMT (e.g., a nerve block or an epidural injection) is not reported separately. However, epidural or nerve block injections unrelated to the OMT may be reported with an OMT code by adding modifier 59.

Example: The osteopathic physician provided osteopathic manipulative treatment to four body regions. Report code 98926.

Chiropractic Manipulative Treatment

Chiropractic manipulative treatment (CMT) is a form of manual treatment to influence joint and neurophysiological function. This treatment may be accomplished using a variety of techniques.

CMT codes include a premanipulation patient assessment. However, additional E/M services may be reported separately by adding modifier 25 if the patient's condition requires a separate E/M service beyond the usual preservice and postservice work associated with the CMT procedure.

For purposes of CMT, the five spinal regions include the following:

- Cervical region (e.g., atlanto-occipital joint)
- Thoracic region (e.g., costovertebral and costotransverse joints)
- Lumbar region
- Sacral region
- Pelvic region (e.g., sacroiliac joint)

The five extraspinal regions include the head (including temporomandibular joint, excluding atlanto-occipital), lower extremities, upper extremities, rib cage (excluding costotransverse and costovertebral joints), and abdomen.

Example: A chiropractor provided chiropractic manipulative treatment to four regions of the spine. Report code 98941.

Education and Training for Patient Self-Management

Education and training for patient self-management is performed by a qualified, nonphysician health care professional who uses a standardized curriculum. The codes are based on the length of time spent face-to-face with one or more patients.

Example: Patient underwent education and training for self-management of the recently diagnosed diabetes mellitus. The nonphysician health care professional spent 30 minutes providing face-to-face instruction. Report code 98960.

Non-Face-to-Face Nonphysician Services

Non-face-to-face nonphysician services that are provided by a qualified health care professional (nonphysician) include the following:

- Telephone services
  - Codes for telephone services are not reported when they result in a patient encounter within 24 hours or at the next available urgent visit appointment. Such telephone services are considered part of the preservice work for the subsequent face-to-face encounter.
  - Telephone service codes are also not reported when the call is related to a service performed and reported by the provider within the past seven days or within the postoperative period of a previously completed procedure.

Example: Patient was out of the country and became concerned about experiencing panic attacks. Patient reached out to the nurse practitioner who initiated a 25-minute telephone call, which included medical discussion evaluation and management services and instructions about proper use of prescribed medication. Report code 98968.

- Qualified nonphysician health care professional digital evaluation and management service in response to a patient's online inquiry using Internet resources to report codes for online medical evaluation services, the qualified nonphysician health care professional must provide a personal, timely response to the inquiry and the encounter must be permanently stored via electronic means or hard copy.

- Remote therapeutic monitoring services (e.g., respiratory system status) includes data review and monitoring of signs, symptoms, and functions to determine a therapeutic response.

- Remote therapeutic monitoring treatment management services use remote therapeutic monitoring results for patient management in accordance with the treatment plan.

Special Services, Procedures, and Reports

Special services, procedures, and reports include the completion of special reports and provision of adjunctive services, which describe special circumstances under which a basic procedure is performed.

> **Example 1:** The physician office handled and conveyed a specimen for transfer to a laboratory. Report code 99000. (If provided, report a service code for obtaining the specimen, such as venipuncture.)

> **Example 2:** A patient was referred to physical therapy after orthopedic surgery. The patient required a 30-day interim visit to the surgeon. Report code 99024 for the surgeon visit. (The code is reported on a claim although the payer does not reimburse for the service provided because its payment was bundled in the previously submitted surgery code. Code 99024 allows for internal tracking of postoperative care services provided by the surgeon during the global surgical period, which reduces the risk of complications of surgery, helps manage side effects of treatment, and supports recovery. Thus, code 99024 supports the quality of care provided to patients.)

Qualifying Circumstances for Anesthesia

Qualifying circumstances for anesthesia codes describe situations that complicate the administration of anesthesia services (e.g., emergencies, extreme age, hypotension, and hypothermia). Codes 99100–99140 are add-on codes, which means that they are reported in addition to the anesthesia service code reported from the Anesthesia section.

> **Example:** An otherwise unusually healthy 84-year-old patient underwent left hip replacement surgery, which required the administration of general anesthesia by the anesthesiologist. Report codes 01214 AA P1 (general anesthesia service) and 99100.

Moderate (Conscious) Sedation

Moderate (conscious) sedation is a drug-induced depression of consciousness that requires no interventions to maintain airway patency or ventilation. CPT specifies that moderate (conscious) sedation does not include pain control, minimal sedation (e.g., anxiolysis), deep sedation, or monitored anesthesia care (MAC). Subsection notes specify services that are included in moderate (conscious) sedation codes (e.g., IV access, administration of agent, and monitoring oxygen saturation). The surgeon who performs the surgical procedure provides moderate (conscious) sedation services. An *independent trained observer* is present during surgery to monitor the patient's sedation. When another physician (e.g., an anesthesiologist) provides general anesthesia, regional anesthesia, or monitored anesthesia care, that other physician reports an appropriate anesthesia code and its modifiers.

Example 1: A 68-year-old patient received 15 minutes of moderate (conscious) sedation services, which were provided by the same physician who removed a superficial orthopedic wire. An independent trained observer was present to monitor the patient's sedation. Report codes 20670 (removal of superficial implant) and 99156.

Example 2: A 19-year-old patient was prepped and draped for brain surgery and received moderate (conscious) sedation in the form of a narcotic called remifentanil (brand name Ultiva) administered in combination with propofol. An independent trained observer was present to monitor the patient's sedation. It was determined that the patient could feel no pain but would be able to communicate with the operating room staff and surgeon during the procedure. Trephination craniectomy and bone flap craniotomy were performed after intraoperative brain magnetic resonance imaging (MRI) confirmed the exact location of the supratentorial tumor. It was noted that the tumor was pressing on the area of the cerebrum that controls the ability to read and speak.

During the procedure, the patient remained heavily sedated but conscious so the surgeon could talk with them while mapping the brain's sensors. The patient read a book aloud during the procedure; when the surgeon pressed on a sensitive region of the brain, the patient's reading was affected, letting the surgeon know which areas to avoid. Upon completion of brain mapping, the risky areas were marked by placing lettered pieces of paper directly onto the brain to identify the areas of risk. The surgeon then opened the brain's outer membrane and, layer by layer, removed the tumor. The patient felt no pain (because the brain has no pain receptors), and the tumor was submitted to pathology for analysis. The patient tolerated the one-hour procedure well and was transported to the recovery room in stable condition. The patient will undergo repeat MRI in 30 days to verify total resection of the tumor. Report codes 61510, 70551, 99156 (first 15 minutes), and 99157, 99157, and 99157 (subsequent 45 minutes). (Code 99156 is reported once for the first 15 minutes of moderate [conscious] sedation. Then, code 99157 is assigned three times for the subsequent 45 minutes of moderate [conscious] sedation.)

Other Services and Procedures

Other services and procedures codes are reported for services and procedures that cannot be coded in another subsection of the Medicine section (e.g., anogenital examination, vision screening by nonoptical professionals, hypothermia treatment).

Example: Patient underwent therapeutic phlebotomy. Report code 99195.

Home Health Procedures/Services

Home health procedures/services codes are reported by nonphysician health care professionals who perform procedures and provide services to the patient in the patient's residence (the patient's home, assisted living facility, or group home). *Home infusion procedures/services* are reported for the provision of home infusion services, and the codes are based on length of infusion time.

Example 1: Patient received a home visit from a registered nurse for mechanical ventilation care. Report code 99504.

Example 2: Patient underwent three hours of home infusion on May 14. Report codes 99601 and 99602.

Medication Therapy Management Services

Medication therapy management services (MTMS) describe face-to-face patient assessments and interventions performed by a pharmacist to

- Optimize the patient's response to medications.
- Manage treatment-related medication interactions or complications.

Documentation of MTMS includes review of the pertinent patient history and medication profile (prescription and nonprescription) as well as recommendations for improving health outcomes and compliance with treatment.

Example: An established patient received 15 minutes of medication therapy management face-to-face services, which was provided by a pharmacist. Report code 99606.

NOTE:

MTMS codes are not reported to describe the provision of product-specific information at the point of dispensing or any other routine dispensing-related activities, such as information provided by a pharmacy about prescribed medications.

Exercise 19.8 – OMT, Chiropractic, Education/Training for Patient Self-Management, Non-Face-to-Face Nonphysician Services, Special Services/Procedures/Reports, Other Services/Procedures, Moderate (Conscious) Sedation, Home Health, Medication Therapy Management Services

Instructions: Assign CPT code(s) to each statement.

1. OSTEOPATHIC MANIPULATIVE TREATMENT: Osteopathic manipulative treatment of the cervical, thoracic, lumbar, and sacral regions.

   _____

2. CHIROPRACTIC MANIPULATIVE TREATMENT: Chiropractic manipulative treatment of the cervical, thoracic, and lumbar spinal regions.

   _____

3. EDUCATION AND TRAINING FOR PATIENT SELF-MANAGEMENT: Education and training for patient self-management using a standardized curriculum, face-to-face with patient, 60 minutes.

   _____

4. NON-FACE-TO-FACE NONPHYSICIAN SERVICES: The nurse practitioner provided 15 minutes of telephone assessment and management services about how the patient was tolerating the switch to a new medication for anxiety and depression.

   _____

5. SPECIAL SERVICES, PROCEDURES, AND REPORTS: The outside laboratory facility picked up a blood specimen from the physician's office and transported it to the lab.

   _____

6. OTHER SERVICES AND PROCEDURES: Automated visual acuity screening test, quantitative, right and left eyes.

   _____

7. OTHER SERVICES AND PROCEDURES: Therapeutic phlebotomy was administered for treatment of hemochromatosis.

   _____

8. HOME HEALTH PROCEDURES/SERVICES: Home visit for newborn care and assessment.

   _____

9. HOME HEALTH PROCEDURES/SERVICES: Home visit for hemodialysis.

   _____

10. MEDICATION THERAPY MANAGEMENT SERVICES: A pharmacist provided face-to-face medical therapy management to a patient, 10 minutes.

   _____

Summary

The Medicine section includes codes for procedures and services that are procedure-oriented, that apply to various medical specialties, and that apply to different types of health care providers. Guidelines located at the beginning of the Medicine section provide instruction about multiple procedures, add-on codes, separate procedures, subsection information, unlisted service or procedure, special reports, and materials supplied by the physician. Instructional notes appear throughout the Medicine section to provide coding clarification and direction. Almost every Medicine subsection contains notes unique to the subsection.

Internet Links

American Chiropractic Association: www.acatoday.org

American Physical Therapy Association (APTA): www.apta.org

Chemotherapy: Go to **www.cancer.gov**, scroll over About Cancer and click on the Treatment link to view types of cancer treatment, including chemotherapy.

National Center for Complementary and Integrative Health (at the National Institutes of Health): www.nccih.nih.gov

Review

19.1 – Multiple Choice

Instructions: Select the most appropriate response.

1. Which is a manual treatment performed to influence joint and neurophysiological function?
    a. Bilevel (biphasic) positive airway pressure (BiPAP)
    b. Chiropractic manipulative treatment (CMT)
    c. Intermittent positive pressure breathing (IPPB)
    d. Osteopathic manipulative treatment (OMT)

2. A physician who specializes in physical medicine and rehabilitation and who treats acute/chronic pain and musculoskeletal disorders is a(n)
    a. doctor of osteopathy.
    b. internist.
    c. psychologist.
    d. physiatrist.

3. Chemotherapy administered in addition to other cancer treatments, such as surgery and/or radiation therapy, is called _____ chemotherapy.
    a. adjacent
    b. adjudicate
    c. adjunct
    d. adjuvant

4. Which uses low-voltage electrodes that are placed on the scalp and target sites to test the nervous system's pathway?
    a. Central motor evoked potential study
    b. Orbicularis oculi (blink) test
    c. Short-latency somatosensory evoked potential study
    d. Visual evoked potential (VEP) test

5. Which is a biofeedback diagnostic test that measures muscle function using a pressure-sensitive tube?
    a. Electrocardiography
    b. Electromyogram
    c. Manometry
    d. Tensilon test

6. Which Medicine subsection includes codes for a drug-induced depression of consciousness that requires no interventions to maintain airway patency or ventilation?
   a. Moderate (Conscious) Sedation
   b. Other Services and Procedures
   c. Photodynamic Therapy
   d. Noninvasive Vascular Diagnostic Studies

7. Which is considered an epicutaneous allergy sensitivity test?
   a. Intradermal test
   b. Patch test
   c. Puncture test
   d. Scratch test

8. End-Stage Renal Disease Services (ESRD) category codes in the Dialysis subsection of the Medicine section are reported monthly to distinguish _____ services, which are related to a patient's ESRD and performed in an outpatient setting.
   a. age-specific
   b. hemodialysis-related only
   c. miscellaneous
   d. unlisted procedure

9. The Medicine section includes codes for procedures and services that are
   a. diagnosis-oriented and apply to a limited number of medical specialties.
   b. disease-oriented and apply to many medical specialties.
   c. process-oriented and apply to a limited number of medical specialties.
   d. procedure-oriented and apply to many medical specialties.

10. Which of the following is identified in the CPT with a plus symbol and usually contains a parenthetical note that identifies the primary procedure to which the code applies?
    a. Add-on code
    b. Multiple or bundled code
    c. Separate procedure code
    d. Unlisted service or procedure code

11. A 42-year-old patient underwent immunization administration of Hepatitis A vaccine. Which CPT codes are assigned?
    a. 90471, 90632   b. 90471, 90636   c. 90471, 90746   d. 90471, 90749

12. Binaural hearing aid check. Which CPT code is assigned?
    a. 92590   b. 92591   c. 92592   d. 92593

13. Cardiovascular stress test, bicycle with continuous electrocardiographic monitoring, interpretation and report only. Which CPT code is assigned?
    a. 93015   b. 93016   c. 93017   d. 93018

14. A 30-day, patient-initiated spirometric recording, including hook-up, reinforced education, data transmission and capture, trend analysis, and periodic recalibration as well as physician review and interpretation. Which CPT code is assigned?
    a. 94010   b. 94014   c. 94015   d. 94016

15. Inhalation bronchial challenge testing with histamine. Which CPT code is assigned?
    a. 95070   b. 95076   c. 95079   d. 95199

16. Comprehensive computer-based motion analysis by videotaping and 3D kinematics with dynamic plantar pressure measurements during walking. Which CPT code is assigned?
    a. 96000   b. 96001   c. 96002   d. 96004

17. Physical therapy re-evaluation. Which CPT code is assigned?
    a. 97161   b. 97162   c. 97163   d. 97164

18. A patient and their spouse received 30 minutes of face-to-face individual education and training from a qualified nurse practitioner for patient self-management of diabetic testing supplies. Which CPT code(s) are assigned?

    a. 98960   **c.** 98961

    b. 98960, 98960 59   **d.** 99078

19. During a therapeutic service, a 15-year-old patient required 15 minutes of moderate (conscious) sedation. The physician who performed the therapeutic service also administered the sedation, and an independently trained observer monitored the patient's level of consciousness and physiological status, which included postservice work. Which CPT code is assigned?

    a. 99151   **b.** 99152   **c.** 99155   **d.** 99156

20. A psychiatrist used dolls to communicate with a 5-year-old patient during a psychiatric diagnostic evaluation. Which CPT code is assigned?

    a. 90791   **b.** 90792   **c.** 90845   **d.** 90847

19.2 – Coding Practice: Medicine Section

Instructions: Assign CPT code(s) to each case.

1. OPHTHALMOLOGY: Based on the patient's prescription for bifocal lens, the patient's anatomical facial characteristics were measured, laboratory specifications documented, and final adjustment of bifocal eyeglasses performed.

   _____

2. CNS ASSESSMENTS/TESTS: The patient had standard cognitive performance testing for one hour done on November 15. This was done on a computer. A neuropsychologist interpreted the results and documented the report.

   _____

3. OPHTHALMOLOGY: The patient arrived at the office for an eye examination. The patient has never been seen in this practice. The patient complains of redness of both eyes and a decrease in visual acuity. After reviewing the patient's medical history, including medications, the patient's eyes are examined with the ophthalmoscope. Using a slit lamp exam, several small healing ulcers of the right and left cornea are seen. The patient is given instructions for eye irrigation and a prescription for steroidal eye drops. Diagnosis: Viral keratitis.

   _____

4. GASTROENTEROLOGY: Patient presented for a Bernstein acid perfusion test, esophagus. After insertion of a nasogastric (NG) tube, a solution was passed through the tube to record any complaints of chest pain. The first solution was saline, and the patient did not report any pain. The second solution was hydrochloric acid, and this solution did elicit a pain response in the patient. The Bernstein test was positive for esophagitis.

   _____

5. NONINVASIVE VASCULAR DIAGNOSTIC STUDIES: Patient underwent a complete transcranial Doppler study of intracranial arteries.

   _____

6. SPECIAL OTORHINOLARYNGOLOGIC SERVICE: A seven-year-old patient presented for visual reinforcement audiometry (VRA) evaluation. After being placed in a sound booth, both voice and lighted toys were used for hearing assessment. An audiogram recorded the findings, which were normal.

   _____

7. PULMONARY: The patient, a 14-year-old with cystic fibrosis, was seen for chest wall cupping as a manipulation procedure of the chest wall to help clear mucous secretion. This initial demonstration was also observed by the patient's mother as a teaching opportunity for home care by the parent.

---

8. CARDIOVASCULAR: Patient received an outpatient cardiac rehabilitation session during the sixth week of the postoperative period. Patient had previously undergone coronary artery bypass graft surgery of four vessels. This session included exercise and a review of diet restrictions with the patient.

---

9. BIOFEEDBACK: Biofeedback training of perineal muscles and urethral sphincter to assist with the patient's urine incontinence, 15 minutes. Manometry and electromyogram (EMG) were used to measure contractions and muscle pressure.

---

10. CARDIOVASCULAR: The patient presented three years' postimplantation for interrogation device evaluation services of a dual-chamber cardiac pacemaker with analysis, including review and report, while the patient was both at rest and on a treadmill. No pacemaker reprogramming was needed.

---

11. CARDIOVASCULAR: After placing the patient in the supine position, complete transthoracic echocardiography was performed to record cardiac function. The patient's ventricular septal defect (VSD), which is a congenital heart condition, was identified. The size of the defect was 2.0 mm. The remainder of the cardiac structures appeared normal in size and function.

---

12. CHIROPRACTIC MANIPULATIVE TREATMENT: After placing the patient on the adjustment table, chiropractic manipulation of C7, T4, and L1 were performed to reduce subluxation and increase blood flow. The patient was scheduled for another appointment in one week's time.

---

13. VACCINES, TOXOIDS: A 40-year-old patient presented for a hepatitis A and hepatitis B vaccine. This combination HepA/HepB immunization was administered by the nursing staff, IM, in the left arm.

---

14. PHYSICAL MEDICINE AND REHABILITATION: A primary care physician provided 30 minutes of activities of daily living training in using adaptive utensils for eating. During the encounter, safety procedures while cooking were also discussed with this patient, who has diagnoses of arthritis and type 2 diabetes mellitus.

---

15. NEUROLOGY AND NEUROMUSCULAR PROCEDURES: Patient was awake when electrodes were placed on the head for recording. An electro-encephalogram (EEG) was performed with extended monitoring during a 90-minute period. The patient was awake for the entire EEG.

---

16. GASTROENTEROLOGY: Gastric electrical activity was measured during diagnostic electrogastrography by placing electrodes transcutaneously over the abdominal cavity. The recording of gastric activity showed that the patient had decreased activity in the large intestine.

---

17. SPECIAL OTORHINOLARYNGOLOGIC SERVICES: The patient presented with facial paralysis of the left side of the lower face. An electroneuronography as part of a facial nerve function study was done to measure nerve conduction. Electrodes were placed over the site of the paralysis. Diagnosis: Bell's palsy.

18. IMMUNE GLOBULINS, SERUM OR RECOMBINANT PRODUCTS: A 25-year-old patient received intramuscular hepatitis B immune globulin (HBIg) (human) injection, which was administered by the nursing staff.

19. PSYCHIATRY: Patient participated in a multifamily group psychotherapy session for a total of 30 minutes. This session was done at a local community hospital in the mental health inpatient unit.

20. CARDIOVASCULAR: After placing electrodes on the patient's chest, the heart's activity was recorded via electrocardiography. The 12-lead strip was reviewed and a report was written by the attending physician.

21. CARDIOVASCULAR: Under adequate anesthesia, incisions were made in the left leg of the patient for access of the femoral catheter. A second site allowed for insertion of the balloon-tipped catheter. After threading the balloon catheter to the heart, the blocked coronary artery was identified. The balloon was inflated, and percutaneous transluminal coronary angioplasty resulted in movement of the arthrosclerosis plaque to the sides of the artery. The balloon catheter was advanced to another branch of the blocked coronary artery. The same inflation method was done for percutaneous transluminal coronary angioplasty with good result. The balloon catheter was withdrawn. The incision sites were closed with sutures and pressure dressings.

22. CARDIOVASCULAR: While the patient was exercising on a stationary bicycle, continuous electrocardiogram (ECG) monitoring and recording was done. The patient's cardiologist was in attendance for the entire 45-minute cardiovascular stress test. At the conclusion of the test, the physician provided a written report on the findings and the interpreted ECG recordings.

23. GASTROENTEROLOGY: Patient underwent gastroesophageal reflux study via esophagus, which included placement of nasal catheter pH electrodes, recording, analysis, and interpretation.

24. HOME HEALTH PROCEDURES/SERVICES: A 15-year-old patient was recently diagnosed with asthma. A home health nurse visited on May 6 to provide home services for respiratory therapy training in the use of bronchodilators for both the patient and guardian.

25. PHYSICAL MEDICINE AND REHABILITATION: A patient is status post left side cerebrovascular accident (CVA) and hypertension. Patient presents for physical therapy evaluation to regain strength and mobility on the left side. The patient underwent moderate complexity physical therapy evaluation.

26. ALLERGY AND CLINICAL IMMUNOLOGY: Using allergen vials specifically kept in the office for a certain patient, a pollen and grass mix was injected into the upper-right arm. Then, a dust mite, cat dander, and feather mixture was injected into the patient's upper-left arm. The patient was observed in the waiting room for 30 minutes postinjection, with no reaction.

_____

27. SPECIAL DERMATOLOGICAL PROCEDURES: Using an Excimer laser, approximately 25 pulses were delivered to a patient's psoriasis lesions on the elbows and forearms. Total area of treatment measured approximately 10 sq cm.

_____

28. IMMUNE GLOBULINS, SERUM OR RECOMBINANT PRODUCTS: Rabies immune globulin was administered intramuscularly (IM) to the patient's upper-left arm.

_____

29. DIALYSIS: ESRD services for a 25-year-old patient for the month of September. Number of visits to a physician for the month totaled four.

_____

30. CHEMOTHERAPY ADMINISTRATION: Intravenous (IV) infusion of chemotherapy drugs, two hours.

_____

Part

VIII

Insurance and Reimbursement Overview

Chapter Outline

Third-Party Payers

Health Care Reimbursement Systems

Impact of HIPAA on Reimbursement

Chapter Objectives

At the conclusion of this chapter, the student should be able to:

1. Define key terms related to insurance and reimbursement.
2. Describe the types of third-party payers.
3. Describe the types of health care reimbursement systems.
4. Describe the impact of HIPAA on health care reimbursement.

Key Terms

ANSI ASC X12N 837

capitation

case mix

charge description master (CDM)

chargemaster

CMS-1450

CMS-1500

commercial payer

electronic data interchange (EDI)

electronic transaction standard

employer self-insurance plan

encounter form

explanation of benefits (EOB)

fee-for-service

flat file

government-sponsored programs

health insurance claim

health insurance policy

HIPAA administrative simplification (AS)

managed care

Medicare administrative contractor (MAC)

Medicare Summary Notice (MSN)

nonparticipating provider (nonPAR)

overpayment

overpayment recovery

participating provider (PAR)

preauthorization

pre-existing medical condition

prospective cost-based rate

prospective payment system (PPS)

prospective price-based rate

remittance advice (remit)

revenue code

roster billing

superbill

UB-04

workers' compensation

Introduction

This chapter includes a discussion of third-party payers, health care reimbursement methodologies, and the impact of HIPAA on health care reimbursement. Third-party payers process health insurance claims to reimburse providers (e.g., physicians, health care facilities) for services provided to patients for covered benefits. Health care reimbursement methodologies were originally developed by the Centers for Medicare & Medicaid Services (CMS) to control health care costs associated with government programs; however, most third-party payers have also adopted them. HIPAA has impacted health care reimbursement as a result of the implementation of federal regulations such as administrative simplification, privacy and security of protected health information, and more.

Third-Party Payers

A third-party payer is an insurance company or other organization (e.g., BlueCross BlueShield) that processes health care claims for reimbursement of procedures and services. Payers also serve as **Medicare administrative contractors (MACs)** by processing claims for physicians (Medicare Part B); health care facilities (Medicare Part A); suppliers of durable medical equipment, prosthetics, orthotics, and supplies (DMEPOS); and home health and hospice agencies. The CMS, an administrative agency in the Department of Health & Human Services (DHHS), selects MACs through a competitive bidding process.

Title IX of the *Medicare Prescription Drug, Improvement, and Modernization Act of 2003 (MMA)* called for the elimination of carriers, fiscal intermediaries (FIs), and durable medical equipment regional carriers (DMERCs) and the creation of Medicare administrative contractors. The MMA limits *indemnification* (insurance against loss) for adverse judgments against MACs and associated legal costs. Providers no longer have a right to choose who will review claims or pay benefits because MACs integrate Medicare Part A and Part B functions into one contract, and providers have a single point of contact for all claims-related activity. MACs have been established in 12 geographic areas (or jurisdictions) throughout the United States, and four of them also process home health and hospice (HH+H) claims. Durable medical equipment (DME) claims are processed by four additional DME MACs, which provide reimbursement for Medicare Durable Medical Equipment, Orthotics, and Prosthetics (DMEPOS) claims according to defined geographic areas (or jurisdictions) that service the DMEPOS suppliers.

 NOTE:

By 2010, Medicare had eliminated the following to create Medicare Administrative Contractors (MACs) that consolidated the administration of Medicare Part A and B benefits so that Medicare beneficiaries have claims processed by one contractor. (Carrier and fiscal intermediary language still appears in some Medicare literature.)

- *Carriers* (processed Medicare Part B claims)
- *Fiscal intermediaries (FIs)* (processed Medicare Part A claims)
- *Durable medical equipment regional carriers (DMERCs)* (processed durable medical equipment, prosthetics, orthotics, and supplies [DMEPOS])

Durable medical equipment, prosthetics, orthotics, and supplies (DMEPOS) claims are processed by DME MACs, and home health and hospice (HH&H) claims are processed by HH&H MACs.

A **health insurance policy** is an agreement between an individual and a third-party payer (or health insurance company) that contains a list of reimbursable medical benefits, or *covered benefits* (which might include office visits, inpatient hospitalizations, laboratory, tests, prescription medications, treatment services, and so on). The policy also lists procedures and services that are *not* covered by the third-party payer, called *noncovered benefits*, and when an individual undergoes procedures or receives services that are not covered by the policy, the individual is responsible for reimbursing the health care provider directly (e.g., cosmetic surgery). A health care provider is a physician or other health care practitioner (e.g., a nurse practitioner) who provides services to patients.

After patient care has been delivered, the provider submits a **health insurance claim** to a payer to request reimbursement for procedures performed or services provided (e.g., CMS-1500, UB-04). The **CMS-1500** (Figure 20-1) is a standard claim submitted by physician offices to third-party payers. The **UB-04** (or **CMS-1450**) (Figure 20-2) is a standard claim submitted by health care institutions to payers for inpatient and outpatient encounters. CMS-1500 and UB-04 claims can also be submitted as electronic data interchange (EDI) transactions using specialized software (Figure 20-3), which is discussed later in this chapter. *Health care clearinghouses* and *third-party administrators (TPAs)* process or facilitate the processing of health information (such as a claim) received from another entity (such as a provider or payer) from a nonstandard into a standard format. (TPAs provide additional operational services, such as contracted employee benefits management.)

Determining which claim to submit, as well as which coding system to use to report codes on the claim, depends on the health care setting (Table 20-1). Noninstitutional providers (e.g., physician offices, independent labs, ambulance companies that are *not* associated with hospitals, ambulatory surgery centers, and independent diagnostic testing facilities) and suppliers (for durable medical equipment, prosthetics, orthotics, and supplies dealers) submit the CMS-1500 claim to third-party payers, and they report ICD-10-CM diagnosis codes and CPT and HCPCS Level II (CPT/HCPCS) procedure and service codes with modifiers. Institutional providers (e.g., hospitals, nursing facilities, comprehensive outpatient rehabilitation facilities, community mental health centers, outpatient physical therapy facilities, rehabilitation agencies, and end-stage renal facilities) submit the UB-04 claim to payers. For inpatient claims, ICD-10-CM diagnosis codes and ICD-10-PCS procedure codes are reported. For outpatient claims (e.g., emergency department, outpatient care), ICD-10-CM diagnosis codes and CPT/HCPCS procedure and service codes with modifiers are reported.

Before delivering health care services to patients, some payers require providers to obtain **preauthorization** (prior approval) of treatment (e.g., procedures/services provided by a specialist) and to submit post-treatment reports. If the provider does not meet the preauthorization requirements, the claim is denied. If the patient's insurance policy contains a *hold harmless clause* that states the patient is not responsible for paying what the insurance plan denies, the health care provider is prohibited from collecting payment from the patient. Claims are also denied if the medical necessity of procedures or services is not established. This means that every procedure or service reported on the claim must be linked to a condition that justifies the necessity for performing that procedure or providing that service. If the procedures or services delivered are determined to be unreasonable or unnecessary, the claim is denied.

Health Insurance Marketplace

The *Patient Protection and Affordable Care Act (PPACA)* was signed into federal law on March 23, 2010, and resulted in the creation of a *Health Insurance Marketplace*® (or *health insurance exchange*), abbreviated as the Marketplace, effective October 1, 2013. The PPACA is abbreviated as the *Affordable Care Act (ACA)*, and it has been nicknamed *Obamacare* (because it was signed into federal law by President Obama). *The Health Insurance Marketplace*® *does NOT replace other health insurance programs (e.g., individual and group commercial health insurance, Medicaid, Medicare, TRICARE)* and allows Americans to purchase health coverage that fits their budget and meets their health care needs. It is a resource where individuals, families, and small businesses can

- Learn about their health coverage options
- Compare health insurance plans based on costs, benefits, and other important features
- Choose a plan
- Enroll in coverage

HEALTH INSURANCE CLAIM FORM

APPROVED BY NATIONAL UNIFORM CLAIM COMMITTEE (NUCC) 02/12

METROPOLITAN
PO BOX 500

BIG CITY IL 606050500

PICA

PICA							

1. MEDICARE (Medicare#) □   MEDICAID (Medicaid#) □   TRICARE (ID#/DoD#) □   CHAMPVA (Member ID#) □   GROUP HEALTH PLAN (ID#) □   FECA BLK LUNG (ID#) □   OTHER (ID#) [X]

1a. INSURED'S I.D. NUMBER (For Program in Item 1)
225120661W

2. PATIENT'S NAME (Last Name, First Name, Middle Initial)
PUBLIC, JOHN, Q

3. PATIENT'S BIRTH DATE   MM **03** DD **09** YY **2000**   SEX M [X] F □

4. INSURED'S NAME (Last Name, First Name, Middle Initial)
PUBLIC, JOHN, Q

5. PATIENT'S ADDRESS (No., Street)
10A SENATE AVENUE

6. PATIENT RELATIONSHIP TO INSURED
Self [X] Spouse □ Child □ Other □

7. INSURED'S ADDRESS (No., Street)
10A SENATE AVENUE

CITY **ANYWHERE**   STATE **NY**

8. RESERVED FOR NUCC USE

CITY **ANYWHERE**   STATE **NY**

ZIP CODE **123451234**   TELEPHONE (Include Area Code) ( )

ZIP CODE **123451234**   TELEPHONE (Include Area Code) ( )

9. OTHER INSURED'S NAME (Last Name, First Name, Middle Initial)

10. IS PATIENT'S CONDITION RELATED TO:

11. INSURED'S POLICY GROUP OR FECA NUMBER

a. OTHER INSURED'S POLICY OR GROUP NUMBER

a. EMPLOYMENT? (Current or Previous)   □ YES [X] NO

a. INSURED'S DATE OF BIRTH   MM **03** DD **09** YY **1945**   SEX M [X] F □

b. RESERVED FOR NUCC USE

b. AUTO ACCIDENT?   □ YES [X] NO   PLACE (State)

b. OTHER CLAIM ID (Designated by NUCC)

c. RESERVED FOR NUCC USE

c. OTHER ACCIDENT?   □ YES [X] NO

c. INSURANCE PLAN NAME OR PROGRAM NAME
METROPOLITAN

d. INSURANCE PLAN NAME OR PROGRAM NAME

10d. CLAIM CODES (Designated by NUCC)

d. IS THERE ANOTHER HEALTH BENEFIT PLAN?
□ YES [X] NO   If yes, complete items 9, 9a, and 9d.

READ BACK OF FORM BEFORE COMPLETING & SIGNING THIS FORM.
12. PATIENT'S OR AUTHORIZED PERSON'S SIGNATURE I authorize the release of any medical or other information necessary to process this claim. I also request payment of government benefits either to myself or to the party who accepts assignment below.

SIGNED **SIGNATURE ON FILE**   DATE

13. INSURED'S OR AUTHORIZED PERSON'S SIGNATURE I authorize payment of medical benefits to the undersigned physician or supplier for services described below.

SIGNED **SIGNATURE ON FILE**

14. DATE OF CURRENT ILLNESS, INJURY, or PREGNANCY (LMP)   MM **01** DD **05** YY   QUAL. **431**

15. OTHER DATE   QUAL.   MM DD YY

16. DATES PATIENT UNABLE TO WORK IN CURRENT OCCUPATION   FROM MM DD YY   TO MM DD YY

17. NAME OF REFERRING PROVIDER OR OTHER SOURCE

17a.
17b. NPI

18. HOSPITALIZATION DATES RELATED TO CURRENT SERVICES   FROM MM DD YY   TO MM DD YY

19. ADDITIONAL CLAIM INFORMATION (Designated by NUCC)

20. OUTSIDE LAB?   □ YES [X] NO $ CHARGES

21. DIAGNOSIS OR NATURE OF ILLNESS OR INJURY Relate A-L to service line below (24E)   ICD Ind. **0**

A. **Z0000**   B. **Z23**   C. ___   D. ___
E. ___   F. ___   G. ___   H. ___
I. ___   J. ___   K. ___   L. ___

22. RESUBMISSION CODE   ORIGINAL REF. NO.

23. PRIOR AUTHORIZATION NUMBER

24. A. DATE(S) OF SERVICE From MM DD YY	To MM DD YY	B. PLACE OF SERVICE	C. EMG	D. PROCEDURES, SERVICES, OR SUPPLIES (Explain Unusual Circumstances) CPT/HCPCS	MODIFIER	E. DIAGNOSIS POINTER	F. $ CHARGES	G. DAYS OR UNITS	H. EPSDT Family Plan	I. ID. QUAL.	J. RENDERING PROVIDER ID. #
1	01 09 YY		11		S0622		AB	150 00	1		NPI	
2	01 09 YY		11		G0010		B	25 00	1		NPI	
3	01 09 YY		11		G0008		B	25 00	1		NPI	
4											NPI	
5											NPI	
6											NPI	

25. FEDERAL TAX I.D. NUMBER   SSN EIN [X]
111234523

26. PATIENT'S ACCOUNT NO.
12-1

27. ACCEPT ASSIGNMENT? (For govt. claims, see back) [X] YES □ NO

28. TOTAL CHARGE $ **200 00**

29. AMOUNT PAID $ **30 00**

30. Rsvd for NUCC Use

31. SIGNATURE OF PHYSICIAN OR SUPPLIER INCLUDING DEGREES OR CREDENTIALS (I certify that the statements on the reverse apply to this bill and are made a part thereof.)

SIGNED **ERIN A HELPER MD**   DATE **MMDDYY**

32. SERVICE FACILITY LOCATION INFORMATION

a.   b.

33. BILLING PROVIDER INFO & PH # (**101**) **1111234**
ERIN A HELPER MD
101 MEDIC DRIVE
ANYWHERE NY 123459874

a. **1234567890**   b.

NUCC Instruction Manual available at: www.nucc.org   **PLEASE PRINT OR TYPE**

CARRIER

PATIENT AND INSURED INFORMATION

PHYSICIAN OR SUPPLIER INFORMATION

FIGURE 20-1 Completed CMS-1500 claim

1 ALFRED STATE MEDICAL CENTER	2		3a PAT. CNTL #	859451562987			4 TYPE OF BILL
548 N MAIN ST			b. MED. REC. #	987654			131
ALFRED NY 14802			5 FED. TAX NO.	6 STATEMENT COVERS PERIOD FROM THROUGH		7	
6075551234 USA			871349061	0505YY	0505YY		

8 PATIENT NAME	a		9 PATIENT ADDRESS	a 15 HILL ST				
b PUBLIC JOHN Q			b ALFRED			c NY	d 14802	e

10 BIRTHDATE	11 SEX	12 DATE	ADMISSION 13 HR 14 TYPE 15 SRC	16 DHR	17 STAT	18 19 20 21	CONDITION CODES 22 23 24 25 26 27 28	29 ACDT STATE	30
08051970	M	0505YY		7	01				

31 OCCURRENCE CODE DATE	32 OCCURRENCE CODE DATE	33 OCCURRENCE CODE DATE	34 OCCURRENCE CODE DATE	35 OCCURRENCE SPAN CODE FROM THROUGH	36 OCCURRENCE SPAN CODE FROM THROUGH	37
a						
b						

38		39 VALUE CODES CODE AMOUNT	40 VALUE CODES CODE AMOUNT	41 VALUE CODES CODE AMOUNT
	a			
	b			
	c			
	d			

42 REV. CD.	43 DESCRIPTION	44 HCPCS / RATE / HIPPS CODE	45 SERV. DATE	46 SERV. UNITS	47 TOTAL CHARGES	48 NON-COVERED CHARGES	49
1 0324	MRA WITH CONTRAST, CHEST	C8909	0505YY	1	850 50		1
2							2
3							3

PAGE 001 OF 001   CREATION DATE 0505YY   TOTALS ▶   850 50

50 PAYER NAME	51 HEALTH PLAN ID	52 REL INFO	53 ASG BEN	54 PRIOR PAYMENTS	55 EST. AMOUNT DUE	56 NPI	987654321
A AETNA	1265891895	Y				57	
B						OTHER	
C						PRV ID	

58 INSURED'S NAME	59 P.REL	60 INSURED'S UNIQUE ID	61 GROUP NAME	62 INSURANCE GROUP NO.
A PUBLIC JOHN Q	18	524856254	COMMERCIAL	495G
B				
C				

63 TREATMENT AUTHORIZATION CODES	64 DOCUMENT CONTROL NUMBER	65 EMPLOYER NAME
A		
B		
C		

66 DX	C3411					68
0						

69 ADMIT DX	70 PATIENT REASON DX		71 PPS CODE	C3411	72 ECI	73

74 PRINCIPAL PROCEDURE CODE DATE	a. OTHER PROCEDURE CODE DATE	b. OTHER PROCEDURE CODE DATE	75	76 ATTENDING NPI 1265891895	QUAL
c. OTHER PROCEDURE CODE DATE	d. OTHER PROCEDURE CODE DATE	e. OTHER PROCEDURE CODE DATE		LAST SMITH FIRST JOHN	
				77 OPERATING NPI LAST FIRST	QUAL

80 REMARKS	81CC a	78 OTHER NPI	QUAL
AETNA	b	LAST FIRST	
PO BOX 650	c	79 OTHER NPI	QUAL
CANANDAIGUA NY 14424	d	LAST FIRST	

UB-04 CMS-1450   APPROVED OMB NO.   NUBC National Uniform Billing Committee LIC9213257   THE CERTIFICATIONS ON THE REVERSE APPLY TO THIS BILL AND ARE MADE A PART HEREOF.

FIGURE 20-2 Completed UB-04 claim

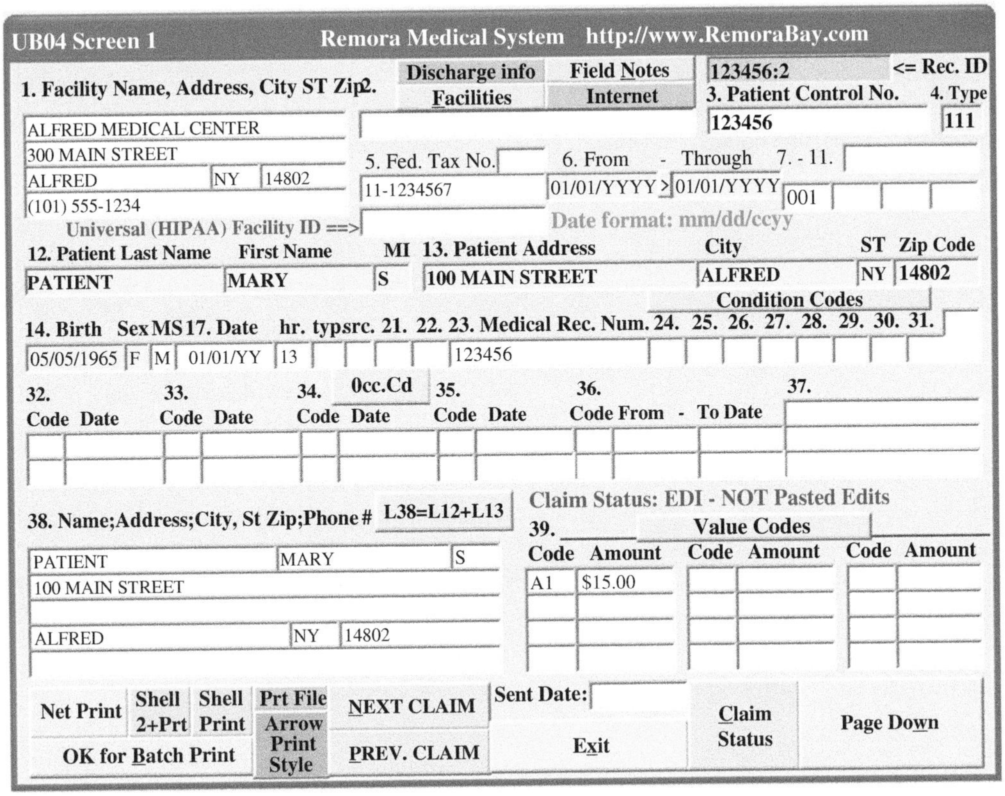

FIGURE 20-3 Sample UB-04 software screen

The Marketplace includes information about programs to help people with low to moderate income and resources pay for health coverage. Information includes ways to save on the monthly premiums and out-of-pocket costs of coverage available through the Marketplace along with information about other programs, including Medicaid and the state Children's Health Insurance Program (CHIP). The Marketplace encourages competition among private health plans, and it is accessible through websites, call centers, and in-person assistance. In some states it is run by the state, and in others it is run by the federal government.

Example: The *Advance Premium Tax Credit (APTC)* is a tax credit that eligible individuals take in advance to lower monthly health insurance premiums. When applying for coverage at the Health Insurance Marketplace®, the expected income for the year is estimated. If the individual qualifies for a premium tax credit based on that estimate, they can use any amount of the credit in advance to lower their premium. At the end of the year, the insured is required to "reconcile tax credits" by filing an appropriate federal tax form as part of their tax return. The IRS determines if too many (or too few) tax credits were applied by comparing the amount on the submitted tax form against their modified adjusted gross income. The tax amount due or refund is adjusted to either collect excess tax credits or deposit the deficit of tax credits.

Most individuals who do not currently have health insurance through their place of work or otherwise are eligible to use the Health Insurance Marketplace (**www.healthcare.gov**) to compare and choose a plan. To be eligible for health coverage through the marketplace, individuals must

- Be a U.S. citizen or national (or be lawfully present)
- Live in the United States
- Not be incarcerated

TABLE 20-1 Claims and Coding Systems According to Type of Health Care Setting

Claim	Codes Reported	Health Care Setting
CMS-1491	ICD-10-CM and HCPCS Level II	Ambulance services
CMS-1500	ICD-10-CM CPT, and HCPCS Level II	Noninstitutional providers and suppliers • Ambulatory surgery centers[1] • Anesthesiologists who administer hospital-based inpatient and outpatient anesthesia • Certified portable x-ray services • Home health agencies and hospices[2] • Independent clinical laboratories located at physician offices, group practices, hospitals, nursing facilities, end-stage renal disease facilities, pharmacies, home health agencies, rural health clinics, health fairs, anatomical testing laboratories, and nuclear medicine providers • Independent diagnostic testing facilities (e.g., certified mammography center) • Physician, chiropractor, optometrist, and podiatrist offices • Privately practicing occupational therapists and physical therapists • Roster billing[3] for flu and pneumonia vaccinations
UB-04	ICD-10-CM and ICD-10-PCS	Institutional providers (inpatient) • Acute care hospitals • Long-term care facilities • Psychiatric hospitals • Rehabilitation facilities • Short-term hospitals • Hospices (inpatient respite care)[4]
UB-04	ICD-10-CM, CPT, and HCPCS Level II	Institutional providers (outpatient) • Hospital emergency departments • Hospital outpatient departments
UB-04	ICD-10-CM, CPT, HCPCS Level II, and HIPPS	Noninstitutional providers (outpatient) • Home health agencies[5] • Hospices (home care)[5]

[1]Some ambulatory surgery centers submit the UB-04 claim instead of the CMS-1500 claim.

[2]Some home health agencies and hospices submit the UB-04 claim instead of the CMS-1500 claim.

[3]**Roster billing** is a simplified process available to public health clinics and other noninstitutional entities that offer mass immunization programs. Hospices also submit claims for the administration of pneumococcal pneumonia, influenza virus, and hepatitis B vaccines.

[4]Respite care includes services that provide primary caregivers (e.g., the spouse of a terminally ill person) with temporary relief from tasks associated with caregiving (e.g., in-home assistance, short hospital or nursing facility stays, adult day care).

[5]Physicians who are not employees of the HHA and/or hospice and who provide professional home care services for home health agencies and hospices submit claims with ICD-10-CM diagnosis codes and CPT and HCPCS Level II procedure/service codes.

Types of Third-Party Payers

Third-party payers include the following:

- BlueCross and BlueShield (BCBS)
- Commercial insurance companies

- Employer self-insurance plans
- Government-sponsored programs (e.g., Medicare)
- Managed care (e.g., HMO)
- Workers' compensation

NOTE:

Patient demographic data; ICD-10-CM/PCS, CPT, and HCPCS Level II codes; and other information (e.g., dates of service) are entered in the hospital's computer system to populate the UB-04 claim. Then, the hospital's billing department reviews the completed UB-04 claim for accuracy and submits it to third-party payers.

When third-party payers deny a claim, the billing department collaborates with the health information department to re-review the submitted claim to correct data entry and coding errors. If codes submitted were correct, the billing department and health information department collaborate to write an appeal to the third-party payer, which may include supporting patient record documentation.

BlueCross and BlueShield (BCBS)

BlueCross and BlueShield (BCBS) payers cover the costs of hospital care and physician services. BlueCross initially covered just hospital care, and BlueShield covered just physician services; today, both offer a full range of health care coverage. While each independent BCBS plan serves its local community, its membership in the BCBS Association allows it to link with other local plans so that regional and national employers can be served (e.g., an employee can receive health care services while traveling).

NOTE:

In some states (e.g., California, Idaho, and Washington), BCBS payers are organized as two separate insurance companies. In other states (e.g., Missouri, New York, and Pennsylvania), BCBS payers are organized as multiple insurance companies according to region.

Commercial Payers

Commercial payers include private health insurance and employer-based group health insurance. Private health insurance usually consists of an indemnity plan, which covers individuals for certain health care expenses. The insurance company reimburses the patient or the provider, depending on the contract language. Individuals pay annual premiums (with predetermined rates).

Employer-based group health insurance is often provided as an employee benefit. The employer typically pays 80 percent of insurance premiums, and the employee pays the remaining 20 percent. The employer generally contracts with a commercial health insurance plan (e.g., Aetna).

Employer Self-Insurance Plans

For **employer self-insurance plans**, an employer accepts direct responsibility (or the risk) for paying employees' health care without purchasing health insurance and creates an employer self-insurance plan. Usually, the plan contracts with a third-party administrator (TPA), which is an organization that provides the following services to employers (and insurance companies):

- *Benefit design*: Medical services covered by the plan
- *Claims administration*: Processing claims to reimburse services
- *Utilization review or utilization management*: Reviewing medical care for appropriateness, necessity, and quality (e.g., preadmission authorization)

Government-Sponsored Programs

Government-sponsored programs include

- CHAMPVA
- Federal Employee Health Benefits Program (FEHBP or FEP)
- Indian Health Service (IHS)
- Medicaid and CHIP
- Medicare
- Military Health System (MHS)
- Programs of All-inclusive Care for the Elderly (PACE)
- TRICARE

The *Civilian Health and Medical Program of the Department of Veterans Affairs (CHAMPVA)* program provides health care benefits to dependents of veterans who

- Are rated as 100 percent permanently and totally disabled as a result of service-connected conditions
- Died as a result of service-connected conditions
- Died on duty with fewer than 30 days of active service

The *Federal Employee Health Benefits Program (FEHBP or FEP)* is a voluntary health care program that covers federal employees, retirees, and their dependents and survivors. The *Indian Health Service (IHS)* is a DHHS agency that provides federal health care services to American Indians and Alaska natives.

Medicaid (Title XIX of the Social Security Act Amendments of 1965) is a joint federal and state program that provides health care coverage to low-income populations and certain older adults and individuals with disabilities. It is an entitlement program that is jointly financed by state governments and the federal government, with federal spending levels determined by the number of participants and services provided. The state *Children's Health Insurance Plan (CHIP)* was established to provide health assistance to uninsured, low-income children either through separate programs or through expanded eligibility under state Medicaid programs.

Medicare (Title XVIII of the Social Security Act Amendments of 1965) provides health care coverage to older adults and persons with disabilities; federal spending is funded by the Medicare Trust Fund (payroll tax). Medicare administrative contractors review local coverage determinations (LCDs) and national coverage determinations (NCDs) to specify under what clinical circumstances a service is covered, considered to be reasonable and necessary, and correctly coded. The *Programs of All-inclusive Care for the Elderly (PACE)* are community-based Medicare and Medicaid programs that provide integrated health care and long-term care services to older adult persons who require a nursing-facility level of care.

The *Military Health System (MHS)* provides and maintains readiness to provide health care services and support to members of the Uniformed Services during military operations. It also provides health care services and support to members of the Uniformed Services, their family members, and others entitled to Department of Defense health care.

TRICARE is the uniformed services health care program for active duty service members, active duty family members, National Guard and Reserve members and their family members, retirees and retiree family members, survivors, and certain former spouses worldwide. The health care resources of the Military Health System (e.g., military hospitals and clinics) and a civilian health care network of professionals, institutions, pharmacies, and suppliers provide health for members. TRICARE was formerly called CHAMPUS (Civilian Health and Medical Program of the United States).

NOTE:

The Recovery Audit Contractor (RAC) program evaluates individual provider compliance to (1) identify overpayments (and underpayments) made by Medicare and Medicaid and (2) recover overpayments made to durable medical equipment (DME) providers, health care facilities, and physician practices. For example, RACs use proprietary software to detect errors in codes reported on CMS-1500 claims.

Medicare's Comprehensive Error Rate Testing (CERT) program operates parallel to the RAC program to evaluate Medicare administrative contractors' (MAC) program performance. For example, CERT assesses the ability of a MAC to detect errors that are considered fraudulent.

CMS uses competitive measures to award MAC contracts and has established Zone Program Integrity Contractors (ZPICs) to perform program integrity functions in the newly established MAC jurisdictions (or zones). ZPICs are expected to perform program integrity functions for Medicare Parts A through D, DME, home health, hospice, and Medi-Medi programs.

Managed Care

Managed care combines the financing and delivery of health care services to replace conventional fee-for-service health insurance plans with more affordable care for consumers and providers who agree to certain restrictions (e.g., patients receive care from participating providers). (Managed care plans range from structured closed-panel staff model health maintenance organizations to less structured preferred provider organizations.) For example, a *health maintenance organization (HMO)* is an alternative to traditional group health insurance coverage that provides comprehensive health care services to voluntarily enrolled members on a prepaid basis. It provides preventive care services to promote "wellness" or good health, thus reducing the overall cost of medical care.

A **participating provider (PAR)** is a member of a managed care plan, while a **nonparticipating provider (nonPAR)** is not a member of the plan. (PAR and nonPAR providers are also associated with traditional health insurance plans. Patients may incur higher out-of-pocket costs when receiving care from nonPARs.)

Fee-for-service plans reimburse providers for individual health care services rendered, while managed care is financed according to a method called **capitation**. *Capitation* is the term used when providers accept preestablished payments for providing health care services to enrollees over a period of time, usually one year. If the managed care physician provides services that cost less than the capitation amount, the physician keeps any profits. If services provided cost more than the capitation amount, the physician loses money. Patients who subscribe to managed care plans receive care from *their primary care provider (PCP)*, the physician responsible for supervising and coordinating health care services, for preauthorizing referrals to specialists, and for inpatient hospital admissions, except in emergencies.

NOTE:

In managed care, the primary care provider receives a *capitation* payment and is responsible for managing all of an individual's health care, which includes reimbursing health care expenses provided by other caregivers (e.g., lab tests, specialists).

Risk Adjustment Coding

The implementation of a *risk adjustment program* to lessen or eliminate the influence of risk selection on premiums charged by health plans uses a *risk adjustment model software* (e.g., CMS-HCC, HHS-HCC, ESRD, RxHCC), which provides payments to health plans that disproportionately attract higher-risk enrollees (e.g., individuals with chronic conditions). *Risk adjustment* uses statistical data models to adjust health plan contractual bids, and resultant payments are based on enrollees' expected health care costs.

(Statistical data models measure incremental predictive costs of an enrollee's demographic, disease, and financial characteristics.) It determines the impact of enrollees' health status on health care spending by assessing patient outcomes and actual health care costs. The risk adjustment model uses an actuarial tool to predict health care costs based on the relative actuarial risk of enrollees in risk adjustment covered health plans. Each model organizes ICD-10-CM codes into diagnostic groups (DXGs) and condition categories (CCs) that are clinically related and have similar predicted costs. The resultant hierarchical condition categories (HCCs) are based on disease severity so that risk scores reflect the most severe and costly category of a condition. For example, Affordable Care Act Marketplace managed care plans use the *HHS-Hierarchical Condition Categories (HHS-HCC) risk adjustment model* to summarize ICD-10-CM codes along with demographic and financial data into levels of severity for calculating risk scores. Other risk adjustment models focus on rates associated with Medicare Advantage (CMS-HCC), end-stage renal disease (ESRD), and Medicare Part D prescription drug plans (RxHCC). Federal legislation, such as the 21st Century Cures Act of 2016, requires changes to risk adjustment models to add ICD-10-CM codes (e.g., mental health and substance abuse disorders).

Risk adjustment coding and the consideration of demographic (e.g., age, sex) and financial characteristics allow patients to be assigned a *risk adjustment factor (RAF) score*, which is used to predict health care costs. For example, a patient with an acute health condition would be expected to incur average medical costs for a single episode of care (that includes multiple encounters). However, a patient who requires the medical management of multiple chronic conditions is expected to require increased utilization of services and resultant higher health care costs. It is the *medical complexity of care* that increases health care costs, and a risk adjustment program based on ICD-10-CM codes and demographic/financial data allows reimbursement to be risk adjusted based on enrollees' health conditions.

Risk adjustment coders depend on accurate and complete documentation to assign accurate ICD-10-CM codes. They must review all documentation to verify existing codes, capture new codes, and correct erroneous codes based on official coding guidelines and the following risk adjustment concepts:

- MEAT (measure, evaluate, assess, treat)

- TAMPER (treatment, assessment, monitor/medicate, plan, evaluate, referral)

Thus, valid documentation substantiates and supports the capture of ICD-10-CM codes. If documentation is missing, the ICD-10-CM code cannot be captured, and it becomes important to implement provider training about documentation needed to support ICD-10-CM codes.

The risk adjustment program's *risk transfer formula* is used to transfer funds from health plans with relatively lower risk enrollees to health plans that enroll relatively higher risk individuals, protecting such health plans against adverse selection. Enrollee risk scores are based on demographic and health status information, and they are calculated as the sum of demographic and health factors, weighted by estimated marginal contributions to total risk and calculated relative to average expenditures. Thomson Reuters MarketScan® data is the primary source for risk adjustment model calibration, and its database includes data from all 50 states.

> **Example:** An average risk score is 1.0, and the formula for calculating the *total risk score is demographic risk factor + health status risk factor.* If a 57-year-old female has a 0.5 demographic risk factor and a 0.7 health status risk factor, the total risk score is 1.2, resulting in the health plan receiving higher payments for care provided because the patient's risk score is greater than the average. This provides an incentive for the health plan to enroll individuals with higher demographic and health status risk factors. To monetize this example, if the value of 1.0 is $1,000, this patient's risk score monetary average is calculated as $(0.5 \times \$1,000) + (0.7 \times \$1,000) = \$500 + \$700 = \$1,200$.

Workers' Compensation

Workers' compensation is a state-mandated insurance program that reimburses health care costs and lost wages if an employee suffers a work-related disease or injury. Qualified employees and their dependents are eligible for reimbursement.

Exercise 20.1 – Third-Party Payers

Instructions: Complete each statement.

1. Medicare claims are processed by MACs, which is the abbreviation for Medicare administrative _____.

2. CMS selects payers to process Medicare claims through a competitive _____ process.

3. The UB-04 claim is used by health care _____ to obtain reimbursement for inpatient hospitalizations and outpatient procedures and services.

4. Organizations that process or facilitate the processing of claims information received from another entity from a nonstandard into a standard format are called a health care _____ and a third-party administrator.

5. If the patient's insurance policy contains a statement that the patient is not responsible for paying what the insurance plan denies, the health care provider is prohibited from collecting payment from the patient. This statement is called a(n) _____ harmless clause.

6. Private health insurance and employer-based group health insurance companies are considered _____ payers.

7. The joint federal and state program that provides health care coverage to low-income populations and certain older adults and individuals with disabilities is called _____.

8. The government-sponsored health program that provides health care coverage to older adults and persons with disabilities is called _____.

9. The combined financing and delivery of health care services to replace conventional fee-for-service health insurance plans with more affordable care for consumers and providers who agree to certain restrictions is called _____ care.

10. The type of plan that reimburses providers for individual health care services rendered is called _____ -for-service.

Health Care Reimbursement Systems

Prior to implementation of major government-sponsored health programs (e.g., Medicare and Medicaid) in 1965, health care services were reimbursed by the following payers:

- BlueCross and BlueShield (private and group health plans)
- Commercial health insurance (private)
- Employer-based group health insurance and self-insurance plans
- Government-sponsored programs, limited to the following:
  - Indian Health Service (limited eligibility)
  - Dependents' medical care program (health care for dependents of active military personnel)
- Prepaid health plans (forerunner of managed care)
- Self-pay (patients paid cash)
- Workers' compensation (limited eligibility)

Payers (except prepaid or managed care plans) typically reimbursed physicians on a fee-for-service basis, which is a retrospective payment system that billed payers after health care services were provided to the patient. Hospital reimbursement was generated on a *per diem* basis (Latin meaning "by the day"), which meant payers used a retrospective payment system to issue payment that was based on actual daily charges.

Example: Payers typically reimbursed providers for 80 percent of charges submitted, and patients paid the remaining 20 percent (coinsurance). Thus, a provider who submitted a charge of $120 was paid $96 by the payer and $24 by the patient. (Government programs, such as Medicare, establish a physician fee schedule for services provided. The physician is reimbursed 80 percent of the fee schedule.)

Prospective Payment Systems, Fee Schedules, and Exclusions

Health care costs increased dramatically with implementation of government-sponsored health programs in 1965. This led to the creation and implementation of prospective payment systems and fee schedules (Table 20-2) for government health programs. The purpose was to control costs by reimbursing facilities with preestablished rates for inpatient care provided. Shortly after passage of Medicare and Medicaid legislation in 1965, Congress began investigating prospective payment systems. A **prospective payment system (PPS)** is a reimbursement methodology that establishes predetermined rates based on patient category or type of facility (with annual increases based on an inflation index and a geographic wage index). The CMS manages implementation of Medicare prospective payment systems, fee schedules, and exclusions according to

- Prospective cost-based rates
- Prospective price-based rates

Prospective cost-based rates are based on reported health care costs (e.g., charges) from which a prospective *per diem* rate is determined. Annual rates are usually adjusted using actual costs from the prior year. This method may be based on the facility's case mix (patient acuity that determines level of health care resources required, such as intensive care). Prospective payment systems based on this reimbursement methodology include ambulance fee schedules.

Prospective price-based rates are associated with a particular category of patient (e.g., inpatients), and rates are established by the payer (e.g., Medicare) prior to the provision of health care services. PPSs based on this reimbursement methodology include diagnosis-related groups (DRGs) for inpatient care.

TABLE 20-2 Prospective Payment Systems and Fee Schedules, Year Implemented, and Rate Type

Prospective Payment Systems and Fee Schedules	Year	Type
Ambulance Fee Schedule	2002	Cost-based
Ambulatory Surgical Center (ASC) Payment System	1994	Price-based
Clinical Laboratory Fee Schedule	1985	Cost-based
Durable Medical Equipment, Prosthetics, Orthotics, and Supplies (DMEPOS) Fee Schedule	1989	Cost-based
End-Stage Renal Disease Prospective Payment System (ESRD PPS)	2011	Price-based
Federally Qualified Health Center Prospective Payment System (FQHC PPS)	2014	Price-based
Home Health Prospective Payment System (HH PPS)	2000	Price-based
Hospice Payment System	1983	Cost-based
Hospital Inpatient Prospective Patient System (IPPS)	1983	Price-based
Hospital Outpatient Prospective Payment System (OPPS)	2000	Price-based
Inpatient Psychiatric Facility Prospective Payment System (IPF PPS)	2004	Cost-based
Inpatient Rehabilitation Facility Prospective Payment System (IRF PPS)	2002	Price-based
Long-Term (Acute) Care Hospital Prospective Payment System (LTC PPS)	2001	Price-based
Medicare Physician Fee Schedule (MPFS)[1]	1992	Cost-based
Skilled Nursing Facility Prospective Payment System (SNF PPS)	1998	Price-based

[1]MPFS was originally implemented as the Resource-Based Relative Value Scale (RBRVS) System.

Typically, third-party payers adopt prospective payment systems, fee schedules, and exclusions after Medicare has implemented them; payers modify them to suit their needs. A *fee schedule* is cost-based, fee-for-service reimbursement methodology that includes a list of maximum fees and corresponding procedures/services, which payers use to compensate providers for health care services delivered to patients. *Exclusions* are "Medicare PPS Excluded Cancer Hospitals" (e.g., Roswell Park Memorial Institute in Buffalo, New York) that applied for and were granted waivers from mandatory participation in the hospital inpatient PPS.

Example: Prior to 1983, acute care hospitals generated invoices based on total charges for an inpatient stay. In 1982, an eight-day inpatient hospitalization at $225 per day (including ancillary service charges) would be billed $1,800. This *per diem* reimbursement rate actually discouraged hospitals from limiting inpatient lengths of stay. In 1983, a PPS rate of $950 would be reimbursed for the same inpatient hospitalization, regardless of length of stay (unless the case qualified for additional reimbursement as an outlier). The PPS rate encourages hospitals to limit inpatient lengths of stay because any reimbursement received in excess of the actual cost of providing care can be retained by the facility. (In this example, if the $950 PPS rate had been paid in 1980, the hospital would have absorbed the $850 loss.)

Inpatient Prospective Payment System (1983)

The *Tax Equity and Fiscal Responsibility Act of 1983 (TEFRA)* legislated implementation of the hospital *inpatient prospective payment system (IPPS)*, which uses Medicare severity diagnosis-related groups (MS-DRGs) to reimburse short-term hospitals a predetermined rate for Medicare inpatient services. (Other payers have adopted the IPPS.)

 NOTE:

Certain cancer hospitals that applied and received waivers from CMS are considered excluded hospitals, which means that they do not participate in the IPPS.

Diagnosis-related groups (DRGs) (Figure 20-4) organize inpatient hospital cases into groups that are expected to consume similar hospital resources.

- Each DRG has a payment weight assigned to it that is based on the average resources used to treat Medicare patients in that DRG.
- DRGs are organized into *major diagnostic categories (MDCs)*, which are mutually exclusive categories that are loosely based on body systems (e.g., nervous system).
- Inpatient cases that are unusually costly are called *outliers*, and the IPPS payment is increased to protect the hospital from large financial losses due to unusually expensive cases.

To determine an IPPS (DRG or MS-DRG) payment, hospitals submit a UB-04 claim for each inpatient to a *Medicare administrative contractor (MAC)*, which is a third-party payer that contracts with Medicare to carry out the operational functions of the Medicare program.

- Based on the information provided on the UB-04, the case is categorized into a DRG, which determines the reimbursement provided to the hospital.
- DRG payments are then adjusted to accommodate the wage index applicable to the area where the hospital is located, a cost-of-living adjustment factor for hospitals located in Alaska and Hawaii, a percentage add-on payment for hospitals that serve a disproportionate share of low-income patients, and/or a percentage add-on payment if the hospital is an approved teaching hospital.
- In addition, if a case is categorized as an outlier, additional payments are added to the DRG-adjusted base payment rate.

Medicare Severity Diagnosis-Related Groups (MS-DRGs)
MDC 02 – Diseases and Disorders of the Eye

CC = complication(s) and/or comorbidity(ies)
MCC = major complication(s) and/or comorbidity(ies)

MS-DRG	Description
113	Orbital procedures w CC/MCC

MS-DRG: 113
Title: Orbital procedures w CC/MCC
Type: SURG
Major Diagnostic Category (MDC): 02 DISEASES & DISORDERS OF THE EYE
Relative Weight: 2.1321
Geometric Mean Length of Stay (days): 4.2
Arithmetic Mean Length of Stay (days): 5.8

Related Codes

MS-DRG	Title	Relative Weight	Length of Stay
113	Orbital procedures w CC/MCC	1.4141	3.8
114	Orbital procedures w/o CC/MCC	1.0292	2.0
115	Extraocular procedures except orbit	1.1185	3.3
116	Intraocular procedures w CC/MCC	0.8891	2.2
117	Intraocular procedures w/o CC/MCC	0.7094	1.5

Crosswalk of CMS-DRG to MS-DRG

CMS-DRG	MDC	MS-DRG
037 - ORBITAL PROCEDURES	02	113 - Orbital procedures w CC/MCC

MS-DRG	Description
114	Orbital procedures w/o CC/MCC
115	Extraocular procedures except orbit
116	Intraocular procedures w CC/MCC
117	Intraocular procedures w/o CC/MCC
121	Acute major eye infections w CC/MCC
122	Acute major eye infections w/o CC/MCC
123	Neurological eye disorders
124	Other disorders of the eye w MCC
125	Other disorders of the eye w/o MCC

FIGURE 20-4 Medicare severity diagnosis-related groups (MS-DRGs), major diagnostic category 02

Costs not considered when calculating the Medicare DRG-adjusted base payment rates are as follows:

- *Direct costs* of medical education for interns and residents, which are based on a per-resident payment amount

- *Reasonable costs* for (1) hospital bad debts attributable to nonpayment of the Medicare deductible and coinsurance, and (2) heart, liver, lung, and kidney acquisition costs incurred by an approved transplant facility

The *IPPS 3-day payment window* (or *IPPS 72-hour rule*) requires outpatient procedures and services provided by a hospital on the day of or during the three days prior to a patient's inpatient admission to be covered by the IPPS DRG payment and reported on the UB-04 with ICD-10-CM and ICD-10-PCS codes for

- Diagnostic services (e.g., lab testing)
- Therapeutic (or nondiagnostic) services

Diagnostic services include examinations and procedures provided to the patient or that were performed as the result of hospital outpatient procedure or service and that aided in the assessment of a medical condition or identified a disease. Examples include diagnostic laboratory services, such as hematology and chemistry, diagnostic x-rays, isotope studies, electrocardiograms, pulmonary function studies, thyroid function tests, psychological tests, and other tests provided to determine the nature and severity of an ailment or injury.

 NOTE:

- Services that are distinct from and unrelated to the inpatient admission are separately billed by the hospital *if documentation supports that the service is unrelated to the inpatient admission*.
- However, hospitals must bundle technical components of all outpatient diagnostic services and related non-diagnostic services (e.g., therapeutic services) with the claim for an inpatient stay when services are furnished to a Medicare beneficiary during the three days preceding an inpatient admission.
- The following hospital and hospital units are subject to a 1-day payment window (instead of the 3-day payment window): cancer hospitals, children's hospitals, inpatient rehabilitation hospitals and units, long-term care hospitals, and psychiatric hospitals and units.

Medicare also requires that physician services clinically related to an inpatient admission and provided within 72 hours of the admission be paid at the lower facility rate (instead of the usually greater office or nonfacility rate). CMS requires that HCPCS Level II modifier PD (diagnostic or related nondiagnostic item or service provided in a wholly owned or wholly operated entity to a patient who is admitted as an inpatient within three days) be added to CPT codes to identify claims for related services provided within 72 hours of an inpatient admission. As a result of this new requirement

- Physician office claims must be held for at least three days prior to submission, and CMS requires hospitals to notify physician offices about related inpatient admissions.
- Modifier PD must be added to CPT and HCPCS Level II codes that are reported on CMS-1500 claims for any inpatients who received physician office services within 72 hours prior to admission.

In practice, physician offices need to implement a process to ensure that claims submission is delayed by three days. Also, an office staff member needs to review daily list(s) of inpatient admissions received from local hospital(s) to identify patients whose claims need to be modified by adding -PD to CPT codes.

Example: A 79-year-old established Medicare patient receives physician office evaluation and management (E/M) services (99214) for complaints of chest pain and shortness of breath. The general practitioner (GP) performs a 12-lead ECG (93000), which indicates the patient is currently experiencing a myocardial infarction (MI). The patient is immediately transported by ambulance to the local hospital and admitted to the intensive care unit. Because the patient is admitted within 72 hours of the office visit, the E/M services (99214 PD) are paid to the physician at the lesser facility rate (instead of the physician office rate), and only the professional component rate of the ECG (93010 PD) is paid to the physician (instead of the higher global procedure rate). (CPT code 93010 is reported for the professional component of the ECG, not 93000 which is reported for the global service.)

According to CMS, all nondiagnostic services (other than ambulance and maintenance renal dialysis services) furnished by a hospital on the date of admission or during the three-day payment window are deemed to be related to the admission and, therefore, must be bundled with the inpatient stay if the services were provided on the day of or during the three days prior to a patient's inpatient admission. The exception to the rule is when a hospital determines, attests, and documents that the service furnished during the three-day payment window is *clinically distinct or independent from the reason for the patient's admission.* Hospitals are required to report condition code 51 with the nondiagnostic service CPT or HCPCS Level II code on the outpatient UB-04.

 NOTE:

> Medicare implemented *Medicare severity diagnosis-related groups (MS-DRGs)* in 2007 to organize inpatient hospital cases into groups according to similar resource utilization. Hospitals receive a predetermined payment according to MS-DRG for treating Medicare patients. Like the original DRGs, the MS-DRGs are based on diagnoses, procedures, other demographic information, and the presence of complications or comorbidities (CCs). However, hospital inpatients are distinguished according to those with no CCs, CCs, or major CCs (MCCs). This allows Medicare to distinguish "sick patients" from "very sick patients" and to reimburse hospitals accordingly. As such, the number of MS-DRGs expanded to 745 (as compared to 538 original DRGs). MS-DRGs also emphasize the importance of proper documentation of patient care, relating it to reimbursement optimization (e.g., increased diagnosis specificity to justify more severe illnesses resulting in increased reimbursement). Facilities implement clinical documentation improvement (CDI) programs to ensure thorough and accurate documentation in patient records. (*To optimize reimbursement* means to legally enhance reimbursement from payers to providers, such as assigning specific codes based on documentation in the patient record.)
>
> Other systems developed for payment purposes (based on CMS's DRG system) include the following:
>
> * *All Patient DRGs (AP-DRGs),* which organize the non-Medicare population, especially newborns and children
>
> * *All Patient Refined DRGs (APR-DRGs),* which organize the non-Medicare population, such as HIV patients, neonates, and pediatric patients
>
> * *International Refined DRGs (IR-DRGs),* which were created by other countries that adapted DRGs for their own use, comparing resource usage across health care facilities and regions and incorporating the concept of severity of illness adjustments using multiple levels of comorbid and complication (CC) conditions
>
> * *Yale Refined Diagnosis-Related Groups (RDRGs),* which refined the original DRGs to incorporate a measure of severity, expanding the number of DRGs to 1,263 RDRGs

An *IPPS transfer rule* states that any patient with a diagnosis associated with 1 to 10 CMS-determined DRGs who is discharged to a post-acute provider is treated as a transfer case. This means that hospitals are paid a graduated *per diem* rate for each day of the patient's stay, not to exceed the prospective payment DRG rate. (Outliers are also recognized for extraordinarily high-cost cases.) CMS identified 10 high-volume DRGs that contain a disproportionate percentage of discharges to post-acute care settings (e.g., DRG 14—Specific Cerebrovascular Disorders Except Transient Ischemic Attack). CMS defines the following as post-acute care settings:

* Hospitals or distinct units excluded from the prospective payment system

* Skilled nursing facilities

* Patient's home under a written plan of care for the provision of home health services from a home health agency if the services begin within three days of discharge

The Department of Health & Human Services, Office of Inspector General (OIG) monitors hospital readmissions and transfers that seem to focus on revenue generation rather than medical necessity when determining DRGs. A *hospital readmission* on the day of discharge is treated as a *continuous episode of care,* which means the new admission is combined with the previous admission and the hospital receives one DRG payment. A *hospital transfer* is also considered a *continuous episode of care,* which means the transfer to the second hospital is combined with the first hospital admission and both hospitals cost-split one DRG payment. To convince the OIG that the hospital is properly classifying readmissions and transfers, consider implementing software that flags same-day readmissions for review, ensure that hospital discharge planners accurately assess the patient's condition upon discharge, and remind providers to document the fact that patients were discharged in a timely manner.

Hospital Value-Based Purchasing Program

Hospital *pay-for-performance (P4P)* quality initiatives link reimbursement to performance criteria to improve the efficiency, overall value, and quality of health care provided, resulting in optimal patient outcomes. Traditionally, payment was based on the *process* of care. P4P strategies promote the *right care for every patient every time* and define the *right care* as being effective, efficient, equitable, patient centered, safe, and timely. This means that despite the patient's ethnicity, gender, geographic location, and socioeconomic status, patients receive "right care." The hospital *value-based purchasing (VBP)* program is a P4P quality initiative that is part of a long-standing CMS effort to link Medicare's inpatient prospective payment system (IPPS) to a value-based system for the purpose of improving health care quality, including the quality of care provided in the inpatient hospital setting, which affects payment for inpatient stays to over 3,500 hospitals. Participating hospitals are paid for inpatient acute care services based on quality of care, not just quantity of services provided. The inpatient hospital VBP was authorized by the Patient Protection and Affordable Care Act (PPACA). A hospital quality data reporting infrastructure was developed as part of the Hospital Inpatient Quality Reporting (IQR) Program, as authorized by the Medicare Prescription Drug, Improvement, and Modernization Act of 2003 (MMA).

The *Hospital Inpatient Quality Reporting (Hospital IQR) program* was developed to equip consumers with quality of care information so they can make more informed decisions about health care options. The Hospital IQR program requires hospitals to submit specific quality measures data about health conditions common among Medicare beneficiaries and that typically result in hospitalization. Eligible hospitals that do not participate in the Hospital IQR program will receive an annual market basket update with a 2.0 percentage point reduction.

The *hospital readmission reduction program (HRRP)* requires CMS to reduce payments to IPPS hospitals with excess readmissions, and utilizes readmission measures established by CMS (e.g., hospital inpatient admission within 30 days of discharge from the same hospital). CMS also established payment adjustment policies to determine which hospitals are subject to the HRRP, the methodology to calculate the hospital readmission payment adjustment factor, the portion of the IPPS payment used to calculate readmission payment adjustment amounts, and a process for hospitals to review readmission information and submit corrections before readmission rates are publicized.

Skilled Nursing Facility Prospective Payment System (1998)

The *skilled nursing facility prospective payment system (SNF PPS)* uses a *patient-driven payment model (PDPM)* as a case-mix reimbursement system that connects payment to patients' conditions and care needs instead of the volume of services provided. (In addition to IRFs, the PDPM applies to long-term acute care facility and skilled nursing facility payments.) The PDPM classification methodology uses a combination of six payment components to derive payment, five of which are case-mix adjusted to cover utilization of SNF resources that vary according to patient characteristics. The sixth non-case-mix adjusted component addresses utilization of resources that do not vary by patient. A resident assessment instrument (RAI) completed on each SNF patient captures the *minimum data set (MDS)* according to the following schedule: 5, 14, 30, 60, and 90 days after admission. *Resident Assessment Validation and Entry (RAVEN)* software, developed by CMS, is a data entry system that allows SNFs to capture and transmit the MDS.

 NOTE:

Medicare introduced the first prospective payment system (PPS) to pay for inpatient hospital care, and other prospective payment systems were adopted in subsequent years (e.g., SNF PPS). Under the inpatient prospective payment system (IPPS), inpatients are discharged once the acute phase of illness has passed and hospitals are reimbursed according to diagnosis-related groups. The patients are often transferred to other types of health care, such as outpatient care, skilled care facilities, rehabilitation hospitals, and home health care. The transfer facilities provide an appropriate level of health care in a safe and cost-effective manner after the patient's attending physician (with the assistance of discharge planners, case managers, social workers, nurses, and others) has determined which facility is best by evaluating the patient's medical condition, special needs, and treatment goals.

CMS adopted an *SNF all-cause all-condition hospital readmission measure* and an *SNF Value-Based Purchasing (VBP) Program* to promote higher quality and more efficient health care for Medicare beneficiaries as well as value-based incentive payments for qualified SNFs.

Each component of the *patient-driven payment model (PDPM) payment* is calculated by multiplying the case-mix index (CMI) that corresponds to the patient's case-mix group (CMG) by the wage-adjusted component base payment rate. (The specific day in the variable *per diem* adjustment schedule is also factored in, when applicable.) PDPM components are then totaled together along with the non-case-mix component payment rate to create a patient's total SNF PPS (PDPM) *per diem* rate.

Home Health Prospective Payment System (2000)

The *home health prospective payment system (HH PPS)* uses the *home health patient-driven groupings model (HH PDGM)* to provide reimbursement for Medicare home health care services based on clinical characteristics and other patient information, placing home health periods of care into meaningful payment categories. The PDGM also eliminated the use of therapy service thresholds. As a result of PDGM implementation, the unit of home health payment was reduced from a 60-day episode to a 30-day period.

 NOTE:

> Medicare does not reimburse durable medical equipment (DME) during the initial 30 days that a patient receives home care services. DME is reimbursed according to a fee schedule during this period.

Rates for each 30-day episode of HHA care are adjusted by case-mix methodology based on entry of data elements from the outcome and assessment information set (OASIS) into Java-based *Home Assessment Validation and Entry (HAVEN)* (also referred to as jHAVEN) data entry software. The HHA clinician (such as a registered nurse) conducts a comprehensive assessment and collects OASIS data elements to capture clinical severity factors, functional severity factors, and service utilization factors that influence case mix. Each data element is assigned a score value, and scores are totaled (by HAVEN software) to determine the HIPPS rate code and case-mix weight (and resultant total reimbursement).

Hospice Payment System

Medicare's hospice program authorizes coverage for hospice care for terminally ill beneficiaries and established a fee-for-service payment rate system. The *Patient Protection and Affordable Care Act of 2010* reformed the hospice payment rate system (Table 20-3) to implement aggregate expenditures to control Medicare hospice costs.

Medicare pays a daily rate for each day a patient is enrolled in the hospice benefit, regardless of the number of services provided on a given day. Payments are made based on the *level of care* required to meet the patient's and family's needs, including

- Routine home care
- Continuous home care
- Inpatient respite care
- General inpatient care

 NOTE:

> Routine home care payments are made at a higher payment rate for the first 60 days of hospice care, and a reduced payment rate for hospice care for 61 days and over.

TABLE 20-3 Sample Hospice Payment System Rates

Level of Hospice Care	Hospice Payment Rate
Routine home care (Days 1–60)	$191 per day
Routine home care (Days 61+)	$150 per day
Continuous home care	$965 per day or $40 per hour
Inpatient respite care	$171 per day
General inpatient care	$734 per day
Aggregate reimbursement cap per beneficiary served	$28,500
Inpatient days cap	20% of total days of hospice service

A service intensity add-on (SIA) payment in addition to the per diem routine home care rate is made for services furnished during the last seven days of a patient's life. SIA eligibility criteria include the following:

- The day is a routine home care level of care day.
- The day occurs during the last seven days of the patient's life, and the patient is discharged expired.
- Direct patient care is furnished by a registered nurse (RN) or social worker, respectively, that day.

The SIA payment is equal to the continuous home care hourly payment rate multiplied by the amount of direct patient care furnished by an RN or social worker during the seven-day period for a minimum of 15 minutes and up to four hours total per day.

Daily hospice payment rates are adjusted for differences in wage rates among markets. Each level of hospice care's base rate has a labor share (adjusted by the hospice wage index) and a nonlabor share. Base rates are updated annually, based on the hospital market basket update.

Two caps affect Medicare payments under the hospice benefit.

- *Inpatient cap* (number of days of inpatient care furnished is limited to not more than 20 percent of total patient care days)
- *Aggregate* cap (limits the amount of Medicare payments a provider may receive in an accounting year, and it is calculated by multiplying the number of hospice beneficiaries during the accounting year by a per-beneficiary *cap amount*)

There are two methods for counting beneficiaries.

- *Patient-by-patient proportional method* (counts only that fraction which represents the portion of a patient's total days of care in all hospices and all years that was spent in that hospice in that cap year)
- *Streamlined method* (counts those beneficiaries who received care from a single hospice during the initial year the hospice elected this method only)

When a beneficiary receives care from more than one hospice, the patient-by-patient proportional method is used. The aggregate payment cap is then compared with actual aggregate payments made to the hospice during the cap year; any payments in excess of the cap are considered overpayments and must be refunded to Medicare by the hospice.

Outpatient Prospective Payment System (2000)

The Balanced Budget Act of 1997 legislated implementation of the hospital *outpatient prospective payment system (OPPS)*, which uses *ambulatory payment classifications (APCs)* to reimburse hospital outpatient services. Outpatient health care services are organized clinically and according to resources required.

A reimbursement rate is established for each APC (Figure 20-5) and, depending on services provided, hospitals can be paid for more than one APC per encounter, with second and subsequent APCs discounted at 50 percent (if they are designated with status indicator "T").

Each CPT and HCPCS Level II code is assigned a *status indicator (SI)* as a payment indicator to identify how each code is paid (or not paid) under the OPPS. For example, status indicator "S" refers to "significant procedures for which the multiple procedure reduction does not apply." This means that the CPT and/or HCPCS Level II code is paid the full APC reimbursement rate. OPPS status indicator "T" refers to "services to which the multiple procedure payment reduction applies." (CPT modifier 51 is not added to codes reported for OPPS payment consideration.) This means that the reported CPT and HCPCS Level II code will be paid a discounted APC reimbursement rate when reported with other procedures on the same claim.

 NOTE:

The OPPS does not cover payment of professional services, which are reported on the CMS-1500 claim and reimbursed according to a fee schedule, such as the Medicare Physician Fee Schedule (MPFS). Hospitals report outpatient encounters on the UB-04 (or CMS-1450) claim using ICD-10-CM for diagnoses and CPT and HCPCS Level II for procedures and services.

Outpatient Prospective Payment System (OPPS) Formula

(APC Weight × Conversion Factor × Wage Index) + Add-On Payments = Payment

NOTE: When a patient undergoes multiple procedures and services on the same day, multiple APCs are generated and payments are added together. APC software automatically discounts multiple APC payments when appropriate (e.g., bilateral procedure).

EXAMPLE: Using the sample data below, the OPPS payment for a patient who underwent percutaneous breast biopsy procedure using stereotactic guidance with placement of breast localization device in Buffalo, New York is calculated as $1,253.73. (NOTE: Add-on payments do not apply to this example, and APC payments were not discounted.)

$$(22.98 \times \$54.561 \times 0.8192) + (0.78 \times \$54.561 \times 0.8192) + (4.29 \times \$54.561 \times 0.8192)$$

$$\$1,027.12 + \$34.86 + \$191.75 = \$1,253.73$$

Conversion Factor = $54.561
Wage Index = 0.8192

HCPCS Code	Description	APC	APC Weight
C7501	Percutaneous breast biopsies	5073	22.98
Q9965	Low osmolar contrast material	1446	0.78
C8903	MRI with contrast, breast	5571	4.29

FIGURE 20-5 Formula for determining OPPS payments

The unit of payment for the OPPS is an outpatient visit or encounter. An *outpatient encounter* (or outpatient visit) includes all outpatient procedures and services (e.g., same-day surgery, x-rays, laboratory tests, and so on) provided during one day to the same patient. Thus, a patient who undergoes multiple outpatient procedures and receives multiple services on the same day will be assigned to one or more outpatient groups (called APCs). Each APC is weighted and has a prospective payment amount associated with it; if a patient is assigned multiple APCs, the payments are totaled to provide reimbursement to the hospital for the encounter. (APC payments may be discounted when certain procedures or services are provided, such as bilateral procedures.) A *wage index* adjusts payments to account for geographic variations in hospitals' labor costs.

APC grouper software is used to assign an APC to each CPT and HCPCS Level II code reported on an outpatient claim, as well as appropriate ICD-10-CM codes. Outpatient code editor (OCE) software is used in conjunction with the APC grouper to identify Medicare claims edits and assign APC groups to reported codes.

 NOTE:

Add-ons that can increase OPPS payments include pass-through payments that provide additional reimbursement to hospitals that use innovative (new and improved) biologicals, drugs, and technical devices. During committee meetings, health care personnel routinely discuss "pass-through payments" due to new technology, such as innovative medical devices (e.g., using surgical glue instead of stitches) and new drugs and vaccines (e.g., human papillomavirus [HPV] vaccine). Other add-ons include outlier payments for high-cost services, hold harmless payments for certain hospitals, and transitional payments to limit losses under the OPPS. The hospital profits if the payment rate is higher than the cost of care provided, and the hospital loses money if the payment rate is lower than the cost of care provided.

Example: OCE software reviews "to/from" dates of service to identify and reject claims that are submitted for reimbursement as hospital-based outpatient care when, in fact, the claim should be processed as inpatient care.

NOTE:

A Medicare patient's coinsurance amount is initially calculated for each APC based on 20 percent of the national median charge for services in the APC. The coinsurance amount for an APC does not change until the amount becomes 20 percent of the total APC payment, and no coinsurance amount can be greater than the hospital inpatient deductible in a given year.

NOTE:

New York State has implemented ambulatory patient groups (APGs) as a payment methodology for most Medicaid outpatient services (e.g., outpatient clinic, ambulatory surgery, and emergency department services). APGs result in

- Higher payments for higher intensity services and lower payments for lower intensity services
- The transition of funds from inpatient to outpatient services to support quality outpatient care and to address the problem of avoidable hospitalizations

Inpatient Psychiatric Facility Prospective Payment System (2004)

The *inpatient psychiatric facility prospective payment system (IPF PPS)* uses a *per diem* patient classification system that reflects differences in patient resource use and costs. The IPF PPS replaced a reasonable cost-based payment system and affected approximately 2,000 facilities; its purpose is to promote long-term cost control and utilization management. Licensed psychiatric facilities and hospital-based psychiatric units were reimbursed according to the new PPS, which was phased in over a three-year period beginning in 2004.

Health information department coders use ICD-10-CM to assign codes to inpatient behavioral health diagnoses and ICD-10-PCS to assign procedure codes. Coders then enter data into DRG software to calculate the IPF PPS DRG. Inpatient psychiatric facilities are reimbursed according to a *per diem* payment that is calculated using DRG data, wage-adjusted rates, and facility-level adjusters. (IPPS MS-DRGs reimburse acute care hospitals a flat payment based on ICD-10-CM/PCS codes and other data.) Providers use the *Diagnostic and Statistical Manual of Mental Disorders (DSM)*, which is published by the American Psychiatric Association. Although *DSM* codes do not affect IPF PPS rates, the manual contains diagnostic assessment criteria that are used as tools to identify psychiatric disorders. The *DSM* includes psychiatric disorders and codes, provides a mechanism for communicating and recording diagnostic information, and is used in the areas of research and statistics. (Currently, *DSM-5* is in use.)

Inpatient Rehabilitation Facility Prospective Payment System (2002)

The *inpatient rehabilitation facility prospective payment system (IRF PPS)* utilizes information from a patient assessment instrument (IRF PAI) to classify patients according to the *patient-driven payment model* (also adopted for SNFs and LTCHs).

The *IRF PPS 1-day payment window* (or *IRF PPS 24-hour rule*) requires that outpatient preadmission services provided by an IRF up to one day prior to a patient's inpatient admission be covered by the IRF PPS payment.

The *IRF PPS transfer rule* is similar to the IPPS transfer rule, except that for the IRF, the rule covers all patient diagnoses. If a patient is transferred from an IRF to another rehabilitation facility, an acute inpatient hospital, a long-term care hospital, or a nursing home that accepts payment under Medicare or Medicaid, the patient's length of stay must be reviewed. A patient who is discharged to home, outpatient therapy, home health, or a day rehabilitation program is not considered a transfer. If a patient remains in the IRF for more than three days—which is the defining length of stay for a short stay carrying its own payment classification, but fewer days than defined by the case-mix group (CMG)—the transfer payment methodology is triggered. The transfer payment methodology reimburses a *per diem*–based payment for the number of days of care in the facility prior to a transfer.

Long-Term (Acute) Care Hospital Prospective Payment System (2001)

The *long-term (acute) care hospital prospective payment system (LTCH PPS)* uses information from long-term acute care hospital patient records to classify patients into distinct *Medicare severity long-term (acute) care diagnosis-related groups (MS-LTC-DRGs)* based on the *patient-driven payment model* (also adopted for SNFs and LTCHs). The *LTCH PPS 1-day payment window* (or *LTCH PPS 24-hour rule*) requires that outpatient preadmission services provided by a long-term acute care hospital up to one day prior to a patient's inpatient admission be covered by the MS-LTCH-DRG payment.

 NOTE:

Do not confuse the LTCH PPS with the SNF PPS, discussed previously in this chapter. Long-term acute care hospitals are categorized as short-term hospitals, while skilled nursing facilities (SNFs) are considered long-term care facilities (LTCFs) (e.g., nursing facilities). Medicare even certifies long-term acute care hospitals as "short-term acute care hospitals."

Clinical Laboratory Fee Schedule (1985)

The *clinical laboratory fee schedule* is a data set of outpatient clinical diagnostic laboratory services. Medicare reimburses laboratory services the lowest of actual charges, local or state fee schedule amount, or national limitation amount (NLA) for the HCPCS Level II code submitted.

Durable Medical Equipment, Prosthetics, Orthotics, and Supplies Fee Schedule (1989)

The *durable medical equipment, prosthetics, orthotics, and supplies (DMEPOS) fee schedule* is released annually and updated quarterly to implement fee schedule amounts for new codes and to revise any amounts for existing codes that were calculated in error. A Medicare competitive acquisition process is used for certain items to determine DME payment amounts, which creates incentives for suppliers to provide quality items and services in an efficient manner and at a reasonable cost.

Resource-Based Relative Value Scale System (1992)

The *Medicare physician fee schedule (MPFS)* reimburses providers according to predetermined rates assigned to services, and it is revised by CMS each year. All services are standardized to measure the value of a service as compared with other services provided. These standards, called *relative value units (RVUs)*, are payment components consisting of the following:

- *Physician work*, which reflects the physician's time and intensity in providing the service (e.g., judgment, technical skill, and physical effort)
- *Practice expense*, which reflects overhead costs involved in providing a service (e.g., rent, utilities, equipment, and staff salaries)
- *Malpractice expense*, which reflects malpractice expenses (e.g., costs of liability insurance)

 NOTE:

Most third-party payers, including state Medicaid programs, have adopted aspects of the MPFS. Thus, the MPFS contains fees for services not commonly provided to Medicare patients (e.g., obstetrical services).

Payment limits were also established by adjusting the RVUs for each locality by geographic adjustment factors (GAF), called *geographic cost practice indices (GPCIs)*, so that Medicare providers are paid differently in each state and also within each state (e.g., New York State has five separate payment localities). An annual *conversion factor* (dollar multiplier) converts RVUs into payments using a formula (Figure 20-6).

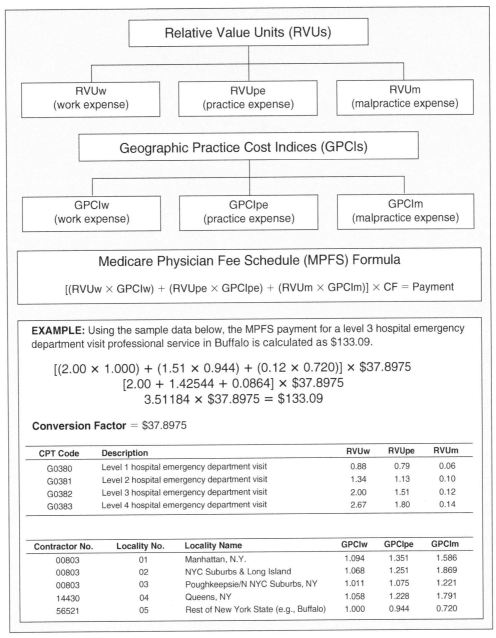

Relative Value Units (RVUs)

| RVUw (work expense) | RVUpe (practice expense) | RVUm (malpractice expense) |

Geographic Practice Cost Indices (GPCIs)

| GPCIw (work expense) | GPCIpe (practice expense) | GPCIm (malpractice expense) |

Medicare Physician Fee Schedule (MPFS) Formula

$$[(RVUw \times GPCIw) + (RVUpe \times GPCIpe) + (RVUm \times GPCIm)] \times CF = Payment$$

EXAMPLE: Using the sample data below, the MPFS payment for a level 3 hospital emergency department visit professional service in Buffalo is calculated as $133.09.

$$[(2.00 \times 1.000) + (1.51 \times 0.944) + (0.12 \times 0.720)] \times \$37.8975$$
$$[2.00 + 1.42544 + 0.0864] \times \$37.8975$$
$$3.51184 \times \$37.8975 = \$133.09$$

Conversion Factor = $37.8975

CPT Code	Description	RVUw	RVUpe	RVUm
G0380	Level 1 hospital emergency department visit	0.88	0.79	0.06
G0381	Level 2 hospital emergency department visit	1.34	1.13	0.10
G0382	Level 3 hospital emergency department visit	2.00	1.51	0.12
G0383	Level 4 hospital emergency department visit	2.67	1.80	0.14

Contractor No.	Locality No.	Locality Name	GPCIw	GPCIpe	GPCIm
00803	01	Manhattan, N.Y.	1.094	1.351	1.586
00803	02	NYC Suburbs & Long Island	1.068	1.251	1.869
00803	03	Poughkeepsie/N NYC Suburbs, NY	1.011	1.075	1.221
14430	04	Queens, NY	1.058	1.228	1.791
56521	05	Rest of New York State (e.g., Buffalo)	1.000	0.944	0.720

FIGURE 20-6 Formula for determining Medicare physician fee schedule payments

Ambulatory Surgical Centers Payment System (1994)

The *Ambulatory Surgical Center Payment System* uses ambulatory payment classification (APC) groups and relative payment weights to reimburse ASCs for surgical procedures performed. (The payment weights are multiplied by an ASC conversion factor to calculate ASC payment rates.)

ASC relative payment weights are updated each year using the national OPPS relative payment weights for that calendar year and, for office-based procedures, the practice expense payments under the physician fee schedule will also be updated for that calendar year. Medicare plans to make the relative payment weights budget neutral to ensure that changes in the relative payment weights from year to year do not cause the estimated amount of expenditures to ASCs to increase or decrease as a function of those changes. Medicare also maintains and updates an "exclusionary list of procedures" for which an ASC facility fee is not paid (because those procedures are included on the OPPS inpatient list).

Ambulance Fee Schedule (2002)

The *Balanced Budget Act of 1997* legislated implementation of an *ambulance fee schedule*, which reimburses ambulance service providers a preestablished fee for each service provided. Characteristics of the fee schedule consist of the following:

- Seven categories of ground ambulance services, ranging from basic life support to specialty care transport, and two categories of air ambulance services are established.

- Payment for each category is based on the relative value assigned to the service, adjusted to reflect wage differences in different parts of the country (mileage also will affect payment levels).

- Ambulance providers will not be allowed to charge beneficiaries more than their deductible and 20 percent of Medicare's fee for the service. (Under the old payment system, providers could charge beneficiaries higher rates.)

- The fee schedule allows for increased payments when an ambulance service is provided in rural areas.

The *Medicare Ground Ambulance Data Collection System (GADCS)* collects cost, revenue, utilization, and other information from selected ground ambulance organizations. Users report data collected over a continuous 12-month period, and data is submitted to the *Medicare Payment Advisory Commission (MedPAC)* for analysis and reporting to Congress.

End-Stage Renal Disease Prospective Payment System (ESRD PPS) (2011)

The *end-stage renal disease prospective payment system (ESRD PPS)* provides a single, per-treatment payment to ESRD facilities to cover all resources used when providing an outpatient dialysis treatment. CMS adjusts the ESRD PPS base rate to reflect patient and facility characteristics that contribute to higher per-treatment costs.

The ESRD PPS includes *Consolidated Billing (CB) requirements* for limited Medicare Part B services as part of the ESRD facility's bundled payment. (The *CB payment rate system* bundles ESRD drugs and related laboratory tests with the composite rate payments, resulting in one reimbursement amount paid for ESRD services provided to patients.) Lists of items and services subject to Part B CB requirements are periodically updated, at which time they are no longer separately payable when provided to ESRD beneficiaries *by providers other than ESRD facilities*.

Federally Qualified Health Centers Prospective Payment System (FQHC PPS) (2014)

Federally Qualified Health Centers (FQHCs) are safety net providers that primarily provide services typically furnished in an outpatient clinic (e.g., community health centers). The FQHC PPS for medically necessary primary health services and qualified preventive health services furnished by an FQHC practitioner is the basis for reimbursement. The FQHC PPS base payment rate has been updated annually using the FQHC *market basket*, which replaced the *Medicare Economic Index* as the index for establishing Medicare values for reimbursement.

Case-Mix Analysis, Severity of Illness (SI), and Intensity of Services (IS) Systems

Implementation of Medicare PPS resulted in health care facilities analyzing their **case mix** (patient acuity) to

- Forecast health care trends unique to their individual settings.
- Ensure that they continue to provide appropriate services to their patient populations.
- Recognize that different patients require different resources for care.

Example: Upon review of Sunnyvale Hospital's case mix, the greatest number of patients receive cardiovascular services. Wheaton Hospital's case mix indicates that the majority of its patients receive labor and delivery services. Knowing the case mix allows the hospitals to customize services required for their respective patient populations.

In addition, Medicare and other payers are interested in reviewing case-mix data because they recognize that some facilities may serve caseloads that include disproportionate shares of patients with above-average (or below-average) care needs.

Multiple possible payment rates based on patients' anticipated care needs allow payment systems to decrease the average difference between the preestablished payment and each patient's actual cost to the facility (called a *case-mix adjustment*). This also results in a reduced risk to facilities and to payers, and facilities are also willing to admit high-resource cases because higher payments can be anticipated. It creates a disincentive for facilities to admit large volumes of low-need, low-cost patients, which will result in lower payments.

Health care facilities use case-mix, intensity of service, and severity of illness software to analyze and measure standards of patient care to assess quality, including the following:

- Acute Physiological and Chronic Health Evaluation (APACHE)
- Atlas Outcomes/MediQual Systems (formerly Medical Illness Severity Grouping System, or MEDISGRPS)
- Comprehensive Severity Index (CSI)
- Patient Management Categories (PMCs)
- Severity of Illness Index (SOII)

Severity of illness (SI) is the physiologic complexity that comprises the extent and interaction of a patient's disease(s) as presented to medical personnel. Severity of illness scores are based on physiologic measures (not just ICD-10-CM codes) of the degree of abnormality of individual signs and symptoms of a patient's disease(s). The more abnormal the signs and symptoms, the higher the score.

 NOTE:

Severity of illness and intensity of services are commonly abbreviated as SI/IS or SIIS.

A health care facility's utilization management (UM) team determines whether a patient's illness is severe enough to require the current or proposed level of care by evaluating the documentation of objective clinical indicators of illness (e.g., sign, symptoms, laboratory findings). In addition, the UM team also determines *intensity of services (IS)*, which involves determining whether provided services are appropriate for the patient's current or proposed level of care (e.g., intravenous medications, heart monitoring, surgical interventions). The ultimate goal is to ensure that patients receive the appropriate level of care. If the patient's severity of illness and/or intensity of services do not meet criteria for the level of care provided, the patient is transferred to the appropriate level of care.

Example: A patient was admitted as a hospital inpatient from the facility's emergency department after work up for severe chest pain. Upon initial review of patient record documentation, the patient's laboratory results revealed positive cardiac enzymes, positive electrocardiogram (EKG) suggestive of ischemia, and continued chest pain. Thus, *severity of illness* for inpatient hospitalization was met. Upon further review of the patient record, documentation indicated the patient received intravenous nitroglycerin for chest pain and underwent cardiac catheterization, which revealed two blocked coronary arteries. Patient underwent surgical placement of stents in the blocked arteries. Thus, *intensity of services* for inpatient hospitalization was also met.

Risk management tools that identify the risk of dying include the following:

- Acute Physiological and Chronic Health Evaluation (APACHE)
- Medicare Mortality Predictor System (MMPS)

Example: The Health Data Institute created MMPS software to capture data on Medicare patients admitted with stroke, pneumonia, myocardial infarction, and congestive heart failure. The purpose was to predict death within 30 days of hospital admission because these conditions accounted for 13 percent of discharges and 31 percent of 30-day mortality for Medicare patients over age 64 prior to 1988. The MMPS system was "calibrated on a stratified, random sample of 5,888 discharges (about 1,470 for each condition) from seven states, with stratification by hospital type to make the sample nationally representative," and predictors were abstracted from the patient record. The organization determined that "risk-adjusted predicted group mortality rates may be useful in interpreting information on unadjusted mortality rates, and patient-specific predictions may be useful in identifying unexpected deaths for clinical review."

Source: "Predicting hospital-associated mortality for Medicare patients: A method for patients with stroke, pneumonia, acute myocardial infarction, and congestive heart failure," by J. Daley, S. Jencks, D. Draper, G. Lenhart, N. Thomas, and J. Walker, Baxter Healthcare Corp., Health Data Institute, Lexington, Mass. *Journal of the American Medical Association* 260, no. 24 (December 23, 1988).

Medical Necessity of Medicare Part A Hospital Inpatient Admissions

Physicians are responsible for documenting the medical necessity of an inpatient admission, which CMS calls *physician certification*. Physician documentation includes authentication of the admission order, reason for inpatient services (including the data points physicians use to reach their conclusion that the patient requires inpatient admission), estimated or actual length of time the beneficiary requires inpatient status in the hospital, and plans for posthospital care. In addition, physicians must clearly document any unexpected change in patient status (e.g., improvement) specific to the clinical issues in the case. CMS recommends that such documentation be included in the discharge order.

The CMS *2-Midnight Rule* specifies that the decision to admit a hospital inpatient should generally be based on the physician's reasonable expectation of a length of stay spanning two or more midnights, taking into account complex medical factors that must be documented in the medical record. Under the rule, surgical procedures, diagnostic tests, and other treatments (in addition to services designated as inpatient-only) are generally appropriate for inpatient hospital admission and payment under Medicare Part A when the physician expects the beneficiary to require a stay that crosses at least two midnights and admits the beneficiary to the hospital based upon that expectation. (The rule was published as a response to facilities' and beneficiaries' concerns about increasingly long stays as outpatients, such as observation care, due to hospital uncertainties about payment.) Because the decision to admit a hospital inpatient is based upon the physician's expectation, as opposed to a retroactive determination based on actual length of stay, unforeseen circumstances that result in a shorter stay than the physician's reasonable expectation may still result in a hospitalization that is appropriately considered inpatient.

As enumerated in the final rule, CMS anticipates that most of these situations will arise in the context of beneficiary death, transfer, or departure against medical advice. However, CMS does recognize that on occasion there may be situations in which the beneficiary improves much more rapidly than the physician's reasonable expectation. Such instances must be clearly documented and the initial expectation of a hospital stay spanning two or more midnights must have been reasonable in order for this circumstance to be an acceptable inpatient admission payable under Part A.

CMS further clarifies that the more usual situation would be the one in which the physician's initial expectation of the beneficiary's length of stay is uncertain. If the physician is uncertain whether the beneficiary will be able to be discharged after one midnight in the hospital or whether the beneficiary will require a second midnight of care, the initial day should be spent in observation until it is clearly expected that a second midnight would be required, at which time the physician may order inpatient admission. If the physician believes that a rare and unusual circumstance exists in which an inpatient admission is warranted, but does not expect the beneficiary to require two or more midnights in the hospital, the physician may admit the beneficiary to inpatient status but should thoroughly document why inpatient admission and Medicare Part A payment is appropriate.

Critical Pathways

Critical pathways are interdisciplinary guidelines developed by hospitals to facilitate management and delivery of quality clinical care due to constrained resources. They allow for the planning of provision of clinical services that have expected time frames and resources targeted to specific diagnoses and/or procedures. The targeted clinical services are frequently those that are high in volume and resource use and, therefore, are costly. Critical pathways are usually interdisciplinary in focus, merging medical and nursing plans of care with other disciplines (e.g., physical therapy, nutrition, and mental health). Critical pathways essentially can be viewed as interdisciplinary practice guidelines with predetermined standards of care. They provide opportunities for collaborative practice and team approaches that can maximize the expertise of multiple disciplines.

 NOTE:

Originally, critical pathways began with admission and ended with discharge from the hospital. Now that they are being implemented in other health care settings, there is potential for pathways to be focused more on the full range of an episode of care.

Revenue Cycle Management

Revenue cycle management is the process by which health care facilities and providers ensure their financial viability by increasing revenue, improving cash flow, and enhancing the patient's experience. In a physician practice, revenue cycle management is also called *accounts receivable management*. Hospitals use a chargemaster to record encounter data about ambulatory care provided to patients. The **chargemaster**, or **charge description master (CDM)** (Figure 20-7), is a document that contains a computer-generated list of procedures, services, and supplies, as well as corresponding revenue codes along with charges for each. A **revenue code** is a four-digit UB-04 code that is assigned to each procedure, service, or supply to indicate the location or type of service provided to an institutional patient, such as radiology or laboratory. Physician offices and clinics use an **encounter form**, or **superbill** (Figure 20-8), to record encounter data about office procedures and services provided to patients.

Chargemaster and encounter form data are entered in a patient accounting system, and charges are automatically posted to the insurance claim (UB-04 or CMS-1500, depending on the health care setting). The claim is submitted to the third-party payer to generate payment for services provided (e.g., emergency department, laboratory, physician office, or radiology). Chargemasters and encounter forms allow for accurate and efficient billing of services rendered.

Chargemaster

A chargemaster usually contains the following:

- *Department code*: Refers to the specific ancillary department where the service is performed
- *Service code*: Internal identification of specific service rendered
- *Service description*: Narrative description of the service, procedure, or supply
- *Revenue code*: Four-digit UB-04 code assigned to each procedure, service, or supply that indicates the location or type of service provided to a patient
- *Charge amount*: Dollar amount the facility charges for each procedure, service, or supply
- *Relative value units (RVUs)*: Numeric value assigned to a procedure that is based on difficulty and time consumed

A *chargemaster review process* is routinely conducted by designated hospital personnel (e.g., coding specialists) to ensure accurate reimbursement by updating CPT and HCPCS Level II codes and linking each to appropriate UB-04 revenue codes. These designated individuals must have knowledge of proper revenue and

(A)

Revenue Codes and the Chargemaster

> NOTE: Before 2002, revenue codes consisted of only three digits.

Revenue Codes are four-digit codes preprinted on a facility's chargemaster to indicate the location or type of service provided to an institutional patient. (They are also reported in FL 42 of the UB-04.)

EXAMPLE: **REVENUE CODES**

Code	Complete description	Abbreviated description
0270	Medical/surgical supplies	MED-SURG SUPPLIES
0450	Emergency department services	EMER/FACILITY CHARGE
0981	Emergency department physician fee	EMER/PHYSICIAN FEE

The *chargemaster* (or *charge description master, CDM*) is a document that contains a computer-generated list of procedures, services, and supplies with charges for each. Chargemaster data are entered in the facility's patient accounting system, and charges are automatically posted to the patient's bill (UB-04). The bill is submitted to the payer to generate payment for ancillary and other services (e.g., emergency department, laboratory, radiology, and so on). The chargemaster allows the facility to accurately and efficiently bill for the patient services rendered, and it usually contains the following:

- Department code (refers to the specific ancillary department where the service is performed)
- Service code (internal identification of specific service rendered)
- Service description (narrative description of the service, procedure, or supply)
- Revenue code (UB-04 revenue code that is assigned to each procedure, service, or product)
- Charge amount (dollar amount facility charges for each procedure, service, or supply)
- Relative value units (RVUs) (numeric value assigned to a procedure; based on difficulty and time consumed)

(B)

EXAMPLE: **CHARGEMASTER**

GOODMEDICINE HOSPITAL   Printed on
ANYWHERE US 12345   04/15/YYYY

DEPARTMENT CODE: 01.855

DEPARTMENT: Radiology

SERVICE CODE	SERVICE DESCRIPTION	REVENUE CODE	HCPCS CODE	CHARGE	RVU
8550001	MRI, breast	0324	C8937	375.50	4.70
8550002	MRI, cardiac stress imaging	0324	C9763	525.50	5.95
8500025	PET imaging, whole body	0350	G0219	899.50	8.73
8500026	PET imaging, any site	0350	G0235	999.50	11.10

FIGURE 20-7 Revenue codes and the chargemaster (A) Explanation of revenue codes (B) Sample portion of hospital chargemaster

expense matching to the Medicare cost center report (e.g., revenue codes) and must be willing to spend the time necessary on an extremely detailed and time-consuming task. Because it results in generation of gross revenue for the health care facility, all who use the chargemaster must be educated about its proper use and its impact on the facility's financial status.

NOTE:

Chargemasters (and encounter forms) are usually developed using database software that allows for the entry of thousands of items and potential charges. Each item includes an accounting code number, a HCPCS code, and a brief narrative description.

Commercial software helps health care facilities maintain an accurate and complete chargemaster for billing and compliance purposes. The result is fewer claims denials and more accurate outpatient reimbursement.

ENCOUNTER FORM

YUE REIS, M.D. • 101 MAIN STREET • ANYWHERE, NEW YORK 12345

(101) 555-1234 (OFFICE) • (101) 555-2234 (FAX)

EIN: 14-8526547 • NPI: 9876543210

PATIENT AND ENCOUNTER INFORMATION		FINANCIAL INFORMATION	
Patient Name		Account Number	
Patient Number	Date of Birth	Total Charge $	Amount Paid $
Date of Encounter / /	Date of Follow-up Encounter / /	Paid by ❏ Cash ❏ Check ❏ Credit Card ❏ Other	

PROCEDURES AND SERVICES

EVALUATION AND MANAGEMENT SERVICES			VACCINATIONS		OFFICE PROCEDURES	
	NEW	**ESTABLISHED**	❏ Hep A	_____	❏ Venipuncture	_____
❏ Level 1	_____	_____	❏ Hep B	_____	❏ Electrocardiogram	_____
❏ Level 2	_____	_____	❏ HPV	_____	❏ Allergy testing	_____
❏ Level 3	_____	_____	❏ Flu	_____	❏ Acupuncture	_____
❏ Level 4	_____	_____	❏ DTaP-IPV	_____	❏ Osteopathic Rx	_____
❏ Level 5	_____	_____	❏ MMRV	_____	❏ Education & training	_____
❏ Other	_____	_____	❏ Administration	_____	❏ Other	_____

DIAGNOSES AND CONDITIONS

❏ Abdominal pain	_____	❏ Diabetes mellitus	_____	❏ Syncope	_____
❏ Anxiety & depression	_____	❏ Hyperlipidemia	_____	❏ URI	_____
❏ Arrhythmia	_____	❏ Hypertension	_____	❏ UTI	_____
❏ Back pain	_____	❏ Hypothyroidism	_____	❏ Vaccination	_____
❏ Cough	_____	❏ Otitis media	_____	❏ Well child visit	_____
❏ Other: _____	_____	❏ Other: _____	_____	❏ Other: _____	_____

FIGURE 20-8 Portion of sample encounter form (superbill)

Encounter Form

Encounter form data are entered in the office's medical practice management software to generate the CMS-1500 claim that is submitted to the payer. (Many physician offices still complete paper-based CMS-1500 claims, which are submitted to health care clearinghouses to be converted to a standardized format. The health care clearinghouse submits the standardized claims data to the payer, where they are processed to generate physician reimbursement.) Similar to the chargemaster review process, the encounter form should be assigned to one individual in the physician's office who will take responsibility for reviewing and updating it twice a year when codes (e.g., ICD-10-CM, ICD-10-PCS, CPT, and HCPCS Level II codes) are added, deleted, and revised. (This process used to be conducted just once each year until 2004, when federal regulations required that code changes be issued twice each year.)

Claims Management

The health insurance claims cycle begins when providers generate CMS-1500 claims using medical practice management software (e.g., Medisoft) and health care facilities generate UB-04 (CMS-1450) claims using system-wide integrated software (e.g., Meditech). Claims are submitted to payers, clearinghouses, or third-party administrators electronically for processing. Then, patients receive an *explanation of benefits* and providers and facilities receive a *remittance advice*, both of which contain details about claims adjudication (e.g., payments made; deductibles, coinsurance, copayments required). For *denied claims* (e.g., lack of preauthorization, missing or incorrect data, procedure/serviced deemed medically unnecessary), providers and facilities submit corrected claims or letters of appeal. Payers conduct a *peer review*, which evaluates appeals to determine whether to reverse or uphold a claims denial. (The *Original Medicare Appeals Process* for Medicare Parts A and B contains five levels, which begins after an initial determination about Medicare reimbursement is made by the Medicare administrative contractor.) (The *Understanding Health Insurance* textbook contains detailed content about claims management.)

NOTE:

Intelligent automation uses robotic process automation (RPA bots) and artificial intelligence (AI) algorithms to perform repetitive tasks and improve revenue cycle management. For example, RPA bots complete and submit claims, reducing claims processing time and minimizing claims denials (fewer human errors), while AI algorithms analyze historical claims data, identifying claims denial and fraud/abuse patterns so procedures can be implemented to prevent future denials.

Revenue Cycle Management

Revenue cycle management includes the following features, typically in this order:

- *Physician order* for inpatient admission or outpatient services is documented by responsible physician.

- *Patient registration*: Patient is admitted as an inpatient or scheduled for outpatient services.
  - Appropriate consents for treatment and release of information are obtained.
  - Patient demographic and insurance information is collected.
  - Patient's insurance coverage is validated and utilization management is performed (e.g., clinical reviews) to determine medical necessity.
  - Preadmission clearance (e.g., precertification, preauthorization, screening for medical necessity).

- *Charge capture (or data capture)*: Providers use chargemasters or encounter forms to select procedures or services provided (ancillary departments, such as the laboratory, use automated systems that link to the chargemaster).

- *Diagnosis and procedure coding*: Assignment of appropriate ICD-10-CM, ICD-10-PCS, and/or CPT/HCPCS codes, typically performed by health information management personnel, to assign APCs, DRGs, and so on.

- *Patient discharge processing*: Patient information is verified, discharge instructions are provided, patient follow-up visit is scheduled, consent forms are reviewed for signatures, and patient policies are explained to the patient.

- *Billing and claims processing*: All patient information and codes are input into the billing system, and CMS-1500 or UB-04 claims are generated and submitted to third-party payers.

- *Resubmitting claims*: Before reimbursement is received from third-party payers, late charges, lost charges, or corrections to previously processed CMS-1500 or UB-04 claims are entered, and claims are resubmitted to payers—this may result in payment delays and claims denials.

- *Third-party payer reimbursement posting*: Payment from third-party payers is posted to appropriate accounts, and rejected claims are resubmitted with appropriate documentation; this process includes electronic remittance, which involves receiving reimbursement from third-party payers electronically.

- *Appeals process*: Analysis of reimbursement received from third-party payers identifies variations in expected payments or contracted rates and may result in submission of appeal letters to payers.

- *Patient billing*: Self-pay balances are billed to the patient; these include deductibles, copayments, and non-covered charges.

- *Self-pay reimbursement posting*: Self-pay balances received from patients are posted to appropriate accounts.

- *Collections*: Payments not received from patients in a timely manner result in collections letters being mailed to patients until payment is received; if payment is still not received, the account is turned over to an outside collections agency.

- *Collections reimbursement posting*: Payments received from patients are posted to appropriate accounts.

- *Auditing process*:
  - *Compliance monitoring*: Level of compliance with established managed care contracts is monitored; provider performance per managed care contractual requirements is monitored; compliance risk is monitored.
  - *Denials management*: Claims denials are analyzed to prevent future denials; rejected

(continues)

claims are resubmitted with appropriate documentation.

○ *Tracking of resubmitted claims and appeals for denied claims*: Resubmitted claims and

appealed claims are tracked to ensure payment by payers.

○ *Posting lost charges and late charges*: Late claims are submitted.

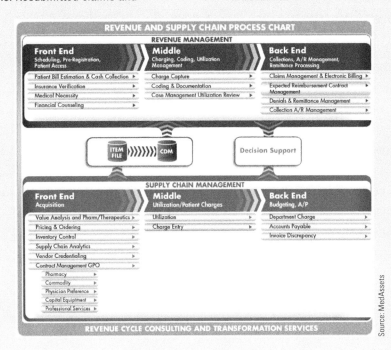

Source: MedAssets

Exercise 20.2 – Health Care Reimbursement Systems

Exercise 20.2A – Health Care Reimbursement

Instructions: Complete each statement.

1. A payer reimburses a provider 80 percent of charges submitted, and the patient is responsible for paying the remaining 20 percent coinsurance amount. Kai Allen underwent an office procedure, for which the physician billed the payer $1,500. The payer reimburses the provider the amount of $1,200, and the patient reimburses the provider the amount of $ _____.

2. Two patients each undergo a four-day inpatient stay at an acute care hospital for treatment of a myocardial infarction (heart attack). One patient has Aetna commercial insurance company and can expect the hospital to be reimbursed 80 percent of the *per diem* charge. The Medicare patient can expect the hospital to be reimbursed the MS-DRG prospective payment rate. Daily charges incurred for the four-day stay were $1,400 per day. The MS-DRG prospective payment rate for a myocardial infarction is $4,500. Aetna will reimburse the hospital $4,480. Medicare will reimburse the hospital $ _____.

3. Designated hospital personnel routinely conduct a _____ review process to ensure accurate reimbursement by updating CPT and HCPCS Level II codes and linking each to appropriate UB-04 revenue codes.

(continues)

Exercise 20.2 – **continued**

4. MS-DRGs are used as the reimbursement method for the _____ hospital PPS.

5. The outpatient hospital PPS establishes a payment rate for outpatient care by using APCs to organize similar health care services clinically and according to _____ (e.g., procedures, services) required.

Exercise 20.2B – Health Care Payment Systems

Instructions: For each payment system, select the appropriate type of prospective rate.

1. The ambulance fee schedule uses a _____ rate type.
   a. cost-based
   b. price-based

2. The ambulatory surgical center payment system uses a _____ rate type.
   a. cost-based
   b. price-based

3. The home health prospective payment system uses a _____ rate type.
   a. cost-based
   b. price-based

4. The long-term (acute) care hospital prospective payment system uses a _____ rate type.
   a. cost-based
   b. price-based

5. The Medicare physician fee schedule uses a _____ rate type.
   a. cost-based
   b. price-based

Impact of HIPAA on Reimbursement

The Health Insurance Portability and Accountability Act of 1996 (HIPAA) amended the Internal Revenue Code of 1986 to improve portability and continuity of health insurance coverage in the group and individual markets; to combat waste, fraud, and abuse in health insurance and health care delivery; to promote the use of medical savings accounts; to improve access to long-term care services and coverage; to simplify the administration of health insurance by creating unique identifiers for providers, health plans, employers, and individuals; to create standards for electronic health information transactions; and to create privacy and security standards for health information.

 NOTE:

The Federal False Claims Act provides CMS with regulatory authority to enforce fraud and abuse statutes for the Medicare program, and HIPAA extends that authority to all federal and state health care programs.

HIPAA legislation is organized according to five titles.

- Title I—Health Care Access, Portability, and Renewability
- Title II—Preventing Health Care Fraud and Abuse, Administrative Simplification, and Medical Liability Reform
- Title III—Tax-Related Health Provisions

- Title IV—Application and Enforcement of Group Health Plan Requirements
- Title V—Revenue Offsets

Health Care Access, Portability, and Renewability

HIPAA provisions were designed to improve the portability and continuity of health coverage by limiting exclusions for **pre-existing medical conditions**, which are illnesses or injuries that required treatment during a prescribed period of time (e.g., six months) prior to the insured's effective date of coverage under a new insurance policy. HIPAA provisions require that individuals be granted credit for prior health coverage and that a process be implemented to transmit certificates and other information concerning prior coverage to a new group health plan or issuer. Individuals will also be allowed to enroll in health coverage when they lose other health coverage, change from group to individual coverage, or gain a new dependent. HIPAA prohibits discrimination practices associated with health coverage enrollment eligibility and the establishment of premiums (for employees and their dependents) based on health status. The availability of health insurance coverage is also guaranteed to employees of small companies, and both small and large group markets are guaranteed renewability of health insurance coverage. HIPAA preserves the traditional role of individual states in regulating health insurance, and states are provided with flexibility to require greater protection.

 NOTE:

This section will cover health care access, portability and renewability, prevention of health care fraud and abuse, administrative simplification, and medical liability reform issues.

Preventing Health Care Fraud and Abuse

HIPAA defines *fraud* as "an intentional deception or misrepresentation that someone makes, knowing it is false, that could result in an unauthorized payment." The attempt itself is considered fraud, regardless of whether it is successful. Fraud is an act that represents a crime against payers or other health care programs (e.g., Medicare), including attempts or conspiracies to commit those crimes. *Abuse* "involves actions that are inconsistent with accepted, sound, medical, business, or fiscal practices." Abuse includes actions that result in unnecessary costs to payers and government programs (e.g., Medicare), reimbursement for services not medically necessary, or that fails to meet professionally recognized standards for health care services. The difference between fraud and abuse is the individual's intent; however, both have the same impact in that they steal valuable resources from the health care industry.

Examples of fraud include the following:

- Billing Medicare for services or supplies not provided
- Entering another person's Medicare number on a claim to obtain reimbursement for a patient not eligible for Medicare
- Unbundling codes reported on claims (reporting multiple codes to increase reimbursement, when a single combination code should be reported)
- Upcoding claims submitted to payers (reporting codes not supported by documentation in the patient record to increase reimbursement)
- Misrepresenting the diagnosis to justify payment
- Soliciting, offering, or receiving a kickback
- Falsifying plans of treatment and medical records to justify payment

 NOTE:

According to the Department of Health & Human Services, Office of Inspector General, providers are not subject to criminal, civil, or administrative penalties for innocent or negligent errors. The False Claims Act covers offenses committed with actual knowledge of the falsity of the claim, reckless disregard, or deliberate ignorance of the falsity of the claim. The False Claims Act does not cover mistakes, errors, or negligence. The Civil Monetary Penalties Law is an administrative remedy that is similar in scope and effect to the False Claims Act, and it also has exactly the same standard of proof.

Example: The medical review of claims submitted to Medicare by a physician group practice that contains mental health providers identified a pattern of psychiatric services billed on behalf of nursing facility patients with a medical history of dementia. Review of patient record documentation at the nursing facility revealed no mental health care physician orders or plans of treatment. This is considered billing for services not furnished, and it is an example of fraud.

Examples of abuse include the following:

- Mistakenly billing a Medicare patient using a higher fee schedule rate than the one used for non-Medicare patients and not correcting the billing error

- Mistakenly submitting claims to Medicare when Medicare is not the beneficiary's primary payer and not correcting the claims submission

- Mistakenly submitting excessive charges for services or supplies and not correcting the excessive charges error

- Mistakenly submitting claims for services that are not medically necessary and not correcting the claims submission to appropriately link procedure/service CPT/HCPCS Level II codes to ICD-10-CM codes

- Violating Medicare's participating (PAR) provider agreements with payers and not implementing a process to correctly follow PAR provider agreements

- Improper billing practices that result in payment by a government program when the claim is the legal responsibility of another payer and not correcting the erroneous claims submission

 N O T E :

Medical necessity requires the documentation of services or supplies that are proper and are needed for the diagnosis or treatment of a medical condition; are provided for the diagnosis, direct care, and treatment of a medical condition; meet the standards of good medical practice in the local area; and are not mainly for the convenience of the physician.

Example: During the first 30 days on the job, Ellis Adams mistakenly submitted CMS-1500 claims to Medicare instead of the patients' workers' compensation payers. The error was identified, the supervisor was notified, and the Medicare administrative contractors were immediately contacted to cancel processing of the submitted claims. Ellis then correctly submitted the CMS-1500 claims to the workers' compensation payers. Submitting claims to Medicare when Medicare is not the beneficiary's primary payer is an example of abuse if not corrected.

DRG Creep

Health Care Fraud and Abuse: Diagnosis Related Group (DRG) Creep, by W. McKay Henderson, Partner, Price Waterhouse Coopers, Health Care Fraud and Abuse Practice. (Permission to reuse granted by W. McKay Henderson, Price Waterhouse, Inc.)

What is it? *DRG creep* focuses on the medical necessity and billing patterns of DRG coding to determine whether the claims that hospitals submit

accurately reflect the care required or given to the patient. The intent is to prevent hospitals from maximizing Medicare reimbursements by choosing diagnosis codes that result in higher payments.

What separates a simple miscoding error from a false claim? The Office of Inspector General (OIG) contends that fraudulent upcoding maximized reimbursement revenue by hiring consultants or

(continues)

investing in sophisticated computer packages to help increase their reimbursements. And the DOJ and OIG put a stop to it. (*To maximize revenue* means to fraudulently increase reimbursement from payers to providers, such as reporting codes not supported by documentation that increase the DRG payment rate.)

How does upcoding happen? It is speculated that the government believes the upcoding trend is due to either computer software packages that assign the link between ICD-10-CM/PCS codes and DRGs, and/or to consultants who have trained the hospital staff who assign DRG codes. As part of its investigation, the DOJ requested hospitals to provide not only medical records and hospital documentation but also audit results, analyses of computer programs, and all consultants' reports. Those hospitals and medical centers that voluntarily disclose overpayments related to DRG miscoding may receive a reduction in fines and penalties levied against them.

Deterring Fraud and Abuse

CMS employs a four-part strategy to deter fraud and abuse, which focuses on prevention, early detection, coordination, and enforcement.

- Prevention involves paying the claim correctly the first time, and it is the most desirable approach. It is also the best way to guarantee initial accuracy of claims and payments, and it avoids the requirement to "pay and chase" providers, which is a lengthy, uncertain, and expensive process.

- Early detection identifies patterns of fraudulent activity by using data to monitor unusual billing patterns and other indicators of the integrity and financial status of providers, promptly identifying and collecting overpayments, and making appropriate referrals to law enforcement. If CMS finds errors, repayment is pursued and further action may be warranted depending on the facts and circumstances of each case.

- Coordination with partners is another important way by which CMS maximizes its success in preventing fraud; information and tactics for fighting fraud and abuse are shared with individual states, the DOJ, and the private sector.

- When fraudulent providers are discovered, enforcement action is taken against them (e.g., suspension of payment, referral to OIG for potential exclusion from Medicare program, disenrollment, collection of overpayments, and imposition of civil monetary penalties). Investing in prevention, early detection, and enforcement has a proven record of returns to the Medicare Trust Fund; the Medicare Integrity Program originally saved an estimated $7.5 billion in fiscal year 1997, mostly by preventing inappropriate payments through audits, medical reviews, and ensuring that Medicare does not pay for claims owed by private insurers. The Correct Coding Initiative (CCI) was implemented to reduce Medicare program expenditures by detecting inappropriate coding on claims and denying payment for them.

The Health Insurance Association of America (HIAA) conducts surveys that report statistics about the following health care fraud activities:

- Billing patients for services already paid for and accepting kickbacks for patient referrals

- Committing mail or wire fraud

- Falsifying patient's diagnosis to justify tests, surgeries, or other procedures

- Misrepresenting noncovered treatments as medically necessary covered treatments for the purpose of obtaining higher insurance payments

- Performing medically unnecessary services

- Performing procedures for the sole purpose of producing insurance payments

- Sales of durable medical equipment that is not needed or unnecessary

Regulating Fraud and Abuse

The following federal fraud and abuse laws are enforced by the Department of Justice, Department of Health & Human Services Office of Inspector General (OIG), and Centers for Medicare & Medicaid Services (CMS). Legislation covers civil fines; criminal penalties, prosecution, and imprisonment; exclusion from federal health care programs; and loss of professional license. (Cengage's *Understanding Health Insurance* contains details about each law.)

- Anti-Kickback Statute (AKS)
- Civil False Claims Act (FCA)
- Civil Monetary Penalties Law (CMPL)
- Health Insurance Portability and Accountability Act (HIPAA)
- Physician Self-Referral Law (Stark statute)

 NOTE:

By law, providers are not subject to civil, criminal, or administrative sanction penalties for innocent errors, or even for negligence.

Example: A provider bills Medicare for services provided to a patient that are not documented in the patient record. The charges submitted on the claim total $95. If found guilty of fraud, the provider would be required to pay a fine in an amount that is three times the fraudulent charge plus a significant penalty ($11,803 × an applicable inflation factor). The False Claims Act fine is rounded to the nearest dollar, and in 2022 would be calculated as ($11,803 × 1.0622) + ($95 × 3) = $12,822.

The DHHS Office of the Inspector General (OIG) developed a series of provider-specific *compliance guidances*, which identify risk areas and offer concrete suggestions to improve and enhance an organization's internal controls so that billing practices and other business arrangements are in compliance with Medicare's rules and regulations. Voluntary compliance guidelines have been established for the following:

- Ambulance industry
- Ambulance suppliers
- Clinical laboratories
- Durable medical equipment, prosthetics, orthotics, and supply industry
- Home health agencies
- Hospices
- Hospital industry
- Hospitals
- Individual and small-group physician practices
- Nursing facilities
- Medicare Advantage organizations
- Pharmaceutical manufacturers
- Third-party medical billing companies

A voluntary compliance program helps providers avoid generating erroneous and fraudulent claims by ensuring that submitted claims are true and accurate, expediting and optimizing proper payment of claims, minimizing billing mistakes, and preventing conflicts with self-referral and anti-kickback statutes.

Example: If a coder determines that a physician's documentation is unclear or conflicting, the coder should generate a physician query to obtain clarification. In some facilities, the policy is to have the coder contact the physician directly. In others, the coder works with a clinical documentation specialist (CDI) who contacts the physician.

The *National Correct Coding Initiative (NCCI) program* was developed by CMS to promote national correct coding methodologies, eliminate improper coding, and reduce Medicare program expenditures by detecting inappropriate codes on claims and denying payment for them. The principles of the NCCI are to ensure that the service

- Represents the standard of care in accomplishing the overall procedure
- Is necessary to successfully accomplish the comprehensive procedure (and that failure to perform the service may compromise the success of the procedure)
- Does not represent a separately identifiable procedure unrelated to the comprehensive procedure planned

NCCI program *mutually exclusive edits and procedure-to-procedure (PTP) code pair edits* are automated prepayment edits that prevent improper payment when certain codes are submitted together for Part B-covered services. Mutually exclusive edits apply when one procedure or service could not reasonably be performed with the other (Figure 20-9). When clinical circumstances do justify reporting both codes, add a modifier to either code of the code pair so that payment of both codes might be allowed.

Procedure-to-procedure (PTP) code pair edits are code pairs (or edit pairs) for which one code is a component (column 1) of a more comprehensive code (column 2), and only the comprehensive code is paid (Figure 20-10). When clinical circumstances justify reporting both codes, a modifier is added to either code of the code pair for payment consideration. They are used by Medicare administrative contractors to adjudicate provider claims for physician services, outpatient hospital services, and outpatient therapy services; they are not applied to facility claims for inpatient services.

The HCPCS Level II and CPT coding systems are used by physicians and others to describe services rendered. CCI edits are based on HCPCS Level II and CPT coding principles along with current standards of medical and surgical coding practice, input from specialty societies, and analysis of current coding practice.

The federal *False Claims Act (FCA)* also imposes civil liability on those who submit false/fraudulent claims to the government for payment and can exclude violators from participation in government programs (e.g., Medicaid and Medicare).

NATIONAL CORRECT CODING INITIATIVE MUTUALLY EXCLUSIVE EDITS					
Column 1	Column 2	* = In existence prior to 1996	Effective Date	Deletion Date * = no data	Modifier 0 = not allowed 1 = allowed 9 = not applicable
10060	G0127		19990401	*	1
10060	G0456		20130701	20141231	1
10060	G0457		20130701	20141231	1
10060	G0471		20150701	*	1

FIGURE 20-9 Sample of NCCI mutually exclusive edits

NATIONAL CORRECT CODING INITIATIVE COLUMN 1/COLUMN 2 EDITS					
Column 1	Column 2	* = In existence prior to 1996	Effective Date	Deletion Date * = no data	Modifier 0 = not allowed 1 = allowed 9 = not applicable
11010	G0428		20110701	*	1
15771	G0429		20200101	*	1
16000	G0456		20130701	20141231	1
16025	G0457		20130701	20141231	1

FIGURE 20-10 Sample of NCCI procedure-to-procedure code pair edits

NOTE:

Qui tam provisions of the FCA encourage and reward private individuals (sometimes called *whistle-blowers*) who are aware of fraud being committed against the government to report that information. In addition, the FCA only covers offenses that are committed with actual knowledge of the falsity of the claim, or reckless disregard or deliberate ignorance of the truth or falsity of a claim. The FSA does not penalize mistakes, errors, or negligence. The OIG has stated that it is mindful of the difference between innocent errors (e.g., erroneous claims) and reckless or intentional conduct (e.g., fraudulent claims).

The *Federal Anti-Kickback Statute* prohibits the offer, payment, receipt, or solicitation of compensation for referring Medicaid/Medicare patients and imposes a fine per violation, plus imprisonment. Civil penalties may also be imposed, and violators can be excluded from participation in government programs (e.g., Medicaid and Medicare). *Safe harbor regulations* were also implemented, which specify various payment and business practices that, although potentially capable of inducing referrals of business reimbursable under federal health care programs, would not be treated as criminal offenses under the anti-kickback Statute.

> **Example:** The DHHS implemented a safe harbor for the waiver or reduction of coinsurance or deductible amounts (cost-sharing amounts) for inpatient hospital services reimbursed under the PPS. For full or partial waivers to be protected, three standards had to be met: (1) the hospital could not claim waived amounts as bad debt or otherwise shift the cost of the waivers; (2) the hospital could not discriminate in offering waivers or reductions based on the patient's reason for admission; and (3) the waivers or reductions could not result from an agreement between the hospital and a third-party payer. The DHHS concluded that waivers of cost-sharing amounts for inpatient hospital services that complied with these standards would not increase costs to the Medicare program, shift costs to other payers, or increase patient demand for inpatient hospital services.

Subtitle A of the Health Insurance Portability and Accountability Act of 1997 (HIPAA) authorized implementation of a fraud and abuse control program, which coordinates federal, state, and local law enforcement programs to control fraud and abuse with respect to health plans; conducts investigations, audits, evaluations, and inspections relating to delivery of and payment for health care in the United States; facilitates enforcement of health care fraud and abuse provisions; provides for modification and establishment of safe harbors; and issues advisory opinions and special fraud alerts to provide for reporting and disclosure of certain final adverse actions against health care providers, suppliers, or practitioners.

The *Federal Claims Collection Act of 1966* established uniform procedures for government agencies to follow in the collection, compromise, suspension, termination, or referral for litigation of debts owed to the government. This means that MACs (as agents of the federal government) are responsible for attempting to collect **overpayments**, which are funds that a provider or beneficiary receives in excess of amounts due and payable under Medicare and Medicare statutes and regulations. Any review conducted by the MAC for overpayment recovery must be done within three calendar years after the year in which the overpayment was made. Once a determination of overpayment has been made, the amount so determined is a debt owed to the U.S. government.

NOTE:

The Federal Claims Collection Act of 1966 does not apply where there is an indication of fraud, for which such cases are submitted to the Office of Inspector General (OIG) for review and referral to the Department of Justice (DOJ).

Examples of overpayments include the following:

- Payment based on a charge that exceeds the reasonable charge
- Duplicate processing of charges and/or claims
- Payment made to the wrong payee (e.g., payment made to a provider on a nonassigned claim, or payment made to a beneficiary on an assigned claim)

- Payment for noncovered items and services, including medically unnecessary services
- Incorrect application of the deductible, coinsurance, or copayment
- Payment for items or services rendered during a period of nonentitlement
- Primary payment for items or services for which another entity is the primary payer
- Payment for items or services rendered after the beneficiary's date of death (postpayment reviews are conducted to identify and recover payments with a billed date of service that is after the beneficiary's date of death)

Once a Medicare administrative contractor determines that an overpayment was made, it proceeds with recovery by issuing an overpayment demand letter (Figure 20-11) to the provider. The letter contains information about the review and statistical sampling methodology used, as well as corrective actions to be taken. Corrective actions include payment suspension, imposition of civil monetary penalties, institution of prepayment or postpayment review, and additional edits.

 NOTE:

A provider is not liable for overpayments received if found to be without fault as determined by the MAC, such as when reasonable care was exercised in billing and accepting payment and the provider had a reasonable basis for assuming that payment was correct. In addition, if the provider had a reason to question the payment and promptly brought the question to the attention of the MAC, the provider may be found without liability.

EMPIRE MEDICARE ADMINISTRATIVE CONTRACTOR
P.O. Box 1000 • Albany, NY 12246 • (800) 555-1234

June 15, YYYY

Patient Billing Department
Alfred State Medical Center
100 Main Street
Alfred NY 14802

RE: PATIENT: Mary Sue Patient
     SSN: 123-45-6789
     CLAIM #:   987654321
     DATE OF SERVICE: April 5, YYYY

Dear Provider,

Please be advised that an overpayment of benefits has been made for the above named patient. In order to resolve this matter, we are asking you to make repayment. Please make your check payable to:

EMPIRE MEDICARE ADMINISTRATIVE CONTRACTOR

in the amount of:

$995.00

and forward it to:

**EMPIRE MAC
P.O. Box 1000
Albany, NY 12246**

We are requesting this refund due to the following reason:

CLAIM WAS PROCESSED IN DUPLICATE.

If you have any questions, please feel free to contact us.

Sincerely,

Mary Louse Smith
Claims Analysis (39-392)

FIGURE 20-11 Sample overpayment recovery letter

The *Payment Error and Prevention Program (PEPP)* identifies and reduces improper Medicare payments, resulting in a reduction in the Medicare payment error rate. It also participates in **overpayment recovery** by collecting overpayments made by Medicare, Medicaid, and other payers.

The *Stark I physician self-referral law* prohibits a physician from referring Medicare patients to clinical laboratory services where they or a member of their family have a financial interest. (The financial interest includes both ownership/investment interests and compensation arrangements.) By 1994, because some providers routinely waived coinsurance and copayments, the DHHS OIG issued the following fraud alert:

> Routine waiver of deductibles and copayments by charge-based providers, practitioners or suppliers is unlawful because it results in (1) false claims, (2) violations of the anti-kickback statute, and (3) excessive utilization of items and services paid for by Medicare.

(The only exception to the alert is waiving deductibles and copayments for financial hardship cases, but this *cannot be done on a routine* basis.)

In 1995, the *Stark II physician self-referral law* expanded the Stark I law by including referrals of Medicare *and* Medicaid patients for the following designated health care services (DHCS):

- Clinical laboratory services
- Durable medical equipment and supplies
- Home health services
- Inpatient and outpatient hospitalization services
- Occupational therapy services
- Outpatient prescription drugs
- Parenteral and enteral nutrients, equipment, and supplies
- Physical therapy services
- Prosthetics, orthotics, and prosthetic devices and supplies
- Radiation therapy services and supplies
- Radiology services, including MRIs, CT scans, and ultrasound services

Medicare Part A reimburses health care facilities for costs associated with training residents. The *Physicians at Teaching Hospitals (PATH) initiative* resulted from the discovery that some health care organizations were billing Medicare Part B for services that were already paid under Part A. The PATH initiative requires a national review of teaching hospitals' compliance with reimbursement rules and training of physicians who provide services at teaching facilities.

Administrative Simplification

The purpose of **HIPAA administrative simplification (AS)** provisions is to develop standards for the maintenance and transmission of health information required to identify individual patients. These standards are designed to improve efficiency and effectiveness of the health care system by standardizing the interchange of electronic data for specified administrative and financial transactions. In addition, the intent is to protect the security and confidentiality of electronic health information. HIPAA provisions require compliance by all health care organizations that maintain or transmit electronic health information. The penalty structure for HIPAA violations is based on the following tiers, and the annual maximum fine is almost $2 million for an organization.

- Tier 1: Lack of knowledge (minimum $100 fine per violation and maximum fine of $50,000)
- Tier 2: Reasonable cause (minimum $1,000 fine per violation and maximum fine of $50,000)
- Tier 3: Willful neglect (minimum $10,000 fine per violation and maximum of up to $50,000)
- Tier 4: Willful neglect not corrected within 30 days (minimum $50,000 per violation)

NOTE:

HIPAA established the *Designated Standard Maintenance Organization (DSMO)*, which is made up of organizations that agree to maintain the electronic transactions standards adopted by the Secretary of DHHS and to develop or modify adopted standards. Approved DSMOs include the Accredited Standards Committee X12, Dental Content Committee of the American Dental Association, Health Level Seven (HL7), National Council for Prescription Drug Programs, National Uniform Billing Committee, and National Uniform Claim Committee.

Unique Identifiers

HIPAA administrative simplification provisions require the following national identifiers to be established:

- *National standard employer identifier number (EIN).* The IRS's federal tax identification number was adopted as the national employer identifier, retaining the hyphen after the first two numbers (e.g., 12-3456789). The EIN is assigned to employers who, as sponsors of health insurance for their employers, must be identified in health care transactions.

- *National provider identifier (NPI).* HIPAA provisions require hospitals, doctors, nursing homes, and other health care providers to obtain a unique identifier consisting of 10 numeric digits (e.g., 1234567890) for filing electronic claims with public and private insurance programs. Providers apply for the NPI once and keep it if they relocate or change specialties. Currently, health care providers are assigned different ID numbers by each health plan, which results in slower payments, increased costs, and a lack of coordination.

NOTE:

A *check digit* is a one-digit character, alphabetic or numeric, that is used to verify the validity of a unique identifier.

- *National health plan identifier (HPID).* The HPID is assigned to third-party payers, and it contains 10 numeric positions including a check digit in the tenth position (e.g., 1234567890). (The HPID was formerly called the PlanID and the PAYERID.)

- *National individual identifier (patient identifier).* The HIPAA provision for a national individual identifier (or patient identifier) has been withdrawn. Although HIPAA included a requirement for the assignment of a unique personal health care identifier to each person in the United States, Congress is proposing legislation that would eliminate the requirement to establish a national individual identifier.

Electronic Health Care Transactions

HIPAA requires payers to implement **electronic transaction standards**, a uniform language for electronic data interchange. **Electronic data interchange (EDI)** is the computer-to-computer transfer of data between provider and third-party payer (or provider and health care clearinghouse) in a data format agreed upon by the sending and receiving parties. HIPAA's administrative simplification provisions directed the federal government to adopt national electronic standards for the automated transfer of certain health care data among health care payers (e.g., Medicare administrative contractors), payers (e.g., BCBS), and providers (e.g., hospitals and physicians). The provisions enable the entire health care industry to communicate electronic data using a single set of standards, eliminating all nonstandard formats currently in use. The standards allow a health care provider to submit a standard transaction for eligibility, authorization, referrals, claims, or attachments containing the same standard data content to any payer. This "simplifies" clinical, billing, and other financial applications, and it reduces costs.

Computer-generated paper claims are not considered EDI. Providers that generate paper-based claims submit them to health care clearinghouses, which convert them to a standardized electronic format for submission to payers. A health care clearinghouse performs centralized claims processing for providers and health care plans; it receives claims from providers, transmits claims to payers, receives remittance

```
ABC INSURANCE COMPANY
100 MAIN STREET
ALFRED NY 14802
1-800-555-1234                              REMITTANCE ADVICE

DAVID MILLER, M.D.                                          PROVIDER #: 123456
101 NORTH STREET                                           PAGE #: 1 OF 1
                                                           DATE: 04/05/YY
ALFRED, NY 14802                                           CHECK/EFT#: 000235698

PERF PROV  SERV DATE  POS NOS  PROC  MODS BILLED  ALLOWED DEDUCT    COINS GRP/RC AMT PROV PD
_____
NAME BAKER, JENNY   HIC 235962541      ACNT BAKE1234567-01      ICN 1235626589651   ASG Y MOA MA01
236592ABC  0405 0405YY 11  1 G0463     150.00   65.00  0.00     0.00  CO-42 15.00   65.00
PT RESP  10.31         CLAIM TOTALS     150.00   65.00  0.00     0.00        15.00

                                                                     NET   50.00
_____
TOTALS: # OF   BILLED   ALLOWED   DEDUCT   COINS   TOTAL   PROV PD  PROV    CHECK
        CLAIMS  AMT       AMT      AMT     RC AMT   AMT    ADJ AMT   AMT     AMT
          1    150.00    50.00     0.00    15.00    65.00   50.00   0.00    50.00
```

FIGURE 20-12 Sample remittance advice (single claim)

advice and payment instructions from payers, and transmits that information to providers (all in a HIPAA-compliant format). A health care clearinghouse also conducts eligibility and claim status queries in the format prescribed by HIPAA.

A **remittance advice (remit)** (Figure 20-12) is a statement sent by the payer to the provider, which details how submitted claims were processed and contains reimbursement amounts. If a claim is denied, an explanation of denial is included on the remittance advice. Providers may receive an electronic remittance advice (ERA) or a paper-based statement, called a standard paper remittance (SPR). The remittance advice includes the following information: patient name, health insurance claim number (HICN), provider's name, date(s) of service, type of service, procedure codes and modifiers, charges (both submitted and allowed), reimbursement amount including any deductions (e.g., copayments), reason and/or remark codes (e.g., explanation of denial), and an indication that the claim has been forwarded to a supplemental carrier for processing, if applicable.

> **Example:** Health care providers submit electronic claims data to payers on computer tape, diskette, or by computer modem or fax. The payer receives the claim, processes the data, and sends the provider the results of processing electronic claims (an electronic remittance advice).

An **explanation of benefits (EOB)** (Figure 20-13A) is sent to the patient by the payer, and it contains the same information as the remittance advice but it is in an easy-to-read format. Medicare patients receive a **Medicare Summary Notice (MSN)** (Figure 20-13B) (instead of an EOB), which is an easy-to-read monthly statement that clearly lists health insurance claims information.

 NOTE:

The MSN replaced the Explanation of Medicare Benefits (EOMB), the Medicare Benefits Notice (Part A), and benefit denial letter.

Electronic claims are processed by Medicare administrative contractors if they are not in an electronic format. Advantages of EDI include the following:

- Claim status and eligibility information in 24 hours or less
- Cost effectiveness and reduction in opportunity for error
- Electronic funds transfer of accounts receivable into the provider's bank
- Electronic remittances sent to a provider-preferred location
- Faster payment of electronic claims
- Lower administrative, postage, and handling costs

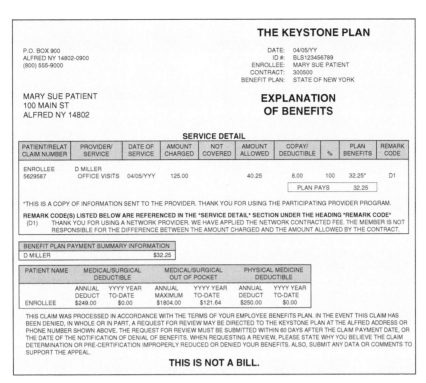

FIGURE 20-13A Sample explanation of benefits (EOB)

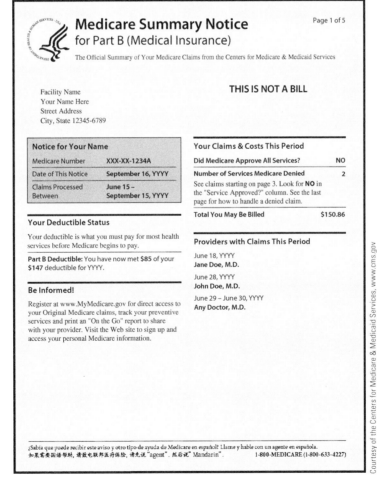

FIGURE 20-13B Sample Medicare Summary Notice (MSN)

- Online receipt or acknowledgment
- Standardized electronic claims submission, coordination of benefits exchange, and remittance receipts reduce system costs.

Health care transactions include claims, claim payments, and (provider) referrals. Three electronic formats are supported for health care transactions, including the UB-04 flat-file format (Figure 20-14), the National Standard Format (NSF) (Figure 20-15), and the **ANSI ASC X12N 837** electronic format (American National Standards Institute, Accredited Standards Committee, Insurance Subcommittee X12N, claims validation table 837) (Figure 20-16).

> **NOTE:**
>
> A **flat file** consists of a series of fixed-length records (e.g., eight spaces for the patient's date of birth). The UB-04 flat file is used to bill institutional services (e.g., hospitals), and the National Standard Format (NSF) flat file is used to bill physician and noninstitutional services (e.g., the physician's office). ANSI ASC X12N 837 is a variable-length file format that is used to bill institutional, professional, dental, and drug claims. The flat-file formats were developed for use in claims processing software application programs because the ANSI ASC X12N 837 format is not suitable for use in an application program, and it must be translated into a flat-file format prior to claims processing.
>
> Medicare administrative contractors do not accept flat-file format transactions for claims submission. Medicare administrative contractors also do not send electronic remittance advices in the flat-file format or exchange electronic eligibility queries/responses in any version not adopted as a national standard in the final rules for the HIPAA Administrative Simplification transaction standards. However, providers can use health care clearinghouses to translate outgoing and/or incoming electronic transactions, which will convert flat-file formats to the ANSI ASC X12N 837 format. Providers who do not use a health care clearinghouse must install software that can send and receive files in the ANSI ASC X12N 837 format.

```
MSG_HDR BCBS ECM_Y06 SndApp SndFac RcApp RcFac 200601052369 56941
INS_CLM 562697 20060105 20060110 ADL05691125.00
PRV_DT1M_P Smith DKSL23659
PRV_DT1M_H Jones DLEP65915
PAT_IDF DCB5432 Green 19941205
CRD_STS YYN
SRV_CMN GM 20060105 50.00
SRV_FEE CP 45.00
SRV_FEE CK 12.00
SRV_CMN GM 20060106 55.00
SRV_FEE CO 10.00
SRV_FEE RK
```

FIGURE 20-14 Sample UB-04 electronic flat-file format

```
ELECTRONIC MEDIA CLAIMS NATIONAL STANDARD FORMAT
RECORD NAME: CLAIM HEADER RECORD "PATIENT DATA"          RECORD TYPE: CA0
```

FIELD NUMBER	FIELD NAME	FIELD LENGTH	FIELD TYPE	FIELD POSITIONS FROM	TO
01.0	RECORD ID "CA0"	3	X	01	03
02.0	RESERVED (CA0-02.0)	2	X	04	05
03.0	PATIENT CONTROL NUMBER	17	X	06	22
04.0	PATIENT LAST NAME	20	X	23	42
05.0	PATIENT FIRST NAME	12	X	43	54
06.0	PATIENT MIDDLE INITIAL	1	X	55	55
07.0	PATIENT GENERATION	3	X	56	58
08.0	PATIENT DATE OF BIRTH	8	X	59	66
09.0	PATIENT GENDER	1	X	67	67
10.0	PATIENT TYPE OF RESIDENCE	1	X	68	68

FIGURE 20-15 Portion of electronic medical claims National Standard Format (NSF)

UB-04 data elements in ANSI ASC X12N 837 format	Description of data elements
ST*837*123456~ BHT*0019*00*A98765*YYYY0504*0830~	Header
NM1*41*2*GOODMEDICINE HOSPITAL*****54*888229999~	Submitter name
NM1*40*2*CAPITAL BLUE CROSS*****54*16000~	Receiver name
HL*1**20*1~	Service provider hierarchical level for submitter
NM1*85*2*GOODMEDICINE HOSPITAL*****54*888229999~ REF*1J*898989~	Service provider name
HL*2*1*22*1~ SBR*P********BL~	Subscriber (patient) hierarchical level
NM1*IL*1*PUBLIC*JOHN*Q**MI*GRNESSC1234~ N3*1247 HILL STREET~ N4*ANYWHERE*US*12345~ DMG*D8*19820805*M**::RET:3::RET:2~ REF*SY*150259874~	Subscriber (patient) name
NM1*PR*2*CAPITAL BLUE CROSS*****PI*00303~	Payer name
CLM*ABH123456*5015***11:A:1~ DTP*096*TM*1200~ DTP*434*RD8*YYYY0504-YYYY0510~ DTP*435*DT*YYYY05101100~ CL1*2*1*01~ HI*BK:66411*BJ:66411~ HI*BF:66331:::::::Y*BF:66111:::::::N*BF:V270:::::::N~ HI*BR:7569:D8:YYYY0510~	Claim information
SE*91*123456~	Trailer

FIGURE 20-16 Portion of UB-04 data submitted in ANSI ASC X12N 837 electronic format

HIPAA administrative simplification provisions also require the following code sets to be used:

- *Current Dental Terminology (CDT)*: Dental services
- *International Classification of Diseases, 10th Revision, Clinical Modification (ICD-10-CM)*: All diagnoses
- *International Classification of Diseases, 10th Revision, Procedure Classification System (ICD-10-PCS)*: Hospital inpatient procedures and services only
- *Current Procedural Terminology (CPT)*: Outpatient hospital and physician procedures and services
- *Health Care Common Procedure Coding System, Level II (National codes)*: Outpatient hospital and physician procedures and services, and institutional/professional pharmacy transactions
- *National Drug Code (NDC)*: Retail pharmacy transactions

 NOTE:

No standard code set was adopted for nonretail pharmacy drug claims.

Privacy and Security Rules

Any information communicated by a patient to a health care provider is considered *privileged communication*, which means that it is private. Patients have the right to *confidentiality*, which is the process of keeping privileged communication secret and means that information cannot be disclosed without the patient's authorization. (Exceptions include information released via *subpoena duces tecum*, court order, and according to statutory reporting requirements.) A *breach of confidentiality* occurs when patient information is *disclosed* (or released) to other(s) who do not have a right to access the information. In this situation, the disclosing provider failed to obtain patient authorization to release privileged communication; this results in violation of federal law (HIPAA).

According to HIPAA privacy and security provisions, patients have the right to an expectation of *privacy* regarding their privileged communication, which means information cannot be disclosed without their authorization. *Security* safeguards also must be implemented to ensure that facilities, equipment, and patient information are safe from damage, loss, tampering, theft, and unauthorized access.

 NOTE:

HIPAA is the first federal law that governs the privacy of health information nationwide. If security policies and procedures are not established and enforced, concerns might be raised about the security of patient information during legal proceedings. This could result in questions about the integrity of the medical record.

The HIPAA *privacy rule* provisions protect the confidentiality of protected health information (PHI). Because the use and disclosure of health information is inconsistently protected by state laws, patients' privacy and confidentiality is also inconsistently protected. The HIPAA privacy rule establishes standards to protect the confidentiality of individually identifiable health information maintained or transmitted electronically in connection with certain administrative and financial transactions (e.g., electronic transfer of health insurance claims). The rule provides new rights for individuals with respect to protected health information (PHI) and mandates compliance by *covered entities*, which are private and public sector organizations that must follow HIPAA provisions. For the privacy rule, covered entities include health care providers that conduct certain transactions in electronic forms, health plans, and health care clearinghouses.

Protected health information (PHI) is information that is identifiable to an individual (or individual identifiers) such as name, address, telephone number, date of birth, Medicaid ID number and other medical record numbers, Social Security number (SSN), and name of employer. In most instances, covered entities are required to obtain an individual's authorization prior to disclosing the individual's health information, and HIPAA has established specific requirements for an authorization form. All medical records and other individually identifiable health information used or disclosed by a covered entity in any form, whether electronically, paper-based, or verbally, are covered by the privacy rule.

The HIPAA *security rule* contains standards and safeguards for PHI that is collected, maintained, used, and transmitted electronically. Covered entities impacted by this rule include health plans, health care clearinghouses, and certain health care providers. CMS is responsible for overseeing compliance with and complaints about security rules.

The standard for electronic signature is *digital*, which applies a mathematical function to the electronic document resulting in a unique bit string (computer code) called a message digest, which is encrypted and appended to the electronic document. (*Encrypt* means to encode a computer file, making it safe for electronic transmission so unauthorized parties cannot read it.) The recipient of the transmitted electronic document *decrypts* (decodes) the message digest and compares the decoded digest to the transmitted version. If they are identical, the message is unaltered and the identity of the signer is proven.

The DHHS Medicare Program, other federal agencies operating health plans or providing health care, state Medicaid agencies, private health plans, health care providers, and health care clearinghouses must assure their customers (e.g., patients, insured individuals, providers, and health plans) that the integrity, confidentiality, and availability of electronic PHI they collect, maintain, use, or transmit are protected. The confidentiality of health information is threatened not only by the risk of improper access to stored information, but also by the risk of interception during electronic transmission of the information. The purpose of the *security rule* is to adopt national standards for safeguards to protect the confidentiality, integrity, and availability of electronic PHI. Prior to publication of the *security rule*, no standard measures existed in the health care industry to address all aspects of the security of electronic health information while being stored or during the exchange of that information between entities. In general, security provisions should include the following procedures:

- Define authorized users of patient information to control access.
- Implement a tracking procedure to sign out records to authorized personnel.
- Limit record storage access to authorized users.
- Lock record storage areas at all times.
- Require the original medical record to remain in the facility at all times (except when a court order requires the original medical record to be submitted to the court clerk).

Although security and privacy are linked, be sure you do not confuse the purpose of each rule. The *security rule* defines administrative, physical, and technical safeguards to protect the availability, confidentiality, and integrity of PHI. The standards require covered entities to implement basic safeguards to protect electronic PHI from unauthorized access, alteration, deletion, and transmission. In contrast, the *privacy rule* establishes standards for how PHI should be controlled; it also establishes what uses (e.g., continuity of care) and disclosures (e.g., third-party reimbursement) are authorized or required, as well as what rights patients have with respect to their health information (e.g., patient access).

Medical Liability Reform

The threat of excessive awards in medical liability cases has increased providers' liability insurance premiums, which has resulted in increases in health care costs. Because of this, some providers have stopped practicing medicine in areas of the country where liability insurance costs are highest, and the direct impact on individuals and communities across the country has been reduced access to quality medical care. Although medical liability reform was included in HIPAA legislation, no final rule was published. Individual states, such as Ohio, have passed medical liability reform, and the Department of Health and Human Services (HHS) has investigated ways to improve medical liability while increasing patient safety.

The Agency for Healthcare Research and Quality (AHRQ), an administrative agency that is part of HHS, established a Medical Liability Reform & Patient Safety Initiative to conduct research designed to help individual states and health care systems test models to reform medical liability and patient safety while meeting the following goals: putting patient safety first and work to reduce preventable injuries; fostering better communication between doctors and their patients; ensuring that patients are compensated in a fair and timely manner for medical injuries while also reducing the incidence of frivolous lawsuits; and reducing liability premiums. Individual states implemented medical liability laws, such as medical liability immunity statutes related to COVID-19, damage caps that limit damages in medical liability actions (e.g., lawsuits), licensing provisions and liability laws for senior and volunteer physicians, and other liability reforms in certain states (e.g., limiting attorney fees, statute of limitations on time period for initiating medical malpractice lawsuits).

Exercise 20.3 – Impact of HIPAA on Reimbursement

Exercise 20.3A – Fraud and Abuse

Instructions: Select the term that best describes the example provided.

1. Submitting excessive charges for services or supplies is _____.
   a. abuse
   b. fraud

2. Unbundling codes reported on claims to increase reimbursement is _____.
   a. abuse
   b. fraud

3. Billing Medicare for services or supplies that were not provided to patients is _____.
   a. abuse
   b. fraud

4. Submitting a claim for services that are not medically necessary is _____.
   a. abuse
   b. fraud

5. Violating Medicare participating provider agreements with payers is _____.
   a. abuse
   b. fraud

(continues)

Exercise 20.3 – continued

Exercise 20.3B – Reimbursement Terminology

Instructions: Complete each statement.

1. HIPAA provisions require health care providers to obtain a national provider _____, which contains 10 numeric digits, for filing electronic claims with public and private insurance programs.

2. The statement sent by payer to provider that details how submitted claims were processed and contains reimbursement amounts is called the remittance _____ (or remit).

3. When protected health information is disclosed to others who do not have a right to access the information, a breach of _____ has occurred.

4. The computerized exchange of health information between provider and payer in a format agreed upon by the sending and receiving parties is called EDI, which is the abbreviation for electronic data _____.

5. HIPAA requires the implementation of standards and safeguards to protect health information that is collected, maintained, used, or transmitted electronically, which is called the _____ rule.

Summary

A third-party payer is an insurance company or other organization (e.g., a Medicare administrative contractor) that processes health care claims for reimbursement of procedures and services. Third-party payers include BlueCross and BlueShield (BCBS), commercial insurance companies, employer self-insurance plans, government-sponsored programs (e.g., Medicaid, Medicare, and TRICARE), managed care plans (e.g., a health maintenance organization), and workers' compensation. A health insurance policy is an agreement between an individual and a third-party payer (or insurance company) that contains a list of reimbursable medical benefits (or covered benefits) (e.g., office visits, inpatient hospitalizations, laboratory, tests, prescription medications, and treatment services). Health reform was implemented as a result of the Patient Protection and Affordable Care Act (PPACA). This resulted in the creation of the Health Care Marketplace®.

Government programs reimburse providers according to prospective cost-based rates and prospective payment systems. Typically, third-party payers adopt prospective payment systems, fee schedules, and exclusions after Medicare has implemented them; payers modify them to suit their needs.

The Health Insurance Portability and Accountability Act of 1996 (HIPAA) amended the Internal Revenue Code of 1986 to improve portability and continuity of health insurance coverage in the group and individual markets; combat waste, fraud, and abuse in health insurance and health care delivery; promote the use of medical savings accounts; improve access to long-term care services and coverage; simplify the administration of health insurance by creating unique identifiers for providers, health plans, employers, and individuals; create standards for electronic health information transactions; and create privacy and security standards for health information.

Internet Links

Accredited Standards Committee X12N (ASC X12N): www.x12.org

Centers for Medicare & Medicaid Services: www.cms.gov

Health Level Seven (HL7): www.hl7.org

Health Reform: Go to **www.healthcare.gov** to learn more about the *Health Insurance Marketplace*.

Medicare Payment Systems: Go to **www.cms.gov**, click on the Medicare link, and then click on one or more of the topics below the Medicare Fee-for-Service Payment heading.

National Uniform Billing Committee: www.nubc.org

National Uniform Claim Committee: www.nucc.org

Office of Inspector General of the U.S. Department of Health & Human Services: www.oig.hhs.gov

Workgroup for Electronic Data Interchange (WEDI): www.wedi.org

Review

Multiple Choice

Instructions: Select the most appropriate response.

1. An insurance policy is an agreement between an insurance policy and a(n)
    a. health care facility.
    b. health care provider.
    c. individual.
    d. third-party payer.

2. Which of the following prohibits the health care provider from collecting payment from the patient for claims that the insurance plan has denied?
    a. Hold harmless clause
    b. Indemnification
    c. Medical necessity
    d. Preauthorization

3. Under an employer self-insurance plan, who would be responsible for payment of the employees' health care?
    a. Employee
    b. Employer
    c. Third-party payer
    d. Workers' compensation

4. A cancer hospital that has been granted a waiver from mandatory participation in the hospital inpatient prospective payment system is called a(n) _____ by CMS.
    a. exception   b. exclusion   c. pardon   d. release

5. The IPPS payment window for outpatient preadmission services provided by a long-term (acute) care hospital is _____ hours.
    a. 24   b. 36   c. 48   d. 72

6. Case-mix adjustments
    a. allow payment systems to increase preestablished payments.
    b. create an incentive for facilities to admit large volumes of low-cost patients.
    c. result in fewer possible payment rates based on anticipated care needs.
    d. result in higher anticipated payments for high-resource cases.

7. Severity of illness (SI) scores are based on
    a. DRG assignment.
    b. ICD-10-CM codes.
    c. physiologic measures, signs, and symptoms.
    d. the admission diagnosis.

8. Monitoring unusual billing patterns and other indicators is an example of which of the strategies used by CMS to deter fraud and abuse?
    a. Coordination   b. Early detection   c. Enforcement   d. Prevention

9. A person found guilty of Medicare fraud faces
    a. administrative sanction penalties.
    b. civil penalties.
    c. criminal, civil, and administrative sanction penalties.
    d. criminal penalties.

10. From an NCCI program perspective, which is the *lesser* procedure or service when reported with another code?
    a. Code combination
    b. Component code
    c. Comprehensive code
    d. Mutually exclusive code

11. Which HIPAA standards and safeguards were implemented to protect health information that is collected, maintained, used, or transmitted electronically?
    a. Confidentiality rule
    b. Disclosure rule
    c. Privacy rule
    d. Security rule

12. Which is a statement sent by the payer to the provider that contains reimbursement amounts and details how submitted claims were processed?
    a. Electronic data interchange (EDI)
    b. Explanation of benefits (EOB)
    c. Remittance advice
    d. Transaction for eligibility

13. The threat of excessive awards in medical liability cases has resulted in
    a. decreased health care costs.
    b. increased access to quality medical care.
    c. increased liability insurance premiums for providers.
    d. increased numbers of practicing providers.

14. Medicare's Comprehensive Error Rate Testing (CERT) program was implemented to evaluate
    a. individual provider compliance with Medicare regulations.
    b. Medicare administrative contractor (MAC) program performance.
    c. reimbursement made to hospitals serving more acutely ill patients.
    d. the transition from CMS-DRGs to MS-DRGs throughout the country.

15. Which claim is reported for noninstitutional providers and suppliers, such as physician offices?
    a. CMS-1491
    b. CMS-1495
    c. CMS-1500
    d. UB-04

Books and Manuals

American Medical Association. (2024). *CPT*. Chicago, IL: Author.

Centers for Medicare & Medicaid Services. (2023). *Internet-only manuals*. Washington, DC: Department of Health and Human Services.

Colbert, B. A., James A., & Katrancha, E. (2023). *Essentials of pharmacology for health occupations*. Clifton Park, NY: Cengage.

Ehrlich, A., Schroeder, C. L., Ehrlich, L., & Schroeder, K. (2022). *Medical terminology for health professionals*. Clifton Park, NY: Cengage.

Green, M. A. (2024). *Understanding health insurance: A guide to billing and reimbursement: 2022*. Clifton Park, NY: Cengage.

Green, M. A., & Bowie, M. J. (2019). *Essentials of health information management: Principles and practices*. Clifton Park, NY: Cengage.

Merriam-Webster. (2006). *Merriam-Webster's medical desk dictionary*. Clifton Park, NY: Cengage.

Neighbors, M., & Tannehill-Jones, R. (2023). *Human diseases*. Clifton Park, NY: Cengage.

Optum. (2024). *HCPCS level II*. Salt Lake City, UT: Author.

Optum. (2024). *ICD-10-CM*. Salt Lake City, UT: Author.

Optum. (2024). *ICD-10-PCS*. Salt Lake City, UT: Author.

Rizzo, D. C. (2016). *Fundamentals of anatomy and physiology*. Clifton Park, NY: Cengage.

Scott, A., & Fong, E. (2019). *Body structures & functions*. Clifton Park, NY: Cengage.

Journals and Newsletters

Coding clinic for HCPCS. Chicago, IL: American Hospital Association.

Coding clinic for ICD-10-CM and ICD-10-PCS. Chicago, IL: American Hospital Association.

CPT assistant. Chicago, IL: American Medical Association.

For the record. Spring City, PA: Great Valley Publishing Co., Inc.

Healthcare business monthly. Salt Lake City, UT: AAPC.

Journal of the American Health Information Management Association. Chicago, IL: American Health Information Management Association.

Internet-Based Resources

CMS Medicare Manuals
https://www.cms.gov

Find-A-Code Medical Coding and Billing Database
https://www.findacode.com

Medline Plus Encyclopedia
https://medlineplus.gov

Optum Coding
https://www.optumcoding.com

World Health Organization
https://www.who.int

Software

Optum. (2023). *Encoder Pro Expert*. Salt Lake City, UT: Author.

Glossary

Note: The chapter in which each term appears as a key term is indicated in parentheses.

2-midnight rule (7) surgical procedures, diagnostic tests, and other treatments (in addition to services designated as inpatient-only) are generally appropriate for inpatient hospital admission and payment under Medicare Part A *when the physician expects the beneficiary to require a stay that crosses at least two midnights and admits the beneficiary to the hospital based upon that expectation.*

A

acute care facility (ACF) (7) hospital that provides health care services to patients who have serious, sudden, or acute illnesses or injuries and/or who need certain surgeries.

acute care hospital (7) *see* short-term hospital.

add-on code (9) reported when another procedure is performed in addition to the primary procedure during the same operative session; modifiers -50 (bilateral procedure) and -51 (multiple procedures) are *not* used with add-on codes.

adjacent tissue transfer and rearrangement (12) closure of defects by relocating a flap of adjacent normal, healthy tissue to a defect.

adjuvant (18) substance administered with an antigen that enhances the response to the antigen.

adjuvant chemotherapy (19) chemotherapy administered in addition to other cancer treatments, such as surgery and/or radiation therapy.

adjuvant technique (14) additional procedure or technique that may be required during a lower extremity bypass graft procedure.

admitting diagnosis (7) provisional or tentative diagnosis entered in a field on the inpatient face sheet by admissions office staff; it is often a sign or symptom.

advance beneficiary notice (ABN) (8) waiver signed by the patient acknowledging that because medical necessity for a procedure, service, or supply cannot be established, the patient accepts responsibility for reimbursing the provider or DMEPOS dealer for costs associated with the procedure, service, or supply.

advance care planning (10) face-to-face services between physician or other qualified health care professional and patient, family member, or surrogate for the purpose of counseling and discussing advance directives, with or without completing relevant legal forms (e.g., health care proxy).

airway management (11) ensuring an open airway to the patient's lungs.

aliquot (18) portion of a specimen used for testing.

allergen (19) allergy-causing substances to which a patient reacts.

allergen immunotherapy (19) small amounts of allergens administered to increase a patient's tolerance to allergens.

allergy sensitivity test (19) performed on skin (cutaneous) and mucous membranes to identify the source of a patient's allergies.

allogenous (13) graft that involves tissue organ transplanted from one person to another.

ambulatory care (5) *see* outpatient care.

ambulatory patient (5) patient who is treated and released the same day and who does not stay overnight in the hospital.

ambulatory surgery patient (5) patient who undergoes procedures that can be performed on an outpatient basis, with the patient treated and released the same day.

analgesia (11) loss of pain sensation without loss of consciousness.

analgesic (11) drug that reduces pain, resulting in analgesia.

analyte (18) substance or chemical compound undergoing analysis.

ancillary service (7) diagnostic and/or therapeutic service provided to inpatients and outpatients.

anesthesia (11) process of inducing a loss of sensitivity to pain in all or part of the body, resulting from the administration of an anesthetic.

anesthesia conversion factor (11) dollar amount assigned to a geographic location.

anesthesia time unit (11) based on total anesthesia time and reported as one unit for each 15 minutes (or fraction thereof) of anesthesia time.

anesthesiologist (11) physician who, after medical school, completes a one-year internship and three-year residency in anesthesia.

anesthetic (11) drug or agent that causes a loss of feeling, awareness, and/or consciousness.

angiography (17) x-ray of a blood vessel after injection of contrast material.

angioscopy (14) microscopic visualization of substances as they pass through capillaries.

anoscopy (15) diagnostic procedure during which anal mucosa and the lower rectum are visualized using an anoscope.

ANSI ASC X12N 837 (20) variable-length file format that is used to bill institutional, professional, dental, and drug claims.

antepartum care (16) begins with conception and ends with delivery, including initial and subsequent history; physical examinations; documentation of weight, blood pressures, and fetal heart tones; routine chemical urinalysis (glucose); monthly visits up to 28 weeks' gestation; biweekly visits to 36 weeks' gestation; and weekly visits until delivery.

anterior approach (16) making an incision overlying the intervertebral disc by cutting through epidermis, dermis, subcutaneous, fascia, and muscle tissue.

anterolateral approach (16) making an incision along (and removing) the rib that corresponds to the vertebra that is located above the compressed intervertebral disk.

anteroposterior projection (17) patient is positioned with his or her back parallel to the film; the x-ray beam travels from front to back, or anterior to posterior.

antibody (18) proteins in the body made by the immune system that fight infection and disease.

antigen (18) foreign substances that elicit the formation of antibodies.

aortography (17) x-ray of the aorta after injection of contrast material.

arterial puncture (18) puncture of an artery with a needle for the purpose of drawing blood.

arthrocentesis (13) procedure done to puncture a joint for fluid removal or medication injection.

arthrodesis (13) surgical fixation of a joint.

arthrography (17) x-ray of a joint after injection of contrast material.

arthroscopy (13) visual examination of the inside of a joint.

artificial ankylosis (13) *see* arthrodesis.

arytenoidectomy (13) excision of an arytenoid cartilage, which is located in the bilateral vocal fold.

arytenoidopexy (13) surgical fixation of arytenoidal cartilage and/or surrounding muscles.

assay (18) measurement of the amount of a constituent in a specimen, such as via laboratory test.

assumption coding (1) inappropriate assignment of codes based on the presumption, from a review of clinical evidence in the patient's record, that the patient has certain diagnoses or received certain procedures/services even though the provider did not specifically document those diagnoses or procedures/services.

augmentation (13) process of enlarging or increasing.

autogenous (13) originating in the patient's body.

autonomic function test (19) evaluates autonomic nervous system functioning.

axis of classification (ICD-10-PCS) (6) the sections, body parts, root operations, and so on that comprise the seven-character ICD-10-PCS code; each axis specifies information about the procedure performed, and within a defined code range, a character specifies the same type of information for that axis of classification.

B

backbench work (13) preparing the cadaver donor heart and/or lung allograft prior to lung transplantation and dissecting allograft from surrounding soft tissues to prepare the aorta, superior vena cava, inferior vena cava, pulmonary artery, left atrium, trachea, pulmonary venous/atrial cuff, and/or bronchus for implantation.

base unit value (11) represents the degree of difficulty associated with providing anesthesia for a surgical procedure.

bed count (7) *see* bed size.

bed size (7) total number of inpatient beds for which a facility is licensed by the state; facility must be equipped and staffed to care for these patient admissions.

behavioral health care hospital (7) health care facility that specializes in treating individuals with mental health diagnoses.

benign (3) not cancerous.

Bethesda System (18) format for reporting cervical/vaginal cytology that includes a state of specimen adequacy, the general category, and a descriptive diagnosis.

Bier block (11) *see* intravenous regional anesthesia.

biofeedback (19) technique that trains the patient to gain some control over autonomic body functions.

biopsy (12) removal and examination of tissue to establish a diagnosis, confirm a diagnosis, or determine the extent of a disease.

bone density study (17) evaluates diseases of the bone; used to assess the response of bone disease to treatment.

bone marrow aspiration (14) use of a needle to remove a sample of the liquid bone marrow for examination under a microscope.

bone marrow biopsy (14) boring a small hole into a long bone and using a large, hollow needle to remove bone marrow for examination under a microscope.

bronchoscopy (13) visual examination of the interior of the bronchus.

brushing (13) combing the mucous lining of the trachea or bronchus with a bronchial brush to collect cells.

burr hole (16) small opening in the skull made with a surgical drill.

C

cadaver donor cardiectomy with or without pneumonectomy (14) harvesting the allograft (heart with or without lung tissue) and preserving the allograft with cold preservation solution and cold maintenance.

cadaver donor pneumonectomy (13) harvesting the allograft (lung tissue) and preserving the allograft with cold preservation solution and cold maintenance.

capitation (20) provider accepts a preestablished contracted payment for providing health care services to enrollees over a period of time, usually one year.

capnography (11) monitoring carbon dioxide levels.

carcinoma (Ca) *in situ* (3) malignant tumor that is localized, circumscribed, encapsulated, and noninvasive, but has not spread to deeper or adjacent tissues or organs.

cardiac ablation (14) stops atrial or ventricular fibrillation by using radiofrequency waves (modified electrical energy) to create small scars on the heart's surface.

cardiac blood pool imaging (17) use of a gamma camera for sampling, which is performed repetitively over several hundred heartbeats during the transition of the radionuclide through the central circulation.

cardiac catheterization (19) invasive diagnostic medical procedure that includes several components, beginning when the physician introduces one or more catheters into peripheral arteries and/or veins.

cardiography (19) diagnostic procedure that records the heart's electronic activity with a cardiograph and produces a cardiogram (or electrocardiogram, ECG or EKG).

cardiopulmonary bypass (14) procedure to divert blood from the heart to the aorta, using a pump oxygenator.

care plan oversight services (10) cover the physician's time supervising a complex and multidisciplinary care treatment program for a specific patient who is under the care of a home health agency, hospice, or nursing facility.

case management (10) process in which a physician or another qualified health care professional is responsible for direct care of a patient and for the coordination and control of access to or initiation and/or supervision of other health care services needed by the patient.

case mix (20) types and categories of patients cared for by a health care facility.

category (2) three-character ICD-10-CM disease code within a section.

category I code (9) traditional five-character CPT code and descriptor for a procedure or service, which is organized within one of six sections.

category II code (9) optional CPT "performance measurements" alphanumerical tracking code that contains a letter in the last field.

category III code (9) temporary "emerging technology" alphanumerical code that contains a letter in the last field; reported for data collection purposes and is archived after five years if not assigned a CPT category I code.

caudal anesthesia (11) local anesthetic injected into the caudal canal, which is the sacral portion of the spinal canal.

cell washing (13) flushing fluid into an area and removing the fluid, using aspiration technique to collect cells.

Centers for Medicare & Medicaid Services (CMS) (1) administrative agency in the federal Department of Health & Human Services.

certified anesthesiologist assistant (CAA) (11) has obtained a specialty master's degree from an accredited program, is trained as a nonphysician anesthesia care practitioner, has passed the National Commission for the Certification of Anesthesiologist Assistants (NCCAA) certification exam, and works under the direction of a licensed anesthesiologist to provide anesthesia care.

certified registered nurse anesthetist (CRNA) (11) licensed registered nurse (RN) who has obtained at least one year of acute care nursing experience (e.g., intensive care unit), completed an accredited nurse anesthesia program leading to a doctoral degree, and passed the National Board of Certification and Recertification for Nurse Anesthetists (NBCRNA) national certification exam.

charge description master (CDM) (20) *see* chargemaster.

chargemaster (20) document that contains a computer-generated list of procedures, services, and supplies and corresponding revenue codes along with charges for each.

chemotherapy (19) treatment of cancer with drugs that serve to destroy cancer cells or slow the growth of cancer cells and keep cancer from spreading to other parts of the body, preventing recurrence of the cancer.

Chemstrip automated urine analyzer (18) *see* reagent strip automated urine analyzer.

chiropractic manipulative treatment (CMT) (19) manual treatment performed to influence joint and neurophysiological function.

cholecystectomy (15) surgical removal of the gallbladder.

classification system (1) *see* coding system.

clinical documentation improvement (CDI) (1) helps ensure accurate and thorough patient record documentation and identifies discrepancies between provider documentation and codes to be assigned.

clinical documentation integrity (CDI) (1) see clinical documentation improvement.

Clinical Laboratory Improvement Act of 1988 (CLIA) (18) certification that is required to perform certain pathology and laboratory tests (and to submit claims to Medicare and Medicaid).

clinic outpatient (5) patient who receives scheduled diagnostic and therapeutic care.

closed fracture (4) type of fracture that is contained beneath the skin and has intact ligaments and skin.

closed fracture treatment (13) fracture site that is not surgically opened or exposed.

CMS-1450 (1) (20) *see* UB-04.

CMS-1500 (1) (20) standard claim submitted by physicians' offices to third-party payers.

cochlear implant (16) implanted electronic device for treatment of sensory deafness.

code (1) numerical and alphanumerical characters that are reported to health plans for health care reimbursement and to external agencies (e.g., state departments of health) for data collection, in addition to being reported internally (e.g., acute care hospital) for education and research.

coder (1) acquires a working knowledge of coding systems (e.g., CPT, HCPCS Level II, ICD-10-CM, and ICD-10-PCS), coding principles and rules, government regulations, and third-party payer requirements to ensure that all diagnoses (conditions), services (e.g., office visit), and procedures (e.g., surgery and x-ray) documented in patient records are coded accurately for reimbursement, research, and statistical purposes.

coding (1) assignment of codes to diagnoses, services, and procedures based on patient record documentation.

coding conventions (ICD-10-CM) (2) general rules used in the ICD-10-CM classification system that are independent of coding guidelines.

abbreviations (2) use of NEC (not elsewhere classifiable) and NOS (not otherwise specified) in the ICD-10-CM index and tabular list. (NEC and NOS abbreviations do *not* appear in ICD-10-PCS.)

> **NEC (not elsewhere classifiable) (2)** equivalent of "other specified"; identifies codes that are to be assigned when information needed to assign a more specific code cannot be located in the coding manual.

> **NOS (not otherwise specified) (2)** equivalent of "unspecified"; identifies codes that are to be assigned when information needed to assign a more specific code cannot be obtained from the provider.

and (2) interpreted as meaning "and/or."

boxed note (2) defines terms, provides coding instruction, and lists fifth-digit subclassifications for categories that use the same fifth digits; Index to Procedures boxed notes also provide coding instruction and list fourth-digit subclassifications for categories that use the same fourth digits. (Boxed notes do not appear in ICD-10-CM or ICD-10-PCS.)

code also (2) ICD-10-CM note that provides instruction that two codes may be required to fully describe a condition; this note does *not* provide sequencing direction.

cross references (2) instruction to refer to another entry in the index (e.g., *see*, *see also*, *see* condition) or tabular list (e.g., *see* category) to assign the correct code.

> ***see* (2)** instructional term that directs the coder to refer to another term in the index.

> ***see also* (2)** instructional term that is located after a main term or subterm in the index and directs the coder to another main term (or subterm) that may provide additional useful index entries.

> ***see* category (2)** instructional term that directs the coder to the tabular list, where a code can be selected from the options provided there.

> ***see* condition (2)** instructional term that directs the coder to the main term in the index for a condition.

default code (2) ICD-10-CM code listed next to a main term in the index; represents that condition that is most commonly associated with the main term, or is the unspecified code for the condition.

due to (2) index subterm (in alphabetical order) that indicates the presence of a cause-and-effect (or causal) relationship between two conditions.

eponym (2) disease, syndrome, or procedure named for a person.

etiology and manifestation convention (2) includes the following in the tabular list: code first underlying disease; code, if applicable, any causal condition first; in diseases classified elsewhere; and use additional code.

> **code first underlying disease (2)** tabular list instructional note that assists with proper sequencing of codes.

> **code, if applicable, any causal condition first (2)** tabular list instructional note that requires causal conditions to be sequenced first, if present.

> **in diseases classified elsewhere (2)** indicates that manifestation codes are a component of the etiology/manifestation coding convention.

> **use additional code (2)** instructional note that assists in proper sequencing of the codes.

excludes1 note (2) appears below codes in the ICD-10-CM tabular list to direct the coder to another location in the tabular list to classify conditions that are excluded from the code—code either the original code or the code to which the excludes1 note directs you.

excludes2 note (2) appears below codes in the ICD-10-CM tabular list to direct the coder to another location in the tabular list to classify conditions that are excluded from the code; both the original code and the code to which the excludes2 note directs you can be reported if documentation supports both conditions.

format (2) for ease of reference, index subterms are indented two spaces below a main term; second, third, and fourth qualifiers are indented two, four, and six spaces, respectively, below the subterm.

in (2) index subterm (in alphabetical order) that indicates the presence of a cause-and-effect (or causal) relationship between two conditions.

includes note (2) appears immediately below tabular list codes to further define terms or provide examples.

inclusion term (2) listed below certain codes in the tabular lists; includes conditions or procedures for which that code number is to be assigned; can be synonyms of the code title or, for "other" codes, a list of conditions or procedures assigned to that code.

manifestation (2) condition that occurs as the result of another condition; a manifestation code is always reported as a secondary code.

modifier (2) additional term included after the colon in the ICD-10-CM tabular lists that is to be included in the statement to classify a condition or procedure.

other code (2) when this word appears in an ICD-10-CM code description, the code is assigned when patient record documentation provides detail for which a specific code does not exist.

other specified code (2) when this phrase appears in an ICD-10-CM code description, the code is assigned when patient record documentation provides detail for which a specific code does not exist.

punctuation (2) brackets, parentheses, and colons.

> **brackets (2)** used in the index to enclose manifestation codes; used in the tabular list to enclose synonyms, abbreviations, alternative wording, and explanatory phrases.

> **colon (2)** used after an incomplete term in the tabular list when one or more additional terms (called modifiers) after the colon must be documented in the diagnostic or procedural statement to classify a condition or procedure.

> **parentheses (2)** used in the index and tabular list to enclose non-essential modifiers, which are supplementary words that may be present in or absent from the physician's statement of a disease or procedure without affecting the code number to which it is assigned.

syndrome (2) association of clinically recognizable features such as signs, symptoms, and characteristics that often occur together, so that the presence of one or more features alerts the health care provider as to the possible presence of the others; coders should follow ICD-10-CM index guidance when assigning codes to a syndrome; in the absence of index guidance, assign codes for the documented manifestations of the syndrome.

tables (2) index feature that organizes subterms, second qualifiers, and third qualifiers and their codes in columns and rows to make it easier to select the proper code. (Tables also appear in ICD-10-PCS, which facilitate assignment of values to create the seven-character code.)

trust the index (2) concept that inclusion terms listed in the Tabular List of Diseases are not meant to be exhaustive and that additional terms found only in the Index to Diseases (but not in the Tabular List of Diseases) may also be assigned to a code.

typeface (2) for ease of reference, index main terms are boldfaced and manifestation codes are italicized.

unspecified code (2) when patient record documentation is insufficient to assign a more specific code, this (unspecified) code is assigned.

with (2) index term that is located immediately below the main term, *not in alphabetical order*.

coding conventions (ICD-10-PCS) (6) general rules used in the ICD-10-PCS classification system that are independent of coding guidelines.

> **cross reference (6)** instruction in the ICD-10-PCS index that directs coders to alternate terms in the index (*see*) or tables (*use*) for proper code assignment.

> > ***see* (6)** cross reference that provides direction to another main term in the ICD-10-PCS index.

> > ***use* (6)** cross-reference that provides direction to alternate terms in an ICD-10-PCS table.

coding system (1) organizes a medical nomenclature according to similar conditions, diseases, procedures, and services; it contains codes for each.

colectomy (15) removal of part or all of the large intestine.

colonoscopy (15) visual examination of the entire colon, from the rectum to the cecum, and may include the terminal ileum.

colostomy (15) removal of a portion of the colon or rectum; the remaining colon is brought to the abdominal wall.

combination code (2) single code used to classify two diagnoses (or procedures), a diagnosis with an associated secondary process (manifestation), or a diagnosis with an associated complication.

commercial payer (20) private health insurance company or employer-based group health insurance company.

commissurotomy (14) narrowed valve leaflets are widened by carefully opening the fused leaflets with a scalpel.

comorbidity (7) coexisting condition (e.g., diabetes mellitus) that is treated during the same encounter as or impacts the medical management of another condition (e.g., myocardial infarction).

complex fistulectomy (15) excision of multiple fistulas.

complication (7) condition that occurs during the course of an inpatient hospital episode.

component coding (17) reporting a radiology procedure code and a surgical procedure code to completely describe the service provided.

composite graft (14) vein and synthetic graft material or segments of veins from two or more locations.

compound fracture (4) *see* open fracture.

computed axial tomography (CT) (CAT) (17) x-ray of horizontal and vertical cross-sectional views or "slices" of the body that are computer-processed to create three-dimensional, or 3D, images.

computed tomography angiography (CTA) (17) x-rays of different angles to create cross-sectional images of organs, bones, and tissues that visualize blood flow in arterial and venous vessels throughout the body.

computer-assisted coding (CAC) (1) uses computer software to analyze the electronic health record or electronic medical record (EMR) to generate codes for documented terms and phrases; uses "natural language processing" theories to generate codes that are reviewed and validated by coders for reporting on third-party payer claims.

concurrent care (10) provision of similar services, such as hospital inpatient care, to the same patient by more than one physician or other qualified health care professional on the same day.

concurrent coding (1) review of records and/or use of encounter forms and chargemasters to assign codes during an inpatient stay or an outpatient encounter; typically performed for outpatient encounters because encounter forms and chargemasters are completed in "real time" by health care providers as part of the charge-capture process.

concurrent medically directed anesthesia procedure (11) maximum number of procedures an anesthesiologist or a CRNA medically directs within the context of a single procedure when the procedures overlap.

conization (16) removal of a cone-shaped piece of tissue.

consultation (10) examination of a patient by a health care provider, usually a specialist, for the purpose of advising the referring or attending physician in the evaluation and/or management of a specific problem with a known diagnosis.

contiguous sites (3) adjacent locations as in cancer of multiple sites that overlap or border each other (e.g., nasopharynx and oropharynx cancer).

contrast agent (17) radiopaque substances (solid or liquid) that obstruct the passage of x-rays, making the structure containing the agent appear white on radiographic film; administered to provide better radiographic visualization of organs studied.

contrast material (17) *see* contrast agent.

Cooperating Parties for the ICD-10-CM/PCS (2) AHA, AHIMA, CMS, and NCHS.

coronal plane (17) divides the body into anterior or ventral and posterior or dorsal portions at a right angle to the sagittal plane, separating the body into front and back; also called ventral or dorsal plane.

coronary artery bypass graft (CABG) (14) procedure performed to improve flow of blood to the heart.

coronary endarterectomy (14) removal of the inner layer of coronary arteries that contain cholesterol plaques.

corpectomy (16) removal of a portion of the vertebra and adjacent intervertebral disks.

costovertebral approach (16) procedure performed where the ribs articulate with thoracic vertebrae.

counseling (10) as related to CPT E/M coding, a discussion with a patient and/or family concerning one or more of the following areas: diagnostic results, impressions, and recommended diagnostic studies; prognosis; risks and benefits of management (treatment) options; instructions for management (treatment) and follow-up; importance of compliance with chosen management (treatment) options; risk factor reduction; and patient and family education.

CPT appendices (9) located after CPT category III codes and provide additional guidance for proper code assignment.

CPT instructional notes (9) appear throughout CPT sections to clarify the assignment of codes.

CPT Symbols (9)

● bullet located to the left of a code number identifies new CPT procedures and services.

▲ triangle located to the left of a code number identifies a revised code description.

►◄ horizontal triangles surround new and revised guidelines and notes. *This symbol is not used for revised code descriptions.*

; semicolon saves space in CPT so that some code descriptions are not printed in their entirety next to a code number; the entry is indented and the coder refers back to the common portion of the code description located before the semicolon.

+ plus symbol identifies add-on codes for procedures that are commonly, but not always, performed at the same time and by the same surgeon as the primary procedure.

⊘ forbidden symbol identifies codes that are not to be appended with modifier -51.

⦰ flash symbol indicates that a code is pending FDA approval but that it has been assigned a CPT code.

\# number symbol precedes CPT codes that appear out of numerical order.

⊃ green reference symbol indicates that the coder should refer to the *CPT Assistant* monthly newsletter.

⊃ blue reference symbol indicates that the coder should refer to the *CPT Changes: An Insider's View* annual publication, which contains all coding changes for the current year.

⊃ red reference symbol indicates that the coder should refer to the *Clinical Examples in Radiology* quarterly newsletter.

★ star symbol precedes CPT codes that are reported for synchronous telemedicine services and require addition of modifier -95.

◄ the loudspeaker symbol is used to identify codes that may be used to report audio-only telemedicine services when appended with modifier 93.

⊬ PLA symbol identifies duplicate proprietary laboratory analyses (PLA) tests.

⇅ double arrow symbol identifies CPT category I PLA codes.

critical access hospital (CAH) (7) located more than 35 miles from any hospital or another CAH; state certified as being a necessary provider of health care to area residents.

critical care (10) delivery of medical care services to critically ill or injured patients who require the full, exclusive attention of the physician.

cross-over vein graft (14) making an incision to expose the vein's incompetent valve, dividing that section of the vein, and connecting it to a nearby vein that has functioning valves.

***Current Procedural Terminology* (CPT) (1)** coding system used by physicians and outpatient health care settings to assign CPT codes for reporting procedures and services on health insurance claims; considered Level I of the Healthcare Common Procedure Coding System (HCPCS); published and updated by the American Medical Association (AMA) to classify procedures and services; listing of descriptive terms and identifying codes for reporting medical services and procedures; provides a uniform language that describes medical, surgical, and diagnostic services to facilitate communication among providers, patients, and third-party payers.

cutdown (14) a procedure whereby a catheter is inserted directly into a vein through an incision.

cystography (17) x-ray of the urinary bladder after injection of contrast material.

cystoscopy (15) allows for direct visual examination of urinary bladder and urethra.

cystourethroscopy (15) *see* cystoscopy.

cytogenetics (18) study of the cell and its heredity-related components, including chromosomes.

cytopathology (18) study of diseased cells.

 D

Data Elements for Emergency Department Systems (DEEDS) (5) collection of data reported by hospital-based emergency departments for the purpose of reducing incompatibility in emergency department records.

defect (12) wound that is the result of surgical intervention or trauma.

definitive identification (18) specialized testing performed for identification at the genus or species level.

delivery/birthing room attendance and resuscitation services (10) services provided for attendance at delivery, initial stabilization of the newborn, and delivery/birthing room resuscitation.

delivery services (16) services from patient admission to the hospital through delivery of the placenta.

descriptive qualifiers (9)   terms that clarify the assignment of a CPT code by altering its description; may be located in the code description, in parentheses, or after a semicolon.

destruction (12)   ablation of benign, premalignant, or malignant tissues by any method.

Diagnostic and Statistical Manual (DSM) of Mental Disorders (1)   manual published by the American Psychiatric Association that contains diagnostic assessment criteria used as tools to identify psychiatric disorders; DSM includes psychiatric disorders and codes, provides a mechanism for communicating and recording diagnostic information, and is used in the areas of research and statistics.

Diagnostic Coding and Reporting Guidelines for Outpatient Services (5)   developed by the federal government and approved for use by hospitals and providers for coding and reporting hospital-based outpatient services and provider-based office visits.

diagnostic endoscopy (15)   use of instrumentation for surgical visualization to determine extent of disease.

diagnostic mammography (17)   assessment of suspected disease of breasts.

diagnostic procedure (12)   laboratory, radiographic, and other tests performed to evaluate the patient's complaints or symptoms and to establish the diagnosis.

dipstick (18)   small strip of plastic that is infused with a chemical; reacts to products in urine by changing color.

direct aneurysm repair (14)   surgical suture of the sac of an aneurysm and may also include partial or total excision with or without patch graft.

direct laryngoscopy (13)   insertion of a flexible (fiberoptic) or rigid laryngoscope to visualize throat structures.

discectomy (16)   removal of an intervertebral disc.

dislocation (13)   total displacement of bone from its joint.

DME MAC medical review policies (8)   local coverage determinations and national coverage determinations.

donor site (12)   anatomical site from which healthy skin is removed.

Doppler ultrasonography (17)   evaluates movement by measuring changes in the frequency of echoes reflected from moving structures.

dosimetry (17)   measurement and calculation of radiation treatment doses.

downcoding (1)   routinely assigning lower-level CPT codes as a convenience instead of reviewing patient record documentation and the coding manual to determine the proper code to be reported.

dual energy x-ray absorptiometry (DEXA) (17)   bone density study that uses two x-ray beams with different levels of energy pulsing alternately to create the image.

duplex scan (19)   noninvasive test that is performed to evaluate a vessel's blood flow.

durable medical equipment, prosthetics, orthotics, and supplies (DME-POS) (8)   include items such as artificial limbs, braces, medications, surgical dressings, and wheelchairs.

durable medical equipment, prosthetics, orthotics, and supplies (DME-POS) dealer (8)   supplies patients with durable medical equipment.

E

echocardiography (19)   diagnostic procedure that uses ultrasound to obtain two-dimensional images of the heart and/or great arteries (aorta and vena cavae).

electrocardiography (19)   *see* cardiography.

electromyography (19)   test used to detect nerve function by measuring the electrical activity generated by muscles.

electronic data interchange (EDI) (20)   computer-to-computer transfer of data between provider and third-party payer (or provider and health care clearing house) in a data format agreed upon by the sending and receiving parties.

electronic transaction standard (20)   uniform language for electronic data interchange.

embolectomy (14)   surgical removal of an embolus.

emergency department service (10)   provided in a hospital, and open 24 hours a day for the purpose of providing unscheduled episodic services to patients who require immediate medical attention.

emergency patient (5)   patient treated for urgent problems and either released the same day or admitted to the hospital as an inpatient.

employer self-insurance plan (20)   employer accepts direct responsibility for (or the risk of) paying employees' health care without purchasing health insurance.

en bloc **(14)**   as a whole.

encoder (1)   software that automates the coding process; software search features facilitate the location and verification of diagnosis and procedure codes.

encoding (1)   process of standardizing data by assigning numeric values (codes or numbers) to text or other information.

encounter (2)   face-to-face contact between a patient and a health care provider who assesses and treats the patient's condition; Medicare uses the term *encounter* in the guidelines for coding and reporting to indicate all health care settings, including inpatient hospital admissions.

encounter form (20)   document used to record encounter data about office procedures and services provided to patients.

endoscopic retrograde cholangiopancreatography (ERCP) (15)   passing an endoscope through the esophagus, stomach, and duodenum to the ducts of the biliary tree and pancreas.

endoscopy (12)   procedure performed to visualize a body cavity, using a medical instrument that consists of a long tube that can be inserted into the body, either through a small incision or a natural opening.

endotracheal tube (ET) (11)   artificial airway used for short-term airway management or mechanical ventilation due to potential or actual respiratory system insufficiency.

endovascular aneurysm repair (14)   placement of grafts to repair defects.

enterectomy (15)   resection of small bowel segments.

enterolysis (15)   freeing of intestinal adhesions.

enucleation of the eye (16)   severing of the eyeball from extraorbital muscles and the optic nerve and its removal.

epidural anesthesia (11)   local anesthetic injected into the epidural space, where it acts primarily on spinal nerve roots; anesthetized area includes the abdomen or chest to large regions of the body.

esophagogastroduodenoscopy (EGD) (15)   use of a fiberoptic endoscope to visualize the esophagus, stomach, and proximal duodenum.

esophagogastroscopy (15)   *see* upper GI endoscopy.

esophagoscopy (15)   visualization of the esophagus, using an endoscope.

essential modifier (2)   *see* subterm.

established patient (10)   one who *has* received professional services within the past three years from the physician or from another physician of the same exact specialty or subspecialty who belongs to the same group practice.

etiology (2)   cause of disease.

evidence-based coding (1)   clicking on codes that CAC software generates to review electronic health record documentation (evidence) used to generate the code; when it is determined that documentation supports the CAC-generated code, the coding auditor clicks to accept the code; when documentation does not support the CAC-generated code, the coding auditor replaces it with an accurate code.

evidence-verification coding (1)   *see* evidence-based coding.

evisceration of ocular contents (16)   removal of the contents of the eyeball; the sclera remains intact.

evocative (18)   causing a specific response; this term is used to describe various tests intended to cause production of hormones or other secretions.

excision (12)   removal of a portion or all of an organ or another tissue, using a scalpel or another surgical instrument.

exenteration of the orbit (16)   removal of orbital contents; may also include removal of bone, muscle, and/or the myocutaneous flap.

explanation of benefits (EOB) (20)   statement sent by the payer to the patient that contains the same information as a remittance advice but in an easy-to-read format.

external fixation device (13)   hardware inserted through bone and skin that is held rigid with cross-braces outside of the body; external fixation is always removed after the fracture has healed.

extracapsular cataract extraction (ECCE) (16)   removal of lens and anterior portion of capsule.

extracorporeal life support (ECLS) (14)   *see* extracorporeal membrane oxygenation (ECMO).

extracorporeal membrane oxygenation (ECMO) (14)   provides cardiac and/or respiratory support to the heart and/or lungs, which allow them to rest and recover when patients are sick or injured.

F

face-to-face time (10) amount of time the physician or other qualified health care professional spends with the patient, family, or caregiver.

fee-for-service (20) method of reimbursing providers for individual health care services rendered.

field block (11) subcutaneous injection of local anesthetic in area bordering the field to be anesthetized.

fine-needle aspiration (FNA) (12) procedure in which a thin needle is inserted through a mass several times to remove fluid from a cyst or cells from a solid mass; suction is applied as the needle is withdrawn to obtain strands of single cells for cytological diagnosis.

first-listed diagnosis (5) diagnosis, condition, problem, or other reason for encounter/visit documented in the patient record to be chiefly responsible for the services provided.

flap (12) relocation of a mass of tissue (usually skin) that has been partially removed from one part of the body so it retains its own blood supply.

flat file (20) fixed-length file format that was developed for use in claims processing (because the ANSI ASC X12 837 variable-length file format is not suitable for use in an application program and must be translated into a flat file format prior to claims processing).

fluorescence *in situ* hybridization (FISH) (18) test performed to detect submicroscopic changes in chromosomes (e.g., genetic disorders such as Williams syndrome) or to identify unknown chromosomal material.

fluoroscopy (17) procedure in which a continuous x-ray beam generates a movie-like image that is viewed on a monitor; used for invasive procedures such as intravenous/intra-arterial catheterization and extracorporeal shock wave lithotripsy.

fracture (4) break in a bone resulting from injury or a disease process.

functional modifier (9) pricing or payment modifier that a third-party payer considers when determining reimbursement.

G

gamma globulin (19) *see* immune globulin.

gastrectomy (15) removal of all or a portion of the stomach.

general anesthesia (11) administration of anesthetic agents that are inhaled or administered intravenously.

general hospital (7) acute care facility that provides emergency care, general surgery, and inpatient admission services based on licensing by the state.

global period (12) time established (0, 10, or 90 days) for each surgical procedure.

global service (17) combined technical and professional components.

global surgical package (12) defined by CMS as including preoperative and postoperative visits, intra-operative services, treatment for surgical complications, postsurgical pain management, supplies (except for identified exclusions), and miscellaneous services.

global surgery (12) *see* global surgical package.

government-sponsored programs (20) include CHAMPVA, Federal Employee Health Benefits Program, Indian Health Service, Medicaid, Medicare, Military Health System, Programs of All-inclusive Care for the Elderly, and TRICARE.

graft (12) any tissue or organ used for implantation or transfer, which involves moving healthy tissue from one site to another to replace diseased or defective tissue.

Gram stain (18) method of classifying all bacteria as gram positive or gram negative.

gross examination (18) evaluating a specimen visually, with the naked eye.

guidelines (9) define terms and clarify the assignment of codes for procedures and services that are located in a particular section of the CPT.

H

harvesting (13) removing tissue for transplantation.

HCPCS Level I (8) five-digit Current Procedural Terminology (CPT) codes developed and published by the American Medical Association (AMA).

HCPCS Level II (1) coding system managed by the Centers for Medicare & Medicaid Services (CMS) that classifies medical equipment, injectable drugs, transportation services, and other services not classified in the CPT.

HCPCS Level II miscellaneous codes (8) include *miscellaneous/not otherwise classified* codes that are reported when a DMEPOS dealer submits a claim for a product or service for which there is no existing HCPCS Level II code.

HCPCS Level II modifiers (8) two-digit alpha or alphanumeric codes added to any HCPCS Level I (CPT) or II (national) code to provide additional information regarding the product or service reported.

HCPCS Level II permanent national codes (8) maintained by the HCPCS National Panel, which unanimously makes decisions about additions, revisions, and deletions.

HCPCS Level II temporary codes (8) maintained by the CMS and other members of the HCPCS National Panel, independent of permanent level II codes, and allow payers the flexibility to establish codes that are needed before the next January 1 annual update.

HCPCS national codes (1) *see* HCPCS Level II.

Healthcare Common Procedure Coding System (HCPCS) (1) includes Level I codes (CPT) and Level II codes (HCPCS Level II national codes).

health insurance claim (20) electronic transmission or paper-based document submitted by the provider to an insurance plan to request reimbursement for procedures performed or services provided.

health insurance policy (20) agreement between an individual and a third-party payer (or insurance company) that contains a list of reimbursable medical benefits.

Health Insurance Portability and Accountability Act of 1996 (HIPAA) (1) federal legislation that amended the Internal Revenue Code of 1986 to improve portability and continuity of health insurance coverage in the group and individual markets, combat waste/fraud/abuse in health insurance and health care delivery, promote the use of medical savings accounts, improve access to long-term care services and coverage, simplify the administration of health insurance by creating unique identifiers for providers/health plans/employers, create standards for electronic health information transactions, and create privacy/security standards for health information.

hematology (18) study of the function and disorders of blood.

hemodialysis (19) process of removing waste products, toxins, and excess fluids from the blood; patient's blood is diverted into a dialyzer, where it is treated and returned to the patient's circulation by another tube inserted into a different blood vessel.

hepatotomy (15) open drainage of abscess or cyst.

HIPAA administrative simplification (AS) (20) developed standards for the maintenance and transmission of health information required to identify individual patients; designed to improve efficiency and effectiveness of the health care system by standardizing the interchange of electronic data for specified administrative and financial transactions.

home or residence services (10) provided to individuals and families in their place of residence to promote, maintain, or restore health and/or to minimize the effects of disability and illness, including terminal illness.

hospital-acquired condition (HAC) (7) medical conditions that patients develop *during* an inpatient hospitalization, which were *not* present on admission.

hospital inpatient and observation care service (10) provided to hospital inpatients and indicated when the patient's condition requires services and/or procedures that cannot be performed in any other place of service without putting the patient at risk.

hysteroscopy (16) visualization of the cervical canal and uterine cavity using a hysteroscope.

I

ICD-10 Coordination and Maintenance Committee (2) NCHS and CMS Department of HHS federal agencies that are responsible for overseeing all changes and modifications to ICD-10-CM (NCHS) and ICD-10-PCS (CMS).

ICD-10-CM Official Guidelines for Coding and Reporting (2) rules developed to accompany and complement official conventions and instructions provided in ICD-10-CM.

ICD-10-PCS Official Guidelines for Coding and Reporting (6) rules developed to accompany and complement official conventions and instructions provided in ICD-10-PCS.

ileostomy (15) removal of the colon and rectum with the small intestine brought to the abdominal wall.

immobilize (13) *see* stabilize.

immune globulin (Ig) (19)   sterilized solution obtained from pooled human blood plasma, which contains immunoglobulins (or antibodies) that protect against infectious agents that cause various diseases.

immune serum globulin (19)   *see* immune globulin.

immunoglobulin (18)   protein produced by plasma cells that help fight infection; antibody that protects against infectious agents that cause various diseases.

immunology (18)   study of the immune system.

incision (12)   a cut made with a knife, electrosurgical unit, or laser especially for surgical purposes (e.g., on body tissue).

incision and drainage (I&D) (12)   cutting open a lesion and draining its contents.

inconclusive diagnosis (5) *see* qualified diagnosis.

indemnification (20)   insurance against loss.

Index (6)   organizes ICD-10-PCS main terms in alphabetical order, providing the first 3–4 characters (and sometimes all 7 characters) of a code as well as direction to a specific location in the ICD-10-PCS Tables. Also contained in CPT as an alphabetical list of main terms, subterms, and codes.

Index to Diseases and Injuries (2)   alphabetical listing of ICD-10-CM main terms and their codes; subdivided into Index to Diseases and Injuries (includes a Table of Neoplasms and a Table of Drugs and Chemicals) and Index of External Causes of Injury; main terms are boldfaced, and subterms and qualifiers are indented below main terms.

indirect laryngoscopy (13)   insertion of a small hand mirror in the patient's mouth at the back of the throat while the physician wears headgear that contains a mirror and light source; the mirror worn by the physician reflects light into the patient's mouth, allowing the physician to visualize the patient's throat.

inferred words (9)   used to save space in the CPT index when referencing subterms.

infiltration anesthesia (11)   topical injection of local anesthetic into tissue.

informational modifier (9)   clarifies aspects of the procedure or service provided for the payer.

inpatient (7)   patient who remains overnight in a facility for 24 or more hours and who is provided with room and board and nursing services.

inpatient neonatal and pediatric critical care and intensive service (10)   provided to critically ill neonates and infants by a physician.

institutional coding (1)   captures severity of illness (ICD-10-CM) and intensity of services (ICD-10-PCS), both of which are used to justify an inpatient facility admission.

internal fixation device (13)   pins, screws, and/or plates inserted through or within a fracture area to stabilize and immobilize the injury; often called open reduction with internal fixation, or ORIF.

International Classification of Diseases for Oncology, Third Edition (ICD-O-3) (1)   implemented in 2001 to classify a tumor according to primary site (topography) and morphology (histology, behavior, and aggression of tumor).

***International Classification of Diseases, 11th Revision* (1CD-11) (1)**   developed by the World Health Organization (WHO) and released in 2018 for a planned implementation by member states on January 1, 2022, ICD-11 was revised for the purpose of recording, reporting, and analyzing health information; ICD-11 contains improved usability, which means it contains more clinical detail and requires less training time, classification of all clinical detail, eHealth readiness for the electronic health record, linkage to other classifications and terminologies (e.g., SNOMED-CT), multilingual support, and updated scientific content.

International Classification of Diseases, Tenth Revision, Clinical Modification (ICD-10-CM) (1)   developed by the Centers for Medicare & Medicaid Services (CMS) to classify all diseases and injuries.

International Classification of Diseases, Tenth Revision, Procedure Coding System (ICD-10-PCS) (1)   developed by the National Center for Health Statistics (NCHS) to classify inpatient procedures and services.

International Classification of Functioning, Disability and Health (ICF) (1)   classifies health and health-related domains that describe body functions and structures, activities, and participation; complements ICD-10, looking beyond mortality and disease.

intersex surgery (16)   performed as a series of staged procedures to transform the normal adult genitalia of one sex to that of the other sex; also called genital reconstructive surgery or sex reassignment surgery.

interventional radiologic procedure (17)   use of percutaneous or minimally invasive techniques under imaging guidance to diagnose and treat conditions.

intracapsular cataract extraction (ICCE) (16)   removal of lens and surrounding capsule.

intradermal test (intracutaneous) (19)   injection of purified allergen extracts into skin to test for allergy to suspected insect venom or penicillin.

intravenous push (19)   injection administered by a health care professional who is in constant attendance to administer the injection and observe the patient.

intravenous regional anesthesia (11)   insertion of IV cannula into the extremity on which the procedure is to be performed and a tourniquet applied to interrupt blood circulation; then a large volume of local anesthetic injected into a peripheral vein, anesthetizing the extremity.

introduction (12)   procedures that inject, insert, puncture, or scope.

J

jamming (1)   routinely assigning an unspecified ICD-10-CM disease code instead of reviewing the coding manual to select the appropriate code number.

L

laminectomy (16)   excision of the entire posterior arch or lamina of a vertebra.

laminotomy (16)   removal of part of the lamina from one side of the vertebra.

laparoscopy (15)   examination of the peritoneal contents using a laparoscope that is inserted through the abdominal wall.

laryngoscopy (13)   visualization of the back of the throat, including the larynx and vocal cords.

laser-assisted uvulopalatoplasty (15)   procedure that uses a laser technique to remove tissue from the uvula, soft palate, and pharynx.

lateral extracavitary approach (LECA) (16)   making a midline incision in the area of the affected vertebral segment, which is inferiorly curved out to the lateral plane.

laterality (2)   in ICD-10-CM, whether the condition occurs on the left, the right, or is bilateral; in CPT, whether the procedure is performed bilaterally; in CPT, when laterality is not indicated in the procedure description for paired organs or body parts, add HCPCS Level II modifier -LT or -RT to indicate the left or right side, respectively.

lateral projection (17)   positioning patient at a right angle to the film, so the x-ray beam travels through the side of the body.

LEEP electrodissection conization (16)   superficial dissection of the cervix.

lithotripsy (15)   *see* percutaneous lithotomy.

local anesthesia (11)   applying a topical agent on the body's surface or injecting a local anesthetic agent for the purpose of numbing a small part of the body; appropriate for minor surgeries.

local coverage determinations (LCDs) (8)   define coverage criteria, payment rules, and documentation required as applied to DMEPOS claims processed by DME MACs for frequently ordered DMEPOS equipment, services, and supplies; formerly called local medical review policies (LMRPs).

Logical Observation Identifiers Names and Codes (LOINC®) (1)   electronic database and universal standard used to identify medical laboratory observations and for the purpose of clinical care and management.

LOINC® (1)   *see* Logical Observation Identifiers Names and Codes (LOINC).

long-term acute care hospital (LTACH) (7)   health care facility designed specifically for patients who need functional restoration and/or rehabilitation and medical management for an average of three to six weeks; LTAC hospitals have an average inpatient length of stay of more than 25 days and provide extended medical and rehabilitative care for patients who are clinically complex and may suffer from multiple acute or chronic conditions.

long-term hospital (7)   *see* long-term acute care (LTAC) hospital.

loop electrodissection conization (16)   deep dissection of the cervix.

lumpectomy (12)   partial mastectomy.

luxation (13)   *see* dislocation.

M

magnetic resonance angiography (MRA) (17)   noninvasive diagnostic study that is used to evaluate disorders of arterial and venous structures.

magnetic resonance imaging (MRI) (17)   noninvasive x-ray procedure that uses an external magnetic field to produce a two-dimensional view of an internal organ or structure such as the brain or spinal cord.

main term (2)   printed in boldfaced type and followed by the ICD-10-CM code number.

malignant (3) cancerous.

malunion (4) failure of the ends of a fractured bone to heal (unite).

mammography (17) radiological examination of the soft tissue and internal structures of the breast.

managed care (20) combines financing and delivery of health care services; replaces conventional fee-for-service health insurance plans with more affordable care for consumers and providers who agree to certain restrictions.

manipulation (13) realignment of bones.

manometry (19) diagnostic test that measures muscle function using a pressure-sensitive tube.

mass spectrometry (11) monitoring proper levels of the anesthetic.

mastectomy (12) surgical removal of all or a portion of the breast.

maximizing reimbursement (7) reimbursement that is *not* permitted because it involves selecting and reporting as principal diagnosis the ICD-10-CM code that results in the highest level of reimbursement for the facility whether that diagnosis meets the criteria for selection or not; it also includes assigning a higher-paying ICD-10-CM code to a diagnosis (or ICD-10-CM or CPT/HCPCS code to a procedure) even if patient record documentation does not support that code selection.

Maze procedure (14) stops atrial fibrillation or atrial flutter by using incisions in heart tissue to stop abnormal heart rhythm.

medical decision making (MDM) (10) refers to the complexity of establishing a diagnosis and/or selecting a management option as measured by the number of diagnoses or management options, the amount and/or complexity of data to be reviewed, and the risk of complications and/or morbidity or mortality.

medical necessity (1) determination that a service or procedure rendered is reasonable and necessary for the diagnosis or treatment of an illness or injury.

medical nomenclature (1) includes clinical terminologies and clinical vocabularies that are used by health care providers to document patient care; *clinical terminologies* include designations, expressions, symbols, and terms used in the field of medicine, and *clinical vocabularies* include clinical phrases or words along with their meanings.

Medicare administrative contractor (MAC) (20) processes claims for physicians, health care facilities, and suppliers of durable medical equipment, prosthetics, orthotics, and supplies.

Medicare Benefit Policy Manual **(8)** provides direction about services and procedures to be reimbursed by the Medicare administrative contractor.

Medicare National Coverage Determinations Manual **(8)** indicates whether a service is covered or excluded under the Medicare program.

Medicare Prescription Drug, Improvement, and Modernization Act (MMA) (1) federal legislation that requires all code sets to be valid at the time services are provided; eliminated carriers, fiscal intermediaries, and durable medical equipment regional carriers, and created Medicare administrative contractors.

Medicare Pricing, Data Analysis, and Coding (PDAC) contractor (8) assists suppliers and manufacturers in determining HCPCS codes to be used; previously called the Statistical Analysis Durable Medical Equipment Regional Carrier (SADMERC).

Medicare Summary Notice (MSN) (20) an easy-to-read monthly statement sent to Medicare beneficiaries, which clearly lists health insurance claims information.

metastatic cancer (3) *see* secondary malignancy.

microbiology (18) study of microbes.

microtechnique (18) one of three types of micromanipulation techniques that may be used for the preparation of an embryo for transfer.

midsagittal plane (17) vertically divides the body through the midline into two equal left and right halves.

minimally invasive procedure (19) includes percutaneous access.

moderate (conscious) sedation (11) moderate sedation or analgesia that results in a drug-induced depression of consciousness.

modality (6) describes a method of treatment.

modified Maze procedure (14) *see* cardiac ablation.

modifying unit (11) part of anesthesia formula that recognizes added complexities associated with the administration of anesthesia, including physical factors and difficult circumstances.

Mohs microsurgery (12) technique of excising skin tumors by removing tumor tissue layer by layer, examining the removed portion microscopically for malignant cells, and repeating the procedure until the entire tumor is removed.

monitored anesthesia care (MAC) (11) administration of varying amounts of local, regional, and certain mind-altering drugs by an anesthesiologist or a CRNA during a patient's diagnostic or therapeutic procedure.

multiaxial structure (6) a value from each of seven hierarchies (positions) is assigned to construct an ICD-10-PCS code.

multihospital system (7) two or more hospitals owned, managed, or leased by a single organization; these may include acute, long-term, pediatric, rehabilitation, or psychiatric care facilities.

multiple codes (2) more than one ICD-10-CM code that is assigned to completely classify the elements of a complex diagnosis (or procedure) statement.

multiple sleep latency (19) observation of a patient during at least a six-hour period of sleep and includes assessment of sleep latency (dormancy) and/or wakefulness after the sleep period.

myringotomy (16) surgical incision of the tympanic membrane; usually performed to release pressure or fluid.

N

narcosynthesis (19) form of psychotherapy that is provided when the patient is under the influence of a drug, such as a sedative or narcotic.

National Correct Coding Initiative (NCCI) program (9) implemented by the Centers for Medicare & Medicaid Services (CMS) to promote national correct coding methodologies and to control the improper assignment of codes that results in inappropriate reimbursement of Medicare Part B claims.

national coverage determinations (NCDs) (8) define coverage criteria, payment rules, and documentation required as applied to DMEPOS claims processed by DME MACs for frequently ordered DMEPOS equipment, services, and supplies.

National Drug Codes (NDC) **(1)** contains prescription drugs and a few selected over-the-counter (OTC) products, which pharmacies use to report transactions and some health care professionals use for reporting on claims.

necropsy (18) autopsy.

needle electromyography (19) inserting needle electrodes into skeletal muscles and observing electrical activity of those muscles using an oscilloscope and a loudspeaker.

neoplasm (3) new growth, or tumor, in which cell reproduction is out of control.

nephrectomy (15) surgical removal of a kidney.

neuroplasty (16) freeing or decompression of an intact nerve from scar tissue.

neurorrhaphy (16) repair of nerves.

neurostimulator (16) electrode and pulse generator that are implanted along the spine to alleviate pain or control spasms.

newborn care services (10) include services provided to newborns in a variety of health care settings.

newborn patient (7) patient who receives infant care upon birth and, if necessary, receives neonatal intensive care (either within a hospital or as the result of transfer to another hospital).

new patient (10) one who has *not* received any professional services within the past three years from the physician or from another physician of the same exact specialty or subspecialty who belongs to the same group practice.

Nissen fundoplasty (15) mobilizing the lower end of the esophagus by suturing the fundus of the stomach around the circumference of the lower esophagus at the esophagogastric junction.

nonessential modifier (2) qualifying word contained in parentheses after the main term in the ICD-10-CM Index to Diseases and Injuries that does not have to be included in the diagnostic or procedural statement for the code number listed after the parentheses to be assigned.

non-face-to-face time (10) time the physician or other qualified health care professional spends performing activities that require their participation; it does not include activities that are normally performed by clinical staff.

noninvasive procedure (19) requires no surgical incision or excision; not an open procedure.

nonparticipating provider (nonPAR) (20) health care provider (e.g., physician) who is not a member of a health care plan; nonPAR providers do not receive reimbursement directly from a payer; the reimbursement is sent to the patient, and the nonPAR provider must collect payment for services rendered from the patient.

non-segmental instrumentation (13) fixation at each end of the construct (structure) that may span several vertebral segments without attachment to the intervening segments.

nonselective vascular catheterization (14) introduction of a catheter into a vessel without further advancement past the punctured vessel *or* introduction of a catheter into any portion of the aorta or vena cava from any approach (e.g., axillary, brachial, femoral, jugular).

nontunneled (14) not implanted under the skin, such as a short-term intravenous catheter that is inserted directly into a large vein.

nonunion (4) *see* malunion.

Notice of Exclusions from Medicare Benefits (NEMB) (9) document signed by patient prior to undergoing a procedure or service that is not covered by Medicare.

nuclear imaging (17) noninvasive x-ray procedure that creates an image by measuring radiation emission, or radiation "uptake," of body areas after the administration of a radionuclide.

nuclear medicine (17) use of radioactive elements for diagnostic imaging and radiopharmaceutical therapy.

O

oblique projection (17) positioning the patient with the body slanted sideways toward the film, halfway between a parallel and right-angle position; the x-ray beam travels through this angle of the body.

observation patient (5) patient who receives services furnished on a hospital's premises that are ordered by a physician (or another authorized individual), including use of a bed and periodic monitoring by nursing or other staff, and that are reasonable and necessary to evaluate the outpatient's condition or determine the need for possible admission as an inpatient.

observation care service (10) includes use of a bed and at least periodic monitoring by a hospital's nursing or other staff that is reasonable and necessary to evaluate a patient's condition or determine the need for possible admission to the hospital as an inpatient.

obturator (13) object used to close a gap.

ocular implant (16) inserted inside the muscular cone.

office or other outpatient services (10) provided in a physician's office, a hospital outpatient department, or another ambulatory care facility.

omentectomy (16) surgical removal of the omentum.

one-lung ventilation (OLV) (11) isolation of the right or left lung so that one lung is ventilated and the other is allowed to collapse.

oophorectomy (16) surgical removal of an ovary or ovaries.

open fracture (4) type of fracture that has an associated open wound.

open fracture treatment (13) surgically opening a fracture site or exposing it so treatment can be provided.

operating microscope (16) used during a surgical procedure to perform microsurgery techniques.

optimizing reimbursement (7) determining which of several diagnoses to report as the principal diagnosis when multiple diagnoses equally meet the criteria for selection as the principal diagnosis.

orbital implant (16) inserting an implant outside the muscular cone into the eye socket, and placing an intraocular lens (IOL).

orthotics (8) branch of medicine that deals with the design and fitting of orthopedic (relating to bone disorders) devices.

oscilloscope (19) device that displays electrical waveforms on a monitor.

osteogenesis (13) bone growth.

osteopathic manipulative treatment (OMT) (19) manual treatment performed by a physician during which emphasis is placed on normal body mechanics and manipulative methods to detect and correct structure.

osteophytectomy (16) removal of bone spurs to relieve compression of the spinal cord or nerve roots.

osteotomy (13) surgical incision into bone.

ostomy (15) surgically creating an opening in the body for the discharge of body wastes.

other (additional) diagnoses (7) any condition that coexists at the time of admission, that develops subsequently, or that affects the treatment received and/or the length of stay.

other significant procedure (7) surgical in nature, carries an operative or anesthetic risk, requires highly trained personnel, or requires special facilities or equipment; also called a secondary procedure.

Outcome and Assessment Information Set (OASIS) (5) core set of comprehensive assessments for adult home care patients used to measure patient outcomes for Outcome-Based Quality Improvement (OBQI); conduct patient assessment, patient care planning, and internal HHA performance improvements; and generate agency-level case mix reports that contain aggregate statistics about various patient characteristics such as demographic, health, or functional status at start of care; HHAs use Home Assessment and Validation and Entry (HAVEN) data entry software to report OASIS data.

outpatient (5) *see* ambulatory patient.

outpatient care (5) any health care service provided to a patient who is not admitted to a facility.

overcoding (1) reporting codes for signs and symptoms associated, in addition to an established diagnosis code.

overlapping sites (3) *see* contiguous sites.

overpayment (20) reimbursement a provider or beneficiary receives in excess of amount due.

overpayment recovery (20) collecting excess payments made by Medicare, Medicaid, and other payers.

P

palatopharyngoplasty (15) surgical resection of excess tissue from the uvula, soft palate, and pharynx to open the airway.

parenterally (17) administered other than by mouth or rectum, such as implantation, infusion, or injection.

paring and curettement (12) removal of growths or other material from the wall of a cavity or another surface.

participating provider (PAR) (20) health care provider (e.g., physician) who is a member of a health care plan; PAR providers receive reimbursement directly from the payer.

patch test (epicutaneous) (19) applying an allergen to a patch, which is placed on skin; the test is performed to identify substances that cause contact dermatitis, such as latex, medications, fragrances, preservatives, hair dyes, metals, and resins.

payment modifier (9) *see* functional modifier.

pediatric critical care patient transport (10) includes the physical attendance and direct face-to-face care provided by a physician during the interfacility transport of a critically ill or critically injured patient aged 24 months or younger.

percutaneous lithotomy (15) two-stage procedure that requires a percutaneous nephrostomy and dilation of the nephrostomy tract.

percutaneous needle biopsy (13) insertion of a long needle through the skin and into other tissue (e.g., chest wall, lung, or mediastinum) to obtain tissue for diagnostic evaluation.

percutaneous skeletal fixation (13) use of an external or internal fixation device to stabilize and immobilize a fracture; types include external fixation and internal fixation.

percutaneous vertebroplasty (13) process of injecting material (e.g., cement) into vertebral body to reinforce that body using image guidance.

pericardiectomy (14) removal of part of the pericardium (to treat chronic pericarditis).

pericardiocentesis (14) insertion of a needle to withdraw fluid from the pericardial sac.

pericardiotomy (14) requires thoracotomy as incision for pericardial drainage, fluid collection, or foreign body removal.

perinatal period (4) interval of time occurring before, during, and up to 28 days following birth.

peripherally (14) access via a peripheral vein, such as a catheter that is inserted into a peripheral vein using a needle or trocar.

peripheral nerve block (11) injection of local anesthetic in the vicinity of a peripheral nerve to anesthetize that nerve's area of innervation.

peritoneal dialysis (19) insertion of soft catheter into abdominal cavity and infusion of dialysate fluid at intermittent times.

peritoneoscopy (15) *see* laparoscopy.

pharmacologic management (19) evaluation of a patient's medications for effect, proper dosage, and renewal of prescribed medications.

phlebotomy (18) *see* venipuncture.

physiatrist (19) physician who specializes in physical medicine and rehabilitation and treats acute/chronic pain and musculoskeletal disorders.

physical medicine and rehabilitation (19) branch of medicine that focuses on the prevention, diagnosis, and treatment of disorders of the musculoskeletal, cardiovascular, and pulmonary systems that may produce temporary or permanent impairment.

physical status modifier (11) added to each reported anesthesia code to indicate the patient's condition at the time anesthesia was administered.

physician query process (1) contacting the responsible physician to request clarification about documentation and codes to be assigned; the process is activated when the coder notices a problem with documentation quality.

placeholder (2) use of the letter X in certain ICD-10-CM codes to allow for future expansion; it is used when a code contains fewer characters than needed to assign a fifth-, sixth-, or seventh-character.

place of service (POS) (10) the physical location where health care is provided to patients.

plane of view (17) terminology used when performing a radiology procedure.

plexus anesthesia (11) injection of local anesthetic in the vicinity of a nerve plexus.

pneumocentesis (13) puncture of the pleural space with a transthoracic needle to drain fluid or to obtain material for diagnostic study.

pneumonectomy (13) removal of the entire lung or one or more lobes of the lung.

polysomnography (19) sleep study that includes sleep staging with additional parameters of sleep.

positron emission tomography (PET) (17) producing x-ray images of the body after administering radioisotopes, which tracks metabolism or blood flow, not anatomy.

postanesthesia evaluation (11) evaluation of the patient during recovery from anesthesia, as well as evaluation, treatment, and follow-up of possible anesthesia-related complications.

posteroanterior (PA) projection (17) positioning the patient as facing the film and parallel to it; the x-ray beam travels from back to front, or posterior to anterior.

postoperative pain management (11) administration of epidural or subarachnoid medications on the date(s) of service after the date of surgery.

postpartum care (16) begins after vaginal or cesarean section delivery and includes the recovery room visit; any uncomplicated inpatient hospital and outpatient postpartum visits; episiotomy; and repair of cervical, vaginal, or perineal lacerations.

preadmission testing (PAT) (5) occurs after a surgical patient registers with a facility's admitting department, when the patient undergoes preoperative nursing assessment and receives preanesthesia evaluation by an anesthesiologist.

preanesthesia evaluation (11) assessing information from the patient's record, interviewing the patient, conducting a physical examination, evaluating preoperative test results, and ensuring that informed anesthetic consent has been obtained.

preauthorization (20) prior approval.

pre-existing medical condition (20) illness or injury that required treatment during a prescribed period of time prior to the insured's effective date of coverage under a new insurance policy.

present on admission (POA) (7) conditions that are present at the time an order for inpatient hospital admission occurs; conditions that develop during an outpatient hospital encounter (including emergency department, observation care, or outpatient surgery) are considered POA.

present on admission (POA) indicator (7) assigned to each diagnosis and external cause of injury code that is coded and reported on inpatient UB-04 or 837 Institutional (electronic) claims.

presumptive identification (18) identification by colony morphology, growth on selective media, or Gram stains.

preventive medicine services (10) include routine examinations or risk management counseling for children and adults who exhibit no overt signs or symptoms of a disorder while presenting to the medical office for a preventive medical physical.

pricing modifier (9) see functional modifier.

primary care (5) acute care and preventive services provided as outpatient care and referred to as the *point of first contact*.

primary care provider (PCP) (5) manages and coordinates the patient's care, including referring the patient to a medical specialist for consultation and a second opinion; physician responsible for supervising and coordinating health care services and preauthorizing referrals to specialists and for overseeing inpatient hospital admissions, except in emergencies.

primary defect (12) wound resulting from initial surgical intervention (e.g., excision of lesion) or trauma (e.g., deep abrasions).

primary malignancy (3) original tumor site.

principal diagnosis (7) condition established after study to be chiefly responsible for occasioning the admission of the patient to the hospital for care.

principal procedure (7) performed for definitive treatment rather than for diagnostic or exploratory purposes, necessary to treat a complication, or is most closely related to the principal diagnosis.

proctectomy (15) surgical removal of the rectum.

proctosigmoidoscopy (15) visual examination of the rectum and sigmoid colon.

professional coding (1) captures the complexity and intensity of procedures performed and services provided (CPT and HCPCS Level II) during an outpatient or physician office encounter.

professional component (17) services provided by the physician, which include supervising the performance of a diagnostic imaging procedure, interpreting imaging films, and documenting the imaging report.

prolonged services (10) physicians' services involving patient contact that are considered beyond the usual service in either an inpatient or an outpatient setting.

prospective cost-based rate (20) based on reported health care costs from which a prospective *per diem* rate is determined; annual rate is usually adjusted using actual costs from the prior year; may be based on the facility's case mix (patient acuity).

prospective payment system (PPS) (20) reimbursement methodology that establishes predetermined rates based on patient category or type of facility, with annual increases based on an inflation index and a geographic wage index.

prospective price-based rate (20) associated with a particular category of patient; rate is established by the payer prior to the provision of health care services.

prosthetics (8) branch of medicine that deals with the design, production, and use of artificial body parts.

psychotherapy (19) treatment of mental and emotional disorders by having patients talk about their condition(s) and related issues with a mental health physician or therapist.

pulse oximetry (11) monitoring arterial oxyhemoglobin saturation.

puncture, prick, or scratch test (percutaneous) (19) procedure in which tiny drops of purified allergen extracts are pricked or scratched into the skin's surface; performed to identify allergies to pollen, mold, pet dander, dust mites, foods, insect venom, and penicillin.

Q

qualified diagnosis (5) diagnosis documented as probable, suspected, questionable, rule out, or working diagnosis.

qualifying circumstance (11) coded when anesthesia services are provided during situations or circumstances that make anesthesia administration more difficult.

qualitative assay (18) detects whether a particular substance is present.

quantitative assay (18) detects the amount of a substance in a specimen.

R

radiation oncology (17) specialty of medicine that utilizes high-energy ionizing radiation in the treatment of malignant neoplasms and certain nonmalignant conditions.

radiographic projection (17) describes the path that the x-ray beam travels through the body, from entrance to exit.

radiological supervision and interpretation (17) term for the radiological portion of a procedure when two different physicians perform the surgical and radiological components of a procedure.

radiologic guidance (17) performed during a procedure to visualize access to an anatomical site to guide the placement, replacement, or removal of a catheter, central venous access device (CVAD), or needle.

radiologist (17) physician who has undergone specialized training to interpret diagnostic x-rays, perform specialized x-ray procedures, and administer radiation for the treatment of disease.

radiology (17) branch of medicine that uses imaging techniques to diagnose and treat disease.

radionuclide (17) radioactive material, such as an isotope of iodine.

radiopharmaceutical therapy (17) destroys diseased tissue, such as a malignant neoplasm.

range of codes (9) code numbers separated by a dash or a series of codes separated by commas in the CPT index.

reagent strip automated urine analyzer (18) instrumentation used to determine various components in the urine.

recipient heart with or without lung allotransplantation (14) removal (harvesting) of heart with or without lung tissue; includes transplantation of the allograft and care of the recipient.

recipient lung allotransplantation (13) transplantation of a single or double lung allograft and care of the recipient.

recipient site (12) anatomical site to which healthy skin is attached.

reconstruction (12) surgical rebuilding of a body part, such as the breast or the knee joint.

reconstruction of the vena cava (14) surgical procedure performed to correct a congenital defect or to repair the vena cava when the patient sustains trauma or the vena cava is damaged due to long-term drug therapy.

reduction (13) *see* manipulation.

referred outpatient (5) patient who receives diagnostic or therapeutic care because such care is unavailable in the primary care provider's office.

regional anesthesia (11) anesthesia agents injected into or near the spinal fluid and around a nerve or network of nerves to block the nerve supply to a specific part of the body.

rehabilitation hospital (7) health care facility that admits patients who are diagnosed with trauma or disease and who need to learn how to function.

remittance advice (remit) (20) statement sent by the payer to the provider that details how submitted claims were processed and contains reimbursement amounts.

removal (12) procedures performed to eliminate tissue (e.g., amputations) or take something out (e.g., removal of implants, such as buried wire, pins, or screws).

renal dialysis (19) artificial removal of toxic waste products from the body when the patient's kidneys are unable to perform this function due to disease or deterioration.

repair (12) procedure performed to surgically improve improperly functioning parts of the body.

replantation (13) surgical reattachment of a finger, a hand, a toe, a foot, a leg, or an arm that has been completely severed from a person's body.

residual effect (2) condition produced (sequela) after the acute phase of an illness or injury has terminated.

revenue code (20) four-digit UB-04 code that is assigned to each procedure, service, or supply to indicate the location or type of service provided to an institutional patient, such as radiology or laboratory.

revision (12) surgical modification of a previous procedure or a device.

rhinoplasty (15) repair of a skin defect of the nose using harvested tissue or plastic surgery to change the nose's shape or size.

root operation (6) describes the intent or objective of an ICD-10-PCS procedure.

root type (6) describes the purpose of an ICD-10-PCS procedure or service.

roster billing (20) simplified claims submission process available to public health clinics and other noninstitutional entities that offer mass immunization programs.

rule of nines (12) divides total body surface area (BSA) into nine segments by percentage.

RxNorm (1) provides normalized names for clinical drugs and links its names to many of the drug vocabularies commonly used in pharmacy management and drug interaction software, including those of First Databank, Micromedex, MediSpan, Gold Standard Drug Database, and Multum; by providing links among these vocabularies, RxNorm can mediate messages among systems that do not use the same software and vocabulary.

S

saddle block anesthesia (11) *see* caudal anesthesia.

sagittal plane (17) vertically divides the body into unequal left and right portions.

salpingo-oophorectomy (16) surgical removal of both fallopian tubes and ovaries.

saphenopopliteal vein anastomosis (14) surgical incision to expose the saphenous vein and connect it to the popliteal vein using end-to-end anastomosis.

screening mammography (17) radiographic (x-ray) of the breast that is performed when a patient presents without signs and symptoms of breast disease.

secondary defect (12) wound resulting from removal of tissue to create flap(s) or graft(s).

secondary malignancy (3) tumor that has metastasized, or spread, to a secondary site either adjacent to the primary site or to a remote region of the body.

secondary procedure (7) *see* other significant procedure.

second-stage fistulectomy/fistulotomy (15) in treatment of anal fistulas, use of a seton to cut through the fistula; the seton is left in place until later removal.

sedation (11) administration of medication into a vein to relieve pain and anxiety, making the patient feel calm.

segmental instrumentation (13) fixation at each end of the construct (structure) and includes at least one additional interposed bony attachment.

selective vascular catheterization (14) insertion and manipulation or guidance of a catheter into the branches of the arterial system (other than the aorta or the vessel punctured) for the purpose of performing diagnostic or therapeutic procedures.

separate procedure (12) performed as an integral component of a total service or procedure.

sequela (2) residual (long-term condition produced) that develops after the acute phase of an illness or injury has ended. (Historically, ICD-9-CM referred to a sequela as a *late effect* of an illness or injury.)

seton (15) large silk suture or rubber bands.

shaving (12) horizontal slicing to remove epidermal and dermal lesions; removal includes scissoring or any sharp method.

short-term hospital (7) average length of stay (LOS) of 4–5 days and a total LOS of fewer than 25 days.

shunting procedure (14) performed to move blood from one area to another for conditions such as atrial septal defect (ASD), coarctation of the aorta, patent ductus arteriosus (PDA), tricuspid atresia, and ventricular septal defect (VSD).

sigmoidoscopy (15) visual examination of the entire rectum and sigmoid colon and may include a portion of the descending colon.

simple fracture (4) *see* closed fracture.

single code (9) single code number listed in the CPT index.

single hospital (7) hospital that is self-contained and not part of a larger organization.

single-path coding (1) combines professional and institutional coding to improve productivity and ensure the submission of clean claims, leading to improved reimbursement.

single photon emission computerized tomography (SPECT) (17) three-dimensional x-ray images of internal organs produced after administration of a radioactive material, which visualize anatomy and function.

skeletal traction (13) exerts a pulling force on the affected limb to realign bone or joint.

sleep laboratory (19) area in a hospital facility that is managed by a sleep technologist who explains and performs the sleep studies.

sleep staging (19) during a sleep study (polysomnography), involves the use of a 1-4 lead electroencephalogram (EEG), electro-oculogram (EOG), and submental electromyogram (EMG).

sleep study (19) evaluation of adult and pediatric patients during sleep by monitoring brain waves, heart rate, and eye movements; performed to diagnose sleep disorders, which include breathing, movement, and neurologic disorders that occur at night.

SNOMED CT (1) *see Systemized Nomenclature of Medicine Clinical Terms.*

special evaluation and management services (10) provided for establishment of baseline information prior to life or disability insurance certificates being issued and for examination of a patient with a work-related or medical disability problem.

special report (9) document that must accompany the claim to describe the nature, extent, and need for the procedure or service when an unlisted procedure or service code is reported.

specialty coders (1) individuals who have obtained advanced training in medical specialties (e.g., anesthesia, obstetrics) and who are skilled in that medical specialty's compliance and reimbursement areas.

specialty hospital (7) health care facility that delivers care to a particular population of patients or type of disease.

specimen (18) tissue submitted for laboratory or pathological evaluation; also the unit of service used to report surgical pathology codes.

spinal anesthesia (11) local anesthetic injected into cerebrospinal fluid at the lumbar spine, where it acts on spinal nerve roots and part of the spinal cord; anesthetized area extends from the legs to the abdomen or chest.

splenoportography (14) radiographic visualization of the splenic and portal veins.

stabilize (13) to secure bone in a fixed position.

stab phlebectomy (14) multiple tiny incisions made over varicose vein sites; at each stab site the varicosity is extracted and then the varicose segment is removed.

standby service (10) physician, or other qualified health care professional, spending a prolonged period of time *without patient contact* waiting for an event to occur that will require the physician's or professional's service.

statistical modifier (9) *see* informational modifier.

stented valve (14) includes framework on which the replacement heart valve is mounted to provide support for the valve's leaflets.

stentless valve (14) an actual heart valve obtained from either a human donor (homograft) or a pig; it does not contain framework.

stereotactic localization (12) use of specialized three-dimensional imaging to target a nonpalpable lesion.

stereotaxis (16) use of a stereotactic guidance system to allow the physician to determine three-dimensional coordinates in order to create a lesion on the spinal cord (to alleviate chronic pain in a particular part of the body); to stimulate the spinal cord percutaneously (to create a lesion that will block pain); or to facilitate the biopsy, aspiration, or excision of a spinal cord lesion.

stoma (15) surgically created opening between ureter, small intestine, or large intestine, through to abdominal wall.

stroma (12) supporting tissue (matrix) of an organ.

subacute care patient (7) receives specialized services such as chemotherapy, injury rehabilitation, ventilator support, wound care, and other types of health care services provided to seriously ill patients.

subcategory (2) ICD-10-CM codes that contain four, five, six, or seven characters; subcategory codes that require additional characters are invalid if the fifth, sixth, or seventh character(s) is absent.

subcutaneous fistulectomy (15) removal of an anal fistula, without division of the sphincter muscle.

subglottic stenosis (13) narrowing of the airway below the vocal cords, adjacent to the cricoid cartilage.

subluxation (13) partial displacement of a bone from its joint.

submuscular fistulectomy (15) removal of an anal fistula, including division of the sphincter muscle.

subterm (2) qualifying word listed below the main term in the ICD-10-CM Index to Diseases and Injuries; list of alternate sites, etiology, or clinical status.

superbill (20) *see* encounter form.

surface anesthesia (11) topical application of local anesthetic cream, solution, or spray to skin or mucous membranes.

surgical endoscopy (15) performed when anything in addition to visualization is done, such as the removal of a foreign body.

surgical package (12) defined by CPT as including a variety of services provided by a surgeon to include surgical procedure performed; local infiltration, metacarpal/metatarsal/digital block anesthesia; one related E/M service on the date immediately prior to or date of the procedure (including history and physical); immediate postoperative care; and typical postoperative follow-up care.

suture (12) closure of a wound using catgut, glue, silk thread, wire, or other materials.

swing bed (7) allows a rural hospital to admit a nonacute care patient.

sympathectomy (14) excision of a segment of the sympathetic nerve.

***Systematized Nomenclature of Medicine, Clinical Terms* (SNOMED CT) (1)** comprehensive and multilingual clinical terminology of body structures, clinical findings, diagnoses, medications, outcomes, procedures, specimens, therapies, and treatments.

systemic radiation therapy (17) unsealed radioactive materials that travel throughout the body.

T

Tables (6) used to construct a complete and valid ICD-10-PCS code; contain terms (and definitions) and rows that contain values (characters) needed to construct a valid code.

Tabular List of Diseases and Injuries (2) chronological list of ICD-10-CM codes, divided into 21 chapters based on body system or condition.

technical component (17) use of equipment and supplies as well as the employment of radiological technologists to perform diagnostic imaging examinations and administer radiation therapy treatments.

telemedicine (9) provision of remote medical care an interactive audio and video telecommunications system that permits real-time communication between the provider, at the distant site, and the patient, at the originating site, as an alternative to in-person face-to-face encounters.

tenosynovitis (16) swollen tendon sheaths.

therapeutic apheresis (14) removal of blood components, cells, or plasma solute and retransfusion of the remaining components into the patient.

therapeutic port film (17) x-rays taken during delivery of radiation treatment that utilize the treatment beam of the machine.

therapeutic surgical procedure (12) performed to treat specific conditions or injuries; includes the procedure itself and normal, uncomplicated follow-up care.

thoracentesis (13) surgical puncture of the chest wall with a needle to obtain fluid from the pleural cavity.

thoracoscopy (13) visual examination of the pleural cavity; provides an alternative to open lung or thoracotomy procedures to treat pleural disorders surgically.

thrombectomy (14) surgical removal of a thrombus.

thromboendarterectomy (14) surgical excision of a thrombus and atherosclerotic inner lining from an obstructed artery.

tissue approximation (12) method of replacing sutures with material or substance (e.g., surgical glue), which facilitates enhanced cosmetic results and faster healing of defects.

tracheobronchoscopy (13) visual examination of the interior of the trachea and bronchus.

transfer of care (10) occurs when a provider who is managing some or all of a patient's problems relinquishes that responsibility to another provider who explicitly agrees to accept this responsibility and who, from the initial encounter, is *not* providing consultative services; the provider transferring care no longer manages these problems but may continue to manage other conditions.

transitional pass-through payment (8) temporary additional payment (over and above the OPPS payment) made for certain innovative medical devices, drugs, and biologicals provided to Medicare beneficiaries.

transmyocardial revascularization (TMR) (14) procedure that uses a high-powered laser to create small channels in the heart muscle to increase blood supply to the myocardium.

transpedicular approach (16) performed through and inside pedicle (segment between transverse process and vertebral body) of thoracic vertebra to access thoracic disc, and it does not require retraction of spinal cord but may involve removal of the lamina and facet joint.

transurethral resection of the prostate (TURP) (15) resection of the prostate gland via transurethral approach using an electrosurgical device.

transurethral ureteroscopic lithotripsy (15) procedure in which a cystoscope is inserted through the urethra into the bladder and a ureteroscope is passed into the ureters.

transverse plane (17) horizontally divides the body into superior and inferior portions.

triage (5) organized method of identifying and treating patients according to urgency of care required.

tube pericardiostomy (14) insertion of a tube for drainage or specimen collection.

tunneled (14) implanted catheter that is inserted under the skin and into a vein.

tympanoplasty (16) repair or reconstruction of the eardrum.

tympanostomy (16) *see* myringotomy.

type 1 diabetes mellitus (3) a condition in which the patient's body is unable to produce insulin.

type 2 diabetes mellitus (3) a condition in which the patient's body is unable to properly use insulin produced.

type of service (TOS) (10) refers to the kind of health care services provided to patients, including critical care, consultation, initial hospital care, subsequent hospital care, and confirmatory consultation.

U

UB-04 (20) standard claim submitted by health care institutions to payers for inpatient and outpatient services.

ultrasonography (17) *see* ultrasound.

ultrasound (17)   high-frequency sound waves that bounce off internal organs and create echoes; the echo pattern is displayed on the ultrasound machine monitor.

UMLS (1)   *see* Unified Medical Language System (UMLS).

unbundling (1)   reporting multiple codes to increase reimbursement when a single combination code should be reported.

uncertain behavior (3)   subsequent morphology or behavior that cannot be predicted based on the submitted specimen; the tissue appears to be in transition, and the pathologist cannot establish a definitive diagnosis.

undermining (12)   process of using a surgical instrument to separate skin and mucosa from its underlying stroma so that the tissue can be stretched and moved to overlay a defect.

Unified Medical Language System (UMLS) (1)   set of files and software that allows many health and biomedical vocabularies and standards to enable interoperability among computer systems; used to enhance or develop applications, including electronic health records, classification tools, dictionaries and language translators; used to link health information, medical terms, drug names, and billing codes across different computer systems.

Uniform Ambulatory Care Data Set (UACDS) (5)   established by the federal government as a standard data set for ambulatory care facility records.

Uniform Hospital Discharge Data Set (UHDDS) (7)   established by the federal government to define data collected for inpatient hospitalizations.

unlisted procedure (9)   code assigned when the provider performs a procedure or service for which there is no CPT code.

unlisted service (9)   *see* unlisted procedure.

unspecified behavior (3)   neoplasm is identified, but the results of pathology examination are not available; thus, there is no indication as to histology or nature of the tumor.

upcoding (1)   reporting codes that are not supported by documentation in the patient record for the purpose of increasing reimbursement.

upper GI endoscopy (15)   direct visualization of the esophagus and the stomach.

ureterolithotomy (15)   surgical removal of stones from the ureter.

urethroplasty (15)   surgical repair of the urethra.

V

vaginal birth after cesarean (VBAC) (16)   planned vaginal birth after previous cesarean section.

values (6)   term associated with ICD-10-PCS characters, which are selected from tables.

valvuloplasty (14)   open-heart surgery during which the surgeon removes the damaged valve and replaces it with a prosthetic, homograft or allograft, stented, or stentless valve.

valvulotomy (14)   open-heart surgery in which an incision is made into a valve to repair valvular damage.

vascular family (14)   group of vessels that is accessed by the same first-order vessel and is supplied by the same primary branch from the aorta.

venipuncture (18)   puncture of a vein with a needle for the purpose of drawing blood; most common method of collecting blood specimens.

venography (17)   x-ray of a vein after injection of contrast material.

venous valve transposition (14)   surgical procedure performed to treat chronic deep venous insufficiency.

ventricular assist device (VAD) (14)   provides temporary support for the heart by substituting for left or right heart function.

vertebral augmentation (13)   process of creating a cavity in a vertebral body followed by injecting material (e.g., cement) under image guidance.

view (17)   patient's position in relation to the x-ray camera.

W

Whipple procedure (15)   surgical removal of the pancreas, duodenum, bile duct, and stomach with reconstruction.

workers' compensation (20)   state-mandated insurance program that reimburses health care costs and lost wages if an employee suffers a work-related disease or injury.

X

x-ray (17)   radiographic visualization or imaging of internal body structures using low-dose high-energy radiation.

Index

Notes

Notes

Notes

Notes

Notes